Pediatric Cardiac Surgery

Pediatric Cardiac Surgery

FOURTH EDITION

Editor

Constantine Mavroudis MD
Director, Congenital Heart Institute, Florida Hospital for Children
Site Director, Johns Hopkins Children's Heart Surgery, Florida Hospital for Children
Orlando, FL, USA

Associate Editor

Carl L. Backer MD
Division Head, Cardiovascular-Thoracic Surgery
Ann & Robert H. Lurie Children's Hospital of Chicago, formerly Children's Memorial Hospital
Professor of Surgery
Department of Surgery
Northwestern University Feinberg School of Medicine
Chicago, IL, USA

With illustrations by Rachid F. Idriss

WILEY-BLACKWELL
A John Wiley & Sons, Ltd., Publication

Library of Congress Cataloging-in-Publication Data
Pediatric cardiac surgery. – 4th ed. / edited by Constantine Mavroudis and Carl L. Backer.
p. ; cm.
Includes bibliographical references and index.
ISBN-13: 978-1-4051-9652-9 (hard cover : alk. paper)
ISBN-10: 1-4051-9652-1
I. Mavroudis, Constantine. II. Backer, Carl.
[DNLM: 1. Cardiac Surgical Procedures. 2. Heart Defects, Congenital–surgery. 3. Child. 4. Infant.
WS 290]
LC classification not assigned
617.4'12059–dc23

2011030347

A catalogue record for this book is available from the British Library.

Wiley also publishes its books in a variety of electronic formats. Some content that appears in print may not be available in electronic books.

Cover images: From left to right: courtesy of Rachid F. Idriss, courtesy of C. Mavroudis, iStock © John Barnett, courtesy of C. Backer, courtesy of C. Backer.

Cover design by Fortiori Design

Set in 9.25/12pt Palatino by Toppan Best-set Premedia Limited
Printed and bound in Malaysia by Vivar Printing Sdn Bhd

3 2013

Contents

List of Contributors

Robert H. Anderson BSc, MD, FRCPath
Emeritus Professor
University College
London, UK
Visiting Professor
University of Newcastle
Newcastle, UK
Visiting Professor of Pediatrics
Medical University of South Carolina
Charleston, SC, USA

Janine Arruda, MD
Staff, Pediatric Cardiology
Center for Pediatric and Congenital Heart Disease
Cleveland Clinic Children's Hospital
Cleveland, OH, USA

Carl L. Backer, MD
Division Head, Cardiovascular-Thoracic Surgery
Ann & Robert H. Lurie Children's Hospital of Chicago, formerly
Children's Memorial Hospital
Professor of Surgery
Department of Surgery
Northwestern University Feinberg School of Medicine
Chicago, IL, USA

Nancy Benson, MSN
Center for Congenital Heart Surgery
Cleveland Clinic Children's Hospital
Cleveland, OH, USA

Darryl H. Berkowitz, MD
Attending Physician
Society Hill Anesthesia Consultants
Pennsylvania Hospital
Philadelphia, PA, USA

Pierre-Luc Bernier, MD, FRCSC
Attending Surgeon
Division of Cardiovascular Surgery
The Montreal Children's Hospital
McGill University
Montreal, QC, Canada

Edward L. Bove, MD
Helen and Marvin Kirsh Professor of Surgery
Chair, Department of Cardiac Surgery
C.S. Mott Children's Hospital at the University of Michigan
Ann Arbor, MI, USA

John W. Brown, MD
Harris B. Shumacker Professor Emeritus of Surgery
Indiana University School of Medicine
Indianapolis, IN, USA

Morgan L. Brown, MD
Research Fellow
Cardiovascular Surgery
Mayo Clinic
Rochester, MN, USA

Christopher A. Caldarone, MD
Professor and Chair, Division of Cardiac Surgery
University of Toronto
Staff Cardiovascular Surgeon
Labatt Family Heart Center
The Hospital for Sick Children
Toronto, ON, Canada

Paul J. Chai, MD
Associate Medical Director
All Children's Hospital Heart Center
Thoracic and Cardiovascular Surgeon
Johns Hopkins Children's Heart Surgery, All Children's Hospital
Saint Petersburg, FL, USA

John P. Cheatham, MD, FAAP, FACC, FSCAI
George H. Dunlap Endowed Chair in Interventional Cardiology
Director, Cardiac Catheterization & Interventional Therapy
Co-Director, The Heart Center
Nationwide Children's Hospital
Professor, Pediatrics & Internal Medicine, Cardiology Division
The Ohio State University
Columbus, OH, USA

David R. Clarke, MD
Clinical Professor of Cardiothoracic Surgery
School of Medicine
University of Colorado Denver
Aurora, CO, USA

John M. Costello, MD, MPH
Medical Director, Regenstein Cardiac Care Unit
Ann & Robert H. Lurie Children's Hospital of Chicago, formerly
Children's Memorial Hospital
Associate Professor of Pediatrics
Northwestern University Feinberg School of Medicine
Chicago, IL, USA

Lara Danziger-Isakov, MD, MPH
Staff, Center for Pediatric Infectious Diseases
Director for Pediatric Clinical Research
Cleveland Clinic Children's Hospital
Assistant Professor of Pediatrics
Cleveland Clinic Lerner College of Medicine of Case Western
Reserve University
Cleveland, OH, USA

Jeffrey R. Darst, MD
Assistant Professor, Pediatrics
Section of Cardiology
Children's Hospital Colorado
Aurora, CO, USA

Denise Davis, RN, MSN, CPNP-AC/PC
Center for Congenital Heart Surgery
Cleveland Clinic Children's Hospital
Cleveland, OH, USA

Barbara J. Deal, MD
Division Head, Cardiology
Getz Professor of Cardiology
Ann & Robert H. Lurie Children's Hospital of Chicago, formerly
Children's Memorial Hospital
Professor of Pediatrics
Northwestern University Feinberg School of Medicine
Chicago, IL, USA

Joseph A. Dearani, MD
Professor of Surgery
Cardiovascular Surgery
Mayo Clinic
Rochester, MN, USA

Danny Del Duca, MD
Resident, Cardiac Surgery
McGill University
Montreal, QC, Canada

Ralph E. Delius, MD
Vice Chief, Department of Cardiovascular Surgery
Children's Hospital of Michigan
Associate Professor of Surgery
Wayne State University School of Medicine
Detroit, MI, USA

Eric J. Devaney, MD
Associate Professor of Surgery
University of California, San Diego
Rady Children's Hospital at the University of California
San Diego, CA, USA

Konstantinos Dimopoulos, MD, MSc, PhD, FESC
Consultant Cardiologist
Adult Congenital Heart Centre and Centre for Pulmonary
Hypertension
Royal Brompton Hospital
National Heart & Lung Institute
Imperial College London
London, UK

Ali Dodge-Khatami, MD, PhD
Chief of Pediatric Cardiac Surgery
Program Head for Congenital Heart Disease
University Heart Center
Professor of Cardiac Surgery
University of Hamburg-Eppendorf School of Medicine
Hamburg, Germany

Brian W. Duncan, MD, MBA
BioEnterprise
Arboretum Ventures
Cleveland, OH, USA

Osama Eltayeb, MD
Fellow in Pediatric Cardiothoracic Surgery
Indiana University School of Medicine
Indianapolis, IN, USA

Charles D. Fraser Jr, MD
Chief of Congenital Heart Surgery and Cardiac Surgeon In-Charge
Texas Children's Hospital
Baylor College of Medicine
Houston, TX, USA

Stephanie Fuller, MD
Assistant Professor
Division of Cardiothoracic Surgery
The Children's Hospital of Philadelphia
University of Pennsylvania School of Medicine
Philadelphia, PA, USA

Mark Galantowicz, MD
Chief, Department of Cardiothoracic Surgery
Murray D. Lincoln Chair of Cardiothoracic Surgery
Co-Director, The Heart Center
Nationwide Children's Hospital
Professor of Surgery
The Ohio State University
Columbus, OH, USA

Michael A. Gatzoulis, MD, PhD, FACC, FESC
Professor of Cardiology, Congenital Heart Disease and Consultant
Cardiologist
Adult Congenital Heart Centre and Centre for Pulmonary
Hypertension
Royal Brompton Hospital
National Heart & Lung Institute
Imperial College London
London, UK

J. William Gaynor, MD
Associate Professor of Surgery
The Children's Hospital of Philadelphia
Philadelphia, PA, USA

Peter J. Gruber, MD, PhD
D. Rees and Eleanor T. Jenson Presidential Chair in Surgery
Investigator, University of Utah
Molecular Medicine (U2M2) Program
Eccles Institute of Human Genetics
Chief, Section of Pediatric Cardiothoracic Surgery
Primary Children's Medical Center
Salt Lake City, UT, USA

Thomas Günther, MD
Department of Cardiovascular Surgery
German Heart Center
Technische Universität München
Munich, Germany

Frank L. Hanley, MD
Professor of Cardiothoracic Surgery – Pediatric Cardiac Surgery
Director, Children's Heart Center
Lucile Packard Children's Hospital
Stanford University Medical Center
Falk CV Research Center
Stanford, CA, USA

Jeffrey S. Heinle, MD
Surgical Director, Heart and Lung Transplant Program
Texas Children's Hospital
Associate Professor of Surgery and Pediatrics
Baylor College of Medicine
Houston, TX, USA

Samantha Hill, MD, MSc, FRCSC
Resident, Cardiac Surgery
McGill University
Montreal, QC, Canada

Sharon L. Hill, MSN, ACNP-BC
Interventional Nurse Practitioner
The Heart Center, Nationwide Children's Hospital
College of Nursing
The Ohio State University
Columbus, OH, USA

Jennifer C. Hirsch, MD, MS
Assistant Professor, Department of Surgery and Pediatrics
Surgical Director, Pediatric Cardiac Intensive Care Unit
Division of Pediatric Cardiovascular Surgery
C.S. Mott Children's Hospital at the University of Michigan School
of Medicine
Ann Arbor, MI, USA

Ralf J. Holzer, MD, MSc, FSCAI
Assistant Director, Cardiac Catheterization & Interventional
Therapy
The Heart Center, Nationwide Children's Hospital
Assistant Professor of Pediatrics
The Ohio State University
Columbus, OH, USA

Fejeania Hunter, RN, BSN, CPNP
Center for Congenital Heart Surgery
Cleveland Clinic Children's Hospital
Cleveland, OH, USA

Jeffrey P. Jacobs, MD, FACS, FACC, FCCP
Surgical Director of Heart Transplantation and Extracorporeal Life
Support Programs
All Children's Hospital Heart Center
Thoracic and Cardiovascular Surgeon
Johns Hopkins Children's Heart Surgery, All Children's Hospital
Clinical Professor
Department of Surgery
University of South Florida (USF)
Saint Petersburg, FL, USA

Marshall L. Jacobs, MD
Center for Congenital Heart Surgery
Cleveland Clinic Children's Hospital
Cleveland, OH, USA

Richard A. Jonas, MD
Chief, Cardiac Surgery
Codirector, Children's National Heart Institute
Cohen Funger Professor of Cardiac Surgery
Children's National Medical Center
Washington, DC, USA

Jason M. Kane, MD, MS
Associate Professor of Pediatrics
Northwestern University Feinberg School of Medicine
Director, Regenstein Cardiac Care Unit
Division of Cardiology
Ann & Robert H. Lurie Children's Hospital of Chicago, formerly
Children's Memorial Hospital
Chicago, IL, USA

John M. Karamichalis, MD
Clinical Instructor in Surgery
Division of Pediatric Cardiothoracic Surgery
University of California, San Francisco
San Francisco, CA, USA

Sunjay Kaushal, PhD, MD
Attending Surgeon
University of Maryland
Baltimore, MD, USA

Ergin Kocyildirim, MD
Assistant Professor
Department of Cardiothoracic Surgery
McGowan Institute for Regenerative Medicine
University of Pittsburgh
Pittsburgh, PA, USA

Steven W. Kubalak, PhD
Associate Professor
Department of Regenerative Medicine and Cell Biology
Cardiovascular Developmental Biology Center
Medical University of South Carolina
Charleston, SC, USA

John J. Lamberti, MD
Professor of Surgery
University of California San Diego
Eugene and Joyce Klein Director of the Heart Institute
Children's Hospital of San Diego
Rady Children's Hospital
San Diego, CA, USA

Rüdiger Lange, MD, PhD
Director Department of Cardiovascular Surgery
German Heart Center
Technische Universität München
Munich, Germany

Richard Lorber, MD
Staff, Pediatric Cardiology
Center for Pediatric and Congenital Heart Disease
Cleveland Clinic Children's Hospital
Cleveland, OH, USA

Richard D. Mainwaring, MD
Clinical Associate Professor of Surgery
Cardiothoracic Surgery–Pediatric Cardiac Surgery
Stanford University School of Medicine
Stanford, CA, USA

George B. Mallory Jr, MD
Pediatric Pulmonologist
Director, Pediatric Lung Transplantation Program
Texas Children's Hospital
Professor of Pediatrics
Baylor College of Medicine
Houston, TX, USA

Constantine Mavroudis, MD
Director, Congenital Heart Institute, Florida Hospital for Children
Site Director, Johns Hopkins Children's Heart Surgery, Florida
Hospital for Children
Orlando, FL, USA

Max B. Mitchell, MD
Professor of Surgery
School of Medicine
University of Colorado Denver Health Sciences Center
Children's Hospital Colorado Heart Institute
Aurora, CO, USA

David L.S. Morales, MD
Congenital Heart Surgery
Director of Mechanical Circulatory Support
Associate Professor of Surgery and Pediatrics
Texas Children's Hospital
Baylor College of Medicine
Houston, TX, USA

Victor O. Morell, MD
Codirector, University of Pittsburgh Medical Center Heart and
Vascular Institute
Vice Chair and Director of Cardiovascular Services
Department of Cardiothoracic Surgery
McGowan Institute for Regenerative Medicine
Chief, Pediatric Cardiothoracic Surgery
Children's Hospital of Pittsburgh
Associate Professor of Surgery
Pittsburgh, PA, USA

Muhammad Ali Mumtaz, MD
Medical Director and Chief, Children's Cardiothoracic Surgery
Children's Hospital of the King's Daughters
Norfolk, VA, USA

Ashok Muralidaran, MD
Clinical Instructor
Cardiothoracic Surgery–Pediatric Cardiac Surgery
Stanford University School of Medicine
Stanford, CA, USA

Richard G. Ohye, MD
Associate Professor, Department of Surgery
Division of Pediatric Cardiovascular Surgery
C.S. Mott Children's Hospital at the University of Michigan School
of Medicine
Ann Arbor, MI, USA

Vincent F. Olshove, BS, CCP, CCT, FPP
Director, Cardiovascular Perfusion
The Heart Center, Nationwide Children's Hospital
Clinical Instructor, Circulation Technology
The Ohio State University
Columbus, OH, USA

Noritaka Ota, MD
Cardiac Surgeon
Department of Cardiovascular Surgery
Mt. Fuji Shizuoka Children's Hospital
Shizuoka, Japan

Mario Petrou, PhD, FRCS
Consultant Cardiothoracic Surgeon
Departments of Thoracic Surgery and Adult Cardiac Surgery
Royal Brompton Hospital
London, UK

Alistair Phillips, MD, FACC, FACS
Surgical Director, Pediatric Heart Transplantation and Mechanical
Circulatory Support
Surgical Director, Adult Congenital Heart Disease
Associate Professor, Division of Pediatric Surgery
Cincinnati Children's Hospital Medical Center
Cincinnati, OH, USA

Stamatia Prapa, MD
Clinical Research Fellow
Imperial College London
Royal Brompton Hospital
London, UK

Tamar J. Preminger, MD
Staff, Pediatric Cardiology
Center for Pediatric and Congenital Heart Disease
Cleveland Clinic Children's Hospital
Cleveland, OH, USA

Lourdes R. Prieto, MD
Director, Cardiac Catheterization
Center for Pediatric and Congenital Heart Disease
Cleveland Clinic Children's Hospital
Associate Professor
Cleveland Clinic Lerner College of Medicine of Case Western
Reserve University
Cleveland, OH, USA

H. Jay Przybylo, MD
Attending Anesthesiologist
Department of Anesthesia
Ann & Robert H. Lurie Children's Hospital of Chicago, formerly
Children's Memorial Hospital
Associate Professor of Anesthesiology
Northwestern University Feinberg School of Medicine
Chicago, IL, USA

Athar Qureshi, MD
Assistant Professor
Cleveland Clinic Lerner College of Medicine of Case Western
Reserve University
Staff, Center for Pediatric and Congenital Heart Disease
Cleveland Clinic Children's Hospital
Cleveland, OH, USA

Vadiyala Mohan Reddy, MD
Associate Professor of Cardiothoracic Surgery and Pediatrics
Chief, Division of Pediatric Cardiac Surgery
Lucile Packard Children's Hospital
Stanford University
Stanford, CA, USA

Dewei Ren, MD
Congenital Heart Surgery
Texas Children's Hospital
Houston, TX, USA

W. Steves Ring, MD
Professor, Department of Cardiovascular and Thoracic Surgery
University of Texas Southwestern Medical Center
Children's Medical Center of Dallas
Dallas, TX, USA

Mark D. Rodefeld, MD
Associate Professor of Surgery
Indiana University School of Medicine
Indianapolis, IN, USA

Joseph W. Rossano, MD
Assistant Professor of Pediatrics
Texas Children's Hospital
Baylor College of Medicine
Houston, TX, USA

Mark Ruzmetov, MD
Fellow in Pediatric Cardiothoracic Surgery
Indiana University School of Medicine
Indianapolis, IN, USA

Marcy L. Schwartz, MD
Staff, Pediatric Cardiology
Center for Pediatric and Congenital Heart Disease
Cleveland Clinic Children's Hospital
Cleveland, OH, USA

Darryl F. Shore, MD, FRCS
Consultant Cardiac Surgeon
Adult Congenital Heart Center
Royal Brompton Hospital
National Heart & Lung Institute
Imperial College London
London, UK

Thomas L. Spray, MD
Chief, Division of Cardiothoracic Surgery
The Children's Hospital of Philadelphia
Professor of Surgery
University of Pennsylvania School of Medicine
Philadelphia, PA, USA

Richard Sterba, MD
Staff, Pediatric Cardiology
Center for Pediatric and Congenital Heart Disease
Cleveland Clinic Children's Hospital
Cleveland, OH, USA

Robert D. Stewart, MD, MPH
Interim Chair
Center for Congenital Heart Surgery
Cleveland Clinic Children's Hospital
Cleveland, OH, USA

Christo I. Tchervenkov, MD, FRCSC, FACS
Director
Division of Cardiovascular Surgery
The Montreal Children's Hospital
Tony Dobell Professor of Pediatric Surgery
McGill University
Montreal, QC, Canada

Kim Teknipp, MSN
Center for Congenital Heart Surgery
Cleveland Clinic Children's Hospital
Cleveland, OH, USA

Jamie Thomas, RN, MSN, CPNP-AC/PC
Pediatric Nurse Practitioner
Pediatric Intensive Care Unit
Cleveland Clinic Children's Hospital
Cleveland, OH, USA

Mark W. Turrentine, MD
Professor of Surgery
Indiana University School of Medicine
Indianapolis, IN, USA

Nicola Viola, MD
Consultant Cardiac Surgeon
Specialist Services Division
Cardiovascular and Thoracic Care Group
Southampton General Hospital
Southampton, UK

Henry L. Walters III, MD
Chief, Department of Cardiovascular Surgery
Children's Hospital of Michigan
Professor of Surgery
Wayne State University School of Medicine
Detroit, MI, USA

Andy Wessels, PhD
Professor
Cardiovascular Developmental Biology Center
Regenerative Medicine and Cell Biology
Medical University of South Carolina
Charleston, SC, USA

Preface

This is the *4th Edition* of *Pediatric Cardiac Surgery*. The first edition was published by Arciniegas in 1985, was followed by the *2nd Edition* in 1994, and the *3rd Edition* in 2003 by the present editors. Timely updates are important for any textbook as scientific intellectual curiosity, sentinel discoveries, and technological improvements have progressed at lightning speed. Even cardiac embryology, a field thought to be constant and thoroughly studied, has emerged with new findings of a second heart field, detailed results of syndromic genomes, and the promise of new paradigms and ontologies. Our readership from around the world has included numerous colleagues comprised of surgeons, cardiologists, intensivists, anesthesiologists, residents, students, perfusionists, and nurses. They have found the book to be well organized, easy to read, and to the point. We have preserved this format for the *4th Edition* and added several chapters that have mirrored the directions and practice of pediatric and congenital heart surgery in the twenty-first century.

Several new chapters by new authors have highlighted the advances of congenital heart surgery. While this textbook emphasizes the pediatric nature of the specialty, it is clear that there are more adults with congenital heart disease living today than there are children with congenital heart disease. This is a testimony to the years of scientific and clinical research that have combined to improve the lot of these patients who now present with medical and surgical problems of their own. The new chapter on adult congenital heart disease reviews these very important issues and serves as an important contribution to the textbook. Several new and updated chapters, written by experts in their field, review advances that have been made in congenital heart surgery such as right ventricular to pulmonary artery conduits, arrhythmia surgery, double-outlet ventricles, and cardiac transplantation, among many others. In some cases, the same authors have updated their previous chapters. In others, new authors have been selected because of their demonstrated expertise.

The *4th Edition* maintains its comprehensive coverage of the breadth of congenital heart surgery and related fields.

Each chapter reviews the embryology, physical findings, diagnostic criteria, and therapeutic choices associated with each disease entity. State-of-the art technology and the latest in surgical techniques are discussed.

As in previous editions of *Pediatric Cardiac Surgery*, the figures have predominantly been illustrated by Rachid Idriss. His drawing techniques are legendary not only because of his artistic talents, but more so for his ability to see an operation in his mind's eye and demonstrate with a few lines the important parts of the relative anatomy and reparative operation. Sutures are clear, pledgets are well placed, and structures are anatomically correct. Hidden intracardiac anatomy is displayed by ghost techniques that transform the image into a three-dimensional living characterization of reality. His contribution to this *4th Edition* cannot be overstated.

This textbook is reflective of the cooperation, expertise, and altruism that the contributing authors have so generously shared with the readership. Simply stated, these chapters are a delight to read. We are sure that the reader will have the same experience. All royalties from the sale of this book will be contributed to the Thoracic Surgery Foundation for Research and Education for the purpose of supporting congenital heart surgery initiatives. We are greatly indebted to the editorial staff at Wiley-Blackwell for their support, in particular, Kate Newell. Important editorial contributions were made by Patricia Heraty and, in particular, Melanie Gevitz who was so instrumental in organizing the successful efforts associated with the *2nd* and *3rd Editions*. In the Orlando Office, we found a jewel, Allison Siegel, who took on this project with an impressive zeal, expertise, and commitment that are rarely found anywhere.

The concluding paragraph in this Preface is quoted from the Preface of the *3rd Edition* because it stands as a timeless dedication to our loved ones and family members who have shown their devotion, calmed the children, and explained our absences on countless occasions without rancor, excuses, or disappointment. It reads, "Finally, as with all surgeons and physicians, our accomplishments are facilitated by the sacrifices made by our families. Every author who wrote a chapter for this textbook, no doubt, has loved ones who have contributed in one way or another to their creativity, stability, and industry. We thank each and every one of these wives, husbands, children, parents, and friends, including our own, which have had the patience, perseverance, and equanimity to stand by."

Constantine Mavroudis, MD
Carl L. Backer, MD

CHAPTER 1

Development of the Heart and Great Vessels

Peter J. Gruber,[1] Andy Wessels,[2] and Steven W. Kubalak[2]

[1]Primary Children's Medical Center, Salt Lake City, UT, USA
[2]Medical University of South Carolina, Charleston, SC, USA

Introduction

Modern cardiac embryology combines molecular and cellular biologic techniques with traditional embryologic morphologic approaches during development. The limited descriptions of human cardiac development are necessarily supplemented by nonhuman models of cardiac development. Avian embryos have traditionally been favored experimental models because of the ease with which they can be observed and manipulated. More recently, the developing mouse has become the preferred model for studying cardiac development because of the strength of genetic and molecular investigative tools available in this species. Where possible, this chapter discusses how results in experimental animal models relate to human cardiac development. Table 1.1 provides a simplified comparison of two widely utilized developmental schemes for developmental staging in chick and mouse embryos [1–7]. The comparison of multiple species provides an important platform for understanding the development of the human heart and the pathogenesis of human disease.

Formation of Cardiac Precursors

All of the cells that will become part of the heart derive from populations of undifferentiated precursors that will be influenced by external signals into their final developmental pathways. In addition to the intellectual challenge of understanding how these acts of differentiation occur, intense activity in this field is also driven by the possibility of controlling cardiac tissue differentiation to replace diseased myocardium in the postnatal heart.

Repeated cell divisions of the fertilized egg form a cell mass that evolves into two distinct layers of cells. The epiblast layer is separated from a second layer of cells, called the hypoblast in the chick or the primitive endoderm in the

mouse and human. The next critical stage of development is gastrulation where widespread cell migration into and reorganization within the blastocoele cavity result in the formation of three germ layers (ectoderm, mesoderm, and endoderm) and the determination of the future body plan of the embryo (Figure 1.1) [7,8].

Gastrulation of precardiac cells is an early event in all species. In the human, gastrulation takes place at the beginning of the third week of development and angioblasts in the cardiogenic region are present shortly thereafter. At the time that precardiac cells gastrulate in chick embryos (Hamburger–Hamilton stage 3), the primitive streak is less than 1mm in length; the portion of the streak through which the precardiac cells ingress extends as a relatively broad swath 0.125–0.75 mm from the anterior limit of the streak [9]. The most anteriorly gastrulating cells contribute to the most anterior portion of the primitive heart tube.

After cells have undergone gastrulation they enter the undifferentiated mesenchyme. Uncommitted precardiac cells enter the primitive streak only to become specified to their cell type or migratory pathways in the mesoderm after leaving the streak [9]. Subsequently, the precardiac cells will move laterally to join the lateral plate mesoderm at the level of Hensen's node. The lateral plate mesoderm then splits into two layers, a splanchnic layer directly above the endoderm and a somatic layer directly below the ectoderm. The anterior endoderm provides signals to splanchnic mesodermal cells to enter the precardiac lineage. Fibroblast growth factors (FGFs)-1, -2, and -4 and bone morphogenetic protein 2 (BMP-2) are proteins that appear to be critical to this process [10]. However, to date no single gene has been identified whose ablation leads to a specific failure of all myocardial differentiation from precardiac mesoderm. This observation may argue the presence of either a considerable genetic redundancy in precardiac myocyte differentiation or an unsuspected diversity of

Table 1.1 Simplified comparison of developmental stages between human, mouse, and chicken embryos.

Human			Mouse	Chicken
			Embryonic days/ (Theiler's stage)[c]	Hamburger/Hamilton stage[d]/(days of incubation)
Carnegie stage[a]	Streeter horizon[b]	Days gestation		
9	IX	20	8–8.5 (12)	7–8 (1.1)
10	X	22	8.5–9 (13)	10 (1.5)
11	XI	24	9–9.5 (14)	11 (1.8)
12	XII	26	9.5–10.25 (15)	14 (2.2)
13	XIII	28	10.25–10.5 (16)	17 (2.6)
14	XIV–XV	32	10.5–10.75 (17)	19 (2.9)
15	XVI	33	11 (18)	20-21 (3.3)
16	XVIII	37	11.5 (19)	24 (4)
17	XX	41	12 (20)	26 (4.8)
18	XXI–XXII	44	12.5 (21)	28 (5.6)
19	XXIII	47	13 (21)	29–30 (6.4)
20		50	14 (22)	31–32 (7.2)
21		52	14 (22)	34 (8)
22		54	14 (22)	35 (8.7)
23		56	14 (22)	36 (9.6)

[a]O'Rahilly R, Muller F, Streeter GL. (1987) Developmental Stages in Human Embryos. Washington, DC: Carnegie Institution of Washington [2].
[b]Streeter GL. (1942) Developmental horizons in human embryos. Description of age group XI, 13–20 somites, and age group XII, 21–29 somites. Contrib Embryol 30, 211–245 [3]; Streeter GL. (1945) Developmental horizons in human embryos. Description of age group XIII, embryos about 4 or 5 millimeters long, and age group XIV, period of indentation of lens cesicle. Contrib Embryol 32, 27–63 [4]; Streeter GL. (1948) Developmental horizons in human embryos. Description of age group XI, 13–20 somites, age group XV, XVI, XVII, and XVII. Contrib Embryol 32, 133–203 [5].
[c]Theiler K. (1989) The House Mouse: Atlas of Embryonic Development. New York, NY: Springer Verlag [6].
[d]Hamburger V, Hamilton HL. (1992) A series of normal stages in the development of the chick embryo. 1951. Dev Dyn 195, 231–272 [1].

precardiac myocyte lineages following independent genetic pathways.

Precardiac cells are found in an epithelial sheet at the cranial end of the splanchnic mesoderm and can be identified at this point by a variety of molecular markers such as the transcription factors NKX2-5, MEF2, HAND1, HAND2, GATA4, TBX5, and ISL1 [11–17]. The region of splanchnic mesoderm expressing precardiac markers is also known as the "heart-forming field" and is larger than the region that will actually contribute cells to the heart tube [18]. In rodent embryos, but not chick embryos, precardiac mesodermal cells exhibit spontaneous contractile activity, indicating a relatively advanced state of differentiation towards the cardiac myocyte lineage [19,20].

The precardiac mesodermal cell mass migrates as a single unit rather than as a collection of independent cells. The precardiac mesodermal sheets on each side of the embryo migrate together towards the midline cranial to the anterior intestinal portal. When the most cranial portions of the bilateral precardiac mesoderm masses meet in the midline, the total premyocardial cell population forms a horseshoe-shaped crescent called the first (primary) heart field. The

cues that enable and promote movement of these cells are provided by a noncardiac tissue, the endoderm, as demonstrated by experimental removal of the endoderm and/or ectoderm. The extracellular matrix molecule fibronectin may be one of the important components of the endodermal surface to which the precardiac cells are responding [21].

Precursors of the endocardium follow similar migratory pathways as the precardiac cells, but there are important differences. Pre-endocardial cells and pre-endothelial cells are known as angioblasts. The endocardial angioblasts are first detectable in the splanchnic mesoderm. Mesodermal cells are induced to enter the angioblast lineage by signals such as transforming growth factor beta (TGFβ) 2–4 and vascular endothelial growth factor (VEGF) signaling from the endoderm [10]. Endocardial angioblasts migrate anteriorly and to the midline with the premyocardial cell mass, but they do so as individual cells.

Formation of the Tube Heart

As the precardiac cell masses of the first heart field move steadily towards the midline, endocardial cells begin to

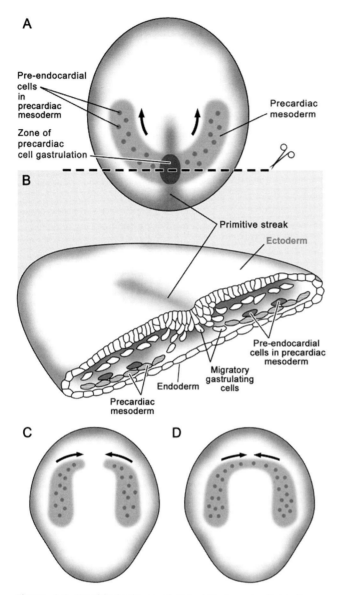

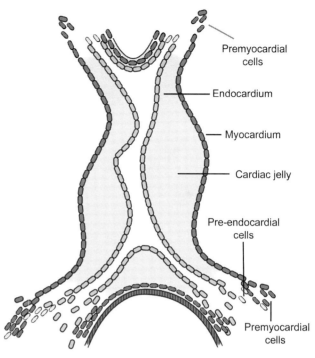

Figure 1.2 Formation of the tube heart is initiated by fusion of the bilateral precardiac mesoderm populations in the midline, resulting in formation of a myocardial tube surrounding an endothelial (endocardial) channel. The myocardial population of the cardiac tube at this stage consists of only the precursors of the future trabeculated portions of the left ventricle. Additional segments are added by ongoing migration of precardiac mesoderm into the tube heart.

Figure 1.1 Simplified schema of gastrulation, precardiac cell migration, and formation of the heart forming fields. **A,** Cells destined to become cardiac cells migrate from the epiblast into the primitive streak through a broad region caudal to the most anterior portion of the primitive streak. The direction of migration of the gastrulated cells, as indicated by the arrows, is away from the midline and anteriorly on each side. **B,** The embryo in cross-section at the level indicated by the dotted line in **A**. The precardiac mesoderm forms an epithelial sheet closely associated with the endoderm. The pre-endocardial cells are scattered throughout the same region and can be distinguished immunohistochemically from the general precardiac mesoderm. **C,** and **D,** The two lateral precardiac mesoderm populations (also known as heart forming fields) will migrate anteriorly before turning towards the midline (**C**). They will meet in the midline, as shown in **D**, at a location immediately anterior to the anterior intestinal portal.

form a network of tiny channels that will coalesce into a complex endocardial network surrounded by a myocardial mantle [22]. If the mesodermal sheets are prevented from meeting in the midline as a consequence of genetic [15] or mechanical manipulation [23], dual heart tubes will be formed that undergo some degree of further independent development. However, in normal development, the endothelial network quickly transforms into a single endothelial channel within a single myocardial tube (Figure 1.2) [7].

The tube heart at the time of its formation is connected to the foregut along its dorsal surface throughout its length by a structure called the dorsal mesocardium [24]. As looping proceeds, the dorsal mesocardium degenerates until it remains connected only at the atrial and arterial poles of the heart. The disintegration of the central portion of the dorsal mesocardium is a key event for looping to proceed normally, while the arterial and venous attachments provide "anchors" for the looping heart tube. The mesenchymal portion of the dorsal mesocardium known as the dorsal mesenchymal protrusion [25,26] protrudes into the atrium posteriorly and is a derivative of the second

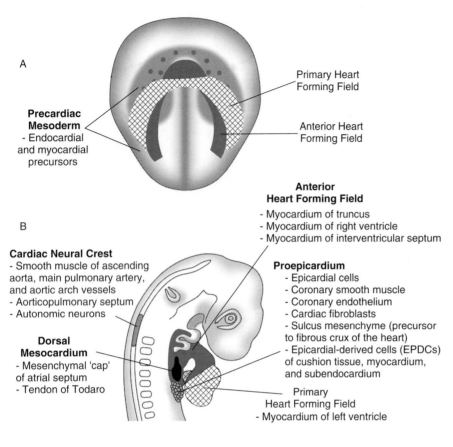

A

**Primary Heart
Forming Field**

**Precardiac
Mesoderm**
- Endocardial
and myocardial
precursors

**Anterior Heart
Forming Field**

B

**Anterior
Heart Forming Field**
- Myocardium of truncus
- Myocardium of right ventricle
- Myocardium of interventricular septum

Cardiac Neural Crest
- Smooth muscle of ascending
aorta, main pulmonary artery,
and aortic arch vessels
- Aorticopulmonary septum
- Autonomic neurons

Proepicardium
- Epicardial cells
- Coronary smooth muscle
- Coronary endothelium
- Cardiac fibroblasts
- Sulcus mesenchyme (precursor
to fibrous crux of the heart)
- Epicardial-derived cells (EPDCs)
of cushion tissue, myocardium,
and subendocardium

**Dorsal
Mesocardium**
- Mesenchymal 'cap'
of atrial septum
- Tendon of Todaro

**Primary
Heart Forming Field**
- Myocardium of left ventricle

Figure 1.3 Normal heart development requires integration of cell populations from multiple sources. **A,** Precardiac mesoderm gives rise to the endocardium and the majority of cardiac cushion cells. Premyocardial cells give rise to the entire spectrum of cardiac myocyte phenotypes. The primary heart forming field will give rise to most of the myocardium of the atria and left ventricle. The anterior heart forming field will give rise to the myocardium of the outflow tract, right ventricle, and interventricular septum. **B,** Multiple extracardiac embryonic tissues provide critical cell populations to normal cardiac development. These cell populations include cardiac neural crest cells as well as cells from the proepicardium and the dorsal mesocardium.

heart field [25]. It is an important contributor to atrioventricular (AV) septation and serves as a conduit for the developing pulmonary veins. The dorsal mesocardium is also a pathway for cellular migrations as development proceeds, including neural crest-derived neural structures [27] and possibly cells derived from the ventral neural tube [28].

Soon after the formation of the cardiac tube the heartbeat is initiated and blood circulation can be observed (embryonic day 8.5 in the mouse and day 20 in the human). With the initiation of circulation the heart becomes the first organ to adopt its essential mature function in the embryo. At this point in cardiac organogenesis, however, the tube heart has not yet obtained its full complement of cell populations necessary for complete cardiac development. Early fate mapping studies [29–31] showed that the primary heart tube is derived from two bilateral fields of precardiac mesoderm, currently called the first heart field; this precardiac mesoderm was long considered the precursor tissue of the heart. Studies by others [32], however, strongly suggested that growth of the heart tube, specifically at the arterial pole, depended on the addition of cardiac tissue from a secondary pool of progenitor cells. It was not until the early twenty-first century that the nature of this additional cell population was elucidated. The combined studies of various laboratories [25,33–36] have provided

significant new insights into the importance of this additional population of cells, called the second heart field, in the elongation and growth of the heart tube and in the formation of a mature four-chambered heart (Figure 1.3) [7]. Thus, these studies have demonstrated that the secondary heart field contributes at the arterial pole to the outflow tract and right ventricle and at the venous pole to parts of the atria and the dorsal mesenchymal protrusion.

The Tube Heart, Segments, and Segmental Identity

Traditionally, the heart tube has been regarded as containing the precursors of all of the cardiac segments. In reality, at the time the heartbeat is initiated the heart tube primarily consists of future left ventricular tissues [37,38]. Immunohistochemical, in situ hybridization, and cell fate tracing techniques have demonstrated that the outflow tract, the right ventricle [32], the AV junction segment [37], the atria [39], and the sinus venosus are added to the heart as looping proceeds. Indeed, these are the structures that are most important in the pathogenesis of the majority of forms of complex human congenital heart disease. Recent studies indicate that the outlet (truncal and conal) primordia [35,40] as well as the right ventricle and much of the interventricular septum [35] and parts of the cardiac venous pole develop from the anterior/secondary heart field.

In prelooping and early looping stages the primitive heart tube consists of circumferential sheets of myocardial cells two to three layers thick surrounding an endothelial tube, these layers being separated by an acellular, extracellular matrix-rich space known as the cardiac jelly. As looping proceeds, the future segments can be distinguished morphologically by their position in the heart tube and by structural features, such as the striking accumulations of cardiac jelly in the AV canal and outflow segments. Segments can be distinguished physiologically by measurement of the differences in their velocity of muscular contraction and relaxation, their rates of spontaneous pacemaker activity, and the speed of electrical impulse conduction.

Segmental differentiation creates the physiological competence of the embryonic heart [41]. Unidirectional antegrade blood flow is maintained by organization of the tube heart into alternating regions of rapid and slow contractile properties [42]. The atrium has the fastest rate of spontaneous contractility and is the site of pacemaker activity. The wave of depolarization spreads from myocyte to myocyte from the atrium to the outflow tract, but the velocity of conduction is not uniform throughout the length of the heart tube. Atrial conduction is rapid, AV conduction is slow, ventricular conduction is rapid, and outlet conduction is slow. The zones of rapid conduction show rapid contraction–relaxation mechanical properties, while the slow zones of conduction demonstrate slow, sustained contractions. The result is a forceful contraction of the atria, followed by a sphincter-like contraction of the AV junction (prior to maturation of AV valves) that prevents the retrograde flow of blood during the forceful ventricular ejection phase. The cardiac cycle of the tube heart is completed by a sphincter-like contraction of the outflow tract (prior to maturation of the semilunar valves) to prevent retrograde blood flow from the aortic arches.

Genetic Determination of Cardiac Segmentation

In addition to functional differences, cardiac segments can also be distinguished by unique patterns of gene expression. However, despite the rapidly increasing number of markers that distinguish segments following heart tube formation, there has been less success in identifying segmental markers in the precardiac mesoderm. Data suggest that the final determination of lineage fate occurs in the precardiac mesoderm [9,31], but the timing and nature of the mechanisms are as yet poorly understood. Perhaps the best-studied determinants of the anterior–posterior axis in the gastrulating embryo are retinoids [43,44]. Retinoids are products of vitamin A metabolism, and manipulation of retinoid signaling pathways results in significant abnor-

malities in axial patterning in general and cardiac development in particular [45–49]. Abnormal development of atrial segments and systemic venous structures are observed in conditions of retinoid deficiency [50–52]. Excess retinoids create cardiac malformations, often involving the outflow tract [53,54], and result in ventricular expression of several genes that are normally largely restricted to the atria at these stages of normal development [55–57]. The spatial and temporal patterns of retinoid signaling in early cardiac development are highly correlated with the presence of retinaldehyde dehydrogenase 2 (RALDH2), a key enzyme in the retinol (vitamin A) to retinoic acid pathway [58–60]. Retinoid signaling pathways are clearly key mechanisms of segmental differentiation within the heart, but it is likely that other pathways yet to be determined are also involved.

Transgenic mice provide some of the most interesting data regarding differences between the genetic pathways regulating different regions of the heart. In these experiments, regulatory portions from one gene are used to drive the expression of a second gene whose product can readily be detected in the tissues. The DNA resulting from the combined portions of the two genes is injected into the male pronucleus of fertilized mouse eggs, and frequently the DNA is incorporated into the mouse nuclear DNA. The eggs are implanted in a female mouse and generally allowed to proceed through development until birth. The newborn animals bearing the new DNA (the "transgene") can be identified by analysis of their DNA. If the transgene is present, the animal will be bred and its offspring analyzed for the pattern of expression of the transgene.

Use of this technology has demonstrated several features of segmental and regional gene expression in the heart [61]. The genetic elements that determine regional patterns of gene expression are modular, in that genes expressed widely in the heart often have discrete portions of their regulatory DNA responsible for subsets of the overall pattern. For instance, a transgene driven by a 10-kilobase (kb) segment of the *Gata6* gene exhibits expression throughout the atria, AV junction, and left and right ventricles, excluding only the outflow tract; a smaller 2.3-kb fragment of the same gene drives expression only in the AV junction (Figure 1.4) [7,62]. The segmental and regional boundaries of gene expression determined by a specific genetic element may be variable during development, and transgenes expressed widely in the primitive tube heart can be restricted in their expression in the adult heart. Finally, the fact that some transgenes are differentially activated spatially and temporally in the heart is a striking confirmation of the nonequivalence of these tissues at the most basic level of gene regulation (Figure 1.4) [7].

Gene knockout experiments in mice also provide insight into the genetic regulatory networks critical to segmental differentiation. The requirement of the transcription factor HAND2 for normal development of the primitive right

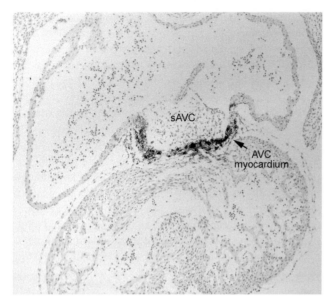

Figure 1.4 Section of an 11.75 embryonic day mouse embryo from a line carrying a transgene that expresses the LacZ reporter gene under the control of a portion of the GATA-6 promoter. At this stage of development expression of the LacZ gene, which produces the dark-staining cells indicated, is limited to atrioventricular canal myocardium. (sAVC, superior atrioventricular endocardial cushion; AVC, atrioventricular canal.) (Courtesy of A. Wessels and J. Burch.)

ventricle in mice is an especially compelling example of the apparent dependence of specific segments on specific genetic regulatory pathways [63].

A relatively new transgenic technique that has revolutionized the understanding of the developing heart is the use of Cre-lox mouse model systems [64]. In this approach mice are generated that contain the coding sequence for the Cre recombinase enzyme under the regulation of a gene sequence of interest. When these Cre mice are crossed with mice that carry sequences flanked by lox P sites, one can specifically delete these "Floxed" sequences and, depending on the nature of the Cre and Flox constructs, achieve, for instance, tissue-specific gene deletions [65] or cell fate tracing [25].

It is beyond the scope of this chapter to discuss in detail how each of the above techniques has advanced our insight into normal and abnormal cardiac development. For the interested reader there are some excellent recent reviews that discuss the use of these strategies [66,67].

Looping

As the heart tube extends due to addition of cardiac tissue to the arterial and venous poles, the heart tube bends to the right. As morphogenesis continues, the loop becomes more

complex. The left ventricle moves inferior and anterior to the atrium, the right ventricle slightly anterior and to the right of the left ventricle. The bending of the heart tube is the first morphologic demonstration that the left and right sides of the embryo will not be morphologic mirror images, inextricably linking cardiac development to the correct establishment of the three body axes [68,69].

All vertebrate and most invertebrate body plans demonstrate fundamental asymmetries about the three body axes of anterior–posterior (A–P), dorsal–ventral (D–V), and left–right (L–R). At the molecular level, the axes are determined by asymmetric propagation of signaling events occurring very early in development. The process of L–R axis determination as it concerns heart development has been recently reviewed and broadly conceptualized as requiring three steps involving the initiation, elaboration, and interpretation of the sidedness signal [70,71]. The first step requires initiation of polarity along the A–P, D–V, and L–R axes. The initiating signals for these events are unknown in mammalian embryos. The second step is an elaboration and amplification of the initial L–R asymmetry through a variety of cellular signaling mechanisms. As is true in general for developmental processes, most of the molecules involved in elaborating the L–R signaling process in mice have easily recognized counterparts in birds. However, in a remarkable twist on that theme, some of the molecules required for left-sidedness in mice are determinants of right-sidedness in birds [72]. The molecules responsible for these processes in humans are poorly understood. The third step is the interpretation of the asymmetric signals elaborated in the second step by the cells and tissues of developing organs. The developmental fates of paired structures as to whether to form with mirror symmetries (such as the limbs), or as paired but unequal structures (such as the cardiac atria) is thus the result of both proper signal delivery to the organ primordia and proper reaction of the organ primordia to the signal.

As a measure of the complexity of the impact of genetic mechanisms on L–R axis determination on cardiac development, many genetic models of abnormal cardiac looping have now been described in mice [73]. Some are primarily models of abnormal directionality of looping, while others also show perturbation of the alignment of cardiac segments. Mouse models of globally randomized situs [74,75], situs inversus [76], situs defects affecting different embryonic organs to different degrees [77], and situs defects with preferential bilateral right- or left-sidedness have all been described [73]. Many of the genes implicated in the mouse models are candidate genes for heterotaxies in the human population [78].

The left and right atria have their molecular identities determined by L–R signaling mechanisms. Molecular distinctions between left and right atria are established early after the atrial segment appears and are genetically dependent on L–R signaling mechanisms [79–81]. It is interesting to note, however, that there is often an increased incidence of transposition of the great arteries in mouse models of abnormal L–R axis determination [73], suggesting a possible element of L–R signaling in normal outflow development.

The mechanisms by which genetic signals result in regulated bending of the heart tube are unknown. Looping movements are intrinsic to the heart and will occur if the heart is isolated from the embryo, with or without beating [82,83]. The deformation of the straight heart tube into a looped structure likely results from some type of mechanical force [84]. However, the source of the required deforming force is not known. A simple explanation would be that myocytes replicate faster in the larger curvature of the loop and more slowly in the lesser curvature, and data suggesting a contribution of regional differences in growth have been presented [85,86]. However, cytochalasin B, an inhibitor of actin polymerization and therefore an inhibitor of cytoskeletal rearrangements, is also capable of either abolishing looping or reversing the direction of looping, according to whether it has been universally applied or selectively applied [87]. This suggests that the required asymmetric mechanical tension may be generated within the cells of the tube heart in response to as yet unknown regulatory signals.

Looping, Convergence, and Septation – Key Landmarks

Looping determines not only the sidedness of the heart but also the correct relationship of the segments of the heart to each other. Imaginary but useful divisions can be assigned to the morphogenetic steps leading from the more-or-less straight heart tube to the looped but still tubular heart, and from the looped heart to the heart poised for septation. Therefore, in this chapter, looping describes the initial period of growth, bending, and twisting of the heart tube. Looping begins and ends with the AV junction connected solely to the left ventricle and the outflow tract connected only to the right ventricle. The second phase of looping, sometimes called convergence, is the process of bringing the right atrial inflow over the right ventricle and the aortic outflow tract over the left ventricle, in the process aligning the outflow septal ridges for fusion with the primitive muscular septum and AV cushions. Ventricular septation is the process of closing the primary interventricular foramen while bringing the interventricular septum into continuity with the conus septum. Descriptions of these processes require recognition of a relatively small number of critical landmarks present in the embryonic heart during the looping and convergence stages of development (Figure 1.5) [7,88].

The looped heart has an inner curvature and an outer curvature. By nature of the tight angulation of the inner curvature the primitive atrial, AV, ventricular, and outflow segments are in close proximity for the remainder of cardiac development. As the region where the right ventricle acquires its inflow and the left ventricle acquires its outflow, the inner curvature of the heart is arguably the most critical, complex, and dynamic site in normal cardiac development.

On the lumenal surface of the heart, the fold in the heart at the inner curvature results in a small muscular ridge inside the heart between the AV junction and the outflow tract called the ventriculoinfundibular flange or ridge. Other key landmarks are the two major endocardial cushions of the AV junction and the two endocardial ridges of the outflow tract. The inferior endocardial cushion is attached to the dorsal AV myocardium and the superior endocardial cushion is attached to the ventral atrioventricular myocardium. As convergence proceeds, small right and left lateral AV endocardial cushions will become visible. The two outflow tract endocardial cushions form extended spiral ridges from the end of the truncus distally to the body of the right ventricle caudally. The endocardial cushion ridge ending in the anterior right ventricle is called the septal endocardial ridge. The endocardial ridge terminating posteriorly in the right ventricle is called the parietal endocardial ridge. The parietal endocardial ridge makes contact with the right lateral endocardial cushion, which itself will become continuous with the superior endocardial cushion. The septal endocardial ridge will make contact with the inferior endocardial cushion. As the endocardial cushions fuse during normal septation, they create, together with the mesenchymal cap of the primary atrial septum and the dorsal mesenchyme protrusion, the central AV mesenchymal complex extending from the AV junction to the distal extent of the myocardial outflow tract. At the most basic level the process of fusion of mesenchymal tissues can be thought of as a tissue zipper that septates the heart [26]. The reason that the endocardial cushion tissues of the conus septum cannot be found on inspection of the mature heart is that these mesenchymal structures are replaced by myocardium in the process known as myocardialization [89]. With respect to human congenital heart disease, this is a critical series of events, as disease phenotypes such as complex transposition, truncus arteriosus, and a number of tetralogy phenotypes all derive from aberrations of these normal developmental steps.

The left and right ventricular lumens are in continuity through the primary interventricular foramen. From the right ventricle, blood passes into the outflow tract of the heart. A myocardial cuff extends along the outflow tract to the junction with the aortic sac at the level of the pericardial reflection.

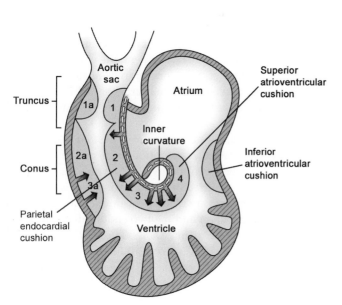
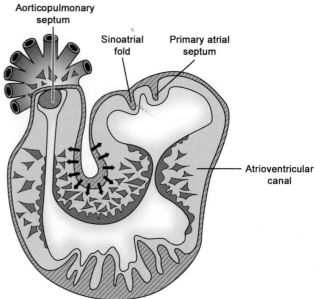

Figure 1.5 Highly simplified representation of key cardiac landmarks in early cardiac development. On the left, the cartoon illustrates the relative positions of the endocardial cushions at approximately HH stage 24. The truncal cushions are indicated as 1 and 1a, the distal conal cushions by 2 and 2a, the proximal conal cushions by 3 and 3a, and the superior atrioventricular cushion by 4. The arrows indicate the future sites of myocardialization. At the inner curvature, normal development results in loss of the myocardial sleeve and retention of the primitive fibrous continuity between the parietal endocardial cushion and the superior atrioventricular cushion. This is reflected by the fibrous continuity of the mitral valve and the aortic valve observed in the normal mature heart. In the cartoon on the right, the myocardialization of the inner curvature is indicated by the arrows; the mesenchymal invasion of the endocardial cushions is indicated by the polygonal cells. (After Mjaatvedt CH, Yamamura H, Wessels A, Ramsdell A, Turner D, *et al.* (1999) Mechanisms of segmentation, septation, and remodeling of the tubular heart: endocardial cushion fate and cardiac looping. In: Harvey RP, Rosenthal N, editors. *Heart Development*. San Diego: Academic Press. pp. 159–175 [88].)

During convergence, the angle of the inner curvature of the heart becomes more acute. The right AV junction is formed by rightward expansion of the AV junction, while at the same time the major (or midline) AV endocardial cushions are approaching each other in the center of the lumen of the AV junction. The outflow endocardial ridges, although unfused, define distinct aortic and pulmonary channels. The aortic channel moves leftward and anterior of its original position. Because of the combined rightward expansion of the AV orifice and the leftward movement of the aortic outflow tract the acute angle of the inner curvature now defines the region where the AV junction and the outflow tract are in continuity. These same morphogenetic movements result in rotation of the outflow ridges to a plane that is closer to parallel to that of the growing muscular septum.

Endocardial Cushion Development and Myocardialization

When the tube heart initially forms, the myocardial and endocardial cell layers are separated by an acellular substance traditionally called "cardiac jelly" [90]. Cardiac jelly can be regarded as a basement membrane, as it lies between two juxtaposed epithelia (the myocardium and the endocardium) and contains traditional basement membrane proteins. The initial production and distribution of these molecules is largely controlled by factors produced by the associated AV myocardium [91,92]. Cardiac jelly condenses into opposing swellings at the outflow and AV regions of the early, looped heart. The resulting endocardial cushions function in combination with the specialized contractile properties of the AV junction and outflow tract myocardium to prevent reversal of blood flow [93]. The AV endocardial cushions also function as the substrate for the formation of the mesenchymal tissues of the crux of the heart, including the AV valves and central fibrous body [94]. Endocardial cushions of the embryonic outflow tract participate in the formation of the aorticopulmonary septum, semilunar valves, and conus septum [95]. During morphogenesis of the endocardial cushions, the mesenchymal cell population that populates the originally acellular cardiac jelly is derived from the endothelial cells of the heart [67,96] along with a population of epicardially derived cells that also migrates into the AV cushions, but not the outflow tract cushions [97].

Endothelial invasion of the cardiac jelly results in a true transdifferentiation of cell phenotype, from a cell within a typical epithelium to an independently migratory, fibroblast-like mesenchymal cell [98–100]. This process has been compared to cellular changes during malignant transformation and is at least partially under the control of TGFβ-mediated signaling processes [101,102]. Only endocardium from the outflow tract and AV cushions are competent to undergo transformation, and only outflow tract and AV junction myocardium are able to induce transformation [101,103]. Not all the endocardial cells of the AV and conotruncal regions participate in these changes; as migration proceeds, residual endocardial cell populations undergo divisions to replenish their numbers. The mesenchymal cells also replicate actively to populate the cushions [99]. Recent data suggest that a similar process may result in an endothelial-to-mesenchymal transformation contributing to the neointima of atheromatous plaques [104].

Myocardialization is the process in which the mesenchyme of the endocardial cushions is replaced by myocardium [89]. All of the septal structures inside the heart – the interventricular septum, the atrial septum, and the conal septum – are created in part by fusion of nonmyocardial mesenchymal cushions. Myocardialization is responsible for the formation of the myocardial conus septum and the inlet and anterior outlet portions of the interventricular septum. In humans, the AV membranous septum is the only nonmyocardial septal structure derived from endocardial cushion tissue. The myocardialization of the conal cushions appears, based on Cre-lox cell fate studies, to primarily involve myocardial cell invasion of the cushion tissue. The mechanisms controlling this process are unclear [89,105,106].

Atrial Septation

Atrial septation and connection of the common pulmonary vein to the left atrium are closely related events in the normal heart [81]. Recent investigations in mouse, chick, and human embryos highlight the importance of the dorsal mesocardium to these events. At the site where the dorsal mesocardium is in continuity with the atrium (approximately the level of the lung buds) there is a protrusion of mesenchymal tissue into the atrium. This tissue has been recognized for many years and by a variety of names, including "spina vestibuli," "endocardial proliferation of the dorsal mesocardium," "sinus venosus tissue," and, most recently, the "dorsal mesenchymal protrusion" – the terminology adopted herein. Unlike other mesenchymal tissues in the AV junction, the dorsal mesenchymal protrusion is not derived from an epithelial-to-mesenchymal transformation, but rather is a derivative of the second

heart field [25,26]. The dorsal mesenchymal protrusion extends into the atrial cavity and is contiguous with the mesenchymal cap on the leading edge of the septum primum. Together with the two major atrioventricular cushions, the dorsal mesenchymal protrusion and the cap eventually fuse to form the atrioventricular mesenchymal complex. This process is essential for normal atrioventricular septation (Figure 1.6) [7,81]. Recent papers strongly suggest that perturbation of the development of the dorsal mesenchymal protrusion might be one of the major mechanisms in the pathogenesis of atrioventricular septal defects.

Based on the expression of several molecular markers that distinguish between left and right atrial myocardium [81], the myocardial portion of the septum primum is derived from left atrial myocardium. Growth of the septum primum occurs by lengthening of its myocardial portion. As described above, the mesenchymal cap on the leading edge of the septum primum is mesenchymal, the cells being derived by endothelial-to-mesenchymal transformation similar to that seen in the endocardial cushions [67]. As growth of the septum primum proceeds, it brings the mesenchymal cap of the septum, as well as the dorsal mesenchymal protrusion into contact with the two major AV endocardial cushions (Figure 1.7) [25,26]. The primary interatrial foramen is closed by fusion of these mesenchymal tissues as they form the AV mesenchymal complex [26]. Knowledge of this process is critical towards understanding the pathogenesis of complete common AV canal, as well as understanding the tissue relationships relevant to its repair.

Before the closure of the primary interatrial foramen occurs, the foramen secundum appears in the body of the septum primum. In humans, this process is initiated by the appearance of small fenestrations that increase in number and size until they coalesce into a definitive foramen secundum [81].

The septum secundum forms as an infolding of the atrial roof in the intervalvar space between the left venous valve of the sinus venosus and the septum primum. The septum secundum also marks the site of boundary between left atrial and right atrial tissues. As a result, the left atrial myocardium of the septum secundum exhibits left atrial markers while the right atrial myocardial surface of the septum secundum exhibits right atrial markers [81].

Interventricular Septation

As the primary interventricular foramen initially provides all of the inflow to the right ventricle and the entire outflow for the left ventricle, its correct closure is critical to normal cardiac development. Closure of the primary interventricular foramen is accomplished through coordinated growth of the muscular interventricular septum and fusion of

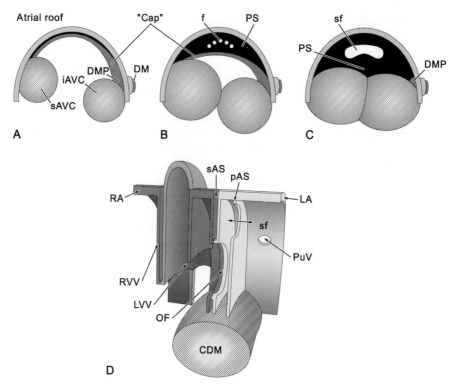

Figure 1.6 Sequence of events in atrial septation in human development. **A,** Heart at approximately 4.5 weeks of development. The leading edge of the septum primum is covered by a mesenchymal cap that is in continuity with the protrusion of the dorsal mesocardium into the atrial cavity. The superior and inferior atrioventricular cushions (sAVC and iAVC) are also in continuity with the mesenchymal cap. (DM, dorsal mesocardium; DMP, dorsal mesocardial protrusion.) **B,** Heart at ~6 weeks development. The septum primum with its mesenchymal cap is approaching the fusing inferior atrioventricular cushion and superior atrioventricular cushion. Fenestrations (f) are appearing in the muscular septum primum (PS). **C,** At ~6–7 weeks of development the fusion of the sAVC, iAVC, and cap of the septum primum is complete. The multiple fenestrations in the septum primum coalesce, forming the secondary foramen (sf). **D,** The secondary atrial septum (sAS) is created by infolding of myocardium at the junction of left and right atrial myocardium. Use of molecular markers distinguishing different populations of sinoatrial myocardial cells shows that the right-sided fold of the sAS and left venous valve (LVV) are derived from right atrial (RA) myocardium, while the left-sided fold of the sAS and primary atrial septum (pAS) are derived from left atrial (LA) myocardium. The right venous valve (RVV) is formed by infolding at the site of juncture of sinus venosus (SV) myocardium and RA myocardium, resulting in an RA molecular phenotype on the atrial surface and a SV molecular phenotype on the luminal surface. (CDM, endocardial cushion-derived mesenchyme; PuV, common pulmonary vein; OF, foramen ovale.) (After Wessels A, Anderson RH, Markwald RR, *et al.* (2000) Atrial development in the human heart: an immunohistochemical study with emphasis on the role of mesenchymal tissues. Anat Rec 259, 288–300 [81].)

endocardial cushions in the AV junction and the outflow tract.

Growth of the muscular interventricular septum is closely associated with dynamic changes in patterning of the ventricular myocardium [107]. When the heart tube initially forms and early after looping, its myocardial layers are but a few cells thick. After looping, the ventricular chambers enlarge caudally in a pouch-like fashion. The pouches are located on the greater curvature of the looped heart and quickly develop a series of circumferential ridges on their internal surfaces (Figure 1.8) [7,107].

The myocytes of the primitive trabecular ridges differ from the subjacent compact myocardium in that the myo-cytes of the compact myocardium are actively proliferating, while the trabecular myocytes have withdrawn from the cell cycle and are not dividing [107]. The "germinal layer" of compact myocardium provides increases in the numbers of ventricular wall myocytes, but the initial major increases in myocardial mass occur through increase in the trabecular component of the myocardium [107]. The compact myocardium "feeds" cells into the ventricular junctions of the developing trabeculae; this is a relationship that persists throughout embryonic myocardial growth [107].

The primitive trabecular ridges become fenestrated and sheet-like as they expand. Trabeculae are believed to

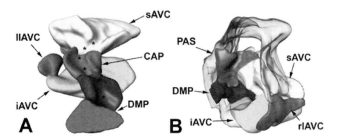

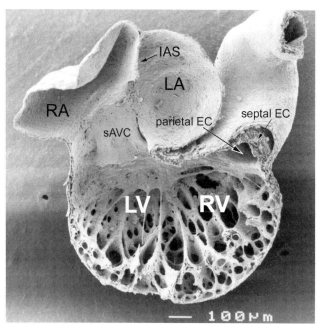

Figure 1.7 Three-dimensional reconstructions demonstrating the spatiotemporal relationships of the atrioventricular mesenchymal tissues during mouse heart development. Computer-generated three-dimensional reconstructions (AMIRA software) based on stained serial sections of mouse hearts **A** at embryonic day 11.5 and **B** at embryonic day 13. These panels show how the respective bodies of mesenchyme fuse with each other to accomplish atrioventricular septation. **A,** The mesenchymal tissues are viewed from above, while all other cardiac tissues are digitally removed to facilitate the study of the relationship of the mesenchymal components. At this stage, the individual mesenchymal components have not fused completely yet. The asterisks mark the groove within these tissues where the myocardial part of the septum primum is located (removed for reconstruction). **B,** The AV tissues are viewed as if one was standing in the right atrium. At this stage, all the mesenchymal tissues have fused. This panel demonstrates how the dorsal mesenchymal protrusion forms a wedge between the major AV cushions at the same time forming the base of the septum primum. At this stage the atrial cap cannot be distinguished any longer from the other endocardially derived mesenchymal tissues (for more detailed description see Snarr et al. [25,26]. (CAP, mesenchymal cap on the primary atrial septum; DMP, the dorsal mesenchymal protrusion; iAVC, inferior AV cushion; llAVC, left lateral AV cushion; PAS, primary atrial septum [septum primum]; rlAVC, right lateral AV cushion; sAVC, superior AV cushion.) (Reproduced with permission from Snarr et al. [26].)

Figure 1.8 Scanning electron micrograph of a section through the right and left ventricles of an embryonic chick heart. The pleat-like ridges characteristic of early myocardial trabeculum formation are easily appreciated. At this stage, the inner curvature of the heart separates the atrioventricular inflow from the right ventricle and the outflow tract from the left ventricle. (EC, endocardial cushion; IAS, interatrial septum; LA, left atrium; RA, right atrium; sAVC, superior atrioventricular cushion.) (Courtesy of David Sedmera.)

assume several physiologic functions in the primitive heart. They enhance contractile function of the ventricles [108]. The surface area of the endocardium is greatly increased by the presence of trabeculae, which is believed to improve nutrient and gas exchange with the developing myocardium before the development of a true coronary vasculature [109]. The trabeculae have been asserted to be the conduction system equivalent to (and possibly precursors to) the distal bundle branches and Purkinje fibers in the developing heart [42]. Trabeculae also help to direct the flow of blood in the preseptated heart [110]. Thus, the infrequent, yet important echocardiographic finding of ventricular noncompaction bears important implications.

In the chick heart, the primitive muscular septum is initially formed by a coalescence of trabeculae. In the mammalian heart, the primitive muscular septum appears to be the product of infolding of the compact myocardium pro-

duced by growth of the ventricular apices. Perhaps as a consequence, the interventricular groove is a more distinctive feature of mammalian hearts than avian hearts. The leading edge of the primitive muscular septum in humans is readily identified by the HNK1-Leu7 antibody that characterizes the primary ring (Figure 1.9) [7,111,112]. Use of this antibody in human embryos clearly demonstrates that the myocardial precursors of the right ventricle and right ventricular septum, including the inflow segment, are derived in their entirety from myocardial cell populations distal to the original primary interventricular foramen [113].

The primitive muscular interventricular septum is initially a crescent-shaped structure that extends at its posterior limit to the inferior endocardial cushion and at its anterior limit to the superior endocardial cushion. Part of the process of closure of the primary interventricular foramen consists of expansion of the superior and inferior endocardial cushions towards each other, where they will make contact and fuse at approximately 6 weeks' gestation in the human. The mechanism of fusion of the endocardial cushions in spite of the continuous mechanical activity of the heart is not known, but certainly deserves respect.

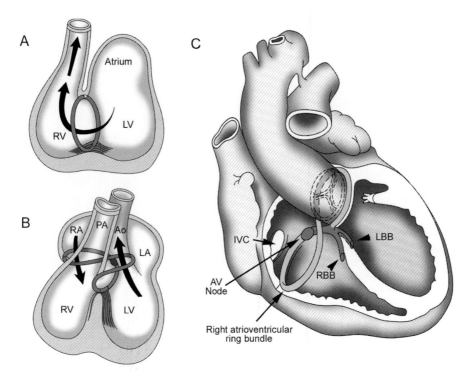

Figure 1.9 These diagrams demonstrate the development of the conduction system from a ring of myocardium detected in human embryonic heart by their expression of a carbohydrate epitope recognized by the antibodies Gln2, HNK1, and Leu7. **A,** Human heart at roughly 5 weeks' gestation. A ring of myocardium surrounding the primary interventricular foramen is detected. Note that the superior aspect of the ring is at the junction of atrioventricular (AV) myocardium and ventricular myocardium. **B,** In the human heart of roughly 7 weeks' development, convergence has resulted in expansion of the small segment of AV junctional myocardium to the right, accompanying the rightward expansion of the AV inlet. The leftward movement of the outlet results in the looping of the ring around the aortic root. As the muscular ventricular septum begins to grow, strands of ring tissue can be found extending from the major aspect of the ring on the crest of the septum down the septal walls towards the expanding apices of the right and left ventricles. **C,** The mature cardiac conduction system of AV node, bundle of His, and right bundle branch (RBB) and left bundle branch (LBB) is derived from the primitive ring tissue. In addition, remnants of the primitive ring in the adult heart can be found on the atrial side of the tricuspid valve fibrous annulus as well as in retroaortic myocardium. (RV; right ventricle, LV, left ventricle; RA, right atrium; LA, left atrium; PA, pulmonary artery; Ao, aorta; IVC, inferior vena cava.) (After Wessels A, Vermeulen JL, Verbeek FJ, *et al.* (1992) Spatial distribution of "tissue-specific" antigens in the developing human heart and skeletal muscle. III. An immunohistochemical analysis of the distribution of the neural tissue antigen G1N2 in the embryonic heart; implications for the development of the atrioventricular conduction system. Anat Rec 232, 97–111 [111]; and Moorman AFM, Lamers WH (1999) Development of the conduction system of the vertebrate heart. In: Harvey RP, Rosenthal N, editors. *Heart Development.* San Diego: Academic Press. pp. 195–207 [112].)

Further growth of the interventricular muscular septum results in fusion of the crest of the septum with the fused cushion. The boundaries between the original muscular septum and endocardial cushion-derived portions of the septum become obscured by myocardialization except for the membranous septum between the left ventricle and right atrium. Normal inlet septum development is primarily determined by interactions between the inferior endocardial cushion-derived tissue and the muscular ventricular septum, while the smooth anterior interventricular septum is derived from interactions between the superior endocardial cushion and the muscular septum. The membranous septum is the approximate site of final union between the muscular septum and the superior and inferior endocardial cushions [114].

The Atrioventricular Junction Segment and Atrioventricular Valve Development

The electrophysiologic and physiologic properties of the junctional myocardium between the primitive atria and ventricles are critical to the preseptated heart, as previously discussed. However, myocardial continuity between the AV junctional myocardium, the atrial myocardium, and the ventricular myocardium must be interrupted for the development of the fibrous crux of the heart and the correct function of the conduction system. This is accomplished by formation of a layer of fibrous insulation called the annulus fibrosis that will completely interrupt myocardial continuity between the AV myocardium and the ventricular myocardium, with the exception of the penetrating bundle of His specialized myocardium. In the mature heart the remnants of AV junction myocardium become incorporated into the myocardium of the definitive atrium [94].

Fibrous interruption of AV myocardial continuity results from the fusion of mesenchymal cell populations of the AV endocardial cushions with a mesenchymal cell population found in the atrioventricular sulcus on the external surface of the looped heart. Atrioventricular sulcus mesenchyme cells are brought to the heart in the course of the epicardial cell migration (see Figure 1.3) [7], as discussed in greater detail later in this chapter in connection with coronary artery development. Morphologic studies suggest that the sulcus mesenchyme actively invaginates into the endocardial cushions [115]; the mechanisms driving mesenchymal invagination and the parting of the myocardial layer are unknown. Interruption of myocardial continuity begins at 52 to 60 days of gestation in the human heart and is normally "complete" by the fourth month of gestation [94]. Failure to form the insulating tissues of the AV junction may underlie clinical pre-excitation syndromes. Interestingly, isolated myocytes possibly representing remnants of the embryonic junctional myocardium, originally present between the sulcus mesenchyme and the endocardial cushion mesenchyme, have been identified bridging the fibrous insulation of normal neonatal hearts [116]. This location is different from that noted for parietal accessory atrioventricular bundles [117], which are described as subepicardial and, therefore, seem to represent a different myocardial path through the sulcus mesenchyme-derived fibrous tissue. No structures similar to parietal accessory AV connections are noted in the course of normal development. Thus, the possibility that these accessory connections develop postnatally should be considered. The relationship between pre-excitation pathways in general and normal morphologic events requires further investigation.

Atrioventricular valve development may be tied to the process of sulcus tissue ingrowth, as the hinge points of the definitive leaflets are normally found at the point of juncture between the endocardial cushion tissues and the invaginating sulcus tissue. Atrioventricular valve leaflets are formed by separation of endocardial cushion tissue and myocardium from the ventricular walls in the poorly understood process of delamination [105,118,119]. Other events occurring at the same time that certainly influence normal valvar morphogenesis and may contribute to the delamination process include coarsening of the ventricular trabeculae, incorporation of trabeculae into the compact myocardium, and apical expansion of the ventricular cavity.

At the time of delamination, the atrial surfaces of the valve leaflets are composed of endocardial cushion tissue while the ventricular surfaces are primarily myocardial. The myocardial layer provides continuity with the evolving subvalvar tension apparatus. As leaflet morphogenesis proceeds, the myocardial component is eliminated by unknown processes. Initially, the ends of the AV leaflets are connected to the compact ventricular myocardium either directly or via trabecular outgrowths of the myocardium. As development proceeds, papillary muscles are derived by two mechanisms: from initially independent, pre-existing trabeculae coalescing together to form papillary muscles; and from delamination of myocardium into myocardial structures that join with trabeculae or form of themselves the papillary muscles. The mitral valve papillary muscles are derived from a single large trabecula that then separates into the two independent papillary supports [119]. Thus the surgically challenging group of patients with parachute mitral valve derivatives are likely due to deficiencies in this process. Tricuspid valve papillary muscles develop independently from each other and via different mechanisms; the anterior papillary muscle of the tricuspid derives from an early coalescence of trabeculae detectable at 6 weeks' gestation, the septal leaflet papillary muscle is a product of delamination during the tenth to twelfth week of gestation, and the posterior papillary muscle complex is still a relatively indistinct structure at 12 weeks' gestation [105]. Chordae are formed by progressive fenestration and fibrous differentiation of trabeculae and/or the initially solid individual valve leaflets; there is disagreement with respect to the derivation of chordae from myocardium or endocardial cushion tissue [105,107,118].

As previously noted, there are four endocardial cushions in the AV junction. The superior and inferior cushions are the most prominent endocardial cushion masses from their first appearance, but there are also important contributions from the lateral endocardial cushions, which are visible only after Carnegie Stage 17 (approximately 42 days) [94,118]. The left lateral cushion contributes to the posterior (mural) leaflet of the mitral valve. The right lateral cushion, which becomes continuous anteriorly with the septal endocardial cushion of the outflow tract, contributes to the formation of the anterior and inferior leaflets of the tricuspid valve.

Atrioventricular valve morphogenesis is one of the most prolonged aspects of human cardiac development. Recognizable elements of the tricuspid valve begin formation at 5–6 weeks' gestation. The AV endocardial cushions are actively reconfiguring at this time, with fusion of the superior and right lateral AV endocardial cushions to each other. The conal cushions are also completing their fusion during this time. The fused outflow septum then expands apically to reach the inner curvature of the heart, anterior to the fusing superior and right lateral endocardial cushions. In this position the fused outflow cushions will become adherent to the myocardium of the ventriculoinfundibular fold, establishing the anterior position of the conus septum with respect to the atrioventricular valvular structures, and also forming the crista supraventricularis [105]. Despite the overall advanced stage of cardiac morphogenesis at this point, the tricuspid valve leaflets are still very primitive in appearance and not freely mobile. The inferior leaflet is fully delaminated by the end of the eighth week of gestation, the anterior leaflet by the eleventh week, and the septal leaflet in the twelfth week. The commissure separating the anterior and septal leaflets is not complete until the septal leaflet is fully delaminated [105].

In development of the mitral valve, the inferior and superior AV cushions begin to fuse at roughly 5 weeks' gestation; even before fusion, the enlarged trabecular complex that will evolve into the two mitral papillary muscles can be seen connecting the superior and inferior cushions [118,119]. The left lateral cushion, the precursor to the posterior leaflet, is visible by the seventh week of gestation. At approximately this time initial delamination of the mitral valve structures becomes detectable and continues until the tenth week of development. Between the tenth and fourteenth weeks of development myocardial elements of the leaflets are eliminated, papillary muscles achieve their adult appearance, and chordae differentiate [118,119].

Development of the Conduction System

The sinoatrial node first becomes detectable at approximately 10.5 days in mouse development, roughly equivalent to Carnegie stage 14 (approximately 32 days) of human development, at the medial wall of the right common cardinal vein and extending cranially to the junction of the anterior and common cardinal veins. This corresponds to what will become the portion of the superior vena cava between the orifice of the azygous vein and the right atrium in the adult [120].

In the human embryo the AV node becomes detectable histologically at approximately Carnegie stage 15 (approximately 33 days) [121]. It is located in the posterior portion of the AV canal in the myocardium under the ventricular margin of the inferior endocardial cushion and is included in the primary ring [94]. The primitive AV node is in direct continuity with the AV and ventricular myocardium. From the earliest stages a cellular tract destined to become the bundle of His can be noted extending from the main mass of AV nodal tissue to the ventricular subendocardium. The AV sulcus mesenchyme will invaginate to make contact with the endocardial cushion mesenchyme inferiorly to the main mass of the developing AV node while encasing the future bundle of His in the fibrous insulating tissue at the crux of the heart [94].

The proximal bundle branches are detected in the human by antibodies to the primary ring antigen Gln2/HNK1/Leu7 (Figure 1.9) [7,111,112]. Differentiation of conduction tissue in the ventricles appears to occur by a process of recruitment of "working" myocardium into the conduction lineage and to be associated with withdrawal from the cell cycle [122,123]. Numerous observations support the contention that the trabeculae of the primitive heart are the initial conduction pathways connecting the proximal bundle branches with the ventricular free walls [124]. Subsets of trabeculae probably remain as elements of the conduction tissue in the mature heart.

The cellular morphology of Purkinje fibers is extremely variable between species [125]. In some species intramural Purkinje fibers are very difficult to distinguish by morphologic criteria. Molecular markers that unambiguously identify intramural Purkinje fibers across species are not known [124]. However, in all animals in which they have been studied, intramural Purkinje fibers are late-appearing structures in comparison to the central AV node–His bundle–bundle branch conduction tissues. In the developing sheep heart, where Purkinje fibers are easily distinguished by morphologic criteria from "working" ventricular myocytes, intramural Purkinje fibers are not seen until 60 days' gestation, while the AV node becomes visible as early as 27 days' gestation [126]. In this species, morphologic differentiation of the conduction tissue clearly progresses outward from the AV node.

Purkinje fibers in the chick embryo myocardium can be recognized by specific expression of the gap junction protein Cx42. Use of this marker shows that chick embryo Purkinje fibers are only detectable at day 10 of chicken development. In this model ventricular myocytes are recruited to differentiate into Purkinje cells only in the vicinity of developing coronary arteries [123]. Data suggest that endothelin signaling may be an important determinant of this process [127].

Morphogenesis of the Outflow Tract

Landmarks in the Outflow Tract

The morphologic terminology for the outflow tract used in this chapter follows that proposed by Pexieder [128]. The outflow tract is relatively short in the early phases of looping, after which it becomes elongated, with a distinct bend. The site of the bend is the primary external landmark dividing the truncus from the conus portions of the outflow tract: separate structures. The external landmarks for the entire region are the ventriculoinfundibular fold proximally and the aortic sac distally. The aortic sac–outflow junction is identified by flaring of the root of the aortic sac, the reflection of the pericardium, and the distal limit of the cardiac jelly and myocardium. The proximal end of the outflow tract lumen is marked by myocardial ridge on the inner surface of the ventriculoinfundibular fold, the ventriculoinfundibular flange. The septal outflow ridge and parietal outflow ridge spiral from the right ventricle to the distal outflow tract, with a distinct change in their direction noted at the site of the bend in the outflow tract. As septation proceeds, the myocardial outflow tract shortens.

At the base of the heart the conal ridges are continuous with the AV endocardial cushions. During remodeling of the conus the mesenchymal (fibrous) continuity of the cushions will be retained between the mitral and aortic valves but will be lost between the tricuspid and pulmonary valves. The mechanisms through which outflow tract remodeling occurs are of great interest but remain largely undetermined. It is precisely these mechanisms that are of particular importance in understanding the pathogenesis of a large number of clinically challenging congenital heart disease phenotypes. Indeed, the normal processes of outflow tract remodeling are easily disrupted via pharmacologic, genetic, or experimental microsurgical manipulations, often resulting in persistence of a complete myocardial conus for both semilunar valves and a ventricular septal defect – double-outlet right ventricle (DORV) [129,130]. In one experimental model in which a clip was placed on a vitelline vein, the resulting malformation appeared to be secondary to altered embryonic blood flow; however, this model of altered blood flow does not explain the vast majority of congenital heart disease phenotypes [129,131,132]. Indeed, different teratogenic models are capable of resulting in different forms of conal abnormalities within the spectrum of DORV [129]. The frequency with which DORV is observed in experimental models pre-sumably points to the requirement for integration of multiple processes for the embryonic heart to proceed beyond the "default" relationship of having both great arteries arising from the right ventricle. It also points out that the terminology "DORV" may undesirably lump an etiologically disparate group of defects into one final common pathway lesion. Thus, careful analysis of vessel morphology is required to accurately determine the cardiac phenotype. Alternatively, varieties of DORV may be forms of developmental arrest that represent final common morphologic pathways for a multitude of initial insults [130].

Aorticopulmonary Septation

The aorticopulmonary septum is initially formed as a condensation of mesenchyme in the roof of the aortic sac, between the fourth and sixth aortic arches (Figure 1.10) [7,130]. The extracardiac origin of this mesenchyme had been well recognized since the late 1970s [133] and in 1983 was identified by Kirby to be a population of neural crest cells [134]. Two prongs of mesenchymal condensations penetrate into the endocardial cushion ridges at the truncal end of the outflow tract. Septation moves towards the heart and is accomplished by fusion of the prongs of neural crest-derived mesenchyme. As the septum forms, the arterial trunks thus become separated by neural crest-derived smooth muscle cells [106]. As aorticopulmonary septation proceeds towards the heart and the trunks of the aorta and pulmonary artery become distinct, the distal extent of the myocardial sleeve remains at or below the septation complex. There is very little apoptosis detected in the distal

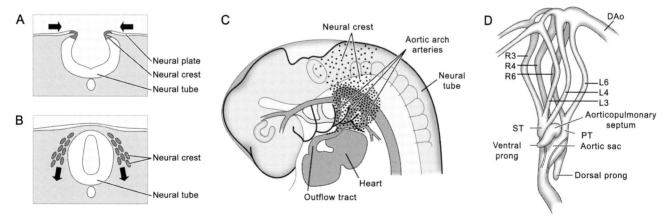

Figure 1.10 Features of the neural crest contribution to normal cardiac development. **A,** and **B,** The neural crest is a population of cells that is released to migrate throughout the embryo by fusion of the lateral neural plates to form the closed neural tube. **C,** The cardiac neural crest migrates via the aortic arch arteries into the outflow tract of the heart. **D,** The neural crest cells that form the aorticopulmonary septum form a condensed mass of cells between the fourth and sixth aortic arch vessels with two "prongs" that penetrate into the conal and truncal endocardial cushions. (PT, pulmonary trunk; ST, systemic trunk; DAo, descending aorta.) (Reproduced with permission from Kirby [130]. Contribution of neural crest to heart and vessel development. In: Harvey RP, Rosenthal N, eds. *Heart Development*. pp. 179–193. Copyright © 1999 Elsevier.)

truncal myocardium, so it is probable that the myocardium is not simply dying away [106]. It remains a topic of active debate whether subaortic conal myocardium retracts towards the heart or transdifferentiates into smooth muscle cells in the roots of the aorta and pulmonary artery [106,135,136]. In the absence of the aorticopulmonary septum, the outlet of the heart communicates with a common arterial trunk such as that seen in truncus arteriosus or in incomplete forms such as aorticopulmonary window.

Development of the Semilunar Valves

The semilunar valves develop at the juncture between the aorticopulmonary septum and the conus septum. They are derived from the parietal and septal conal ridges, the small intercalated ridges that form between the conal endocardial ridges, and the mesenchymal prongs of neural crest-derived mesenchyme that penetrate into the conal endocardial ridges. In the mouse, the neural crest cells of the mesenchymal prongs are marked by expression of the protein α-smooth muscle actin (ASMA) [106,137]. Cardiac neural crest cells can also be visualized using a variety of transgenic mouse model systems, the most frequently used being the Wnt1-cre mouse in combination with the Rosa26R-lacZ reporter mouse [67]. Fusion of the endocardial ridges occurs by contact of the ridges followed by disappearance of the endothelial cells at the site of contact. The ridges are then connected to each other by a whorl or knot-like structure of ASMA-positive cells, which is the forming aorticopulmonary septum.

Semilunar valve leaflet development begins shortly after septation. In mice, the initial process is outgrowth of unexcavated cusps of tissue corresponding to the future leaflets from the arterial surface of the distal endocardial ridges and intercalated cushions [138]. Valve sinuses are formed by active endothelial excavation of the outlet surface of the leaflets. The initial valve leaflets are thickened structures filled with an abundant extracellular ground substance densely populated with endocardial-derived mesenchymal cells bordered by a cuboidal endothelium on the arterial surface and a flattened, streamlined endothelium on the ventricular surface [139]. After the sinuses are fully excavated, the leaflets remodel into the delicate fibrous tissue characterizing mature semilunar valves [139]. Valve remodeling is a slow process that may be histologically incomplete at the time of birth [138,140]. The mechanisms of these processes are largely unexplored. The neural crest does not play as prominent a role as in aorticopulmonary septum formation – the only ASMA-positive neural crest-derived cells present in the semilunar valve leaflets as they develop are at the junctures of the leaflet commissures and the arterial wall of the great vessels [106]. These locations may hint at links between neural crest abnormalities and abnormalities of valve commissure formation or location.

A mouse model of both aortic and pulmonary valve aplasia secondary to ablation of the *Nfatc* gene has been described [141,142]. NFAT proteins are transcription factors known to be important mediators of intracellular calcium signaling in the immune system, nervous system, myocardium, and skeletal muscle [143]. NFAT signaling is initiated by calcineurin, the primary intracellular target of cyclosporine and FK506. During heart development, expression of the *Nfatc* gene is limited to a subset of cells in the endocardium, but beyond this observation the mechanism of contribution of NFATc to semilunar valve development is unknown. Although rare, aplasia of both semilunar valves has been described in humans as well [144,145]. Additionally, single semilunar valve dysplasia is one of the most common forms of congenital heart disease, either seen in isolation (e.g., bicuspid aortic valve) or in conjunction with other defects such as tetralogy of Fallot, tetralogy of Fallot with absent pulmonary valve syndrome, pulmonary atresia, and a wide variety of left ventricular outflow tract defects that include aortic valvar hypoplasia with hypoplastic left heart syndrome as its most severe manifestation.

A more complex model of abnormal semilunar valvulogenesis is found in mice deficient for *Sox4* [146]. These animals die in mid-gestation with semilunar valve insufficiency (as do NFATc-deficient embryos) and have been demonstrated to suffer from a spectrum of cardiovascular defects ranging from isolated lack of the infundibular septum to complete failure of conotruncal and aorticopulmonary septation. Additional extracardiac defects noted include tracheoesophageal fistulae. The outflow tract malformations noted in this model are hypothesized to result from abnormalities in signaling between neural crest (see below) and the outflow tract endocardial cushion cell populations. Unlike the models of common trunk associated with "pure" neural crest defects, *Sox4*-deficient mice exhibit variably severe defects in the numbers and relative differentiation of semilunar valve cusps.

Conus Septation

Formation of the conus septum is a multistep process. Initially the conal endocardial ridges are "simple" structures consisting of cardiac jelly bounded by endocardium and myocardium. As in the AV cushions, a subset of endocardial cells transdifferentiates into mesenchymal cells that then invade the cardiac jelly. The conal endocardial ridges subsequently enlarge and, with each sphincter-like contraction of the conal myocardium, are brought into apposition [93]. Fusion of the endocardial ridges, another poorly understood process, proceeds temporally from the distal conus to the base of the heart and results in an initially mesenchymal conus septum. When the proximal conal cushions fuse they complete the separation of the subaortic and subpulmonary outflow tracts. The endocardial cushion tissue is then replaced by myocardial tissue in a process that is initially completed at the proximal conus septum and is last completed at the distal conus septum. The myocardialization of the conal cushions results in the formation of the supraventricular crest and the muscular outflow septum.

Mesenchymal neural crest prongs of the aorticopulmonary septation complex extend into the conal endocardial ridges, but unlike their role in aorticopulmonary septation they do not form the conal septum. The neural crest cells in the conal ridges disappear, possibly by an apoptotic mechanism, and their presence is speculated to be important in some way for regulating the subsequent process of myocardialization [147].

Morphogenesis of the Great Vessels and Coronary Circulation

The Neural Crest and Cardiac Development

Neural crest cells migrate into the heart through the aortic arches and are necessary for aorticopulmonary septation, outflow tract septation, and formation of the tunica media of the third, fourth, and sixth aortic arch vessels [130,134,148]. An additional population of neural crest cells differentiates into the entirety of the autonomic innervation of the heart. Other neural crest-derived structures in proximity to the developing heart and great vessels include the thymus, thyroid, and parathyroid glands.

The neural crest is a transient structure in vertebrate development originating in the dorsal-most region of the neural tube (Figure 1.10) [7,130,148,149]. The cells of the neural crest reside on the lateral margins of the neural plate and the right- and left-sided populations are brought into apposition by the folding of the neural plate into the neural tube. The cells then disperse and migrate along precise pathways to their multiple destinations. As with closure of the neural tube, this process is initiated cranially and extends caudally [148]. Specific regions of the neural crest seed cells via specific pathways to specific structures [150]. The neural crest cells that reach the outflow tract of the early heart migrate via the third, fourth, and sixth aortic arch vessels. The region of the neural crest contributing to cardiac and fourth aortic arch morphogenesis is sometimes called the "cardiac" neural crest [130,148].

Experimental ablation of the cardiac neural crest results in structural heart defects including DORV, truncus arteriosus, tetralogy of Fallot, and ventricular septal defects [149]. The most consistent impact of experimental neural crest ablation on the cardiovascular system in chick embryos is aberrant patterning of the aortic arch arteries, although no specific malformation of the aortic arch vessels is predominant in this model [130]. There are strong similarities between lesions observed following neural crest ablations in the chick embryo and the spectrum of cardiovascular anomalies in the DiGeorge syndrome [151,152]. Several cardiac teratogens in experimental animals have spectra of defects that are also comparable, such as bis-diamine in rats [153], alcohol in mice [154], nimustine hydrochloride in fetal rats and chick embryos [155,156], endothelin A blockade in chick embryos [157], and retinoic acid in humans [158]. Mouse genetic models of abnormal neural crest function include the Splotch mouse, caused by loss of the transcription factor PAX3 [159]. Endothelin signaling is particularly important in cardiac neural crest functioning, as demonstrated by the presence of aortic arch abnormalities and other neural crest-associated defects in mice bearing targeted disruptions of endothelin 1 (ET-1) [160,161], endothelin converting enzyme-1 (ECE-1) [162], and the endothelin-A (ETA) receptor [163,164]. Additional mouse models exhibiting cardiovascular features of cardiac neural crest deficiency include the trisomy 16 mouse and mice with targeted multigene deletions comparable to human chromosome 22q11 microdeletions [137,165].

Origins of the Outflow Tract Endothelium

In common with the endothelium of the aortic arch vessels, outflow tract endothelium is derived from precursors in lateral and paraxial mesoderm of the cranial region [166] corresponding to cells of the second heart field [35]. Similarly, the epicardium of the distal portion of the outflow tract is derived from a separate population of precursor cells than that of the remainder of the heart [167]. As previously noted, the outflow tract myocardium, the myocardium of the right ventricle, and interventricular septum originate from the second heart field [35]. Taken together, these data suggest a distinct developmental origin of the entirety of the cardiac outflow tract.

Epicardial Cell Migration and Development of the Coronary Arteries

The development of the epicardium is a relatively late event in the development of the heart, but its proper formation is essential for normal development of the coronary arteries, valves, and the interstitial fibroblast population of the myocardium. The epicardium migrates over the surface of the heart from villous projections in the region of the septum transversum in mammals [168–171]. The precursor tissue is histologically and functionally complex and has been called the proepicardium or proepicardial organ [172]. It is a transitory embryonic structure that gives rise to the epicardial cell layer and is also the source of the nonmyocardial mesenchymal cells (i.e., fibroblasts, coronary smooth muscle cells) of the heart. The migrating cells eventually flatten over the surface of the myocardium and develop morphologic characteristics compatible with primitive epithelial cells. The flattening process also causes cells to occupy a greater surface area, bringing adjacent clusters of cells into contact with each other until a continuous sheet results. In the rodent, where the process is well studied, these events occur between days 9 and 11 of embryonic life, and the villous projections are markedly diminished by day 10.5 [171,172]. This is poorly understood in human development; while these important processes in rodent development are complete just before mid-gestation, in the human most are shifted towards the first 2 months of development (see [173] for comparison of developmental landmarks between human and mouse).

As the epicardial layer of cells extends over the heart, an extensive acellular extracellular matrix layer appears between the epicardium and the myocardium. If migration from the proepicardial organ is physically disrupted in chick embryos, then no epicardium develops and there is failure of the subepicardial extracellular matrix to form as well [174]. The subepicardial space becomes populated by mesenchymal subepicardial cells generally accepted to provide the precursors of cardiac fibroblasts, coronary vascular smooth muscle cells, and coronary endothelial cells. Recent publications using transgenic mouse models that allow the tracing of cells derived from the epicardium have also suggested that these cells may give rise to a population of myocytes localized in the interventricular septum [175,176]. The subepicardial extracellular matrix accumulates to its greatest degree in the AV groove. In addition to being a key site for coronary vasculogenesis, the mesenchymal cells that come to populate the AV groove matrix will form the majority of the fibrous insulating ring between the atria and the ventricles [94]. All of the cell populations just described as invading the myocardium and/or subepicardial extracellular matrix have come to be known as epicardial-derived cells (EPDCs) [97]. As identified by lineage markers, EPDCs migrate into the sulcus matrix and subsequently into the AV endocardial cushions. In addition to entering the AV cushions, EPDCs also migrate into the myocardium and subendocardium. Specific possible morphogenetic roles of the myocardial and subendocardial EPDCs have not been determined, but abnormalities of the compact myocardium, AV cushions, and coronary vasculature have all been documented in their absence [167].

The subepicardial space is the site of origin of the vascular plexus of the coronary vessel precursors. There are three sequential and overlapping phases of nutrient delivery to the myocardium during embryogenesis of the heart [109,177]. The first phase is associated with the development of an extensive network of intratrabecular sinusoids lined by endocardial cells through which nutrient flow to the myocardium likely occurs. The second phase is the development of a subepicardial plexus of endothelial-lined channels that penetrate the myocardium. A subset of these channels will communicate with the intratrabecular sinusoids. The third stage is regression and coalescence of the vascular subepicardial network into muscular arterial channels. As soon as the vessels are readily identifiable they are noted to penetrate into the ventricular and atrial walls, where they establish a mid-myocardial network. The vessels spread to the ventral surface of the heart and follow the sulci (especially the AV sulcus) to the outflow tract where they form a plexus in the myocardial sheath surrounding the truncus arteriosus. Coalescence of vessels and capillary outgrowth from the peritruncal plexus results in penetration of the wall of the aorta by the definitive proximal coronary arteries [172,177–179]. Abnormalities of this process likely contribute to the pathogenesis of a number of surgically important disease phenotypes including intramural coronary ostia, abnormalities of coronary positioning in both normally related and transposed great vessels, and anomalous left coronary artery from the pulmonary artery syndrome.

Development of the Aortic Arch

The great vessels are the conduit for blood to flow from the heart to the body and, therefore, must be formed and functional at the time of initiation of embryonic circulation (approximately day 20–22 in humans). The vessels of the embryo are formed by a process called vasculogenesis. Vasculogenesis occurs by aggregation of pre-endothelial cells (angioblasts) into networks of small endothelial channels (in contrast to the process of building vessels by sprouting growth or branching, called angiogenesis). The dorsal aorta and aortic arches are created by fusion of independently formed regional vasculogenic networks. After communications between the networks are established the definitive lumen is formed through merging of the small endothelial passages into larger channels [180,181]. The channels are functional vessels composed of only endothelial cells. Mesenchymal cells in the descending aorta and neural crest cells in the aortic arch region will then be recruited to form the smooth muscle cells of the media of the developing arteries by an obscure process [182–184]. These enveloping events require signaling through extracellular proteins known as angiopoietins via the Tie1 (TIE) and Tie2 (TEK) receptors in endothelial cells [185]. The transcription factor KLF2 (LKLF) has also been shown to be necessary for formation of the tunica media in embryonic vessels [186].

The initial embryonic arterial circulation is morphologically bilaterally symmetric and consists of multiple pairs of aortic arch vessels connecting the heart outflow to the paired dorsal aortae. The dorsal aortae are initially paired for the full length of the embryo. Fusion of the paired aortae into a single structure begins distally and progresses retrograde to the seventh somite. As development proceeds, the paired first, second, third, fourth, and sixth aortic vessels and the dorsal aortae undergo an intricate series of transformations. The first and second aortic arch vessels regress, remaining patent only as capillary structures. The dorsal aorta between the third and fourth aortic arch vessels (the carotid duct) regresses completely, leaving no remnant, resulting in the paired third aortic arch vessels becoming the only source of blood flow from the aortic sac/truncus complex to the head of the embryo. The third aortic arch vessels become the precursors of the definitive common carotid arteries. The right dorsal aorta completely regresses at the site of dorsal aortic bifurcation; this leaves the right fourth aortic arch vessel to become a short stub connecting the right seventh intersegmental (future subclavian) artery to the aortic sac/truncus complex. The right sixth aortic arch vessel becomes the right pulmonary artery. The left sixth aortic arch vessel becomes the left pulmonary artery and the ductus arteriosus connecting the pulmonary plexus-derived distal main pulmonary artery and left pulmonary artery to the left dorsal aorta at the junction of the left dorsal aorta and the left fourth arch vessel. The left dorsal aorta remains widely patent throughout its length but remodels so that the definitive left fourth aortic arch vessel, the ductus arteriosus, and the left seventh intersegmental artery (future left subclavian artery) all connect to the left dorsal aorta within a very short span. Understanding these developmental concepts and relationships is important in planning repair of great vessel abnormalities as well as vascular rings. Despite the generally superb imaging (echocardiography, computed tomography angiography, or magnetic resonance imaging) that accompanies patients with aortic patterning defects, one is occasionally surprised by intraoperative findings. A facile knowledge of great vessel developmental derivatives can help troubleshoot an intraoperative surprise and potentially limit the dissection required to reveal the relevant operative anatomy.

The vertebral arteries are derived from anastomoses between the seven cervical intersegmental arteries. After continuity is established between the intersegmental arteries their connections to the dorsal aorta regress (with the exception of the connection of the seventh intersegmental vessel that becomes the subclavian artery) creating the subclavian origin of the definitive vertebral arteries.

Neural crest cells are critical to the normal pattern of regression or maintenance of aortic arch vessel patency (Figure 1.10) [7,130]. When neural crest cells are physically ablated in chick embryos, vascular patterning is abnormal in 100% of experiments, although the specific pattern of ablation-induced abnormalities is not predictable [181]. Neural crest cells invade and replace the original tunica media of the aortic arch vessels, but it is not known by what subsequent mechanisms neural crest cells determine the future vascular pattern.

Several genetic models of abnormal aortic vessel patterning that are not yet linked to neural crest abnormalities have been identified in mouse and zebra fish. Knockout experiments in mice involving the closely related transcription factors mesoderm/mesenchyme forkhead 1 (MF1) and mesenchyme forkhead 1 (MFH1) demonstrate cardiovascular phenotypes that include coarctation of the aorta, interruption of the aortic arch, ventricular septal defects, and in the case of MF1, thickening and partial fusion of semilunar valve leaflets [187].

Development of the Pulmonary Veins

The earliest evidence of the formation of the common pulmonary vein in the embryo is the presence of a strand of endothelial cells in the dorsal mesocardium. The endothelial strand forms a lumen and initially is a midline structure. As the dorsal mesenchymal protrusion is developing and projecting into the atrial cavity on the right side of the primitive pulmonary vein, the relative position of the pulmonary vein changes as it occupies a position to the left of the middle [67]. The continued development of the dorsal mesenchymal protrusion, the myocardialization of this mesenchyme, and the concomitant growth of the septum primum eventually result in the connection of the pulmonary vein to the left atrium in normal development [81]. Therefore, the development of the pulmonary vein does not result from an outgrowth of the atrial wall. The remodeling of the original single common pulmonary vein orifice into the four separate orifices characteristic of the mature heart is a topic deserving of additional study. Initially, the walls of the pulmonary veins are not muscular. However, as development proceeds, myocardial sleeves are formed around these veins. Recent studies have revealed some of the molecular pathways that underlie this mechanism [188]. As pulmonary myocardium is a frequent site initiating atrial fibrillation, advancing our knowledge of this event is of high importance.

Development of the Systemic Veins

The embryonic systemic veins are also formed by vasculogenesis. Initially there are three bilaterally symmetric venous drainages: the vitelline, umbilical, and cardinal venous systems [189]. The vitelline veins drain the embryonic gastrointestinal tract and gut derivatives. The umbilical veins bring oxygenated blood from the placenta to the heart. The cardinal venous system returns blood from the embryonic head, neck, and body wall. All three of these drainages enter into the sinus venosus of the primitive heart tube. The adult venous pattern is established through complex patterns of regression, remodeling, and replacement of these embryonic venous systems and their connections to the sinus venosus [190,191].

The sinus venosus is initially bilaterally symmetric, with right and left "horns" that provide connection for the right and left common cardinal veins, umbilical veins, and vitelline veins. However, the connections of the left-sided cardinal, vitelline, and umbilical venous systems with the left horn of the sinus venosus normally regress. This results in the coronary sinus remaining as the primary structural derivative of the left horn of the sinus venosus in the normal fetal and postnatal heart. When embryonic venous connections with the left venous horn fail to regress, persistence of the left superior vena cava is observed. The right horn of the sinus venosus normally accommodates the entirety of the systemic venous drainage except the portion from the heart returned via the coronary sinus. In addition, the portion of the mature right atrium between the orifices of the vena cavae is derived from the right horn of the sinus venosus.

The right and left vitelline veins are connected to each other via a plexus of veins that become the liver sinusoids. The left vitelline vein regresses after it loses connection with the left horn of the sinus venosus. Therefore, the entire venous system of the embryonic gut normally drains to the heart through the right vitelline vein. The connection of the right vitelline vein to the right sinus venosus persists into fetal and adult life as the terminal portion of the inferior vena cava.

The left umbilical vein also loses its connection with the left horn of the sinus venosus, but it is the right umbilical vein that regresses as a distinct structure. The left umbilical vein forms anastomoses with the ductus venosus (derived from the liver plexus of the vitelline veins). No derivatives of the embryonic umbilical venous drainage connect to the heart or persist following the closure of the ductus venosus in adult life.

The cardinal venous system initially consists of bilateral anterior cardinal veins and bilateral posterior cardinal veins. Fusion of the anterior and posterior cardinal veins at the level of the sinus venosus forms the common cardinal veins. The left anterior cardinal vein loses its connection with the left horn of the sinus venosus, but a small remnant on the surface of the heart normally persists as a passage of coronary venous blood to the coronary sinus and is known as the oblique vein of the left atrium. Another portion of the left anterior cardinal vein persists as the left internal jugular vein. As the left anterior cardinal vein loses connection with the heart it becomes connected to the right anterior cardinal vein via the intercardinal anastomosis that forms between the thyroid vein and the thymic vein; this connection will persist as the left brachiocephalic vein. The portion of the right anterior cardinal vein between the right atrium and the drainage of the left anterior cardinal vein proximally (via the intercardinal anastomosis) becomes the normal right superior vena cava.

The posterior cardinal veins are the only portions of the embryonic venous drainage that are destined to have a symmetrical fate. Both posterior cardinal veins will regress throughout most of their length and lose their direct connections with the sinus venosus. The posterior cardinal veins originally drain the body wall, gonadal, and renal structures. Their function in venous drainage of the body wall is supplanted by the supracardinal venous plexus, while the gonadal and renal venous drainage is captured by the subcardinal venous plexus.

The posterior cardinal, supracardinal, and subcardinal venous beds contribute the segments that form the definitive inferior vena cava (IVC) to the level of the vitelline vein-derived segment connecting to the right atrium origin. Remnants of the posterior cardinal veins in the fetal and adult circulation are limited to the most distal portion of the IVC (formed by anastomosis of the right and left posterior cardinal veins) and the common iliac veins. The posterior cardinal vein-derived IVC connects to the supracardinal segment of the IVC. The supracardinal venous system is the site of origin of the azygous and hemiazygous veins, which ordinarily connect to the IVC between the renal veins and the common iliac veins. The supracardinal segment of the IVC connects to the subcardinal segment of the IVC, which receives the drainage of the gonadal veins and renal veins before connecting to the vitelline venous channel into the heart.

In both the supracardinal and subcardinal venous systems the initial vascular structures are bilaterally symmetric, with the left-sided channels regressing and the right-sided channels persisting, resulting in the typical right sided location of the IVC. The mechanisms through which the definitive systemic venous structures are formed are very poorly understood. The frequency of venous drainage abnormalities in human and animal models of altered left-right axis differentiation [73] makes it clear that the mechanisms of venous morphogenesis are likely dependent on appropriate left-right signaling. This is a particularly important series of developmental relationship that persists in those cases of interrupted IVC with azygous continuation in which the hepatic veins drain directly into the right atrium.

References

1. Hamburger V, Hamilton HL. (1992) A series of normal stages in the development of the chick embryo. 1951. Dev Dyn 195, 231–272.
2. O'Rahilly R, Muller F, Streeter GL. (1987) *Developmental Stages in Human Embryos*. Washington, DC: Carnegie Institution of Washington.
3. Streeter GL. (1942) Developmental horizons in human embryos. Description of age group XI, 13–20 somites, and

age group XII, 21–29 somites. Contrib Embryol 30, 211–245.

4. Streeter GL. (1945) Developmental horizons in human embryos. Description of age group XIII, embryos about 4 or 5 millimeters long, and age group XIV, period of indentation of lens cesicle. Contrib Embryol 32, 27–63.

5. Streeter GL. (1948) Developmental horizons in human embryos. Description of age group XI, 13–20 somites, age group XV, XVI, XVII, and XVII. Contrib Embryol 32, 133–203.

6. Theiler K. (1989) *The House Mouse: Atlas of Embryonic Development*. New York, NY: Springer Verlag.

7. McQuinn T, Wessels A. (2003) Embryology of the heart and great vessels. In: Mavroudis C, Backer CL, editors. *Pediatric Cardiac Surgery* 3rd ed. Philadelphia, PA: Mosby Inc. pp. 1–24.

8. Gilbert SF. (1994) *Developmental Biology*. Sunderland, MA: Sinauer Associates Inc. pp. 202–243.

9. Inagaki T, Garcia-Martinez V, Schoenwolf GC. (1993) Regulative ability of the prospective cardiogenic and vasculogenic areas of the primitive streak during avian gastrulation. Dev Dyn 197, 57–68.

10. Lough J, Sugi Y. (2000) Endoderm and heart development. Dev Dyn 217, 327–342.

11. Black BL, Olson E. (1999) Control of cardiac development by the MEF2 family of transcription factors. In: Harvey M, Rosenthal N, editors. *Heart Development*. San Diego, CA: Academic Press. pp. 131–142.

12. Bruneau BG, Logan M, Davis N, *et al.* (1999) Chamber-specific cardiac expression of Tbx5 and heart defects in Holt–Oram syndrome. Dev Biol 211, 100–108.

13. Harvey RP, Biben C, Elliott DA. (1999) Transcriptional control and pattern formation in the developing vertebrate heart: Studies on NK-2 class homeodomain factors. In: Harvey RP, Rosenthal N, editors. *Heart Development*. San Diego, CA: Academic Press. pp. 111–129.

14. Horb ME, Thomsen GH. (1999) Tbx5 is essential for heart development. Development 126, 1739–1751.

15. Parmacek MS. (1999) GATA transcription factors and cardiac development. In: Harvey M, Rosenthal N, editors. *Heart Development*. San Diego, CA: Academic Press. pp. 291–306.

16. Srivastava D. (1999) Segmental regulation of cardiac development by the basic helix-loop-helix transcription factors dHAND and eHAND. In: Harvey M, Rosenthal N, editors. *Heart Development*. San Diego, CA: Academic Press. pp. 143–155.

17. Prall OW, Menon MK, Solloway MJ, *et al.* (2007) An Nkx2-5/Bmp2/Smad1 negative feedback loop controls heart progenitor specification and proliferation. Cell 128, 947–959.

18. Mohun TJ, Leong LM. (1999) Heart formation and the heart field in amphibian embryos. In: Harvey M, Rosenthal N, editors. *Heart Development*. San Diego, CA: Academic Press. pp. 37–49.

19. Baldwin HS, Jensen KL, Solursh M. (1991) Myogenic cytodifferentiation of the precardiac mesoderm in the rat. Differentiation 47, 163–172.

20. Goss CM (1942) The physiology of the embryonic mammalian heart before circulation. Am J Physiol 137, 146–152.

21. Linask KK, Lash JW (1988) A role for fibronectin in the migration of avian precardiac cells. I. Dose-dependent effects of fibronectin antibody. Dev Biol 129, 315–323.

22. De Ruiter M, Poelmann R, VanderPlas-de Vries I, *et al.* (1992) The development of the myocardium and endocardium in mouse embryos. Anat Embryol 185, 461–473.

23. De Haan RL. (1959) Cardia bifida and the development of pacemaker function in the early chicken heart. Dev Biol 1, 586–602.

24. Webb S, Brown NA, Anderson RH, *et al.* (2000) Relationship in the chick of the developing pulmonary vein to the embryonic systemic venous sinus. Anat Rec 259, 67–75.

25. Snarr BS, O'Neal JL, Chintalapudi MR, *et al.* (2007) Isl1 expression at the venous pole identifies a novel role for the second heart field in cardiac development. Circ Res 101, 971–974.

26. Snarr BS, Wirrig EE, Phelps AL, *et al.* (2007) A spatiotemporal evaluation of the contribution of the dorsal mesenchymal protrusion to cardiac development. Dev Dyn 236, 1287–1294.

27. Verberne ME, Gittenberger-de Groot AC, van Iperen L, *et al.* (2000) Distribution of different regions of cardiac neural crest in the extrinsic and the intrinsic cardiac nervous system. Dev Dyn 217, 191–204.

28. Sohal GS, Ali MM, Ali AA, *et al.* (1999) Ventrally emigrating neural tube cells differentiate into heart muscle. Biochem Biophys Res Comm 254, 601–604.

29. Rawles ME. (1943) The heart-forming ares of the early chick blastoderm. Physiol Zool 16, 22–42.

30. Rosenquist GC, De Haan RL. (1966) Migration of precardiac cells in the chick embryo: a radioautographic study. *Contributions to Embryology*. Washington, DC: Carnegie Institute of Washington. pp. 111–121.

31. Stalsberg H, DeHaan RL. (1969) The precardiac areas and formation of the tubular heart in the chick embryo. Dev Biol 19, 128–159.

32. de la Cruz MV, Sanchez Gomez C, Arteaga MM, *et al.* (1977) Experimental study of the development of the truncus and the conus in the chick embryo. J Anat 123, 661–686.

33. Kelly RG, Brown NA, Buckingham ME. (2001) The arterial pole of the mouse heart forms from Fgf10-expressing cells in pharyngeal mesoderm. Dev Cell 1, 435–440.

34. Mjaatvedt CH, Nakaoka T, Moreno-Rodriguez R, *et al.* (2001) The outflow tract of the heart is recruited from a novel heart-forming field. Dev Biol 238, 97–109.

35. Verzi MP, McCulley DJ, De Val S, *et al.* (2005) The right ventricle, outflow tract, and ventricular septum comprise a restricted expression domain within the secondary/anterior heart field. Dev Biol 287, 134–145.

36. Waldo KL, Kumiski DH, Wallis KT, *et al.* (2001) Conotruncal myocardium arises from a secondary heart field. Development 128, 3179–3188.

37. de la Cruz MV, Sanchez-Gomez C, Palomino MA. (1989) The primitive cardiac regions in the straight tube heart (Stage 9) and their anatomical expression in the mature heart: an experimental study in the chick embryo. J Anat 165, 121–131.

38. Patten BM, Kramer TC. (1933) The initiation of contraction in the embryonic chick heart. Am J Anatomy 53, 349–375.

39. Castro-Quezada A, Nadal-Ginard B, de la Cruz MV. (1972) Experimental study of the formation of the bulboventricular loop in the chick. J Embryol Exp Morphol 27, 623–637.

40. Markwald RR, Trusk T, Moreno-Rodriguez R. (1998) Formation and septation of the tubular heart integrating the dynamics of morphology with emerging molecular concepts. In: de la Cruz MV, Markwald RR, editors. *Living Morphogenesis of the Heart*. Boston, MA: Birkhauser. pp. 43–84.

41. Moorman AF, Lamers WH. (1998) Molecular anatomy of the developing heart. Trends Cardiovasc Med 4, 257–264.

42. de Jong F, Opthof T, Wilde AA, *et al.* (1992) Persisting zones of slow impulse conduction in developing chicken hearts. Circ Res 71, 240–250.

43. Conlon RA, Rossant J. (1992) Exogenous retinoic acid rapidly induces anterior ectopic expression of murine Hox-2 genes in vivo. Development 116, 357–368.

44. Ruiz i Altaba A, Jessell T. (1991) Retinoic acid modifies mesodermal patterning in early *Xenopus* embryos. Genes Dev 5, 175–187.

45. Conlon RA. (1995) Retinoic acid and pattern formation in vertebrates. Trends Genet 8, 314–319.

46. Kastner P, Grondona JM, Mark M, *et al.* (1994) Genetic analysis of RXRα developmental function: convergence of RXR and RAR signaling pathways in heart and eye morphogenesis. Cell 78, 987–1003.

47. Osmond MK, Butler AJ, Voon FCT, *et al.* (1991) The effects of retinoic acid on heart formation in the early chick embryo. Development 113, 1405–1417.

48. Smith S, Dickman ED. (1997) New insights into retinoid signaling in cardiac development and physiology. Trends Cardiovasc Med 7, 324–329.

49. Gruber PJ, Kubalak SW, Pexieder T, *et al.* (1996) RXRα deficiency confers genetic susceptibility for aortic sac, conotruncal, atrioventricular cushion, and ventricular muscle defects in mice. J Clin Invest 98, 1332–1343.

50. Dersch H, Zile MH. (1993) Induction of normal cardiovascular development in the vitamin A-deprived quail embryo by natural retinoids. Dev Biol 160, 424–433.

51. Heine UI, Roberts AB, Munoz EF, *et al.* (1985) Effects of retinoid deficiency on the development of the heart and vascular system of the quail embryo. Virchows Archives (Cell Pathology) 50, 135–152.

52. Twal W, Roze L, Zile MH. (1995) Anti-retinoic acid monoclonal antibody localizes all-trans-retinoic acid in target cells and blocks normal development in early quail embryo. Dev Biol 168, 225–234.

53. Dickman ED, Smith SM. (1996) Selective regulation of cardiomyocyte gene expression and cardiac morphogenesis by retinoic acid. Dev Dyn 206, 39–48.

54. Pexieder T, Blanc O, Pelouch V, *et al.* (1995) Late fetal development of retinoic acid induced transposition of the great arteries. In: Clark MR, Takas A, editors. *Developmental Mechanisms of Heart Disease*. Armonk, NY: Futura Publishing Company. pp. 297–307.

55. Kostetskii I, Jiang Y, Kostetskaia E, *et al.* (1999) Retinoid signaling required for normal heart development regulates GATA-4 in a pathway distinct from cardiomyocyte differentiation. Dev Biol 206, 206–218.

56. Liberatore CM, Searcy-Schrick RD, Yutzey KE. (2000) Ventricular expression of tbx5 inhibits normal heart chamber development. Dev Biol 223, 169–180.

57. Yutzey KE, Rhee JT, Bader D. (1994) Expression of the atrial-specific myosin heavy chain AMHC1 and the establishment of anterior polarity in the developing chicken heart. Development 120, 871–883.

58. Means A, Gudas L. (1995) The roles of retinoids in vertebrate development. Annu Rev Biochem 64, 201–233.

59. Moss JB, Xavier-Neto J, Shapiro MD, *et al.* (1998) Dynamic patterns of retinoic acid synthesis and response in the developing mammalian heart. Dev Biol 199, 55–71.

60. Xavier-Neto J, Shapiro MD, Houghton L, *et al.* (2000) Sequential programs of retinoic acid synthesis in the myocardial and epicardial layers of the developing avian heart. Dev Biol 219, 129–141.

61. Kelly RG, Franco D, Moorman AF, *et al.* (1999) Regionalization of transcriptional potential in the myocardium. In: Harvey RP, Rosenthal N, editors. *Heart Development*. San Diego, CA: Academic Press. pp. 333–355.

62. He CZ, Burch JB. (1997) The chicken GATA-6 locus contains multiple control regions that confer distinct patterns of heart region-specific expression in transgenic mouse embryos. J Biol Chem 272, 28550–28556.

63. Srivastava D, Thomas T, Lin Q, *et al.* (1997) Regulation of cardiac mesodermal and neural crest development by the bHLH transcription factor, dHAND. Nat Gen 16, 154–160.

64. Akagi K, Sandig V, Vooijs M, *et al.* (1997) Cre-mediated somatic site-specific recombination in mice. Nucleic Acids Res 25, 1766–1773.

65. McCulley DJ, Kang JO, Martin JF, *et al.* (2008) BMP4 is required in the anterior heart field and its derivatives for endocardial cushion remodeling, outflow tract septation, and semilunar valve development. Dev Dyn 237, 3200–3209.

66. Moon A. (2008) Mouse models of congenital cardiovascular disease. Cur Top Dev Biol 84, 171–248.

67. Snarr BS, Kern CB, Wessels A. (2008) Origin and fate of cardiac mesenchyme. Dev Dyn 237, 2804–2819.

68. Manner J. (2000) Cardiac looping in the chick embryo: A morphological review with special reference to terminological and biomechanical aspects of the looping process. Anat Rec 259, 248–262.

69. Manner J. (2009) The anatomy of cardiac looping: a step towards the understanding of the morphogenesis of several forms of congenital cardiac malformations. Clin Anat 22, 21–35.

70. Yost HJ. (1999) Establishing cardiac left-right asymmetry. In: Harvey RP, Rosenthal N, editors. *Heart Development*. San Diego, CA: Academic Press. pp. 373–389.

71. Bakkers J, Verhoeven MC, Abdelilah-Seyfried S. (2009) Shaping the zebrafish heart: from left-right axis specification to epithelial tissue morphogenesis. Dev Biol 330, 213–220.

72. Meyers EN, Martin GR. (1999) Differences in left–right axis pathways in mouse and chick: functions of FGF8 and SHH. Science 285, 403–406.

73. McQuinn TC, Miga DE, Mjaatvedt CH, *et al.* (2001) Cardiopulmonary malformations in the inv/inv mouse. Anat Rec 263, 62–71.

74. Icardo JM, Sanchez de Vega MJ. (1991) Spectrum of heart malformations in mice with situs solitus, situs inversus, and associated visceral heterotaxy. Circulation 84, 2547–2558.

75. Layton WM, Jr. (1976) Random determination of a developmental process: reversal of normal visceral asymmetry in the mouse. J Hered 67, 336–338.

76. Yokoyama T, Copeland NG, Jenkins NA, *et al.* (1993) Reversal of left-right asymmetry: a situs inversus mutation. Science 260, 679–682.

77. Tan SY, Rosenthal J, Zhao XQ, *et al.* (2007) Heterotaxy and complex structural heart defects in a mutant mouse model of primary ciliary dyskinesia. J Clin Invest 117, 3742–3752.

78. Casey B, Hackett BP. (2000) Left–right axis malformations in man and mouse. Curr Opin Genet Dev 10, 257–261.

79. Franco D, Kelly R, Lamers WH, *et al.* (1997) Regionalized transcriptional domains of myosin light chain 3f transgenes in the embryonic mouse heart: morphogenetic implications. Dev Biol 188, 17–33.

80. Kitamura K, Miura H, Miyagawa-Tomita S, *et al.* (1999) Mouse Pitx2 deficiency leads to anomalies of the ventral body wall, heart, extra- and periocular mesoderm and right pulmonary isomerism. Development 126, 5749–5758.

81. Wessels A, Anderson RH, Markwald RR, *et al.* (2000) Atrial development in the human heart: an immunohistochemical study with emphasis on the role of mesenchymal tissues. Anat Rec 259, 288–300.

82. Manasek FJ, Monroe RG. (1972) Early cardiac morphogenesis is independent of function. Dev Biol 27, 584–588.

83. Manning A, McLachlan JC. (1990) Looping of chick embryo hearts in vitro. J Anat 168, 257–263.

84. Taber LA. (2006) Biophysical mechanisms of cardiac looping. Int J Dev Biol 50, 323–332.

85. Sissman NJ. (1966) Cell multiplication rates during development of the primitive cardiac tube in the chick embryo. Nature 210, 504–507.

86. Stalsberg H. (1969) The origin of heart asymmetry: right and left contributions to the early chick embryo heart. Dev Biol 19, 109–127.

87. Itasaki N, Nakamura H, Sumida H, *et al.* (1991) Actin bundles on the right side in the caudal part of the heart tube play a role in dextro-looping in the embryonic chick heart. Anat Embryol (Berl) 183, 29–39.

88. Mjaatvedt CH, Yamamura H, Wessels A, *et al.* (1999) Mechanisms of segmentation, septation, and remodeling of the tubular heart: endocardial cushion fate and cardiac looping. In: Harvey RP, Rosenthal N, editors. *Heart Development.* San Diego, CA: Academic Press. pp. 159–175.

89. van den Hoff MJ, Moorman AF, Ruijter JM, *et al.* (1999) Myocardialization of the cardiac outflow tract. Dev Biol 212, 477–490.

90. Davis CL. (1924) The cardiac jelly of the chick embryo. Anat Rec 27, 201.

91. Kitten GT, Markwald RR, Bolender DL. (1987) Distribution of basement membrane antigens in cryopreserved early embryonic hearts. Anat Rec 217, 379–390.

92. Markwald RR, Krug EL, Runyan RB, *et al.* (1985) Proteins in cardiac jelly which induce mesenchyme formation. In: Ferrans VA, Rosenquist GC, Weinstein C, editors. *Cardiac Morphogenesis.* New York, NY: Elsevier. pp. 60–68.

93. Patten BM, Kramer TC, Barry A. (1948) Valvular action in the embryonic chick heart by localized apposition of endocardial masses. Anat Rec 102, 299–311.

94. Wessels A, Markman MW, Vermeulen JL, *et al.* (1996) The development of the atrioventricular junction in the human heart. Circ Res 78, 110–117.

95. Van Mierop LH, Alley RD, Kausel HW, *et al.* (1962) The anatomy and embryology of endocardial cushion defects. J Thorac Cardiovasc Surg 43, 71–83.

96. Bolender DL, Markwald RR. (1979) Epithelial–mesenchymal transformation in chick atrioventricular cushion morphogenesis. Scan Electron Microsc, 313–321.

97. Gittenberger-de Groot AC, Vrancken Peeters MP, Mentink MM, *et al.* (1998) Epicardium-derived cells contribute a novel population to the myocardial wall and the atrioventricular cushions. Circ Res 82, 1043–1052.

98. Fitzharris TP. (1981) Endocardial shape change in the truncus during cushion tissue formation. In: Pexieder T, editor. *Mechanisms of Cardiac Morphogenesis and Teratogenesis.* New York, NY: Raven Press. pp. 227–235.

99. Markwald RR, Fitzharris TP, Manasek FJ. (1977) Structural development of endocardial cushions. Am J Anat 148, 85–120.

100. Pexieder T. (1981) Prenatal development of the endocardium: a review. Scan Electron Microsc, 223–253.

101. Nakajima Y, Krug EL, Markwald RR. (1994) Myocardial regulation of transforming growth factor-beta expression by outflow tract endothelium in the early embryonic chick heart. Dev Biol 165, 615–626.

102. Nakajima Y, Yamagishi T, Nakamura H, *et al.* (1998) An autocrine function for transforming growth factor (TGF)-β3 in the transformation of atrioventricular canal endocardium into mesenchyme during chick heart development. Dev Biol 194, 99–113.

103. Runyan RB, Markwald RR. (1983) Invasion of mesenchyme into three-dimensional collagen gels: a regional and temporal analysis of interaction in embryonic heart tissue. Dev Biol 95, 108–114.

104. De Ruiter MC, Poelmann RE, VanMunsteren JC, *et al.* (1997) Embryonic endothelial cells transdifferentiate into mesenchymal cells expressing smooth muscle actins in vivo and in vitro. Circ Res 80, 444–451.

105. Lamers WH, Virágh S, Wessels A, *et al.* (1995) Formation of the tricuspid valve in the human heart. Circulation 91, 111–121.

106. Ya J, Vandenhoff MJB, Deboer PAJ, *et al.* (1998) Normal development of the outflow tract in the rat. Circ Res 82, 464–472.

107. Sedmera D, Pexieder T, Vuillemin M, *et al.* (2000) Developmental patterning of the myocardium. Anat Rec 258, 319–337.

108. Challice CE, Viragh S. (1974) The architectural development of the early mammalian heart. Tissue Cell 6, 447–462.

109. Tokuyasu KT. (1985) Development of myocardial circulation. In: Ferrans VJ, Rosenquist G, Weinstein C, editors. *Cardiac Morphogenesis.* Amsterdam, Netherlands: Elsevier. pp. 226–237.

110. Hogers B, DeRuiter MC, Baasten AM, *et al.* (1995) Intracardiac blood flow patterns related to the yolk sac circulation of the chick embryo. Circ Res 76, 871–877.

111. Wessels A, Vermeulen JL, Verbeek FJ, *et al.* (1992) Spatial distribution of "tissue-specific" antigens in the developing human heart and skeletal muscle. III. An immunohisto-chemical analysis of the distribution of the neural tissue antigen G1N2 in the embryonic heart; implications for the development of the atrioventricular conduction system. Anat Rec 232, 97–111.

112. Moorman AFM, Lamers WH. (1999) Development of the conduction system of the vertebrate heart. In: Harvey RP, Rosenthal N, editors. *Heart Development.* San Diego, CA: Academic Press. pp. 195–207.

113. Lamers WH, Wessels A, Verbeek FJ, *et al.* (1992) New findings concerning ventricular septation in the human heart. Implications for maldevelopment. Circulation 86, 1194–1205.

114. de la Cruz MV, Markwald RR. (1998) Embryological development of the ventricular inlets: septation and atrioventricular valve apparatus. In: de la Cruz MV, Markwald RR, editors. *Living Morphogenesis of the Heart.* Boston, MA: Birkhauser. pp. 131–155.

115. Manner J. (1999) Does the subepicardial mesenchyme contribute myocardioblasts to the myocardium of the chick embryo heart? A quail-chick chimera study tracing the fate of the epicardial primordium. Anat Rec 255, 212–226.

116. Wessels A, Mijnders TA, de Gier-de Vries C, *et al.* (1992) Expression of myosin heavy chain in neonate human hearts. Cardiol Young 2, 318–334.

117. Anderson RH, Becker AE, Brachenmacher C, *et al.* (1972) Ventricular preexcitation: a proposed nomenclature for its substrates. Euro J Cardiol 3, 27–36.

118. Oosthoek PW, Wenink AC, Vrolijk BC, *et al.* (1998) Development of the atrioventricular valve tension apparatus in the human heart. Anat Embryol (Berl) 198, 317–329.

119. Oosthoek PW, Wenink AC, Wisse LJ, *et al.* (1998) Development of the papillary muscles of the mitral valve: morphogenetic background of parachute-like asymmetric mitral valves and other mitral valve anomalies. J Thorac Cardiovasc Surg 116, 36–46.

120. Van Mierop LH, Gessner IH. (1970) The morphologic development of the sinoatrial node in the mouse. Am J Cardiol 25, 204–212.

121. Domenech-Mateu JM, Arno-Palau A, Martinez-Pozo A. (1991) Study of the development of the atrioventricular conduction system as a consequence of observing an extra atrioventricular node in the normal heart of a human fetus. Anat Rec 230, 73–85.

122. Cheng G, Litchenberg WH, Cole GJ, *et al.* (1999) Development of the cardiac conduction system involves recruitment within a multipotent cardiomyogenic lineage. Development 126, 5041–5049.

123. Gourdie RG, Mima T, Thompson RP, *et al.* (1995) Terminal diversification of the myocyte lineage generates Purkinje fibers of the cardiac conduction system. Development 121, 1423–1431.

124. Moorman AF, de Jong F, Denyn MM, *et al.* (1998) Development of the cardiac conduction system. Circ Res 82, 629–644.

125. Viragh S, Challice CE. (1973) The impulse generation and conduction system of the heart. In: Challice CE, Viragh S, editors. *Ultrastructure of the Mammalian Heart.* New York, NY: Academic Press. pp. 43–89.

126. Canale E, Smolich JJ, Campbell GR. (1987) Differentiation and innervation of the atrioventricular bundle and ventricular Purkinje system in sheep heart. Development 100, 641–651.

127. Gourdie RG, Wei Y, Kim D, *et al.* (1998) Endothelin-induced conversion of embryonic heart muscle cells into impulse-conducting Purkinje fibers. Proc Natl Acad Sci U S A 95, 6815–6818.

128. Pexieder T (1995) Overview: conotruncus and its septation at the advent of the molecular biology era. In: Clark EB, Markwald RR, Takao A, editors. *Developmental Mechanisms of Heart Disease.* Armonk, NY: Futura Publishing Co., Inc. pp. 227–247.

129. Gittenberger-de Groot AC, Poelmann RE. (1997) Principles of abnormal cardiac development. In: Burggren W, Keller B, editors. *Development of Cardiovascular Systems.* New York, NY: University Press. pp. 259–267.

130. Kirby ML. (1999) Contribution of neural crest to heart and vessel development. In: Harvey RP, Rosenthal N, editors. *Heart Development.* San Diego, CA: Academic Press. pp. 179–193.

131. Hogers B, DeRuiter MC, Gittenberger-de Groot AC, *et al.* (1997) Unilateral vitelline vein ligation alters intracardiac blood flow patterns and morphogenesis in the chick embryo. Circ Res 80, 473–481.

132. Hogers B, DeRuiter MC, Gittenberger-de Groot AC, *et al.* (1999) Extraembryonic venous obstructions lead to cardiovascular malformations and can be embryolethal. Cardiovasc Res 41, 87–99.

133. Thompson RP, Fitzharris TP. (1979) Morphogenesis of the truncus arteriosus of the chick embryo heart: the formation and migration of mesenchymal tissue. Am J Anat 154, 545–556.

134. Kirby ML, Gale TF, Stewart DE. (1983) Neural crest cells contribute to normal aorticopulmonary septation. Science 220, 1059–1061.

135. Bartelings MM, Gittenberger-de Groot AC. (1988) The arterial orifice level in the early human embryo. Anat Embryol (Berl) 177, 537–542.

136. Thompson RP, Fitzharris TP. (1985) Division of cardiac flow. In: Ferrans VA, Rosenquist GC, Weinstein C, editors. *Cardiac Morphogenesis.* New York, NY: Elsevier. pp. 169–180.

137. Waller BR, McQuinn T, Phelps AL, *et al.* (2000) Conotruncal anomalies in the Trisomy 16 mouse: an immunohistochemical analysis with emphasis on the involvement of neural crest. Anat Rec 260, 279–293.

138. Hurle JM, Colvee E, Blanco AM. (1980) Development of mouse semilunar valves. Anat Embryol (Berl) 160, 83–91.

139. Maron BJ, Hutchins GM. (1974) The development of the semilunar valves in the human heart. Am J Pathol 74, 331–344.

140. Hyams VJ, Manion WC. (1968) Incomplete differentiation of the cardiac valves. A report of 197 cases. Am Heart J 76, 173–182.

141. de la Pompa JL, Timmerman LA, Takimoto H, *et al.* (1998) Role of the NF-ATc transcription factor in morphogenesis of cardiac valves and septum. Nature 392, 182–186.

142. Ranger AM, Grusby MJ, Hodge MR, *et al.* (1998) The transcription factor NF-ATc is essential for cardiac valve formation. Nature 392, 186–190.

143. Crabtree GR (1999) Generic signals and specific outcomes: signaling through Ca2+, calcineurin, and NF-AT. Cell 96, 611–614.

144. Hartwig NG, Vermeij-Keers C, De Vries HE, *et al.* (1991) Aplasia of semilunar valve leaflets: two case reports and developmental aspects. Pediatric Cardiol 12, 114–117.

145. Miyabara S, Ando M, Yoshida K, *et al.* (1994) Absent aortic and pulmonary valves: investigation of three fetal cases with cystic hygroma and review of the literature. Heart Vessels 9, 49–55.

146. Ya J, Schilham MW, de Boer PA, *et al.* (1998) Sox4-deficiency syndrome in mice is an animal model for common trunk. Circ Res 83, 986–994.

147. Poelmann RE, Mikawa T, Gittenberger-de Groot AC. (1998) Neural crest cells in outflow tract septation of the embryonic chicken heart: differentiation and apoptosis. Dev Dyn 212, 373–384.

148. Gilbert SF. (1994) *Developmental Biology* 4th ed. Sunderland, MA: Sinauer Associates Inc. pp. 272–288.

149. Kirby ML, Turnage KL 3rd, Hays BM. (1985) Characterization of conotruncal malformations following ablation of "cardiac" neural crest. Anat Rec 213, 87–93.

150. Phillips MT, Kirby ML, Forbes G. (1987) Analysis of cranial neural crest distribution in the developing heart using quail-chick chimeras. Circ Res 60, 27–30.

151. Nishibatake M, Kirby ML, Van Mierop LH. (1987) Pathogenesis of persistent truncus arteriosus and dextroposed aorta in the chick embryo after neural crest ablation. Circulation 75, 255–264.

152. Van Mierop LH, Kutsche LM. (1986) Cardiovascular anomalies in DiGeorge syndrome and importance of neural crest as a possible pathogenetic factor. Am J Cardiol 58, 133–137.

153. Ikeda T, Matsuo T, Kawamoto K, *et al.* (1984) Bis-diamine induced defects of the branchial apparatus in rats. In: Nora JJ, Takao A, editors. *Congenital Heart Disease: Causes and Processes.* Mt Kisco, NY: Futura. pp. 223–236.

154. Daft PA, Johnston MC, Sulik KK. (1986) Abnormal heart and great vessel development following acute ethanol exposure in mice. Teratology 33, 93–104.

155. Miyagawa S, Ando M, Takao A. (1988) Cardiovascular anomalies produced by nimustine hydrochloride in the rat fetus. Teratology 38, 553–558.

156. Miyagawa S, Kirby ML. (1989) Pathogenesis of persistent truncus arteriosus induced by nimustine hydrochloride in chick embryos. Teratology 39, 287–294.

157. Kempf H, Linares C, Corvol P, *et al.* (1998) Pharmacological inactivation of the endothelin type A receptor in the early chick embryo: a model of mispatterning of the branchial arch derivatives. Development 125, 4931–4941.

158. Lammer E, Chen D, Hoar R, *et al.* (1985) Retinoic acid embryopathy. N Engl J Med 313, 837–841.

159. Conway SJ, Henderson DJ, Copp AJ. (1997) Pax3 is required for cardiac neural crest migration in the mouse: evidence from the *splotch* (Sp^{2H}) mutant. Development 124, 505–514.

160. Kurihara Y, Kurihara H, Oda H, *et al.* (1995) Aortic arch malformations and ventricular septal defects in mice deficient in endothelin-1. J Clin Invest 96, 293–300.

161. Yanagisawa H, Hammer RE, Richardson JA, *et al.* (1998) Role of endothelin-1/endothelin-A receptor-mediated signaling pathway in the aortic arch patterning in mice. J Clin Invest 102, 22–33.

162. Yanagisawa H, Yanagisawa M, Kapur RP, *et al.* (1998) Dual genetic pathways of endothelin-mediated intercellular signaling revealed by targeted disruption of endothelin converting enzyme-1 gene. Development 125, 825–836.

163. Clouthier DE, Hosoda K, Richardson JA, *et al.* (1998) Cranial and cardiac neural crest defects in endothelin-A receptor-deficient mice. Development 125, 813–824.

164. Clouthier DE, Williams SC, Yanagisawa H, *et al.* (2000) Signaling pathways crucial for craniofacial development revealed by endothelin-A receptor-deficient mice. Dev Biol 217, 10–24.

165. Lindsay EA, Botta A, Jurecic V, *et al.* (1999) Congenital heart disease in mice deficient for the DiGeorge syndrome region. Nature 401, 379–383.

166. Noden DM. (1991) Origins and patterning of avian outflow tract endocardium. Development 111, 867–876.

167. Gittenberger-de Groot AC, Peeters M, Bergwerff M, *et al.* (2000) Epicardial outgrowth inhibition leads to compensatory mesothelial outflow tract collar and abnormal cardiac septation and coronary formation. Circ Res 87, 969–971.

168. Ho E, Shimada Y. (1978) Formation of the epicardium studied with the scanning electron microscope. Dev Biol 66, 579–585.

169. Shimada Y, Ho E. (1980) Scanning electron microscopy of the embryonic chick heart: formation of the epicaridium and surface structure of the four heterotypic cells that constitute the embryonic heart. In: Van Praagh R, Takao A, editors. *Etiology and Morphogenesis of Congenital Heart Disease.* Mt Kisco, NY: Futura.

170. Shimada Y, Ho E, Toyota N. (1981) Epicardial covering over myocardial wall in the chicken embryo as seen with the scanning electron microscope. Scan Electr Microsc, 275–280.

171. Komiyama M, Ito K, Shimada Y. (1987) Origin and development of the epicardium in the mouse embryo. Anat Embryol 176, 183–189.

172. Viragh S, Gittenberger-de Groot AC, Poelmann RE, *et al.* (1993) Early development of quail heart epicardium and associated vascular and glandular structures. Anat Embryol (Berl) 188, 381–393.

173. Sissman NJ. (1970) Developmental landmarks in cardiac morphogenesis: comparative chronology. Am J Cardiol 25, 141–148.

174. Manner J. (1993) Experimental study on the formation of the epicardium in chick embryos. Anat Embryol 187, 281–289.

175. Cai CL, Martin JC, Sun Y, *et al.* (2008) A myocardial lineage derives from Tbx18 epicardial cells. Nature 454, 104–108.

176. Zhou B, Ma Q, Rajagopal S, *et al.* (2008) Epicardial progenitors contribute to the cardiomyocyte lineage in the developing heart. Nature 454, 109–113.

177. Waldo KL, Willner W, Kirby ML. (1990) Origin of the proximal coronary artery stems and a review of ventricular vascularization in the chick embryo. Am J Anat 188, 109–120.

178. Bogers AJ, Gittenberger-de Groot AC, Poelmann RE, *et al.* (1989) Development of the origin of the coronary arteries, a matter of ingrowth or outgrowth? Anat Embryol (Berl) 180, 437–441.

179. Waldo KL, Kumiski DH, Kirby ML. (1994) Association of the cardiac neural crest with development of the coronary arteries in the chick embryo. Anat Rec 239, 315–331.

180. Drake CJ, Hungerford JE, Little CD. (1998) Morphogenesis of the first blood vessels. Ann N Y Acad Sci 857, 155–179.

181. Waldo K, Kirby M. (1998) Development of the great arteries. In: de la Cruz MV, Markwald RR, editors. *Living Morphogenesis of the Heart*. Boston, MA: Birkhauser. pp. 187–217.

182. Hungerford JE, Little CD. (1999) Developmental biology of the vascular smooth muscle cell: building a multilayered vessel wall. J Vasc Res 36, 2–27.

183. Hungerford JE, Owens GK, Argraves WS, *et al.* (1996) Development of the aortic vessel wall as defined by vascular smooth muscle and extracellular matrix markers. Dev Biol 178, 375–392.

184. Takahashi Y, Imanaka T, Takano T. (1996) Spatial and temporal pattern of smooth muscle cell differentiation during development of the vascular system in the mouse embryo. Anat Embryol (Berl) 194, 515–526.

185. Suri C, Yancopolous GD. (1999) Growth factors in vascular morphogenesis: insights from gene knockout studies in mice. In: Little CD, Mironov V, Sage H, editors. *Vascular Morphogenesis: In Vivo, In Vitro, In Mente*. Boston, MA: Birkhauser. pp. 65–72.

186. Kuo CT, Veselits ML, Barton KP, *et al.* (1997) The LKLF transcription factor is required for normal tunica media formation and blood vessel stabilization during murine embryogenesis. Genes Dev 11, 2996–3006.

187. Winnier GE, Kume T, Deng K, *et al.* (1999) Roles for the winged helix transcription factors MF1 and MFH1 in cardiovascular development revealed by nonallelic noncomplementation of null alleles. Dev Biol 213, 418–431.

188. Douglas YL, Mahtab EA, Jongbloed MR, *et al.* (2009) Pulmonary vein, dorsal atrial wall and atrial septum abnormalities in podoplanin knockout mice with disturbed posterior heart field contribution. Pediatric Res 65, 27–32.

189. Evans HM. (1909) On the development of the aortae, cardinal and umbilical veins, and other blood vessels of vertebrate embryos from capillaries. Anat Rec 3, 498.

190. Larsen WJ. (1993) *Human Embryology*. New York, NY: Churchill Livingston.

191. McClure CFW, Butler EG. (1925) The development of the vena cava inferior in man. Am J Anat 35, 331–383.

CHAPTER 2

Nomenclature and Classification of Pediatric and Congenital Heart Disease

Jeffrey P. Jacobs

All Children's Hospital, Saint Petersburg, FL, USA

Background

Over the past five decades, tremendous progress had been made in the diagnosis and treatment of patients with pediatric and congenital cardiac malformations. Survival is now expected for many patients with lesions previously considered untreatable. In parallel with these advances, the science of nomenclature and classification of pediatric and congenital heart disease has also rapidly evolved. Part of this evolution of the science of Nomenclature and Classification is closely related to the rapid advancement in the science of analytical outcomes of the treatments of patients with pediatric and congenital cardiac malformations [1–124].

In the current era, research into nomenclature and classification is closely linked to research about databases that track outcomes. The nomenclature and classification is indeed the fundamental building block of any database designed to track outcomes. In order to perform meaningful multi-institutional analyses, it has been documented that any database must incorporate the following six essential elements:

1. use of a common language and nomenclature [3–36, 40,42–49,51,53,56,57,62–64,66,67,69,72,73,78-80,82–84, 96–108];
2. use of a database with an established uniform core data set for collection of information [1-36,38,40-43,49,53,55–57, 62,63,65,69,70,73,74,76,78–81,85–91,96–108,110,111,113, 116–124];
3. incorporation of a mechanism of evaluating case complexity [37,39,50,52–54,56–59,63,68,69,71,73,75,78–80,92,93, 109,112,115];
4. availability of a mechanism to assure and verify the completeness and accuracy of the data collected [60,61,63,69,73, 78–80,94];
5. collaboration between medical and surgical subspecialties [69,73,78–80];
6. standardization of protocols for life-long follow-up [73,77–80,95,114].

The aforementioned six elements are all based on utilization and implementation of a standardized international and universal system of nomenclature and classification. This system has been created and is named the International Pediatric and Congenital Cardiac Code (IPCCC) [82]. The IPCCC will be described in this chapter.

Although nomenclature and databases are separate topics, they are very closely related. Furthermore, many of the recent advances in the science of nomenclature and classification have been stimulated by the recent rapid advances in computer science and database development [42,62]. Although the concepts of nomenclature and database are closely and practically linked, the remainder of this chapter will focus specifically on the nomenclature and classification of pediatric and congenital heart disease.

Nomenclature is defined as the system of names used in a branch of learning or activity [125]. Classification is defined as an arrangement, according to some systematic division, into classes or groups based on some factor common to each [125]. Aristotle was the first known biologist to attempt to classify living things. In 1735, Linnaeus first published *Systema Naturae*, a work that eventually led to our currently used binomial nomenclature system for the classification of living species. With the Linnaean method, well over 1 million species are systematically divided in a hierarchical manner into kingdom, phylum, class, order, family, genus, and species [126].

To describe the heart, this chapter proposes the use of a ternary system composed of three elements:

Pediatric Cardiac Surgery, Fourth Edition. Edited by Constantine Mavroudis and Carl L. Backer.
© 2013 Blackwell Publishing Ltd. Published 2013 by Blackwell Publishing Ltd.

1. the segmental anatomy of the heart;
2. the classification of the cardiac lesion;
3. the description of the cardiac lesion.

First, the segmental anatomy is described by the relations of the cardiac chambers to one another and the mechanism by which these chambers are connected. Second, the given cardiac lesion is classified according to major lesion type. Third, the cardiac lesion is described, fully or in part, according to the hierarchical nomenclature system developed by the IPCCC.

Segmental Anatomy

In order to properly describe any heart, it is essential to provide a description of both the relations of structures within the heart, and the manner in which they are joined together or connected. The first feature accounts for the broad interspatial relations between the various structures. This feature, nonetheless, is not always concordant with the fashion in which two cardiac structures are joined to each other, or in some instances, not joined together [127]. It is the structure of the cardiac components, and their relations, that form the basis of the segmental approach of Van Praagh and Vlad [128–130]. The sequential segmental approach of Anderson added junctional morphology to these considerations [127,131–133]. Others have now sought to combine the approaches, and advocate complete description of both relations and connections [67,72,134].

The Meaning of Left and Right

When discussing the morphology of the atria and the ventricles, and their connections and spatial relationships, the words "left" and "right" can be confusing [44,48,72]. In this chapter, we adhere to the following previously published rules that can be used to provide consistency and accuracy when describing anatomical phenotypes regarding the words "left" and "right." These rules are required, to provide consistency and accuracy when describing anatomical phenotypes [44,48,72].

For cardiac chambers, irrespective of the system of nomenclature utilized, unless otherwise stated, "left" refers to morphologically left, and "right" refers to morphologically right. In other words, "left" refers to those chambers that, in the normal individual, are positioned on the left side of the body, and "right" to those that, in the normal person, are right-sided. Thus, left ventricle means the morphologically left ventricle, left atrium refers to the morphologically left atrium, and right atrial appendage refers to the morphologically right atrial appendage, and so on. When discussing cardiac chambers, the words "left" and "right" do not imply sidedness or position. If one wishes to describe the position or sidedness of a cardiac chamber, it is necessary to use terms such as left-sided ventricle. The term left ventricle, therefore, merely means the morphologically left ventricle, and does not mean or imply left-sidedness or right-sidedness. Similarly, it does not imply connections to the right or left atrium, or the pulmonary or systemic circulations.

In contrast, when describing structures that are not cardiac chambers, such as the superior vena cava, and using the prefix "left" or "right," it is now the spatial position that is being described, rather than any other connection or phenotypic variation that may exist.

Cardiac Relations and Cardiac Connections (or Cardiac Alignments)

A description of both cardiac relations and cardiac connections is integral to a depiction of the segmental anatomy of the heart. Cardiac relations describe the broad interspatial relations between the various cardiac structures. Cardiac connections describe the specific mechanism by which two cardiac structures connect to each other regardless of their interspatial relations [127]. Cardiac relations and cardiac connections can be characterized according to the segmental approach of Van Praagh and Vlad [128–130], the sequential segmental approach advocated by Anderson and colleagues [127,131–133], or both [67,72,134].

The essence of the original segmental approach of Van Praagh was analysis of the topological arrangement, or cardiac relations, of the atrial chambers, the ventricular mass, and the arterial trunks [72,135]. When Anderson and colleagues [136] sought to further develop this innovative methodology, they also emphasized the importance of describing the manner in which the basic segments were united, or joined together, across their junctions; in other words, the cardiac connections or alignments [72]. Very rarely the segmental topological arrangements do not correspond with the way the chambers and arterial trunks are united across their junctions [137]. It is essential, therefore, that any system of nomenclature distinguishes between segmental topologies and junctional variations [67,72,137]. This goal is important for all hearts, and especially those found in patients with heterotaxy. It may be accomplished either via the European approach of Anderson and colleagues, or the Bostonian approach developed by Van Praagh and his colleagues, as long as care is taken to specify both these features [26,67,72].

The Segmental Approach of Van Praagh

The segmental approach developed by Van Praagh and colleagues [128–130], documents the anatomy of the cardiac components, and the relations of the three major cardiac segments, namely, the atrial chambers, the ventricles, and the arterial trunks, in a venoarterial sequence. Letters are coded in braces, also known as curly brackets "{}" to describe the segments as follows:

1. the atrial "situs" (the sidedness of the atrial chambers);
2. the ventricular "loop" (the ventricular topology);
3. the relationship of the arterial trunks in space.

In this system, the atrial situs is coded with a single letter code:
- "S" for "situs solitus," otherwise known as normal arrangement;
- "I" for "situs inversus," or the mirror-imaged arrangement;
- "A" for "situs ambiguus";
- "X" for unknown.

"Situs ambiguus is defined as an abnormality in which there are components of situs solitus and situs inversus in the same person. Situs ambiguus, therefore, can be considered to be present when the thoracic and abdominal organs are positioned in such a way with respect to each other as to be not clearly lateralized and thus have neither the usual, or normal, nor the mirror-imaged arrangements [72]."

"Heterotaxy is synonymous with 'visceral heterotaxy' and 'heterotaxy syndrome.' Heterotaxy is defined as an abnormality where the internal thoraco-abdominal organs demonstrate abnormal arrangement across the left–right axis of the body. By convention, heterotaxy does not include patients with either the expected usual or normal arrangement of the internal organs along the left–right axis, also known as 'situs solitus,' nor patients with complete mirror-imaged arrangement of the internal organs along the left–right axis also known as 'situs inversus' [72]."

The ventricular loop is also coded with a single letter code dependent on the topology and chirality, or handedness, of the ventricular mass:
- "D" for D-loop;
- "L" for L-loop;
- "X" for those instances where the looping cannot be determined.

The relationship of the arterial trunks is also coded with a single letter code:
- "S" for normally related great arteries;
- "I" for inverted, or mirror-imaged normally related great arteries;
- "D" for D-transposed or D-malposed great arteries, with the aorta to the right of the pulmonary trunk;
- "L" for L-transposed or L-malposed great arteries, with the aorta to the left of the pulmonary trunk;
- "A" for the aorta directly anterior to the pulmonary trunk.

In this system, a normal heart is coded {S,D,S}. This coding system employing three letters does not specify the way the cardiac chambers within the segments are joined together, a feature that many describe as the type of "atrioventricular and ventriculoarterial connections." This feature, known in the school using the approach of Van Praagh as "atrioventricular and ventriculo-arterial alignments" [67], is separately specified.

The Sequential Segmental Approach of Anderson
The sequential segmental approach developed by Anderson and colleagues [127,131–133], documents the anatomy of the cardiac components, as well as the connections (or junctions) between them.

The atrial chambers, on the basis of the morphology of their appendages, are classified as one of four types. "Isomerism" describes the situation in which morphologically right structures, or morphologically left structures, are found on both sides of the body in the same individual:
- usual or normally arranged;
- mirror-imaged;
- isomerism of the morphologically left atrial appendages;
- isomerism of the morphologically right atrial appendages.

The arrangements at the atrioventricular junctions are classified by both types of atrioventricular connections and modes of atrioventricular connections. Types of atrioventricular connections describe how the atrial and ventricular chambers are joined together:
- concordant;
- discordant;
- biventricular and mixed;
- double-inlet left ventricle;
- double-inlet right ventricle;
- absent right atrioventricular connection;
- absent left atrioventricular connection.

Modes of atrioventricular connections describe the structure of the valve, or valves, guarding the junctions:
- two perforate valves;
- one single perforate valve with an absent atrioventricular connection;
- one perforate along with one imperforate valve;
- a common atrioventricular valve;
- an absent valve with an unguarded orifice.

An imperforate valve is a structure formed by union of valvar leaflets so as to block completely the existing junction between adjacent structures, either an atrium and a ventricle, or a ventricle and an arterial trunk. Such an imperforate valve is different from a muscular wall of a chamber, because perforating the valve recreates the initial channel present between the adjacent structures. Either an atrioventricular valve or an arterial valve can be imperforate. In addition, either or both atrioventricular valves may override or straddle the ventricular septum.

The arrangements at the ventriculoarterial junctions are also classified by both types of ventriculoarterial connections and modes of ventriculoarterial connections. Types of ventriculoarterial connections describe how the ventricular chambers and great arteries are joined together:
- concordant;
- discordant (transposition);
- double-outlet right ventricle;
- double-outlet left ventricle;
- single outlet–common arterial trunk;
- single outlet–solitary aortic trunk with pulmonary atresia;

- single outlet–solitary pulmonary trunk with aortic atresia;
- single outlet–solitary arterial trunk.

Modes of ventriculoarterial connections describe the structure of the valve, or valves, guarding the junctions:

- two perforate valves;
- one single perforate valve with an absent ventriculoarterial connection;
- one perforate along with one imperforate valve;
- a common ventriculoarterial valve (truncal valve);
- an absent valve with an unguarded orifice.

An imperforate valve is a structure formed by union of valvar leaflets so as to block completely the existing junction between adjacent structures, either an atrium and a ventricle, or a ventricle and an arterial trunk. Such an imperforate valve is different from a muscular wall of a chamber, because perforating the valve recreates the initial channel present between the adjacent structures. Either an atrioventricular valve or an arterial valve can be imperforate. In addition, either or both ventriculoarterial valves may override the ventricular septum.

Although Anderson did not include the side of the aortic arch in his analysis, many physicians have used an "L" (left aortic arch) or "R" (right aortic arch) descriptor to incorporate the aortic arch side in the sequential segmental approach. Although use of abbreviations is not part of the traditional Andersonian approach, a normal heart could be described as [SCCL] (situs solitus, concordant atrioventricular connection, concordant ventricular arterial connection, left aortic arch). Specification of the arrangement of the atrial appendages, the atrioventricular connections, and the ventriculoarterial connections, does not specify nor imply the ventricular topology, or the relationships of the cardiac chambers or great arteries in space. These variables are separately specified.

Atrial Situs

The development of morphologically right-sided structures on one side of the body, and morphologically left-sided structures on the other side, is termed lateralization. Normal lateralization, the usual arrangement, is also known as "situs solitus." The mirror-imaged arrangement is also known as "situs inversus." The term "visceroatrial situs" is often used to refer to the situs of the viscera and atria when their situs is in agreement. The arrangement of the organs themselves, and the arrangement of the atrial chambers, is not always the same [127,129]. When the sidedness of the atrial chambers and the sidedness of the remaining organs are not harmonious, the sidedness of the organs and atrial chambers must be separately specified.

When considering the arrangement of the organs, the school of nomenclature that developed using the teachings of Van Praagh recognizes three patterns: situs solitus is the usual arrangement, situs inversus is the mirror-imaged variant of solitus, and the third pattern is situs ambiguus, which is defined as any situation where a combination of situs solitus and situs inversus occurs in the same individual.

In the normal atrial arrangement, or "atrial situs solitus," the morphologically right atrium is on the right, and the morphologically left atrium is on the left. In the mirror-imaged atrial arrangement, or "atrial situs inversus," the morphologically left atrium is on the right, and the morphologically right atrium is on the left. In terms of overall morphology, it is usually easy to differentiate the morphologically right atrium from the morphologically left atrium. This distinction can generally be made on the basis of the anatomy of the atrial appendages, the morphology of the atrial septum, and the drainage of the supradiaphragmatic portion of the inferior vena cava.

Typically, the morphologically right atrial appendage is broad and blunt, whereas the morphologically left atrial appendage is narrow, pointed, and fingerlike. Uemura and colleagues [138] showed that the extent of the pectinate muscles relative to the vestibules of the right- and left-sided atrioventricular junctions distinguished between the morphologically right and left atrial appendages. In the normal morphologically right atrium, which of course is right-sided, the pectinate muscles extend all round the vestibule, and reach to the cardiac crux. In the normal left-sided morphologically left atrium, these pectinate muscles are confined within the tube-like left atrial appendage, and the smooth vestibule is confluent with the smooth-walled body of the left atrium. In patients with mirror-imaged arrangement, or "situs inversus," this morphological pattern is itself mirror-imaged.

The morphologically right side of the atrial septum contains the rim of the oval fossa, or "limbus of the fossa ovalis," whereas the morphologically left side of the interatrial septum is made up of the flap valve of the oval fossa. When the organs themselves are lateralized, the supradiaphragmatic termination of the inferior caval vein provides an extremely reliable landmark for the morphologically right atrium [127]. During echocardiographic examinations, the arrangement of the atrial chambers, also known as "atrial situs," is often inferred by documenting the location of the inferior vena cava within the abdomen, specifically by determining its relationship to the descending thoracic aorta in subcostal short and long axis views. In the normal atrial arrangement, or atrial "situs solitus," the aorta and inferior vena cava typically lie apart, on opposite sides of the spine, with the aorta on the left. This arrangement is mirror-imaged in atrial "situs inversus," with the aorta on the right and the inferior vena cava on the left. The rules as stated above, however, are reliable only in the setting of usual or mirror-imaged arrangements. In the setting of heterotaxy, these relationships do not pertain [139]. When there is isomerism of the right atrial appendages, or "asplenia syndrome," the aorta and inferior vena cava are almost always on the same side of the spine, with the vein slightly anterior. In the setting of isomerism of the left atrial appendages, or "polysplenia syndrome," the inferior vena cava usually does not connect directly with the right atrium, its suprarenal course often being interrupted, with the blood returning to the heart through the azygos or hemiazygos veins, such that the aorta is midline and the azygos vein is located in a posterolateral position [139].

"Isomerism" describes the situation in which morphologically right structures, or morphologically left structures, are found on both sides of the body in the same individual. In chemistry, two compounds can have the same chemical structure, but be mirror images of each other. These compounds are called enantiomers, or isomers, giving the arrangements of enantiomerism, or stereoisomerism. Such isomerism has long been known to exist in the lungs of patients with heterotaxy. Evidence of such isomerism also has been noted in the heart. Van Mierop and colleagues [140,141] described the existence of right isomerism in the setting of asplenia syndrome, while Moller and colleagues [142] pointed to the presence of bilateral left-sidedness in the setting of polysplenia syndrome.

The presence of isomerism of the appendages within the atrial chambers, therefore, can be determined by the examination of the extent of the pectinate muscles relative to the atrioventricular junctions. The atrial chambers as a whole, however, are not isomeric. It is erroneous to describe "atrial isomerism," although this incorrect term is used widely and loosely. It is only the appendages that are isomeric in the setting of heterotaxy.

Some cardiac morphologists, however, do not accept the concept of isomerism of the atrial appendages. They prefer to use the term atrial situs ambiguus to describe this subset of patients. Furthermore, in the living patient, it may be difficult to document the extent of the pectinate muscles relative to the atrioventricular junctions. Because of this difficulty, it should be noted that, in heterotaxy, bronchopulmonary anatomy usually is consistent with the structure of the appendages, and can aid in the documentation of heterotaxy. Most patients with heterotaxy, also have splenic abnormalities and the anatomy and structure of the spleen are often used to stratify patients with heterotaxy. Splenic anatomy, however, shows less correlation with the arrangement of the atrial appendages when compared with bronchopulmonary anatomy.

The morphology of the lungs, and the relation between the bronchial tree and the pulmonary arteries, therefore, are useful in determining "situs." The arrangement of the atrial appendages is highly consistent with bronchopulmonary morphology [127,143]. In the majority of patients with heterotaxy, when attention is paid to the lungs and bronchial tree, the left-sided structures are seen to be the mirror-images of their right-sided counterparts. A morphologically right lung typically has three lobes, and a morphologically left lung typically has two lobes. Furthermore, the right side tends to have an eparterial bronchus, whereas the bronchus on the left side is typically hyparterial. An eparterial bronchus is one that branches superior to the first lobar division of the pulmonary artery, in contrast to a hyparterial bronchus that branches inferior to the first lobar division of the respective pulmonary artery. Tracheobronchial anatomy can be assessed from examination of the chest radiograph [127,144,145]. Isomerism is consistent with a ratio of less than 1 to 1.6 between the lengths of the two main bronchi, whereas lateralization has a ratio of more than 1 to 1.6. Examination of chest radiographs, therefore, may provide one of the simplest techniques for differentiating isomerism from lateralization in a living patient, albeit that this can now be shown with even greater detail using tomographic techniques. Bronchial tomography has been used to measure bronchial length, and comparison of measured bronchial length with the age of the patient has been used to determine the presence of right versus left bronchial isomerism [127,143,146]. Nevertheless, although the correlation between bronchial morphology and the structure of the atrial appendages is highly consistent, it is not absolute. In patients with heterotaxy, the anatomy of the atrial appendages does not always correspond with the bronchial arrangement [147–149].

Splenic anatomy is often used to stratify patients with heterotaxy [142,150]. In most instances, right isomerism is associated with absence of the spleen, and left isomerism is associated with multiple spleens. This association between splenic anatomy and the arrangement of the atrial appendages, however, is weaker than the correlation between the arrangement of the atrial appendages and bronchial morphology. Moreover, absence of the spleen, or presence of multiple spleens, is not always easily documented. Multiple spleens are not always easy to differentiate from one spleen with spleniculi [142,150,151]. A rudimentary spleen cannot easily be differentiated from one that is absent [152]. Splenic anatomy can be difficult to determine both clinically and at autopsy [127].

Although not all patients with multiple spleens have isomerism of the left atrial appendages, and not all patients with absence of the spleen have isomerism of the right atrial appendages, it has become customary for many pediatric cardiologists to stratify heterotaxy into the subsets of "asplenia syndrome" and "polysplenia syndrome" [142,150]. Because a syndrome includes a constellation of findings, each of which may not be present in all instances, and because the splenic arrangement does not always fit with the expected patterns of the remaining thoracoab-dominal organs, investigators may at times be comfortable with describing the presence of the spleen in patients known to have "asplenia syndrome" [142].

Ventricular Loop

The morphologically right ventricle typically possesses coarse trabeculations in its apical component, while the morphologically left ventricle typically exhibits fine apical trabeculations. Ventricular topology, or "looping of the heart," describes the chirality, or handedness, of the ventricular mass. With right hand ventricular topology, or "D-loop," the right ventricle wraps around the left ventricle such that the palmar surface of the right hand can be placed on the septal surface of the right ventricle with the thumb in the inlet and the fingers in the outlet. With left hand ventricular topology, or "L-loop," it is the palmar surface of the left hand that fits on the right ventricular septum in this fashion.

The concept of looping refers to the formation of the ventricular loop in the embryo. The loop normally rotates to form a D-loop. In order to describe the fashion in which the atrial chambers are joined to the ventricular mass, this being the feature known variously as the atrioventricular connections or alignments, it is essential in any given patient; first, to note the atrial arrangement, and second, to describe the specific ventricular topology.

Atrioventricular Connection

The term "atrioventricular connections," or "atrioventricular alignments," refers to the mechanism of union between the atrial and the ventricular myocardium. As already discussed, in any patient, in order to describe the fashion in which the atrial chambers are joined to the ventricular mass, it is essential to first, note the atrial arrangement, and second, to describe the specific ventricular topology.

The arrangements at the atrioventricular junctions are classified by both types of atrioventricular connections and modes of atrioventricular connections. Types of atrioventricular connections describe how the atrial and ventricular chambers are joined together. Modes of atrioventricular connections describe the structure of the valve, or valves, guarding the junctions. The atrial chambers can be joined to the ventricles in biventricular or univentricular fashion. Biventricular atrioventricular connections can be of the following types:
- concordant;
- discordant;
- biventricular and mixed.

Univentricular atrioventricular connections can be of the following types:
- double-inlet left ventricle;
- double-inlet right ventricle;
- absent right atrioventricular connection;
- absent left atrioventricular connection.

The right atrium is connected to the right ventricle, and the left atrium to the left ventricle in *concordant atrioventricular connections*. In *discordant atrioventricular connections*, the right atrium is connected to the left ventricle, and the left atrium to the right ventricle.

When both atria connect to one ventricle, the term double-inlet atrioventricular connection is used. Absent right atrioventricular connection and absent left atrioventricular connection refer to absence of one atrioventricular connection.

In cases of heterotaxy (isomerism of the atrial appendages or situs ambiguus) in the setting of univentricular atrioventricular connections, the description of the atrioventricular connection is exactly the same as for patients without heterotaxy (those patients with usual or mirror-imaged arrangement of the atrial appendages). In cases of heterotaxy (isomerism of the atrial appendages or situs ambiguus) in the setting of biventricular atrioventricular connections, the atrioventricular connection was previously described as *ambiguous*. This terminology was utilized because a biventricular atrioventricular connection is by definition ambiguous in cases of isomerism or situs ambiguus. In the setting of heterotaxy, when the atrial chambers are joined to the ventricles in biventricular fashion, this anatomical phenotype is unique. When the appendages are isomeric, and the atria are joined to the ventricles in biventricular fashion, then irrespective of whether the isomeric appendages are morphologically left or right, and irrespective of the ventricular topology, half of the heart will be joined in concordant fashion, and the other half joined together in discordant fashion. In the setting of heterotaxy, therefore, biventricular atrioventricular connections or alignments are, of necessity, mixed. In the past, biventricular atrioventricular connections in the setting of heterotaxy were described as ambiguous; in the current era, biventricular atrioventricular connections in the setting of heterotaxy are described as *biventricular and mixed*.

Analysis of the way the atrial myocardium is joined to the ventricular mass gives only half of the necessary information concerning the morphology of the atrioventricular junctions. It is also necessary to take account of the structure of the valve or valves guarding the junctions; in other words, the mode of the atrioventricular connection or alignment.

Ventriculoarterial Connection

The arrangements at the ventriculoarterial junctions are classified by both types of ventriculoarterial connections and ventriculoarterial modes of connections. Types of ventriculoarterial connections describe the ventricular chambers and the manner in which the great arteries are joined together. Modes of ventriculoarterial connections describe the structure of the valve, or valves, guarding the junctions.

In concordant ventriculoarterial connections, the right ventricle is connected to the pulmonary artery and the left ventricle to the aorta. In discordant ventriculoarterial connections, the right ventricle is connected to the aorta and the left ventricle to the pulmonary artery. Both great vessels arise entirely or predominately from one ventricle in double-outlet ventriculoarterial connection [27,28]. In single-outlet connection, only one great artery is connected to the heart.

Modes of ventriculoarterial connection include two perforate valves, a single perforate valve, one perforate and one imperforate valve, and a common (truncal) valve. The distinction between a single perforate valve, one perforate valve, and one imperforate valve is best understood by considering the example of pulmonary atresia with ventricular septal defect (PA-VSD). If the right ventricle is in continuity with the pulmonary artery but the pulmonary valve is imperforate, the ventriculoarterial connection type is concordant, and the mode is one perforate and one imperforate valve. If there is no pulmonary trunk (or only a fibrous remnant of the pulmonary trunk), the ventriculoarterial connection type is single-outlet–solitary aortic trunk with pulmonary atresia, and the mode is single perforate valve [127].

The Position of the Heart and the Orientation of Its Apex

The position of the heart in the chest, and the orientation of the cardiac apex, must also be described separately, because these features can vary independently from each other, and have no definitive relationship to other cardiac relations and connections. The ventricular mass may be right-sided, left-sided, or midline. The cardiac apex may also be right-sided, left-sided, or midline. These features take on added importance when planning the route or pathway of an extracardiac Fontan connection. The terms "dextrocardia," "levocardia," "mesocardia," "dextroversion," and "levoversion" have been used over the years in various fashions by various authors [153].

"Dextrocardia" is usually considered synonymous with a right-sided ventricular mass, while "dextroversion" is frequently defined as a configuration where the ventricular apex points to the right. In a patient with the usual atrial arrangement, or situs solitus, dextroversion, therefore, implies a turning to the right of the heart. In the same context, "levocardia" has most often been used synonymously with a left-sided ventricular mass, and "levoversion" is frequently defined as a configuration where the

ventricular apex points to the left. "Mesocardia" is the term used to account for the ventricular mass occupying the midline. One must be cautious, however, about the use of such terms, because others have used variations of this terminology, suggesting terms such as "dextrorotation," "mixed dextrocardia," or "pivotal dextrocardia" in attempts to compress all the information into a single term. These variations are not universally understood, and should be avoided. The proper description of a heart, irrespective of the system used, should include a description of the position of the heart in the chest and the orientation of the cardiac apex. These features can vary significantly in heterotaxy, and they are not always in harmony. For example, one might encounter a patient where the cardiac mass may be located predominantly in the right chest, but with its apex pointing to the left, in other words, "dextrocardia with levoversion." The separate description of the location of the cardiac mass and the direction of the cardiac apex is not merely an academic exercise, as these features can profoundly impact planned surgical interventions.

Classification of Cardiac Lesions

The description of the segmental anatomy of the heart includes a complete description of the following variables:
1. situs;
2. ventricular topology (ventricular loop);
3. atrioventricular connections (type and mode);
4. ventriculoarterial connections (type and mode);
5. the relationships of the arterial trunks in space;
6. the position of the heart and the orientation of its apex.

After the description of the segmental anatomy of the heart, the cardiac lesions must be classified and ultimately described. Cardiac lesions historically have been classified by incidence [154–157] (Table 2.1) [134] and by differentiation of cyanotic and acyanotic lesions (Table 2.2) [134]. Table 2.2 provides information useful in conceptualizing a classification system for congenital heart lesions [134]. Only seven major lesion groups compose approximately 80% of congenital heart disease, a fact to be considered in developing a congenital heart disease nomenclature and classification system. The incidence of any given lesion, however, varies from center to center depending on a variety of factors, including institutional expertise and institutional acuity level. The classification of lesions into cyanotic and acyanotic groupings can be further refined by subdivision of the major groups into subsets based on underlying pathophysiological mechanisms (Table 2.3) [134]. In the cyanotic group, right-to-left shunting with decreased pulmonary blood flow and intracardiac mixing of oxygenated and desaturated blood are two causative mechanisms of cyanosis. The two most common pathophysiological entities in acyanotic congenital heart

Table 2.1 Common lesions in congenital heart disease and approximate incidence.

Ventricular septal defect (20%)
Atrial septal defect (10%)
Patent ductus arteriosus (10%)
Coarctation of the aorta (10%)
Congenital aortic stenosis (10%)
Tetralogy of Fallot (10%)
Pulmonary stenosis (10%)
Transposition of the great arteries (5–8%)
Pulmonary atresia (5%):
　with intact ventricular septum
　with ventricular septal defect
Atrioventricular septal defect (2–5%)
Tricuspid atresia (3%)
Truncus arteriosus (3%)
Total anomalous pulmonary venous connection (2%)
Hypoplastic left heart syndrome (2%)
Interrupted aortic arch (1%)
Ebstein anomaly (0.5%)
Mitral stenosis (rare)
Aortopulmonary window (rare)

Table 2.2 Acyanotic versus cyanotic lesions in congenital heart disease and approximate incidence.

Acyanotic

Ventricular septal defect (20%)
Atrial septal defect (10%)
Patent ductus arteriosus (10%)
Coarctation of the aorta (10%)
Congenital aortic stenosis (10%)
Atrioventricular septal defect (2–5%)
Aortopulmonary window (rare)
Interrupted aortic arch (1%)
Mitral stenosis (rare)

Cyanotic

Tetralogy of Fallot (10%)
Pulmonary stenosis (10%)
Transposition of the great arteries (5–8%)
Pulmonary atresia (5%):
　with intact ventricular septum
　with ventricular septal defect
Tricuspid atresia (3%)
Truncus arteriosus (3%)
Total anomalous pulmonary venous connection (2%)
Hypoplastic left heart syndrome (2%)
Ebstein anomaly (0.5%)

Table 2.3 Pathophysiological classification of lesions in congenital heart disease and approximate incidence.

Acyanotic

Left-to-right shunts
Ventricular septal defect (20%)
Atrial septal defect (10%)
Patent ductus arteriosus (10%)
Atrioventricular septal defect (2–5%)
Aortopulmonary window (rare)

Left-sided obstructive lesions
Coarctation of the aorta (10%)
Congenital aortic stenosis (10%)
Interrupted aortic arch (1%)
Mitral stenosis (rare)

Cyanotic

Right-to-left shunts
Tetralogy of Fallot (10%)
Pulmonary stenosis (10%)
Pulmonary atresia (5%):
　with intact ventricular septum
　with ventricular septal defect
Tricuspid atresia (3%)
Ebstein anomaly (0.5%)

Complex mixing defects
Transposition of the great arteries (5–8%)
Total anomalous pulmonary venous connection (2%)
Truncus arteriosus (3%)
Hypoplastic left heart syndrome (2%)

disease are left-to-right shunting and left-sided obstructive lesions.

Although traditionally popular, the classification systems shown in Tables 2.2 and 2.3 are problematic [134]. In many lesions, the direction of shunting changes gradually, often with changes in pulmonary vascular resistance. Furthermore, cyanosis can evolve gradually; several lesions that initially are acyanotic can become cyanotic. For example, ventricular septal defect is initially associated with acyanosis with left-to-right shunting; however, as pulmonary vascular resistance gradually increases, the direction of shunting can change to right-to-left, and the patient can become cyanotic. Furthermore, the common physiological characterization of tetralogy of Fallot (TOF) as either cyanotic ("blue") or acyanotic ("pink") is of limited usefulness because it describes the condition of a patient at a point in time, rather than the cardiac malformation itself. In most infants with tetralogy and adequate or generous antegrade pulmonary blood flow, with the acquisition of right ventricular hypertrophy, progressive or periodic cyanosis eventually develops [13].

Because of the aforementioned limitations, alternative classification systems must be considered. The lesions of congenital heart disease can be classified with a segmental system that starts with the great veins and proceeds to the great arteries. This segmental system can accommodate the incidence of various lesions and can meet the needs of surgeons, cardiologists, and pathologists. All lesions of congenital heart disease are distributed into one of the six segments listed in Table 2.4 [134] (and further subdivided in Table 2.5) [134]. Almost any given cardiac lesion in congenital heart disease can be placed into one of these subdivisions, as shown in Table 2.6 [134], which classifies the most common congenital cardiac lesions. Certain lesions involve more than one subdivision or even segment; the system functions by placing the lesion in the subdivision most involved.

Description of Cardiac Lesions

After being classified into a major group of lesions, a cardiac lesion may be further described according to the hierarchical nomenclature system developed and maintained by The International Society for Nomenclature of Paediatric and Congenital Heart Disease (ISNPCHD) [80,82]. This system is named the International Paediatric and Congenital Cardiac Code (IPCCC) [80,82] and was developed to fill the need for a standardized nomenclature to be used in databases worldwide, allowing for shared meaningful data. Its form is driven by the need to be inclusive of extant classification systems, rather than exclusive. Furthermore, the system is hierarchical in nature, so that it allows user centers to choose a level of detail applicable to the center's needs but allows data sharing with other centers that choose to code with a higher or lower level of detail.

During the 1990s, both The European Association for Cardio-Thoracic Surgery (EACTS) and The Society of Thoracic Surgeons (STS) created databases to assess the outcomes of congenital cardiac surgery. Beginning in 1998, these two organizations collaborated to create the International Congenital Heart Surgery Nomenclature and Database Project [3–36]. By 2000, a common nomenclature, along with a common core minimal data set, were adopted by The European Association for Cardio-Thoracic Surgery and The Society of Thoracic Surgeons, and published in the Annals of Thoracic Surgery [3–36]. In 2000, The International Nomenclature Committee for Pediatric and Congenital Heart Disease was established. This committee eventually evolved into the International Society for Nomenclature of Paediatric and Congenital Heart Disease. The working component of this international nomenclature society has been The International Working Group for Mapping and Coding of Nomenclatures for Paediatric and Congenital Heart Disease, also known as the Nomenclature Working Group. By 2005, the Nomenclature Working Group cross-mapped the nomenclature of the International Congenital Heart Surgery Nomenclature and Database Project of The European Association for Cardio-Thoracic Surgery and The Society of Thoracic Surgeons with the European Paediatric Cardiac Code of the Association for European Paediatric Cardiology, and therefore created the International Paediatric and Congenital Cardiac Code, which is available for free download from the internet at http://www.IPCCC.net [80,82].

The initial hierarchical nomenclature levels of the IPCCC for the more common lesions shown in Table 2.6 [134] are displayed in Table 2.7 [134]. Most lesions have several

Table 2.4 Segmental system of classification of lesions of congenital heart disease: level 1.

I. Great veins
II. Atria
III. Atrioventricular junction
IV. Ventricles
V. Ventriculoarterial junction
VI. Great arteries

Table 2.5 Segmental system of classification of lesions of congenital heart disease: level 2.

I. Great veins
Systemic veins
Pulmonary veins
II. Atria
Right atrium
Atrial septum
Left atrium
III. Atrioventricular junction
Right atrioventricular valve
Common atrioventricular valve
Left atrioventricular valve
IV. Ventricles
Right ventricle
Ventricular septum
Left ventricle
Single ventricle
V. Ventriculoarterial junction
Right ventriculoarterial valve
Common ventriculoarterial valve
Left ventriculoarterial valve
Both ventriculoarterial valves
VI. Great arteries
Pulmonary artery
Aorta
Both great arteries
Coronary arteries

Table 2.6 Segmental system of classification of lesions of congenital heart disease: level 3.

I. Great veins	**V. Ventriculoarterial junction**

I. Great veins

Systemic veins
  Systemic venous anomaly, superior vena cava
  Systemic venous anomaly, inferior vena cava
Pulmonary veins
  Total anomalous pulmonary venous connection
  Partial anomalous pulmonary venous connection
  Cor triatriatum
  Pulmonary venous stenosis

II. Atria

Right atrium
Atrial septum
  Atrial septal defect
Left atrium

III. Atrioventricular junction

Right atrioventricular valve
  Tricuspid stenosis
  Tricuspid regurgitation
  Ebstein anomaly of the tricuspid valve
Common atrioventricular valve
  Atrioventricular canal defect (atrioventricular septal defect)
Left atrioventricular valve
  Mitral stenosis
  Mitral regurgitation

IV. Ventricles

Right ventricle
  Tetralogy of Fallot
  Double-chamber right ventricle
Ventricular septum
  Ventricular septal defect
Left ventricle
  Single ventricle
  Single ventricle, double-inlet left ventricle
  Single ventricle, double-inlet right ventricle
  Single ventricle, mitral atresia
  Single ventricle, tricuspid atresia
  Single ventricle, unbalanced atrioventricular canal defect
  Single ventricle, heterotaxia syndrome
  Single ventricle, other
  Hypoplastic left heart syndrome

V. Ventriculoarterial junction

Right ventriculoarterial valve
  Pulmonary stenosis
  Pulmonary insufficiency
  Pulmonary atresia with intact ventricular septum
  Pulmonary atresia with ventricular septal defect
Common ventriculoarterial valve
  Truncus arteriosus
Left ventriculoarterial valve
  Aortic stenosis
  Aortic insufficiency
  Aortic atresia
  Sinus of Valsalva aneurysm
  Aortic-left ventricular tunnel
Both ventriculoarterial valves
  Transposition of the great arteries
  Double-outlet right ventricle
  Double-outlet left ventricle

VI. Great arteries

Pulmonary artery
  Pulmonary arterial stenosis
  Pulmonary artery sling
Aorta
  Aortic coarctation
  Interrupted aortic arch
Both great arteries
  Patent ductus arteriosus
  Aortopulmonary window
  Vascular ring
  Pulmonary arterial origin from ascending aorta (hemitruncus)
Coronary arteries
  Anomalous origin of coronary artery from pulmonary artery

further levels of hierarchical analysis and description; these are published in the April 2000 supplement to the Annals of Thoracic Surgery [3–36] and on the Internet at http://www.IPCCC.net. The myriad of detailed coding choices presented in this system appear daunting in print but are manageable with computer-generated coding, in which only short lists of coding possibilities (two hierarchical levels) are seen at any given time.

Consensus Definitions

In addition to developing and maintaining the IPCCC, the ISNPCHD has published consensus definitions for several complex congenital cardiac malformations, including the functionally univentricular heart [64], hypoplastic left heart syndrome [66], congenitally corrected transposition [67], and heterotaxy [72]. On 9 July 2007, the ISNPCHD created two new committees so that the Society now has the following three committees:

1. The International Working Group for Mapping and Coding of Nomenclatures for Paediatric and Congenital Heart Disease, also known as the Nomenclature Working Group (NWG);

2. The International Working Group for Defining the Nomenclatures for Paediatric and Congenital Heart Disease, also known as the Definitions Working Group (DWG);

Table 2.7 Segmental system of classification and nomenclature of lesions of congenital heart disease: level 4.

I. GREAT VEINS

Systemic veins
  Systemic venous anomaly, SVC
    Abnormal RSVC
    Absent RSVC
    Bilateral SVC
    CS ostial atresia or stenosis (CS draining cephalad through LSVC)
    Levoatrial-cardinal vein
    Other (specify)
    Retroaortic innominate vein
    SVC occlusion
    SVC stenosis
  Systemic venous anomaly, IVC
    Abnormal RIVC
    Biatrial drainage of IVC
    Cor triatriatum dexter
    IVC occlusion
    IVC stenosis
    LIVC
    Other (specify)
    Separate entry of hepatic veins (RIVC to right-sided atrium)
Pulmonary veins
  Total anomalous PV connection
    Type 1 (supracardiac)
    Type 2 (cardiac)
    Type 3 (infracardiac)
    Type 4 (mixed)
  Partial anomalous PV connection
    Nonscimitar
    Scimitar
  Cor triatriatum
    Accessory atrial chamber receives all PV and communicates with LA
    Accessory atrial chamber receives all PV and does not communicate with LA
    Accessory atrial chamber receives part of the PV (subtotal cor triatriatum)
  Pulmonary venous stenosis
    Congenital
      Congenital, diffusely hypoplastic
      Congenital, long segment focal (tubular) stenosis
      Congenital, discrete stenosis
    Acquired
      Acquired, postoperative
      Acquired, not postoperative

II. ATRIA

Right atrium
Atrial septum
  Atrial septal defect
    Common atrium (single atrium)
    Coronary sinus
    PFO
    Primum
    Secundum
    Sinus venosus
Left atrium

III. ATRIOVENTRICULAR JUNCTION

Right AV valve
  Tricuspid stenosis
    Congenital
      Valvar hypoplasia
      Abnormal subvalvar apparatus
      Double-orifice valve
      Parachute deformity
      Other
    Acquired
      Status post cardiac surgery
  Tricuspid regurgitation
    Congenital
      Primary annular dilatation
      Prolapse
      Leaflet underdevelopment
      Absent papillary muscle or chordae
      Other
    Acquired
      Status post cardiac surgery
  Ebstein anomaly of the tricuspid valve
    Ebstein anomaly, type I
    Ebstein anomaly, type II
    Ebstein anomaly, type III
    Ebstein anomaly, type IV
    Ebstein anomaly, "left-sided" Ebstein anomaly
    Ebstein anomaly, atypical Ebstein-like anomalies associated with hypoplastic right heart syndrome
    Ebstein anomaly, other
Common AV valve
  AV canal defect (AVSD)
    AVC (AVSD), partial (incomplete) (PAVSD) (ASD, Primum)
    AVC (AVSD), intermediate (transitional)
    AVC (AVSD), complete (CAVSD)
Left atrioventricular valve
  Mitral stenosis
    Congenital
      Subvalvar
      Valvar
      Supravalvar
      Mixed
      Other
    Acquired
      Status post cardiac surgery
  Mitral regurgitation
    Congenital
      Subvalvar
      Valvar
      Mixed
      Other
    Acquired
      Status post cardiac surgery

(Continued)

Table 2.7 (*Continued*)

IV. VENTRICLES

Right ventricle
  Tetralogy of Fallot
    TOF, pulmonary stenosis
    TOF, pulmonary atresia
    TOF, common atrioventricular canal (TOF/CAVSD)
    TOF, absent pulmonary valve
  Double-chamber right ventricle
    DCRV, no VSD
    DCRV, VSD
      VSD to lower RV chamber
      VSD to upper RV chamber
      VSD to lower and upper RV chamber
Ventricular septum
  VSD
    VSD, multiple
    VSD, type 1 (subarterial) (supracristal) (conal septal defect) (infundibular)
    VSD, type 2 (perimembranous) (paramembranous) (conoventricular)
    VSD, type 3 (inlet) (AV canal type)
    VSD, type 4 (muscular)
    VSD, type: Gerbode type (LV-RA communication)
Left ventricle
Single ventricle
  Single ventricle, double-inlet left ventricle
    DILV {S,L,L}, outlet chamber (bulboventricular foramen)
    DILV {S,D,D}, outlet chamber (bulboventricular foramen)
    DILV {S,D,N} (Holmes heart)
    DILV, DOLV
    DILV, DORV
  Single ventricle, double-inlet right ventricle
    DIRV, DORV
    DIRV, outlet chamber (bulboventricular foramen)
    DIRV, other
  Single ventricle, mitral atresia
    Mitral atresia, DORV
    Mitral atresia, {S,D,N}
    Mitral atresia, {S,L,L} (corrected transposition)
  Single ventricle, tricuspid atresia
    Type 1a (no TGA, pulmonary atresia)
    Type 1b (no TGA, pulmonary hypoplasia, small VSD)
    Type 1c (no TGA, no pulmonary hypoplasia, large VSD)
    Type 2a (D-TGA, pulmonary atresia)
    Type 2b (D-TGA, pulmonary or subpulmonary stenosis)
    Type 2c (D-TGA, large pulmonary artery)
    Type 3a (L-TGA, pulmonary or subpulmonary stenosis)
    Type 3b (L-TGA, subaortic stenosis)
  Single ventricle, Unbalanced AV canal defect
    Single ventricle, unbalanced AV canal, right dominant
    Single ventricle, unbalanced AV canal, left dominant
  Single ventricle, heterotaxia syndrome
    Heterotaxia syndrome, DORV, CAVC (CAVSD), Asplenia
    Heterotaxia syndrome, DORV, CAVC (CAVSD), Polysplenia
    Heterotaxia syndrome, single LV
  Heterotaxia syndrome, other

  Single ventricle, other
    Single ventricle, other, mostly LV
    Single ventricle, other, mostly RV
    Single ventricle, other, indeterminate
  Hypoplastic left heart syndrome
    HLHS, aortic atresia + mitral atresia
    HLHS, aortic atresia + mitral stenosis
    HLHS, aortic atresia + VSD (well developed mitral valve and LV)
    HLHS, aortic stenosis + mitral atresia
    HLHS, aortic stenosis + mitral stenosis
    HLHS, aortic stenosis + mitral valve hypoplasia
    HLHS, hypoplastic AV + MV + LV (HLHC)

V. VENTRICULOARTERIAL JUNCTION

Right ventriculoarterial valve
  Pulmonary stenosis
    Pulmonary stenosis, subvalvar
    Pulmonary stenosis, valvar
    Pulmonary stenosis, supravalvar
  Pulmonary insufficiency
  Pulmonary atresia with intact ventricular septum
    No coronary fistulas/sinusoids
    Coronary fistulas/sinusoids: non-RV-dependent coronary circulation
    Coronary fistulas/sinusoids: RV-dependent coronary circulation
  Pulmonary atresia with VSD
    Type A (native PAs present, no MAPCA)
    Type B (native PAs present, MAPCA present)
    Type C (no native PAs, MAPCA present)
Common ventriculoarterial valve
  Truncus arteriosus
    With confluent or near confluent PAs (large aorta type) (Van Praagh A1, A2;
    Colette and Edwards I, II, III)
    With absence of one PA (large aorta type with absence of one PA) (Van Praagh A3)
    With interrupted aortic arch or coarctation (large PA type) (Van Praagh A4)
Left ventriculoarterial valve
  Aortic stenosis
    Aortic stenosis, subvalvar
    Aortic stenosis, valvar
    Aortic stenosis, supravalvar
  Aortic insufficiency
    Congenital
    Acquired
  Aortic atresia
  Sinus of Valsalva aneurysm
    Sinus of Valsalva aneurysm, Left sinus
    Sinus of Valsalva aneurysm, Right sinus
    Sinus of Valsalva aneurysm, Non-coronary sinus
  Aortic-LV tunnel
    Type I: simple tunnel
    Type II: aortic wall aneurysm
    Type III: intracardiac aneurysm
    Type IV: aortic wall aneurysm and intracardiac aneurysm

Table 2.7 (*Continued*)

Both ventriculoarterial valves
  Transposition of the great arteries
    TGA: IVS
    TGA: IVS, LVOTO
    TGA: VSD
    TGA: VSD, LVOTO
  Double-outlet right ventricle
    DORV, VSD type
      Subaortic VSD + no PS
      Doubly committed VSD + no PS
    DORV, TOF type
      Subaortic VSD + PS
      Doubly committed VSD + PS
    DORV, TGA type
      Subpulmonary VSD + no PS (Taussig-Bing)
      Subpulmonary VSD + PS
      DORV, remote VSD (uncommitted VSD)
      Common atrioventricular canal (CAVSD) + PS
      Common atrioventricular canal (CAVSD) + no PS
      No CAVSD + PS
      No CAVSD + no PS
    DORV, IVS
  Double-outlet left ventricle
    DOLV, subaortic VSD
    DOLV, subpulmonary VSD
    DOLV, doubly committed VSD
    DOLV, noncommitted VSD
    DOLV, IVS
    DOLV, Ebstein anomaly

VI. GREAT ARTERIES

Pulmonary artery
  PA stenosis
    PA stenosis (hypoplasia), main (trunk)
    PA stenosis (hypoplasia), branch
  PA sling
    With tracheal stenosis
    With tracheomalacia
    With tracheal stenosis and tracheomalacia
    Without tracheal stenosis or tracheomalacia

Aorta
  Aortic coarctation
    COA, isolated
    COA, with VSD
    COA, with complex intracardiac anomaly
  Interrupted aortic arch
    Type A: interruption distal to the left subclavian artery
    Type B: interruption between the left carotid and left subclavian arteries
    Type C: interruption between the innominate and left carotid arteries
Both great arteries
  Patent ductus arteriosus
    PDA, normal origin and insertion
    PDA, abnormal origin and insertion
  Aortopulmonary window
    Type 1 proximal defect
    Type 2 distal defect
    Type 3 total defect
    Intermediate type
  Vascular ring
    Double aortic arch
    Right aortic arch – left ligamentum or left PDA
    Innominate artery compression
    Vascular ring, other
    PA origin from ascending aorta (hemitruncus)
      Left PA
      Right PA
Coronary arteries
  Anomalous origin of coronary artery from PA
    Anomalous left coronary from the PA (ALCAPA)
    Anomalous right coronary from the pulmonary artery (ARCAPA)
    Anomalous circumflex from the pulmonary artery (ACxPA)
    Anomalous left and right coronaries from the pulmonary artery (both) ALCAPA and ARCAPA)

ASD, atrial septal defect; AV, atrioventricular; CAVSD, complete atrioventricular septal defect; COA, coarctation of the aorta; CS, coronary sinus; DCRV, double-chamber right ventricle; DILV, double-inlet left ventricle; DIRV, double-inlet right ventricle; DOLV, double-outlet left ventricle; DORV, double-outlet right ventricle; HLHC, hypoplastic left heart complex; HLHS, hypoplastic left heart syndrome; IVC, inferior vena cava; IVS, intact ventricular septum; LA, left atrium; LIVC, left inferior vena caval; LSVC, left superior vena cava; LV, left ventricle; LVOTO, left ventricular outflow tract obstruction; MAPCA, major aortopulmonary collateral arteries; MV, mitral valve; PA, pulmonary artery; PAVSD, partial atrioventricular septal defect; PDA, patent ductus arteriosus; PFO, patent foramen ovale; PS, pulmonary stenosis; PV, pulmonary vein; RA, right atrium; RIVC, right inferior vena cava; RSVC, right superior vena cava; RV, right ventricle; {S,D,D}, {S,D,N}, {S,L,L}, Van Praagh descriptors of segmental anatomy – see text for detailed explanation; SVC, superior vena cava; TGA, transposition of the great arteries; TOF, tetralogy of Fallot; VSD, ventricular septal defect.

3. The International Working Group for Archiving and Cataloguing the Images and Videos of the Nomenclatures for Paediatric and Congenital Heart Disease, also known as the Archiving Working Group (AWG), and the Congenital Heart Archiving Research Team (CHART).

The NWG will continue to maintain, preserve, and update the IPCCC, as well as provide ready access to it for the international pediatric and congenital cardiology and cardiac surgery communities, related disciplines, the healthcare industry, and governmental agencies, both electronically and in published form. The DWG will write definitions for the terms in the International Paediatric and Congenital Cardiac Code, building on the previously published definitions from the NWG [64,66,67,72]. The AWG will enable the linkage of images and videos to the IPCCC. The images and videos will be acquired from cardiac morphologic specimens and imaging modalities such as echocardiography, angiography, computerized axial tomography, and magnetic resonance imaging, as well as intraoperative images and videos. An image and video archive will be created, based on the IPCCC, and this archive will be linked to CTSNet (http://www.ctsnet.org), and the new Congenital Portal of CTSNet (http://www.ctsnet.org/portals/congenital/index.html).

Examples of some of the consensus definitions of nomenclature developed by the ISNPCHD are provided below. By the time the next edition of this book is published, the DWG will have developed consensus definitions for the majority of terms in the nomenclature of pediatric and congenital cardiac disease.

The term "functionally univentricular heart" describes a spectrum of congenital cardiovascular malformations in which the ventricular mass may not readily lend itself to partitioning that commits one ventricular pump to the systemic circulation, and another to the pulmonary circulation.

A heart may be functionally univentricular because of its anatomy or because of the lack of feasibility or lack of advisability of surgically partitioning the ventricular mass. Common lesions in this category typically include double inlet right ventricle (DIRV), double inlet left ventricle (DILV), tricuspid atresia, mitral atresia, and hypoplastic left heart syndrome. Other lesions which sometimes may be considered to be a functionally univentricular heart include complex forms of atrioventricular septal defect, double outlet right ventricle, congenitally corrected transposition, pulmonary atresia with intact ventricular septum, and other cardiovascular malformations. Specific diagnostic codes should be used whenever possible, and not the term "functionally univentricular heart". See The International Society for Nomenclature of Paediatric and Congenital Heart Disease (ISNPCHD) http://www.ipccc.net/.

The version of the IPCCC derived from the International Congenital Heart Surgery Nomenclature and Database Project of the EACTS and STS uses the term "single ventricle" as synonymous for the functionally univentricular heart [24,64].

The consensus of the EACTS and STS Congenital Heart Surgery Database Committees was that the nomenclature proposal for single ventricle hearts would encompass hearts with double-inlet atrioventricular connection (both DILV and DIRV, hearts with absence of one atrioventricular connection (mitral atresia and tricuspid atresia), hearts with a common atrioventricular valve and only one completely well developed ventricle (unbalanced common atrioventricular canal defect), hearts with only one fully well developed ventricle and heterotaxia syndrome (single ventricle heterotaxia syndrome), and finally other rare forms of univentricular hearts that do not fit in one of the specified major categories [24,64].

In the version of the IPCCC derived from the nomenclature of the International Congenital Heart Surgery Nomenclature and Database Project of the EACTS and the STS, patients classified in this section of the nomenclature, therefore, include all those who would be coded using the Short List for "Single Ventricle," specifically [24,64]:

- Single ventricle;
- Single ventricle, DILV;
- Single ventricle, DIRV;
- Single ventricle, heterotaxia syndrome;
- Single ventricle, mitral atresia;
- Single ventricle, tricuspid atresia;
- Single ventricle, unbalanced AV canal.

Despite the recognition that hypoplastic left heart syndrome is a common form of functionally univentricular heart, with a single or dominant ventricle of right ventricular morphology, the EACTS-STS version of the IPCCC includes an entirely separate section for consideration of hypoplastic left heart syndrome. Also, it is recognized that a considerable variety of other structural cardiac malformations, such as pulmonary atresia with intact ventricular septum, biventricular hearts with straddling atrioventricular valves, and some complex forms of double-outlet right ventricle (DORV), may at times be best managed in a fashion similar to that which is used to treat other functionally univentricular hearts. Nomenclature for description of those entities, however, is not included in this Single Ventricle section of the EACTS-STS version of the IPCCC [24,64].

"Hypoplastic left heart syndrome is synonymous with the term hypoplasia of the left heart and is defined as a spectrum of cardiac malformations with normally aligned great arteries without a common atrioventricular junction, characterized by underdevelopment of the left heart with significant hypoplasia of the left ventricle including atresia, stenosis, or hypoplasia of the aortic or mitral valve, or both valves, and hypoplasia of the ascending aorta and aortic arch." [66]

"Hypoplastic left heart syndrome without intrinsic valvar stenosis or atresia is synonymous with the term hypoplastic left heart complex and is defined as a cardiac malformation at the milder end of the spectrum of hypoplastic left heart syndrome with normally aligned great arteries without a common atrioventricular junction, characterized by underdevelopment of the left heart with significant hypoplasia of the left ventricle and hypoplasia of the aortic or mitral valve, or both valves, in the absence of intrinsic valvar stenosis or atresia, and with hypoplasia of the ascending aorta and aortic arch." [66]

"The Norwood operation is synonymous with the term 'Norwood (Stage 1)' and is defined as an aortopulmonary connection and neoaortic arch construction resulting in univentricular physiology and pulmonary blood flow controlled with a calibrated systemic-to-pulmonary artery shunt, or a right ventricle to pulmonary artery conduit, or rarely, a cavopulmonary connection." [66]

"Congenitally corrected transposition is synonymous with the terms 'corrected transposition' and 'discordant atrioventricular connections with discordant ventriculo-arterial connections,' and is defined as a spectrum of cardiac malformations where the atrial chambers are joined to morphologically inappropriate ventricles, and the ventricles then support morphologically inappropriate arterial trunks." [67]

"Heterotaxy is synonymous with 'visceral heterotaxy' and 'heterotaxy syndrome.' Heterotaxy is defined as an abnormality where the internal thoraco-abdominal organs demonstrate abnormal arrangement across the left-right axis of the body. By convention, heterotaxy does not include patients with either the expected usual or normal arrangement of the internal organs along the left-right axis, also known as "situs solitus," nor patients with complete mirror-imaged arrangement of the internal organs along the left-right axis also known as "situs inversus." [72]

"Isomerism in the context of the congenitally malformed heart is defined as a situation where some paired structures on opposite sides of the left–right axis of the body are, in morphologic terms, symmetrical mirror images of each other." [72]

"Left isomerism in the context of the congenitally malformed heart is defined as a subset of heterotaxy where some paired structures on opposite sides of the left–right axis of the body are symmetrical mirror images of each other, and have the morphology of the normal left-sided structures." [72]

"Right isomerism in the context of the congenitally malformed heart is defined as a subset of heterotaxy where some paired structures on opposite sides of the left–right axis of the body are symmetrical mirror images of each other, and have the morphology of the normal right-sided structures." [72]

"Isomerism of the left atrial appendages is a subset of heterotaxy where the atrial appendages on both sides of the body have the appearance of the morphologically left atrial appendage." [72]

"Isomerism of the right atrial appendages is a subset of heterotaxy where the atrial appendages on both sides of the body have the appearance of the morphologically right atrial appendage." [72]

"Situs ambiguus is defined as an abnormality in which there are components of situs solitus and situs inversus in the same person. Situs ambiguus, therefore, can be considered to be present when the thoracic and abdominal organs are positioned in such a way with respect to each other as to be not clearly lateralized and thus have neither the usual, or normal, nor the mirror-imaged arrangements." [72]

"Asplenia literally means absent spleen." [72]

"Asplenia syndrome can be defined as a subset of heterotaxy with components of bilateral right-sidedness, usually associated with absence of the spleen." [72]

"Polysplenia literally means multiple spleens." [72]

"Polysplenia syndrome can be defined as a subset of heterotaxy with components of bilateral left-sidedness, usually associated with multiple spleens." [72]

"Ivemark syndrome is a term that, historically, is synonymous with asplenia syndrome." [72]

The NWG was consulted by the World Health Organization (WHO) Disease Classification Revision Committee to provide definitions of Eisenmenger for The International Classification of Diseases. The NWG provided definitions of the following four related terms:

- Eisenmenger defect is a membranous ventricular septal defect with anterior malalignment of the conal septum without outflow tract obstruction, as described by Eisenmenger in 1897. This terminology is no longer in common usage and many cardiologists would not be able to define the precise defect to which the term refers.
- Eisenmenger syndrome could briefly be described as, acquired severe pulmonary vascular disease associated with congenital heart disease.
- The term, Eisenmenger complex, represents an acquired condition that is the combination of an Eisenmenger defect (malalignment membranous VSD) with severe pulmonary hypertension and a right-to-left shunt. It may at times be used synonymously (incorrectly) with the term, Eisenmenger syndrome, the latter meaning severe pulmonary vascular disease associated with a VSD and/or other cardiac malformations. Other than for historical purposes however, the phrase, Eisenmenger complex, should be dropped as its definition is not widely agreed on or known.
- The term, Eisenmenger disease, may be used by some to be synonymous with Eisenmenger complex or Eisenmenger syndrome. The term is not used widely and should not be retained because of its ambiguity.

Nomenclature, Definitions, and Classification Controversies

Some cardiac lesions remain difficult to assign to one or another subset. Among the lesions subject to debate were:
1. ostium primum atrial septal defect;
2. tetralogy of Fallot–pulmonary atresia (TOF-PA);
3. double-outlet right ventricle (DORV);
4. single ventricle;
5. transposition of the great arteries (TGA).

Reasonable consensus has been achieved; however, it is likely that as the initiative for a comprehensive standardized nomenclature system progresses, continuing debate by surgeons, cardiac pathologists, and pediatric cardiologists will assure that the system will evolve to achieve a uniform nomenclature that crosses geographic boundaries and specialty preferences [5].

Ostium Primum Atrial Septal Defect (Partial Atrioventricular Canal)

Ostium primum atrial septal defect (partial atrioventricular canal) is defined as a crescent-shaped hole in the inferior portion of the atrial septum just above the atrioventricular valve with varying degrees of left atrioventricular valve regurgitation owing to a cleft in the anterior leaflet of the mitral valve [6,8]. The controversy surrounding this lesion revolves not around the definition or the moniker but in how to classify the lesion as it relates to surgical outcome and long-term disability [158,159]. Most surgeons believe repair of an ostium primum defect with a cleft anterior mitral leaflet (partial atrioventricular canal with a cleft of the left atrioventricular valve or partial atrioventricular septal defect with cleft of the left atrioventricular valve) has potential consequences regarding mitral valve function and cardiac arrhythmia. Therefore, including ostium primum atrial septal defect (partial atrioventricular canal) with other forms of atrial septal defect for the purpose of risk stratification yields a disparate analysis. Ostium primum atrial septal defect (partial atrioventricular canal) is consequently best analyzed with the other atrioventricular canal defects (complete atrioventricular canal and intermediate atrioventricular canal) when risk stratification models or outcome reports are considered. Subsets of analysis can be developed for each of the subtypes of atrioventricular canal: complete, intermediate or transitional, and partial or incomplete.

Tetralogy of Fallot with Pulmonary Atresia Versus Pulmonary Atresia with Ventricular Septal Defect

The distinction between TOF-PA and PA-VSD can be arbitrary and has led to nomenclature and identification controversies. The surgical considerations and outcomes, however, are very similar regardless of the name given this entity. For the most part, these lesions are repaired by closure of the VSD and placement of a right ventricle-to-pulmonary artery conduit. Postoperative complications are related to right ventricular dysfunction, residual VSDs, residual pulmonary stenosis, and the need for replacement of the conduit. The Congenital Heart Surgery Nomenclature and Database Project decided to group TOF-PA patients with PA-VSD patients, preferring to classify these patients as having PA-VSD [13,15].

Pulmonary atresia, as defined in the context of TOF by the International Congenital Heart Surgery Nomenclature and Database Project [15], is the lack of luminal continuity between the right ventricle and the pulmonary trunk [160]. Pulmonary atresia also occurs with corrected transposition [161]. In that case, there is lack of luminal continuity between the left ventricle and the pulmonary trunk. A broad definition of *pulmonary atresia* [15], therefore, is the lack of luminal continuity and the absence of blood flow from a ventricle or a rudimentary chamber to the pulmonary artery. In the severe form of pulmonary atresia, the pulmonary arteries are partially or completely absent. Pulmonary atresia can occur in biventricular hearts with an intact ventricular septum or VSD and in hearts with a univentricular atrioventricular connection. That pulmonary atresia can occur with almost any form of congenital heart disease is supported by the results of the classic studies by Van Praagh and associates [161,162]. *Ventricular septal defect* is defined as an opening or hole in the interventricular septum [7,163,164]. From these two definitions, it follows that *PA-VSD* is a group of congenital cardiac malformations in which there is lack of luminal continuity and absence of blood flow from either ventricle to the pulmonary artery in a biventricular heart that has an opening or

a hole in the interventricular septum. In the severe form of PA-VSD, the native pulmonary arteries are partially or completely absent [15].

Because the term PA-VSD has been frequently used interchangeably with TOF-PA, it is useful to define the latter [15]. *Tetralogy of Fallot–pulmonary atresia* is a congenital cardiac malformation characterized by the following features: (1) extreme underdevelopment of the right ventricular infundibulum, (2) a large-outlet, subaortic VSD, (3) marked anterior and leftward displacement of the infundibular septum, which often is fused with the anterior wall of the right ventricle; the result is complete obstruction of blood flow into the pulmonary artery [15,160]. Tetralogy of Fallot–pulmonary atresia, therefore, is a specific type of PA-VSD with the intracardiac malformation more accurately defined [15]. The presence or absence of multiple aortopulmonary collateral arteries does not change these definitions. Other types of intracardiac anatomy in PA-VSD include DORV and TGA with complete atrioventricular septal defect [165].

In most cases of PA-VSD, the intracardiac anatomical features are those of TOF. A rudimentary infundibulum may be identified with careful inspection; this structure is partially or completely fused with the anterior wall of the right ventricle. This configuration usually is the case in the presence of a main pulmonary artery. The presence of a main pulmonary artery can serve as a guide to intracardiac diagnosis depending on to which ventricle the artery is attached and whether the structure found has a lumen or is a fibrous cord. If the main pulmonary artery or fibrous cord originates from the right ventricle and the aorta also arises entirely or predominately from the right ventricle, the diagnosis is DORV with pulmonary atresia (DORV-PA). If, on the other hand, the main pulmonary artery or fibrous cord originates from the left ventricle along with the aorta, the defect is double-outlet left ventricle with pulmonary atresia. If the main pulmonary artery or fibrous cord originates from the left ventricle and the aorta arises from the right ventricle, the defect is TGA with pulmonary atresia (TGA-PA). In many patients with PA-VSD, however, no main pulmonary artery or fibrous cord originates from the heart. In these cases, the precise intracardiac diagnosis cannot be made with certainty. For example, if no main pulmonary artery or fibrous cord originates from the heart and the aorta arises entirely from the right ventricle, it is impossible to establish whether DORV-PA or TGA-PA is present. In these situations, the malformation is simply called by its general name, PA-VSD.

Tetralogy of Fallot Versus Double-Outlet Right Ventricle

Another area of controversy centers on differentiation of TOF and DORV [13]. Some authors [166,167] use the term DORV when the pulmonary artery arises from the right ventricle and more than 50% of the aorta arises from the right ventricle. Other authors [168] use the term DORV only when the pulmonary artery arises from the right ventricle and 90% or more of the aorta arises from the right ventricle. Still others [169] use the term DORV only when there is absence of fibrous continuity between the aortic and mitral valves. Double-outlet right ventricle is defined by the International Congenital Heart Surgery Nomenclature and Database Project [27] as a type of ventriculoarterial connection in which both great vessels arise entirely or predominately from the right ventricle. In a commentary on the difficulties encountered by the nomenclature project in achieving consensus, Marshall Jacobs stated, "It is inescapable that some hearts will be called TOF at some centers and DORV at other centers [13]."

Double-Outlet Right Ventricle Versus Transposition of the Great Arteries

Double-outlet right ventricle with subpulmonary VSD and TGA-VSD can be differentiated from one another by site of origin of the pulmonary artery [27]. Because DORV is a type of ventriculoarterial connection in which both great vessels arise entirely or predominantly from the right ventricle [170], hearts with DORV and subpulmonary VSD are considered a subset of DORV. If the aorta arises entirely or predominately from the right ventricle, the pulmonary artery arises entirely or predominately from the left ventricle, and there is a subpulmonary VSD, the defect is considered a subset of TGA-VSD [171,172].

Double-outlet right ventricle with subpulmonary VSD is further delineated by the presence or absence of associated pulmonary stenosis. Hearts with DORV and subpulmonary VSD without pulmonary stenosis are considered to be Taussig–Bing type (Taussig–Bing syndrome). The very rare hearts with DORV and subpulmonary VSD and pulmonary stenosis are not of the Taussig–Bing type. In surgical series of DORV [172,173], subpulmonary VSDs are present in approximately 30% of patients. These VSDs are usually unrestrictive, lie anteriorly and superiorly beneath the pulmonary valve in the interventricular septum, and are within the limbs of the septomarginal trabecula.

Single Ventricle

The commonly used terms, *single ventricle* and *univentricular heart*, are debated by anatomists and pathologists. In an attempt to derive a classification useful and relevant to surgical therapy, the Nomenclature and Database Project limited hearts considered univentricular or as single ventricles to be those in which the atrial chambers connect to only one well developed, dominant ventricle. The well developed ventricle has an inlet portion that supports the subvalvar tensor apparatus, a trabecular zone, and an outlet portion to a great artery. Also often present is an incomplete, rudimentary, or hypoplastic ventricle that may lack an atrioventricular connection [24].

In 2000, The International Congenital Heart Surgery Nomenclature and Database Project defined single-ventricle anomalies as cardiac malformations characterized by the lack of two completely well developed ventricles. Anderson prefers the term *functionally single ventricle* rather than *single ventricle* because these hearts generally have a functional single ventricle and a diminutive or hypoplastic ventricle.

In 2006, the NWG of the ISNPCHD addressed the definition of single ventricle as well [64]. The following five paragraphs are taken directly from their manuscript titled: "Classification of the Functionally Univentricular Heart: Unity from mapped codes" and document the rich history behind the terms single ventricle and functionally univentricular heart:

"The debate about the proper nomenclature for the functionally univentricular heart goes back several decades. The approach taken at Boston Children's Hospital from the 1970s is summarized by the following passage, authored by Donald C. Fyler, in the textbook 'Nadas' Pediatric Cardiology:[1'] [174]

'At Boston Children's Hospital, a single ventricle is defined as the presence of two atrioventricular valves with one ventricular chamber or a large dominant ventricle associated with a diminutive opposing ventricle.[2-4] The term double-inlet ventricle is also used to describe this group of anomalies. While the concept of a univentricular heart[5-8] fits the physiologic idea of a common mixing chamber and has pathologic merits as well, lumping patients with mitral atresia, tricuspid atresia, and others into one category adds confusion rather than contributing to classification. The easy distinction between a single atrioventricular valve and two atrioventricular valves has been a reproducible basis for clinical impressions extending over many years. To change nomenclature would require significant benefits that are not apparent at the present time.'" [175–181]

"The concept of the 'univentricular heart' as discussed above by Fyler is essentially the one evolved by a group of European morphologists and clinicians, albeit with strong support from Freedom in Toronto.[5-7] The evolution of their system, however, depended on emphasizing that, in the hearts under discussion, it was the atrioventricular connection, rather than the heart itself, which was truly univentricular. Thus, in one of the cited works,[8] the situation was summarized as follows:

'In most hearts with double-inlet connection it is not the ventricles that are univentricular; it is the AV connection. The concept of a univentricular AV connection, then, appropriately groups hearts with double-inlet along with those having absence of one AV connection. It distinguishes this entire group from those other hearts with biventricular AV connections (each atrium connected to its own ventricle). The term "univentricular AV connection" is thus a collective one for all those hearts in which the atria connect to only one ventricle.'" [178–181]

"With ongoing experience, it has now become clear that many of these hearts with biventricular atrioventricular connections can also lead to a situation which, in terms of physiology, is functionally univentricular. Thus, in the initial review of this supplement, Jacobs and Anderson[9] explain how the term 'functionally univentricular heart' allows for the grouping together of hearts in which 'one chamber was incapable independently of supporting either the pulmonary or the systemic circulation.' This approach is based upon the concept of '*appreciating that the entire ventricular mass was functionally univentricular whenever one or other ventricle was incapable, for whatever reason, of supporting either the systemic or the pulmonary circulation."⁹* The endpoint of this evolutionary journey, therefore, is an approach that permits description of the patients possessing functionally univentricular hearts based upon a clear understanding of the cardiac phenotype, and a detailed description of this cardiac phenotype." [64,182]

Therefore, as stated previously, the functionally univentricular heart is defined as a spectrum of congenital cardiovascular malformations in which the ventricular mass may not readily lend itself to partitioning that commits one ventricular pump to the systemic circulation, and another to the pulmonary circulation. The version of the IPCCC derived from the International Congenital Heart Surgery Nomenclature and Database Project of the EACTS and STS uses the term "single ventricle" as synonymous for the functionally univentricular heart.

Transposition of the Great Arteries

Malposition of the great arteries is defined as all defects with abnormal position of the great vessels regardless of the ventricular origin. Transposition of the great arteries (TGA) is defined as right ventricular origin of the aorta and left ventricular origin of the pulmonary artery [26,183]. The term *transposition* is synonymous with either *ventriculoarterial discordance* or *discordant ventriculoarterial connection* [26,184,185]. Subtypes of malposition of the great arteries include the following lesions:

1. double-outlet right ventricle (DORV);
2. double-outlet left ventricle (DOLV);
3. anatomically corrected malposition (concordant ventriculoarterial connections with parallel great arteries) [26];
4. physiologically uncorrected TGA (atrioventricular concordance with ventriculoarterial discordance);
5. corrected TGA (atrioventricular discordance with ventriculoarterial discordance) [25,183].

Transposition of the great arteries as a subset of malposition includes both corrected TGA and physiologically uncorrected TGA because the great arteries arise from the wrong ventricles in both lesions [25].

The term congenitally corrected TGA was introduced in 1961 to differentiate the naturally occurring condition from surgically repaired transposition [186]. Congenitally corrected TGA is probably the most accepted term in current use for this anatomic complex, but inclusion of the modifier "congenitally" makes it cumbersome, and acceptance is by no means universal [26]. Acceptable synonyms include *corrected TGA, atrioventricular and ventriculoarterial discordance, atrioventricular discordance with transposition, double discordance,* and *discordant transposition.*

In 2000, the Nomenclature and Database Project defined *corrected TGA* [26] as a malformation in which (1) the two ventricles are connected inappropriately to the atria and (2) the great arteries are transposed. Thus the systemic venous atrium (right atrium) is connected to the morphologically left ventricle and the pulmonary venous atrium (left atrium) is connected to the morphologically right ventricle. In addition, the aorta originates from the right ventricle and the pulmonary artery from the left ventricle. As a result of the abnormal (discordant) connections at both levels, the defect is "physiologically corrected" with systemic venous blood flow to the pulmonary circulation and pulmonary venous blood flow to the systemic circulation. In clinical practice, because of frequently associated defects (e.g., VSD, left ventricular outflow tract obstruction, left atrioventricular [tricuspid] valve abnormalities [typically regurgitation], PA-VSD, and conduction abnormalities), corrected transposition often is far from physiologically correct. The term *physiologically corrected transposition* is therefore of little practical use [26].

In 2006, the NWG of the ISNPCHD published the following definition: "Congenitally corrected transposition is synonymous with the terms 'corrected transposition' and 'discordant atrioventricular connections with discordant ventriculo-arterial connections', and is defined as a spectrum of cardiac malformations where the atrial chambers are joined to morphologically inappropriate ventricles, and the ventricles then support morphologically inappropriate arterial trunks." [67].

Use of the term *d-TGA* to refer to physiologically uncorrected TGA is not precise, not acceptable, and should be discouraged [25]. Likewise, use of the term *l-TGA* to refer to corrected TGA is not precise, not acceptable, and should be discouraged [25,26]. The terms *d-TGA, a-TGA,* and *l-TGA* define the spatial arrangements of the great arteries and should not be used to define transposition. The term *d-TGA* refers only to hearts in which the aortic valve is to the right of the pulmonary valve. In *l-TGA* the aortic valve is to the left of the pulmonic valve, and in *a-TGA* the aortic valve is directly anterior to the pulmonic valve.

Many clinicians incorrectly use the terms *TGA, d-TGA,* and *complete transposition* synonymously. The term *d-TGA* refers only to hearts with TGA in which the aortic valve is to the right of the pulmonary valve. This anatomic arrangement is the most common variant of TGA, found in more than 80% of cases reported by Van Praagh [25]. The terms *complete transposition* and *incomplete transposition* are obsolete. In the past, double-outlet right or left ventricle was termed incomplete transposition. All malpositions of the great arteries now classified as transposition are "complete" transpositions. Thus complete transposition may refer to either physiologically uncorrected TGA or corrected TGA, because in both cases the great arteries arise from the wrong ventricle and thus are completely transposed. Used as a modifier, "complete" is redundant and should be avoided [25].

Although *d-TGA* represents the most common spatial relation of the great arteries in uncorrected TGA, all cases of *d-TGA* are not physiologically uncorrected TGA, and not all cases of physiologically uncorrected TGA are *d-TGA*

[25]. Physiologically uncorrected TGA includes hearts with the segmental anatomy {S,D,D}, {S,D,A}, and {S,D,L} as well as {I,L,L} and {I,L,D}. Van Praagh stated that in hearts in which one is not able to define the atrial situs, it is impossible to say whether there is atrioventricular concordance. Yet many cases of situs ambiguus – {A,L,L} or {A,D,D} – behave as physiologically uncorrected TGA and are managed with arterial switch [25].

The term *l-TGA* typically has been used synonymously with corrected TGA; however, not all cases of *l-TGA* are physiologically corrected TGA [25]. Furthermore, corrected TGA includes hearts with the segmental anatomy {S,L,L}, {S,L,D}, and {I,D,D}. Van Praagh and colleagues [187] introduced the term *l-TGA* in the 1960s to describe TGA with a left-sided (usually anterior) aorta. In most cases, this situation coexists with atrioventricular discordance with an L-loop ventricular arrangement in which the morphologically left ventricle is right-sided and the morphologically right ventricle is left-sided. Because the association of *l-TGA* with an L-loop is so close, many clinicians incorrectly believe that the presence of *l-TGA* is indicative of *corrected TGA*. Since the terms *l-TGA* and *corrected TGA* were introduced, many morphologists and clinicians have tended to use the terms as though they are synonymous. Some patients with corrected TGA and an L-loop, however, have an aorta that lies anterior and to the right of the pulmonary artery {S,L,D}. Furthermore, patients with corrected TGA and situs inversus also can have an aorta that lies anterior and to the right of the pulmonary artery {I,D,D} [25,26].

The terms *d-TGA*, *a-TGA*, and *l-TGA* cannot be used to imply or define the presence of corrected TGA or uncorrected TGA. They merely define the spatial arrangements of the great arteries in TGA. They are important modifiers, however, because the spatial relations of the great vessels may closely correlate with the anatomic features of the coronary arteries [25].

"Regardless of the original intent of these terms, many people use *'d-transposition'* to refer to the combination of d-looped ventricles and transposition, and *'l-transposition'* to imply the combination of l-looped ventricles and transposition, without reference to the position of the arterial roots. In this use, {S,D,L} transposition is a form of d-transposition, and {I,L,D} is form of l-transposition. Using this interpretation, the terms, 'd-transposition' and 'l-transposition' refer to d-loop transposition and l-loop transposition. This usage adds even more confusion, because it is apparent that universal agreement does not exist as to whether or not the 'd' and 'l' refer to arterial position or ventricular looping. This point alone potentially represents the worst problem with the terms 'd-transposition' and 'l-transposition,' and further justifies the recommendation to avoid these terms." [67]

Summary

This chapter provides a ternary system for describing any heart. First, the segmental anatomy of the heart is described.

Second, all cardiac lesions are classified as to their major lesion type. Third, each lesion is further described according to the hierarchical nomenclature system initially developed by the International Congenital Heart Surgery Nomenclature and Database Project [3–36] and subsequently unified with other nomenclature systems including the European Paediatric Cardiac Code to become refined by the International Paediatric and Congenital Cardiac Code (IPCCC) [80,82].

Further debate by surgeons, anatomists, and pediatric cardiologists is expected to result in nomenclature changes and continued evolution of this nomenclature system. We are now closer than ever to achieving the goal of establishing a uniform nomenclature system that crosses geographic boundaries and specialty preferences.

References

1. Mavroudis C (Chairman) and Congenital Database Subcommittee: Backer CL, Bove E, Burke RP, *et al.* (1998) *Data analyses of the Society of Thoracic Surgeons National Congenital Cardiac Surgery Database, 1994–1997.* Summit Medical, Minnetonka, MN, September 1998.
2. Mavroudis C, Gevitz M, Ring WS, *et al.* (1999) The Society of Thoracic Surgeons National Congenital Cardiac Surgery Database. Ann Thorac Surg 68, 601-624.
3. Mavroudis C, Jacobs JP. (2000) The International Congenital Heart Surgery Nomenclature and Database Project. Ann Thorac Surg 69(suppl 4), 1–372.
4. Mavroudis C, Jacobs JP. (2000) Introduction. Ann Thorac Surg 69(suppl 4), S1.
5. Mavroudis C, Jacobs JP. (2000) Overview and minimum dataset. Ann Thorac Surg 69(suppl 4), S2–S17.
6. Jacobs JP, Quintessenza JA, Burke RP, *et al.* (2000) Atrial septal defect. Ann Thorac Surg 69(suppl 4), S18–S24.
7. Jacobs JP, Burke RP, Quintessenza JA, *et al.* (2000) Ventricular septal defect. Ann Thorac Surg 69(suppl 4), S25–S35.
8. Jacobs JP, Burke RP, Quintessenza JA, *et al.* (2000) Atrioventricular canal defect. Ann Thorac Surg 69(suppl 4), S36–S43.
9. Jacobs JP, Quintessenza JA, Gaynor JW, *et al.* (2000) Aortapulmonary window. Ann Thorac Surg 69(suppl 4), S44–S49.
10. Jacobs M. (2000) Congenital heart surgery nomenclature and database project: truncus arteriosus. Ann Thorac Surg 69(suppl 4), S50–S55.
11. Herlong JR, Jaggers JJ, Ungerleider RM. (2000) Pulmonary venous anomalies. Ann Thorac Surg 69(suppl 4), S56–S69.
12. Gaynor JW, Weinberg P, Spray T. (2000) Systemic venous anomalies. Ann Thorac Surg 69(suppl 4), S70–S76.
13. Jacobs M. (2000) Tetralogy of Fallot. Ann Thorac Surg 69 (suppl 4), S77–S82.
14. Lacour-Gayet F. (2000) Right ventricular outflow tract obstruction–intact ventricular septum. Ann Thorac Surg 69(suppl 4), S83–S96.
15. Tchervenkov CI, Roy N. (2000) Pulmonary atresia–ventricular septal defect. Ann Thorac Surg 69(suppl 4), S97–S105.

16. Dearani JA, Danielson GK. (2000) Ebstein's anomaly and tricuspid valve disease. Ann Thorac Surg 69(suppl 4), S106–S117.

17. Nguyen KH. (2000) Aortic valve disease. Ann Thorac Surg 69(suppl 4), S118–S131.

18. Mitruka SN, Lamberti JJ. (2000) Mitral valve disease. Ann Thorac Surg 69(suppl 4), S132–S146.

19. Ring WS. (2000) Aortic aneurysm, sinus of valsalva aneurysm, and aortic dissection. Ann Thorac Surg 69(suppl 4), S147–S163.

20. Myers JL, Mehta SM. (2000) Aortico-left ventricular tunnel. Ann Thorac Surg 69(suppl 4), S164–S169.

21. Tchervenkov CI, Jacobs M, Tahta SA. (2000) Hypoplastic left heart syndrome. Ann Thorac Surg 69(suppl 4), S170–S179.

22. Delius RE. (2000) Pediatric cardiomyopathies and end-stage congenital heart disease. Ann Thorac Surg 69(suppl 4), S180–S190.

23. Myers JL, Mehta SM. (2000) Diseases of the pericardium. Ann Thorac Surg 69(suppl 4), S191–S196.

24. Jacobs M, Mayer JE. (2000) Single ventricle. Ann Thorac Surg 69(suppl 4), S197–S204.

25. Jaggers JJ, Cameron DE, Herlong JR, et al. (2000) Transposition of the great arteries. Ann Thorac Surg 69(suppl 4), S205–S235.

26. Wilkinson JL, Cochrane AD, Karl TR. (2000) Congenital heart surgery nomenclature and database project: corrected (discordant) transposition of the great arteries (and related malformations). Ann Thorac Surg 69(suppl 4), S236–S248.

27. Walters III HW, Mavroudis C, Tchervenkov CI, et al. (2000) Double outlet right ventricle. Ann Thorac Surg 69(suppl 4), S249–S263.

28. Tchervenkov CI, Walters III HW, Chu VF. (2000) Double outlet left ventricle. Ann Thorac Surg 69(suppl 4), S264–S269.

29. Dodge-Khatami A, Mavroudis C, Backer CL. (2000) Anomalies of the coronary arteries. Ann Thorac Surg 69 (suppl 4), S270–S297.

30. Backer CL, Mavroudis C. (2000) Patent ductus arteriosus, coarctation of the aorta, and interrupted aortic arch. Ann Thorac Surg 69(suppl 4), S298–S307.

31. Backer CL, Mavroudis C. (2000) Vascular rings, tracheal stenosis, and pectus excavatum. Ann Thorac Surg 69(suppl 4), S308–S318.

32. Deal BJ, Jacobs JP, Mavroudis C. (2000) Arrhythmias. Ann Thorac Surg 69(suppl 4), S319–S331.

33. Rocchini AP. (2000) Therapeutic cardiac catheter interventions. Ann Thorac Surg 69(suppl 4), S332–S342.

34. Gaynor JW, Bridges ND, Spray T. (2000) End-stage lung disease. Ann Thorac Surg 69(suppl 4), S343–S357.

35. Mehta SM, Myers JL. (2000) Cardiac tumors. Ann Thorac Surg 69(suppl 4), S358–S368.

36. Joffs C, Sade RM. (2000) Palliation, correction, or repair. Ann Thorac Surg 69(suppl 4), S369–S372.

37. Lacour-Gayet F. (2002) Risk stratification theme for congenital heart surgery. Semin Thorac Cardiovasc Surg Pediatr Card Surg Annu 5, 148–152.

38. Lacour-Gayet F, Maruszewski B, Mavroudis C, et al. (2000) Presentation of the international nomenclature for congenital heart surgery – the long way from nomenclature to collection of validated data at the EACTS. Eur J Cardiothoracic Surg 18, 128–135.

39. Mavroudis C, Jacobs JP. (2002) Congenital heart disease outcome analysis: methodology and rationale. J Thorac Cardiovasc Surg 123, 6–7.

40. Maruszewski B, Lacour-Gayet F, Elliott MJ, et al. (2002) Congenital Heart Surgery Nomenclature and Database Project: update and proposed data harvest. Eur J Cardiothoracic Surg 21, 47–49.

41. Mavroudis C, Gevitz M, Elliott MJ, et al. (2002) Virtues of a worldwide congenital heart surgery database. Semin Thorac Cardiovasc Surg Pediatr Card Surg Annu 5, 126–131.

42. Jacobs JP. (2002) Software development, nomenclature schemes, and mapping strategies for an international pediatric cardiac surgery database system. Semin Thorac Cardiovasc Surg Pediatr Card Surg Ann 5, 153–162.

43. Gaynor JW, Jacobs JP, Jacobs ML, et al. (2002) Congenital heart surgery nomenclature and database project: update and proposed data harvest. Ann Thorac Surg 73, 1016–1018.

44. Franklin RCG, Jacobs JP, Tchervenkov CI, et al. (2002) Bidirectional crossmap of the short lists of the European Paediatric Cardiac Code and the International Congenital Heart Surgery Nomenclature and Database Project. Cardiol Young 12(suppl 2), 18–22.

45. Franklin RCG, Jacobs JP, Tchervenkov CI, et al. (2002) European Paediatric Cardiac Code Short List crossmapped to STS/EACTS short list with ICD-9 & ICD-10 crossmapping. Cardiol Young 12(suppl 2), 23–49.

46. Franklin RCG, Jacobs JP, Tchervenkov CI, et al. (2002) STS/EACTS Short List mapping to European Paediatric Cardiac Code Short List with ICD-9 & ICD-10 crossmapping. Cardiol Young 12(suppl 2), 50–62.

47. Béland M, Jacobs JP, Tchervenkov CI, et al. (2002) Report from the Executive of the International Working Group for Mapping and Coding of Nomenclatures for Paediatric and Congenital Heart Disease. Cardiol Young 12, 425–430.

48. Franklin RCG, Jacobs JP, Tchervenkov CI, et al. (2002) Bidirectional crossmap of the Short Lists of the European Paediatric Cardiac Code and the International Congenital Heart Surgery Nomenclature and Database Project. Cardiol Young 12, 431–435.

49. Kurosawa H, Gaynor JW, Jacobs JP, et al. (2002) Congenital heart surgery nomenclature and database project: update and proposed data harvest. Jpn J Thorac Cardiovasc Surg 50, 498–501.

50. Lacour-Gayet FG, Clarke D, Jacobs JP, et al. (2004) The Aristotle score for congenital heart surgery. Semin Thorac Cardiovasc Surg Pediatr Card Surg Annu 7, 185–191.

51. Béland MJ, Franklin RCG, Jacobs JP, et al. (2004) Update from the international working group for mapping and coding of nomenclatures for paediatric and congenital heart disease. Cardiol Young 14, 225–229.

52. Lacour-Gayet FG, Clarke D, Jacobs JP, et al. (2004) The Aristotle score: a complexity-adjusted method to evaluate surgical results. Eur J Cardiothoracic Surg 25, 911–924.

53. Jacobs JP, Mavroudis C, Jacobs ML, *et al.* (2004) Lessons learned from the data analysis of the second harvest (1998–2001) of the society of thoracic surgeons (STS) congenital heart surgery database. Eur J Cardiothoracic Surg 26, 18–37.

54. Welke KF, Jacobs JP, Jenkins KJ. (2005) Evaluation of quality of care for congenital heart disease. Semin Thorac Cardiovasc Surg Pediatr Card Surg Annu 8, 157–167.

55. Jacobs JP, Elliott MJ, Anderson RH. (2005) Creating a database with cardioscopy and intra-operative imaging. Cardiol Young 15 (suppl 1), 184–189.

56. Jacobs JP, Maruszewski B, Tchervenkov CI, *et al.* (2005) The current status and future directions of efforts to create a global database for the outcomes of therapy for congenital heart disease. Cardiol Young 15 (suppl 1), 190–198.

57. Jacobs JP, Lacour-Gayet FG, Jacobs ML, *et al.* (2005) Initial application in the STS congenital database of complexity adjustment to evaluate surgical case mix and results. Ann Thorac Surg 79, 1635–1649.

58. Lacour-Gayet F, Clarke DR, Aristotle Committee. (2005) The Aristotle method: a new concept to evaluate quality of care based on complexity. Curr Opin Pediatr 17, 412–417.

59. Lacour-Gayet F, Jacobs JP, Clarke DR, *et al.* (2005) Performance of surgery for congenital heart disease: shall we wait a generation or look for different statistics? J Thorac Cardiovasc Surg 130, 234–235.

60. Maruszewski B, Lacour-Gayet F, Monro JL, *et al.* (2005) An attempt at data verification in the EACTS Congenital Database. Eur J Cardiothorac Surg 28, 400–406.

61. Jacobs ML. (2005) Editorial comment. Eur J Cardiothorac Surg 28, 405–406.

62. Jacobs JP, Maruszewski B, and The European Association for Cardio-Thoracic Surgery (EACTS) and The Society of Thoracic Surgeons (STS) Joint Congenital Heart Surgery Nomenclature and Database Committee. (2005) Computerized outcomes analysis for congenital heart disease. Curr Opin Pediatr 17, 586–591.

63. Jacobs JP, Jacobs ML, Maruszewski B, *et al.* (2005) Current status of the European Association for Cardio-Thoracic Surgery and the Society of Thoracic Surgeons Congenital Heart Surgery Database. Ann Thorac Surg 80, 2278–2284.

64. Jacobs JP, Franklin RCG, Jacobs ML, *et al.* (2006) Classification of the functionally univentricular heart: unity from mapped codes. Cardiol Young 16 (suppl 1), 9–21.

65. Jacobs JP, Mavroudis C, Jacobs ML, *et al.* (2006) What is operative mortality? Defining death in a surgical registry database: a report from the STS Congenital Database Task Force and the Joint EACTS-STS Congenital Database Committee. Ann Thorac Surg 81, 1937–1941.

66. Tchervenkov CI, Jacobs JP, Weinberg PM, *et al.* (2006) The nomenclature, definition and classification of hypoplastic left heart syndrome. Cardiol Young 16, 339–368.

67. Jacobs JP, Franklin RCG, Wilkinson JL, *et al.* (2006) The nomenclature, definition and classification of discordant atrioventricular connections. Cardiol Young 16 (suppl 3), 72–84.

68. Al-Radi OO, Harrell FE Jr, Caldarone CA, *et al.* (2007) Case complexity scores in congenital heart surgery: a comparative study of the Aristotle basic complexity score and the Risk Adjustment in Congenital Heart Surgery (RACHS-1) system. J Thorac Cardiovasc Surg 133, 865–875.

69. Jacobs JP, Mavroudis C, Jacobs ML, *et al.* (2007) Nomenclature and databases – the past, the present, and the future: a primer for the congenital heart surgeon. Pediatr Cardiol 28, 105–115.

70. Lacour-Gayet F, Jacobs ML, Jacobs JP, *et al.* (2007) The need for an objective evaluation of morbidity in congenital heart surgery. Ann Thorac Surg 84, 1–2.

71. Lacour-Gayet FG, Jacobs JP, Clarke DR, *et al.* (2007) Evaluation of quality of care in congenital heart surgery: contribution of the Aristotle complexity score. Adv Pediatr 54, 67–83

72. Jacobs JP, Anderson RH, Weinberg P, *et al.* (2007) The nomenclature, definition and classification of cardiac structures in the setting of heterotaxy. Cardiol Young 17 (suppl 2), 1–28.

73. Jacobs JP, Wernovsky G, Elliott MJ. (2007) Analysis of outcomes for congenital cardiac disease: can we do better? In: Supplement to *Cardiology in the Young: Controversies and Challenges Facing Paediatric Cardiovascular Practitioners and their Patients.* (Jacobs JP, Wernovsky G, Gaynor JW, Anderson RH, editors.) Cardiol Young 17 (suppl 2), 145–158.

74. Jacobs JP, Jacobs ML, Mavroudis C, *et al.* What is operative morbidity? Defining complications in a surgical registry database: a report from the STS Congenital Database Task Force and the Joint EACTS-STS Congenital Database Committee. Ann Thorac Surg 84, 1416–1421.

75. O'Brien SM, Jacobs JP, Clarke DR, *et al.* (2007) Accuracy of the Aristotle basic complexity score for classifying the mortality and morbidity potential of congenital heart surgery procedures. Ann Thorac Surg 84, 2027–2037.

76. Curzon CL, Milford-Beland S, Li JS, *et al.* (2008) Cardiac surgery in infants with low birth weight is associated with increased mortality: analysis of the Society of Thoracic Surgeons Congenital Heart Database. J Thorac Cardiovasc Surg 135, 546–551.

77. Jacobs JP, Haan CK, Edwards FH, *et al.* (2008) Editorial for the annals of thoracic surgery: the rationale for incorporation of HIPAA compliant unique patient, surgeon, and hospital identifier fields in the STS database. Ann Thorac Surg 86, 695–698.

78. Jacobs JP. (2008) Databases and the assessment of complications associated with the treatment of patients with congenital cardiac disease. Prepared by: The Multi-Societal Database Committee for Pediatric and Congenital Heart Disease. Cardiol Young 18 (suppl 2), S1–S530.

79. Jacobs JP. (2008) Introduction – databases and the assessment of complications associated with the treatment of patients with congenital cardiac disease. Cardiol Young 18 (suppl 2), S1–S37.

80. Jacobs JP, Jacobs ML, Mavroudis C, *et al.* (2008) Nomenclature and databases for the surgical treatment of congenital cardiac disease – an updated primer and an analysis of opportunities for improvement. Cardiol Young 18 (suppl 2), S38–S62.

81. Tchervenkov CI, Jacobs JP, Bernier P-L, *et al.* (2008) The improvement of care for paediatric and congenital cardiac disease across the World: a challenge for the World Society

for Pediatric and Congenital Heart Surgery. Cardiol Young 18 (suppl 2), S63–S69

82. Franklin RCG, Jacobs JP, Krogmann ON, et al. (2008) Nomenclature for congenital and paediatric cardiac disease: Historical perspectives and the international pediatric and congenital cardiac code. Cardiol Young 18 (suppl 2), S70–S80.

83. Jacobs JP, Benavidez OJ, Bacha EA, et al. (2008) The nomenclature of safety and quality of care for patients with congenital cardiac disease: a report of the Society of Thoracic Surgeons Congenital Database Taskforce Subcommittee on patient safety. Cardiol Young 18 (suppl 2), S81–S91.

84. Strickland MJ, Riehle-Colarusso TJ, Jacobs JP, et al. (2008) The importance of nomenclature for congenital cardiac disease: implications for research and evaluation. Cardiol Young 18 (suppl 2), S92–S100.

85. Jacobs ML, Jacobs JP, Franklin RCG, et al. (2008) Databases for assessing the outcomes of the treatment of patients with congenital and paediatric cardiac disease – the perspective of cardiac surgery. Cardiol Young 18 (suppl 2), S101–S115.

86. Jenkins KJ, Beekman RH 3rd, Bergersen LJ, et al. (2008) Databases for assessing the outcomes of the treatment of patients with congenital and paediatric cardiac disease – the perspective of cardiology. Cardiol Young 18 (suppl 2), S116–S123.

87. Vener DF, Jacobs JP, Schindler E, Maruszewski B, Andropoulos D. (2008) Databases for assessing the outcomes of the treatment of patients with congenital and paediatric cardiac disease – the perspective of anaesthesia. Cardiol Young 18 (suppl 2), S124–S129.

88. LaRovere JM, Jeffries HE, Sachdeva RC, et al. (2008) Databases for assessing the outcomes of the treatment of patients with congenital and paediatric cardiac disease – the perspective of critical care. Cardiol Young 18 (suppl 2), S130–S136.

89. Welke KF, Karamlou T, Diggs BS. (2008) Databases for assessing the outcomes of the treatment of patients with congenital and paediatric cardiac disease – a comparison of administrative and clinical data. Cardiol Young 18 (suppl 2), S137–S144.

90. O'Brien SM, Gauvreau K. (2008) Statistical issues in the analysis and interpretation of outcomes for congenital cardiac surgery. Cardiol Young 18 (suppl 2), S145–S151.

91. Hickey EJ, McCrindle BW, Caldarone CA, et al. (2008) Making sense of congenital cardiac disease with a research database: the Congenital Heart Surgeons' Society Data Center. Cardiol Young 18 (suppl 2), S152–S162.

92. Jacobs ML, Jacobs JP, Jenkins KJ, et al. (2008) Stratification of complexity: the risk adjustment for congenital heart surgery. 1 Method and the Aristotle complexity score – past, present, and future. Cardiol Young 18 (suppl 2), S163–S168.

93. Clarke DR, Lacour-Gayet F, Jacobs JP, et al. (2008) The assessment of complexity in congenital cardiac surgery based on objective data. Cardiol Young 18 (suppl 2), S169–S176.

94. Clarke DR, Breen LS, Jacobs ML, et al. (2008) Verification of data in congenital cardiac surgery. Cardiol Young 18 (suppl 2), S177–S187.

95. Morales DLS, McClellan AJ, Jacobs JP. (2008) Empowering a database with national long-term data about mortality: the use of national death registries. Cardiol Young 18 (suppl 2), S188–S195.

96. Bacha EA, Cooper D, Thiagarajan R, et al. (2008) Cardiac complications associated with the treatment of patients with congenital cardiac disease: consensus definitions from the Multi-Societal Database Committee for Pediatric and Congenital Heart Disease. Cardiol Young 18 (suppl 2), S196–S201.

97. Deal BJ, Mavroudis C, Jacobs JP, Gevitz M, Backer CL. (2008) Arrhythmic complications associated with the treatment of patients with congenital cardiac disease: consensus definitions from the Multi-Societal Database Committee for Pediatric and Congenital Heart Disease. Cardiol Young 18 (suppl 2), S202–S205.

98. Shann KG, Giacomuzzi CR, Harness L, et al. (2008) Complications relating to perfusion and extracorporeal circulation associated with the treatment of patients with congenital cardiac disease: consensus definitions from the Multi-Societal Database Committee for Pediatric and Congenital Heart Disease. Cardiol Young 18 (suppl 2), S206–S214.

99. Cooper DS, Jacobs JP, Chai PJ, et al. (2008) Pulmonary complications associated with the treatment of patients with congenital cardiac disease: consensus definitions from the Multi-Societal Database Committee for Pediatric and Congenital Heart Disease. Cardiol Young 18 (suppl 2), S215–S221.

100. Welke KW, Dearani JA, Ghanayem NS, et al. (2008) Renal complications associated with the treatment of patients with congenital cardiac disease: consensus definitions from the Multi-Societal Database Committee for Pediatric and Congenital Heart Disease. Cardiol Young 18 (suppl 2), S222–S225.

101. Checchia PA, Karamlou T, Maruszewski B, et al. (2008) Haematological and infectious complications associated with the treatment of patients with congenital cardiac disease: consensus definitions from the Multi-Societal Database Committee for Pediatric and Congenital Heart Disease. Cardiol Young 18 (suppl 2), S226–S233.

102. Bird GL, Jeffries HE, Licht DJ, et al. (2008) Neurological complications associated with the treatment of patients with congenital cardiac disease: consensus definitions from the Multi-Societal Database Committee for Pediatric and Congenital Heart Disease. Cardiol Young 18 (suppl 2), S234–S239.

103. Ghanayem NS, Dearani JA, Welke KF, et al. (2008) Gastrointestinal complications associated with the treatment of patients with congenital cardiac disease: consensus definitions from the Multi-Societal Database Committee for Pediatric and Congenital Heart Disease. Cardiol Young 18 (suppl 2), S240–S244.

104. Walters HL 3rd, Jeffries HE, Cohen GA, et al. (2008) Congenital cardiac surgical complications of the integument, vascular system, vascular-line(s), and wounds: consensus definitions from the Multi-Societal Database Committee for Pediatric and Congenital Heart Disease. Cardiol Young 18 (suppl 2), S245–S255.

105. Dickerson H, Cooper DS, Checchia PA, *et al.* (2008) Endocrinal complications associated with the treatment of patients with congenital cardiac disease: consensus definitions from the Multi-Societal Database Committee for Pediatric and Congenital Heart Disease. Cardiol Young 18 (suppl 2), S256–S264.

106. Jeffries H, Bird G, Law Y, *et al.* (2008) Complications related to the transplantation of thoracic organs: consensus definitions from the Multi-Societal Database Committee for Pediatric and Congenital Heart Disease. Cardiol Young 18 (suppl 2), S265–S270.

107. Vener DV, Tirotta CF, Andropoulos D, *et al.* (2008) Anaesthetic complications associated with the treatment of patients with congenital cardiac disease: consensus definitions from the Multi-Societal Database Committee for Pediatric and Congenital Heart Disease. Cardiol Young 18 (suppl 2), S271–S281.

108. The Multi-Societal Database Committee for Pediatric and Congenital Heart Disease. (2008) Part IV – the dictionary of definitions of complications associated with the treatment of patients with congenital cardiac disease. Cardiol Young 18 (suppl 2), S282–S530.

109. Jacobs JP, Shahian DM, Jacobs ML, *et al.* (2009) Invited commentary of "Monitoring risk-adjusted outcomes in congenital heart surgery: does the appropriateness of a risk model change with time?" by Tsang VT, Brown KL, Synnergren MJ, *et al.* Ann Thorac Surg 87, 587–588.

110. Jacobs JP, Cerfolio RJ, Sade RM. (2009) The ethics of transparency: publication of cardiothoracic surgical outcomes in the lay press. Ann Thorac Surg 87, 679–686.

111. Welke KF, O'Brien SM, Peterson ED, *et al.* (2009) The complex relationship between pediatric cardiac surgical case volumes and mortality rates in a national clinical database. J Thorac Cardiovasc Surg 137, 1133–1140.

112. O'Brien SM, Clarke DR, Jacobs JP, *et al.* (2009) An empirically based mortality index for analyzing outcomes of congenital heart surgery. J Thorac Cardiovasc Surg 138, 1139–1153.

113. Jacobs JP, Quintessenza JA, Burke RP, *et al.* (2009) Analysis of regional congenital cardiac surgical outcomes in Florida using the Society of Thoracic Surgeons Congenital Heart Surgery Database. Cardiol Young 19, 360–369.

114. Dokholyan RS, Muhlbaier LH, Falletta J, *et al.* (2009) Regulatory and ethical considerations for linking clinical and administrative databases. Am Heart J 157, 971–982.

115. Jacobs JP, Jacobs ML, Lacour-Gayet FG, *et al.* (2009) Stratification of complexity improves utility and accuracy of outcomes analysis in a multi-institutional congenital heart surgery database – application of the RACHS-1 and Aristotle systems in the STS congenital heart surgery database. Pediatr Cardiol 30, 1117–1130.

116. Jacobs JP, Jacobs ML, Mavroudis C, *et al.* (2002) Executive summary: The Society of Thoracic Surgeons congenital heart surgery database – second harvest – (1998–2001) beta site test. The Society of Thoracic Surgeons (STS) and Duke Clinical Research Institute (DCRI), Duke University Medical Center, Durham, North Carolina, United States, Fall 2002 Harvest.

117. Jacobs JP, Jacobs ML, Mavroudis C, *et al.* (2003) Executive Summary: The Society of Thoracic Surgeons Congenital Heart Surgery Database – Third Harvest – (1998–2002). The Society of Thoracic Surgeons (STS) and Duke Clinical Research Institute (DCRI), Duke University Medical Center, Durham, North Carolina, United States, Spring 2003 Harvest.

118. Jacobs JP, Jacobs ML, Mavroudis C, *et al.* (2004) Executive Summary: The Society of Thoracic Surgeons Congenital Heart Surgery Database – Fourth Harvest – (2002–2003). The Society of Thoracic Surgeons (STS) and Duke Clinical Research Institute (DCRI), Duke University Medical Center, Durham, North Carolina, United States, Spring 2004 Harvest.

119. Jacobs JP, Jacobs ML, Mavroudis C, *et al.* (2005) Executive Summary: The Society of Thoracic Surgeons Congenital Heart Surgery Database – Fifth Harvest – (2002–2004). The Society of Thoracic Surgeons (STS) and Duke Clinical Research Institute (DCRI), Duke University Medical Center, Durham, North Carolina, United States, Spring 2005 Harvest.

120. Jacobs JP, Jacobs ML, Mavroudis C, *et al.* (2006) Executive Summary: The Society of Thoracic Surgeons Congenital Heart Surgery Database – Sixth Harvest – (2002–2005). The Society of Thoracic Surgeons (STS) and Duke Clinical Research Institute (DCRI), Duke University Medical Center, Durham, North Carolina, United States, Spring 2006 Harvest.

121. Jacobs JP, Jacobs ML, Mavroudis C, *et al.* (2007) Executive Summary: The Society of Thoracic Surgeons Congenital Heart Surgery Database — Seventh Harvest – (2003–2006). The Society of Thoracic Surgeons (STS) and Duke Clinical Research Institute (DCRI), Duke University Medical Center, Durham, North Carolina, United States, Spring 2007 Harvest.

122. Jacobs JP, Jacobs ML, Mavroudis C, *et al.* (2008) Executive Summary: The Society of Thoracic Surgeons Congenital Heart Surgery Database – Eighth Harvest – (January 1, 2004 – December 31, 2007). The Society of Thoracic Surgeons (STS) and Duke Clinical Research Institute (DCRI), Duke University Medical Center, Durham, North Carolina, United States, Spring 2008 Harvest.

123. Jacobs JP, Jacobs ML, Mavroudis C, *et al.* (2008) Executive Summary: The Society of Thoracic Surgeons Congenital Heart Surgery Database – Ninth Harvest – (July 1, 2004 – June 30, 2008). The Society of Thoracic Surgeons (STS) and Duke Clinical Research Institute (DCRI), Duke University Medical Center, Durham, North Carolina, United States, Fall 2008 Harvest.

124. Jacobs JP, Jacobs ML, Mavroudis C, *et al.* (2009) Executive Summary: The Society of Thoracic Surgeons Congenital Heart Surgery Database – Tenth Harvest – (January 1, 2005 — December 31, 2008). The Society of Thoracic Surgeons (STS) and Duke Clinical Research Institute (DCRI), Duke University Medical Center, Durham, North Carolina, United States, Spring 2009 Harvest.

125. *Webster's New World Dictionary of the American Language*, college ed. (1957) New York, NY: World Publishing.

126. Jaques HE. (1947) *Living Things: How to Know Them*. Dubuque, IA: Wm Brown.

127. Macartney FJ. (1994) Classification and nomenclature of congenital heart defects. In: Stark J, deLeval M, eds. *Surgery for Congenital Heart Defects*, 2nd ed, Philadelphia, PA: WB Saunders.

128. Van Praagh R. (1972) The segmental approach to diagnosis in congenital heart disease. Birth Defects Original Article Series 8, 4–23.

129. Van Praagh R. (1977) Terminology of congenital heart disease: glossary and commentary. Circulation 56, 139–143.

130. Van Praagh R, Vlad P. (1978) Dextrocardia, mesocardia, and levocardia: the segmental approach in congenital heart disease. In: Keith JD, Rowe RD, Vlad P, eds. *Heart Disease in Infancy and Childhood*, 3rd ed. New York, NY: Macmillan.

131. Anderson RH, Becker AE, Freedom RM, *et al.* (1984) Sequential segmental analysis of congenital heart disease. Pediatr Cardiol 5, 281–287.

132. Wilcox BR, Anderson RH. (1992) *Surgical anatomy of the heart*, 2nd ed. London: Gower Medical Publishing.

133. Anderson RH, Ho SY. (1997) Sequential segmental analysis – description and categorization for the millennium. Cardiol Young 7, 98–116.

134. Jacobs JP. (2003) Nomenclature and classification for congenital cardiac surgery. In: Mavroudis C, Backer CL, eds. *Pediatric Cardiac Surgery*, 3rd ed. Philadelphia, PA: Mosby.

135. Van Praagh R, Van Praagh S, Vlad P, *et al.* (1964) Anatomic types of congenital dextrocardia. Diagnostic and embryologic implications. Am J Cardiol 13, 510–531.

136. Shinebourne EA, Macartney FJ, Anderson RH. (1976) Sequential chamber localization – logical approach to diagnosis in congenital heart disease. Br Heart J 38, 327–340.

137. Anderson RH, Smith A, Wilkinson JL. (1987) Disharmony between atrioventricular connections and segmental combinations: unusual variants of "crisscross" hearts. JACC 10, 1274–1277.

138. Uemura H, Ho SY, Devine WA, *et al.* (1995) Atrial appendages and venoatrial connections in hearts with patients with visceral heterotaxy. Ann Thorac Surg 60, 561–569.

139. Huhta JC, Smallhorn JF, Macartney FJ. (1982) Two dimensional echocardiographic diagnosis of situs. Br Heart J 48, 97–108.

140. Van Mierop LHS, Wiglesworth FW. (1964) Isomerism of the cardiac atria in the asplenia syndrome. Lab Invest 11, 1303–1315.

141. Van Mierop LHS, Patterson PR, Reynolds RW. (1964) Two cases of congenital asplenia with isomerism of the cardiac atria and the sinoatrial nodes. Am J Cardiol 13, 407–412.

142. Moller JH, Nakib A, Anderson RC, *et al.* (1967) Congenital cardiac disease associated with polysplenia: a developmental complex of bilateral "left-sidedness". Circulation 36, 789–799.

143. Macartney FJ, Anderson RH, Smallhorn JF, *et al.* (1980) Segmental analysis in practice. In: Becker AE, Marcelletti C, Losekoot TG, eds. *Paediatric Cardiology* Volume 3. Edinburgh: Churchill Livingstone.

144. Macartney FJ, Partridge JB, Shinebourne EA, *et al.* (1978) Identification of atrial situs. In: Anderson RH, Shinebourne EA, eds. *Paediatric Cardiology*, Edinburgh: Churchill Livingstone.

145. Van Mierop LH, Eisen S, Schiebler GL. (1970) The radiographic appearance of the tracheobronchial tree as an indicator of the visceral situs. Am J Cardiol 26, 432–435.

146. Partridge JB, Scott O, Deverall PB, *et al.* (1975) Visualization and measurement of the main bronchi by tomography as an objective indicator of thoracic situs in congenital heart disease. Circulation 51, 188–196.

147. Brandt PW, Calder AL. (1977) Cardiac connections: the segmental approach to radiologic diagnosis in congenital heart disease. Curr Probl Diagn Radiol 7, 1–35.

148. Stanger P, Rudolph AM, Edwards JE. (1977) Cardiac malpositions: an overview based on study of sixty-five necropsy specimens. Circulation 56, 159–172.

149. Caruso G, Becker AE. (1979) How to determine atrial situs? Considerations initiated by 3 cases of absent spleen with a discordant anatomy between bronchi and atria. Br Heart J 41, 559–567.

150. Van Mierop LHS, Gessner IH, Schiebler GL. (1972) Asplenia and polysplenia syndromes. In: Bergsma D, ed. *Birth Defects: Atlas and Compendium*. Baltimore, MD: Williams & Wilkins.

151. Landing BH, Lawrence TY, Payne Jr. VC, *et al.* (1971) Bronchial anatomy in syndromes with abnormal visceral situs, abnormal spleen and congenital heart disease. Am J Cardiol 28, 456–462.

152. Layman TE, Levine MA, Amplatz K, *et al.* (1967) "Asplenic syndrome" in association with rudimentary spleen. Am J Cardiol 20, 136–140.

153. Wilkinson JL, Acerete F. (1973) Terminological pitfalls in congenital heart disease. Reappraisal of some confusing terms, with an account of a simplified system of basic nomenclature. Br Heart J 35, 1166–1177.

154. Ferencz C, Rubin JD, McCarter RJ, *et al.* (1985) Congenital heart disease: prevalence at livebirth: the Baltimore-Washington Infant Study. Am J Epidemiol 121, 31–36.

155. Spencer FC: Congenital heart disease. (1989) In: Schwartz SI, Shires GT, Spencer FC, eds. *Principles of Surgery*, 5th ed. New York, NY: McGraw-Hill.

156. Treasure T. (2000) Commentary: rational decision-making about paediatric cardiac surgery. Lancet 355, 1004–1007.

157. Gardiner K, Pemberton PJ, Ramsey J. (1998) The aftermath of the Bristol case: supraregional neonatal cardiac surgery works in Western Australia. BMJ 317, 814.

158. Bharati S, Lev M. (1973) The spectrum of common atrioventricular orifice (canal). Am Heart J 86, 553–561.

159. Levy MJ, Salomon J, Vidne BA. (1974) Correction of single and common atrium, with reference to simplified terminology. Chest 66, 444–446.

160. Kirklin JW, Barratt-Boyes BG. (1993) Ventricular septal defect and pulmonary stenosis or atresia. In: *Cardiac Surgery: Morphology, Diagnostic Criteria, Natural History, Techniques, Results, and Indications*, 2nd ed. New York, NY: Churchill-Livingstone.

161. Van Praagh R, Ando M, Van Praagh S, *et al.* (1976) Pulmonary atresia: anatomic considerations. In: Kidd BSL, Rowe RD, eds. *The Child with Congenital Heart Disease after Surgery*. Mt Kisco, NY: Futura.

162. Bharati S, Paul MH, Idriss FS, *et al.* (1975) The surgical anatomy of pulmonary atresia with ventricular septal defect: pseudotruncus. J Thorac Cardiovasc Surg 69, 713–721.

163. Tchervenkov CI, Shum-Tim D. (1996) Ventricular septal defect. In: Baue AE, Geha AS, Hammond GL, *et al.*, eds. *Glenn's Thoracic and Cardiovascular Surgery*, 6th ed. Stamford, Conn, Appleton & Lange.

164. Mavroudis C, Backer CL, Idriss FS. (1994) Ventricular septal defect. In: Mavroudis C, Backer CL, eds. *Pediatric Cardiac Surgery*, 2nd ed. St. Louis, MO: Mosby-Year Book.

165. Tchervenkov CI, Salasidis G, Cecere R, *et al.* (1997) One-stage midline unifocalization and complete repair in infancy versus multiple-stage unifocalization followed by repair for complex heart disease with major aortopulmonary collaterals, J Thorac Cardiovasc Surg 114, 727–735.

166. Pacifico AD, Kirklin JW, Bargeron LM. (1973) Complex congenital malformations: surgical treatment of double-outlet right ventricle and double-outlet left ventricle. In: Kirklin JW, ed. *Advances in Cardiovascular Surgery*. New York, NY: Grune & Stratton.

167. Stark J. (1994) Double outlet ventricles. In: Stark J, deLeval M, eds. *Surgery for Congenital Heart Defects*, 2nd ed. Philadelphia, PA: WB Saunders.

168. Kirklin JW, Barrat-Boyes BG, eds. (1986) *Cardiac Surgery: Morphology, Diagnostic Criteria, Natural History, Techniques, Results, and Indications*. New York, NY: John Wiley & Sons, Inc.

169. VanPraagh S, Davidoff A, Chin A, *et al.* (1982) Double outlet right ventricle: anatomic types and developmental implications based on a study of 101 autopsied cases. Coeur 13, 389–440.

170. Anderson RH, Pickering D, Brown R. (1975) Double outlet right ventricle with l-malposition and uncommitted ventricular septal defect. Eur J Cardiol 32, 133–142.

171. Piccoli G, Pacifico AD, Kirklin JW, *et al.* (1983) Changing results and concepts in the surgical treatment of double-outlet right ventricle: analysis of 137 operations in 126 patients. Am J Cardiol 52, 549–554.

172. Kirklin JW, Pacifico AD, Blackstone EH, *et al.* (1986) Current risks and protocols for operations for double-outlet right ventricle: derivation from an 18 year experience. J Thorac Cardiovasc Surg 92, 913–930.

173. Musumeci F, Shumway S, Lincoln C, *et al.* (1988) Surgical treatment for double-outlet right ventricle at the Brompton Hospital, 1973 to 1986. J Thorac Cardiovasc Surg 96, 278–287.

174. Fyler DC. (1992) Single ventricle. In: *Nadas' Pediatric Cardiology*. St. Louis, MO: Mosby-Year Book. pp. 649–658.

175. VanPraagh R, Ongley PA, Swan HJC. (1964) Anatomic types of single or common ventricle in man: morphologic and geometric aspects of 60 necropsied cases. Am J Cardiol 13, 367–386.

176. vanPraagh R, Plett JA, vanPraagh S. (1979) Single ventricle. Pathology, embryology, terminology and classification. Herz 4, 113–150.

177. van Praagh R, David I, van Praagh S. (1982) What is a ventricle? The single-ventricle trap. Pediatr Cardiol 2, 79–84.

178. Anderson RH, Becker AE, Freedom RM, *et al.* (1979) Problems in the nomenclature of the univentricular heart. Herz 4, 97–106.

179. Wilkinson JL, Becker AE, Tynan M, *et al.* (1979) Nomenclature of the univentricular heart. Herz 4, 107–112.

180. Anderson RH, Macartney FJ, Tynan M, *et al.* (1983) Univentricular atrioventricular connection: the single ventricle trap unsprung. Pediatr Cardiol 4, 273–280.

181. Anderson RH, Becker AE, Tynan M, *et al.* (1984) The univentricular atrioventricular connection: getting to the root of a thorny problem. Am J Cardiol 54, 822–828.

182. Jacobs M, Anderson RH. (2006) Nomenclature of the functionally univentricular heart. Cardiol Young 16 (suppl 1), 3–8.

183. Van Praagh R, Perez-Trevino C, Lopez-Cuellar M, *et al.* (1971) Transposition of the great arteries with posterior aorta, anterior pulmonary artery, subpulmonary conus and fibrous continuity between aortic and atrioventricular valves. Am J Cardiol 28, 621–631.

184. Van Praagh R, Van Praagh S. (1966) Isolated ventricular inversion: a consideration of the morphogenesis, definition and diagnosis of nontransposed and transposed great arteries. Am J Cardiol 17, 395–406.

185. Shinebourne EA, Macartney FJ, Anderson RH. (1976) Sequential chamber localization: logical approach to diagnosis in congenital heart disease. Br Heart J 38, 327–340.

186. Schiebler GL, Edwards JE, Burchell HB, *et al.* (1961) Congenital corrected transposition of the great vessels: a study of 33 cases. Pediatrics 27, 849–888.

187. Van Praagh R, Van Praagh S, Vlad P, *et al.* (1964) Anatomic types of congenital dextrocardia: diagnostic and embryologic implications. Am J Cardiol 13, 510–531.

CHAPTER 3

Physiology of the Fetal and Neonatal Circulations and Fetal Cardiac Surgery

Ashok Muralidaran,[1] Vadiyala Mohan Reddy,[2] and Frank L. Hanley[1]

[1]Stanford University School of Medicine, Stanford, CA, USA
[2]Lucile Packard Children's Hospital, Stanford University, Stanford, CA, USA

Fetal Circulation

Blood flow in a normal adult is in series, a sequential flow of blood from the systemic venous system to the right heart, to the lungs, and to the left heart where well oxygenated blood is eventually pumped back into the systemic circulation. In the fetus, the right and left hearts control different proportions of the total blood volume, thus acting in a parallel fashion. The total fetal cardiac output is thus a sum of both of the ventricles' output – the combined ventricular output (CVO) or the biventricular output. The general pattern favors the streaming of well oxygenated blood from the placenta to the heart and the brain; and the less oxygenated blood streams into the umbilical arteries and, finally, back to the placenta.

Fetal Intra- and Extracardiac Shunts

Three important shunts help accomplish the streaming of blood that we previously described: the ductus venosus, the foramen ovale, and the ductus arteriosus. This is illustrated in Figure 3.1 [1].

A good fraction of the oxygenated placental blood returning via the umbilical vein (UV) is diverted directly into the inferior vena cava (IVC) via the ductus venosus (DV), thus bypassing the liver parenchyma [2]. When this well oxygenated blood reaches the right atrium it is preferentially shunted across to the left atrium via the foramen ovale, thus making its way via the left ventricle to the coronary and cerebral circulations. The venous return from these circulations and the upper body drains via the superior vena cava into the right atrium, streaming directly into the right ventricle with almost no blood traversing the foramen ovale [2]. The right ventricle then pumps this deoxygenated blood into the main pulmonary artery, the majority of it flowing into the descending aorta via the ductus arteriosus, supplying the abdominal viscera, the lower body, and the umbilical arteries with reoxygenation at the placenta. The lower body venous return is via the IVC to the right atrium, being split between the shunt across the foramen ovale and the normal flow via the tricuspid valve to the right ventricle [3]. Figure 3.2 illustrates the flows in the main vessels, shunts, and chambers as a proportion of the biventricular output [1]. Note the minimal flow to the lungs in the fetus later transitioning to support a full cardiac output in the neonate.

Venous Return

The richly oxygenated UV blood splits in half as it enters the liver, being distributed equally between the DV and the liver parenchyma [4]. The DV blood flows into the IVC streaming dorsal and leftward to that of the blood returning from the lower body, facilitating its preferential route into the left atrium (LA) and hence, the brain and myocardium [5]. The other half that enters the liver does so preferentially via the left portal vein, contributing to about 80% of the total hepatic blood flow. The remaining 20% is split between the portal vein (15%) and the hepatic arteries (5%) [4].

The crista dividens – the lower border of the septum secundum – forms the cephalad margin of the foramen ovale (FO) lying to the right of the atrial septum, overriding the IVC orifice. It splits the IVC stream into an anterior and rightward portion flowing into the right atrium (RA) and

Pediatric Cardiac Surgery, Fourth Edition. Edited by Constantine Mavroudis and Carl L. Backer.
© 2013 Blackwell Publishing Ltd. Published 2013 by Blackwell Publishing Ltd.

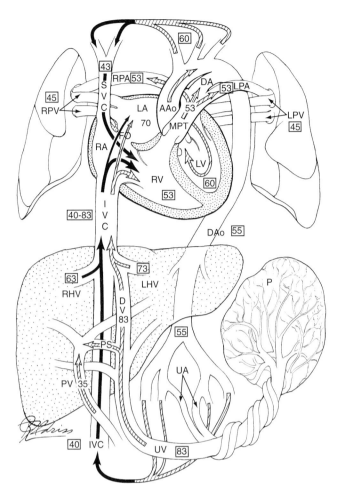

Figure 3.1 Diagrammatic representation of normal fetal circulation, major flow patterns, and blood hemoglobin oxygen saturations. (AAo, ascending aorta; DAo, descending aorta; DV, ductus venosus; FO, foramen ovale; IVC, inferior vena cava; LA, left atrium; LHV, left hepatic vein; LPA, left pulmonary artery; LPV, left pulmonary veins; LV, left ventricle; MPT, main pulmonary trunk; P, placenta; PS, portal sinus; PV, portal vein; RA, right atrium; RHV, right hepatic vein; RPA, right pulmonary artery; RPV, right pulmonary veins; RV, right ventricle; UA, umbilical arteries; UV, umbilical vein).

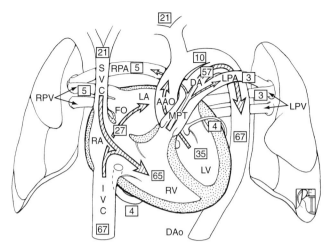

Figure 3.2 Representative values for percentages of fetal cardiac output (combined ventricular output) returning to and leaving the heart in normal fetal lambs. (AAo, ascending aorta; DAo, descending aorta; DV, ductus venosus; FO, foramen ovale; IVC, inferior vena cava; LA, left atrium; LHV, left hepatic vein; LPA, left pulmonary artery; LPV, left pulmonary veins; LV, left ventricle; MPT, main pulmonary trunk; P, placenta; PS, portal sinus; PV, portal vein; RA, right atrium; RHV, right hepatic vein; RPA, right pulmonary artery; RPV, right pulmonary veins; RV, right ventricle; UA, umbilical arteries; UV, umbilical vein).

Cardiac Output, Oxygenation, and Distribution

The RV is the dominant ventricle in the fetus. It predominantly perfuses the lower body, the abdominal organs, and the placenta. As illustrated in Figure 3.2 [1], the RV contributes approximately 65% and the LV, 35% of CVO [6]. Composed of the SVC, the coronary sinus and the predominantly lower body return from the IVC, this overwhelmingly deoxygenated blood is pumped by the RV mostly to the descending aorta via the ductus arteriosus, with only 8% of the RV output reaching the lungs. This preferentially distributes the deoxygenated blood for reoxygenation in the placenta.

The LV perfuses the ascending aorta, resulting in 21% of the CVO reaching the brain and upper body and 10% reaching the descending aorta via the isthmus. As shown in Figure 3.1 [1], the blood streaming into the LV has a relatively high saturation rate of 60%. Hence, there is some saturated blood from the LV entering the descending aorta that may perfuse the placenta contributing to the physiological "left-to-right" shunt equivalent in the fetus [7]. Individual organ blood flows are shown in Figure 3.3 [2] as proportions of the CVO.

Table 3.1 [1] shows some representative fetal blood gas values. Although the systemic arterial partial pressure of oxygen (pO$_2$) of the fetus is low, because of the fetal hemoglobin and the consequent left shift of the hemoglobin–oxygen dissociation curve, hemoglobin O$_2$ saturation (or

a posterior and leftward stream that flows into the LA. The latter stream is predominantly composed of the UV return that flowed via the DV. Intermixing does occur, in that some DV blood flows into the RA and some deoxygenated IVC blood flows into the LA, but the left atrium has a significantly higher saturation than the right (Figure 3.1) [1].

Blood returning to the heart via the SVC is preferentially streamed into the tricuspid orifice by the crista interveniens situated in the posterolateral wall of the RA. The coronary sinus flow is also directed toward the tricuspid valve and hence, the right ventricle (RV). The pulmonary venous return is to the LA, mixing with the blood crossing the FO.

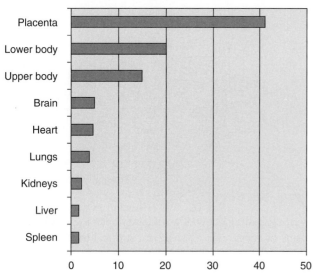

Figure 3.3 Average combined cardiac output distributed to different organs or parts in eight different fetal animals. (Adapted with permission from Rudolph, *et al.* [2].)

Table 3.1 Normal fetal pH and blood gas data. Reproduced with permission from Heymann [1].

	Umbilical vein	Descending aorta	Ascending aorta
pH	7.40–7.45	7.35–7.40	7.37–7.42
pO_2 (torr)	28–33	20–24	22–26
pCO_2 (torr)	45–50	48–53	46–51

at the same hemoglobin saturation, the oxygen content) is higher in the fetus than the adult. Fetal O_2 consumption is significantly less as the work of breathing is absent and thermoregulation requirements *in utero* are far less [8].

Intracardiac and Vascular Pressures

Fetal vascular pressures (shown in Figure 3.4 [1]) also reflect the preferential streaming patterns described previously. The high flow from the placenta results in the UV having a 3–5 mmHg higher pressure than the IVC. The RA pressure is higher than the LA and along with the kinetic energy of blood streaming via the IVC, contributes to the shunting of blood across the FO [3]. The ductus arteriosus offers little resistance to flow and pressures in the main pulmonary trunk; the pulmonary arteries and the RV are only slightly higher (1–2 mmHg) than the aorta and the LV.

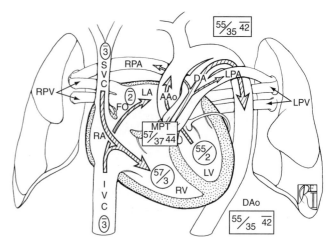

Figure 3.4 Representative values for vascular pressures in normal fetal lambs. (AAo, ascending aorta; DAo, descending aorta; DV, ductus venosus; FO, foramen ovale; IVC, inferior vena cava; LA, left atrium; LHV, left hepatic vein; LPA, left pulmonary artery; LPV, left pulmonary veins; LV, left ventricle; MPT, main pulmonary trunk; P, placenta; PS, portal sinus; PV, portal vein; RA, right atrium; RHV, right hepatic vein; RPA, right pulmonary artery; RPV, right pulmonary veins; RV, right ventricle; UA, umbilical arteries; UV, umbilical vein).

Circulatory Changes at Birth

The Transition

At birth, the pattern of circulation changes from the fetal "parallel" type to the adult "series" type, leading to more efficient oxygen uptake and delivery [9]. This happens with rapid establishment of pulmonary circulation, loss of placental circulation, and the closure of the ductus venosus, the foramen ovale, and eventually the ductus arteriosus. There is a rapid increase in O_2 consumption probably related to the work of breathing and thermoregulation, with an increase in cardiac output, a decrease in pulmonary vascular resistance, and an increase in pulmonary blood flow. The consequent increase in pulmonary venous return to the LA coupled with a decrease in IVC flow to the RA from cessation of placental UV return reverses the pressure difference between the LA and the RA, closing the flap valve of the FO. Pressures are also reversed across the DA, with a left-to-right flow reversal being established before it closes.

Closure of the Ductus Arteriosus

In the fetus, the patency of the ductus arteriosus is maintained by prostaglandin E2 (PGE_2) and prostacyclin (PGI_2) [10]. The initial functional closure which occurs within 12 hours of birth is thought to be mediated by the increase in systemic pO_2, though other vasoactive substances may also be contributory [11]. A reduction in circulating prostaglandin levels is implicated in persistent ductal closure. Eventually there is fibrous replacement of the musculature of the ductus arteriosus with formation of the ligamentum arteriosum.

Pulmonary Circulation

The high fetal pulmonary vascular resistance (PVR) is attributed to vasoconstriction in the thick medial layer of the small branches [12]. With increasing gestation, there is growth of new arteries, an increase in the cross-sectional area of the vascular bed, a drop in the PVR, and a slight increase in pulmonary blood flow [12]. Hypoxia is a major vasoconstrictive factor, as are acidosis and the leukotrienes [13,14].

A diverse group of vasoactive substances causes fetal and perinatal pulmonary vasodilatation – bradykinin, histamine, acetylcholine, PGE_1, PGE_2, prostaglandin D2 (PGD2), PGI_2, and catecholamines, to name a few [15]. Their effects are mediated by the endothelial release of secondary substances like nitric oxide (NO). A baseline relaxation of the fetal pulmonary vasculature has been attributed to NO [16].

Ventilation causes a mechanical stretch-induced production of PGI_2 in the fetal lung, with a drop in PVR that is accentuated with oxygen [17]. A calcium-dependent potassium channel activation has been hypothesized to mediate this effect of oxygen [18]. At birth, a combination of ventilatory stretch, increased alveolar oxygen tension, local NO, and PGI_2 production blend to produce a dramatic fall in PVR and a resultant striking increase in pulmonary blood flow. A role for ventilation-induced local mast cell degranulation and release of histamine and PGD_2 has also been suggested in contributing to postnatal pulmonary vasodilation [19].

Myocardial Performance

The immature fetal myocardium displays significant structural and hence functional differences from that of the adult. Not only are myocardial cells smaller, smooth, and rounded as opposed to being rod-shaped as in the adult, the cytoplasm has proportionately more water and lower myofibril content and they are not all arranged parallel to the cellular axis [20]. This may account for the differences in force generation and in the fetal myocardium being stiffer and less compliant.

The Frank-Starling mechanism is intact in the fetus at least at low atrial pressures but studies have differed on ventricular performance at higher atrial filling pressures [21–24]. Increases in arterial pressure significantly depress cardiac function in the fetus [24]. It does appear that in the fetus the preload and afterload are interrelated. The

enhancement in stroke volume occurring after increasing the filling pressure by volume loading is stifled by a simultaneous augmentation in the afterload.

It is a matter of great interest how the neonatal left ventricle transitions from a low-pressure, low-output chamber to functioning at systemic pressures controlling a full cardiac output abruptly at birth. Changes in contractility, increase in beta adrenergic receptor density, and postnatal thyroid hormone changes have been suggested to aid in this transition [25,26].

Fetal Surgery

With expanding knowledge of fetal physiology and mechanisms of congenital lesions, fetal surgical therapy was the next logical clinical step. A succinct review of the initial two decades of fetal surgery with particular respect to the San Francisco center is provided by Dr. Harrison in a personal perspective [27].

Currently for congenital diaphragmatic hernia, the management strategy has shifted away from open fetal surgery to open or endoscopic tracheal occlusion to hasten lung growth and maturity. Endoscopic laser ablation of the communicating vessels is offered in select cases of twin-to-twin transfusion syndrome. Trials are being conducted comparing conventional postnatal care and intrauterine treatment of meningomyelocele [28]. The EXIT procedure stands for *ex utero* intrapartum treatment, where fetuses with certain congenital pulmonary lesions or prenatally diagnosed neck tumors are carefully managed at birth. During a controlled surgical delivery, the umbilical-placental circulation is maintained while the airway is secured, or the neonate is placed on extracorporeal membrane oxygenation (ECMO). A detailed discussion of fetal surgery in general is beyond the scope of this chapter.

Fetal Cardiac Surgery

Animal Models of Congenital Lesions

Advances in fetal echocardiography provided early and accurate information about structural cardiac defects and the attendant physiological derangements [29]. Thus, a flurry of research began in the 1970s exploring the possibilities of intrauterine cardiac repair. Dr. Rudolph's group pioneered the research in fetal cardiovascular physiology by creating models of cardiac lesions in fetal lambs that included banding of the aorta to simulate stenosis and placing an inflated balloon in the left atrium to create an inflow limitation [30]. A combination of these resulted in a lesion similar to hypoplastic left heart syndrome (HLHS). Turley and associates performed a banding model of aortic and pulmonary stenosis and attempted intrauterine repair

[31]. A model of pulmonary stenosis and intrauterine repair with improvement in fetal hemodynamics was also reported [32]. These studies were performed without cardiopulmonary bypass. Not only was placing the fetus on cardiopulmonary bypass essential to further advance research in fetal cardiac surgery; but equally important was addressing the issues of the nature of the bypass circuit, the fetus' systemic reaction to extracorporeal circulation, the placental and fetal-maternal interactions during bypass, and fetal cardioplegia.

Cardiopulmonary Bypass and the Placenta

In one of the early attempts at establishing fetal extracorporeal circulation, Hawkins and associates placed fetal lambs on bypass at hypo- and normothermia and conducted the study at varying flow rates [33]. Placental dysfunction evidenced by a combined metabolic and respiratory acidosis was manifest on bypass and this remains a formidable barrier to success to date. The exact mechanism of post-bypass placental failure is yet to be elucidated, but has stimulated much research.

Understanding Placental Hemodynamics

To better comprehend the placental vasculature, Assad, Lee, and Hanley placed the isolated *in situ* lamb placenta on bypass and studied the placental vascular resistance and compliance to varying flow rates [34,35]. They quantified the large capacitance of the placental vessels and calculated the precise perfusion rates and pressures required to create, and hence, avoid increased placental vascular resistance. In their studies, a high flow rate was required to sustain placental function, and hence, as a corollary, lower flow induced dysfunction.

A fetal lamb model testing this hypothesis revealed high bypass flow rates (300–400 mL/kg/min) as being relatively better than low rates (100–125 mL/kg/min) in offsetting placental dysfunction, although it eventually occurred in all animals [36]. The normal fetal lamb cardiac output is approximately 400 mL/kg/min and in most studies the small cannula sizes in the circuit and slow gravity venous drainage limited high flow rates. A novel use of a vacuum-assisted venous drainage in fetal bypass has been studied with improvement in bypass flows but with a modest overall result [37].

The Fetal Stress Response

Bradley, Hanley and associates performed a seminal study which demonstrated altered organ perfusion during fetal bypass documenting significantly deranged flows to the placenta correlating with the observed increase in placental vascular resistance [38]. A role for the fetal stress response

with a humoral etiology for placental dysfunction was postulated and tested in further studies. Adding indomethacin to the bypass prime significantly abated the increase in placental vascular resistance suggesting the role for vasoactive prostaglandins [39,40]. In addition, when high spinal anesthesia was also administered to the fetal lamb, an abrogation of the fetal stress release of catecholamines was achieved, and in a study, resulted in acceptable placental perfusion during bypass [41]. With the previously mentioned techniques, fetal lambs have survived up to term in a chronic study [42]. Procedural complications of high spinal anesthesia and an adverse reaction to indomethacin in certain vascular beds preclude the application of this model to the human context. A recent study established a strong association of rising vasopressin (a known placental vasoconstrictor) levels with placental dysfunction during bypass thus underscoring the importance of the fetal stress response [43].

Role of the Endothelium in Placental Dysfunction

Champsaur and coworkers evaluated the various beneficial effects of pulsatile flow during fetal lamb bypass as opposed to the conventional continuous flow obtained with roller pumps. In their earliest study, they documented higher pump flows and placental flow with decreased systemic vascular resistance in the pulsatile pump group [44]. A role for shear stress in inducing the release of NO was postulated as the reason behind the beneficial effects of pulsatility in better preserving placental flow during bypass [45]. The group further demonstrated higher endothelin-1 levels and plasma renin concentration in fetuses on continuous flow bypass as opposed to the pulsatile flow in fetuses, suggesting a major role for endothelial dysfunction mediated by the renin-angiotensin system in placental insufficiency [46]. Reddy and associates provided further evidence for endothelial dysfunction as an etiological factor for placental insufficiency by documenting selective impairment of endothelial-dependent vasodilation post-bypass in the lamb fetus, linking it to a combination of decreased NO levels and elevated circulating endothelin-1 levels acting via vasoconstrictive endothelin-A receptors [47]. A recent study revisited this issue confirming altered placental NO pathway correlating with post-bypass placental dysfunction [48].

Understanding the Fetal Bypass Circuit

The conventional fetal bypass circuits had a volume of about 150 mL, which were primed with crystalloids and/or maternal blood. Large crystalloid volumes caused fetal hemodilution, and maternal blood in amounts sufficient to replace the fetal blood volume (especially in small fetuses), may impair fetal tissue and placental oxygenation [49]. It is well known that the extracorporeal circuit triggered a systemic inflammatory reaction by the activation of complement and eicosanoids in adults and children [50,51]. This was also shown by Reddy and associates in the fetal setting in a study that revealed significantly elevated IL-6 levels post-bypass [52]. Along these lines, attempts were made to suppress the inflammatory reaction by maternal and fetal glucocorticoid administration and by introducing in-line hemofiltration during fetal bypass with modest results [53].

Reddy and colleagues also tested a novel in-line axial flow pump, the Hemopump, that minimized extracorporeal surface area and used no priming volume. This system demonstrated significantly higher placental flow and reduced placental resistance during and after bypass compared to a conventional circuit [54]. This pump was also used on long-term studies of fetal survival to term post-bypass and proved the technical feasibility of such an undertaking [55]. In further studies comparing the Hemopump with the conventional roller pump, they found significantly increased neutrophil degranulation accompanying placental dysfunction in the fetuses on roller pumps further underscoring the necessity to minimize extracorporeal surface area during fetal bypass [56]. The pump, however, was overly simplistic and lacked a mechanism to deal with inadvertent air embolism. Lombardi and associates used a similar miniaturized circuit with a centrifugal pump for placing immature fetal sheep on bypass [57].

Fetal Myocardial Protection

The fetal myocardial ultrastructure differs substantially from that of the mature myocardium, spawning significant differences in fetal cardiac function, as discussed earlier in this chapter. The fetal cardiac myocyte also has a reduced sarcoplasmic reticular content, with depreciated calcium storage and transport capacity [58]. These factors necessitate tailoring the myocardial protection strategies to the fetal context.

To this end Malhotra and associates compared the efficacy of cardioplegia solutions with varying calcium concentrations in preserving myocardial function on an isolated fetal sheep heart preparation [59]. They documented improved post-ischemia recovery and better preservation of myocardial function with solutions that had a reduced calcium concentration as opposed to normocalcemic or hypercalcemic cardioplegia preparations. In another study with a similar preparation, the group documented no difference in post-arrest cardiac function between normothermic fibrillation and hypothermic normocalcemic cardioplegia [60]. The latter study was performed to circumvent the theoretical difficulty of maintaining fetal hypothermia *in utero.*

Miscellaneous Factors

Eghtesady and colleagues report on maternal hemodynamic responses to fetal cardiac bypass in sheep [61]. They noted significant fluctuation in uterine arterial flow independent of the overall maternal hemodynamic status but associated with specific events during fetal bypass correlating with worsening fetal blood gases. In a recent study, the group quantified the fluid shifts occurring in a fetal lamb model emphasizing the possible role for extensive postoperative fetal fluid resuscitation [62]. These studies add a new dimension to the parameters that contribute to success in fetal cardiac surgery.

Future Directions

Most of the research in fetal cardiac bypass has been performed on lamb fetuses, and it is commonly believed by most researchers in the field that the sheep uterus is actually resilient to any manipulation. Hence, the principles gleaned in these years of research have to be prudently applied to primate models before their ultimate translation to human benefit. The first such primate model was reported by Ikai and associates, demonstrating the technical feasibility of placing baboon fetuses less than 1000 g on bypass [63]. Less invasive procedures (i.e., balloon angioplasty of the stenosed aortic valve, left atrial decompression for a restrictive atrial septum) have been reported as options for fetal hypoplastic left heart syndrome [64,65]. However, the case for open fetal cardiac surgery exists, if not for early correction of select severe lesions, at least to halt the progression of severe flow impairments, providing an enhanced probability for a postnatal biventricular repair. A deeper understanding of the placental microcirculation, the maternal, and fetal response to surgical stress, methods for myocardial protection, and advances in fetal extracorporeal support enriched by a molecular perspective would facilitate its translation from the laboratory to a clinical reality.

References

1. Heymann MA. (2003) Physiology of the fetal and neonatal circulations. In: Mavroudis C, Backer CL, eds. *Pediatric Cardiac Surgery*, 3rd ed. Philadelphia PA: Mosby.
2. Rudolph AM, Heymann MA. (1967) The circulation of the fetus in utero. Methods for studying distribution of blood flow, cardiac output and organ blood flow. Circ Res 21, 163–184.
3. Anderson DF, Bissonnette JM, Faber JJ, *et al.* (1981) Central shunt flows and pressures in the mature fetal lamb. Am J Physiol 241, H60–H66.
4. Edelstone DI, Rudolph AM, Heymann MA. (1978) Liver and ductus venosus blood flows in fetal lambs in utero. Circ Res 42, 426–433.

5. Edelstone DI, Rudolph AM. (1979) Preferential streaming of ductus venosus blood to the brain and heart in fetal lambs. Am J Physiol 237, H724–H729.

6. Rudolph AM. (1985) Distribution and regulation of blood flow in the fetal and neonatal lamb. Circ Res 57, 811–821.

7. Reuss ML, Rudolph AM. (1980) Distribution and recirculation of umbilical and systemic venous blood flow in fetal lambs during hypoxia. J Dev Physiol 2, 71–84.

8. Lister G, Walter TK, Versmold HT, et al. (1979) Oxygen delivery in lambs: cardiovascular and hematologic development. Am J Physiol 237, H668–H675.

9. Iwamoto HS, Teitel D, Rudolph AM. (1987) Effects of birth-related events on blood flow distribution. Pediatr Res 22, 634–640.

10. Coceani F, Olley PM, Lock JE. (1980) Prostaglandins, ductus arteriosus, pulmonary circulation: current concepts and clinical potential. Eur J Clin Pharmacol 18, 75–81.

11. Heymann MA, Rudolph AM. (1975) Control of the ductus arteriosus. Physiol Rev 55, 62–78.

12. Levin DL, Rudolph AM, Heymann MA, et al. (1976) Morphological development of the pulmonary vascular bed in fetal lambs. Circulation 53, 144–151.

13. Rudolph AM, Yuan S. (1966) Response of the pulmonary vasculature to hypoxia and H+ ion concentration changes. J Clin Invest 45, 399–411.

14. Soifer SJ, Loitz RD, Roman C, et al. (1985) Leukotriene end organ antagonists increase pulmonary blood flow in fetal lambs. Am J Physiol 249, H570–H576.

15. Rudolph AM. (2003) Fetal circulation and cardiovascular adjustments after birth. In: Rudolph CD, Rudolph AM, Hostetter MK, et al., eds. Rudolph's Pediatrics, 21st ed. New York: McGraw-Hill, pp. 1749–1753.

16. Shaul PW. (1997) Ontogeny of nitric oxide in the pulmonary vasculature. Semin Perinatol 21, 381–392.

17. Leffler CW, Hessler JR, Green RS. (1984) The onset of breathing at birth stimulates pulmonary vascular prostacyclin synthesis. Pediatr Res 18, 938–942.

18. Cornfield DN, Reeve HL, Tolarova S, et al. (1996) Oxygen causes fetal pulmonary vasodilation through activation of a calcium-dependent potassium channel. Proc Natl Acad Sci U S A 93, 8089–8094.

19. Heymann MA. (1987) Postnatal regulation of the pulmonary circulation: a role for lipid mediators? Am Rev Respir Dis 136, 222–224.

20. Mahoney L. (2008) Development of myocardial structure and function. In: Allen HD, Driscoll DJ, Feltes TF, eds. Moss and Adam's Heart Disease in Infants, Children, and Adolescents, 7th ed. Philadelphia: Lippincott Williams & Wilkins, pp. 573–591.

21. Kirkpatrick SE, Pitlick PT, Naliboff J, et al. (1976) Frank–Starling relationship as an important determinant of fetal cardiac output. Am J Physiol 231, 495–500.

22. Thornburg KL, Morton MJ. (1983) Filling and arterial pressures as determinants of RV stroke volume in the sheep fetus. Am J Physiol 244, H656–H663.

23. Thornburg KL, Morton MJ. (1986) Filling and arterial pressures as determinants of left ventricular stroke volume in fetal lambs. Am J Physiol 251, H961–H968.

24. Hawkins J, Van Hare GF, Schmidt KG, et al. (1989) Effects of increasing afterload on left ventricular output in fetal lambs. Circ Res 65, 127–134.

25. Anderson PA, Glick KL, Manring A, et al. (1984) Developmental changes in cardiac contractility in fetal and postnatal sheep: in vitro and in vivo. Am J Physiol 247, H371–H379.

26. Breall JA, Rudolph AM, Heymann MA. (1984) Role of thyroid hormone in postnatal circulatory and metabolic adjustments. J Clin Invest 73, 1418–1424.

27. Harrison MR. (2004) The University of California at San Francisco Fetal Treatment Center: a personal perspective. Fetal Diagn Ther 19, 513–524.

28. Fichter MA, Dornseifer U, Henke J, et al. (2008) Fetal spina bifida repair – current trends and prospects of intrauterine neurosurgery. Fetal Diagn Ther 23, 271–286.

29. Silverman NH, Golbus MS. (1985) Echocardiographic techniques for assessing normal and abnormal fetal cardiac anatomy. J Am Coll Cardiol 5, 20S–29S.

30. Fishman NH, Hof RB, Rudolph AM, et al. (1978) Models of congenital heart disease in fetal lambs. Circulation 58, 354–364.

31. Turley K, Vlahakes GJ, Harrison MR, et al. (1982) Intrauterine cardiothoracic surgery: the fetal lamb model. Ann Thorac Surg 34, 422–426.

32. Bical O, Gallix P, Toussaint M, et al. (1987) Intrauterine creation and repair of pulmonary artery stenosis in the fetal lamb. Weight and ultrastructural changes of the ventricles. J Thorac Cardiovasc Surg 93, 761–766.

33. Hawkins JA, Paape KL, Adkins TP, et al. (1991) Extracorporeal circulation in the fetal lamb. Effects of hypothermia and perfusion rate. J Cardiovasc Surg (Torino) 32, 295–300.

34. Assad RS, Lee FY, Bergner K, et al. (1992) Extracorporeal circulation in the isolated in situ lamb placenta: hemodynamic characteristics. J Appl Physiol 72, 2176–2180.

35. Assad RS, Lee FY, Hanley FL. (2001) Placental compliance during fetal extracorporeal circulation. J Appl Physiol 90, 1882–1886.

36. Hawkins JA, Clark SM, Shaddy RE, et al. (1994) Fetal cardiac bypass: improved placental function with moderately high flow rates. Ann Thorac Surg 57, 293–296; discussion 296–297.

37. Lubbers WC, Baker RS, Sedgwick JA, et al. (2005) Vacuum-assisted venous drainage during fetal cardiopulmonary bypass. Asaio J 51, 644–648.

38. Bradley SM, Hanley FL, Duncan BW, et al. (1992) Fetal cardiac bypass alters regional blood flows, arterial blood gases, and hemodynamics in sheep. Am J Physiol 263, H919–H928.

39. Sabik JF, Assad RS, Hanley FL. (1992) Prostaglandin synthesis inhibition prevents placental dysfunction after fetal cardiac bypass. J Thorac Cardiovasc Surg 103, 733–741; discussion 741–742.

40. Sabik JF, Heinemann MK, Assad RS, et al. (1994) High-dose steroids prevent placental dysfunction after fetal cardiac bypass. J Thorac Cardiovasc Surg 107, 116–124; discussion 124–125.

41. Fenton KN, Heinemann MK, Hickey PR, et al. (1994) Inhibition of the fetal stress response improves cardiac

output and gas exchange after fetal cardiac bypass. J Thorac Cardiovasc Surg 107, 1416–1422.

42. Fenton KN, Zinn HE, Heinemann MK, *et al.* (1994) Long-term survivors of fetal cardiac bypass in lambs. J Thorac Cardiovasc Surg 107, 1423–1427.

43. Lam CT, Sharma S, Baker RS, *et al.* (2008) Fetal stress response to fetal cardiac surgery. Ann Thorac Surg 85, 1719–1727.

44. Champsaur G, Parisot P, Martinot S, *et al.* (1994) Pulsatility improves hemodynamics during fetal bypass. Experimental comparative study of pulsatile versus steady flow. Circulation 90, 1147–1150.

45. Champsaur G, Vedrinne C, Martinot S, *et al.* (1997) Flow-induced release of endothelium-derived relaxing factor during pulsatile bypass: experimental study in the fetal lamb. J Thorac Cardiovasc Surg 114, 738–744; discussion 744–745.

46. Vedrinne C, Tronc F, Martinot S, *et al.* (2000) Better preservation of endothelial function and decreased activation of the fetal renin–angiotensin pathway with the use of pulsatile flow during experimental fetal bypass. J Thorac Cardiovasc Surg 120, 770–777.

47. Reddy VM, McElhinney DB, Rajasinghe HA, *et al.* (1999) Role of the endothelium in placental dysfunction after fetal cardiac bypass. J Thorac Cardiovasc Surg 117, 343–351.

48. Lam C, Baker RS, McNamara J, *et al.* (2007) Role of nitric oxide pathway in placental dysfunction following fetal bypass. Ann Thorac Surg 84, 917–924; discussion 924–925.

49. Itskovitz J, Goetzman BW, Roman C, *et al.* (1984) Effects of fetal–maternal exchange transfusion on fetal oxygenation and blood flow distribution. Am J Physiol 247, H655–660.

50. Chenoweth DE, Cooper SW, Hugli TE, *et al.* (1981) Complement activation during cardiopulmonary bypass: evidence for generation of C3a and C5a anaphylatoxins. N Engl J Med 304, 497–503.

51. Greeley WJ, Bushman GA, Kong DL, *et al.* (1985) Effects of cardiopulmonary bypass on eicosanoid metabolism during pediatric cardiovascular surgery. J Thorac Cardiovasc Surg 95, 842–849.

52. Reddy VM, McElhinney DB, Rajasinghe HA, *et al.* (1998) Cytokine response to fetal cardiac bypass. J Matern Fetal Investig 8, 46–49.

53. Carotti A, Emma F, Picca S, *et al.* (2003) Inflammatory response to cardiac bypass in ewe fetuses: effects of steroid administration or continuous hemodiafiltration. J Thorac Cardiovasc Surg 126, 1839–1850.

54. Reddy VM, Liddicoat JR, Klein JR, *et al.* (1996) Fetal cardiac bypass using an in-line axial flow pump to minimize extracorporeal surface and avoid priming volume. Ann Thorac Surg 62, 393–400.

55. Reddy VM, Liddicoat JR, Klein JR, *et al.* (1996) Long-term outcome after fetal cardiac bypass: fetal survival to full term and organ abnormalities. J Thorac Cardiovasc Surg 111, 536–544.

56. Parry AJ, Petrossian E, McElhinney DB, *et al.* (2000) Neutrophil degranulation and complement activation during fetal cardiac bypass. Ann Thorac Surg 70, 582–589.

57. Lombardi J, Sedgwick J, Schenbeck J, *et al.* (2006) Cardiopulmonary bypass in the immature fetus through novel use of a mini-centrifugal pump. Perfusion 21, 185–191.

58. Friedman WF, Pool PE, Jacobowitz D, *et al.* (1968) Sympathetic innervation of the developing rabbit heart. Biochemical and histochemical comparisons of fetal, neonatal, and adult myocardium. Circ Res 23, 25–32.

59. Malhotra SP, Thelitz S, Riemer RK, *et al.* (2003) Fetal myocardial protection is markedly improved by reduced cardioplegic calcium content. Ann Thorac Surg 75, 1937–1941.

60. Malhotra SP, Thelitz S, Riemer RK, *et al.* (2003) Induced fibrillation is equally effective as crystalloid cardioplegia in the protection of fetal myocardial function. J Thorac Cardiovasc Surg 125, 1276–1282.

61. Eghtesady P, Sedgwick JA, Schenbeck JL, *et al.* (2006) Maternal–fetal interactions in fetal cardiac surgery. Ann Thorac Surg 81, 249–255; discussion 255–256.

62. Baker RS, Lam CT, Heeb EA, *et al.* (2009) Dynamic fluid shifts induced by fetal bypass. J Thorac Cardiovasc Surg 137, 714–722.

63. Ikai A, Riemer RK, Ramamoorthy C, *et al.* (2005) Preliminary results of fetal cardiac bypass in nonhuman primates. J Thorac Cardiovasc Surg 129, 175–181.

64. Tworetzky W, Marshall AC. (2004) Fetal interventions for cardiac defects. Pediatr Clin North Am 51, 1503–1513, vii.

65. Vida VL, Bacha EA, Larrazabal A, *et al.* (2007) Hypoplastic left heart syndrome with intact or highly restrictive atrial septum: surgical experience from a single center. Ann Thorac Surg 84, 581–585; discussion 586.

4

Preoperative Diagnostic Evaluation

Lourdes R. Prieto,[1,2] Marcy L. Schwartz,[1] Richard Sterba,[1] Janine Arruda,[1] and
Tamar J. Preminger[1]

[1]Cleveland Clinic Children's Hospital, Cleveland, OH, USA
[2]Cleveland Clinic Lerner College of Medicine of Case Western Reserve University, Cleveland, OH, USA

Introduction

Evaluation of the preoperative patient with congenital heart disease demands a thorough understanding of the anatomy and the physiology of each cardiac anomaly. Technical evolution of imaging modalities allows increasingly exact definition of anatomic detail, but such detail must be interpreted in the context of a clinical scenario that takes into account the patient's physiologic state. The art of interpreting and synthesizing information gathered from the history, physical examination, and adjunctive diagnostic tests remains the mainstay of clinical excellence. The exercise of this art is a crucial process that must be vigilantly undertaken for each patient in whom a cardiac surgical procedure is planned. This chapter will describe each of the components of a preoperative evaluation, from a detailed history to the delineation of complex anatomy and physiology by all the currently available tools.

History

A significant number of newborns are diagnosed with congenital heart disease before birth with the widespread use of fetal echocardiography [1]. The presence of a murmur, resting cyanosis, or exertional cyanosis account for most other referrals. Severe left-sided obstructive lesions can progress to shock as the presenting manifestation, with a history of rapid breathing, pallor, poor feeding, and lethargy typically preceding.

Infants with lesions that result in increased pulmonary blood flow begin to display symptoms after several days of life as the physiologic decrease in pulmonary resistance occurs. A history of rapid breathing, poor feeding, failure to thrive, and diaphoresis is typically elicited. Lack of symptoms in the first few months of life in an infant with unrestricted pulmonary blood flow should signal persistently elevated pulmonary resistance, and alert the clinician to the possibility of early onset pulmonary vascular disease. Duskiness around the lips or in the nail beds is usually observed in infants with cyanotic heart disease, and it is most pronounced with crying or feeding. Inconsolable crying and irritability in the first few weeks of life as pulmonary resistance decreases should raise the possibility of anomalous origin of the coronary artery from the pulmonary artery.

The onset of symptoms, such as exercise intolerance or chest pain, attributable to progression of obstructive lesions in a previously asymptomatic child, is almost always an indication to relieve the obstruction. Dizziness or syncope in a patient with congenital heart disease should call for a thorough investigation looking for the presence of atrial or ventricular arrhythmias. In the postsurgical patient, the presence of ventricular arrhythmias or refractory atrial arrhythmias may be an indication for surgical intervention, as in the patient with repaired tetralogy of Fallot (TOF) and chronic pulmonary regurgitation [2] or the Fontan patient who may benefit from Fontan revision and surgical cryo-ablation [3].

A family history of congenital or acquired heart disease should always be obtained [4]. Maternal illness or drug exposure during pregnancy, albeit infrequently, is associated with some forms of congenital heart disease [5]. Medications, previous surgical procedures, and any anes-

Pediatric Cardiac Surgery, Fourth Edition. Edited by Constantine Mavroudis and Carl L. Backer.
© 2013 Blackwell Publishing Ltd. Published 2013 by Blackwell Publishing Ltd.

thetic complications should be reviewed in the preoperative interview.

Physical Examination

The presence of dysmorphic features can be associated with some forms of congenital heart disease and should be noted. General visual inspection of a patient can reveal the effects of chronic congestive heart failure: failure to thrive affecting preferentially weight but also height. In infants respiratory effort is increased, displayed by excessive use of abdominal and thoracic muscles. Pallor is seen in patients with low cardiac output, as in severe left-sided obstruction or ventricular dysfunction. Clubbing is a sign of long-standing cyanosis, and peripheral edema is seen in older patients with decompensated right or biventricular failure.

Vital signs, including oxygen saturation, and growth measurements should be part of every preoperative cardiac examination. The precordium should be examined in sequence: inspection, palpation, percussion, and auscultation. Cardiac impulse displacement is palpated with chamber enlargement. A hyperdynamic precordium is observed in large left-to-right shunt lesions or severe valvar insufficiency, while a sternal "tap" is felt with right ventricular hypertension. A thrill is caused by high velocity flow across a pressure drop, as in a stenotic valve or restrictive ventricular septal defect (VSD).

Palpation of the pulses in all extremities can be diagnostic of coarctation of the aorta (CoA), with diminished or absent lower extremity pulses, and a significant delay between the radial and femoral pulsations. In CoA with anomalous origin of the right subclavian artery from the descending aorta, the left arm pulses are normal and the rest diminished. Bounding pulses are felt with aortic insufficiency or aortic run-off lesions, such as patent ductus arteriosus (PDA).

Careful auscultation cannot only differentiate one lesion from another, but also assess severity. Each part of the cardiac cycle should be evaluated, listening for abnormal heart sounds, clicks or murmurs. A widely split second heart sound, along with a systolic ejection murmur in the pulmonary area, is diagnostic of an atrial septal defect (ASD). A pansystolic, high frequency murmur in the left mid to lower sternal border is typical of a VSD. Lower frequency systolic ejection murmurs at the base, sometimes accompanied by a click, are heard with valvar stenosis, and the duration and peak of the murmur vary with severity. A high frequency, early diastolic murmur of aortic insufficiency can be differentiated from the lower frequency apical diastolic rumble of severe mitral insufficiency or a large left-to-right shunt. A continuous murmur is characteristic of a patent ductus, but can also be because of an aortopulmonary shunt in the postsurgical patient, or to aortopulmonary collateral vessels in patients with TOF and pulmonary atresia. Relatively soft to and fro murmurs are typical of repaired TOF patients with severe pulmonary insufficiency. To and fro murmurs can also be heard in newborns with truncus arteriosus and truncal valve insufficiency, or TOF with absent pulmonary valve.

Palpation and percussion of the abdomen reveal hepatomegaly, and sometimes also splenomegaly, in patients with congestive heart failure or right heart dysfunction. Ascites or total body anasarca can be seen in patients with failed Fontan physiology, particularly in the presence of protein-losing enteropathy. Upper body edema is characteristic of patients with elevated superior vena cava pressure, as in superior systemic baffle obstruction following atrial switch for transposition of the great arteries (TGA), or cavo-pulmonary artery anastomosis with elevated pulmonary artery pressure.

Chest Radiography

The chest radiograph can demonstrate various cardiac and extracardiac abnormalities that can be helpful in the anatomic and physiologic evaluation of the patient with congenital heart disease [6]. Abdominal situs, position of the aortic arch, size and shape of the cardiac silhouette and pulmonary vascularity are all important clues in the preliminary evaluation of a patient suspected of having a congenital cardiac anomaly. Pulmonary parenchymal and skeletal abnormalities visible on a chest radiograph are associated with some forms of congenital heart disease. The chest radiograph is also a useful tool in the follow-up of a patient with a left-to-right shunt lesion, as changes in pulmonary vascular resistance will be reflected in changes in the degree of pulmonary vascularity.

Abdominal Situs

The position of the cardiac apex, stomach bubble, and liver is normal in the majority of patients with congenital heart disease, but frequently abnormal in patients with heterotaxy syndromes, asplenia, and polysplenia. Asplenia patients uniformly have complex congenital cardiac lesions, and about 75% of polysplenia patients have complex heart disease. Isolated dextrocardia is often associated with congenital heart disease, while situs inversus totalis has a low incidence of cardiac anomalies. Malposition of the heart can also result from lung hypoplasia, as in patients with Scimitar syndrome.

Cardiac Silhouette

The cardiac silhouette is enlarged with volume loading lesions, such as left-to-right shunts or valvar insufficiency. A boot-shaped heart is typically seen in patients with TOF, and results from up-turning of the cardiac apex resulting from right ventricular hypertrophy, and absence or decrease in size of the pulmonary artery segment. A narrow mediastinum is characteristic of d-transposition of the great arteries (d-TGA) owing to the anterior-posterior orientation of the aorta and pulmonary artery. Severe Ebstein anomaly with severe tricuspid insufficiency gives the classic appearance of right atrial enlargement as a diffuse bulge of the right cardiac border and marked cardiomegaly. Total anomalous pulmonary venous return without obstruction is associated with the "snowman" or "figure of eight" sign attributable to enlargement of the right atrium and ventricle and a large left vertical vein.

Aortic Arch

The finding of a right-sided aortic arch should raise the suspicion of a conotruncal defect, such as TOF or truncus arteriosus, but can also be seen in the absence of congenital heart disease.

Lung Parenchyma

Pulmonary vascularity may be normal, increased, or decreased depending on the ratio of pulmonary to systemic blood flow. Lesions with a left-to-right shunt result in cardiomegaly and increased pulmonary vascular markings. Pulmonary edema with normal cardiac size is the classic finding in patients with obstructed total anomalous pulmonary venous return below the diaphragm (Figure 4.1). The lung fields have a ground-glass appearance as seen in newborns with respiratory distress syndrome. Pulmonary edema is also seen in patients with left heart failure.

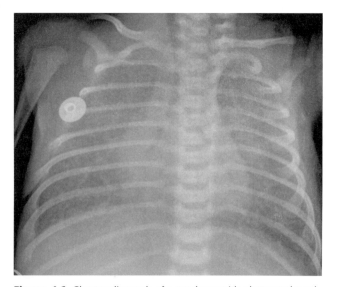

Figure 4.1 Chest radiograph of a newborn with obstructed total anomalous pulmonary venous return below the diaphragm. Note the presence of pulmonary edema with a ground-glass appearance, but normal cardiac silhouette.

Electrocardiography

The 12-lead EKG has always been considered an integral tool in evaluation of patients with suspected congenital heart disease. However, even in Helen Taussig's book *Congenital Malformations of the Heart*, she states that "although the electrocardiogram is a useful adjunct in the analysis of various malformations of the heart….it is of diagnostic value in only a few instances [7,8]." In the current era, the EKG is most helpful in: 1) identifying arrhythmias or potential conduction system disorders; 2) finding a previously unsuspected myocardial abnormality; or 3) its use as a reference point to identify changes that occur during the intracardiac repair or postoperative care.

Although few would argue that a cyanotic infant with left axis deviation would most likely have tricuspid atresia, none would omit further evaluation with echocardiography or some other imaging modality. Many structural congenital heart defects can have typical or classical findings on the EKG that may aid in making a correct diagnosis.

An EKG is the noninvasive tool to investigate the initiation and propagation of electrical wave fronts through cardiac tissue. Assuming the clinician knows the cardiac position, the P-wave axis and morphology can assess sinus node position and help assess its chronotropic adequacy. The lack of the expected normal P-wave axis can be seen in some congenital heart defects such as dextrocardia or sinus venosus ASDs. In some patients with sinus node bradycardia and dysfunction, a low atrial or junctional rhythm may be seen. These patients may need preoperative evaluation to assess the adequacy of sinus node function, so that if permanent pacing is needed and an epicardial pacing system required that system could be implanted at the reparative operation.

Patients with abnormal atrioventricular (AV) node conduction presenting either with second- or third-degree heart block will need careful preoperative evaluation. In our experience, patients with third-degree heart block and significant congenital heart disease will need a permanent pacemaker system. Patients with first- or second-degree heart block will benefit from either noninvasive monitoring with a 24-hour ambulatory monitor, stress test, or perhaps an invasive electrophysiologic study.

Patients whose electrocardiograms show a short PR interval and delta wave consistent with ventricular pre-excitation are not uncommonly seen when the underlying diagnosis is Ebstein anomaly of the tricuspid valve, or with AV and ventriculoarterial discordance. One should always remember that ventricular pre-excitation can be seen in almost any type of congenital heart disease patient. Many, perhaps most, will need ablation to avoid potentially hazardous arrhythmias such as supraventricular tachycardia or atrial fibrillation in the postoperative period [9]. It may be decided to perform an intraoperative ablation in selected cases.

EKG changes occur frequently after repair of congenital heart defects. The preoperative EKG provides a starting point from which we can evaluate new conduction system disturbances such as a change in AV conduction, or intra-ventricular conduction (i.e., right bundle branch block). Some new conduction system abnormalities seen postoperatively, such as second-degree heart block, may lead to further invasive investigation. Abnormalities in myocardial perfusion may be shown as new postoperative ischemia, perhaps in infants who have undergone an arterial switch to correct TGA.

Both 24-hour ambulatory monitoring (Holter) and stress testing are "EKG-based" studies that can be helpful to evaluate a patient preoperatively. When there is a question of sinus node adequacy, the clinician may use Holter tests to look for significant sinus bradycardia or long sinus pauses that can occur while the patient is in a restful state, and would be unaware of such occurrences. Likewise, a stress test would be able to assess the adequacy of the sinus node to increase appropriately when the patient is exercising.

We are including the topic of invasive electrophysiologic testing in this section, but we do not have the ability in this space to provide a complete review of its benefits [10]. Patients with ventricular pre-excitation or a pattern of Wolff-Parkinson-White on their EKG will benefit from at least an electrophysiologic evaluation to assess the conduction properties of the accessory connection. Many will need ablation. When easy access to the ablation site will be "lost" because of the type of surgical repair, ablation should be seriously considered if there is an inducible supraventricular arrhythmia, or if the accessory connection has the potential for rapid antegrade conduction. The electrophysiologic test also has value in patients returning for a repeat operation when there is a suspicion of intra-atrial re-entry tachycardia or ventricular arrhythmias. In this case the ablation can be performed either in the electrophysiologic laboratory or the electrophysiologic mapping study can help guide the surgeon to perform an intraoperative ablation.

Preoperative Echocardiography

Over the last few decades, advances in ultrasound technology have dramatically expanded the role of echocardiography. These advances not only include higher resolution two-dimensional imaging and M-mode, and improved Doppler interrogation (color, pulsed, high-frequency pulsed, and continuous wave), but also routine use of three-dimensional (3-D), pediatric transesophageal, and fetal echocardiography at many centers. Echocardiography is now the primary modality for diagnosing congenital heart disease. Multiple studies have validated the accuracy of echocardiography as the sole means of presurgical complete anatomic evaluation [11,12].

Full anatomic delineation should be undertaken before operative therapy, whenever possible, for appropriate surgical planning. We believe that incomplete or inaccurate information can be greatly minimized by performance of all echocardiograms for preoperative evaluation of congenital heart disease in a dedicated pediatric echocardiography laboratory. Preoperative evaluation is optimized by ensuring adequate patient cooperation with sedation and/or anesthesia when necessary. Care should be taken to acquire a thorough anatomic survey including pulmonary and systemic venous connections, aortic arch anatomy, and coronary artery origins and proximal courses to ensure discovery of any additional potentially surgical lesions or complicating anatomic abnormalities.

Three-dimensional echocardiography is helpful for better appreciation of complex cardiac geometry and spatial orientation of cardiac structures and lesions [13–15]. It provides unique imaging planes to allow clearer understanding of mechanisms of valvar disease and geometric configurations of septal defects. The reliability of quantitative assessment of ventricular function in complex single ventricular morphologies has been shown to be comparable to cardiac magnetic resonance when imaging windows are adequate [16].

Intraoperative transesophageal echocardiography (TEE) has become standard practice in centers performing repair of congenital heart disease. In one report, the majority of centers surveyed used intraoperative TEE in all open heart cases, while some centers employed TEE more selectively [17]. Intraoperative TEE is useful for obtaining further detail of anatomic lesions and for assessing immediate postoperative results. It is particularly valuable for high risk and complex congenital heart disease or cases involving valve repair, prompting return to cardiopulmonary bypass when residual lesions are found (Figure 4.2). It is also helpful for assessing ventricular function when separating from bypass [18]. Pediatric transesophageal 3-D probes are currently under development and live 3-D imaging holds promise for intraoperative assessment.

Atrial Septal Defects

Atrial septal defects are usually diagnosed in association with other congenital heart defects, but may be seen in isolation. The atrial septum should be examined as part of every complete initial echocardiogram since an ASD can be found incidentally or in the presence of a nonspecific flow murmur. A large atrial level left to right shunt leads to right ventricular volume overload. When right ventricular volume overload is seen on echocardiography, with right ventricular dilation and diastolic ventricular septal flattening (Figure 4.3A), full evaluation of the entire atrial septum and pulmonary venous connections with imaging and color Doppler is especially important.

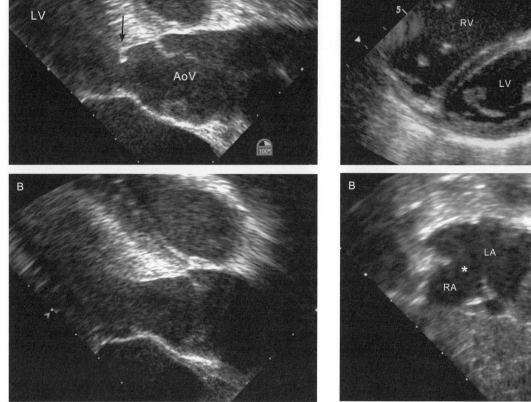

Figure 4.2 This intraoperative transesophageal echocardiogram shows **A,** a prominent subaortic membrane (arrow) before and **B,** following resection. (AoV, aortic valve; LV, left ventricle.)

When evaluating a patient with an ASD for surgery, it is important to understand the natural history of this lesion. Patent foramen ovale and ostium secundum ASDs <8 mm diagnosed in the first 3 months of life spontaneously close in 80% of cases [19], while spontaneous closure is rare after the age of 4 years [20]. The decision to close a secundum ASD by surgery versus catheter device closure depends on the size and anatomy of the defect. Surgery is generally the preferred option for repair of large defects when there are inadequate atrial rims for device closure. Sinus venosus defects and ostium primum ASDs do not close with time and require surgical repair when hemodynamically indicated.

In infants and young children, visualization of the atrial septum is best seen from subcostal views. Right sternal border view may be helpful in older patients. Secundum ASDs are seen in the central portion of the septum (Figure 4.3B). Sinus venosus defects are seen where there is an absence of the septum between the right upper pulmonary vein and the superior vena cava. This physiologically results in partial anomalous pulmonary venous return.

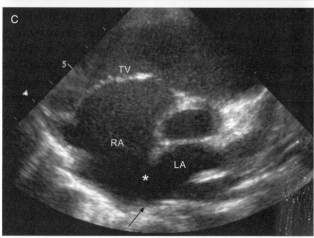

Figure 4.3 A, Parasternal short axis view shows right ventricular volume overload with right ventricular dilation and diastolic ventricular septal flattening. **B,** Subcostal long axis view shows a large secundum atrial septal defect (*).**C,** Parasternal short axis view shows an inferior-type sinus venosus defect (*). No posterior rim of septum is present. The arrow indicates the entrance of the right lower pulmonary vein. (LA, left atrium; LV, left ventricle; RA, right atrium; RV, right ventricle; SVC, superior vena cava.) See also Plate 4.1 (plate section opposite p. 594).

Additional or accessory right pulmonary veins may connect higher in the superior vena cava (SVC). This can often be demonstrated from right sternal border view. Sinus venosus defects are appreciated from subcostal and right sternal border views. As seen with color Doppler, flow is directed away from the orifice of the right upper pulmonary vein where it connects with the left atrium and across the defect into the proximal SVC (Plate 4.1A,B, see plate section opposite p. 594). Inferior type sinus venosus defects are found in the posterior-most portion of the atrial septum. Although the right lower pulmonary vein connection to the left atrium is normal, there is no atrial wall separating the right lower pulmonary vein flow from the right atrium. This is well seen from parasternal short view (Figure 4.3C). Primum ASDs are commonly seen with cleft mitral valve or as a component of common atrioventricular canal defect (CAVC). Primum ASDs are well imaged from apical four-chamber view.

Ventricular Septal Defects

Ventricular septal defects are described by their location (membranous, subpulmonary, conoventricular, or muscular) and their size. Like ASDs, VSDs may be seen in isolation, present with other lesions, or associated with complex congenital heart disease, such as TOF or CAVC. Echocardiographic evaluation is important for assessment of surgical necessity and associated heart defects. The natural history and associated cardiac lesions of each type of VSD may affect timing of surgical repair. Conoventricular malalignment VSDs occur as a result of anterior or posterior deviation of the conal septum and do not regress with time. Anterior malalignment VSDs may be seen alone or as part of TOF. Posterior malalignment VSDs are often seen in conjunction with aortic arch obstructions, such as CoA or interrupted aortic arch, particularly type B [21]. Some membranous VSDs may close spontaneously by growth of tricuspid valve tissue over the defect or be functionally restricted by aortic valve leaflet prolapsing into the defect. Membranous VSDs may occur with double-chambered right ventricular and/or subaortic membranes [22]. Subpulmonary (also called supracristal or intraconal) VSDs are found below the pulmonary valve and do not regress with time. These may be functionally restricted by unsupported aortic valve leaflet prolapsing into the defect. Early repair is usually recommended before aortic valve distortion and regurgitation occur or progress [23]. Many muscular defects become smaller or close with time. Large apical muscular defects can close functionally by hypertrophy of right ventricular muscle bundles or moderator band, such that the right ventricular infundibular apex remains open to the left ventricular apex and restricted from the right ventricular sinus (Figure 4.4A,B) [24].

Indications for surgery include congestive heart failure refractory to medical therapy or defects that do not appear to regress in the presence of pulmonary hypertension and/or left ventricular volume overload. Estimation of right ventricle pressure, using Doppler of the tricuspid regurgitation jet velocity, can be helpful in evaluating for pulmonary hypertension. In addition, systolic flattening of the ventricular septum may indicate elevated right ventricular pressure. Evidence of left ventricular volume overload owing to excessive left-to-right ventricular shunt includes measurement of left ventricular end-diastolic dimension and/or volume, which is compared with normative data relative to patient size (z-scores). Rarely, pulmonary artery banding may be preferable to allow time for potential closure or regression of some large defects or for defects that may be technically difficult for the surgeon to reach. Other indications for VSD repair include aortic valve prolapse resulting in aortic valve distortion with concomitant insufficiency.

VSDs should be imaged from all views to assess location, extent/size, and to find the optimal angle for Doppler interrogation of flow direction and transseptal gradient. Membranous, subpulmonary, and muscular VSDs (Figure 4.4C,D) are well seen from parasternal, subcostal, and apical views. Parasternal long and short axis views are particularly useful for assessing presence of aortic valve prolapse (Figure 4.4E,F). Subpulmonary VSDs should be distinguished from membranous VSDs since the surgical access is different. In parasternal short axis view, membranous VSDs are seen to the right of the aortic root just below the tricuspid valve (Figure 4.4F), while subpulmonary defects are anterior immediately below the pulmonary valve (Figure 4.4G).

Posterior malalignment defects are usually well defined from subcostal views, apical four-chamber view with anterior angulation to the left ventricular outflow tract (LVOT), and parasternal long axis view. Assessment of LVOT obstruction, which may be as surgically pertinent as the VSD, includes measurement of the LVOT diameter and Doppler estimation of the gradient. Anterior malalignment defects and inlet VSDs are discussed separately (TOF and CAVC sections, respectively).

Tetralogy of Fallot

Of the four basic components of TOF, anterior malalignment VSD, right ventricular volume outflow tract obstruction (RVOTO), overriding aortic valve, and right ventricular hypertrophy, the first two are surgically relevant. The VSD must be described with any posterior extension toward the inlet septum and/or the presence of additional VSDs. The severity and level of the RVOTO are variable. Usually subvalvar obstruction is found at the tip of the anteriorly deviated conal septum. There can be additional anterior muscle bundles at the os infundibulum (in the spectrum of double-chambered right ventricle). This is often well seen from subcostal and parasternal short axis views. The length and degree of conal septal thickening are well seen from parasternal views (Figure 4.5A,B). The pulmonary valve

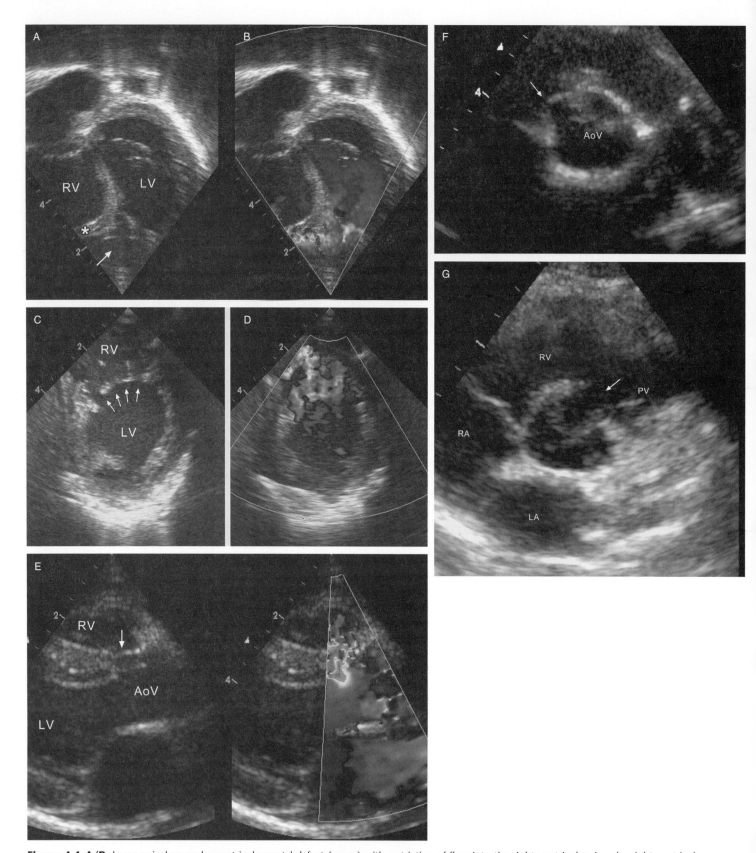

Figure 4.4 A/B, Large apical muscular ventricular septal defect (arrow) with restriction of flow into the right ventricular sinus by right ventricular moderator band/ muscle bundles (*). **C/D,** Parasternal short axis view shows multiple muscular ventricular septal defects (arrows). **E/F,** Parasternal long and short axis views of a membranous VSD with aortic leaflet prolapsing into the defect (arrow). **G,** Parasternal short axis view shows a subpulmonary/ supracristal VSD immediately below the pulmonary valve. (AoV, aortic valve; LA, left atrium; LV, left ventricle; PV, pulmonary valve; RA, right atrium; RV, right ventricle.)

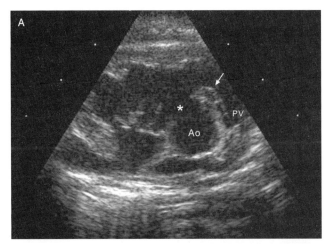

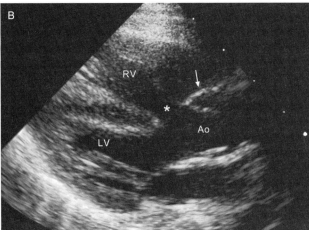

Figure 4.5 Parasternal short (**A**) and long (**B**) axis views of a patient with tetralogy of Fallot shows a thickened anteriorly deviated conal septum (arrow) with large conoventricular septal defect (*). (Ao, aorta; LV, left ventricle; PV, pulmonary valve; RV, right ventricle.)

annulus should be measured and leaflet motion assessed. If the pulmonary valve is adequate, a valve-sparing surgical technique may be possible [25]. An optimal angle for Doppler interrogation of the RVOT gradient can usually be obtained from subcostal short or parasternal views. In addition, the size and confluence of the branch pulmonary arteries need to be seen. In the most extreme form of TOF, or TOF with pulmonary atresia, branch pulmonary arteries may be diminutive with a majority of pulmonary blood flow provided by aortopulmonary collateral arteries. Angiography is often undertaken routinely to examine the extent and distribution of aortopulmonary collateral arteries; however, echocardiographic criteria of branch pulmonary artery size may be helpful in identifying patients who do not require additional diagnostic imaging [26].

The coronary anatomy in TOF should be identified. Echocardiography has been shown to reliably detect coronary abnormalities in TOF [27,28]. In TOF, there is often clockwise rotation of the aortic root such that the right coronary artery originates more leftward and the left coronary artery more posterior than in a normal heart. Of more importance, a significant conal branch or dual left anterior descending from the right coronary artery crossing anterior to the RVOT must be identified to prevent damage if an RVOT patch is required to relieve pulmonary outflow obstruction.

Associated lesions include ASD, PDA, and right aortic arch. TOF may be seen in combination with CAVC.

Truncus Arteriosus

In truncus arteriosus, one great artery is present giving rise to the coronary arteries, pulmonary arteries, and systemic arteries, usually with a conoventricular septal defect [29]. As with many forms of congenital heart disease, the diagnosis can be made by echocardiography from the initial subcostal sweep. A single common trunk with only one semilunar valve and outflow tract is seen (Figure 4.6A). The presence of a main pulmonary artery (type I) or position of the branch pulmonary arteries directly from the trunk (type 2 and 3) determines whether the pulmonary arteries can be excised from the trunk and anastomosed to the right ventricular–pulmonary artery conduit together or separately. Often the branch pulmonary arteries can be seen arising immediately adjacent to each other with minimal or no true main pulmonary artery (so called "type 1½"). The pulmonary artery arrangement from the trunk is usually seen best from parasternal short axis view (Figure 4.6B). The proximity of the main pulmonary artery or the branch pulmonary arteries to the left coronary ostium is well assessed from parasternal long axis view (Figure 4.6C).

The morphology and functional status of the truncal valve should be assessed for stenosis and/or insufficiency which could require valvuloplasty. The most common truncal valve morphologies are bicuspid, tricuspid, and quadricuspid (Figure 4.6D). It is important to evaluate the arch side and structure. Interruption of the aortic arch defines type 4 truncus arteriosus. As with all other diagnoses, other associated lesions such as ASD, additional VSDs, and PDA should be sought.

Common Atrioventricular Canal

Common atrioventricular canal, or atrioventricular septal defect, represents a spectrum of endocardial cushion defects with variations of the three main components. The complete CAVC includes a large primum ASD, large inlet VSD, and a common atrioventricular valve (AVV). A partial AVC includes presence of a primum ASD and cleft mitral valve only, while a transitional AVC includes also a functionally small VSD owing to AVV attachments to the crest of the ventricular septum restricting the ventricular shunt. Full preoperative evaluation, including definition of the size and extent of each component, can usually be accomplished with echocardiography alone [30].

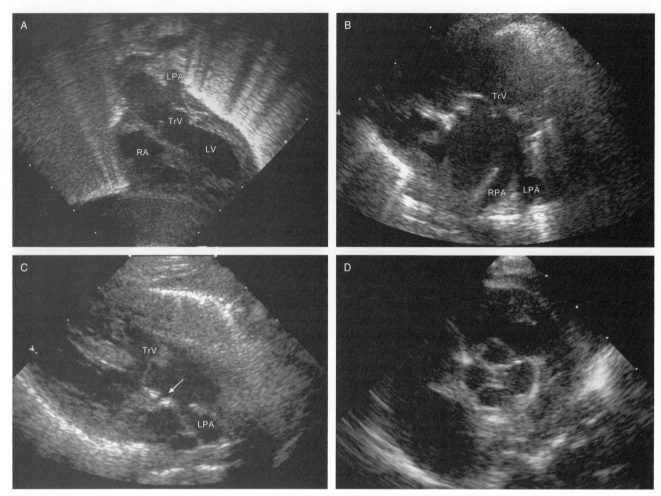

Figure 4.6 A, Subcostal long axis view of a patient with truncus arteriosus shows a single truncal outflow and the left pulmonary artery arising from it. **B,** Parasternal short axis view shows short segment main pulmonary artery arising from the left posterior side of the trunk. There is no evident conal septum seen. **C,** Parasternal long axis view shows the proximity of the left coronary artery ostium (arrow) to the left pulmonary artery takeoff. **D,** Parasternal short axis view shows a quadricuspid truncal valve. (LPA, left pulmonary arteryl; LV, left ventricle; RA, right atrium; RPA, right pulmonary artery; TrV, truncal valve.)

Assessment of ventricular balance of the CAVC defect is an essential part of the initial echocardiogram. CAVC can be well balanced with equal portions of the common AVV sitting over each ventricle or unbalanced with dominance of either right or left ventricle. This is well seen from a subcostal view slightly rotated counter-clockwise from short axis (in-between view) (Figure 4.7A). The number and spacing of the left ventricular papillary muscles should be seen. In cases of significant ventricular dominance (and concomitant hypoplasia of the other ventricle), a two-ventricle surgical approach may not be favorable.

Competency of the common AVV (or left and right AVVs in the case of partial AVC) is of obvious importance. Several views should be used to assess the degree and location of regurgitation jet(s) (Figure 4.7B). Apical four-chamber view also illustrates the apical displacement of the common AVV (Figure 4.7C). Separate AVV annuli are seen at the same level in partial AVC (normally the tricuspid valve is slightly apically offset from the mitral valve). AVV attachments, especially of the inferior bridging leaflet, to the crest of the ventricular septum should be noted. Straddling attachments may complicate the operation. Other hemodynamic preoperative considerations include LVOTO, from AVV attachments to the ventricular septum and/or a subaortic membrane, and pulmonary hypertension, both assessable by Doppler interrogation.

d-Transposition of the Great Arteries

In d-TGA, the aorta arises from the right ventricle and the pulmonary artery from the left ventricle. The pulmonary and systemic circulations in this disease are in parallel (rather than in series) and therefore completely inefficient. Survival depends on bidirectional shunting. An associated

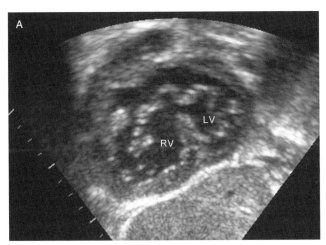

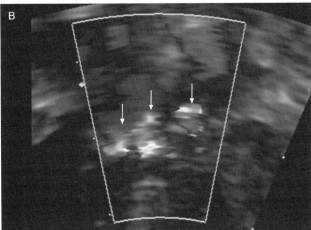

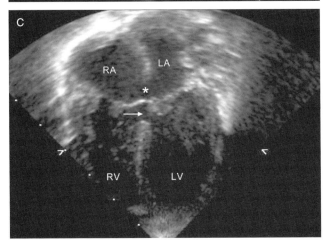

Figure 4.7 A, Subcostal "in-between" view shows a mild right ventricular dominant common atrioventricular canal defect. **B,** Color Doppler in apical four-chamber view shows common atrioventricular valve with multiple regurgitation jets (arrows). **C,** Apical four-chamber view shows a primum atrial septal defect (*) and an inlet VSD (arrow). (LA, left atrium; LV, left ventricle; RA, right atrium; RV, right ventricle.)

VSD, seen in 40–50% of cases, can be of any type or size. A VSD is not usually sufficient for adequate mixing of oxygenated pulmonary venous blood to the systemic circulation. Initially, maintenance of a PDA by administering prostaglandin E is necessary. Most often a balloon atrial septostomy (BAS) is performed for maximal atrial level mixing in order to allow for spontaneous ductal closure until definitive surgery is performed. BAS can now also be performed under echocardiographic guidance. Color and pulsed Doppler are used to ensure the ASD is unrestrictive following BAS.

From subcostal views, the pulmonary artery with its bifurcation is identified arising from the left ventricle. One can appreciate that the arteries arise parallel to each other instead of crossing outflow tracts. This parallel orientation of the great arteries is also well seen from parasternal long axis view (Figure 4.8A). Measurement of the diameters of the great arteries is possible from this view. The aorta is usually anterior and rightward of the PA, but the relationship can be side by side. This orientation is best seen from parasternal short axis view (Figure 4.8B).

Delineation of the coronary anatomy is of obvious preoperative importance before coronary transfer in the arterial switch operation. Echocardiography is now the primary mode of diagnosing coronary anatomy in d-TGA [31,32]. The most useful view for imaging the right and left coronary ostia and proximal segments is parasternal short axis. The bifurcation of the left coronary artery and proximal left anterior descending artery is often seen from leftward angled parasternal long axis [31]. Usually the coronary arteries arise from the right and left sinuses facing the pulmonary valve. The next most common variation is the left circumflex arising from the right coronary artery. Multiple other coronary patterns can be seen, including single coronary and inverted coronary anatomy. Uncommon coronary anatomy pattern, especially involving intramural segments passing between the arterial roots, had in the past been considered to be an operative risk factor for arterial switch operation [33], but more recently does not increase surgical risk at high volume centers [34]. Associated cardiac lesions should be identified. Complex d-TGA with VSD and aortic arch obstruction represents a higher operative risk group [35].

Coarctation of the Aorta

Coarctation of the aorta and other LVOT obstructions should be considered in any infant with clinical evidence of poor cardiac output. Patients beyond infancy with CoA may present with isolated systemic hypertension and decreased femoral pulses. Aortic arch imaging is best accomplished from suprasternal views. The classic finding is a posterior shelf or "3-sign" in the distal aortic arch (Figure 4.9A). In a high percentage of older patients, echocardiographic imaging of the CoA may not be ade-

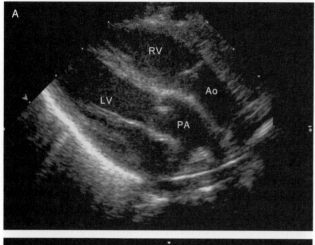

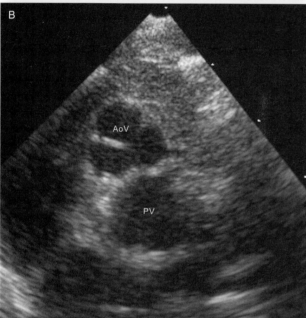

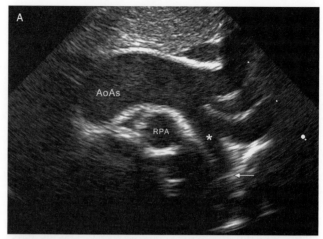

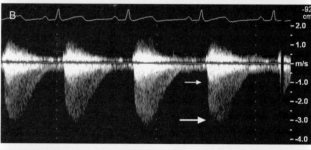

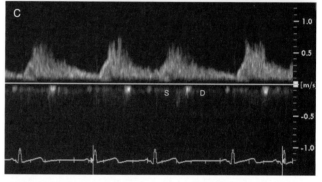

Figure 4.8 A, Parasternal long axis view in a patient with d-transposition of the great arteries shows the parallel orientation of the great arteries. **B,** Parasternal short axis view shows the anterior and rightward position of the aortic valve in relation to the pulmonary valve. Proximal coronary arteries are seen arising from the right and left facing sinuses. (Ao, aorta; AoV, aortic valve; LV, left ventricle; PA, pulmonary artery; PV, pulmonary valve; RV, right ventricle.)

Figure 4.9 A, Suprasternal view of the long axis of the aortic arch shows an elongated hypoplastic transverse arch (*) and discrete posterior shelf at the coarctation site (arrow). **B,** Continuous-wave Doppler in the distal aortic arch shows a double envelope pattern. The small arrow indicates the low velocity proximal envelope and the large arrow indicates the accelerated flow across the coarctation site. **C,** Abdominal aortic Doppler interrogation shows blunted systolic upstroke (S) and continuous antegrade flow through diastole (D). (AoAs, ascending aorta; RPA, right pulmonary artery.)

quate; however, when this region is well seen, results are as reliable as those by magnetic resonance imaging (MRI) [36].

Continuous-wave Doppler across the distal arch reveals a double-envelope pattern, a low proximal velocity signal, and an accelerated flow signal across the coarctation site (Figure 4.9B). The characteristic abdominal aortic Doppler pattern has a blunted systolic upstroke and continuous antegrade flow through diastole (Figure 4.9C). These classic findings may not be readily evident in the newborn with a large PDA. However, an elongated hypoplastic transverse

arch segment or other left-sided cardiac obstructive lesions should heighten suspicion and prompt repeated investigation of the aortic arch as the PDA closes.

Bicommissural aortic valve is associated with CoA in up to 85% of patients. Fusion of the right and left coronary leaflets is most common (70%), while aortic valve disease is more prevalent with fusion of the right and noncoronary leaflets [37].

Hypoplastic Left Heart Syndrome

Hypoplastic left heart syndrome (HLHS) represents a spectrum of congenital heart disease with hypoplastic obstructive left-sided cardiac lesions. It can range from aortic and mitral atresia with an underdeveloped left ventricle to milder forms of left heart obstruction [38,39]. Implied in this diagnosis is left-sided anatomy of insufficient size to sustain cardiac output and dependence on the right ventricle for pulmonary and systemic blood flow (Figure 4.10A,B).

The usual surgical approach to infants with HLHS is staged single ventricular palliation, culminating in the Fontan operation. Cardiac transplantation as a primary treatment for HLHS has lost favor because of donor availability and the long-term complications of chronic rejection. During staged palliation, blood is rerouted through the heart such that the right ventricle and tricuspid valve become the systemic ventricle and AVV, respectively, and the pulmonary artery becomes the neoaorta. Therefore, echocardiographic assessment must focus on the functional status of the pulmonary and tricuspid valves and the right ventricle. The sizes and gradients across the mitral and aortic valves are irrelevant because most of the pulmonary venous return is shunted to the right across the atrial septum. Echocardiographic evaluation of the atrial septum is important in the newborn with HLHS and includes imaging and color and pulsed Doppler interrogation of mean gradient. Mild restriction across the atrial septum is protective from pulmonary overcirculation. However, an intact atrial septum is associated with significant pulmonary hypertension and increased mortality [40]. Likewise, survival is dependent on right-to-left flow across the PDA for perfusion of the descending aorta and retrograde perfusion of the ascending aorta. Severe hypoplasia of the

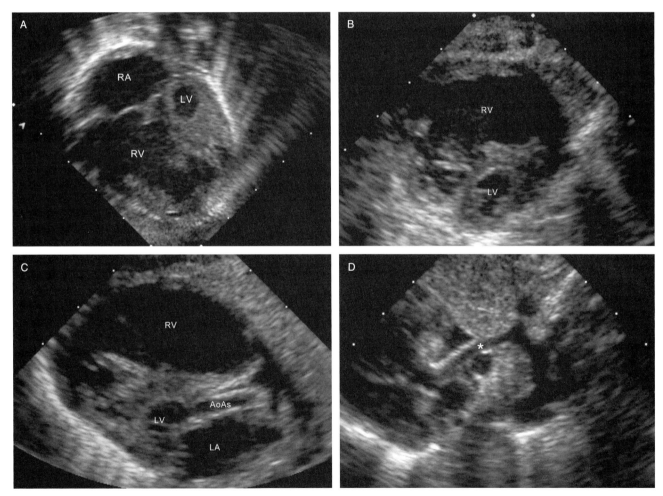

Figure 4.10 In a patient with hypoplastic left heart syndrome. **A,** Apical four-chamber view and **B,** parasternal short axis view show a hypoplastic left ventricle and large right ventricle. **C,** Parasternal long axis view shows a hypoplastic ascending aorta. **D,** Aortic arch image from suprasternal notch shows the size difference between the native ascending aorta (*) and the distal arch. (AoAs, ascending aorta; LA, left atrium; LV, left ventricle; RA, right atrium; RV, right ventricle.)

ascending aorta has been associated with higher stage I mortality risk, likely because of dependence of the coronary perfusion on retrograde flow through the attenuated length of ascending aorta [41]. Measurement of the ascending aortic diameter is usually optimal from parasternal long axis view (Figure 4.10C). Assessment of coronary artery anatomy should be part of all preoperative echocardiographic examinations for HLHS since the surgical approach for HLHS involves the ascending aorta, and coronary injury may result if an anomaly is not identified [42]. Anomalous pulmonary venous connection and drainage has been reported in approximately 6% of patients with HLHS who underwent stage I Norwood procedure. Subcostal and suprasternal imaging and color Doppler flow mapping have been found most helpful for delineating pulmonary venous anatomy [43]. Imaging aortic arch anatomy is of obvious importance before reconstruction and Blalock–Taussig shunt placement (Figure 4.10D).

Cardiac Magnetic Resonance Imaging

Cardiac magnetic resonance imaging (cMRI) has evolved into an excellent noninvasive imaging modality. It complements echocardiography in the diagnosis and preoperative and postoperative assessment of patients with a wide range of congenital heart disease. It is a tomographic technique where images are derived from protons, which are present in abundance in the human body.

Cardiac MRI provides detailed anatomic information with excellent spatial resolution, and it allows for 3-D reconstructions with no limitation of imaging plane. It can be particularly useful in children and adults with complex congenital heart disease, limited acoustic windows, limited vascular access, and in the assessment of extracardiac structures [44]. It has the additional advantage of not exposing patients to ionizing radiation or potentially nephrotoxic iodinated contrast agents, as in computerized tomography (CT) or heart catheterization. Limitations include the fact that it is not portable, it requires sedation in young children, the post-processing is long, and it is contraindicated in patients with certain metal implants. Although monitoring strategies for performing cMRI in patients with pacemakers and implantable cardiac defibrillators have been proposed, the presumed risks are not yet known sufficiently to justify routine cMRI in this group of patients [45].

Applications of Cardiac MRI

Cardiac MRI is considered the best imaging modality when anatomic and functional information are needed and its applications continue to expand. It includes the evaluation of patients with anomalies of the aorta, such as CoA, interrupted aortic arch, and vascular rings, systemic and pulmonary venous abnormalities, functional single ventricles, and arterial and venous collateral vessels. It can be reliably used to quantify shunts (Qp:Qs ratio), vessel-specific blood flow [46,47], regurgitant volumes, and ventricular volumes [48–50]. It has an advantage over echocardiography and CT in tissue characterization and the evaluation of myocardial and pericardial diseases [44].

The basics of MRI are beyond the scope of this chapter. However, some imaging features will be briefly addressed. Special software programs called pulse sequences are used to obtain the MR images. An individual pulse sequence is a combination of radiofrequency pulses, magnetic gradient field switches, and timed data acquisitions, all applied in a precise order. Before starting a study, protocols are predetermined and specific pulse sequences selected based on the question to be answered. Steady-state-free-precession (SSFP) and segmented K-Space gradient echo sequences are the two bright blood cine sequences widely used for cardiac anatomy. SSFP cines are highly reproducible in the measurement of ejection fraction, ventricular volumes and mass [49]. Cine MRI has become the gold standard for the measurements of these parameters [49].

Phase contrast velocity mapping or velocity encoded cine imaging (VENC) is used to measure blood flow velocities in arteries, veins, across cardiac valves, and to quantify cardiac shunts (Qp:Qs). It has been shown to correlate well with oximetry by catheterization [46,47]. VENC is the equivalent of Doppler in echocardiography. The measurement of the Qp:Qs ratio is often important. The ability to quantify Qp:Qs ratio by MRI can be very valuable in medical and surgical planning of selected patients with left-to-right shunt lesions such as ASDs and VSDs and partial anomalous pulmonary venous return.

Contrast-enhanced MR angiography (CE-MRA) is used to delineate arterial and venous structures [51]. Paramagnetic agents such as gadolinium (Gd) are given intravenously as Gd-diethylene-triamine pentaacetic acid (DTPA) and by altering the magnetic properties of tissues allow delineation of vascular structures with excellent spatial resolution [52]. Maximum intensity projection reconstructions allow 3-D visualization of arterial and venous structures. With the use of delayed contrast enhanced cMRI greater contrast can be achieved between normal and abnormal myocardium by a delay in the washout of contrast from the abnormal myocardium [52]. This technique has become the technique of choice to characterize tissues in myocardial and pericardial processes. Gadolinium DTPA has a safety profile superior to the iodinated contrast used in CT and heart catheterizations, but it has been linked to over 200 cases of nephrogenic systemic fibrosis in adults [53]. Thus far, this has not been reported in children.

Intracardiac Shunts

Atrial septal defects and VSDs are common, result in left-to-right shunts and the anatomy is well defined by echocardiography, the imaging modality of choice in young children. Cardiac MRI has been increasingly used in older patients and adults in whom echocardiographic images are often more limited. It can accurately provide anatomic and hemodynamic information by delineating the size, rims [54], direction of blood flow, number of defects in patients with ASD, and associated abnormalities most commonly seen in patients sinus venosus ASDs [55]. It is helpful in determining the suitability for percutaneous versus surgical closure of the defect. In patients with partial anomalous pulmonary venous return, cMRI is a valuable tool in precisely defining the anomalous drainage site and the relationship to adjacent structures, which are very important in the surgical approach to these patients. The Qp:Qs ratio can be determined by VENC by measuring flow in the ascending aorta and pulmonary artery. Gadolinium enhanced MRA is used to delineate the pulmonary and systemic venous anatomy (Figure 4.11).

Tetralogy of Fallot (TOF)

Tetralogy of Fallot is the most common form of cyanotic congenital heart disease and the anatomy can be well defined in infancy by echocardiography. Pulmonary artery branch stenosis is a common associated finding in these patients and SSFP cines and CE-MRA can be used to better delineate the pulmonary artery anatomy. It is important to identify the 5–6% of patients with a major coronary artery crossing the right ventricular outflow tract before surgical repair [28]. A free-breathing navigator gated and ECG triggered 3-D MRA sequence is a noninvasive alternative to define the proximal coronary anatomy [56] when echocardiography is suboptimal. Surgical repair during infancy, which includes a combination of infundibular resection, pulmonary valvotomy, and a transannular patch, often results in pulmonary insufficiency. Repaired TOF patients with a transannular patch often have significant pulmonary insufficiency. Chronic pulmonary insufficiency can lead to progressive right ventricular enlargement, right and left ventricular dysfunction, exercise intolerance, development of atrial and ventricular arrhythmia, and sudden death [57–60]. The long-term effects of restoring pulmonary valve competence by replacing the pulmonary valve are still unknown. Although improvement in ventricular dimensions and function and exercise capacity have been shown to directly correlate with the timing of pulmonary valve replacement (PVR) [61–65] recent data showed that PVR does not result in significant changes in QRS duration, incidence of ventricular tachycardia, or survival, supporting the need to continue to refine the appropriate timing

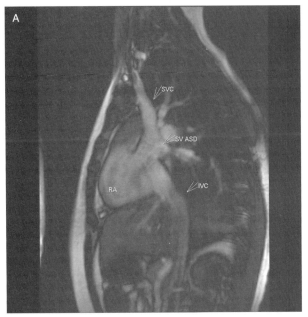

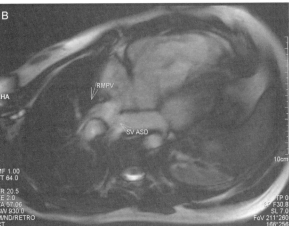

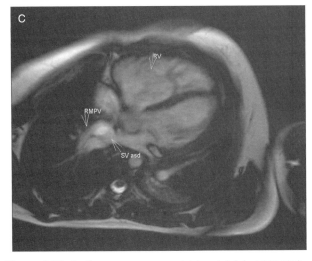

Figure 4.11 A, Cine – sinus venosus atrial septal defect (SV ASD). **B,** Partial anomalous venous return (PAPVR) of the right middle pulmonary vein (RMPV). **C,** Dilated right ventricle (RV). (IVC, inferior vena cava; RA, right atrium; SVC, superior vena cava.)

for PVR [66]. Cardiac MRI has become the gold standard in the evaluation of right ventricular volumes [61] and systolic function and the quantification of pulmonary regurgitation when trying to determine the appropriate timing for PVR. The use of Gd-delayed and enhanced MRI can detect areas of right ventricular and left ventricular fibrosis, which has been found to be a predictor of arrhythmia with potential prognostic implications in terms of morbidity and mortality in repaired TOF patients [67].

Pulmonary Blood Supply in Patients with Pulmonary Atresia

In patients with complex pulmonary valve stenosis or atresia, the pulmonary vascular bed may be supplied by stenotic, hypoplastic, or discontinuous pulmonary arteries. Pulmonary arteries may be absent and segments of the lung supplied by collateral vessels. Defining all sources of pulmonary blood flow, and the presence and distribution of aortopulmonary collateral vessels are very important for patient management [68]. Gadolinium-enhanced 3-D MRA has been shown to accurately define all sources of pulmonary blood flow with good agreement with X-ray angiography and it has been proposed as a noninvasive alternative to cardiac catheterization [69].

Congenital Vascular Abnormalities

Coarctation of the aorta consists of a discrete stenosis usually just distal to the left subclavian artery (Figure 4.12). It is frequently associated with hypoplasia of the aortic arch, anomalies of the brachiocephalic arteries, and mitral and aortic valve abnormalities. The diagnosis is usually made by echocardiography. However, in patients with complex aortic arch anomalies and suboptimal echocardiographic imaging, high resolution anatomic definition can be shown by cMRI using various MR techniques, including SSFP and CE-MRA. The severity of the obstruction can be determined by analyzing the descending aorta flow characteristics such as peak velocity and gradient, blood flow pattern, the presence of collateral vessels and their flow assessment by VENC imaging [70,71]. Cardiac MRI is also useful in the evaluation of left ventricular function, left ventricular mass, and associated lesions.

Vascular rings are rare malformations representing less than 2% of all forms of congenital heart disease. The presenting symptoms result from tracheoesophageal compression and include chronic cough, stridor, wheezing, recurrent pneumonia, cyanosis, and dysphagia. Double aortic arch with a dominant right aortic arch and hypoplasia or atresia of the left aortic arch is the most common form of vascular ring followed by a right aortic arch with anomalous origin of the left subclavian artery from a Kommerell's diverticulum (Figure 4.13). Although pulmonary artery sling and innominate artery compression are not complete anatomic rings, they are included in the

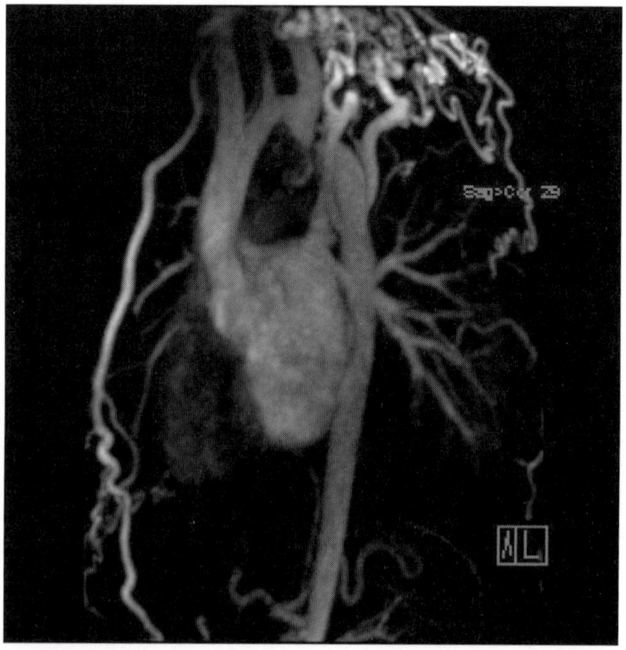

Figure 4.12 Severe coarctation of the aorta (COA) and a very prominent network of collateral arteries.

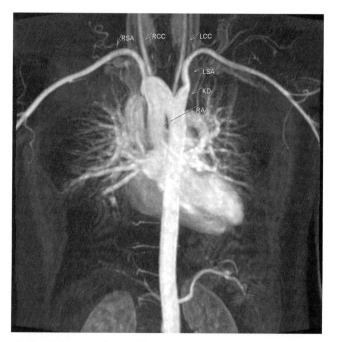

Figure 4.13 Three-dimensional reconstruction in a coronal view of a vascular ring (right aortic arch; RAA) with aberrant origin of the left subclavian artery (LSA) from a Kommerrel's diverticulum (KD). (LCC, left common carotid; RCC, right common carotid; RSA, right subclavian artery.)

description of these vascular abnormalities because of the similarities in presentation, diagnosis, and surgical management. Echocardiography is the initial choice of imaging and it is useful to exclude coexisting intracardiac abnormalities seen in up to 20% of cases [72]. However, cMRI is most useful in providing not only detailed anatomic information of the vascular anomaly but also the relationship to the airways and degree of obstruction, which along with the clinical symptoms will help determine the management choice in these patients. A combination of SSFP, conventional CE-MRA and the whole heart navigator gated 3-D MRA are used in the evaluation of vascular rings. The whole heart navigator gated 3-D MRA does not require the administration of contrast. It provides high spatial resolution images of the vascular anatomy with the ability to perform 3-D reconstructions with no limitation to the plane of imaging [71,73].

Single Ventricle

Patients with single ventricle physiology typically undergo a series of palliative operations. A heart catheterization is performed before the cavopulmonary anastomosis and before the Fontan completion as the standard of care to assess the anatomic and hemodynamic suitability for these procedures. It also provides the opportunity to perform catheter-based interventions such as embolization of arterial and venous collateral vessels and balloon angioplasty of CoA. In selected patients and after echocardiographic screening, cMRI has been shown to be safe, effective, and less costly in the preoperative evaluation of these patients, and it has been proposed as an alternative approach for single ventricle physiology patients [74] (Figure 4.14).

Multislice Computerized Tomography

The development of multidetector CT technology has allowed for extremely fast acquisition with very high spatial resolution. Computed tomography can be considered an alternative to cMRI for anatomic definition and 3-D reconstructions of cardiac and extracardiac structures. Limited functional information can be obtained [75]. Computed tomography has been more often considered an alternative in patients with pacemakers and also to conventional coronary angiography, as it provides valuable detailed anatomic information in patients with anomalous origin of the coronary arteries in terms of the site of origin and course in relationship to the surrounding structures. The short acquisition time and the obviation of the need for sedation are advantageous compared with cMRI, however, there are significant concerns with radiation exposure [76] and the use of potentially nephrotoxic iodinated contrast agents.

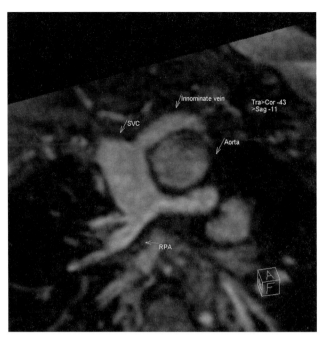

Figure 4.14 Whole heart three-dimensional MRA reconstruction of a widely patent cavopulmonary anastomosis (Glenn shunt) and pulmonary artery branches. (RPA, right pulmonary artery; SVC, superior vena cava.)

Cardiac Catheterization

The role of cardiac catheterization for congenital heart disease in infants, children, and adults has evolved tremendously over the past three decades. While initially utilized as a diagnostic tool to ensure precise definition of anatomy, its role has been transformed into a therapeutic tool and revolutionized the field, forming an even stronger association with the surgeon, be it via preoperative or postoperative intervention (ASD, VSD, aortopulmonary shunt, PDA, paravalvar leak closures, atrial septal angioplasty, valvar, branch pulmonary artery, conduit or aortic coarctation dilations, and/or stent implantations, as well as percutaneous valve implantation). These types of procedures will cause an even greater collaboration between surgeons and interventionalists in the future with the advent of more commonly performed hybrid procedures. Regardless of the type of catheterization, diagnostic or interventional, initial attainment of accurate hemodynamic data is essential.

A fundamental understanding of basic instrumentation and cardiovascular physiology is essential to properly assess hemodynamics in patients with congenital heart disease. While a complete assessment of techniques used to measure physiologic variables in congenital heart disease can be researched in more depth elsewhere, a basic overview to understand the methods follows.

Pressure Measurements

The pressure at the catheter tip is transmitted through the catheter and tubing to a transducer and then converted to an electrical signal, which is passed to a multichannel recorder and then by an optical beam to photographic paper. This entire system must meet certain requirements to accurately display intravascular pressures. Errors can occur in any of these components. These include accommodating for heart rate variations, damping, adjusting the height of the transducer and proper calibration, displaying pressures at different attenuations with display of the mean (time averaged pressure by electronic damping), and the type of catheter selected (stiff, large, and short catheters being ideal in this regard)

The normal right atrial pressure consists of the **a**, **c**, and **v** waves as well as the **x** and **y** descents. The **a** wave reflects atrial contraction at the end of diastole and is typically the prominent wave in the right atrium. The **c** wave represents displacement of the tricuspid valve toward the right atrium in early systole which is noted as the small note on the downslope of the **a** wave. The **v** wave peaks during late systole and reflects the continued atrial filling against the closed tricuspid valve. The **x** descent occurs owing to a decrease in pericardial pressure and movement of the tricuspid valve away from the right atrium during ventricular contraction and is the fall in pressure following the **a** and **c** waves. The **y** descent reflects the decrease in pressure after the **v** wave as the tricuspid valve opens at the start of diastole. Flow in the venae cavae is greatest during the **x** and **y** descents and have similar tracings to the right atrium except in cases of potential obstruction, which can be seen in patients who have undergone a Mustard or Senning procedure or repair of anomalous pulmonary venous connections involving the venae cavae. The normal mean right atrial pressure is 3 mmHg, with typical measurements made at the end of expiration when it is highest [77–79]. The **a** wave is typically larger but may be increased in cases of decreased compliance as a result of right ventricular dysfunction, tricuspid stenosis or atresia, particularly with a restrictive atrial communication. The **v** wave is higher in cases of tricuspid regurgitation.

The left atrial pressures have similar **a**, **c**, **v** waves and **x**, **y** descents but here the **v** wave is dominant. Normal mean left atrial pressure is 8 mmHg [77–79]. Left atrial hypertension occurs in patients with decreased compliance as with left ventricular dysfunction or with obstructive lesions such as mitral stenosis, especially with a restrictive ASD. The **v** wave is increased in mitral regurgitation as well as with large left-to-right shunts, and decreased in total anomalous venous return.

The pulmonary artery wedge pressure reflects the left atrial pressure and is obtained by advancing an end hole catheter with or without a balloon to occlude a pulmonary artery branch. This is often recorded simultaneously with the left ventricular end-diastolic pressure with which there should be no gradient. The capillaries and pulmonary veins cause a delay and relatively damped pressure as compared with direct measurement of the left atrial pressure, but the pulmonary artery wedge pressure is accurate below a mean of 20 mmHg. Normal values in children are a mean of 8 mmHg [77–79].

Pulmonary vein wedge pressure is useful in estimating the pulmonary artery pressure in cases when the pulmonary arteries cannot be entered. The technique is similar to that for the pulmonary artery wedge pressure and is dependent upon careful attention to proper wedging technique as well as transducer calibration. This measurement accurately estimates a pulmonary artery mean pressure of 20 mmHg or less when the mean is less than or equal to 15 mmHg but loses its predictability when elevated further [80].

Right ventricular pressure tracings are characterized by a rapid upstroke during isovolumic contraction, a systolic plateau, and a fall to near zero during isovolumic relaxation. The pressure varies with respiration as the right atrial pressure. The normal right ventricular systolic pressure is less than 30 mmHg and end-diastolic pressure 5 mmHg [77–79]. Right ventricular hypertension is seen in cases of outflow obstruction (valvar or subvalvar pulmonary stenosis, pulmonary artery stenoses, after placement of pulmonary artery bands, and in a double-chambered right ventricle), pulmonary hypertension (primary and secondary), as well as with nonrestrictive VSDs.

The left ventricular pressure wave form is similar to that of the right ventricle but has a more rapid upstroke and flatter systolic plateau. This pressure should be equal to the aortic systolic pressure. The end-diastolic pressure is typically less than 12 mmHg and is slightly higher than the left atrial mean pressure. Left ventricular hypertension associated with congenital heart disease is seen most commonly in valvar and/or subvalvar aortic stenosis or CoA.

The systolic pressure in the pulmonary artery should equal that of the right ventricle and also is subject to respiratory variation. The diastolic pressure is higher because of closure of the pulmonary valve. The normal mean pulmonary artery pressure is less than 20 mmHg.

The aortic pressure varies relative to where it is measured, with the systolic pressure increasing and diastolic pressure decreasing as the catheter is moved more distally toward the descending aorta or iliac arteries because of pulse amplification. In addition to obstructive lesions those with run-off, such as aortic regurgitation, PDA, systemic-to-pulmonary arterial shunts and/or collaterals, as well as arteriovenous malformations, cause an increased pulse pressure.

Pressure gradients are measured to quantify the degree of stenosis across cardiovascular structures and are expressed as a peak systolic ejection gradient, an instantaneous gradient, or a mean gradient. However, as this is dependent on both the cross-sectional area and flow, if there is minimal flow (and/or a low cardiac output) across a severely stenotic area a falsely low gradient may be obtained. The accuracy of gradient data is also compromised when serial obstructions are present.

Saturations and Shunt Measurements

Shunting can occur because of both extracardiac and intracardiac lesions which allow mixing between the pulmonary and systemic circulations. Shunts may be left-to-right, right-to-left or bidirectional. While shunts can be localized by several means including angiography, echocardiography, and/or other indicators, in the catheterization laboratory shunting is quantified by the oxygen content (total amount of oxygen in the blood both as oxyhemoglobin and that dissolved in the plasma) and the saturation of the blood in the various sites. When this is combined with oxygen consumption one can calculate systemic and pulmonary blood flow.

O_2 content = (Hgb or hemoglobin concentration) (1.36) (fractional saturation of blood). The contribution of dissolved O_2 is small and ignored except when 100% oxygen is being administered.

$$\text{Pulmonary blood flow (Qp)} = VO_2 (mL/min)$$

$$= \frac{(\text{oxygen consumption})}{PV\,O_2\,con - PA\,O_2\,con}$$

$$\text{Systemic blood flow (Qs)} = \frac{VO_2 (mL/min)}{SAO_2\,con - MVO_2\,con}$$

$$Qp:Qs = \frac{SAO_2 - MVO_2}{PVO_2\% - PAO_2\%}$$

$$\text{Oxygen consumption} = \frac{PVO_2 - PAO_2}{SAO_2\% - MVO_2\%}$$

The variability in oxygen content is highest in the right atrium (67–87%) owing to variability from inferior vena caval, superior vena caval, and coronary sinus blood flow; therefore in the absence of shunting the pulmonary arterial saturation represents the mixed venous saturation. If a left-to-right shunt is present the mixed venous saturation is obtained from the site proximal to the shunt. As there is normal variation in saturations, an increase of more than 7%, 4%, and 4% is needed to detect a true left-to-right shunt between the superior vena cava and right atrium, right atrium and right ventricle, right ventricle, and pulmonary artery respectively [81]. With a right-to-left shunt pulmonary blood flow is calculated using the oxygen saturation measured proximal to the site of the shunt.

A right-to-left shunt is suspected if the aortic saturation is less than 95% or if there is a 2% or greater stepdown between the left atrial and aortic blood. More commonly, however, left-sided desaturation is secondary to pulmonary venous desaturation from a pulmonary cause and can be diagnosed and corrected with supplemental oxygen.

Cardiac Output Measurements

Cardiac output measures the amount of blood pumped by the heart into the systemic circulation measured in liters per minute, or more commonly in children is expressed as cardiac index where it is corrected for their body surface area ($L/min/m^2$) allowing for patients of different sizes to be compared (see formulas above). In the absence of left-to-right or right-to-left shunts, the pulmonary and systemic flows are equal. In the presence of shunts the pulmonary, systemic and effective blood flows are unequal and therefore their specific measurements important.

Left-to-right shunts can be quantified using the equation:

$$Q\,l - r = Qp - Qs$$

Right-to-left shunts are calculated using the equation:

$$Q\,r - l = Qs - Qp$$

The most common method for measuring cardiac output is via the indicator dilution method, using thermodilution technique where the indicator is cold saline, or the Fick method where the indicator is oxygen; the use of indocyanine green dye is not in current use. With thermodilution, the change in temperature from the iced saline injected into the port in the right atrium to its warming in the pulmonary artery is proportional to the blood flow; this is least accurate when the cardiac output is low. Thermodilution technique is useful when repeat cardiac outputs need to be performed during interventional procedures such as pre- and postdilation of aortic stenosis. The results are less reliable in patients with Fontan operations as a result of lack of thorough mixing of the iced saline bolus as well as in patients with significant tricuspid or pulmonary regurgitation. For the Fick method oxygen consumption can be measured directly or estimated from normograms based on gender, age, and heart rate.

Resistance and Valve Area Measurements

The calculation of vascular resistance, particularly the pulmonary vascular resistance, can be crucial to determining suitability for surgical palliation or repair. Vascular resistance is quantified by the mean pressure change relative to the flow across the vascular circuit with the pulmonary and vascular resistances calculated according to the following formulae:

Pulmonary vascular resistance (PVR)

$$= \frac{\text{meanPA}_P - \text{meanLA}_P \ (\text{PCWp})}{\text{Qp}}$$

Systemic vascular resistance (SVR)

$$= \frac{\text{mean Aop} - \text{mean SVC/RAp}}{\text{Qs}}$$

In children this is most often indexed for body surface area expressed as Woods units (mmHg/L/min/m²).

When the pulmonary vascular resistance is over $4\,\text{WU/m}^2$ pulmonary vasodilators are utilized including 100% oxygen and nitric oxide and repeat hemodynamics obtained in order to determine the reactivity of the pulmonary vascular bed; this is particularly important in cases determining suitability for cardiac transplantation versus need for heart–lung transplantation.

In cases where there is a significant discrepancy in the pulmonary blood flow the resistance in each lung bed should be calculated in addition to the total lung resistance.

Valve areas are calculated using a combination of two basic equations defined by Gorlin and Gorlin in 1951 [82]:

Valve area

$$= \frac{\text{F (flow rate)}}{\text{C(constant)}(44.3)\,\text{h(square root of pressure gradient)}}$$

These equations relate the valve area directly to the flow across the valve and inversely to the square root of the pressure drop. The flow is measured while the valve is open either during diastole for the AVVs or during systole for the semilunar valves with the final formula accounting for this by including a diastolic filling time (DFP sec/beat) or the systolic ejection period (SEP, sec/beat) as well as the heart rate (beats/sec):

$$A\left(\text{area in cm}^2\right) = \frac{\text{CO cm}^3/\text{min}/(\text{DFP or SEP})\text{HR}}{44.3\,\text{C}(0.85 \text{ for MV or 1 for Aov, PV, TV})}$$
$$\text{square root of mean gradient}$$

Calculating valve areas takes into account the gradient relative to the flow. A severe stenosis is present with a valve area of less than $0.5\,\text{cm}^2/\text{m}^2$ for a semilunar valve and less than $1\,\text{cm}^2/\text{m}^2$ for an AVV. In practice, however, the severity of valvar stenoses in young patients is defined by the transvalvar gradients, assuming that the majority of children have relatively normal cardiac outputs.

Angiography

The role of angiography in the anatomic evaluation of many congenital cardiac lesions has been largely supplanted by other less invasive imaging modalities.

Intracardiac anatomy can be discerned in detail by echocardiography and also by cMRI and CT, while extracardiac structures can be well imaged by either MRI or CT [83,84]. Volumetric analysis, such as ventricular volumes and ejection fraction, can be obtained from MRI with high accuracy and reproducibility [85]. Studies have shown a good correlation between MRI and conventional angiography when evaluating larger aortopulmonary collaterals in patients with complex pulmonary anatomy such as TOF with pulmonary atresia [69]. However, because of limitations in spatial resolution in young infants and the inability to accurately define blood supply to lung segments in the presence of small collateral vessels, angiography remains the best imaging modality in this group of lesions, as well as in small patients with stenotic pulmonary veins and coronary artery abnormalities [86].

Another practical consideration in the choice of angiography over other imaging modalities is the need to obtain hemodynamic information or the potential need to perform an intervention, as in the pre-Fontan evaluation of patients with single ventricle complexes. Angiography of the pulmonary arteries is performed in these patients at the time of catheterization, and the site and angles chosen depend on the underlying anatomy and prior surgical procedures. The majority of these patients have had a cavopulmonary anastomosis, and a superior vena cava angiogram in anteroposterior and lateral projections will demonstrate the pulmonary artery anatomy. Visualization of the pulmonary veins is also important in these patients and is typically accomplished by following the contrast as it returns from the pulmonary arteries back to the heart, also known as levophase. If pulmonary vein stenosis is suspected, either a selective injection of contrast in the pulmonary vein, or a pulmonary artery wedge injection of contrast layered with saline will show the pulmonary vein anatomy in detail. To complete the angiographic evaluation of the pre-Fontan patient aortography should be performed to exclude the presence of significant aortopulmonary collaterals that may be occluded in the catheterization laboratory.

Definition of the pulmonary arterial anatomy is important in many patients with congenital heart disease. It is frequently possible to see them well by echocardiography in newborns and infants, but when peripheral stenosis must be excluded, angiography is the procedure of choice. Cranial angulation displays the bifurcation of the right and left branches as they course posteriorly towards the lungs, with the straight lateral projection as the orthogonal view.

Patients with TOF, pulmonary atresia, and major aortopulmonary collaterals need exact definition of the native pulmonary artery and collateral anatomy in order for the surgeon to plan reconstruction of a pulmonary arterial tree [87]. Scouting angiograms should be performed in the

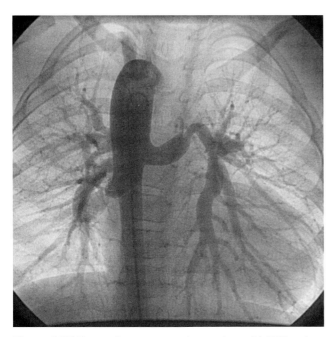

Figure 4.15 Descending aortogram in a patient with TOF and pulmonary atresia showing multiple aortopulmonary collateral vessels perfusing both lungs. The patient had tiny native pulmonary arteries that were opacified with selective injections in each collateral.

ascending and descending aorta, either with an angiographic catheter advanced from a venous approach into the right ventricle and aorta, or an arterial catheter advanced from the femoral artery (Figure 4.15). All the collaterals should be identified from these injections, including any that may arise from less common structures, such as the subclavian arteries or rarely even the coronary arteries. Often, the native pulmonary arteries are also visualized as they fill from one or several of the collaterals, ending blindly as a beak in the direction of the atretic pulmonary valve. Each collateral should then be injected selectively to delineate its origin, course and lung segment(s) perfused, and to evaluate the connections, if present, to the native pulmonary arteries.

In a minority of patients with TOF and pulmonary atresia the native pulmonaries are absent. To be sure, it is sometimes necessary to perform a pulmonary vein wedge injection of contrast layered with saline, which would fill the native pulmonary, if present, in a retrograde fashion.

Coronary Arteries

Patients with pulmonary atresia and intact ventricular septum require exact definition of the coronary artery anatomy to guide surgical management [88]. Echocardiography can be reassuring when the coronary arteries are

seen arising normally from the aorta and there are not extensive sinusoids, but when in doubt aortography or selective coronary angiography must be performed. Right ventricular dependent coronary circulation, defined as right ventricle to coronary artery fistulas plus proximal coronary artery stenoses, is usually present in patients with smaller right ventricles and tricuspid valves, and is an indication for single ventricle palliation. Atresia of the proximal coronary arteries is an indication for cardiac transplantation [89]. Extensive sinusoids without right ventricular dependent coronary circulation calls for a conservative approach to RV decompression in newborns to avoid coronary steal into a low pressure right ventricle.

Preoperative evaluation of the coronary artery anatomy is important in patients with d-TGA in whom an arterial switch is planned. Echocardiography can almost always provide this information, and angiography is not typically performed. In the postoperative arterial switch patient, however, angiography may be necessary if there is any question about coronary insufficiency [90]. An aortic root angiogram should demonstrate the origin and distribution of the translocated coronary arteries. In the most common type D anatomy, both arise anteriorly from the neoaorta following translocation, with the left coronary artery leftward and typically more superior than the right. In these cases, it is preferable to then inject each coronary artery selectively in orthogonal views, to exclude any origin stenosis or kink in the vessel that may have resulted at the time of translocation.

Examination of the coronary arteries is also important in patients with TOF before undergoing complete repair, specifically ascertaining whether the left anterior descending branch originates normally from the left main coronary artery, or from the right coronary artery as in about 5% of patients. In the latter case it would course across the right ventricular outflow tract, and extreme care must be taken by the surgeon to avoid injury. In some cases there is a "dual" left anterior descending system, with a branch arising normally and the other from the right coronary artery, which must also be preserved at the time of surgery. These details can usually be ascertained by echocardiography, but, in TOF patients undergoing preoperative catheterization for other reasons, selective coronary angiography should be considered.

Coronary angiography is mandatory in patients with a history of Kawasaki disease and clinical evidence of myocardial ischemia, and in Kawasaki patients with no symptoms but giant aneurysms by echocardiography (Figure 4.16) [91]. These patients have a significant incidence of coronary artery stenosis that may require bypass grafting [92]. Patients with anomalous origin of the left coronary artery from the pulmonary artery are often diagnosed by echocardiography, but may require angiographic confirmation.

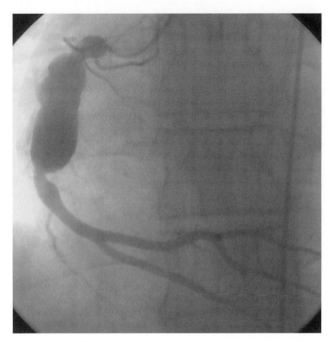

Figure 4.16 Giant right coronary aneurysm in a patient several years after Kawasaki disease.

References

1. McBrien A, Sands A, Craig B, *et al.* (2009) Major congenital heart disease: antenatal detection, patient characteristics and outcomes. J Matern Fetal Neonatal Med 22, 101–105.

2. Therrien J, Siu SC, Harris L, *et al.* (2001) Impact of pulmonary valve replacement on arrhythmia propensity late after repair of tetralogy of Fallot. Circulation 103, 2489–2494.

3. Mavroudis C, Deal BJ, Backer CL. (2002) The beneficial effects of total cavopulmonary conversion and arrhythmia surgery for the failed Fontan. Semin Thorac Cardiovasc Surg Pediatr Card Surg Annu 5, 12–24.

4. Pierpont ME, Basson CT, Benson DW Jr, *et al.* (2007) Genetic basis for congenital heart defects: current knowledge: a scientific statement from the American Heart Association Congenital Cardiac Defects Committee, Council on Cardiovascular Disease in the Young: endorsed by the American Academy of Pediatrics. Circulation 115, 3015–3038.

5. Jenkins KJ, Correa A, Feinstein JA, *et al.* (2007) Noninherited risk factors and congenital cardiovascular defects: current knowledge: a scientific statement from the American Heart Association Council on Cardiovascular Disease in the Young: endorsed by the American Academy of Pediatrics. Circulation 115, 2995–3014.

6. Schweigmann G, Gassner I, Maurer K. (2006) Imaging the neonatal heart – essentials for the radiologist. Eur J Radiol 60, 159–170.

7. Schnitker MA. (1940) *The Electrocardiogram in Congenital Cardiac Disease.* Cambridge, MA: Harvard University Press.

8. Taussig HB. (1947) Methods of diagnosis. In: *Congenital Malformations of the Heart.* London: Oxford University Press, pp. 18–52.

9. Van Hare GF. (1997) Indications for radiofrequency ablation in the pediatric population. J Cardiovasc Electrophysiol 8, 952–962.

10. Walsh EP. (2007) Interventional electrophysiology in patients with congenital heart disease. Circulation 115, 3224–3234.

11. Lopes LM, Damiano AP, Moreira GN, *et al.* (2005) [The role of echocardiography as an isolated method for indicating surgery in patients with congenital heart disease.] Arq Bras Cardiol 84, 381–386.

12. Marek J, Skovranek J, Hucin B, *et al.* (1995) Seven-year experience of noninvasive preoperative diagnostics in children with congenital heart defects: comprehensive analysis of 2,788 consecutive patients. Cardiology 86, 488–495.

13. Hlavacek AM, Crawford FA Jr, Chessa KS, *et al.* (2006) Real-time three-dimensional echocardiography is useful in the evaluation of patients with atrioventricular septal defects. Echocardiography 23, 225–231.

14. Lang RM, Mor-Avi V, Sugeng L, *et al.* (2006) Three-dimensional echocardiography: the benefits of the additional dimension. J Am Coll Cardiol 48, 2053–2069.

15. Marx GR, Sherwood MC. (2002) Three-dimensional echocardiography in congenital heart disease: a continuum of unfulfilled promises? No. A presently clinically applicable technology with an important future? Yes. Pediatr Cardiol 23, 266–285.

16. Soriano BD, Hoch M, Ithuralde A, *et al.* (2008) Matrix-array 3-dimensional echocardiographic assessment of volumes, mass, and ejection fraction in young pediatric patients with a functional single ventricle: a comparison study with cardiac magnetic resonance. Circulation 117, 1842–1848.

17. Stevenson JG. (2003) Utilization of intraoperative transesophageal echocardiography during repair of congenital cardiac defects: a survey of North American centers. Clin Cardiol 26, 132–134.

18. Bezold LI, Pignatelli R, Altman CA, *et al.* (1996) Intraoperative transesophageal echocardiography in congenital heart surgery. The Texas Children's Hospital experience. Tex Heart Inst J 23, 108–115.

19. Radzik D, Davignon A, van Doesburg N, *et al.* (1993) Predictive factors for spontaneous closure of atrial septal defects diagnosed in the first 3 months of life. J Am Coll Cardiol 22, 851–853.

20. Cockerham JT, Martin TC, Gutierrez FR, *et al.* (1983) Spontaneous closure of secundum atrial septal defect in infants and young children. Am J Cardiol 52, 1267–1271.

21. Suzuki T, Ohye RG, Devaney EJ, *et al.* (2006) Selective management of the left ventricular outflow tract for repair of interrupted aortic arch with ventricular septal defect: management of left ventricular outflow tract obstruction. J Thorac Cardiovasc Surg 131, 779–784.

22. Vogel M, Smallhorn JF, Freedom RM, *et al.* (1988) An echocardiographic study of the association of ventricular septal defect and right ventricular muscle bundles with a fixed subaortic abnormality. Am J Cardiol 61, 857–860.

23. Komai H, Naito Y, Fujiwara K, *et al.* (1997) Surgical strategy for doubly committed subarterial ventricular septal defect with aortic cusp prolapse. Ann Thorac Surg 64, 1146–1149.

24. Kumar K, Lock JE, Geva T. (1997) Apical muscular ventricular septal defects between the left ventricle and the right

ventricular infundibulum. Diagnostic and interventional considerations. Circulation 95, 1207–1213.

25. Stewart RD, Backer CL, Young L, *et al.* (2005) Tetralogy of Fallot: results of a pulmonary valve-sparing strategy. Ann Thorac Surg 80, 1431–1438; discussion 1438–1439.

26. Mackie AS, Gauvreau K, Perry SB, *et al.* (2003) Echocardiographic predictors of aortopulmonary collaterals in infants with tetralogy of Fallot and pulmonary atresia. J Am Coll Cardiol 41, 852–857.

27. Jureidini SB, Appleton RS, Nouri S. (1989) Detection of coronary artery abnormalities in tetralogy of Fallot by two-dimensional echocardiography. J Am Coll Cardiol 14, 960–967.

28. Need LR, Powell AJ, del Nido P, *et al.* (2000) Coronary echocardiography in tetralogy of Fallot: diagnostic accuracy, resource utilization and surgical implications over 13 years. J Am Coll Cardiol 36, 1371–1377.

29. Van Praagh R, Van Praagh S. (1965) The anatomy of common aorticopulmonary trunk (truncus arteriosus communis) and its embryologic implications. A study of 57 necropsy cases. Am J Cardiol 16, 406–425.

30. Levine JC, Geva T. (1999) Echocardiographic assessment of common atrioventricular canal. Prog Ped Cardiol 10, 137–151.

31. Pasquini L, Parness IA, Colan SD, *et al.* (1993) Diagnosis of intramural coronary artery in transposition of the great arteries using two-dimensional echocardiography. Circulation 88, 1136–1141.

32. Wernovsky G, Sanders SP. (1993) Coronary artery anatomy and transposition of the great arteries. Coron Artery Dis 4, 148–157.

33. Mayer JE Jr, Sanders SP, Jonas RA, *et al.* (1990) Coronary artery pattern and outcome of arterial switch operation for transposition of the great arteries. Circulation 82, IV139–IV145.

34. Blume ED, Altmann K, Mayer JE, *et al.* (1999) Evolution of risk factors influencing early mortality of the arterial switch operation. J Am Coll Cardiol 33, 1702–1709.

35. Gottlieb D, Schwartz ML, Bischoff K, *et al.* (2008) Predictors of outcome of arterial switch operation for complex D-transposition. Ann Thorac Surg 85, 1698–1702; discussion 1702–1703.

36. Stern HC, Locher D, Wallnofer K, *et al.* (1991) Noninvasive assessment of coarctation of the aorta: comparative measurements by two-dimensional echocardiography, magnetic resonance, and angiography. Pediatr Cardiol 12, 1–5.

37. Fernandes SM, Sanders SP, Khairy P, *et al.* (2004) Morphology of bicuspid aortic valve in children and adolescents. J Am Coll Cardiol 44, 1648–1651.

38. Lev M. (1952) Pathologic anatomy and interrelationship of hypoplasia of the aortic tract complexes. Lab Invest 1, 61–70.

39. Noonan JA, Nadas AS. (1958) The hypoplastic left heart syndrome; an analysis of 101 cases. Pediatr Clin North Am 5, 1029–1056.

40. Rychik J, Rome JJ, Collins MH, *et al.* (1999) The hypoplastic left heart syndrome with intact atrial septum: atrial morphology, pulmonary vascular histopathology and outcome. J Am Coll Cardiol 34, 554–560.

41. Forbess JM, Cook N, Roth SJ, *et al.* (1995) Ten-year institutional experience with palliative surgery for hypoplastic left heart syndrome. Risk factors related to stage I mortality. Circulation 92, II262–II266.

42. Saroli T, Gelehrter S, Gomez-Fifer CA, *el al.* (2008) Anomalies of left coronary artery origin affecting surgical repair of hypoplastic left heart syndrome and Shone complex. Echocardiography 25, 727–731.

43. Seliem MA, Chin AJ, Norwood WI. (1992) Patterns of anomalous pulmonary venous connection/drainage in hypoplastic left heart syndrome: diagnostic role of Doppler color flow mapping and surgical implications. J Am Coll Cardiol 19, 135–141.

44. Constantine G, Shan K, Flamm SD, *et al.* (2004) Role of MRI in clinical cardiology. Lancet 363, 2162–2171.

45. Faris OP, Shein MJ. (2005) Government viewpoint: US Food & Drug Administration: Pacemakers, ICDs and MRI. Pacing Clin Electrophysiol 28, 268–269.

46. Hundley WG, Li HF, Lange RA, *et al.* (1995) Assessment of left-to-right intracardiac shunting by velocity-encoded, phase-difference magnetic resonance imaging. A comparison with oximetric and indicator dilution techniques. Circulation 91, 2955–2960.

47. Powell AJ, Tsai-Goodman B, Prakash A, *et al.* (2003) Comparison between phase-velocity cine magnetic resonance imaging and invasive oximetry for quantification of atrial shunts. Am J Cardiol 91, 1523–1525.

48. Florentine MS, Grosskreutz CL, Chang W, *et al.* (1986) Measurement of left ventricular mass in vivo using gated nuclear magnetic resonance imaging. J Am Coll Cardiol 8, 107–112.

49. Mogelvang J, Stubgaard M, Thomsen C, *et al.* (1988) Evaluation of right ventricular volumes measured by magnetic resonance imaging. Eur Heart J 9, 529–533.

50. Rebergen SA, Chin JG, Ottenkamp J, *et al.* (1993) Pulmonary regurgitation in the late postoperative follow-up of tetralogy of Fallot. Volumetric quantitation by nuclear magnetic resonance velocity mapping. Circulation 88, 2257–2266.

51. Francois CJ, Carr JC. (2007) MRI of the thoracic aorta. Cardiol Clin 25, 171–184.

52. Matsuoka H, Hamada M, Honda T, *et al.* (1993) Precise assessment of myocardial damage associated with secondary cardiomyopathies by use of Gd-DTPA-enhanced magnetic resonance imaging. Angiology 44, 945–950.

53. Daram SR, Cortese CM, Bastani B. (2005) Nephrogenic fibrosing dermopathy/nephrogenic systemic fibrosis: report of a new case with literature review. Am J Kidney Dis 46, 754–759.

54. Durongpisitkul K, Tang NL, Soongswang J, *et al.* (2004) Predictors of successful transcatheter closure of atrial septal defect by cardiac magnetic resonance imaging. Pediatr Cardiol 25, 124–130.

55. Beerbaum P, Parish V, Bell A, *et al.* (2008) Atypical atrial septal defects in children: noninvasive evaluation by cardiac MRI. Pediatr Radiol 38, 1188–1194.

56. Su JT, Chung T, Muthupillai R, *et al.* (2005) Usefulness of real-time navigator magnetic resonance imaging for evaluating coronary artery origins in pediatric patients. Am J Cardiol 95, 679–682.

57. Gatzoulis MA, Elliott JT, Guru V, *et al.* (2000) Right and left ventricular systolic function late after repair of tetralogy of Fallot. Am J Cardiol 86, 1352–1357.

58. Gatzoulis MA, Till JA, Somerville J, *et al.* (1995) Mechanoelectrical interaction in tetralogy of Fallot. QRS prolongation relates to right ventricular size and predicts malignant ventricular arrhythmias and sudden death. Circulation 92, 231–237.

59. Ghai A, Silversides C, Harris L, *et al.* (2002) Left ventricular dysfunction is a risk factor for sudden cardiac death in adults late after repair of tetralogy of Fallot. J Am Coll Cardiol 40, 1675–1680.

60. Murphy JG, Gersh BJ, Mair DD, *et al.* (1993) Long-term outcome in patients undergoing surgical repair of tetralogy of Fallot. N Engl J Med 329, 593–599.

61. Dave HH, Buechel ER, Dodge-Khatami A, *et al.* (2005) Early insertion of a pulmonary valve for chronic regurgitation helps restoration of ventricular dimensions. Ann Thorac Surg 80, 1615–1620; discussion 1620–1621.

62. Doughan AR, McConnell ME, Lyle TA, *et al.* (2005) Effects of pulmonary valve replacement on QRS duration and right ventricular cavity size late after repair of right ventricular outflow tract obstruction. Am J Cardiol 95, 1511–1514.

63. Henkens IR, van Straten A, Schalij MJ, *et al.* (2007) Predicting outcome of pulmonary valve replacement in adult tetralogy of Fallot patients. Ann Thorac Surg 83, 907–911.

64. Therrien J, Provost Y, Merchant N, *et al.* (2005) Optimal timing for pulmonary valve replacement in adults after tetralogy of Fallot repair. Am J Cardiol 95, 779–782.

65. Warner KG, O'Brien PK, Rhodes J, *et al.* (2003) Expanding the indications for pulmonary valve replacement after repair of tetralogy of Fallot. Ann Thorac Surg 76, 1066–1071; discussion 1071–1072.

66. Harrild DM, Berul CI, Cecchin F, *et al.* (2009) Pulmonary valve replacement in tetralogy of Fallot: impact on survival and ventricular tachycardia. Circulation 119, 445–451.

67. Babu-Narayan SV, Kilner PJ, Li W, *et al.* (2006) Ventricular fibrosis suggested by cardiovascular magnetic resonance in adults with repaired tetralogy of Fallot and its relationship to adverse markers of clinical outcome. Circulation 113, 405–413.

68. Reddy VM, McElhinney DB, Amin Z, *et al.* (2000) Early and intermediate outcomes after repair of pulmonary atresia with ventricular septal defect and major aortopulmonary collateral arteries: experience with 85 patients. Circulation 101, 1826–1832.

69. Geva T, Greil GF, Marshall AC, *et al.* (2002) Gadolinium-enhanced 3-dimensional magnetic resonance angiography of pulmonary blood supply in patients with complex pulmonary stenosis or atresia: comparison with x-ray angiography. Circulation 106, 473–478.

70. Riehle TJ, Oshinski JN, Brummer ME, *et al.* (2006) Velocity-encoded magnetic resonance image assessment of regional aortic flow in coarctation patients. Ann Thorac Surg 81, 1002–1007.

71. Soler R, Rodriguez E, Requejo I, *et al.* (1998) Magnetic resonance imaging of congenital abnormalities of the thoracic aorta. Eur Radiol 8, 540–546.

72. Backer CL, Mavroudis C, Rigsby CK, *et al.* (2005) Trends in vascular ring surgery. J Thorac Cardiovasc Surg 129, 1339–1347.

73. Johnson TR, Goldmuntz E, McDonald-McGinn DM, *et al.* (2005) Cardiac magnetic resonance imaging for accurate diagnosis of aortic arch anomalies in patients with 22q11.2 deletion. Am J Cardiol 96, 1726–1730.

74. Brown DW, Gauvreau K, Powell AJ, *et al.* (2007) Cardiac magnetic resonance versus routine cardiac catheterization before bidirectional glenn anastomosis in infants with functional single ventricle: a prospective randomized trial. Circulation 116, 2718–2725.

75. Lin FY, Min JK. (2008) Assessment of cardiac volumes by multidetector computed tomography. J Cardiovasc Comput Tomogr 2, 256–262.

76. Einstein AJ. (2009) Radiation protection of patients undergoing cardiac computed tomographic angiography. JAMA 301, 545–547.

77. Baim DS, Grossman W. (1996) *Cardiac Catheterization, Angiography and Intervention.* Baltimore, MD: Williams and Wilkins.

78. Lock JE, Keane JF, Perry SB. (2000) *Diagnostic and Interventional Catheterization in Congenital Heart Disease.* Boston, MA: Kluwer Academic Publishers.

79. Yang SS, Bentivoglio LG, Maranhao V, *et al.* (1978) *From Cardiac Catheterization Data to Hemodynamic Parameters.* Philadelphia, PA: FA Davis Co.

80. Hawker RE, Celermajer JM. (1973) Comparison of pulmonary artery and pulmonary venous wedge pressure in congenital heart disease. Br Heart J 35, 386–391.

81. Freed MD, Miettinen OS, Nadas AS. (1979) Oximetric detection of intracardiac left-to-right shunts. Br Heart J 42, 690–694.

82. Gorlin R, Gorlin SG. (1951) Hydraulic formula for calculation of the area of the stenotic mitral valve, other cardiac valves, and central circulatory shunts. I. Am Heart J 41, 1–29.

83. Cook SC, Raman SV. (2008) Multidetector computed tomography in the adolescent and young adult with congenital heart disease. J Cardiovasc Comput Tomogr 2, 36–49.

84. Dorfman AL, Geva T. (2006) Magnetic resonance imaging evaluation of congenital heart disease: conotruncal anomalies. J Cardiovasc Magn Reson 8, 645–659.

85. Jahnke C, Nagel E, Gebker R, *et al.* (2007) Four-dimensional single breathhold magnetic resonance imaging using kt-BLAST enables reliable assessment of left- and right-ventricular volumes and mass. J Magn Reson Imaging 25, 737–742.

86. Pourmoghadam KK, Moore JW, Khan M, *et al.* (2003) Congenital unilateral pulmonary venous atresia: definitive diagnosis and treatment. Pediatr Cardiol 24, 73–79.

87. Duncan BW, Mee RB, Prieto LR, *et al.* (2003) Staged repair of tetralogy of Fallot with pulmonary atresia and major aortopulmonary collateral arteries. J Thorac Cardiovasc Surg 126, 694–702.

88. Jahangiri M, Zurakowski D, Bichell D, *et al.* (1999) Improved results with selective management in pulmonary atresia with intact ventricular septum. J Thorac Cardiovasc Surg 118, 1046–1055.

89. Guleserian KJ, Armsby LB, Thiagarajan RR, *et al.* (2006) Natural history of pulmonary atresia with intact ventricular septum and right-ventricle-dependent coronary circulation managed by the single-ventricle approach. Ann Thorac Surg 81, 2250–2257; discussion 2258.

90. Tanel RE, Wernovsky G, Landzberg MJ, *et al.* (1995) Coronary artery abnormalities detected at cardiac catheterization following the arterial switch operation for transposition of the great arteries. Am J Cardiol 76, 153–157.

91. Kato H, Sugimura T, Akagi T, *et al.* (1996) Long-term consequences of Kawasaki disease. A 10- to 21-year follow-up study of 594 patients. Circulation 94, 1379–1385.

92. Mavroudis C, Backer CL, Duffy CE, *et al.* (1999) Pediatric coronary artery bypass for Kawasaki congenital, post arterial switch, and iatrogenic lesions. Ann Thorac Surg 68, 506–512.

CHAPTER 5

Hybrid Procedures for Congenital Heart Disease

Mark Galantowicz,[1] John P. Cheatham,[1] Alistair Phillips,[2] Ralf J. Holzer,[1] Sharon L. Hill,[1] and Vincent F. Olshove[1]

[1]The Heart Center, Nationwide Children's Hospital, The Ohio State University, Columbus, OH, USA
[2]Cincinnati Children's Hospital Medical Center, Cincinnati, OH, USA

Introduction

It is the nature of medical disciplines and therapies to evolve through cycles of association and separation for further refinement or specialization. Over the past decades there have been noteworthy improvements within the specialties of congenital cardiothoracic surgery and interventional cardiology. These advancements have been manifest by falling mortality rates for congenital heart therapies. However, within each discipline there remain certain procedures and patient populations that have suboptimal outcomes. Moreover, with the overall increased survival for congenital heart disease, the importance of morbidity and its impact on the quality of life for our patients has become paramount. At the same time technologic developments seem to be introduced into our surgical/interventional armamentarium at an ever increasing rate. These combined forces have resulted in a closer association between the congenital cardiothoracic surgeon and the interventional cardiologist, along with the teams that support them, in a mutual quest to improve the quantity and quality of life for our patients. This spirit of collaboration is at the core of what we call a "hybrid approach" to congenital heart disease.

A hybrid is often defined as the offspring of two different species. Although this can happen randomly, the purposeful development of a hybrid can optimize the strengths of each species while minimizing the weaknesses of each. One could certainly think of a cardiothoracic surgeon and an interventional cardiologist as different species by the nature of their training, skill sets, expectations, and mannerisms. But more importantly the crafts of surgery and catheterization have areas of strengths and weaknesses that can be optimized by cooperation as a hybrid therapy. These hybrid therapies then develop further with careful planning into a management strategy involving the other services within a heart center, namely the other cardiologists, anesthesiologists, intensive care team, nurses, perfusionists, and even outside services such as neonatology and radiology. This team approach encourages the sharing of ideas, expertise, equipment, and techniques, allowing one to think "outside the box" and to develop novel treatment strategies.

Throughout this chapter we will explore some of the ways that this spirit of collaboration has led to new hybrid therapies for the management of congenital heart disease.

Elements of a Hybrid Program for Congenital Heart Disease

The goals of hybrid therapy are many: 1) to reduce both morbidity and mortality; 2) to reduce the cumulative impact of multiple interventions over a lifetime that are often required to treat those with complex congenital heart disease; 3) to improve the patient's quality of life; 4) to deliver more efficient and cost-effective care; 5) to develop novel treatment strategies; and 6) to encourage teamwork. There are a few key requirements for initiating a successful hybrid program. These requirements are not expensive, do not take up a lot of space, and are within the grasp of all programs; however, without them the likelihood of success is small. Simply put – attitude, respect, and the removal of obstacles to collaboration are the key ingredients to a successful hybrid program. First and foremost, there can be no competition between the surgeon and the interventionalist. There must be mutual respect for each other and the talents and limitations that each possess. It is important that no individual's opinion is weighted more than the other…it is a partnership. We have coined the term "Two Perspectives – Single Focus" to represent this respectful partnership. But this respect needs to be supported by an operational structure that does not put the surgeon and interventionalist in competition with each other for administrative voice, academic advancement, infrastructure and equipment support, or the economics surrounding case volume. Moreover an operational structure for all members of a heart center team (surgery, cardiology, anesthesia, intensive care, perfusion, and nursing) that aligns expectations, outcomes, and awards together, such as a unified service line rather than a collection of separate entities, fosters collaboration. This type of operational structure reflects strong hospital administrative support, another key element for a hybrid program to exist and flourish [1]. Once the obstacles to collaboration are removed, a cultural shift can foster a collective attitude that values and supports innovation through hybrid therapies. Once these key elements are in place, secondary considerations reflecting space, equipment, staff, and training can augment a hybrid program. Nevertheless, a successful hybrid program is clearly more about attitude and collaboration than about a piece of equipment.

Design of a Hybrid Suite

As the collaboration between the cardiothoracic surgeon and interventional cardiologist has increased, and as the lines between surgical and transcatheter treatment have blurred, the need for a therapeutic suite compatible to both disciplines has become apparent. The design of a hybrid suite is a long process that involves many individuals, meetings, and constant monitoring to see the project through to completion.

The initial step in the development of a hybrid suite requires the support and endorsement of hospital administration. The vision, or concept, of the hybrid suite must be presented by the cardiothoracic surgical and interventional cardiology teams, with commitment of the entire heart center team. Once administrative support has been attained and a planning budget established, the design phase can begin.

A design team derived from a variety of clinical and nonclinical areas must be established. Team members should include hospital engineers, architects, building contractors, electrical engineers, administration, and a representative cardiothoracic surgeon, interventional cardiologist, cardiac anesthesiologist, electrophysiologist, echocardiologist, perfusionist, operating room (OR) and catheterization lab nurses and specialists (respiratory therapist [RT], registered cardiovascular invasive specialist [RCIS]), nurse practitioner, and physician assistant). It is important that each member from each group represented takes ownership of the vision and understands that his or her contribution is essential to the end-product of the suite design. The cardiothoracic surgeon and interventional cardiologist must make the time commitment to this process to guarantee that the entire design team understands the vision and purpose of the hybrid suite. It may be necessary to spend time re-selling the vision and maintaining the motivation of the team over the design–implementation phase. It is also extremely important for the design team to be open-minded and creative in finding solutions to problems that will most certainly arise.

The cost associated with the design and construction of a hybrid suite can be significantly greater than a conventional operating or interventional catheterization theater. Consideration must be given to how the suite will be used on a day-to-day basis. Will the suite be used primarily as a cardiothoracic operating theater with cardiopulmonary bypass procedures (Plate 5.1, see plate section opposite p. 594) [2] or principally for interventional catheterization procedures (Plate 5.2, see plate section opposite p. 594)? There are different design considerations, and costs, associated with an interventional catheterization suite compared with an operative suite. While the suite will be used by combined services, it still should have a primary user around whom the designed work-flow and patient-flow should occur. The greatest difference between the two types of rooms, both in design and cost, will be in the selection of the digital radiographic imaging equipment, specifically the need for bi-plane versus single-plane imaging.

As the design phase progresses and equipment is being considered, it is extremely helpful for the entire design team to participate in as many site visits as possible. These in-person site visits reveal both positive and negative aspects to different designs and can be invaluable to the design team. As many members of the design team as possible should attend these visits as the best room design will incorporate input and feedback from all members. These site visits should include as many different centers and equipment variations as possible. Particular attention should be paid to the room layout, imaging equipment and procedure table design and function, boom vendor selection, and audiovisual integration and information management. Pointed questions need to be asked regarding the successes and failures of each site to help understand the issues that will be faced.

Ideally, selection of the vendors for the radiographic imaging equipment, booms, and audiovisual integration would occur early on as these vendors should become part of the design team to assist with additional room design items such as adequate space, heating, ventilation, air conditioning, air exchange, electrical supply (adequate to support the high energy demands of these systems), and even flooring design outlining movement of the C-arms (which can assist staff with equipment placement when the room becomes operational). Additionally, it would be optimal to design a hybrid suite, interventional suite, and cardiothoracic suite all in direct proximity of each other to better optimize the necessary equipment and staff resources.

The types of equipment used, both available today and anticipated for the future, must be considered; space must be allocated for use during the procedure as well as for storage when not in use. The minimum square footage for the procedure area should be 900 ft^2 (84 m^2). Additional space will be necessary for control room (minimum 200 ft^2 [19 m^2]), induction room, pump room, supplies, cold room for radiographic imaging equipment, audiovisual image management router, and equipment storage. The preferred room design is square more than rectangular to allow for ample access on all sides of the patient for all team members.

The choice to design the suite around either the interventional cardiology team or the cardiac surgical team should be determined early. There are two key components to this decision: the digital imaging system (bi-plane versus single-plane) and the procedure table type (traditional interventional versus surgical).

Interventional catheterization procedures are based around the bi-plane imaging system and the ability to see from multiple and complex angulations, with as much as 90% of the procedure time requiring imaging. These bi-plane systems require more floor space and make patient access more difficult depending on the manufacturer and design. Conversely, the cardiothoracic surgical team typically prefers single-plane, ceiling-mounted imaging systems because most of their procedures may involve cardiopulmonary bypass where imaging time may be less than 10% of the total procedure time.

There is not currently a universal hybrid procedure table that performs to all of the specifications of the interventional cardiologist and cardiothoracic surgeon. Interventionalists tend to prefer free-floating, carbon fiber table tops with plenty of width and length for wires and catheters with little concern for table height. Cardiothoracic surgeons, on the other hand, do not typically care about table length but prefer a wide range of table height options, prefer the table top to be as narrow as possible to prevent unnecessary back strain, require Trendelenburg and reverse Trendelenburg, need the table to roll laterally right and left, and frequently have stainless steel rails for attaching auxiliary devices. To meet the need of both operators, table flexibility will need to be taken into consideration. A procedural table with a small, fixed-base footprint and with close to 360-degree rotation is the optimal solution.

One of the most common design features is to get as much off the floor as possible without causing other obstruction and traffic flow problems within the room. One must also consider that while objects on the floor may

be obstructions, so too may the items hanging from the ceiling. So caution in design must be employed when moving objects to the ceiling. Moreover, the ceiling is already challenging considering the rail system for a ceiling mounted C-arm as well as other equipment such as surgical lights, numerous monitors [2–6], injector, gases, and video feeds.

There are a number of different boom designs and manufacturers. Ceiling-mounted telescoping columns are frequently promoted by architects as functional and cost effective, yet tend to create a traffic flow problem in many room designs. If the columns are not located directly over the sources that require the services there will be many cables (electrical, gas, vacuum, video, etc.) running across the floor to where the column is located creating a hazard. Having to pick the exact location of a column leaves little flexibility for adaptation or change of procedures within the suite.

All booms are not created equal, and what may work for one service may not work for the combined needs of the hybrid suite. Slim-line designs with flexibility to raise and lower and the number of joints available for maneuvering into optimal position must all be considered. All boom ceiling mounts need to be located outside the ceiling tracks of the C-arm with adequate length to be able to reach into the area of need. Boom design for anesthesia and perfusion need to be of adequate height and arm length to remain above the equipment they will serve and must allow maneuverability to permit adaptability to change. Figure 5.1 is a typical boom design that shows maneuverability of boom arms within a hybrid OR suite. Reliance on the boom and radiographic imaging vendors to assist in design and placement of the equipment is absolutely necessary. Most vendors have the ability to create three-dimensional graphical displays of the hybrid suite with boom placement, rotation, and movement.

Service to the booms must be sufficient to supply all the equipment. Adequate electrical circuits are needed to supply adequate amperage to the equipment that will be fed by the boom. Appropriate quantity and types of gases (air, CO_2, O_2, N_2, N_2O, anesthetic gas waste, vacuum), composite video, variable-gain amplifier (VGA), electrocardiogram (EKG) synchronization between booms (for synchronized cardioversion, pulsatile perfusion, or echocardiogram [ECHO]), network jacks, etc., all need to be considered. Inadequate planning could result in a very expensive correction.

If an equipment boom is used, special consideration to the number of shelves and the stored equipment is necessary. Electrocautery, defibrillators, video recording equipment, endoscopic equipment, and surgical head lights may all be mounted on this boom if appropriate. Redundant composite video and VGA jacks, network jacks, power, vacuum and additional air, CO_2, O_2, and vacuum should be added. The equipment boom will occupy floor space

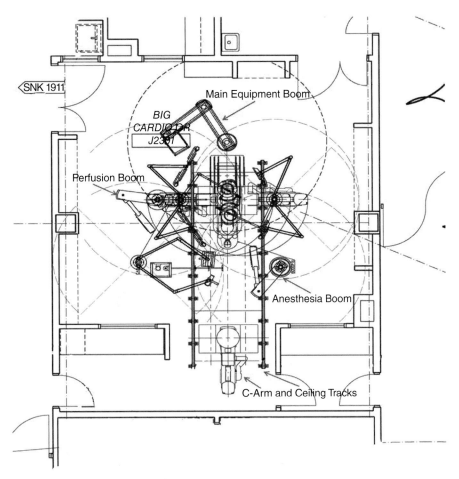

Figure 5.1 Overhead schematic of boom location and movement.

and as such may best be designed to optimize maximal shelves to support future needs.

It is desirable to have monitors of adequate size and number placed about the hybrid suite to allow any personnel within the room to visualize what is occurring during a procedure. A substantial amount of data and images may need to be routed, including angiograms, ECHO imaging, picture archiving and communication system (PACS), physiologic monitor data, live video imaging, etc. Once the decision is made to route and manage the images, the ability to expand in any number of directions is practically endless: images can be routed to or from remote sites on campus, to surgeons' or interventionalists' offices, to the ECHO reading room, or to the conference center, or images and voices can be routed simultaneously between theaters to allow the interventional cardiologist and cardiothoracic surgeon to consult with each other while both are in procedures. Because video integration, routing, and visualization are optimized throughout the room adding additional composite video and VGA jacks on all booms and all walls is a minimal up-front expense that allows any ancillary or

future equipment to be easily and quickly added to the system for routing and image capture.

Once design is completed the construction and installation phase begin. It is imperative that one stay involved at this critical point in the project. It is advisable for at least one clinical team member and physician walk through the room at least weekly to stay informed, to ensure that no unanticipated issues arise, and to make critical decisions on design issues early, while design changes are still relatively easy to implement. If there is not active participation by all team members, the finished product will reflect the design of nonclinical individuals who will not need to function within the finished suite on a daily basis, possibly resulting in suboptimal conditions.

Hybrid Therapy for Vascular Stenoses

The role of Hybrid Vascular Therapy

The treatment of vascular stenoses poses significant challenges to the cardiothoracic surgeon as well as the interventional cardiologist [7]. While surgical patch augmentation has been considered the gold standard for many years, the introduction of endovascular stents into the interventional armamentarium, pioneered by Chuck Mullins, has documented benefits [8–10]. Following the introduction of transcatheter stent therapy, the role of hybrid strategies in the therapy of vascular obstructions has evolved considerably over the last 10 years from a "surgical bailout procedure," to being considered an important alternative treatment strategy for patients with congenital heart disease [2–6,11,12]. As such, current therapeutic options available include surgical patch augmentation, transcatheter balloon angioplasty and stent therapy, or intraoperative hybrid therapy. Each available treatment strategy has advantages and disadvantages (Table 5.1) and an approach that is suitable for one patient may not necessarily be appropriate for another with a similar lesion. Only an understanding of the strengths and limitations of each individual approach will enable the physician to choose the most appropriate treatment strategy for each individual patient.

Selecting the Appropriate Therapy

A variety of factors must be taken into consideration before selecting an individual approach.

Need for Cardiopulmonary Bypass

Intraoperative hybrid therapy under direct vision with or without endoscopic guidance invariably requires the use of cardiopulmonary bypass. Thus, this approach is usually only considered if bypass is required to treat another cardiovascular lesion. Even if cardiopulmonary bypass is used, intraoperative stent placement may in selected cases avoid the need for aortic cross-clamping and reduce the complexity and risk of a surgical procedure [13,14]. However, if a patient does not need cardiac surgical therapy, then vascular lesions are usually better treated in the cardiac catheterization laboratory under angiographic guidance.

Location and Type of the Vascular Stenosis

Very calcified vascular obstructions may benefit from surgical, rather than hybrid therapy [15]. This applies specifically to the proximal branch pulmonary arteries (PAs) where a long-standing, distorted, calcified lesion may require resection and augmentation at the time of conduit or pulmonary valve replacement, rather than transcatheter or hybrid stent delivery. In contrast, stenotic lesions created by vascular folds or external compression are notoriously difficult to address surgically, even with a "perfect" patch repair. In these situations, stent implantation is frequently the most

Table 5.1 Advantages and disadvantages of individual approaches to treat vascular lesions (transcatheter approach, hybrid approach, surgical approach). (CPB, cardiopulmonary bypass).

Approach	Advantages	Disadvantages
Catheter	More accurate measurements and stent positioning Better roadmaps No need for sternotomy or other surgical access No need for cardiopulmonary bypass	Need for stiff wires and large sheaths Use of adult-size stents in small infants often prohibitive Stents have to be used "as is" (cannot be modified) Vascular/technical complications may require surgical bailout Increased hemodynamic instability especially in small children Longer fluoroscopy and procedure times Procedures often technically demanding
Hybrid	No need to minimize delivery system No need to track "curves and bends" No need for stiff wires and long sheaths Use of adult-size stents in small children Potential for stent modification Often hemodynamically better tolerated Better control of vascular and technical complications Shorter fluoroscopy and procedure times Technically less demanding Vascular lesions can be inspected before deciding therapy	Distal wire and stent position more difficult to assess Less suitable to obtain roadmaps Need for sternotomy or other surgical exposure Need for CPB if using direct vision/endoscopy Use of contrast may impact kidney function after CPB
Surgical	Vascular lesions can be inspected before deciding therapy Can often easily be integrated with concomitant surgery Calcified lesions can be resected Surgical patch augmentation adds extra tissue to a vessel No need for fluoroscopy or contrast Hemodynamic stability on CPB Very good control of vascular and technical complications	Some vascular lesions difficult to reach surgically Less suitable to treat kinks and external compressions Need for sternotomy or other surgical exposure Often need for CPB Surgical angioplasty may create focus for recurrent stenosis

appropriate option. Sometimes a combination of surgical resection with patch augmentation followed by stent implantation is required, in which case hybrid stent delivery under direct vision is clearly the treatment of choice.

Not infrequently, though, it is difficult to exactly predict the morphology and type of vascular lesion based solely on angiographic imaging in the cardiac catheterization laboratory. Therefore, in a patient who will require a surgical procedure in the near future (e.g., conduit replacement), final decisions on the extent of surgical resection and the most suitable form of vascular rehabilitation may only be made intraoperatively. In those situations it can be advantageous to defer transcatheter stent placement, especially for proximal PA lesions.

In contrast to the proximal branch PAs or aorta, some vasculature, such as distal branch PAs, cannot easily be reached using surgical techniques and therefore naturally lend themselves to transcatheter therapy. Even though hybrid therapy may occasionally be suitable for isolated distal branch PA lesions, in general the rehabilitation of peripheral branch PA stenoses requires detailed angiographic guidance. As such, treating these lesions in the cardiac catheterization laboratory before any surgical intervention is usually recommended.

The location of a vascular obstruction is very important when planning the most suitable therapeutic approach. The proximal branch PAs are the most common location for intraoperative stent placement [16–23], but are equally amenable to transcatheter or surgical therapy. Pulmonary venous obstructions have a uniformly poor long-term prognosis, whether treated surgically or in the cardiac catheterization laboratory [24–27] but are theoretically amenable to all therapeutic strategies, including a hybrid approach [27–29]. With the exception of infants with associated anomalies, native obstructions of the aortic arch in patients under 10 kg are often better addressed surgically rather than using a transcatheter approach [30,31], whereas transcatheter therapy for recoarctation is usually the primary treatment of choice [32–36]. Patients with more complex arch obstructions can be treated in the catheterization laboratory [37] or may benefit from a hybrid approach to avoid the use of cardiopulmonary bypass [38]. Vascular lesions in superior vena cava (SVC) or inferior vena cava (IVC) are usually easily amenable to all therapeutic strategies.

Other morphologic reasons that may favor a hybrid approach in the OR include extremely hypoplastic vessels or complete vascular obstructions, which are associated with an increased risk of vascular injury or rupture during balloon angioplasty or stent deployment. In these situations, surgical exposure in the OR may allow direct access to the vessel without the use of cardiopulmonary bypass, but with bypass on standby should any complications occur.

Some vascular lesions may be impossible to reach in the cardiac catheterization laboratory due to very steep angulations, protruding stents, or other reasons. In these situations, one approach short of using cardiopulmonary bypass to treat the lesion surgically would be a hybrid approach with surgical exposure through, for example, median sternotomy, with subsequent direct vascular puncture, which may facilitate stent placement or angioplasty in a more direct fashion than using a percutaneous transcatheter route.

Age of the Patient

The younger the patient and the smaller the stenotic vessel, the greater the challenge for transcatheter therapy. Implantation of stents that can be expanded to adult size frequently requires the use of large delivery sheaths and stiff guide wires, which may be poorly tolerated even in otherwise healthy infants. The use of large sheaths may also be prohibitive with standard femoral arterial access in infants with a weight below 10 kg owing to the risk of significant femoral arterial injury. While low-profile, balloon-mounted stents are relatively easy to implant in the cardiac catheterization laboratory and more suitable for small vessels, they cannot be expanded to adult size of the vessel and will therefore create considerable difficulties in the future, especially if a stent has to be removed surgically in a patient that otherwise would not have required a surgical intervention.

Stented vascular obstructions are at risk of developing neointimal proliferation or in-stent stenosis [39–41], the risk of which is further enhanced if stents are implanted into vessels with a very small diameter, an experience learned extensively when placing coronary stents [42]. Balloon angioplasty avoids some of the limitations of stent implantation and has been used intraoperatively in patients undergoing palliative surgery for hypoplastic left heart syndrome (HLHS) [43,44]. However, balloon angioplasty in general, whether in the cardiac catheterization lab or intraoperatively, is associated with a higher recurrence rate and is usually considered only a temporizing measure [33,34,43]. Hybrid stent delivery has considerable advantages in small infants, as it allows implantation of adult-sized stents while avoiding access-related problems and the use of large delivery sheaths and stiff guide wires. Furthermore, stents can be manually shortened in the OR to accommodate shorter vascular lesions [17].

At the other end of the age spectrum, PA rehabilitation in adults can be technically challenging in the cardiac catheterization laboratory. Stents are often required to be expanded to diameters in excess of 20 mm, requiring delivery sheaths that exceed the size of the presently available braided and reinforced sheaths. While transcatheter stent delivery in proximal branch PAs is certainly feasible, the same can frequently be accomplished in a small fraction of the time using hybrid stent delivery under direct vision with endoscopic guidance during concomitant cardiac surgery.

Clinical Status

Sick patients in the early postoperative period are at higher risk of significant hemodynamic instability during transcatheter interventions [45,46]. These procedures are often poorly tolerated because of the use of stiff guide wires and larger delivery sheaths required for stent delivery, which may create hemodynamic instability by holding open the atrioventricular valve and/or arterial valves. However, residual structural pathology after cardiac surgery in itself is poorly tolerated; therefore, these patients require a therapeutic intervention [47]. In these situations, hybrid therapy can offer direct surgical exposure without the use of cardiopulmonary bypass. This allows direct access to a vascular lesion, with balloon angioplasty or stent implantation being performed through a sheath inserted directly into the relevant vascular structure that offers the most appropriate direct exposure. Cardiopulmonary bypass can be readily available if needed, offering an extra safety margin for these procedures.

Previous and Expected Further Surgical and Transcatheter Procedures

Repeated failure to address a vascular lesion using a specific therapeutic strategy should be considered when deciding on a new approach. It is equally important to consider the need for further surgical interventions before implanting endovascular stents in the cardiac catheterization laboratory, as implanted stents subsequently may need to be removed completely or partially, which can be technically challenging or even impossible and may sometimes require patch augmentation [18,48]. As an example, it is advisable to avoid stent implantation to the proximal right PA in a patient who is still expected to undergo Fontan completion. Similarly, stent implantation for an anastomotic SVC stenosis after heart transplantation may interfere with a potential need for retransplantation.

These considerations often vary from patient to patient and between surgical operators. As is the case for all aspects of hybrid therapy, communication between the cardiothoracic surgeon and the interventional cardiologist is essential when considering percutaneous stent implantation in a patient who is expected to require further cardiac surgery. For some lesions, temporizing balloon angioplasty may be preferable to defer stent implantation until the time of surgery, using a hybrid approach.

Setup, Equipment, Stents, and Balloons

While a dedicated hybrid operating and/or cardiac catheterization suite certainly helps in performing complex hybrid therapy [2], it is not an essential requirement for these procedures. The main ingredient to facilitate successful hybrid therapy to treat vascular obstructions is a cooperative environment between cardiac surgical and interventional teams, combined with a high degree of flexibility and the ability to improvise. It is a good practice to discuss with the cardiothoracic surgeon at the time of cardiac catheterization any intended vascular rehabilitation in a patient who is anticipated to undergo open-heart surgery in the near future. Thus, the most appropriate treatment strategy can be defined at a time when all treatment options are available to the patient.

To enable intraoperative hybrid stent delivery, adequate preoperative imaging data are required that allow selection of the appropriate stent and balloon size. In small infants, for example, the distance to vascular side branches is much easier to determine angiographically or by computed axial tomography (CAT) scan than by using direct intraoperative visualization and assessment. The operator should have a very good idea about stent/balloon type and size before stepping into the OR.

It is essential to have a wide variety of stents and balloon catheters available. Table 5.2 lists a variety of stents that can be expanded to adult size and their individual characteristics [49]. Not all of the listed stents have achieved US Food and Drug Administration (FDA) premarket approval, and it is important to note that none of these stents has been approved for use in pediatric patients with congenital vascular lesions, such as branch PA stenosis or coarctation. As such, all these stents are being used on an "off-label" basis [50].

Intraoperative imaging has evolved as an essential component of cardiac surgical procedures [51–53]. While angiography is not always necessary, especially if stent delivery is performed under direct vision with endoscopic guidance, the use of fluoroscopy has a variety of advantages during most stent implantations [54]. Documenting stent expansion on cine-recording or fluoroscopy, allows the operator to detect unequal expansion, maladjustment of the stent from the balloon, or balloon rupture, much more readily than would be noted with direct vision alone. In

Table 5.2 Selected characteristics of some of the most commonly used endovascular stents in congenital heart disease.

Name (Manufacturer)	Material	Max diameter (mm)	Available length (mm)	Flexibility	Shortening	Cells –design
Genesis XD (Cordis)	Stainless steel	18	19, 25, 29, 39, 59	–	–	Closed
Mega LD (EV3)	Stainless steel	18	16, 26, 36	++	++	Open
Max LD (EV3)	Stainless steel	25	16, 26, 36	+	++	Open
CP Stent 8zig (NuMed)	Platinum/iridium, gold	25	22–45	0	–	Closed

addition, if previous "baseline" angiographies are available, these can be used as roadmaps during stent positioning, specifically using fixed objects such as clips or residual wires for orientation. Furthermore, angiographic evaluation of the result in the OR (exit angiography) allows detection of any potential problem or malposition at a time when corrections can still be made relatively easily [53]. A fixed, ceiling-mounted C-arm is a beneficial luxury, but a portable C-arm will work just as well provided the procedure is carefully planned. Patients may have to be positioned in a more unconventional manner so as not to interfere with the operating table itself. Angiographies in larger pediatric patients usually require a power injection; therefore, a portable power injector should be readily available. This alone does not always guarantee optimal image quality, and flow reduction on the cardiopulmonary bypass circuit as well as temporary occlusion of, for example, opposite branch PAs may further enhance image quality.

Techniques available to perform intraoperative stent placement have expanded considerably [17,19,20,55]. In general, two fundamental hybrid techniques, as well as a potential mixture of both techniques, are available for intraoperative stent delivery:

1. stent delivery under direct vision, using endoscopic guidance;

2. perivascular stent delivery through a sheath, using angiographic guidance.

The decision on whether to deploy the stents using direct vision (which invariably requires the use of cardiopulmonary bypass) or using angiographic/fluoroscopic guidance through direct vascular puncture on the beating heart depends on the type of surgical procedure performed, the need for cardiopulmonary bypass, and whether preexisting landmarks are available from previous angiographic imaging.

The majority of patients will have hybrid stent delivery performed under direct vision with the patient on cardiopulmonary bypass (Plate 5.3, see plate section opposite p. 594) [2]. A prerequisite for this technique is the availability of imaging data and measurements of the lesion to be treated. This is usually obtained during prior cardiac catheterization or a CAT scan, but may be obtained through intraoperative angiography before stopping the heart and exposing/opening the vessel. Branch PA stenoses are the most common lesions requiring hybrid therapy [45].

Endoscopy is a very valuable tool to facilitate stent positioning and deployment, as it allows a much more detailed inspection of the relevant lesion, including the distance to any of the side branches (Plate 5.3, see plate section opposite p. 594). For this purpose, the endoscope is advanced across the stenosis until the origin of a side branch can be visualized, which allows one to measure the distance the endoscope has been advanced into the branch PA (Plate 5.3, see plate section opposite p. 594). This provides a good estimate of the maximum stent length that should be used to avoid jailing of a PA side branch and complements the data available from previous imaging. The endoscope further aides in confirming accurate placement of the guide wire. Wire placement in a small PA side branch may lead to stent malposition, jailing of adjacent pulmonary vasculature, and possibly even vascular injury of the side branch during balloon expansion. For the same reason, operators should avoid the temptation to "quickly" deploy a stent without using a guide wire, as the position of the distal balloon tip cannot be reliably assessed during balloon inflation. In contrast to percutaneous stent placement though, hybrid stent delivery does not require stiff guide wires as a rail, and standard soft j-tipped wires are perfectly appropriate. Once the stent is delivered, the result is examined by endoscopy. Stent meshwork that is slightly protruding into the main PA can easily be crimped and folded, as to create a smoother surface and aid subsequent transcatheter interventions (Plate 5.3, see plate section opposite p. 594). Similarly, the OR offers the possibility to even shorten a stent if necessary [17]. Further, hybrid stent delivery is much more forgiving to balloon rupture or stent migration during stent deployment than transcatheter therapy, and a suboptimally deployed or not fully expanded stent can easily be removed under direct vision.

Deploying stents using angiographic guidance is reserved for very specific lesions and circumstances (Plate 5.4, see plate section opposite p. 594) [2]. This approach usually entails performing the procedure without cardiopulmonary bypass and with the surgical team providing access to the vascular lesions [56], be it via sternotomy, thoracotomy, or vascular cut-down. This approach is helpful in hemodynamically unstable patients where the percutaneous use of stiff wires and long sheaths may be poorly tolerated. Similarly, it offers advantages when vascular lesions are very difficult to access using a transcatheter approach because of protruding stents or steep angles. With cardiopulmonary bypass being readily available, this approach may also add an extra safety margin to the therapy of extremely tight or hypoplastic vascular lesions that carry a higher risk of vascular trauma or rupture (Figure 5.2) [2]. With angiographic guidance being the most important part of this procedure, it is important to plan the position of patient as well as the C-arm at the outset of the procedure. To maximize the potential benefit of this approach, the vascular entry point should be directly opposite in a straight line to the lesion that requires treatment. However, care must be taken that the entry side is sufficiently distant from the lesion to allow stent and/or balloon expansion, without the shoulders of the balloon interfering with the entry site. Wire positions and angiographic guidance are very similar to the approach that would be used in the cardiac catheterization laboratory, with the exception that softer materials can be used and that larger, adult-sized stents may be much

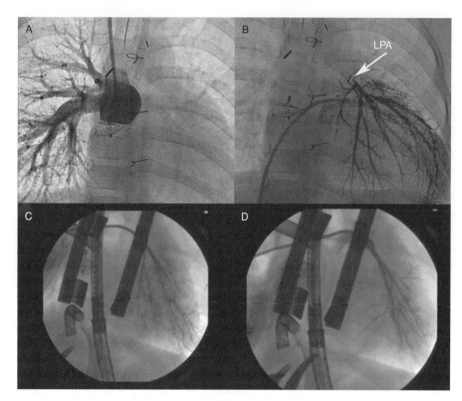

Figure 5.2 3-year-old girl with hypoplastic left heart syndrome and a history of modified Norwood procedure as well as subsequent bidirectional Glenn. Pre-Fontan catheter evaluation documented a disconnected LPA. **A,** Pre-Fontan SVC angiography documenting no filling of an LPA. **B,** Reverse left pulmonary venous angiography documenting a small and hypoplastic LPA. **C,** Intraoperative angiography after advancing a catheter directly into a structure felt to be the LPA, documenting extreme hypoplasia of this vessel. **D,** After deployment of a premounted Genesis stent, this angiography documents improved flow to the distally still severely hypoplastic LPA [2]. (LPA, left pulmonary artery; SVC, superior vena cava.)

better tolerated. With this approach requiring more catheter and wire manipulation when compared to an approach under direct vision, the length of the OR table (if the procedure is performed in the OR) may add an additional challenge, as there will remain less space to hold all wires and equipment in an orderly fashion than an interventional cardiologist is usually accustomed to. Therefore, OR staff and the interventional cardiologist must work closely together and communicate well to avoid wires and other equipment accidentally "dropping" on the floor.

As a summary, hybrid therapy of vascular obstructions neither replaces transcatheter rehabilitation nor surgical angioplasty. However, it adds additional treatment modalities that include aspects of both approaches, which may in combination offer the most beneficial treatment strategy for a selected group of patients. An individualized approach is essential and should be founded on detailed planning and communication between surgical and interventional teams.

Hybrid Closure of Atrial Septal Defects and Ventricular Septal Defects

Hybrid Closure of Atrial Septal Defects

Anatomy
Hybrid closure of an atrial septal defect (ASD) usually entails closure of either patent foramen ovale or secundum ASDs.

Indications
In general most ASDs are able to be closed via percutaneous technique; however, periatrial ASD closure can be safe and effective in small children less than 1 year of age [57]. The approach can also be beneficial during other procedures such as patients with a ventricular septal defect (VSD) being closed via a periventricular approach.

Technique
As with the hybrid closure of VSD, described later, the hybrid closure of ASDs requires a team approach between the interventional cardiologist, the cardiothoracic surgeon, and the echocardiographer. This approach requires placing a purse string in the right atrial appendage and placing a needle across the defect, followed by wire and the delivery of the sheath [58]. Once the sheath is across, the ASD device can be positioned and deployed. This technique is very similar to the periventricular closure of VSD described in greater detail later [58].

A periatrial approach for closure of ASDs can be performed safely with limited morbidity in children. This approach can be useful in patients undergoing other procedures or for children who are smaller and cannot undergo closure via a percutaneous approach [14,57].

Hybrid Closure of Ventricular Septal Defects

Anatomy
The most frequent location is muscular VSDs, with certain apical VSDs being the most challenging to close. The apical

VSD can have inadequate room from the right ventricular (RV) free wall to deploy the RV disc appropriately. There have been reports of closing perimembranous VSDs with the periventricular closure technique.

Indications

The hybrid approach to closure of muscular VSDs was coined "periventricular closure" by Zahid Amin *et al.* [59,60]. Periventricular VSD closure can be beneficial in patients less than 5 kg [61] and either where surgical closure can be difficult to visualize or where cardiopulmonary bypass is not indicated. As with any other hybrid technique, the skills of both the interventional cardiologist and the cardiothoracic surgeon are employed. In addition, however, the guidance of an experienced echocardiographer is crucial with periventricular VSD closure.

Technique

The technique for periventricular closure of muscular VSDs has been detailed in several reports [62–64]. Usually a limited lower midline sternotomy (Plate 5.5, see plate section opposite p. 594) is performed, but a limited anterior thoracotomy can also be used. During the procedure a transesophageal ECHO is performed, but an epicardial ECHO is another option. An appropriate entry point at the RV free wall across from the VSD is selected under echocardiographic guidance, and a purse string is placed. The location should be directly across from the VSD to facilitate placing an 18-gauge, 2-inch needle through the purse string and directed toward the VSD, as depicted in Figure 5.3. Placing a slight bend in the needle facilitates directing the needle more directly toward the VSD. The echocardiographer must find the needle tip, which can be made more echogenic by scratching the tip with a bovie pad, to help align the tip with the VSD [65]. Subsequently, a 0.035-inch angled guide wire is advanced through the needle across

the VSD. The wire position is confirmed by echocardiography. Then a short 7-Fr delivery sheath is advanced over the wire across the VSD. Care must be taken to visualize the tip of the sheath to prevent inadvertent penetration of the left ventricular (LV) free wall. A technique to help avoid this complication is to tie a suture around the sheath before insertion to mark the maximum length to be advanced through the VSD. The VSD device is placed into the loader, attached to the delivery cable, and is de-aired. The loader is placed into the delivery sheath and delivered into the LV. The left-sided disc is deployed in the LV, avoiding pushing against the LV free wall. The sheath and device are pulled back into the VSD (Figure 5.4). Further pulling the sheath into the RV allows the RV disc to deploy. Before releasing the delivery cable, the ECHO is used to ensure that the VSD has no leaks around the device and there is no entrapment of the mitral or tricuspid valve. The delivery cable is released (Figure 5.5).

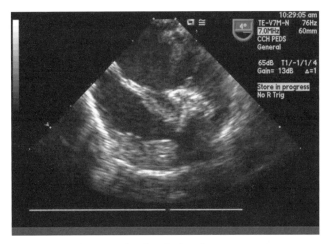

Figure 5.4 Left ventricular disc deployed.

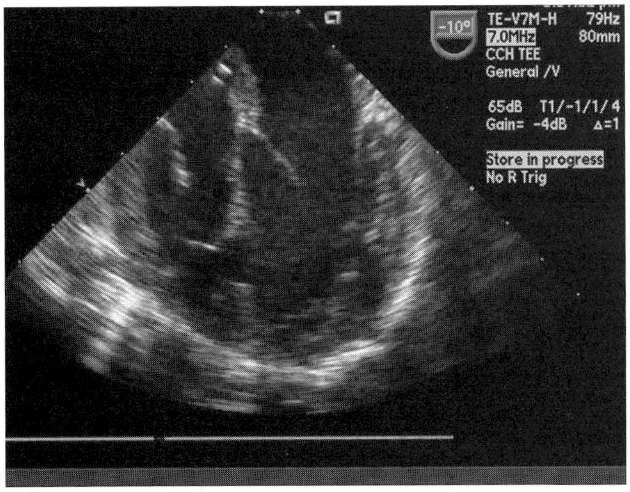

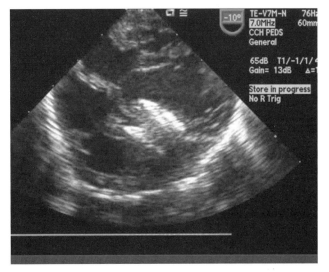

Figure 5.3 Needle across from the ventricular septal defect.

Figure 5.5 Ventricular septal defect closed with the device.

With further development of the techniques, these hybrid procedures will be able to be executed successfully using robotic assistance [66]. Hybrid periventricular approaches are most suited to patients who weigh less than 5 kg and without associated extracardiac anomalies that may increase the risks associated with surgical or transcatheter closure of these defects [65]. Percutaneous closure of mid-muscular VSDs is highly effective; however, reports have documented an increased risk associated with this procedure used for small patients [61]. These smaller patients do not tolerate the valve incompetence created by the wire loop and delivery sheath. Successful device implantation using the Amplatzer muscular VSD device as reported in a multicenter trial was achieved by 86.7% of the procedures, with a closure rate of 92.3% at the 12-month follow-up visit [61]. Patients weighing less than 5 kg had a greater number of major complications than larger patients. Both the periventricular and periatrial approach can be done safely with few complications [57,62,66].

Hybrid Approach for Hypoplastic Left Heart Syndrome

Introduction

The results of staged surgical palliation for HLHS have improved significantly over the years. Nonetheless, the overall morbidity and mortality of the initial Norwood procedure and its impact on the long-term success of the resulting Fontan circulation remain suboptimal [67]. Recent enthusiasm for the use of an RV-PA conduit instead of a modified Blalock-Taussig (BT) shunt during the Norwood procedure has not significantly changed the overall survival [68–70]. Important information about these two options will be forthcoming from the National Heart, Lung, and Blood Institute-sponsored, multicenter, prospective, randomized, clinical trial that is currently underway.

An alternative to the traditional Norwood approach is the hybrid approach for the management of HLHS. The primary goal of the hybrid approach is to create a stable, balanced circulation without the use of open-heart surgery (bypass, cross-clamp, circulatory arrest) with its associated risks in a neonate. The major open-heart surgical procedure is thereby shifted to later in life at an age when a circulation in series can be established with a cavopulmonary anastomosis.

Technique

To date we have experience with more than 100 hybrid stage 1 procedures, 60 comprehensive stage 2 procedures, and 25 Fontan completions in patients treated with this hybrid approach. Now, having developed a reliable, reproducible technique, we may impart some insights that may help lessen the learning curve for other groups adopting this strategy.

Hybrid Stage 1

The goals of initial palliation include: 1) unobstructed systemic output through the patent ductus arteriosus (PDA); 2) balanced pulmonary and systemic blood flows; and 3) an unobstructed ASD. This is currently accomplished by placing bilateral PA bands and a PDA stent via a median sternotomy as one hybrid procedure, followed by a balloon atrial septostomy several days later before discharge (Plate 5.6, see plate section opposite p. 594) [71]. Several lessons learned during this experience have led to our current approach.

Banding. Placing the bands before the stent is important. The PDA stent does not change the patient's hemodynamics or add any stability over an open PDA secondary to prostaglandin. However, adequately placed branch PA bands will improve the hemodynamics by balancing the circulation and improving systemic perfusion, which helps stabilize the patient for any subsequent procedures. Moreover, with the PDA stent in place the left PA is harder to isolate for banding and the stent is at greater risk for distortion while trying to encircle the left PA.

By fashioning the bands from Gore-Tex® (W.L. Gore & Associates, Flagstaff, AZ), some of the historical problems of dense scarring with potential loss of pulmonary segments on band removal have been eliminated. From a standard 3.5-mm tube graft (3 mm for weights <2 kg) an approximately 1 mm wide ring is cut to serve as the PA band. The ring is opened and passed around the right and left PAs. On the right, exposure is straightforward and the band is positioned on the right PA between the ascending aorta and SVC proximal to the right upper PA take-off. Exposure on the left is much more difficult. It is easier to visualize and maneuver a clamp around the left PA with the surgeon standing on the patient's left side, facilitating band placement right at the origin of the left PA. The bands are then tightened by reclosing the band with a 5-0 horizontal mattress suture. An additional stitch is placed through the band and tacked to the local adventitia to resist band migration.

The tightness of the band is an intraoperative decision based on the child's size, PA size, systemic blood pressure, and saturation response to tightening. However, experience has shown that bands closed to approximately 3.3 mm (slightly smaller than the original diameter of the shunt) will adequately balance the circulations and protect the pulmonary bed, while not becoming too tight with resultant cyanosis as the child grows to around 5.5 kg at 6 months of age, when the comprehensive stage 2 procedure is performed.

Stenting. Any transcatheter wire course through the HLHS heart can lead to hemodynamic compromise secondary to acute tricuspid and pulmonary valve insufficiency from wire distortion. This can lead to end-organ damage or, rarely, valve damage. Therefore, we now avoid any wire course through the heart by placing a sheath directly into the main PA above the pulmonary valve, through which the PDA stent can be deployed without crossing any valves. Moreover, by placing the sheath directly into the large main PA, vascular complications from groin access are eliminated, especially in the lower-weight neonates.

After the bands are placed, a 6-Fr sheath is placed in the main PA as proximally as possible just above the sinotubular junction. A silk suture is placed around the distal sheath approximately 2 mm from the tip to serve as an external marker for the surgeon as to how far to insert the sheath. This is important to avoid the sheath being inserted too far into the PA, thereby hindering deployment of the stent to cover the entire length of the PDA. A small hand injection of contrast through the sidearm of the sheath nicely defines the PDA, left PA, descending aorta, and retrograde aortic flow. The PDA length and diameter are measured at the distal, middle, and proximal ends, and the appropriate stent is chosen. Balloon-expandable or self-expandable stents can be used. The key is to be sure the entire length of ductal tissue is covered, which typically spans from the origin of the left PA to past the transverse aortic arch.

Atrial septostomy. Finally, creating an unrestrictive, durable, atrial septal communication in the HLHS heart is more difficult than using a standard balloon septostomy for other anomalies. This has to do with the size and location of the defect, the size of the left atrium, and the stability of the patient. We have varied the timing of the procedure, used other techniques (including static balloon dilatation with and without cutting balloons), and have even placed atrial septal stents. No technique yielded a reliable, reproducible result until our current approach. Now we simply delay the balloon septostomy by nearly a week, which allows some growth of the left atrium, thereby accommodating a 2-cc balloon and yielding a more substantial and durable opening in the atrial septum.

Interstage Monitoring

Close interstage monitoring has been the key to minimizing interstage mortality, as well as perioperative complications at the comprehensive stage 2 procedure. A home monitoring program coupled with a minimum of every-other-week cardiology assessment has been essential to the early detection of treatable problems. Echocardiography is used liberally to monitor for obstruction to flow across the ASD or through the PDA stent, antegrade or retrograde into the transverse aortic arch. Decreased RV function or increased tricuspid regurgitation can serve as another indicator of obstruction. Any evidence of obstruction or decreased ventricular function leads to a catheterization to diagnose and treat the level of obstruction.

Comprehensive Stage 2

This is a formidable operation. Despite the magnitude, the resultant circulation in series rather than in parallel outside of the neonatal period has been well tolerated. Unexpected benefits of the new initial hybrid palliation have been the growth of the native PAs and the transverse aortic arch. Because the transverse arch/innominate artery junction has grown, the aortic cannula can be positioned into the innominate artery during arch reconstruction, thereby removing the need for circulatory arrest with its associated risks. Moreover, much of the procedure can be done with the heart beating on bypass without aortic cross-clamping, thereby minimizing the period of cardiac ischemia.

The open-heart surgery consists of removal of the PDA stent and PA bands, repair of the aortic arch and PAs (if necessary), division of the diminutive ascending aorta with reimplantation into the pulmonary root, main PA to reconstructed aorta anastomosis, atrial septectomy with removal of the atrial stent (if present), and a modified cavopulmonary anastomosis (Plate 5.7, see plate section opposite p. 594) [71].

All of these steps are familiar to a pediatric cardiothoracic surgeon with single-ventricle experience, except for the removal of the PDA stent. This is the most intimidating aspect of the procedure because of the delicate nature of removing the distal part of the stent that continues into the descending thoracic aorta. However, aided by removing the time element of circulatory arrest, a reproducible technique of opening the stent longitudinally with a heavy scissors followed by gently peeling the stent out of the aorta has allowed the stent to be removed every time without injury to the aorta or local nerves. Hopefully, with future stent development specifically designed for this procedure, easier stent removal or, better yet, absorbable stents will make this significant technical hurdle obsolete for surgeons.

Results

Early reports on the initial outcomes of the hybrid approach [72–74] were limited by the impact of the learning curve of this new therapy, small cohorts of patients with mixed diagnoses and risk stratification, as well as short follow-up. Subsequent reports have focused on the use of the hybrid approach in high-risk HLHS patients [75–77]. Importantly, to truly assess the risks of the hybrid approach as compared to the Norwood approach, both stage 1 and 2 results as well as the interstage period must be considered. Recent reports from the groups in Columbus, Ohio and Geissen, Germany, show promising results with this emerging technique [71,78,79].

The goal of our report [71] was to evaluate the benefits and risks of the hybrid approach in a uniform cohort of patients with HLHS, including stage 1 and 2, so that a reasonable comparison can be made to patients treated with the Norwood approach. This is the largest single-institution experience with this hybrid approach, which is offered to all patients with HLHS. The only exclusion criterion is ECHO evidence of restricted flow into the retrograde transverse aorta from the ductus arteriosus. In this report patients with weights >1.5 kg were included even though 2.5 kg is commonly used as the cut-off for high risk.

Our results of the hybrid stage 1 procedure indicate a low-impact, low-risk procedure where 80% of patients are extubated and on enteral feeds within 24 hours, blood usage and inotropic support are rare, delayed sternal closure or extracorporeal membrane oxygenation (ECMO) are not necessary, the intensive care unit (ICU) stay is short, and hospital survival is 97.5%.

Interstage mortality (5%) and reintervention rates (36%) are similar to those reported for the Norwood procedure. Our reintervention rate may be high because we use close interstage monitoring with ECHO and take an aggressive approach to maintaining unrestricted flow through the PDA stent, both antegrade and retrograde, as well as maintaining an unrestricted atrial septal opening.

Only 10% of patients (4 of 40) developed significant retrograde stenosis into the transverse aorta. All were effectively treated by placing an additional retrograde stent and went on to a successful comprehensive stage 2. Given this low incidence we do not recommend a prophylactic reverse central shunt [80]. Moreover, given our experience in three patients with this type of shunt, the unknown physiology it creates with the potential of a coronary steal, and the more complicated postoperative course in patients with this shunt reported in the literature [81] we no longer use a reverse central shunt.

Although the comprehensive stage 2 procedure is a long operation involving essentially all the steps of a traditional Norwood stage 1 and 2 procedure, plus removal of the PDA stent and PA bands, the results show that the postoperative course is more similar to that of a Norwood stage 2 (Glenn) only. Our results indicate that the majority (85%) are extubated within 24 hours, inotropic support greater than the empiric use of milrinone (a cyclic adenosine monophosphate [AMP]-specific phosphodiesterase [PDE] inhibitor) is rare, RV function is preserved, and indicators of overall perfusion are normal by lactate, renal function, lack of seizures, and no ECMO requirements. This is presumably because the patients have a low-risk preoperative profile (normal ventricular function, no end-organ dysfunction, protected pulmonary bed). Then the conduct of the operation minimizes end-organ ischemia with the majority of the procedure performed on bypass with a beating heart and no circulatory arrest time, while the resultant circulation in series with a cavopulmonary shunt is more stable than a circulation in parallel, such as is the case with a Norwood stage 1. In conclusion, our study supports the use of the hybrid approach for the management of HLHS patients with the usual risk profile.

In the 25 patients who have undergone their Fontan completion after starting with a hybrid stage 1 palliation, there have been no deaths, no end-organ dysfunction, and only one patient was fenestrated. These results support the adequacy of branch PA banding in protecting the pulmonary vascular bed for a successful Fontan circulation.

Future

It is clear that this hybrid approach for palliating complex neonatal patients is an additional technique that will only improve over time as experience is accrued. Long-term follow-up and multicenter trials will be important to more clearly define which cohorts of patients gain the most at the lowest risk from this technique. Another area of research and potential benefit of the hybrid stage 1 procedure is the benefit of delaying the necessity of bypass until the brain is more developed. There is a growing body of knowledge that suggests that the developing brain, especially in those with complex congenital heart disease, may be more vulnerable to injury in the neonatal period [82–85]. Hence, a delay in exposure to cardiopulmonary bypass, the associated inflammatory response, and some of the hemodynamic consequences, may have the benefit of better long-term neurologic outcomes.

Completion Angiography in the Cardiac Operating Suite

Postoperative significant residual structural pathology after cardiopulmonary bypass surgery is associated with increased morbidity and poor outcome [45,47]. Intraoperative ECHO imaging has evolved as an essential tool to assess immediate intracardiac and, to some extent, extracardiac surgical repairs [86]. It provides not only important physiologic parameters that may aid in the postoperative management of these patients, but more importantly allows identification of important residual defects at a time when intraoperative surgical or hybrid therapy can still easily be delivered. However, while ECHO is very helpful in assessing ventricular and valvar function and identifying residual septal defects, its use is limited when assessing for residual vascular stenoses within the aorta, coronary, or branch PAs [87,88].

Delayed recognition of residual structural pathology that is not easily identifiable by ECHO, may lead to a compromised and complicated postoperative course. Once a patient deteriorates and has to be taken to the cardiac catheterization laboratory in the postoperative period the prognosis is usually poor [46]. Asoh and colleagues recently reported on 49 children who underwent 62 cardiac catheterization procedures before discharge from ICU and found an overall mortality of 43%, as compared with 5% in patients who did not require cardiac catheterization. Delay to cardiac catheterization of >2–3 weeks was found to be a significant risk factor for death [46].

Angiography may complement the available intraoperative imaging modalities. While completion angiography can be readily performed using a standard C-arm, it is more difficult to obtain when compared with a specifically designed hybrid OR and requires some "planning ahead," with a longer setup and preparation time. A portable C-arm usually needs to be requested in advance, and provisions must be made for adequate archiving of the obtained images. Sufficient space has to be made available when moving in the C-arm. It is much easier to adjust for those requirements at the beginning of a procedure, rather than having to adjust intravenous (IV) poles and drapes in the middle of a case. While most staff can easily step back during image acquisition, the surgeon usually has to remain at the operating table; therefore, some radiation protection must be provided. A lightweight and practical solution is the provision of radiation protection pads that can be attached to the surgical gown using vascular clamps [89]. Obtaining the necessary angiographic projections can be a challenge, especially if using very steep projections where the X-ray tube may impinge on the surgical OR table. To overcome this limitation, one has to tilt the OR table in a way to provide more angulations, without further moving the C-arm.

Once adequately planned, the angiographic evaluation itself is usually fairly straightforward and does not require significant time. In most circumstances, a traditional Berman angiographic catheter is introduced directly through a purse-string suture and positioned by the cardiothoracic surgeon. Alternatively, a hemostatic sheath can be inserted, which facilitates the additional use of guide wires and other catheters, which can be particularly helpful when having to advance a catheter around the aortic arch. The insertion site depends on the vascular structure that requires evaluation. As an example, after a bidirectional Glenn procedure or comprehensive stage 2 palliation for complex single-ventricle physiology, the catheter is placed in the SVC, whereas after repair of tetralogy of Fallot or pulmonary atresia with VSD, the catheter is usually placed in the main PA or RV. Most angiograms are usually performed with low flow, or briefly off cardiopulmonary bypass.

Limited data are available on intraoperative angiography [17,53]. Holzer et al. retrospectively reviewed completion angiography in 15 patients after cardiac surgical procedures performed in a specially designed hybrid operating suite [2]. The underlying surgical repairs included a variety of procedures such as comprehensive stage 2 palliation for HLHS, aortic arch reconstruction, conduit or pulmonary valve replacement, and others. Completion angiograms confirmed expected results in 47% of patients, while 53% identified unexpected abnormalities or residual lesions, and 40% of these underwent hybrid therapy at the same procedure [53]. Figure 5.6 is an example.

It is clear that significant residual structural pathology should be treated as soon as identified, and Zahn et al. have shown interventional therapy can be safely delivered to very fresh suture lines [45]. However, doing so in the OR with cardiopulmonary bypass readily available adds an

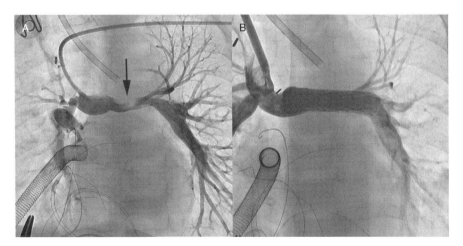

Figure 5.6 6-month-old male infant with HLHS and a past history of hybrid stage 1 palliation. **A,** Comprehensive stage 2 palliation was performed and an intraoperative completion angiogram documented a significant stenosis from a fold in the mid-portion of the LPA (arrow) with some swirling of contrast. **B,** A 25-mm Genesis XD stent was implanted and expanded to 7 mm with excellent angiographic result. (HLHS, hypoplastic left heart syndrome; LPA, left pulmonary artery.)

extra safety margin when compared to a procedure performed in a hemodynamically unstable patient 1 week postoperatively in the cardiac catheterization laboratory. However, despite very strong reasons to avoid residual structural pathology, at this point it is still unclear which lesions require immediate action, which ones can be monitored closely with delayed intervention, and which ones do not require any form of treatment. Angiographic imaging, especially after comprehensive stage 2 palliation, may be misleading, and the combination of an open chest and cardiopulmonary bypass can make interpretation of the images difficult. Equally, it is unclear which surgical repairs may benefit from routine postoperative evaluation. Whether ultimately angiography is routinely performed only in a small group of procedures, such as bidirectional Glenn or PA rehabilitation, or may include a wider spectrum of vascular procedures remains to be defined. Importantly, though, the decision on whether any identified lesion is significant and warrants surgical or hybrid palliation is a collaborative one made by the surgeon and the interventional cardiologist.

In summary, completion angiography complements the available intraoperative imaging modalities and may aid in early identification of significant residual structural pathology. Cooperation between surgical and interventional teams is essential during planning, set-up, and performance of the procedure, as well as during interpretation of the angiographic data. Prospective studies are ongoing to better identify the group of patients that benefit from completion angiography and how to identify pathology that should be treated in the OR.

Hybrid Approach to Valve Replacement

Philip Bonhoeffer's landmark report of the first successful percutaneous implant of a transcatheter pulmonary valve using the NuMED CP stent (NuMED, Inc, Hopkinton, NY) and the Contegra bovine jugular vein graft (Medtronic, Inc, Minneapolis, MN) started a new era in the nonsurgical treatment of congenital heart disease [90]. Within 2 years, Alain Cribier followed with the first successful percutaneous implant of the Cribier–Edwards Transcatheter Heart Valve (later Edwards-SAPIEN THV, Edwards LifeSciences, Irving, CA) in the aortic position [91]. Over the past decade, there have been numerous companies attempting to design and manufacture the "perfect" valve replacement that can be delivered percutaneously through a standard transfemoral vein or artery approach. The delivery systems have steadily decreased in size from 25 Fr to 18 Fr. Currently, the Edwards-SAPIEN THV (Edwards LifeSciences, Irving, CA) and the CoreValve ReValve System (CoreValve, Irving, CA) have gained CE Mark approval in Europe for percutaneous aortic valve replacement, while the Medtronic Melody

Transcatheter Pulmonary Valve (TPV) (Medtronic, Inc, Minneapolis, MN) also has CE Mark approval for percutaneous pulmonary valve replacement in RV-PA conduits. There are currently as many as 17 percutaneous aortic valve replacement prosthesis clinical trials worldwide, with at least seven more with First in Man implant results, and others at different stages of development at this time. There are currently two clinical trials evaluating percutaneous pulmonary valve replacement and two trials evaluating percutaneous aortic valve replacement in the United States as of this writing.

However, what happens when the usual transfemoral artery or vein are not suitable for delivery? In fact, because of the large delivery system required for transfemoral arterial implant of an aortic valve, the cardiac surgeon has been involved in the procedure to provide access via cut down, arteriotomy, and vascular closure. In addition, the surgeon places the patient on cardiopulmonary bypass as needed. However, up until recently, the cardiac surgeon had not participated in the transfemoral venous approach to percutaneous pulmonary valve replacement, although was integrally involved in the clinical trials and valve design.

A hybrid approach using transapical transcatheter aortic valve implantation techniques has been developed recently, especially in those patients with increased age, and many comorbidities such as cerebral vascular disease, low ejection fraction, pulmonary hypertension, respiratory insufficiency, chronic renal failure, and peripheral arterial occlusive disease. The first approved multicenter clinical trial for transapical minimally invasive aortic valve implantation was reported recently [92]. The team consisted of cardiac surgeons and interventional cardiologists using the Bovine Pericardial Xenograft mounted on a balloon expandable low profile stainless steel stent (Edwards-SAPIEN THV, Edwards LifeSciences). Access to the LV apex was gained through a left anterolateral mini thoracotomy in the fifth intercostal space with horizontal opening of the pericardium. Teflon-reinforced purse-string sutures were placed in the LV apex with temporary pacing wires and femoral cannulation for possible cardiopulmonary bypass. A 14-Fr soft sheath was inserted in guide wire position to cross the stenotic aortic valve. Balloon aortic valvuloplasty was performed initially with a 20mm balloon and rapid RV pacing. Afterwards, the sheath was exchanged for a 33-Fr transapical valve delivery system. Either a 23mm or 26mm Edwards-SAPIEN THV was implanted (Plate 5.8, see plate section opposite p. 594). The average EuroScore predicted risk mortality was $27 \pm 14\%$ for the 59 patients in the study. In-hospital mortality was actually only 13.6% without any valve dysfunction. Actuarial survival was $75.7 \pm 5.9\%$ at 110 ± 77 days follow-up.

One of the most important aspects of this multicenter trial was the transnational team approach used by the cardiac surgeons, as well as the excellent collaboration with the interventional cardiologists, anesthesiologists, and perfusionists. Future refinements in sutureless devices are being made, as well as improvement in image guided assistance using three-dimensional computed tomography and transesophageal echocardiography data sets. Miniaturization of the delivery system will continue to evolve and may someday preclude mini thoracotomy. There has also been a recent report of deploying a CoreValve ReValving System through an 18-Fr introducer through the ascending aorta in a hybrid setting [93].

While hybrid delivery has been advocated and useful in the delivery of transcatheter aortic valve implants for all of the previously mentioned reasons, the same cannot be said of transcatheter pulmonary valve implantation. With the venous system able to accommodate a large diameter delivery sheath and the readily accessible femoral, jugular, and subclavian veins, there was no real "urgency" in developing a hybrid approach in the typical patient with a degenerating RV to PA valved conduit. One could even use a transhepatic venous approach if necessary. However, significant pulmonary regurgitation (PR) remains a long-term problem after surgical or percutaneous treatment of numerous congenital cardiac defects. The current Medtronic Melody TPV (18, 20, and 22 mm expanded diameters) delivered percutaneously in degenerating RV-PA conduits, while very effective and safe, only addresses approximately 13% of all affected patients with PR. In addition, delivering in small children may prove problematic. In 2006, 4 years after Dr Bonhoeffer's landmark report, the Shelhigh Injectable Stented Pulmonic Valve (Shelhigh, Inc, Union, NJ) was implanted off-pump by cardiac surgery [94]. In 2008, a multicenter study reported 12 patients ranging from 5.8–53.5 years with severe PR and dilated RV who underwent successful off-pump implant of the above Shelhigh Pulmonic Valve [95]. The prosthesis consists of a porcine pulmonic valve inside a tube of bovine pericardium mounted on a self-expandable Nitinol stent with sizes ranging from 17–31 mm. The valve was delivered through a purse-string suture in the distal RV outflow tract and transmural sutures are used to avoid migration. Also in 2008, a hybrid pulmonary valve implant was reported using the Shelhigh Injectable Stented Pulmonic Valve through the main PA, rather than the RV outflow tract [96].

Two reports in 2009 emphasized the continued interest in developing a hybrid approach to pulmonary valve replacement [97,98]. Feasibility studies using a transapical approach and an RV outflow tract approach in pigs and sheep, respectively, highlighted two new device designs. Both were a modification of the original Bonhoeffer–Medtronic concept using a bovine jugular vein graft (Contegra Pulmonary Valved Conduit, Medtronic, Inc) that was modified with a second endoprosthesis that was based on a self-expandable Nitinol graft. Both studies give promise for further clinical trials in the future. As a matter of fact, Professor Bonhoeffer has recently successfully implanted a (First in Man) modified Melody Transcatheter TPV in the native RV outflow tract using a self-expandable Nitinol graft in a young man in Milan, Italy with severe PR (personal communication with Dr Bonhoeffer).

Summary

Hybrid strategies for complex congenital and structural heart disease are here to stay and will only grow as the collaborative spirit between cardiac surgeons, interventional cardiologists, and other members of the heart center becomes "one voice, one team."

References

1. Cheatham JP. (2009) How to build a hybrid congenital heart disease program. In: Hijazi ZM, Feldman T, Cheatham J, et al., eds. *Complications During Percutaneous Interventions for Congenital and Structural Heart Disease*. Abingdon: Informa Healthcare, pp. 31–40.
2. Holzer RJ, Chisolm JL, Hill SL, et al. (2008) "Hybrid" stent delivery in the pulmonary circulation. J Invasive Cardiol 20, 592–598.
3. Ungerleider RM, Johnston TA, O'Laughlin MP, et al. (2001) Intraoperative stents to rehabilitate severely stenotic pulmonary vessels. Ann Thorac Surg 71, 476–481.
4. Coles JG, Yemets I, Najm HK, et al. (1995) Experience with repair of congenital heart defects using adjunctive endovascular devices. J Thorac Cardiovasc Surg 110, 1513–1519; discussion 1519–1520.
5. Bacha EA, Hijazi ZM, Cao QL, et al. (2005) Hybrid pediatric cardiac surgery. Pediatr Cardiol 26, 315–322.
6. Bacha EA, Hijazi ZM. (2005) Hybrid procedures in pediatric cardiac surgery. Semin Thorac Cardiovasc Surg Pediatr Card Surg Annu 78–85.
7. Bacha EA, Kreutzer J. (2001) Comprehensive management of branch pulmonary artery stenosis. J Interv Cardiol 14, 367–375.
8. Ing FF, Grifka RG, Nihill MR, et al. (1995) Repeat dilation of intravascular stents in congenital heart defects. Circulation 92, 893–897.
9. Mullins CE, O'Laughlin MP, Vick GW 3rd, et al. (1988) Implantation of balloon-expandable intravascular grafts by catheterization in pulmonary arteries and systemic veins. Circulation 77, 188–199.
10. O'Laughlin MP, Perry SB, Lock JE, et al. (1991) Use of endovascular stents in congenital heart disease. Circulation 83, 1923–1939.
11. Bacha EA, Marshall AC, McElhinney DB, et al. (2007) Expanding the hybrid concept in congenital heart surgery. Semin Thorac Cardiovasc Surg Pediatr Card Surg Annu 146–150.
12. Hjortdal VE, Redington AN, de Leval MR, et al. (2002) Hybrid approaches to complex congenital cardiac surgery. Eur J Cardiothorac Surg 22, 885–890.

13. Huebler M, Boettcher W, Koster A, et al. (2007) Hybrid approach facilitates use of a minimized CPB circuit and transfusion free surgery in an extended Norwood stage II procedure. J Card Surg 22, 508–510.

14. Schmitz C, Esmailzadeh B, Herberg U, et al. (2008) Hybrid procedures can reduce the risk of congenital cardiovascular surgery. Eur J Cardiothorac Surg 34, 718–725.

15. Kawata M, Kataoka T, Kuramoto E, et al. (2004) Pulmonary artery stenosis due to external compression by a calcified pericardial band. Jpn Heart J 45, 527–533.

16. Fogelman R, Nykanen D, Smallhorn JF, et al. (1995) Endovascular stents in the pulmonary circulation. Clinical impact on management and medium-term follow-up. Circulation 92, 881–885.

17. Ing FF. (2005) Delivery of stents to target lesions: techniques of intraoperative stent implantation and intraoperative angiograms. Pediatr Cardiol 26, 260–266.

18. Stanfill R, Nykanen DG, Osorio S, et al. (2008) Stent implantation is effective treatment of vascular stenosis in young infants with congenital heart disease: acute implantation and long-term follow-up results. Catheter Cardiovasc Interv 71, 831–841.

19. Mitropoulos FA, Laks H, Kapadia N, et al. (2007) Intraoperative pulmonary artery stenting: an alternative technique for the management of pulmonary artery stenosis. Ann Thorac Surg 84, 1338–1341; discussion 1342.

20. Bokenkamp R, Blom NA, De Wolf D, et al. (2005) Intraoperative stenting of pulmonary arteries. Eur J Cardiothorac Surg 27, 544–547.

21. Chiu KM, Chen JS, Yeh SJ, et al. (2005) Hybrid angioplasty for left pulmonary artery stenosis after total correction of tetralogy of Fallot: report of one case. Acta Paediatr Taiwan 46, 174–177.

22. Menon SC, Cetta F, Dearani JA, et al. (2008) Hybrid intraoperative pulmonary artery stent placement for congenital heart disease. Am J Cardiol 102, 1737–1741.

23. Santoro G, Caianiello G, Rossi G, et al. (2008) Hybrid transcatheter-surgical strategy in arterial tortuosity syndrome. Ann Thorac Surg 86, 1682–1684.

24. Holt DB, Moller JH, Larson S, et al. (2007) Primary pulmonary vein stenosis. Am J Cardiol 99, 568–572.

25. Latson LA, Prieto LR. (2007) Congenital and acquired pulmonary vein stenosis. Circulation 115, 103–108.

26. Devaney EJ, Chang AC, Ohye RG, et al. (2006) Management of congenital and acquired pulmonary vein stenosis. Ann Thorac Surg 81, 992–995; discussion 995–996.

27. Mendelsohn AM, Bove EL, Lupinetti FM, et al. (1993) Intraoperative and percutaneous stenting of congenital pulmonary artery and vein stenosis. Circulation 88, II210–217.

28. Santoro G, Formigari R, Mazzera E, et al. (1996) [Intraoperative stent implantation in congenital stenosis of pulmonary veins.] G Ital Cardiol 26, 201–205.

29. Jhang WK, Chang YJ, Park CS, et al. (2008) Hybrid palliation for right atrial isomerism associated with obstructive total anomalous pulmonary venous drainage. Interact Cardiovasc Thorac Surg 7, 282–284.

30. Ewert P, Peters B, Nagdyman N, et al. (2008) Early and mid-term results with the Growth Stent – a possible concept for transcatheter treatment of aortic coarctation from infancy to adulthood by stent implantation? Catheter Cardiovasc Interv 71, 120–126.

31. Radtke WA, Waller BR, Hebra A, et al. (2002) Palliative stent implantation for aortic coarctation in premature infants weighing <1,500 g. Am J Cardiol 90, 1409–1412.

32. Zabal C, Attie F, Rosas M, et al. (2003) The adult patient with native coarctation of the aorta: balloon angioplasty or primary stenting? Heart 89, 77–83.

33. Rodes-Cabau J, Miro J, Dancea A, et al. (2007) Comparison of surgical and transcatheter treatment for native coarctation of the aorta in patients > or = 1 year old. The Quebec Native Coarctation of the Aorta study. Am Heart J 154, 186–192.

34. Fiore AC, Fischer LK, Schwartz T, et al. (2005) Comparison of angioplasty and surgery for neonatal aortic coarctation. Ann Thorac Surg 80, 1659–1664; discussion 1664–1665.

35. Forbes TJ, Moore P, Pedra CA, et al. (2007) Intermediate follow-up following intravascular stenting for treatment of coarctation of the aorta. Catheter Cardiovasc Interv 70, 569–577.

36. Forbes TJ, Garekar S, Amin Z, et al. (2007) Procedural results and acute complications in stenting native and recurrent coarctation of the aorta in patients over 4 years of age: a multi-institutional study. Catheter Cardiovasc Interv 70, 276–285.

37. Holzer RJ, Chisolm JL, Hill SL, et al. (2008) Stenting complex aortic arch obstructions. Catheter Cardiovasc Interv 71, 375–382.

38. Carrel TP, Berdat PA, Baumgartner I, et al. (2004) Combined surgical and endovascular approach to treat a complex aortic coarctation without extracorporeal circulation. Ann Thorac Surg 78, 1462–1465.

39. McMahon CJ, El-Said HG, Grifka RG, et al. (2001) Redilation of endovascular stents in congenital heart disease: factors implicated in the development of restenosis and neointimal proliferation. J Am Coll Cardiol 38, 521–526.

40. Duke C, Rosenthal E, Qureshi SA. (2003) The efficacy and safety of stent redilatation in congenital heart disease. Heart 89, 905–912.

41. von Schnakenburg C, Fink C, Peuster M. (2002) Histology of a stented aortic segment with critical coarctation 10 months after implantation. Cardiol Young 12, 288–289.

42. Nakatogawa T, Hibi K, Furukawa E, et al. (2004) Impact of peri-stent remodeling on in-stent neointimal proliferation in acute myocardial infarction. Am J Cardiol 94, 769–771.

43. Murphy JD, Sands BL, Norwood WI. (1987) Intraoperative balloon angioplasty of aortic coarctation in infants with hypoplastic left heart syndrome. Am J Cardiol 59, 949–951.

44. Shiraishi I, Yamagishi M, Oka T, et al. (2000) Intraoperative balloon angioplasty for aortic coarctation after Norwood operation. Ann Thorac Surg 70, 289–291.

45. Zahn EM, Dobrolet NC, Nykanen DG, et al. (2004) Interventional catheterization performed in the early postoperative period after congenital heart surgery in children. J Am Coll Cardiol 43, 1264–1269.

46. Asoh K, Hickey E, Dorostkar P, et al. (2008) Outcomes of emergent cardiac catheterization following pediatric cardiac surgery. Catheter Cardiovasc Interv 71, S5 Abstract.

47. Di Russo GB, Martin GR. (2005) Extracorporeal membrane oxygenation for cardiac disease: no longer a mistaken diag-

nosis. Semin Thorac Cardiovasc Surg Pediatr Card Surg Annu 34–40.

48. Holzer R, Hill SL, Chisolm JL, *et al.* (2006) PA rehabilitation using endovascular stenting in children with weight below 15 kg : "stents are for kids, too". Catheter Cardiovasc Interv 68, 461. Abstract.

49. Ing F. (2002) Stents: what's available to the pediatric interventional cardiologist? Catheter Cardiovasc Interv 57, 374–386.

50. Holzer R, Hijazi Z. (2008) The off-versus on-label use of medical devices in interventional cardiovascular medicine?: Clarifying the ambiguity between regulatory labeling and clinical decision making, part III: structural heart disease interventions. Catheter Cardiovasc Interv 72, 848–852.

51. Elliott MJ, Kanani M. (2005) The hows and whys of intraoperative imaging. Cardiol Young 15(Suppl 1), 179–183.

52. Ohye RG, Cohen DM, Wheller JJ, *et al.* (1999) Quantitative digital angiography as an adjunct to the intraoperative placement of endovascular stents in congenital heart disease. J Card Surg 14, 181–184.

53. Holzer R, Hill SL, Chisolm JL, *et al.* (2008) Exit angiography in a dedicated "hybrid OR suite" – initial experience. Catheter Cardiovasc Interv 71, Abstract O21.

54. Brunelli F, Amaducci A, Danzi GB. (2005) Intra-operative stenting of a prosthetic left pulmonary artery stenosis under fluoroscopy. J Invasive Cardiol 17, 98–99.

55. Zartner P, Cesnjevar R, Singer H, *et al.* (2005) First successful implantation of a biodegradable metal stent into the left pulmonary artery of a preterm baby. Catheter Cardiovasc Interv 66, 590–594.

56. Davenport JJ, Lam L, Whalen-Glass R, *et al.* (2008) The successful use of alternative routes of vascular access for performing pediatric interventional cardiac catheterization. Catheter Cardiovasc Interv 72, 392–398.

57. Diab KA, Cao QL, Bacha EA, *et al.* (2007) Device closure of atrial septal defects with the Amplatzer septal occluder: safety and outcome in infants. J Thorac Cardiovasc Surg 134, 960–966.

58. Vasilyev NV, Martinez JF, Freudenthal FP, *et al.* (2006) Three-dimensional echo and videocardioscopy-guided atrial septal defect closure. Ann Thorac Surg 82, 1322–1326; discussion 1326.

59. Amin Z, Gu X, Berry JM, *et al.* (1999) New device for closure of muscular ventricular septal defects in a canine model. Circulation 100, 320–328.

60. Amin Z, Gu X, Berry JM, *et al.* (1999) Perventricular closure of ventricular septal defects without cardiopulmonary bypass. Ann Thorac Surg 68, 149–153; discussion 153–154.

61. Holzer R, Balzer D, Cao QL, *et al.* (2004) Device closure of muscular ventricular septal defects using the Amplatzer muscular ventricular septal defect occluder: immediate and mid-term results of a US registry. J Am Coll Cardiol 43, 1257–1263.

62. Bacha EA, Cao QL, Galantowicz ME, *et al.* (2005) Multicenter experience with perventricular device closure of muscular ventricular septal defects. Pediatr Cardiol 26, 169–175.

63. Bacha EA, Cao QL, Starr JP, *et al.* (2003) Perventricular device closure of muscular ventricular septal defects on the beating heart: technique and results. J Thorac Cardiovasc Surg 126, 1718–1723.

64. Diab KA, Hijazi ZM, Cao QL, *et al.* (2005) A truly hybrid approach to perventricular closure of multiple muscular ventricular septal defects. J Thorac Cardiovasc Surg 130, 892–893.

65. Phillips AB, Green J, Bergdall V, *et al.* (2009) Teaching the "hybrid approach": a novel swine model of muscular ventricular septal defect. Pediatr Cardiol 30, 114–118.

66. Amin Z, Woo R, Danford DA, *et al.* (2006) Robotically assisted perventricular closure of perimembranous ventricular septal defects: preliminary results in Yucatan pigs. J Thorac Cardiovasc Surg 131, 427–432.

67. Ashburn DA, McCrindle BW, Tchervenkov CI, *et al.* (2003) Outcomes after the Norwood operation in neonates with critical aortic stenosis or aortic valve atresia. J Thorac Cardiovasc Surg 125, 1070–1082.

68. Cua CL, Thiagarajan RR, Gauvreau K, *et al.* (2006) Early postoperative outcomes in a series of infants with hypoplastic left heart syndrome undergoing stage I palliation operation with either modified Blalock–Taussig shunt or right ventricle to pulmonary artery conduit. Pediatr Crit Care Med 7, 238–244.

69. Lai L, Laussen PC, Cua CL, *et al.* (2007) Outcomes after bidirectional Glenn operation: Blalock–Taussig shunt versus right ventricle-to-pulmonary artery conduit. Ann Thorac Surg 83, 1768–1773.

70. Tabbutt S, Dominguez TE, Ravishankar C, *et al.* (2005) Outcomes after the stage I reconstruction comparing the right ventricular to pulmonary artery conduit with the modified Blalock Taussig shunt. Ann Thorac Surg 80, 1582–1590; discussion 1590–1591.

71. Galantowicz M, Cheatham JP, Phillips A, *et al.* (2008) Hybrid approach for hypoplastic left heart syndrome: intermediate results after the learning curve. Ann Thorac Surg 85, 2063–2070; discussion 2070–2071.

72. Galantowicz M, Cheatham JP. (2005) Lessons learned from the development of a new hybrid strategy for the management of hypoplastic left heart syndrome. Pediatr Cardiol 26, 190–199.

73. Akintuerk H, Michel-Behnke I, Valeske K, *et al.* (2002) Stenting of the arterial duct and banding of the pulmonary arteries: basis for combined Norwood stage I and II repair in hypoplastic left heart. Circulation 105, 1099–1103.

74. Michel-Behnke I, Akintuerk H, Marquardt I, *et al.* (2003) Stenting of the ductus arteriosus and banding of the pulmonary arteries: basis for various surgical strategies in newborns with multiple left heart obstructive lesions. Heart 89, 645–650.

75. Bacha EA, Daves S, Hardin J, *et al.* (2006) Single-ventricle palliation for high-risk neonates: the emergence of an alternative hybrid stage I strategy. J Thorac Cardiovasc Surg 131, 163–171 e2.

76. Lim DS, Peeler BB, Matherne GP, *et al.* (2006) Risk-stratified approach to hybrid transcatheter-surgical palliation of hypoplastic left heart syndrome. Pediatr Cardiol 27, 91–95.

77. Pizarro C, Murdison KA. (2005) Off pump palliation for hypoplastic left heart syndrome: surgical approach. Semin Thorac Cardiovasc Surg Pediatr Card Surg Annu 66–71.

78. Galantowicz M, Cheatham JP. (2007) A hybrid strategy for the initial management of hypoplastic left heart syndrome: Technical considerations. In: Sievert H, Qureshi SA, Wilson N, *et al.*, eds. *Percutaneous Interventions for Congenital Heart Disease*. Abingdon: Informa Healthcare, pp. 531–538.

79. Akinturk H, Michel-Behnke I, Valeske K, *et al.* (2007) Hybrid transcatheter-surgical palliation: basis for univentricular or biventricular repair: the Giessen experience. Pediatr Cardiol 28, 79–87.

80. Caldarone CA, Benson LN, Holtby H, *et al.* (2005) Main pulmonary artery to innominate artery shunt during hybrid palliation of hypoplastic left heart syndrome. J Thorac Cardiovasc Surg 130(4), e1–2.

81. Li J, Zhang G, Benson L, *et al.* (2007) Comparison of the profiles of postoperative systemic hemodynamics and oxygen transport in neonates after the hybrid or the Norwood procedure; a pilot study. Circulation 116(Suppl 1), 179–187.

82. Wernovsky G, Shillingford AJ, Gaynor JW. (2005) Central nervous system outcomes in children with complex congenital heart disease. Curr Opin Cardiol 20, 94–99.

83. Glauser TA, Rorke LB, Weinberg PM, *et al.* (1990) Congenital brain anomalies associated with the hypoplastic left heart syndrome. Pediatrics 85, 984–990.

84. Licht DJ, Shera DM, Clancy RR, *et al.* (2009) Brain maturation is delayed in infants with complex congenital heart defects. J Thorac Cardiovasc Surg 137, 529–536; discussion 536–537.

85. Mahle WT, Tavani F, Zimmerman RA, *et al.* (2002) An MRI study of neurological injury before and after congenital heart surgery. Circulation 106(suppl 1), 109–114.

86. Balmer C, Barron D, Wright JG, *et al.* (2006) Experience with intraoperative ultrasound in paediatric cardiac surgery. Cardiol Young 16, 455–462.

87. Rosenfeld HM, Gentles TL, Wernovsky G, *et al.* (1998) Utility of intraoperative transesophageal echocardiography in the assessment of residual cardiac defects. Pediatr Cardiol 19, 346–351.

88. Randolph GR, Hagler DJ, Connolly HM, *et al.* (2002) Intraoperative transesophageal echocardiography during surgery for congenital heart defects. J Thorac Cardiovasc Surg 124, 1176–1182.

89. Sawdy JM, Gocha MD, Olshove V, *et al.* (2009) Radiation protection during hybrid procedures: innovation creates new challenges. J Invasive Cardiol 21, 437–440.

90. Bonhoeffer P, Boudjemline Y, Saliba Z, *et al.* (2000) Percutaneous replacement of pulmonary valve in a right-ventricle to pulmonary-artery prosthetic conduit with valve dysfunction. Lancet 356, 1403–1405.

91. Cribier A, Eltchaninoff H, Bash A, *et al.* (2002) Percutaneous transcatheter implantation of an aortic valve prosthesis for calcific aortic stenosis: first human case description. Circulation 106, 3006–3008.

92. Walther T, Simon P, Dewey T, *et al.* (2007) Transapical minimally invasive aortic valve implantation: multicenter experience. Circulation 116(suppl 1), I240–I245.

93. Bauernschmitt R, Schreiber C, Bleiziffer S, *et al.* (2009) Transcatheter aortic valve implantation through the ascending aorta: an alternative option for no-access patients. Heart Surg Forum 12, E63–64.

94. Berdat PA, Carrel T. (2006) Off-pump pulmonary valve replacement with the new Shelhigh Injectable Stented Pulmonic Valve. J Thorac Cardiovasc Surg 131, 1192–1193.

95. Marianeschi SM, Santoro F, Ribera E, *et al.* (2008) Pulmonary valve implantation with the new Shelhigh Injectable Stented Pulmonic Valve. Ann Thorac Surg 86, 1466–1471; discussion 1472.

96. Dittrich S, Gloeckler M, Arnold R, *et al.* (2008) Hybrid pulmonary valve implantation: injection of a self-expanding tissue valve through the main pulmonary artery. Ann Thorac Surg 85, 632–634.

97. Huber CH, Hurni M, Tsang V, *et al.* (2009) Valved stents for transapical pulmonary valve replacement. J Thorac Cardiovasc Surg 137, 914–918.

98. Meng GW, Zhou JY, Tang Y, *et al.* (2009) Off-pump pulmonary valve implantation of a valved stent with an anchoring mechanism. Ann Thorac Surg 87, 597–601.

CHAPTER 6

Anesthesia for the Patient with Congenital Heart Disease

H. Jay Przybylo

Ann & Robert H. Lurie Children's Hospital of Chicago, formerly Children's Memorial Hospital, Northwestern University Feinberg School of Medicine, Chicago, IL, USA

The contemporary era of surgical intervention to correct congenital heart defects began when Robert Gross performed the first successful ligation of a patent ductus arteriosus in 1938 [1]. At that time medications for pediatric anesthesia consisted of volatile general anesthetic agents and narcotic analgesics. Today, more than 70 years after Gross' landmark operation, some of these medications are still an integral part of the anesthetic regimen for pediatric patients undergoing cardiac surgical procedures. Nevertheless, this is an era of great change, in that modern pediatric anesthesiologists continually strive to provide safer operating conditions for the patient. These include monitoring techniques and therapies that limit or prevent complications from the underlying cardiac disease or the techniques used for correction. Currently, we are working on strategies to prevent complications resulting from the inflammatory response to cardiopulmonary bypass and to provide better brain protection during artificial or altered circulation [2]. Also, there has been an expansion of pediatric cardiac anesthesia care outside of the conventional operating room including the cardiac catheterization suite, interventional radiology, computed tomography scanner, and magnetic resonance imaging center [3]. Perhaps the greatest changes we are experiencing are the collection, analysis, and distribution of data. Improvements in speed and storage capability of information technology allow studies of large samples to be easily collected and transmitted worldwide.

Demographics

In recent years a trend has emerged in that there has been an increase in the number of hospital admissions for older patients with a primary diagnosis of congenital heart disease, and at the same time, a decrease in overall mortality in this patient population [4]. As more children with congenital heart disease survive to adulthood many of them will require revision of previous surgical interventions or further diagnostic and therapeutic procedures. The American Heart Association estimates that there are approximately 800 000 people alive in the United States who have had a procedure for a cardiac malformation [5]. We are now anesthetizing patients with congenital heart disease who are in their fifth and sixth decades of life and have the health concerns of adulthood complicating the normal pediatric cardiac anesthesia care [6]. In order to provide care for this growing patient population, anesthesiologists must be knowledgeable in all aspects of congenital heart disease and repair.

The development of ultrasound technology made it possible to not only diagnose congenital heart disease *in utero*; it also provides greater insight into fetal pathophysiology and neonatal cardiac anatomy. This has aided congenital heart surgeons in the selection of patients and timing for early surgical intervention. As heart malformations are the most common congenital defect requiring anesthesia care today, it is expected that members of the cardiac anesthesia team will anesthetize more neonates than any other group of patients who require cardiac procedures. The cardiac anesthesia team therefore will be responsible for the care of patients from extreme prematurity to 50 plus years of age [7].

Our experience has demonstrated approximately one-third of patients who require congenital cardiac anesthesia are less than 1 year of age, one-third are 1–15 years of age, and one-third are adults (some of them in the sixth decade of life). Neonates and infants tend to have malformations that result in abnormal blood flow while older patients are more likely to suffer from heart rhythm disturbances and valve problems. This knowledge is important in developing cardiac anesthesia teams, educational programs, and designing anesthetic protocols [8]. In addition to young age, other variables related to increased morbidity and mortality in anesthesia include increased severity of the illness as measured by physical status and emergency procedures [9,10].

There has been a decrease in overall mortality to less than 5% for all patients with congenital heart disease who underwent an anesthesia-related procedure [11]. Vigilance is ever important for the anesthetist. Anesthesia care provided to children with congenital heart disease entails even greater risk over other children [12]. The demographic considerations clearly demonstrate the wide scope of patient care required by the cardiac anesthetist and the American Academy of Pediatrics has recommended that a pediatric cardiovascular center use the team approach for all aspects of care and intervention for these patients [13]. The quality of life in children after the repair of congenital heart disease is regarded as lower than in other children, the more severe the lesion, the lower the quality of life [14]. The anesthesia team will be charged with developing new modalities of care that will improve on this finding.

Anesthetic Assessment

These complex patients require a thorough evaluation by the anesthesiologist before the procedure. The evaluation will include the present and past history including previous anesthetic experience, family history including prenatal evaluation where necessary, a physical examination, and a review of all studies performed leading to the intended procedure. Our task in anesthesia has become much easier with the electronic medical record. Before the patient visit, it is now possible to review all previous encounters and interventions, be aware of the diagnosis and medical history to date, have a list of all medications, obtain all test results, and review previous anesthetic exposures. In addition, information regarding the specifics of the congenital heart lesion and therapy can be quickly researched via internet access, searching both surgery and anesthesia databases [8,15]. A note of caution that this should be done before actually examining the patient as motivated parents will have this information in hand and issues and questions can be handled in a timely fashion, preventing unnecessary delays searching for pertinent information and building the confidence of parents.

The history should include information specific to the malformation present and the age of the patient, including gestational age for newborns. The prenatal and maternal history should be obtained to balance confounding issues such as prematurity and maternal diabetes. The presence of one congenital defect should always initiate the search for others and the possible presence of a syndrome that could alter the anesthetic management. Cardiac lesions are in the midline groups of congenital defects and are associated with neurological, renal, and intestinal defects in addi-

tion to other organ systems. Altered neurological outcome in children with congenital heart disease is now well recognized, and the history should include specifics of the birth and other indicators of preexisting neurologic impairment [16].

Children can be uncooperative with diagnostic testing and exercise tolerance might not be easily quantitated. The level of physical activity by history can give an indication of cardiac function. Other more subtle indicators include the feeding history and the frequency of respiratory infections. A child with low cardiac reserve may not be able to eat well and be smaller than anticipated while frequent respiratory infections are associated with congestive heart failure. A question of continuing debate regards the child with an upper respiratory tract infection. If multiple symptoms are present the airway might be reactive provoking hypoxemic episodes surrounding the time of anesthesia. The patient's temperature might fluctuate during the anesthesia and airway secretions are increased leading to the possibility of mechanical obstruction of the endotracheal tube. If it is possible the case should be delayed until resolution of the infection [17].

Adult patients, in addition to a complete history of the cardiac malformation and previous interventions, are questioned regarding disease processes related to age. The patient's internist and all other adult specialists caring for the patient should be consulted. The history may help determine cardiac function, but this can also be measured by exercise testing. Some patients with prior repairs develop heart rhythm disturbances over time and this should be investigated.

The patient with functional single ventricle physiology requires special attention. These patients live with passive pulmonary blood flow. Worsening cyanosis can be an indicator of collateral vessel formation or intracardiac shunting. Previous Fontan procedures are associated with protein-losing enteropathy, thromboembolic events, hepatic dysfunction, and thyroid dysfunction as a result of amiodarone therapy for rhythm disturbance [18]. The presence of a single left ventricle (versus right) is beneficial information.

The physical exam by the anesthesiologist is a tool to confirm information obtained by the history and the review of previous records. The physical exam also concentrates on the anatomy of the airway, the ability to gain intravenous access, and an examination of pulses to determine the feasibility of arterial line placement.

Preanesthetic blood testing includes electrolyte levels with special attention to potassium levels potentially altered by or associated with diuretic therapy. Patients with cyanotic heart disease compensate for hypoxemia with polycythemia. There is no agreement at present regarding the upper limit of acceptable hematocrit and the decision to decrease the red cell mass by phlebotomy is generally guided by the presence of associated complications such as thrombosis. Platelet count and coagulation studies should be obtained in patients undergoing cardiopulmonary bypass.

The American Society of Anesthesiologists has developed guidelines for recommended fasting before the induction of anesthesia [19]. These guidelines are intended to provide safe conditions for the induction of anesthesia with the minimum risk of aspiration of gastric contents as the airway reflexes are ablated. The recommendations for fasting balance the concern for preventing dehydration and hypoglycemia while limiting the amount of gastric volume and acid content. Special considerations regarding fasting include the administration of routine medications as prescribed with a small amount of clear, nonfat-containing fluid. Patients with single ventricle physiology are encouraged to maintain normovolemia through oral intake of clear fluids, optimizing pulmonary blood flow at the time of the induction of anesthesia. It is generally safe to allow clear liquids up to 2 hours before the scheduled start of anesthesia.

Anesthetic Management

Most outpatient elective cardiac patients benefit from premedication before being taken to the operating room. Several studies have demonstrated that midazolam and dexmetotomidine decrease anxiety and improve the process of parental separation [20]. Parental presence in the operating room at induction has also been used. Individual preferences, parental cooperation, and the ability to administer and monitor the effects of these medications are determinants as to best practice for the anesthesiologist. In the child with poor or indeterminate cardiac function the use of ketamine may be considered. Concerns of increased pulmonary artery pressures and worsening cyanosis have not been proven [21]. Ketamine can be administered by virtually all routes.

Aside from the standard equipment for the administration of anesthesia special considerations for congenital cardiac anesthesia include the availability of intravenous fluids and various fluid and blood administration sets. Our standard practice for the majority of open heart cases is two peripheral intravenous lines, a double-lumen central line, and a peripheral arterial line. If excessive or brisk blood loss is a potential problem as in reoperations or patients with coagulopathies, rapid infusing devices and infusion pumps should be prepared and determined to be operating appropriately. Distal infusion and low volume injection ports are used to allow prompt administration of medications to the child's circulation. This will also avoid fluid overload in extremely small infants and speed the effects of changes in dosing of medications by continuous infu-

sions. Equipment for airway management should be prepared and checked for function with all necessary devices (especially fiberoptic capability) to ensure safe securing of the airway is readily available for patients with potentially difficult airways.

Resuscitation medications should be prepared based on the patient's weight, accurately labeled, and placed in locations easily available and located in areas that will not cause confusion with other anesthetic medications. For example, heparin for anticoagulation before cardiopulmonary bypass is prepared on a weight basis and placed in a position unique for this drug and away from other medications. Methods for heart rhythm control including the defibrillator should be prepared. Medications used in the process of anesthesia such as antifibrinolytic, inotrope, and vasodilator infusions should be prepared and checked for accuracy. The complexity of caring for these patients is nowhere more obvious than in the number of drugs administered and the different routes by which this is accomplished. The continuous infusion of medications is particularly prone to error. Great care must be taken to assure the concentrations are correct, the infusion pump is programmed appropriately, and the delivery system is connected without error. This is even more critical when caring for extremely small infants. The availability of blood and blood products should be confirmed during the patient "time-out."

The responsibilities for all members of the team should be delineated before starting the induction of anesthesia. Airway management, monitor placement, and venous and arterial access are designated to individual members to ensure expedient preparation of the patient for the procedure. The operation of the defibrillator is also clarified before the beginning of the case.

The induction of anesthesia is primarily directed by the cardiac function. In patients with normal ventricular function, any of the standard anesthetic agents can be safely used for induction. In patients with decreased ventricular contractility ketamine remains a popular choice and can be used by either the intramuscular or intravenous routes. Etomidate administered by intravenous route is useful in older patients potentially avoiding the psychic phenomenon associated with ketamine.

Anesthesiologists often face challenges in establishing vascular access in patients with congenital heart defects. The high number of newborn infants and patients with multiple previous procedures limits available sites for both venous and arterial access. Consideration of these issues before inducing anesthesia allows alternate plans to be developed, adds efficiency to the process, and minimizes anesthesia time. Experience in ultrasound-guided access should be part of the cardiac anesthesiologist's skill set. The use of ultrasound-guided placement has been demonstrated in accessing the central venous compartment via the internal jugular vein. However, in our experience we find children do not tolerate catheters in the neck well and object to the tethering effect of intravenous tubing at this site. Hence, our preference has been for subclavian vein central venous access. Ultrasound-guided access has been shown to decrease the time to successful placement of catheters for venous access [22]. Variable results have been yielded with arterial access [23]. The rate of complications is decreased using guided technology [24]. Another paradigm shift in approaching the patient with difficult vascular access involves a change in technique. In anesthesia we learn to gain venous access using catheter over needle devices. Micropuncture technique and equipment utilizes a guide wire through a narrow guage needle, dilators used as necessary, and the catheter then placed over the guide wire.

Halothane, previously associated with a high incidence of cardiac complications, is no longer available for use. The remaining volatile agents provide essentially equal cardiac stability and all can be used successfully. Of the volatile anesthetic agents currently used in pediatric anesthesia sevoflurane is more easily accepted by children. During induction care must be taken to carefully observe vital signs. There is evidence that all the volatile agents are cardioprotective and decrease mortality in patients anesthetized for heart surgery [25,26].

An anesthetic technique of high-dose narcotics was previously shown as the best technique to prevent the stress response during and after anesthesia for the repair of congenital heart defects in infants [27]. Halothane was the volatile agent used in comparison. More recently, $50\,\mu g/kg$ total fentanyl dose has been demonstrated to be a sufficient amount for anesthesia, higher doses of $100\,\mu g/kg$ were noted to increase the frequency of hypotension without noticeable improvement in the state of anesthesia [28]. In more recent studies the focus has been on the benefits of brain protection and preconditioning of the heart. These studies have demonstrated the benefits of using volatile anesthetic agents during and after bypass maintaining cardiac function after intervention [26,29]. Sevoflurane might depress cardiac function to a greater extent than isoflurane after bypass and the use of all volatile agents in this period should be carefully monitored [30].

Presently a combination of moderate dose fentanyl up to $50\,\mu g/kg$ with sevoflurane before initiating bypass and either desflurane or isoflurane during and after bypass achieve successful results. Patient recall is possible with narcotic technique, and amnestic agents either benzodiazepines or volatile agents at a concentration of one-half minimum alveolar concentration should be administered. Rapid cooling and rewarming is associated with impaired neurologic outcome and weaning from bypass at lower core temperatures utilizing prolonged hypothermic neuroprotection may be warranted [31,32].

It is well recognized that cardiopulmonary bypass results in an inflammatory response. The impact of all facets of anesthesia care on the inflammatory response remains unclear. This includes the use of steroids and volatile agents and the use of ultrafiltration after bypass [33,34].

A method for intraoperative monitoring and clinical correlation after repair entails the use of transesophageal echocardiography (TEE). Care should be exercised after the probe is placed in infants as the immature airway lacks cartilage support and is prone to collapse. Carbon dioxide retention may occur without a concomitant increase in end-tidal levels [35]. In patients with a retroesophageal subclavian artery, passage of the TEE probe may affect the waveform of the arterial line if it is placed in the affected arm.

Three specific cardiac lesions deserve special attention. First, the newborn with hypoplastic left heart syndrome remains a particular clinical challenge. Risk is entailed when these babies are transported from the neonatal intensive care unit to the operating room. These newborns require a high pulmonary vascular resistance to promote systemic perfusion. Extreme caution must be exercised in transporting and caring for these patients before the initiation of bypass. Hypoxic gas mixtures, added low-dose carbon dioxide, and aggressive systemic afterload reduction are necessary to maintain the delicate balance of pulmonary to systemic blood flow [36–38]. Oxygen saturation should be kept at 70–80%; excessive oxygen saturations result in a decrease in pulmonary vascular resistance and excessive pulmonary blood flow at the expense of systemic perfusion. The second condition, the patient with Fontan physiology also requires careful attention to ventilation parameters. Passive pulmonary blood flow is optimized with ventilation that allows negative intrathoracic pressures [39]. Positive-pressure ventilation decreases pulmonary blood flow, and continuous positive airway pressure can have deleterious effects on perfusion, both pulmonary and systemic. Early extubation of these patients is a consideration [40]. A third condition that requires particular attention is the patients having a bidirectional superior cavopulmonary anastomosis. These patients rely on sufficient cerebral blood flow to provide venous return to the pulmonary arteries for optimal arterial oxygen saturation. In these patients hyperventilation is actually detrimental and hypoventilation ($pCO_2 = 50$–$55\,mmHg$) improves oxygenation. Because this is counterintuitive, the anesthesiologist must be aware of this curious physiology [41,42].

Neurologic issues can occur in infants and young children with congenital cardiac defects. A sign of neurologic involvement is evidenced by periventricular leukomalacia (PVL) which has been found to be present in 20% of infants presenting for surgery. The presence of PVL increases to 50% after surgery requiring cardiopulmonary bypass [43]. Signs and symptoms in the child may not be evident early in life but become more apparent on entrance to school. Neuroprotection during cardiopulmonary bypass is a consideration for the anesthesiologist. Variables noted to possibly affect neurologic outcome include the use and length of time of deep hypothermic circulatory arrest (DHCA), the level of hemodilution, acid–base management at deep hypothermia, cerebral blood blow optimization, and the speed of rewarming [31]. Near infrared spectroscopy (NIRS) has recently been used to measure cerebral and somatic regional oxygen saturation. The NIRS probe uses a light source that directs light through bone and tissue which is then sensed by a shallow and deep detector. The absorption data returned to the detectors reflects deoxygenated hemoglobin and total hemoglobin from which regional (cerebral or somatic) oxygenation is calculated. Kussman and colleagues recently reported that perioperative periods of diminished cerebral oxygen delivery, as indicated by rSO(2) <45%, are associated with 1-year Psychomotor Development Index and brain magnetic resonance imaging abnormalities among infants undergoing reparative heart surgery [44,45]. At present methods thought to prevent brain injury include limited use of DHCA, monitoring and responding to regional cerebral perfusion (NIRS), achieving uniform cooling, utilizing pH stat arterial blood gas strategy, and recognizing that hyperglycemia is preferred over hypoglycemia. Raising the hematocrit to 30% during cardiopulmonary bypass appears to result in less neurologic injury [46]. Pharmacologic intervention includes using volatile agents to increase cerebral blood flow and achieve more uniform cooling and rewarming. Medications that have been studied in an effort to reduce neurologic injury include free radical scavengers, antiepileptics, erythropoietin, and anti-inflammatory agents [47]. None have proven unequivocally beneficial to date.

Blood loss after cardiopulmonary bypass continues to be a challenge and subject of debate. Before induction of anesthesia a clear understanding of the desired hematocrit at the end of the procedure will allow adequate preparation of blood and blood products. In general terms for the patient having a two ventricle repair a hematocrit of 30% is adequate. For the functional single ventricle that is still mixing (e.g., Norwood, bidirectional Glenn) a hematocrit of 45% is optimal. After the Fontan procedure a hematocrit of 30–35% is acceptable. In younger patients it is more likely that blood loss will be greater and therefore a higher end hematocrit will be desired [48]. Consideration must be paid to the number of donor exposures each patient will experience. The use of blood products is associated with the potential transfer of pathogens and alloimmunization, both of which may affect the long-term health of the patient [49]. Platelet count and function decreases are frequently encountered [50]. A rational plan for post-cardiopulmonary bypass includes the use of an antifibrinolytic, followed by platelet infusion, cryoprecipitate to increase fibrinogen, and factor VII in increasing order of problematic bleeding [51].

Regional Anesthesia

The use of regional anesthesia techniques for cardiac surgery remains controversial despite its routine use at many pediatric cardiac centers across the country with little if any reports of serious complications. The main objection to the technique (although not supported in the literature) is the theoretical increased risk of epidural hematoma formation with a neuraxial technique followed by systemic anticoagulation. The incidence of spontaneous epidural hematoma has been estimated at 1:150 000 [52]. The estimates of the incidence of epidural hematoma formation after neuraxial anesthesia in cardiac surgery remains speculative and currently very little data exists on which to base a risk–benefit analysis.

Evidence-based data on the use of regional anesthesia in pediatric cardiac surgery is limited. The most common type of regional technique used is a single shot caudal block with morphine, however the duration is usually short and the need for systemic opioids remains [53]. Several reports have been published on the use of neuraxial techniques in congenital cardiac surgery without any adverse events. These studies have all failed to demonstrate a significant objective increased benefit in terms of postoperative recovery [54,55]. Therefore, based on current evidence a neuraxial technique can be used safely, however outcome studies are lacking in terms of the true benefit of the technique. It is recommended that anticoagulation does not occur until 1 hour after the regional block is placed [56].

Fast Tracking and Early Extubation

Many children undergoing cardiopulmonary bypass and congenital cardiac surgery can be rapidly weaned and extubated safely in the operating room or shortly thereafter. In order to fast track patients a multidisciplinary team must be assembled to expedite the patients through the perioperative process. The best way to achieve these common multidisciplinary goals is through clinical pathway algorithms [57,58]. The main goal of the fast track process is early extubation which leads to shorter ICU and hospital stays, with cost savings for both the patient and health care facility. Several studies have proven the effectiveness of employing this strategy in congenital cardiac surgery [59,60]. Many variables need to be considered when one decides on the fast track process that include the following: size of the patient, length of procedure, hemodynamic stability, bleeding, hypothermia, pulmonary dysfunction, and the need for ongoing inotropic support. In the largest series to date of early extubation in children undergoing cardiac surgery with CBP, early extubation was accomplished in 72%, which included 50% of patients less than 1 week of age [61]. Whether it is more advantageous to facilitate endotracheal extubation before the patient leaves the operating room or upon arrival in the ICU has not been determined.

The cardiac anesthesiologist must be vigilant in the pre-planning aspect of the anesthetic approach as the traditional high-dose narcotic, neuromuscular blocker, and inhalational agent technique will prevent a patient from being fast tracked. The narcotic dose and choice of narcotic should be tailored with this goal in mind. Both fentanyl and remifentail can be effective in achieving early extubation in pediatric cardiac fast track patients [62]. Finally, the child must have excellent postoperative analgesia for the fast track process to proceed without incident. Many centers have advocated the use of a combined general anesthesia plus regional anesthesia technique for pediatric cardiac surgery patients with no evidence of epidural hematoma [63]. However, the use of neuraxial analgesia in light of complete anticoagulation remains controversial.

Anesthesia and Cardiac Imaging

Anesthesia for cardiac imaging places responsibility on the anesthesiologist to provide optimum conditions for the acquisition of the best images. The cardiac catheterization laboratory continues to require anesthesia care as interventional transcatheter techniques continue to grow and improve. Anesthesia care is required for procedures ranging from closure of septal defects, to dilation of stenotic valves, to transcatheter valve insertion. The location of the cardiac catheterization laboratory is frequently distant from the traditional operating rooms and requires the development of process and protocols for managing the anesthesia of these patients in remote locations. Malignant hyperthermia is one example that requires prompt therapy to limit morbidity and mortality. Dantrolene must be available so that it can be administered immediately after the diagnosis is made. The logistics of communication with support staff and the attainment of additional assistance, equipment, and therapy before induction of anesthesia in these locations is advised.

Computed tomography (CT) scans of the heart in addition to occurring in a remote location requires anesthesia for procedures of short duration, a brief period of apnea to acquire images without respiratory motion, and slow heart rates to eliminate cardiac motion [64]. Short-acting neuromuscular blockers are utilized and the pharmacologic methods of slowing the heart rate for a brief period of time may be needed. Heart rates near 80 beats per minute yield the best results [65]. Deepening the depth of anesthesia or the use of beta blockers may be requested. A contrast injec-

tion is necessary and this places the added burden of a large bore intravenous catheter being placed in the right arm to provide rapid and direct access to the heart. Magnetic resonance imaging (MRI) of the heart requires multiple lengthy episodes of apnea. Endotracheal intubation is normally required to accomplish this in children. Consideration on methods to secure a difficult airway in remote locations is advised.

Pulmonary Hypertension

The use of inhaled nitric oxide (iNO) in the setting of congenital cardiac surgery has become quite routine. Patients with increased pulmonary blood flow or pulmonary venous obstruction coupled with endothelial injury caused by cardiopulmonary bypass benefit from iNO which is a selective pulmonary vasodilator [66]. Inhaled nitric oxide therapy is an easily administered pulmonary vasodilator added to the anesthesia circuit with no clinically evident systemic vasodilation which can be safely used even in the setting of hemodynamic instability.

When delivered to the respiratory tract, nitric oxide diffuses rapidly across the alveolar–capillary membrane into the smooth muscle layer of the pulmonary vessel. Inhaled nitric oxide catalyzes the formation of cyclic guanosine monophosphate (cGMP) resulting in smooth muscle relaxation. This smooth muscle relaxation is inhibited by the cyclic nucleotide phosphodiesterases (PDE). Of note, PDE5 is inhibited by the phosphodiesterase inhibitor sildenafil, an oral treatment for pulmonary hypertension. Inhaled nitric oxide therapy gains its role as a selective pulmonary vasodilator from nitric oxide's rapid bloodstream deactivation as it combines with hemoglobin to form methemoglobin and nitrate [67]. Methemoglobinemia is measured to determine toxicity. Nitrogen dioxide, another toxic metabolite leads to increased airway reactivity and, later, pulmonary edema [68].

Congenital cardiac anomalies associated with a high risk of elevated pulmonary resistance include atrioventricular septal defect, common arterial trunk, transposition of the great arteries, ventricular septal defects, and total anomalous pulmonary venous connection [69]. Current evidence supports the use of iNO therapy in congenital heart disease both in treatment of pulmonary hypertension and in a prophylactic fashion during surgeries for lesions associated with a high risk of pulmonary hypertension. The effective iNO dose in congenital cardiac surgery rarely exceeds 20 ppm, and this has remained the manufacturer's recommendation for initial administration [70,71]. The prophylactic role of iNO in preventing postoperative pulmonary hypertensive crises and speeding time to extubation has also been established [72]. Nitric oxide therapy needs to be continued during all transports. Future directions will address the role of iNO in combination with intravenous vasodilators, and of the causes of interpatient response variability and its relationship to endothelial biology.

Cardiac Pharmacology

Several drugs used in the conduct of congenital heart procedures warrant mention. Prostaglandin E1 has been infused in newborns for the past 30 years to maintain the patency of the ductus arteriosus in lesions that require continuous flow through this structure to maintain life [73]. Experience continues to demonstrate that this drug is associated with a significant rate of complications divided almost equally between the respiratory system and the heart. Apnea and hypotension are possible and demand careful attention during the transport of these infants [74].

Arginine vasopressin is an antidiuretic hormone (ADH) that is a potent vasoconstrictor. The therapeutic use of this drug includes any form of vasodilatory shock from sepsis to anaphylaxis [75]. Although this drug will likely be used infrequently, it should be considered in conditions of hypotension unresponsive to other mechanisms of support [76].

Pulmonary hypertension is commonly associated with various cardiac malformations. Knowledge of the various pharmacologic approaches to this disease process is needed to provide optimal care. In addition to nitric oxide which must be administered by a metered continuous flow apparatus, oral medications include sildinefil, a phosphdiesterase type 5 inhibitor, the endothelin antagonist bosentan, and the prostenoids, iloprost, a metered inhaled medication, and epoprostenol administered by the intravenous route [77,78]. Patients who require cardiac anesthesia may be taking these agents alone or in combination.

Postanesthesia Process

The transition of patients to the intensive care unit after cardiac surgery involves the physical movement of the patient and equipment, exchange of patient data, and the transfer of responsibility of care. Critical information about the patient is conveyed to the critical care team during a time of significant hemodynamic vulnerability [79]. Elements found critical to the successful transition of a patient include the efficient transition of monitors and equipment, limiting discussions to those related only to the patient, a face-to-face handoff of patient information, and discussion of a plan between all care providers involved, and limited interruptions during the information handover [80–82]. Several studies to date have investigated the standardization of the handover process in pediatric patients after transition from the operating room to the cardiac intensive care unit following cardiac surgery [83,84].

A multidisciplinary team of key stakeholders should be assembled to develop a protocol for the transition of cardiac patients to the intensive care unit following cardiac surgery.

The goal of any transition protocol is to improve patient safety by reducing the number of latent and realized errors that occur during the transition process [85]. Root cause analyses are performed by the team appraising key steps in the process where concerns from performance evaluation have arisen. Actual errors identified are also subject to additional root cause analysis. Ultimately a transition protocol should be developed and tools created to facilitate protocol compliance. After a structured educational period, protocol implementation can begin.

The goal of the transition protocol is that a "sterile team environment" must be maintained throughout the transition process while the anesthesiologist acts as transition team leader until responsibility of care has been transferred. Other highlights of the transition protocol include:
• a critical care team member enters the operating room near the end of the case to receive handoff instructions from the cardiovascular surgeon;
• a focus on the efficient transition of all patient monitors before anesthesia handoff;
• the implementation of a written tool to guide the anesthesiologist's verbal handoff.

Conclusion

The congenital cardiac anesthesiologist must be prepared to care for a wide-ranging group of congenital heart patients from extremely premature infants to patients in the sixth decade of life. The underlying cardiac defects range from cyanotic to acyanotic cardiac malformations as well as disturbances of heart rate and rhythm. The patient with functional single ventricle physiology presents special challenges. This very complex system of disease management entails the potential for numerous errors and the team approach appears to offer the best outcome [86]. This team consists of dedicated anesthesiologists as well as dedicated members from each specialty to develop protocols including standardized methods for transfer of care of these patients.

There is no single regimen of anesthesia that has been demonstrated to be superior, but a balanced technique of narcotics and volatile anesthetic agents appears to provide safety while affording protection for the brain and limiting the inflammatory response for patients undergoing cardiac surgery. Further challenges include providing anesthesia care in remote and isolated locations for nonsurgical procedures including cardiac catheterization and imaging. Transporting these patients before and after anesthetics necessitates specialized equipment such as portable nitric oxide and the ability to deliver hypoxic gas mixtures.

Finally, the anesthesiologist should develop a method of providing pain relief from the end of the procedure until it is no longer an issue. Regional anesthetic techniques may play an important role in the early period after a procedure while patient-controlled analgesia and parent-controlled analgesia for children who are too young to understand will play a pivotal role in the recovery process and improvement of care in these patients.

References

1. Gross RE, Hubbard JH. (1939) Surgical ligation of a patent ductus arteriosus; report of first successful case. JAMA 112, 729–731.
2. Aronson LA, Spaeth JP. (2006) Frontiers in pediatric anesthesia: cardiac anesthesia. Int Anesthesiol Clin 44, 33–49.
3. Marelli AJ, Mackie AS, Ionescu-Ittu R, et al. (2007) Congenital heart disease in the general population: changing prevalence and age distribution. Circulation 115, 163–172.
4. Billett J, Majeed A, Gatzoulis M, et al. (2008) Trends in hospital admissions, in-hospital case fatality and population mortality from congenital heart disease in England, 1994 to 2004. Heart 94, 342–348.
5. Warnes CA, Williams RG, Bashore TM, et al. (2008) ACC/AHA 2008 guidelines for the management of adults with congenital heart disease: a report of the American College of Cardiology/American Heart Association Task Force on Practice Guidelines (writing committee to develop guidelines on the management of adults with congenital heart disease). Circulation 118, e714–e833.
6. Fontan F, Baudet E. (1971) Surgical repair of tricuspid atresia. Thorax 26, 240–248.
7. Mahle WT, Kirshbom PM, Kanter KR, et al. (2008) Cardiac surgery in adults performed at children's hospitals: trends and outcomes. J Thorac Cardiovasc Surg 136, 307–311.
8. Vener DF, Tirotta CD, Andropoulos D, et al. (2008) Anaesthetic complications associated with the treatment of patients with congenital cardiac disease: consensus definitions from the Multi-Societal Database Committee for Pediatric and Congenital Heart Disease. Cardiol Young 18(Suppl 2), 271–281.
9. Murat I, Constant I, Maud'huy H. (2004) Perioperative anaesthetic morbidity in children: a database of 24,165 anaesthetics over a 30-month period. Paediatr Anaesth 14, 158–166.
10. Gobbo Braz L, Braz JR, Módolo NS, et al. (2006) Perioperative cardiac arrest and its mortality in children. A 9-year survey in a Brazilian tertiary teaching hospital. Paediatr Anaesth 16, 860–866.
11. Morray JP, Geiduschek JM, Ramamoorthy C, et al. (2000) Anesthesia-related cardiac arrest in children: initial findings of the Pediatric Perioperative Cardiac Arrest (POCA) Registry. Anesthesiology 93, 6–14.
12. Odegard KC, DiNardo JA, Kussman BD, et al. (2007) The frequency of anesthesia-related cardiac arrests in patients with congenital heart disease undergoing cardiac surgery. Anesth Analg 105, 335–343.
13. American Academy of Pediatrics, Section on Cardiology and Cardiac Surgery. (2002) Guidelines for pediatric cardiovascular centers. Pediatrics 109, 544–549.
14. Uzark K, Jones K, Slusher J, et al. (2008) Quality of life in children with heart disease as perceived by children and parents. Pediatrics 121, e1060–e1067.
15. Gaynor JW, Jacobs JP, Jacobs ML, et al. (2002) Congenital Heart Surgery Nomenclature and Database Project: update and proposed data harvest. Ann Thorac Surg 73, 1016–1018.
16. Majnemer A, Limperopoulos C, Shevell MI, et al. (2009) A new look at outcomes of infants with congenital heart disease. Pediatr Neurol 40, 197–204.
17. Tait AR, Malviya S. (2005) Anesthesia for the child with an upper respiratory tract infection: still a dilemma? Anesth Analg 100, 59–65.
18. Batcher EL, Tang XC, Singh BN, et al.; SAFE-T Investigators. (2007) Thyroid function abnormalities during amiodarone therapy for persistent atrial fibrillation. Am J Med 120, 880–885.
19. American Society of Anesthesiologists Task Force on Preoperative Fasting. (1999) Practice guidelines for preoperative fasting and the use of pharmacologic agents to reduce the risk of pulmonary aspiration: application to healthy patients undergoing elective procedures: a report by the American Society of Anesthesiologist Task Force on Preoperative Fasting. Anesthesiology 90, 896–905.
20. Yuen VM, Hui TW, Irwin MG, et al. (2008) A comparison of intranasal dexmedetomidine and oral midazolam for premedication in pediatric anesthesia: a double-blinded randomized controlled trial. Anesth Analg 106, 1715–1721.
21. Williams GD, Philip BM, Chu LF, et al. (2007) Ketamine does not increase pulmonary vascular resistance in children with pulmonary hypertension undergoing sevoflurane anesthesia and spontaneous ventilation. Anesth Analg 105, 1578–1584.
22. Doniger SJ, Ishimine P, Fox JC, et al. (2009) Randomized controlled trial of ultrasound-guided peripheral intravenous catheter placement versus traditional techniques in difficult-access pediatric patients. Pediatr Emerg Care 25, 154–159.
23. Ganesh A, Kaye R, Cahill AM, et al. (2009) Evaluation of ultrasound-guided radial artery cannulation in children. Pediatr Crit Care Med 10, 45–48.
24. Maecken, T, Grau T. (2007) Ultrasound imaging in vascular access. Crit Care Med 35 (5 Suppl), S178–S185.
25. El Azab SR, Rosseel PM, De Lange JJ, et al. (2002) Effect of VIMA with sevoflurane versus TIVA with propofol or midazolam-sufentanil on the cytokine response during CABG surgery. Eur J Anaesthesiol 19, 276–282.
26. Landoni G, Bignami E, Oliviero F, et al. (2009) Halogenated anaesthetics and cardiac protection in cardiac and non-cardiac anaesthesia. Ann Card Anaesth 12, 4–9.
27. Anand KJ, Hickey PR. (1992) Halothane-morphine compared with high-dose sufentanil for anesthesia and postoperative analgesia in neonatal cardiac surgery. N Engl J Med 326, 1–9.
28. Duncan HP, Cloote A, Weir PM, et al. (2000) Reducing stress responses in the pre-bypass phase of open heart surgery in infants and young children: a comparison of different fentanyl doses. Br J Anaesth 84, 556–564.
29. Yu CH, Beattie WS. (2006) The effects of volatile anesthetics on cardiac ischemic complications and mortality in CABG: a meta-analysis. Can J Anaesth 53, 906–918.
30. Gentry-Smetana S, Redford D, Moore D, et al. (2008) Direct effects of volatile anesthetics on cardiac function. Perfusion 23, 43–47.

31. Halstead JC, Etz C, Meier DM. (2007) Perfusing the cold brain: optimal neuroprotection for aortic surgery. Ann Thorac Surg 84, 768–774.

32. Sahu B, Chauhan S, Kiran U, *et al*. (2009) Neuropsychological function in children with cyanotic heart disease undergoing corrective cardiac surgery: effect of two different rewarming strategies. Eur J Cardiothorac Surg 35, 505–510.

33. Robertson-Malt, S, Afrane B, El Barbary M. (2007) Prophylactic steroids for pediatric open heart surgery. Cochrane Database Syst Rev (4), CD005550.

34. Cho EJ, Yoon JH, Hong SJ, *et al*. (2009) The effects of sevoflurane on systemic and pulmonary inflammatory responses after cardiopulmonary bypass. J Cardiothorac Vasc Anesth 23, 639–645.

35. Stayer SA, Bent ST, Andropoulos DA. (2001) Proper probe positioning for infants with compromised ventilation from transesophageal echocardiography. Anesth Analg 92, 1076–1077.

36. Keidan I, Mishaly D, Berkenstadt H, *et al*. (2003) Combining low inspired oxygen and carbon dioxide during mechanical ventilation for the Norwood procedure. Paediatr Anaesth 13, 58–62.

37. Stieh J, Fischer G, Scheewe J, *et al*. (2006) Impact of preoperative treatment strategies on the early perioperative outcome in neonates with hypoplastic left heart syndrome. J Thorac Cardiovasc Surg 131, 1122–1129.

38. De Oliveira NC, Ashburn DA, Khalid F, *et al*. (2004) Prevention of early sudden circulatory collapse after the Norwood operation. Circulation 110(11 Suppl 1), II133–II138.

39. Lofland GK. (2001) The enhancement of hemodynamic performance in Fontan circulation using pain free spontaneous ventilation. Eur J Cardiothorac Surg 20, 114–119.

40. Morales DL, Carberry KE, Heinle JS, *et al*. (2008) Extubation in the operating room after Fontan's procedure: effect on practice and outcomes. Ann Thorac Surg 86, 576–582.

41. Bradley SM, Simsic JM, Mulvihill DM. (1998) Hyperventilation impairs oxygenation after bidirectional superior cavopulmonary connection. Circulation 98(19 Suppl): II372–II377.

42. Bradley SM, Simsic JM, Mulvihill DM. (2003) Hypoventilation improves oxygenation after bidirectional superior cavopulmonary connection. J Thorac Cardiovasc Surg 126, 1033–1039.

43. Sherlock RL, McQuillen PS, Miller SP. (2009) Preventing brain injury in newborns with congenital heart disease: brain imaging and innovative trial designs. Stroke 40, 327–332.

44. Kussman BD, Wypij D, DiNardo JA, *et al*. (2009) Cerebral oximetry during infant cardiac surgery: evaluation and relationship to early postoperative outcome. Anesth Analg 108, 1122–1131.

45. Kussman BD, Wypij D, Laussen PC, *et al*. (2010) Relationship of intraoperative cerebral oxygen saturation to neurodevelopmental outcome and brain magnetic resonance imaging at 1 year of age in infants undergoing biventricular repair. Circulation 122, 245–254.

46. Jonas RA, Wypij D, Roth SJ, *et al*. (2003) The influence of hemodilution on outcome after hypothermic cardiopulmonary bypass: results of a randomized trial in infants. J Thorac Cardiovasc Surg 126, 1765–1774.

47. Clancy RR. (2008) Neuroprotection in infant heart surgery. Clin Perinatol 35, 809–821.

48. Eisses MJ, Chandler WL. (2008) Cardiopulmonary bypass parameters and hemostatic response to cardiopulmonary bypass in infants versus children. J Cardiothorac Vasc Anesth 22, 53–59.

49. Lauder GR. (2007) Pre-operative predeposit autologous donation in children presenting for elective surgery: a review. Transfus Med 17, 75–82.

50. McEwan A. (2007) Aspects of bleeding after cardiac surgery in children. Paediatr Anaesth 17, 1126–1133.

51. Guzzetta NA, Huch S, Fernandez JD, *et al*. (2009) Use of recombinant factor VIIa for uncontrolled bleeding in neonates after cardiopulmonary bypass. Paediatr Anaesth 19, 364–370.

52. Ho AM, Chung DC, Joynt GM. (2000) Neuraxial blockade and hematoma in cardiac surgery: estimating the risk of a rare adverse event that has not (yet) occurred. Chest 117, 551–555.

53. Rosen KR, Rosen DA. (1989) Caudal epidural morphine for control of pain following open heart surgery in children. Anesthesiology 70, 418–421.

54. Hammer GB, Ngo K, Macario A. (2000) A retrospective examination of regional plus general anesthesia in children undergoing open heart surgery. Anesth Analg 90, 1020–1024.

55. Peterson KL, DeCampli WM, Pike NA, *et al*. (2000) A report of two hundred twenty cases of regional anesthesia in pediatric cardiac surgery. Anesth Analg 90, 1014–1019.

56. Horlocker TT, Wedel DJ, Benzon H, *et al*. (2003) Regional anesthesia in the anticoagulated patient: defining the risks (the second ASRA Consensus Conference on Neuraxial Anesthesia and Anticoagulation). Reg Anesth Pain Med 28, 172–197.

57. Laussen PC, Reid RW, Stene RA, *et al*. (1996) Tracheal extubation of children in the operating room after atrial septal defect repair as part of a clinical practice guideline. Anesth Analg 82, 988–993.

58. Pare DS, Freed MD. (1995) Clinical practice guidelines for quality patient outcomes. Nurs Clin North Am 30, 183–196.

59. Burrows FA, Taylor RH, Hillier SC. (1992) Early extubation of the trachea after repair of secundum-type atrial septal defects in children. Can J Anaesth 39, 1041–1044.

60. Schuller JL, Bovill JG, Nijveld A, *et al*. (1984) Early extubation of the trachea after open heart surgery for congenital heart disease. A review of 3 years' experience. Br J Anaesth 56, 1101–1108.

61. Barash PG, Lescovich F, Katz JD, *et al*. (1980) Early extubation following pediatric cardiothoracic operation: a viable alternative. Ann Thorac Surg 29, 228–233.

62. Friesen RH, Veit AS, Archibald DJ, *et al*. (2003) A comparison of remifentanil and fentanyl for fast track paediatric cardiac anaesthesia. Paediatr Anaesth 13, 122–125.

63. Rosen DA, Rosen KR, Hammer GB. (2002) Pro: regional anesthesia is an important component of the anesthetic technique for pediatric patients undergoing cardiac surgical procedures. J Cardiothorac Vasc Anesth 16, 374–378.

64. Chan FP. (2009) MR and CT imaging of the pediatric patient with structural heart disease. Semin Thorac Cardiovasc Surg Pediatr Card Surg Annu 12, 99–105.

65. Hoffmann MH, Shi H, Manzke R, *et al*. (2005) Noninvasive coronary angiography with 16-detector row CT: effect of heart rate. Radiology 234, 86–97.

66. Wessel DL, Adatia I, Giglia TM, *et al*. (1993) Use of inhaled nitric oxide and acetylcholine in the evaluation of pulmonary hypertension and endothelial function after cardiopulmonary bypass. Circulation 88, 2128–2138.

67. Kawakami H, Ichinose F. (2004) Inhaled nitric oxide in pediatric cardiac surgery. Int Anesthesiol Clin 42, 93–100.

68. Weinberger B, Laskin DL, Heck DE, *et al*. (2001) The toxicology of inhaled nitric oxide. Toxicol Sci 59, 5–16.

69. Bando K, Turrentine MW, Sharp TG, *et al*. (1996) Pulmonary hypertension after operations for congenital heart disease: analysis of risk factors and management. J Thorac Cardiovasc Surg 112, 1600–1609.

70. Russell IA, Zwass MS, Fineman JR, *et al*. (1998) The effects of inhaled nitric oxide on postoperative pulmonary hypertension in infants and children undergoing surgical repair of congenital heart disease. Anesth Analg 87, 46–51.

71. Fullerton DA, Jones SD, Jaggers J, *et al*. (1996) Effective control of pulmonary vascular resistance with inhaled nitric oxide after cardiac operation. J Thorac Cardiovasc Surg 111, 753–763.

72. Miller OI, Tang SF, Keech A, *et al*. (2000) Inhaled nitric oxide and prevention of pulmonary hypertension after congenital heart surgery: a randomised double-blind study. Lancet 356, 1464–1479.

73. Elliott RB, Starling MB, Neutze JM. (1975) Medical manipulation of the ductus arteriosus. Lancet 1, 140–142.

74. Meckler GD, Lowe C. (2009) To intubate or not to intubate? Transporting infants on prostaglandin E1. Pediatrics 123, e25–e30.

75. Levy JH, Adkinson NF Jr. (2008) Anaphylaxis during cardiac surgery: implications for clinicians. Anesth Analg 106, 392–403.

76. Lechner E, Hofer A, Mair R, *et al*. (2007) Arginine-vasopressin in neonates with vasodilatory shock after cardiopulmonary bypass. Eur J Pediatr 166, 1221–1227.

77. Benedict N, Seybert A, Mathier MA. (2007) Evidence-based pharmacologic management of pulmonary arterial hypertension. Clin Ther 29, 2134–2153.

78. Feinstein JA. (2009) Evaluation, risk stratification, and management of pulmonary hypertension in patients with congenital heart disease. Semin Thorac Cardiovasc Surg Pediatr Card Surg Annu 12, 106–111.

79. Tweddell JS, Hoffman GM. (2002) Postoperative management in patients with complex congenital heart disease. Semin Thorac Cardiovasc Surg Pediatr Card Surg Annu 5, 187–205.

80. de Leval MR, Carthey J, Wright DJ, *et al*. (2000) Human factors and cardiac surgery: a multicenter study. J Thorac Cardiovasc Surg 119(4 Pt 1), 661–672.

81. King HB, Kohsin B, Salisbury M. (2003) Systemwide development of medical team training: lessons learned in the Department of Defense. In: Advances for Healthcare Research and Quality and the Department of Defense – Health Affairs. Available: http://www.ahrq.gov/downloads/pub/advances/vol3/King.pdf. Accessed 3/9/2012.

82. Patterson ES, Roth EM, Woods DD, *et al*. (2004). Handoff strategies in settings with high consequences for failure: lessons for health care operations. Int J Qual Health Care 16, 125–132.

83. Catchpole KR, de Leval MR, McEwan A, *et al*. (2007) Patient handover from surgery to intensive care: using Formula 1 pit-stop and aviation models to improve safety and quality. Paediatr Anaesth 17, 470–478.

84. Joy BF, Elliott E, Hardy C, *et al*. (2010) Standardized multidisciplinary protocol improves handover of cardiac surgery patients to the intensive care unit. Pediatr Crit Care Med 12, 304–308.

85. Wilson KA, Burke CS, Priest HA, *et al*. (2005) Promoting health care safety through training high reliability teams. Qual Saf Health Care 14, 303–309.

86. Benavidez OJ, Gauvreau K, Del Nido P, *et al*. (2007) Complications and risk factors for mortality during congenital heart surgery admissions. Ann Thorac Surg 84, 147–155.

Perioperative Care

Carl L. Backer,[1] John M. Costello,[1] Jason M. Kane,[1] and Constantine Mavroudis[2]

[1]Ann & Robert H. Lurie Children's Hospital of Chicago, formerly Children's Memorial Hospital, Chicago, IL, USA
[2]Florida Hospital for Children, Orlando, FL, USA

The improved results after surgical treatment of congenital heart defects in recent years can in part be attributed to the attention now focused on perioperative care. Specific techniques used to accomplish a smooth postoperative course are determined by the patient's age, the nature of the cardiac defect, the child's preoperative clinical condition, and the type of repair performed. Postoperative care of the infant or child following cardiac surgery differs considerably from that of adults. For example, the circulatory response to cardiopulmonary bypass and the anatomy and physiology of the respiratory system vary greatly by age. Postoperative monitoring of infants and children emphasizes noninvasive techniques (especially physical examination) as compared to the routine invasive monitoring of adult cardiac surgery patients. Comorbidities encountered in children also differ vastly from those encountered in adults.

Many different multidisciplinary models are currently used to provide cardiac critical care. Optimal perioperative care requires a multidisciplinary team that includes cardiovascular surgeons, cardiac intensivists, cardiologists, cardiac intensive care unit (ICU) nurses, and respiratory therapists [1,2]. Consultation should be available from all other pediatric subspecialties. The anatomic, physiologic, and electrophysiologic manifestations of many types of congenital and acquired heart disease are complex and often esoteric. A thorough understanding of the subtleties of each cardiac lesion, along with the growing number of diagnostic tools and treatment options used in their management are central to the provision of critical care for this patient population. The cumulative experience and critical mass of the entire team likely contributes to the improved outcomes achieved by centers performing a higher volume of pediatric cardiac surgical procedures [3–6]. To consolidate this experience, many programs now provide care for all critically ill children with cardiac disease in dedicated cardiac ICUs [7]. Regardless of the care model, the cardiac surgeon will have the most intimate knowledge of the intraoperative findings and the adequacy of the repair and thus assumes final responsibility for the patient.

Although many children will have a smooth postoperative course, it is important to maintain a high level of vigilance for early warning signs of possible complications so that the initiation of appropriate therapy is preemptive in nature and not simply a reaction to problems as they arise. Constant attention to detail is essential and prevention of complications (anticipatory rather than reactive care) is the key to optimal postoperative outcomes.

Preoperative Preparation

A smooth operative and postoperative course begins with preparation of the child for surgery. Children undergoing elective surgery should have a careful history and physical examination 1 or 2 days before the procedure. The cardiologist and surgeon should review relevant cardiac diagnostic information to ensure that the evaluation is complete and the surgical plan is clear. Any chronic medical problems that require special attention (e.g., diabetes, seizure disorder, asthma, anticoagulation), or any acute medical illnesses (e.g., pneumonia, upper respiratory infection, otitis media) that would mandate cancellation of elective surgery should be identified [8]. For closed-heart operations (performed without cardiopulmonary bypass [CPB]), routine laboratory evaluations include a chest radiograph, complete blood cell and platelet count, and urinalysis. For open-heart operations we also obtain a prothrombin time, partial thromboplastin time, and serum electrolyte measurement. Blood should be obtained for drug-level assays if the patient is being treated with drugs such as digoxin and phenobarbital. These laboratory tests screen for abnormalities that may have to be corrected before surgery or require special attention during surgery, such as anemia, hypokalemia, and bleeding disorders.

In contrast to older children, the vast majority of neonates who are awaiting cardiac surgery require hospitalization in an ICU. Neonates with critical congenital heart disease may be broadly categorized as having ductal-dependent systemic blood flow, ductal-dependent pulmonary blood flow, transposition physiology, or obstructed pulmonary venous return. Historically, many neonates with critical congenital heart defects who present with shock or severe cyanosis require emergent surgical intervention. However the introduction of prostaglandin E1 (PGE₁) infusions to reopen and maintain patency of the ductus arteriosus in the 1970s has largely eliminated the need for emergency surgery [9]. With the exception of severely obstructed pulmonary venous return, the administration of PGE₁ along with other supportive measures (e.g., judicious use of mechanical ventilation or inotropic support) will allow surgery to be deferred for a few days while awaiting recovery of myocardial and end-organ function. Side effects of PGE₁ include apnea, hypotension, fever, and rash. In patients receiving PGE₁ who develop apnea or those who require interhospital transport of PGE₁, mechanical ventilation has traditionally been initiated. However, the elective initiation of mechanical ventilation in this patient population is associated with a number of side effects and may not be warranted in many cases [10]. A PGE₁ dose of 0.01 μg/kg/minute is effective for maintaining ductal patency, and higher doses are likely associated with more side effects. Aminophylline or caffeine may be safely used to minimize the occurrence of apnea in neonates receiving PGE₁ [11].

Lesions with ductus-dependent systemic blood flow include hypoplastic left heart syndrome and interrupted aortic arch (Table 7.1) [12]. Neonates with these lesions will develop myocardial dysfunction, metabolic acidosis, and hepatic and renal dysfunction as the ductus arteriosus constricts. Systemic perfusion is further compromised as pulmonary vascular resistance falls, leading to preferential shunting to the pulmonary circulation, and volume overload of the systemic ventricle. Preoperative management in these cases is aimed at restoring systemic perfusion and supporting myocardial function. In addition to a PGE₁ infusion, the judicious use of inotropes and afterload reduction may be beneficial to support the volume-overloaded systemic ventricle and augment systemic perfusion. Therapies that further lower pulmonary vascular resistance, such as excessive supplemental oxygen or hyperventilation should be avoided. Additional strategies to improve the balance between systemic and pulmonary blood flow include the use of subambient inspired oxygen and hypoventilation,

Table 7.1 Ductus-dependent lesions.

For pulmonary blood flow

Pulmonary atresia with intact ventricular septum

Tetralogy of Fallot with severe pulmonary stenosis or pulmonary atresia

Critical pulmonary stenosis

Tricuspid atresia with severe pulmonary stenosis

For mixing

Transposition of the great arteries

For systemic blood flow

Hypoplastic left heart syndrome

Interrupted aortic arch

Severe coarctation of the aorta

Critical aortic stenosis

both of which may increase pulmonary vascular resistance. Hypoventilation improves systemic oxygen delivery and thus is the favored approach, but concurrent pharmacological paralysis is required to suppress the patient's respiratory drive [13]. Neonates with ductal-dependent systemic blood flow are at risk for developing necrotizing enterocolitis [14] and many clinicians are reluctant to provide enteral nutrition before surgery.

Ductal-dependent pulmonary blood flow is present in neonates with severe or complete right ventricular outflow tract obstruction (Table 7.1) [12]. These patients present with progressive cyanosis as the ductus arteriosus constricts. A PGE₁ infusion will reliably reopen the ductus arteriosus and improve systemic oxygen saturation levels [15]. In contrast to patients with hypoplastic left heart syndrome or interrupted aortic arch, the ductus in neonates with right ventricular outflow tract obstruction is typically long and tortuous, providing resistance that usually limits pulmonary overcirculation. Such patients generally do not require interventions to balance the circulation, and can tolerate enteral nutrition while awaiting intervention.

In patients with d-transposition of the great vessels, the aorta arises from the right ventricle and the pulmonary artery arises from the left ventricle. Neonates with transposition physiology are dependent on mixing of oxygenated and deoxygenated blood at the ductus arteriosus and through any atrial or ventricular septal defects. In patients with restrictive septal communications, marked cyanosis will be present at birth or will develop with constriction of the ductus arteriosus. PGE₁ is initiated when this diagnosis is suspected followed by an emergent balloon atrial septostomy (BAS), which will facilitate mixing at the atrial level and thus improve systemic oxygenation [16]. Additional benefits of a BAS include a reduction in left atrial pressure, which may facilitate a drop in pulmonary vascular resistance. For these reasons, many centers perform an elective BAS in all patients with d-transposition of the great vessels, unless a sizable secundum atrial septal defect is present.

Patients with obstruction of pulmonary venous return or left atrial egress may present with profound cyanosis within minutes to hours of birth. Neonates with severely obstructed total anomalous pulmonary venous return will not have sustained improvement with medical therapies and require emergent surgical repair. Neonates with hypoplastic left heart syndrome and a severely restrictive or intact atrial septum are at high risk for mortality due to the severity of the heart defect, abnormalities in pulmonary lymphatic development, and late development of pulmonary vein stenosis. Acute stabilization is best achieved by emergent creation of an atrial septal defect in the catheterization laboratory, followed by stage 1 Norwood palliation once pulmonary congestion has improved [17].

Neonates with critical congenital heart defects require preoperative evaluation for noncardiac comorbidities. Major noncardiac structural anomalies (e.g., omphalocele, tracheoesophageal fistula, renal anomalies) are found in approximately 15% of neonates with congenital heart disease [18,19]. An ultrasound scan of the brain should be obtained to rule out intraventricular hemorrhage or other intracranial abnormalities, particularly in neonates who were premature, had a difficult delivery, or presented in shock or with severe cyanosis. Recent literature indicates that the prevalence of central nervous system abnormalities before surgery in newborns with congenital heart defects has been under-appreciated [20]. Preoperative brain magnetic resonance imaging (MRI) examinations obtained in research protocols in term newborns with transposition or single ventricular physiology reveal anatomical and functional characteristics comparable to premature neonates, suggesting abnormal brain development in utero [21,22]. Licht and colleagues have shown that preoperative cerebral blood flow is diminished in neonates with severe congenital heart defects [23]. Microcephaly, periventricular leukomalacia, or stroke may have been seen in approximately one-third of preoperative neonates with complex congenital heart defects [23–25]. The long-term implications of these findings are the subject of ongoing investigations, but they likely contribute to the suboptimal late neurodevelopmental outcomes experienced by some neonates with complex congenital heart disease.

Neonates with congenital heart defects that are associated with syndromes warrant genetic testing and counseling (e.g., interrupted aortic arch and DiGeorge syndrome; atrioventricular septal defect and trisomy 21). This testing is not done to exclude patients from surgery, but rather to help anticipate comorbidities, plan the postoperative care, and facilitate counseling for future pregnancies [26].

Neonates with critical congenital heart disease who are born prematurely are at increased risk for morbidity and mortality and often require extended hospitalization [27]. The care of these patients may be complicated by any of the problems associated with prematurity, including respiratory distress syndrome, necrotizing enterocolitis, and intraventricular hemorrhage. The musculature in the pulmonary arterioles is less well developed, predisposing patients with left-to-right shunting to a rapid decline in pulmonary vascular resistance and overcirculation. In general, attempts to delay surgical or transcatheter intervention while awaiting growth in such patients are likely to be unsuccessful, and early intervention is recommended [28,29].

Intraoperative Care

The monitoring devices to be used in the postoperative period are selected based on the patient's age, heart defect, and anticipated postoperative course. These devices are generally placed in the operating room usually in collaboration with the pediatric cardiac anesthesiologist (see Chapter 6, *Anesthetic Management for Pediatric Cardiac Surgery*). The information obtained from monitoring devices is extremely useful but is only reliable when obtained from appropriately calibrated instruments. The information obtained must be interpreted in the context of known normal values for patient age. Examples of normal resting blood pressure and normal postoperative heart rate for different patient ages are shown in Tables 7.2 and 7.3 [12,30,31].

Electrocardiographic Leads

The electrocardiographic (ECG) leads should be placed on the chest and limbs so that the patient's heart rate, rhythm, and ST segments can be monitored. The leads should be

Table 7.2 Normal values for blood pressure according to age. (Adapted with permission from Nadas *et al.* [31].)

Age (yr)	Systolic/diastolic pressure (mmHg)	Mean value* (mmHg)
Neonate	68/42	51
To 0.5	80/46	57
0.5–1.0	89/60	70
1.0–2.0	99/64	76
2.0–4.0	100/65	77
4.0–12.0	105/65	78
12.0–15.0	118/68	85
>15.0	120/70	87

*Mean arterial blood pressure calculated as diastolic pressure plus one third of pulse pressure.

Table 7.3 Ranges of heart rate during sinus rhythm in normally convalescing patients after open heart surgery. (Adapted with permission from Kirklin *et al.* [30].)

Age	Heart rate (beats/min)
0–1 month	120–190
1–6 months	110–180
6–12 months	100–170
1–3 years	90–160
3–6 years	80–150
6–15 years	80–140
>15 years	70–130

Table 7.4 Average normal ranges of intracardiac and intravascular pressures (mmHg). (Adapted with permission from Rudolph *et al.* [34].)

Location	Infants and children	Newborn period
Right atrium	a, 3–7; v, 2–5; mean, 1–5	Mean, 0–3
Right ventricle	15–30/2–5	35–65/1–5
Pulmonary artery	15–30/5–10 (mean, 10–20)	35–65/20–40 (mean, 25–40)
Pulmonary wedge	a, 3–7; v, 5–15; mean, 5–12	
Left atrium	a, 3–7; v, 5–15; mean, 5–10	Mean, 1–4
Left ventricle	80–130/5–10	

placed away from the area to be prepped and not too close to the electrocautery grounding pad.

Temperature Monitoring

Monitoring of a child's temperature in the operating room and postoperatively is crucial. The high systemic vascular resistance of a hypothermic child can prevent successful weaning from cardiopulmonary bypass. We monitor both the esophageal and rectal or bladder temperatures in all open-heart cases. The use of forced-air warming blankets in the operating room has been very successful in warming patients after hypothermic cardiopulmonary bypass and keeping them warm in a cold operating room [32].

Oxygen Saturation Probe

Use of a probe for monitoring O_2 saturation on a continuous basis is the standard of care for all infants and children undergoing cardiac surgery [33]. An O_2 saturation probe is simple to use, noninvasive, and relays continuous extraordinarily vital and reliable information. A light-emitting diode (LED) readout displays peripheral O_2 saturation at the same time an audible tone is emitted that is synchronized to the saturation percentage. The surgeon can tune in to the tone while the operation is proceeding and know immediately whether the O_2 saturation is decreasing as a result of surgical manipulation. The saturation monitor also gives some information about cardiac output. If the saturation monitor cannot pick up the pulse, either the child is cold and peripherally vasoconstricted or the cardiac output is not sufficient to generate a recognizable pulse waveform – a grave sign. The saturation probe should be used preoperatively, intraoperatively, and postoperatively and is especially valuable during transport.

Arterial Catheter

An indwelling arterial catheter is necessary for all open-heart operations and most major closed-heart procedures.

Use of an arterial catheter allows continuous monitoring of systemic arterial pressure and easy sampling for measurement of arterial blood gases and other laboratory values. A 20- or 22-gauge plastic angiocath catheter can be inserted into the radial or posterior tibial artery percutaneously or with a surgical cutdown. The dorsalis pedis artery and, in the newborn, the umbilical artery are alternative sites. We rarely use the brachial artery because of the risk of hand ischemia; the common femoral artery can be used if no other sites are available.

Venous Catheters

Adequate intravenous access, usually with two 20-gauge peripheral angiocaths, should be obtained before beginning any major cardiac procedure. Central venous access is required for complex procedures and in most neonates to monitor central venous pressure and administer medications (Table 7.4) [12,34]. Percutaneous catheters may be placed in the subclavian, internal jugular, or femoral vein. For over 15 years our practice has relied extensively and reliably on percutaneously placed subclavian venous catheters (usually on the left side). These catheters are easy to insert, are associated with a low incidence of infection, and provide reliable double- or triple-lumen access for the duration of the child's hospitalization. Other centers prefer the use of internal jugular catheters. The use of ultrasound may increase the rate of successful line placement and minimize complications during placement of central lines in the internal jugular veins [35].

Measurement of venous O_2 saturation in the superior vena cava approximates mixed O_2 venous saturation (SvO_2) and is useful for estimating cardiac output. In neonates recovering from single ventricle palliation, venous O_2 saturation will also aid in the calculation of the ratio of pulmonary to systemic blood flow. Postoperative management centered on maximizing SvO$_2$ has been associated with improved survival following stage 1 Norwood palliation in some centers [36]. Thus care should be taken to select the length of a percutaneous catheter such that the tip will be positioned in the superior vena cava. Continuous assessment of superior vena cava O$_2$ saturation is now feasible following congenital heart surgery using oximetric catheters [37].

Atrial Catheters

Right and left atrial lines placed directly at the conclusion of cardiopulmonary bypass (CPB) are useful for measuring central venous pressure and left atrial pressure and are a reliable long-term source of venous access following complex procedures [38–40]. Two complications, however, have led us to abandon use of these lines and instead use percutaneously placed central lines. One complication is bleeding from the atrium at catheter removal. Such bleeding can cause cardiac tamponade that necessitates emergency mediastinal exploration. A second complication is unrecognized migration of the catheter out of the atrium and into the pericardial space. This complication causes infusion of intravenous or hyperalimentation fluid into the pericardium and insidious progressive cardiac tamponade.

With left atrial lines, meticulous attention must be paid to avoiding the introduction of any air or particulate matter into the line. These substances can cause critical coronary or cerebral arterial embolization. The left atrial line should not be used for routine administration of fluid or medications; if obstructed, this line should not be flushed. The left atrial line should be removed with the same precautions for bleeding as in removal of a right atrial line (sedation so the child does not cough or cry, having blood available, and ensuring there are no clotting abnormalities). We have only employed left atrial lines when the sternum is left open and have then removed them at the time of delayed sternal closure 2–3 days later.

Pulmonary Artery Catheter

Pulmonary artery catheters are uncommonly used in the current era following congenital heart surgery, and are generally reserved for patients with an elevated preoperative pulmonary vascular resistance or those in whom residual left-to-right shunting is anticipated (e.g., multiple muscular ventricular septal defects). A flow-directed Swan–Ganz catheter may be passed either through the subclavian vein or internal jugular vein into the pulmonary artery. Alternatively, the catheter can be placed directly into the pulmonary artery through the right ventricular outflow tract or through the right atrium at the time of surgery. The

pulmonary artery catheter can be used for measurement of pulmonary artery pressure and cardiac output, or for quantification of residual left-to-right shunting. If placed directly through the right ventricle free wall, it should be removed 48–72 hours after the procedure, while the mediastinal chest tubes are still in place and while observing similar precautions for bleeding as with the atrial lines. In our clinical practice we use pulmonary artery catheters infrequently. We often use transthoracic echocardiograms to obtain an intermittent, noninvasive assessment of pulmonary artery pressures.

Near-Infrared Spectroscopy

Near-infrared spectroscopy (NIRS) is a noninvasive monitoring technique providing real-time venous weighted regional oxygen saturations. Used as a trend monitor, these data provide validated, surrogate measures of cardiac output in pediatric patients during and after cardiac surgery [41]. The specific value of cerebral NIRS is the ability to obtain noninvasive, real-time information on the cerebral oxygen content that reflects both oxygen delivery and consumption. Alterations in regional somatic oxygen saturation reflect local perfusion changes and may be an earlier, more sensitive indicator of impending multisystem organ injury or low cardiac output [42].

Early recognition of changes in cardiac output by NIRS monitoring has improved timely, critical interventions in the care of our patients in both the operating room and the ICU. In spite of the limitations of NIRS technology, responding to the trended data can have a positive impact on patient outcomes [43]. As a result of our experience, we routinely place cerebral and somatic NIRS probes on all cardiac surgery patients at the beginning of the case, and follow the saturation trends as an early indicator of changes in cardiac output. Changes in the NIRS monitoring trends often occur before or in the absence of any other physiologic changes (Figure 7.1) [12,43].

Pacemaker Wires

Temporary pacing wires have diagnostic and therapeutic utility in complex pediatric cardiac surgical patients. Atrial electrograms may be directly recorded in patients in whom traditional surface electrocardiograms are nondiagnostic. Temporary pacing may be readily employed in patients with sinus node dysfunction or to restore atrioventricular synchrony in patients with junctional ectopic tachycardia or complete heart block. Burst pacing may be used to terminate re-entrant arrhythmias. Complications associated with these wires are rare but include tamponade with removal and retention [44].

Considering the above, at the conclusion of a cardiac procedure we do not routinely place temporary pacing

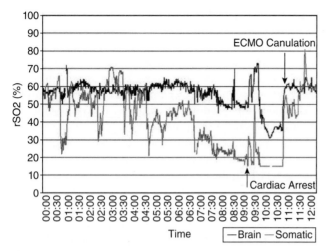

Figure 7.1 Real-time NIRS graph showing 2.5 hours of data that demonstrate acute decrease in rSO2 associated with chest closure in a newborn patient with hypoplastic left heart syndrome and resultant improvement with fluid resuscitation and increased inotropic support. (Reproduced with permission from Kane *et al.* [43].)

wires if the child is in normal sinus rhythm. If a child has evidence of intermittent or complete atrioventricular block, however, temporary atrial and ventricular pacing wires should be placed, typically on the right atrium and the anterior surface of the right ventricle. In certain instances, particularly if the patient is prone to atrial tachycardia or has sinus node dysfunction, the use of temporary atrial pacing wires may be indicated. Temporary pacemaker wires are anchored to the epicardium with fine sutures placed superficially to facilitate removal with minimal risk of hemorrhage. Some other centers agree with this strategy and do not employ routine temporary wires [45]. Other centers advocate routine placement of atrial and ventricular unipolar temporary pacing wires in all patients undergoing CPB [46]. If the patient remains in complete heart block for more than 7–10 days a permanent pacemaker should be placed and the temporary wires removed at that time [47].

Chest Tubes

Drainage catheters appropriate to patient size are left in place after all open and some closed procedures. We do not routinely place chest tubes after simple patent ductus arteriosus ligation or vascular ring division. We recently changed our practice from using rigid thoracotomy tubes with pleurovac drainage to using Blake drains with soft bulb suction except when there is a continuous air leak from the lungs [48]. For a larger child in whom neither pleural space has been entered, a single mediastinal tube

is sufficient. When they are entered, the pleural cavities are drained separately through pleural chest tubes. In small infants, or when there is myocardial swelling, the mediastinal drainage tube can cause coronary arterial or cardiac compression. In this circumstance the mediastinum is best drained with a right pleural tube, which is inserted through the pleural space and then anteriorly into the superior mediastinum. The amount of blood lost through the chest tube(s) should be carefully recorded on an hourly basis.

Nasogastric Tube

The stomach should be routinely decompressed postoperatively with a nasogastric tube in all intubated patients. This step prevents respiratory embarrassment secondary to gastric distention, vomiting, and tracheobronchial aspiration. The nasogastric tube is generally removed when the endotracheal tube is removed.

Urinary Catheter

A urinary catheter is placed in nearly all infants and children undergoing an open cardiac procedure or a complicated closed-heart procedure. The measured urine output per hour is an excellent indicator of the adequacy of renal perfusion and cardiac output. Urinary output should be meticulously recorded on an hourly basis after the operation and should be at least 1 mL/kg/hour in a child with adequate cardiac output and preload. We use urinary catheters with a temperature sensor to avoid placement of rectal temperature probes.

Corticosteroids

Cardiopulmonary bypass is associated with systemic inflammatory response that contributes to dysfunction of multiple organ systems and prolongs postoperative recovery. In a randomized double-blind, placebo-controlled trial conducted at our institution, we demonstrated that the administration of dexamethasone before CPB led to an improved postoperative clinical course and a reduction in the post-bypass inflammatory response as assessed by cytokine levels [49]. We currently administer intravenous dexamethasone (1 mg/kg intravenously, not to exceed 20 mg) in the operating room as soon as the intravenous lines have been placed in all patients who are to undergo CPB. Some form of steroid administration is now used by nearly all pediatric cardiac surgical centers [50].

Routine Postoperative Care

Transport to the Intensive Care Unit

After the procedure the patient must be carefully monitored and transported to the ICU. A formal transition process, derived from Formula One pit stop and aviation models, has been associated with a reduction in technical errors and handover omissions [3]. Before transport, it is helpful for a member of the operating room team to notify the ICU staff of the patient's status. At our center the ICU team receives a "face-to-face" report in the operating room before transport, including a detailed description of the operative findings and repair, the cardiopulmonary bypass, cross-clamp and circulatory arrest times (if any), an assessment of myocardial function coming off bypass, vital signs and filling pressures, and any pressure or O_2 saturation measurements or transesophageal echocardiogram findings. The anesthesia team conveys relevant data about vascular access, the airway and pulmonary function, and the anesthetic. Transportation is facilitated with a portable electrocardiogram and arterial blood pressure monitor along with an O_2 saturation monitor. Oxygen and emergency airway equipment are required for all patients. Battery-operated intravenous pumps are necessary to ensure uninterrupted delivery of fluids and inotropic agents. It is important to avoid hypothermia during transport. On arrival at the ICU, a thorough and systematic approach by trained ICU nurses prevents possible complications and avoids catastrophic situations. The sequence of care of a child is quite important and should begin with attention to the airway and ventilation followed by the cardiovascular system and various subsystems. While the child is being attached to the monitoring systems in the ICU, all staff should observe the patient constantly for signs of difficulties that might require alteration in the normal sequence of events.

Airway and Breathing

Maintaining airway patency and ensuring adequate oxygenation and ventilation are priorities for all patients. Physical examination as soon as the patient arrives in the ICU can reveal clinical signs of desaturation including perioral and/or peripheral cyanosis. Careful inspection for symmetry and adequacy of chest wall expansion and auscultation for bilateral breath sounds should be performed. Other signs of respiratory insufficiency in spontaneously breathing patients include tachypnea, retractions, nasal flaring, grunting, and, of course, apnea. A portable chest radiograph should be obtained for evaluation for pneumothorax, hemothorax, and atelectasis, and for confirmation of the position of the endotracheal tube (ideally in the middle third of the trachea) and the location of central and atrial lines. We obtain routine daily portable chest radiographs for all intubated patients [51]. Continuous pulse oximetry is used in the care of all patients. Selected patients receive continuous end-tidal CO_2 monitoring. Arterial blood gas is always performed.

Patients who are extubated before leaving the operating room are usually placed on supplemental O_2 via nasal cannula or face mask. The initial arterial blood gas for a child who is extubated frequently shows mild CO_2 retention. In the usual case, as the residual effects of anesthesia wear off, the CO_2 tension of arterial blood (PaCO_2) normalizes. If PaCO_2 does not become normal, or if the child starts to show signs of respiratory insufficiency, reintubation should be considered. Careful assessment to identify the cause of respiratory insufficiency may be helpful in avoiding reintubation. Inadequate reversal of muscle relaxants and the sustained effects of narcotics are two situations that are easily managed. Other patients may benefit from noninvasive measures such as continuous positive airway pressure (CPAP) or bilevel positive airway pressure (BiPAP) on a transitional basis. Acute upper-airway edema can be managed with nebulized racemic epinephrine. Some patients may benefit from breathing heliox (helium and O_2 in mixtures) as the edema resolves.

The care of patients who return to the ICU intubated can be complicated. Ensuring a smooth postoperative course requires a thorough understanding of cardiopulmonary interactions [52]. Positive-pressure ventilation and alterations in respiratory mechanics can have a profound effect on hemodynamics, particularly after repair of complex congenital heart defects. Changes in intrathoracic pressure can affect systemic venous return, right ventricular ejection, left atrial filling, and ultimately cardiac output. Appreciation of the unique effects of cardiopulmonary interactions on circulatory physiology following complex congenital heart procedures is essential when selecting ventilator strategy. It is imperative that the physician be present at the time of initiation of ventilatory support. Routine settings simply do not exist. Operating room ventilator and tubing characteristics may differ from those used in the ICU, requiring different settings from those used in the operating room. The presence of a large leak around the endotracheal tube, pleural effusions, chest wall edema, or abdominal distention can dramatically affect the adequacy of delivered breaths. Careful observation and monitoring are critical during this transition phase. In all cases the patient should remain intubated and ventilated until cardiac and respiratory functions are stable.

The usual starting tidal volume is approximately $10\,mL/kg$, and the ventilator rate in general ranges from 24 (newborn) to 8 (adult). A pressure or volume limited mode of ventilation may be used; with either mode, serial blood gases are obtained to monitor the effect of ventilation along with pulse oximetry and end-tidal CO_2 monitoring. Sedation and analgesia, as well as avoidance of patient/ventilator asynchrony and prevention of pulmonary hypertensive crisis, may all be achieved by continuous or intermittent intravenous infusion of morphine and/or midazolam. The importance of patient/ventilator synchrony cannot be overemphasized. In the context of often times minimal cardiac reserve, the demands associated with excessive work of breathing and patient agitation can be deleterious. We commonly use morphine sulfate at 100 μg/kg/hour and midazolam at 50–100 μg/kg/hour. For neonates with delayed sternal closure, limited cardiac reserve, or severe pulmonary hypertension, temporary postoperative paralysis with vecuronium by continuous infusion of 100 μg/kg/hour is frequently used.

Ventilator strategy must be further modified on the basis of each patient's preoperative state and anticipated postoperative physiology. For children with postoperative pulmonary hypertension, ventilator settings are selected to achieve an O_2 tension of arterial blood (Pao$_2$)>100 torr, and a mild respiratory alkalosis. Strong consideration should be given to the early use of inhaled nitric oxide for the treatment of pulmonary hypertension [53]. A 24- to 48-hour period of sedation, paralysis, and full ventilation in our judgment has been associated with less risk of pulmonary hypertensive crisis when the paralysis is stopped and the child is weaned from the ventilator.

For patients who have a single ventricle and shunt-dependent pulmonary blood flow, the goals of mechanical ventilation are different. In these children we try to keep O_2 saturation at 75–80% to maintain a balanced circulation. Excessive ventilation in these patients may reduce pulmonary vascular resistance and lead to pulmonary over-circulation and low systemic output. After a superior cavopulmonary anastomosis (bidirectional Glenn), hyperventilation decreases cerebral blood flow with subsequent decreased blood flow through the superior vena cava to the pulmonary arteries. Therefore mild hypoventilation (Pco$_2$ 48–55 mmHg) has been shown to result in optimal pulmonary blood flow [54,55]. After a Fontan procedure, pulmonary blood flow is passive, and we keep the positive end-expiratory pressure and peak inspiratory pressure at a minimum [56], and aim for early extubation [57]. This strategy minimizes respiratory inhibition of passive pulmonary blood flow.

Most centers are now successfully using protocols that lead to early extubation [58]. For many patients whose condition is stable, weaning can be a quick process. Pressure support and volume support are two ventilator assist modes that are patient triggered and therefore allow assessment of the patient's respiratory drive as well as effort. Flow-sensitive triggering versus pressure-sensitive triggering may facilitate the use of these assist modes in infants. Complex cases require more thought, supervision, and patience. If intubated for a prolonged period, a child may have postextubation vocal cord or subglottic edema. The high negative intrathoracic pressure generated during spontaneous breathing with upper airway obstruction increases afterload, and the increased load may be poorly tolerated by a patient with compromised ventricular function. To minimize such swelling in infants, we often give intravenous dexamethasone before extubation (0.5–1 mg/kg every 6 hours for four doses with the first dose 6 hours before extubation) [59]. Treatment with nebulized racemic epinephrine also is transiently effective in reducing airway edema. Racemic epinephrine (equivalent to 2.25% epinephrine base), 0.125–0.5 mL, is diluted with 2–3 mL water or normal saline solution and is administered by aerosol. Patients should be closely observed for tachyarrhythmias during these treatments and for development of rebound subglottic edema.

Cardiovascular System

The child who had an uncomplicated cardiac procedure with complete correction of the intracardiac defect and adequate myocardial protection should require little extra postoperative manipulation to have a normal convalescence. Standard measures that may be necessary, however, include the following. Blood loss through chest tubes may require replacement during the initial several hours to prevent anemia and hypovolemia. Patients who are hypothermic on admission to the ICU may be peripherally vasoconstricted and may be hypovolemic despite normal systemic arterial and atrial filling pressures. In these patients arterial hypotension should be prevented by adequate volume replacement as the body temperature becomes normal and the peripheral vascular bed dilates. Mild postoperative hypothermia is readily corrected in older children by use of warm blankets and in infants by use of overhead radiant heaters. Hyperthermia increases cardiac workload and O_2 consumption and may lower the threshold for seizure activity. Therefore hyperthermia should be managed early and aggressively with antipyretics (e.g., acetaminophen, ibuprofen, dexamethasone) and surface cooling. An initial 30–40 mg/kg loading dose of acetaminophen is more effective in reducing fever than a 15 mg/kg maintenance dose [60]. Hypovolemia also may be caused by changes in venous capacitance or by protein and fluid leakage into the interstitial, peritoneal, or pleural spaces. This condition should be managed by replacement of the sequestered volume with appropriate amounts of crystalloid, blood, or colloid solution. The standard fluid bolus is 5–10 mL/kg over 5–10 minutes. The hematocrit should be kept greater than 30% during volume administration because anemia decreases the O_2 carrying capacity. Patients who have had palliation only and are still cyanotic require a hematocrit of 40–45%. Care should be taken to avoid over-transfusion as severe polycythemia may increase systemic and pulmonary vascular resistance and interfere with capillary perfusion.

For children who do not follow the anticipated course after cardiac surgery, early consideration must be given to the accuracy of preoperative diagnosis and adequacy of surgical repair. Evaluation begins with an echocardiogram. Cardiac catheterization may be safely performed early after surgery and often will identify residual lesions that are amenable to intervention [61,62].

Fluid and Electrolyte Replacement

Although there is a mild tendency toward sodium and free water retention following CPB, our routine has been to administer standard maintenance fluid therapy after cardiac surgery to help ensure that patients do not become hypovolemic. Extra intravascular fluid is then relatively easily removed with small doses of diuretics (furosemide, 1 mg/kg intravenously every 8 hours). The amount and composition of intravenous fluids may vary depending on the clinical situation and the serum electrolyte levels. For neonates we routinely use dextrose 10% in sodium chloride 0.45% with 20 mEq of potassium chloride per liter. In older children we use dextrose 5% in sodium chloride 0.45% with 20 mEq of potassium chloride/liter.

The formula for maintenance therapy with intravenous fluid is 50 mL of fluid/kg/day in the first 2 days of life. This dosage is increased stepwise to 100 mL/kg/day by the fifth day. For older infants and children, fluid is administered according to the child's weight. Between 0 and 10 kg, infants should receive 100 mL/kg/day. Between 10 and 20 kg, patients should receive 1000 mL/day plus 50 mL/kg/day for each kilogram over 10 kg. Children who weigh 20 kg and more should receive 1500 mL/day plus 10 mL/kg/day for each kilogram over 20 kg (Table 7.5) [12].

Although hypokalemia is known to contribute to ventricular irritability, especially for patients receiving digoxin, this is not as serious a problem in pediatric patients as it is in adults. Hypokalemia should be managed with supplemental intravenous potassium (0.5–1.0 mEq/kg over 2 hours) to keep the serum potassium level normal. However, care should be taken not to administer the potassium too fast or in too concentrated an infusion, or to administer liquid enteral potassium in individual doses exceeding 1 mEq/kg, because doing so can cause a hyperkalemic cardiac arrest. Hyperkalemia typically occurs only in infants and children who have postoperative renal dys-

function. Hyperkalemia should be managed by removing all potassium from intravenous fluids, and oral or rectal administration of sodium polystyrene sulfonate, 1 g/kg every 4 hours may be necessary (Table 7.6) [12]. Should hyperkalemia persist, the patient may need peritoneal dialysis or hemodialysis. Serum magnesium levels should also be monitored postoperatively.

Mild dilutional hyponatremia is almost uniformly present and necessitates no treatment other than diuretic administration and mild restriction of free water intake. Serum sodium levels less than 125 mEq/L may be associated with neurologic symptoms and seizures and should be managed by water restriction and cautious administration of normal saline or 3% normal saline. Hypernatremia is quite rare and usually occurs in patients in renal failure or in infants who have received large amounts of sodium bicarbonate. It should be managed with sodium restriction and liberal fluid intake.

Hypocalcemia occurs mainly in neonates and after transfusion of large amounts of blood products. Myocardial function in neonates is particularly dependent on adequate calcium levels. Serum calcium must be measured frequently and the level maintained within normal limits by intravenous administration of calcium gluconate (50–100 mg/kg intravenously every 6–8 hours) or calcium chloride (20 mg/kg/dose given every 6–8 hours).

Metabolic acidosis usually results from hyperchloremia as a result of fluid administration and ultrafiltration during surgery. However, the most clinically concerning etiology of metabolic acidosis is decreased cardiac output and impaired tissue perfusion resulting in lactic acid production [63,64]. Treatment requires simultaneous correction of the underlying hemodynamic disorder and intravenous administration of sodium bicarbonate (1 mEq/kg/dose). Sodium bicarbonate usually is diluted to 0.5 mEq/mL and administered no faster than 1 mEq/kg/minute. Rapid infusion of sodium bicarbonate has been associated with intraventricular hemorrhage in neonates [65]. Because the buffering action of bicarbonate causes the formation of carbon dioxide, it is important that the infant's ventilatory

Table 7.5 Fluids and electrolytes.

Patient size	mL/kg/hr	mL/kg/day	Type of fluid
Newborns			
Day 1	3	50–75 No electrolytes	D10W, no electrolytes
Day 2–3	4	80–100	D10W 0.45NS with 20 mEq KCl
Day 4–7	4	100	D10W 0.45NS with 20 mEq KCl
Non-newborns			
0–10 kg	4	100	D5 0.45NS with 20 mEq KCl/liter
10–20 kg	2	50 (plus 40 mL/hr for first 10 kg)	D5 0.45NS with 20 mEq KCl/liter
>20 kg	1	20 (plus 60 mL/hr for first 20 kg)	D5 0.45NS with 20 mEq KCl/liter

Table 7.6 Medications and dosages.

ANTIARRHYTHMICS

Amiodarone (Cordarone)	*Cardiac arrest situation:* Infant/child: 5 mg/kg IV bolus, may repeat 3 times Adult: 300 mg IV, may repeat with 150 mg IV in 3–5 minutes, maximum dose 2.2 g IV in 24 h *Non-arrest situation:* Infant/child: 1–2 mg/kg IV over 10–15 minutes, may repeat as needed every 30 minutes, up to 10 mg/kg/day Run IV drip at 5–15 µg/kg/min Adults: 150 mg IV over 10–20 minutes; follow with 250 mg IV over 4 h, then 750 mg IV over next 18 h, then continuous drip 0.5–1 mg/min IV Supplemental bolus doses of 150 mg over 10 minutes may be given for breakthrough ventricular fibrillation or ventricular tachycardia
Lidocaine	Infant/child: 1 mg/1 kg IV bolus, may repeat once, follow with continuous infusion 20–50 µg/kg/min Adults: 1–1.5 mg/kg IV bolus, may repeat doses of 0.5–0.75 mg/kg IV q5 minutes to a total of 3 mg/kg. Follow with continuous infusion, 1–4 mg/min

ANTIHYPERTENSIVES

Esmolol (Brevibloc)	*Postoperative hypertension:* Load: 500 µg/kg/min over 5 minutes with infusion of 125–500 µg/kg/min *SVT* Load: 100–500 µg/kg IV over 5 minutes followed by a continuous infusion 50–500 µg/kg/min
Nicardipine (Cardene)	Infant/child: 0.5–4 µg/kg/min continuous infusion Adult: 5–15 mg/hr continuous infusion
Captopril (Capoten)	Neonates: 0.1 mg/kg/dose PO q8h, titrate to 0.5 mg/kg/dose Infants: 0.1 mg/kg/dose PO q8h, titrate to maximum dose of 2 mg/kg/dose Children: 0.3–0.5 mg/kg/dose PO q8h, titrate to maximum dose of 2 mg/kg/dose
Enalapril (Vasotec)	*Infants and children:* PO: 0.1 mg/kg/day given qd or bid. Titrate as needed up to 0.5 mg/kg/day IV: start at 5–10 µg/kg/dose q8h, titrate to 20 µg/kg/dose *Adolescents and adults:* PO: start at 2.5–5 mg q12h, maximum dose 20 mg q12h IV: 0.625–1.25 mg/dose q8h, titrate as needed (maximum dose 5 mg IV q6h)
Amlodipine (Norvasc)	Children (6–17 yrs): (oral) 2–2.5 mg qd, dosed qd or bid Adults: 2–10 mg/day (oral), dosed qd or bid

DIURETICS

Furosemide (Lasix)	PO: 1–2 mg/kg/dose q6–12h, maximum dose 6 mg/kg/dose IV: 1 mg/kg/dose q6-12 h, maximum dose 4 mg/kg/dose Continuous infusion: <10 kg: 0.1 mg/hr titrate up to 1 mg/hr >10 kg: 1 mg/hr titrate up to 10 mg/hr
Spironolactone (Aldactone)	Neonates: 1–3 mg/kg/day PO q12–24h Children: 1.5–3.3 mg/kg/day PO divided q12–24h (usually q12h) Adults: 25–200 mg/day PO divided q12–24h
Chlorothiazide (Diuril)	Neonates/infants <6 months: IV 2–8 mg/kg/day given bid oral 20–40 mg/kg/day, given bid Infants >6 months and children: IV 4–20 mg/kg/day, divided q6–12h oral 10–40 mg/kg/day, given bid Adults: IV 500–1000 mg IV/day, given bid PO 500–2000 mg/day, given bid

Table 7.6 (*Continued*)

Bumetanide (Bumex)	Neonates: 0.01–0.05 mg/kg/dose IV q24–48° Infants and children: 0.01–0.1 mg/kg/dose IV q6–24° (max 10 mg/day) Infusion (patient >10 kg) 0.02–1.0 mg/hr
Metolazone (Zaroxolyn)	Children: 0.2–0.4 mg/kg/day qd or bid, PO Adults: 5–20 mg/dose qd PO

DIGOXIN (LANOXIN)

Total digitalizing dose (TDD): ½ of TDD administered in the initial dose and then ¼ of TDD given in 2 subsequent doses at 6–12-h intervals.
Infants:
TDD: 25–35 μg/kg PO or 20–30 μg/kg IV
Daily maintenance dose: 6–10 μg/kg PO or 5–8 μg/kg IV divided q12h
1 month-2 years:
TDD: 35–60 μg/kg PO or 30–50 μg/kg IV
Daily maintenance dose: 10–15 μg/kg PO or 7.5–12 μg/kg IV divided q12h
2–5 years:
TDD: 30–40 μg/kg PO or 25–35 μg/kg IV
Daily maintenance dose: 7.5–10 μg/kg/ PO or 6–9 μg/kg IV divided q12h
5–10 years:
TDD: 20–35 μg/kg PO or 15–30 μg/kg IV
Daily maintenance dose: 5–10 μg/kg PO or 4–8 μg/kg IV divided q12h
>10 years
TDD: 10–15 μg/kg PO or 8–12 μg/kg IV
Daily maintenance dose: 2.5–5 μg/kg PO or 2–3 μg/kg IV given once daily
Adults:
TDD: 0.75–1.5 mg PO or 0.5–1 mg IV
Daily maintenance dose: 0.125–0.5 mg PO or 0.1–0.4 mg IV once daily

ANTIBIOTICS

Amikacin (Amikin)	7.5 mg/kg per dose IV q8–12h *UTI:* 5 mg/kg/dose IV q12h *Note:* Measure peak and trough levels if patient has renal dysfunction or if therapy is to last more than 48–72 hours
Amoxicillin	*Endocarditis prophylaxis:* Infants and children: 50 mg/kg PO 1 hour prior to procedure Adults: 2 g PO 1 hour prior to procedure *Asplenia prophylaxis:* 25 mg/kg PO q day
Ampicillin	*Mild to moderate infection:* 50–100 mg/kg/day IV divided q6–8h *Severe infection:* 200–400 mg/kg/day IV divided q4–6h
Ceftriaxone (Rocephin)	50–75 mg/kg/day IV q12–24h
Cephalexin (Keflex)	25–100 mg/kg/day PO divided q6h
Ancef (Cefazolin)	Cephalosporin of choice for surgical prophylaxis Children <40 kg: 50 mg/kg IV Children >40 kg: 25 mg/kg (not to exceed 1 g) IV *Postoperative prophylaxis:* (x48°) 35 mg/kg/dose IV q8°

(*Continued*)

Table 7.6 (*Continued*)

Ceftazidime (Fortaz)	Neonates: 100 mg/kg/day given IV q12° Infants/Children: 100–150 mg/kg/day IV q8° Adult: 1–2 g IV q8–12h
Clindamycin (Cleocin)	15–40 mg/kg/day IV divided, q6–8h 10–30 mg/kg/day PO divided, q6–8h *Surgical prophylaxis for cephalosporin/penicillin allergy:* 10 mg/kg IV, maximum dose 900 mg *Postoperative prophylaxis:* (x48°), 10 mg/kg IV q8°
Gentamicin (Garamycin)	*Systemic infection:* 7 days to 5 years: 2.5 mg/kg/ IV per dose q8–12h >5 years: 2–2.5 mg/kg IV per dose q8h
Oxacillin (Prostaphlin)	100–150 mg/kg IV/day divided q6h
Vancomycin (Vancocin)	10–15 mg/kg/dose IV q6–8h
Meropenem (Merrem)	Neonates: 20 mg/kg/dose IV q12° Infants/Children: 20–40 mg/kg/dose IV q8° Adults: 1–2 g IV q8°

ANALGESICS, SEDATIVES

Acetaminophen w/codeine	0.5–1 mg/kg per dose (as codeine) PO q4–6h prn
Acetaminophen (Tylenol) Chloral hydrate (Noctec)	10–15 mg/kg per dose PO/PR q4-6h prn *Sedation:* 25 mg/kg per dose PO/PR *Hypnosis:* 50–75 mg/kg/dose PO/PR May repeat dose up to a total of 100 mg/kg
Dexmedetomidine (Precedex)	Children: 0.2–0.7 µg/kg/hr
Diazepam (Valium)	IV: 0.05–0.1 mg/kg/dose PO: 0.5 mg/kg/dose
Diphenhydramine HCl (Benadryl)	Children: 2–6 yrs. 6.25 mg PO q6h 6–12 years: 12.5 mg PO q6h >12 years: 25–30 mg PO q6h
Fentanyl (Sublimaze)	IV 0.5–1 mg/kg IV q6°
Hydromorphine (Dilaudid)	1–2 µg/kg per dose IV q1–3h prn
Ibuprofen (Motrin)	Children: 0.015 mg/kg/dose IV q3–6h, continuous infusion 2–3 µg/kg/hr
Ketorolac (Toradol)	Infants and children: 10 mg/kg/dose PO q6–8° Children: IV 0.5 mg/kg IV 6° max dose 15 mg Adults: IV 20–30 mg IV q6° Use for max of 5 days
Lorazepam (Ativan)	0.05–0.1 mg/kg/dose (up to 4 mg) IV
Midazolam (Versed)	0.05–0.2 mg/kg/dose IV 50–150 µg/kg/hr IV
Morphine	0.1 mg/kg/dose IV 50–150 µg/kg/hr IV
Tramadol (Ultram)	Adult dose: 50 mg tab PO q6h prn

Table 7.6 (*Continued*)

ANTIEMETICS

Ondansetron (Zofran)	0.15 mg/kg IV q4–6h
Promethazine (Phenergan)	0.5 mg/kg/dose IV q4–6h

OTHER

Aspirin	10 mg/kg PO or PR qd
Magnesium	25 mg/kg IV
Decadron	CPB dose 1 mg/kg/IV, maximum dose 20 mg Pre-extubation 0.25–2 mg/kg/day divided q6° x24 hr

GASTROINTESTINAL MEDICATIONS

Metoclopramide (Reglan)	0.1–0.2 mg/kg/dose PO/IV qid (maximum dose: 0.8 mg/kg/day)
Ranitidine (Zantac)	<16 years: PO 2–4 mg/kg/day given bid IV 0.5–2 mg/kg/day divided q8h >16 years: 150 mg PO bid or 50 mg IV q8h
Lansoprazole (Prevacid)	Infants: 3–12 months: 0.5–1.5 mg/kg/ PO qd Children <30 kg: 15 mg PO qd Children >30 kg: 30 mg PO qd
Pantoprazole (Protonix)	Children: 20–40 kg: 0.5–1.0 mg/kg/day IV >40 kg: 40 mg/day I
Sodium polystyrene sulfonate (Kayexalate)	1 g/kg PO q6h or PR q2h

status be adequate before administration. Tromethamine (THAM) may be used instead of sodium bicarbonate in patients with impaired ventilation. Other causes of metabolic acidosis include renal tubular acidosis, necrotizing enterocolitis, sepsis, and intraventricular hemorrhage.

Hyperglycemia

The management of hyperglycemia after cardiac surgery in adults and children has been the subject of intense investigation in recent years and remains controversial. In pediatric cardiac surgical patients, observational studies have found associations between hyperglycemia and adverse early postoperative outcomes [66–68]. However, neither intraoperative nor early postoperative hyperglycemia are associated with worse neurodevelopmental outcomes [69]. In a single-center randomized trial involving 700 critically ill children, the majority of whom were recovering from cardiac surgery, patients assigned to the strict glycemic control group had reduced markers of inflammation, shorter ICU length of stay, and lower mortality (3% vs.6%) [70]. Additional trials of glycemic control following pediatric cardiac surgery are ongoing (ClinicalTrials.gov protocol NCT00443599), and these results along with knowledge of neurodevelopmental outcomes are needed before glycemic control can be adopted as standard practice. The use of continuous glucose monitoring may minimize the risk of hypoglycemia in critically ill patients receiving insulin infusions [71].

Renal System

Hourly urine output is a valuable indicator of renal perfusion and cardiac output. Urine output of 1 mL/kg/hour in infants and young children and of 20–40 mL/hour in older children and adults is generally considered adequate. Decreased urine output due to impaired cardiac output is commonly encountered during the first 12–18 hours after complex cardiac surgery, but usually improves as the hemodynamic derangement is corrected and organ perfusion pressure is maintained. The most common cause of persistent poor urine output following congenital heart surgery is inadequate renal perfusion pressure, which is calculated by subtracting the central venous pressure from the mean arterial pressure. Even with adequate cardiac output, in some instances, diuretics are necessary to encourage diuresis and establish a negative fluid balance. Their use does not prevent renal injury or dysfunction [72]. The starting dose of furosemide is 0.5–1.0 mg/kg intravenously per dose at 6–8-hour intervals. The dose then can be sequentially increased to a maximum dose of 10 mg/kg/day until an adequate diuretic response has been obtained or acute renal failure is considered to be present. Additional diuretics that we frequently use are spironolactone and chlorothiazide. In some patients a furosemide infusion (0.1–0.3 mg/kg/hour) establishes more consistent urine output without large fluctuations. A bumetanide drip or the use of fenoldopam (a selective dopamine-1 receptor agonist) are other considerations for patients with marginal urine output [73].

Nutrition

Oral feedings are begun gradually 6–12 hours after removal of the endotracheal tube. The tube is usually removed on the first postoperative day after extracardiac operations and simple open-heart repairs. One exception is coarctation repair, after which feedings are withheld until hypertension is controlled and bowel sounds are clearly active, usually 48–72 hours postoperatively. This strategy helps to prevent reactive mesenteric enteritis and its attendant complications. In infants, feedings are started with small amounts of formula. In the absence of gastric distention, vomiting, and diarrhea, the preoperative feeding formula is slowly resumed (Table 7.7) [12,74]. Older children without evidence of cardiac failure are rapidly advanced to a regular diet. A no-added-salt diet and restricted fluid intake are prescribed for children with signs of congestive heart failure. In Fontan circulation patients we limit free water intake to preserve sodium balance. Early consideration should be given to nasogastric feeding of children unable to resume oral intake within 24–48 hours postoperatively. If enteral feeding is not feasible, parenteral hyperalimentation is indicated (Table 7.8) [12]. Some patients are kept muscle relaxed with vecuronium in the postoperative period. This is not a contraindication to enteral feeding. A number of studies in children have demonstrated that estimates of caloric needs derived from standard equations are often inaccurate. In patients with a prolonged requirement for mechanical ventilation, resting energy expenditure should be periodically measured to avoid overfeeding or underfeeding [75].

Neonates with an umbilical artery line in place should be limited to trophic enteral feedings to reduce the risk of necrotizing enterocolitis (NEC). In contrast, most centers provide full enteral nutrition with a UVC line in place [76].

Table 7.7 Growth, nutrition goals, and caloric content of various formulae.

Calories	Infants	120 kcal/kg/day (should gain approx. 20 g/day)
	Others	1 kcal/mL fluid requirement
Protein	0–1 years	2.5 g/kg/day
	2–13 years	1.5–2 g/kg/day
	13 years	1–1.5 g/kg/day
Fat	0–1 years	0.5 g/kg/day prevents EFA deficiency (0.1 mL/kg/hr 20% IL)
	Infants	Up to 3 g/kg/day
	All others	4 g/kg/day

Caloric content of nutritional solutions

Pedialyte	3 kcal/oz = 0.1 kcal/mL
Pregestimil (hydrolyzed protein, lactose free, contains MCT)	20 kcal/oz = 0.67 kcal/mL
Enfamil, Similac (milk protein based)	20 or 24 kcal/oz = 0.67 kcal/ml or 0.8 kcal/mL
Prosobee, Isomil (soy protein based, lactose free)	20 kcal/oz = 0.67 kcal/mL
Breast milk	22 kcal/oz = 0.7 kcal/mL
Similac Special Care, Enfamil premature	20 or 24 kcal/oz = 0.67 or 0.8 kcal/mL
Portagen (85% fat from MCT)	20 kcal/oz = 0.67 kcal/mL
Pediasure (isoosmolar)	30 kcal/oz = 1.0 kcal/mL
Pediatric Vivonex (hyperosmolar, minimal fat)	24 kcal/oz = 0.8 kcal/mL
Monogen (90% fat from MCT)	22 kcal/oz = 0.73 kcal/mL
Enfaport (84% fat from MCT)	30 kcal/oz = 1.0 kcal/mL
Rice cereal	9 kcal/tbsp
Fat solutions – MCT oil	115 kcal/tbsp = 7.7 kcal/mL
Polycose powder	24 kcal/tbsp = 1.6 kcal/mL

IL = interlipid.
EFA = essential fatty acid.
MCT = medium-chain triglycerides.

Table 7.8 Hyperalimentation: concentrations and goals.

Infants	Goal
Enteral	120 K cal/kg/day = 7.5 mL/kg/h (6 oz/kg/d) 20 kcal formula or 6.25 mL/kg/h (5 oz/kg/d) 24 kcal formula
Parenteral	3.5 mL/kg/h D25 P2.5 plus 0.6 mL/kg/h 20% IL (this combination gives 110 kcals, 2.5 g protein, 3.0 g fat/kg per day)
	Start D12.5 P1.0 plus 0.2 mL/kg/h IL. Increase glucose by 2.5% per day, protein by 0.5 g/day, and IL by 0.1 mL/kg daily

Children	Goal
Enteral	Same number cals as milliliters fluid requirement
Parenteral	Same as above (protein cals not included). Start at D10 P1.0 plus 0.2 mL/kg/h 20% IL and increase as for infants to the following goals

Wt (kg)	15	20	30	40	50	60
Dextrose solution	D25 P2.0	D25 P1.5	D25 P1.5	D25 P1.5	D25 P1.5	D25 P1.5
mL/kg/h	3.2 (4.4)*	2.8 (3.6)*	2.1	1.8	1.6	1.5
20%IL						
mL/kg/hr	0.32 (0.8)*	0.28 (0.8)*	0.21 (0.73)*	0.18 (0.6)	0.16 (0.54)	0.15 (0.48)
= kcal/kg						

Numbers in parentheses are for peripheral total parenteral nutrition with D12.5.
D25 = 25% dextrose.
P2.5 = protein 2.5 gr/kg/day.
*Increased volume and fat.

Signs of NEC include abdominal distention and discoloration, bloody diarrhea or guaiac-positive stools, metabolic acidosis, thrombocytopenia, and pneumatosis intestinalis seen on abdominal radiograph [77]. Treatment includes NPO status, insertion of a nasogastric tube to low intermittent suction, serial blood cultures, administration of broad-spectrum antibiotics, and frequent abdominal radiographs to monitor for perforation. Consultation from a pediatric surgeon should be obtained. Once bowel sounds are heard and the umbilical artery line is removed, enteral nutrition can be initiated, progressing to a goal of 120–150 calories/kg/day. Table 7.7 shows the nutritional goals and caloric content of several formulae [12]. Table 7.8 shows calculations for infant nutrition, both enteral and parenteral [12].

Infection Prophylaxis

Infectious complications are a major source of morbidity following pediatric cardiac surgical procedures. Surgical site infection occurs in 2–5% of children recovering from cardiac surgery. Infants and patients requiring longer cardiopulmonary bypass times, and those needing at least three red blood cell transfusions following surgery are at greatest risk [78]. Published guidelines regarding prevention of surgical site infections emphasize staff education and feedback, the appropriate use of prophylactic antibiotics and skin antiseptics, and the avoidance of razor use for hair removal [79]. Strict adherence to sterile technique during and after the operation is essential in the prevention of infection after cardiac surgery. Broad-spectrum bactericidal antibiotics, given during the perioperative period, have been shown to decrease the risk of infectious complications [80]. We use cefazolin, 50 mg/kg intravenously 30 minutes before the operation and then 50–100 mg/kg/day intravenously divided into 8-hour dosing intervals. Clindamycin (10 mg/kg/dose intravenously every 8 hours) is substituted for patients with known penicillin allergy (Table 7.6) [12]. The first antibiotic dose is given in the operating room as soon as the intravenous lines have been placed, preferably within 30 minutes before incision. We administer cefazolin every 4 hours in the operating room. This is continued on an 8-hour interval regimen until 48 hours postoperatively. Karl and associates performed a worldwide survey of 42 pediatric cardiac surgical units and developed the following conclusions based on the practices at those 42 centers [80]:

1. Perioperative antibiotic prophylaxis in cardiac surgery should be the standard of care.

2. Currently there is no consistent and conclusive evidence of marked superiority of second-generation cephalosporins over first-generation cephalosporins. Cost effectiveness may be the best way to decide.

3. There is consistent evidence indicating that antibiotic prophylaxis of 48 hours duration is effective, a low incidence of infection at the site of surgery being found in all studies using 48 hours of prophylaxis.

4. The duration of antibiotic prophylaxis should not be dependent on catheters, lines, or drains of any type.

5. Currently there is no consistent or conclusive evidence to support the administration of antibiotic prophylaxis in pediatric cardiac surgery for more than 48 hours.

Independent risk factors for bloodstream infections associated with a central line after cardiac surgery include admission weight <5 kg, higher severity of illness score in the first 24 hours after surgery, at least three postoperative red blood cell transfusions, and a requirement for at least 1 week of mechanical ventilation [81]. Staff education and feedback, and adherence to evidence-based guidelines regarding the sterile insertion, access, and maintenance of central lines can prevent many of these infections [82]. Urinary tract infections following cardiac surgery are most effectively prevented by prompt removal of the Foley catheter [83].

Sepsis should be suspected in the postoperative neonate if any of the following symptoms are exhibited: hypoglycemia, thrombocytopenia, acidosis, feeding intolerance, hemodynamic instability, hyperbilirubinemia, or elevated white blood count. Blood, urine, and endotracheal cultures should then be obtained and appropriate antibiotic therapy administered. Patients with asplenia are started on chronic prophylaxis with amoxicillin when their intravenous antibiotics are discontinued.

Postoperative Complications

Low Cardiac Output

Low cardiac output occurs in approximately 25% of newborns within 6–12 hours after surgery [84]. Cardiac output is determined by the product of heart rate and stroke volume, which in turn is determined by preload, afterload, and contractility. Causes of low cardiac output may include one or more of the following: 1) alteration in the heart rate or rhythm; 2) decreased preload from hemorrhage, excessive diuresis, insufficient fluid replacement, or cardiac tamponade; 3) increased afterload from pulmonary hypertension or peripheral vasoconstriction; 4) decreased myocardial contractility from acidosis, electrolyte imbalance, ischemia/reperfusion, a ventriculotomy, or inadequate intraoperative myocardial protection; and 5) suboptimal repair with residual intracardiac shunts, valvular lesions, or excessive pulmonary blood flow. Fluctuations in cardiac output can occur rapidly in the postoperative period, making frequent assessments imperative. Cardiac output assessment includes an evaluation of the child's capillary refill, peripheral pulses, urine output (at least 1 mL/kg/hour), arterial blood pressure, atrial filling pressures, acid–base status, lactate levels, and peripheral and core temperatures. We use cerebral and renal NIRS on all of our postoperative patients as a surrogate for mixed venous O_2 saturation. Initiation of treatment for low cardiac output is based on the identification of the causes.

Heart Rate

Normal postoperative heart rate varies according to the patient's age and size, as shown in Table 7.3 [12,30]. Treatment of neonates for low cardiac output differs from that in older children and adults because of differences in cardiovascular physiology. In neonates ventricular diastolic compliance is diminished and newborn infants have a limited ability to increase their stroke volume [85,86]. This decrease in compliance is related to a greater ratio of non-contractile to contractile mass in the neonatal heart [87]. Stroke volume remains relatively fixed at approximately 1.5 mL/kg. Because of the limited ability of the neonatal heart to increase stroke volume, cardiac output is rate dependent [88]. Sinus tachycardia with a heart rate up to 200 beats/minute is well tolerated in newborns and increases cardiac output. Heart rate may be optimized by pacing or intravenous infusion of chronotropic agents such as dopamine, dobutamine, and epinephrine. In our clinical practice we have found the combination of dopamine and dobutamine very effective in increasing heart rate and cardiac output in a child with intact atrioventricular conduction. In selected cases we have added epinephrine for further augmentation of heart rate. For patients with either complete or intermittent postoperative heart block, ventricular or preferably atrioventricular pacing at an appropriate rate is necessary to increase the cardiac output. Patients with sick sinus syndrome or sinus node dysfunction may benefit from atrial pacing.

Preload

Ensuring adequate circulating blood volume is essential to maintaining good postoperative cardiac output. Hypovolemia results in decreased ventricular filling and low cardiac output. Conversely, augmenting the end-diastolic volume increases the number of interactions between actin and myosin and results in a larger stroke volume and thus higher cardiac output. This is known as the Frank–Starling mechanism (Figure 7.2) [12,89]. Volume replacement therapy should be provided with close attention to filling pressure, arterial pressure, and physical signs such as liver distention and fontanelle depression. The filling pressure required to achieve the same degree of preload will change as myocardial dysfunction improves over time. Certain cardiac lesions will predictably require a higher filling pressure to overcome early diastolic dysfunction (e.g., tetralogy of Fallot, aortic stenosis, etc.). The type and amount of fluid replacement should be based on the hemoglobin level, hematocrit, albumin level, and percentage of volume loss. Transfusion should be considered when more than 10% of the child's blood volume has been removed, as in blood testing for neonates or chest tube loss for older children. Normal circulating blood volume for an infant is 95 mL/kg

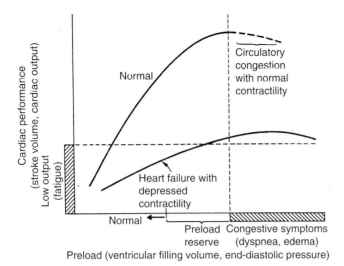

Figure 7.2 The Frank–Starling mechanism dictates that increasing preload will enhance cardiac stroke volume and thus cardiac output. Excessive preload will cause pulmonary congestion and decreased stroke volume. This relationship exists in normal hearts and in those with depressed contractility. (Reproduced with permission from Friedman *et al.* [89].)

and for an older child 75 mL/kg. Boluses of fluid are given in increments of 5–10 mL/kg over several minutes. However, increasing the filling volume to a left atrial pressure greater than 14–16 mmHg rarely produces additional increase in cardiac output, and a left atrial pressure greater than 20 mmHg can cause pulmonary edema [90]. Because of the large venous capacitance of infants, right atrial pressures may not necessarily reflect the volume administered and should not be used solely as an index of adequate volume replacement. In particular, if a child has evidence of facial puffiness, peripheral edema, or a full fontanelle, adequate volume replacement has probably been achieved. In neonates recovering from tetralogy of Fallot or truncus arteriosus repair, preload to the left ventricle, and thus cardiac output, may be maintained by routinely leaving a small atrial communication to allow right-to-left atrial shunting. This principle also applies to the use of fenestration in children undergoing Fontan surgery [91].

Afterload

Afterload is the sum of forces that oppose systolic performance. It is best estimated by systolic wall stress and vascular impedance, both of which are difficult to measure at the bedside. Afterload can be estimated by the resistance of the vascular bed (systemic or pulmonary) against which the ventricle is pumping. An increase in systemic vascular resistance or pulmonary vascular resistance can significantly reduce both stroke volume and the extent and velocity of wall shortening; the result is decreased cardiac output

and ventricular function. Increased vascular resistance is common after CPB in neonates [84] and adults [92]. Physiologic factors such as hypoxia, acidosis, hypothermia, and pain can increase systemic and pulmonary vascular resistance. Such factors are more important in the care of newborn infants who have a very reactive pulmonary vascular bed. Elimination of these vasoconstricting factors is important in reducing afterload. Conversely, increased afterload may be a compensatory response necessary to maintain blood pressure in the setting of decreased cardiac contractility. Increased afterload also may be secondary to residual right or left ventricular outflow tract obstruction.

Regardless of cause, afterload can be pharmacologically decreased by vasodilatation of the vascular bed. For the past 15 years we have been routinely using milrinone after most complex procedures. Milrinone is a phosphodiesterase inhibitor that increases intracellular levels of cyclic adenosine monophosphate (AMP) which causes vasodilation of the systemic and pulmonary vascular beds. Milrinone also has inotropic and lusitropic (myocardial relaxation) properties [93]. Milrinone has been show in a multicenter trial to reduce the occurrence of low cardiac output syndrome following complex two ventricular repairs in infants and children [94]. Milrinone has been used successfully at doses of 0.25–1.0 μg/kg/minute titrated for effect. Peripheral vascular resistance (and systemic blood pressure) is also effectively lowered by intravenous infusion of the calcium channel blocker nicardipine, infused at 0.5–4.0 μg/kg/minute. Nitroglycerin is another direct smooth-muscle relaxant and potent coronary arterial vasodilator. Nitroglycerin is administered in a drip concentration of 1.0–5.0 μg/kg/minute and is titrated by observation of resultant blood pressure. Nitroprusside is another nitric oxide donor that may be used to lower vascular resistance. With the use of any of these vasodilators, volume replacement may be necessary to fill the expanded vascular space and maintain adequate preload. Severe hypotension can result from the use of these drugs. If hypotension occurs, the infusion should be reduced or stopped until adequate preload can be given. These vasodilators should only be used when the patient's arterial pressure is being continuously monitored with an arterial line.

In some patients decreased systemic vascular resistance after CPB leads to hypotension [95]. Risk factors may include preoperative heart failure and longer cross-clamp times. The cause of this state is unclear but may be related to release of inflammatory mediators or relative vasopressin deficiency. Published experience in the care of children [96] and adults [97] suggests that vasopressin infusion of 0.0003–0.002 units/kg/minute may be beneficial.

Positive-pressure ventilation has important effects on afterload of both the systemic and pulmonary ventricle. The increase in mean airway pressure will lead to reduced transmural wall stress and thus decreased afterload of the systemic ventricle. This can be beneficial in patients with poor myocardial function or a volume-overloaded ventricle. In contrast, the elevated intrathoracic pressure associated with positive-pressure ventilation will increase afterload on the right ventricle which may be poorly tolerated in patients with dysfunction of the pulmonary ventricle or regurgitation of the right-sided atrioventricular valve or pulmonary valve.

Contractility

Cardiac contractility is the load-independent ability of the myocardium to generate force. Contractility may be chronically impaired preoperatively by pressure or volume overload related to the specific cardiac lesion. Contractility may be depressed intraoperatively by drugs, anesthesia, myocardial ischemia, extensive ventriculotomy, or myocardial resection. Contractility may be affected postoperatively by hypoxia, acidosis, and pharmacologic agents. In recent

years, the use of modified ultrafiltration after CPB has been shown to improve intrinsic left ventricular systolic function, improve diastolic compliance, increase blood pressure, and decrease inotropic drug use in the early postoperative period [98]. In children the cardiac index tends to be lower 4 hours after the operation than it is soon after discontinuing CPB; it begins to increase to normal value after 9–12 hours [99]. If a child has evidence of low cardiac output after heart rate, preload, and afterload are optimized, myocardial contractility should be enhanced by pharmacologic means. In the care of most patients who have undergone a major cardiac surgical procedure our policy is to start pharmacologic support in the operating room while weaning from bypass rather than waiting for the signs of low output to appear. Several inotropic agents are currently available and each has its own characteristic effects that may be more suitable for use in various clinical situations. These medications and dosages are listed in Table 7.9 [12].

Table 7.9 Dosages of medications for inotropic support, afterload reduction, paralysis, and sedation.

Agent	Dosage
INOTROPIC SUPPORT	
Dobutamine	Range: 5–20 µg/kg/min; concentration: 600 mg/L in D10.2NS*
Dopamine	Range: 2.5–20 µg/kg/min; concentration: 600 mg/L in D10.2NS*
Epinephrine	Range: 0.01–0.4 µg/kg/min; concentration: 10 mg/L D10.2NS*
Isoproterenol	Range: 0.01–0.2 µg/kg/min; concentration: 10 mg/L D10.2NS*
VASODILATORS†	
Milrinone	Range: 0.2–0.7 µg/kg/min; concentration: 1 mL–5 µg/kg/min in 0.45 NS (compatible with other medications if mixed at site).* Double concentration at higher dose range
Nipride	Range: 1–5 µg/kg/min; concentration: 100 mg/L D10 W (protect metriset and IV tubing from light). Monitor liver enzymes*
Nitroglycerin	Range: 1–5 µg/kg/min; concentration: 1 mL–1 µg/kg/min (use nonpolyvinylchloride tubing) in D10.2NS*
PARALYSIS AND SEDATION	
Chloral hydrate	Range: 30–50 µg/kg/dose PR
Fentanyl	Range: 2–20 µg/kg/hr in D10.2NS, continuous infusion
Morphine	Range: 50–100 µg/kg/hr IV in D10.2NS, continuous infusion
Pavulon	Bolus 0.1 mg/kg Infusion 100 µg/kg/hr
Vecuronium	Bolus 0.1 mg/kg Infusion 100 µg/kg/min
Versed	Range: 50–100 µg/kg/hr IV in D10.2NS, continuous infusion
Tylenol	Range: 10–20 mg/kg/dose PR

*Concentration should be doubled or tripled according to hemodynamic status and/or fluid restriction.
†Nitroglycerin and Nipride are not compatible with other medications in this table.

Dopamine has both α-adrenergic and β-adrenergic receptor effects on the myocardium, depending on the dosage used. Doses in the range of 2–5 μg/kg/minute preferentially dilate mesenteric and renal vessels and increase renal blood flow. Doses in the β range (5–10 μg/kg/minute) tend to increase cardiac output with a slight increase in heart rate [100]. Dopamine at α ranges (10–20 μg/kg/minute) is usually avoided because of an increase in pulmonary vascular resistance. It appears that the myocardium of the neonate might be less sensitive than that of older children to the effects of dopamine. Dobutamine, another synthetic catecholamine, acts primarily on myocardial β-adrenergic receptors [101]. A benefit of dobutamine is that it increases contractility with little to no increase in systemic vascular resistance. The usual starting dose of dobutamine is 2.5–5 μg/kg/minute; the dose is then titrated to the desired effect. We have found that some patients respond to dobutamine with an unwanted increase in heart rate.

Isoproterenol, another β agonist, improves cardiac output mainly by increasing heart rate but also has its own direct inotropic effects. Milrinone, which acts mainly by afterload reduction, also exerts an inotropic effect independently. Patients who have marked myocardial dysfunction may respond to intravenous epinephrine at 0.05 μg/kg/minute. Such dosing primarily activates β_1 cardiac receptors, causing increased inotropism, and β_2 peripheral receptors, causing reduced afterload. Epinephrine is not frequently used at doses higher than 0.2 μg/kg/minute because of its marked α-adrenergic action at these doses and adverse effect on renal perfusion. However for some neonates high-dose epinephrine may be required for a short time. Calcium is a strong inotropic agent, but its action is brief. Neonates often require supplemental calcium on a scheduled basis or as an infusion. Digoxin improves cardiac contractility and can be used in patients who appear to require long-term inotropic support. The digitalizing intravenous dose is 40 μg/kg for children younger than 1 year, and 30 μg/kg for those older than 1 year (3 doses divided over a 24-hour period). The daily maintenance dose is one-fourth the total digitalizing dose: 10 μg/kg/day given in two divided doses (Table 7.6) [12].

There is good evidence that critically ill neonates on a high dose of inotropes benefit from supplemental hydrocortisone treatment [102,103]. Suominen and colleagues demonstrated that most of the hemodynamically compromised neonates who were unresponsive to high doses of inotropic agents and fluid resuscitation after heart surgery responded to hydrocortisone with improvement of hemodynamic parameters and a decrease in inotropic requirements [104]. The use of "stress dose steroids" for the patient who is not responding appropriately to inotropic support is now routine at our institution. We use 100 mg/m²/day of hydrocortisone administered intravenously every 6 hours.

When medical therapy is ineffective in supporting cardiac output as evidenced by continued oliguria, hypotension, decreased mixed venous O_2, and increased lactate, the use of a mechanical circulatory assist device such as venoarterial bypass or left ventricular assist device is indicated.

In our practice the most useful mechanical assist device has been extracorporeal membrane oxygenation (ECMO). This modality was originally developed for neonatal respiratory failure but may be used for postcardiotomy cardiogenic shock in children or as a bridge to cardiac transplantation [105–107]. Survival rates of up to 60% have been reported [108]. ECMO provides effective support for postoperative cardiac and pulmonary failure refractory to medical management. Early institution of ECMO may decrease the incidence of cardiac arrest and end-organ damage, thus increasing survival in these critically ill patients [109]. Patients who are within approximately 10 days of surgery are cannulated via the sternotomy incision, whereas patients who are more remote from surgery tend to be cannulated from the neck. The femoral vessels may also be used for cannulation in patients weighing more than 10 kg. Despite full heparinization, the incidence of bleeding complications after ECMO in the support of these patients is relatively low. Use of ECMO as an adjunct to cardiopulmonary resuscitation is now becoming more widely used. In one multicenter study extracorporeal cardiopulmonary resuscitation resulted in hospital survival in 42% of infants and children with heart disease [110].

Left ventricular assist devices are useful in supporting patients with isolated left ventricular failure after cardiac surgery, particularly those who cannot be weaned from CPB after anomalous left coronary artery repair [111]. The Biomedicus (Medtronic, Minneapolis, MN) centrifugal pump can be used with left atrial and aortic cannulation [112]. Ventricular assist devices can also be used to provide longer term mechanical support in patients who require bridge to cardiac transplantation. We currently use two paracorporeal pneumatically driven devices. Thoratec Laboratories (Pleasanton, CA) produces such a device that can be used in patients as small as 25 kg. The Berlin Heart system offers a wide selection of blood pumps and cannulas specifically designed for infants and small children [113,114]. The Berlin Heart has been used in a 2.2 kg infant. In children requiring a bridge to transplantation, EXCOR (Berlin Heart, Inc. The Woodlands, TX) provided substantially longer support times than ECMO, without a significant increase in the rates of stroke or multisystem organ failure. Survival to transplant and long-term survival was higher with the Berlin Heart [115].

Cardiac Arrhythmias

Disturbances of the heart rhythm and rate are common after complex congenital heart surgery and may rapidly result in low cardiac output [116]. The cardiac rhythm cannot always reliably be determined by examination of the electrocardiogram tracing produced by routine bedside monitors, and if there is any concern that the patient is not in sinus rhythm, a 12-lead electrocardiogram should be obtained. Temporary pacing wires may be used to obtain an atrial electrogram; alternatively a transesophageal pacing electrode may be placed. Establishing the correct diagnosis is essential to direct therapy. Consultation from a pediatric cardiac electrophysiologist is routinely obtained in our center for cardiac arrhythmias.

Supraventricular tachycardia (SVT) includes sinus tachycardia, atrial fibrillation, atrial flutter, automatic atrial tachycardia (AAT), orthodromic reciprocating tachycardia (ORT), antidromic reciprocating tachycardia (ART), junctional ectopic tachycardia (JET), and atrioventricular node reentry tachycardia (AVNRT). Sinus tachycardia may be secondary to hypovolemia, pain, anemia, or administration of inotropic drugs. It may also result from low cardiac output due to impaired myocardial contractility or cardiac tamponade. Identification of the etiologic factors guides appropriate therapy.

First-line treatment for most tachyarrhythmias includes correction of any electrolyte abnormalities, decreasing exogenous and endogenous catecholamines, and treatment of fever. Burst pacing via an esophageal pacing electrode or temporary atrial wires or a dose of adenosine (0.1 mg/kg IV) may acutely terminate many types of supraventricular reentrant arrhythmia. If these measures fail, reentrant SVT may also be acutely terminated by synchronized electrical cardioversion (0.5–1.0 J/kg). For persistent supraventricular arrhythmias, amiodarone or procainamide may be useful. JET is more difficult to manage because it does not respond to the various forms of cardioversion noted above [117]. For patients with temporary pacing wires, atrial pacing should be initiated at rates just faster than the junctional rate to restore atrioventricular synchrony. The rate of JET often slows with reduction in temperature to normal or even the use of mild hypothermia [118,119]. Amiodarone or procainamide may be useful in patients with refractory JET [119,120]. Our practice is to load with amiodarone 5 mg/kg IV in 1 mg/kg aliquots. Intravenous amiodarone may cause acute bradycardia and myocardial depression and care must be taken when administering intravenous boluses of this drug [121]. We have not used intravenous propranolol in the immediate postoperative period because of the danger of severe myocardial depression and cardiac arrest. If a beta blocker is considered necessary, intravenous esmolol is our current drug of choice because of its very short half-life.

Premature ventricular contractions (PVCs) may result from myocardial irritability in association with hypokalemia or hypomagnesemia and may be eliminated by correcting these electrolyte abnormalities. Infrequent unifocal PVCs are usually benign and may be observed. Persistent ventricular ectopy (more than six ectopic beats/minute) should be treated by an intravenous bolus of lidocaine (1 mg/kg) followed if necessary by continuous lidocaine drip (20–40 μg/kg/minute). Short runs of ventricular tachycardia are frequently controlled by lidocaine; however when ventricular tachycardia is persistent or associated with systemic arterial hypotension, it should be managed promptly with defibrillation. Persistent ventricular tachycardia is an ominous sign of impending cardiovascular collapse (often secondary to coronary insufficiency) and emergent evaluation is necessary. Long-term control of ventricular tachyarrhythmia may require administration of procainamide, amiodarone, or mexiletine.

Atrioventricular dissociation results in a loss of atrioventricular synchrony and a 20–30% decrease in end-diastolic filling, stroke volume, and cardiac output. Temporary epicardial pacemaker wires will allow sequential atrioventricular pacing, which may prove lifesaving to such patients. Sinus bradycardia and second-degree atrioventricular block may be similarly managed by atrial or atrioventricular sequential pacing. Complete heart block is treated acutely by temporary pacing. A permanent pacemaker should be inserted if normal sinus rhythm has not returned within 7–10 days of surgery [47]. We have favored the use of epicardial pacing in children who will require a lifetime of pacing with conversion to a transvenous system when the patient reaches adulthood. This strategy has been strengthened by the development of steroid-eluting epicardial leads that have been shown to have the same longevity as conventional endocardial leads [122].

Bleeding

Excessive postoperative bleeding occurs in 1–2% of patients undergoing congenital heart surgery. It is somewhat more frequent in severely cyanotic patients, polycythemic patients, and patients who are undergoing a reoperation [123]. Alterations in the normal hemostatic mechanisms occur during CPB. These changes may be attributed to oxygenator platelet adherence and mechanical trauma to the platelets and blood components by cardiotomy suction. Postoperative bleeding can result from inadequate heparin neutralization, thrombocytopenia, or perfusion-related dilution of clotting factors. More rarely it is caused by protamine overdose, fibrinolysis, or disseminated intravascular clotting. Disseminated intravascular clotting is usually associated with postoperative bacteremia and prolonged low cardiac output states. A surgical bleeding point may always be a possibility. Management of bleeding requires correction of the underlying cause, management of systemic hypertension, and simultaneous replacement of platelets and other deficient clotting factors. Underneutralized circulating heparin causes prolongation of the partial thromboplastin time and is corrected by administration of additional protamine. Thrombocytopenia (<50 000 platelets/mm^2) necessitates transfusion of platelets. Platelets should not be administered too rapidly because of the risk of acute pulmonary hypertension with right ventricular failure. Surgical re-exploration is indicated whenever the hourly chest drainage in the absence of clotting abnormalities exceeds 3 mL/kg body weight/hour for 3 consecutive hours after surgery or if there is a sudden, marked increase in chest tube drainage of 5 mL/kg/hour in any 1 hour. Procrastination may result in fatal cardiac tamponade or further transfusion-related clotting abnormalities. At reoperation all suture lines and raw surfaces should be explored for the origin of bleeding. We have used fibrin glue with some success for suture line bleeding [124]. This "glue" is made by mixing cryoprecipitate and thrombin directly in the field at the site of bleeding but is now commercially available (Baxter Healthcare Corp., Westlake Village, CA). The product mixes human plasma, thrombin, and calcium, and it is sprayed in a thin layer on the affected suture lines.

The use of fresh whole blood has been shown to reduce the incidence of postoperative bleeding, particularly when multiple suture lines are involved, such as after the arterial switch procedure [125,126]. If fresh whole blood is not available (e.g., because of testing requirements for human immunodeficiency virus etc.), it is useful to have fresh frozen plasma, cryoprecipitate, and platelets available after CPB so that these factors can be administered before chest closure. Thus the neonatal population may achieve the greatest benefit from post-bypass fresh whole blood therapy [127].

For many years we used aprotinin (antifibrinolytic serine protease inhibitor) to reduce bleeding and the need for blood product use after pediatric cardiopulmonary bypass [128]. Because of concerns for renal failure and myocardial infarction in adults the FDA requested marketing suspension which prompted Bayer to remove the drug from the marketplace [129,130]. We now use epsilon-aminocaproic acid (Amicar) in all cardiopulmonary bypass patients. Amicar has recently been shown to be as effective as Aprotinin without the concerning complications [131] (Table 7.9) [12]. In cases with severe uncontrolled postoperative bleeding we have selectively used recombinant activated factor VII [129].

Cardiac Tamponade

Early postoperative cardiac tamponade results from persistent (usually excessive) surgical bleeding not properly drained by the chest tubes. Cardiac tamponade must be strongly suspected when chest tube drainage abruptly decreases or stops in a patient with previous significant bleeding. This complication can occur even when the pericardium has been removed or left wide open during the operation. External cardiac compression by blood or blood clots causes impaired diastolic filling, elevated venous pressure, paradoxic neck vein distention, systemic arterial hypotension, and a narrow pulse pressure. Arterial pres-

sure decreases characteristically and shows a minimal response to volume administration. Cardiac tamponade demands prompt surgical re-exploration for evacuation of the pericardial hematoma and control of bleeding. For patients with a rapidly deteriorating hemodynamic situation the sternotomy may have to be opened in the ICU for removal of clots and relief of cardiac compression. An assessment can then be made about closing the chest at the bedside, leaving the chest open with a silicone skin patch (Silastic; Dow Corning Corp, Midland, MI), or returning the patient to the operating room. With the ready availability of echocardiography, any child with evidence of low cardiac output who has a suspected diagnosis of cardiac tamponade can quickly have this complication detected. The use of echocardiography helps prevent unnecessary opening of the chest of a patient who has low cardiac output because of myocardial dysfunction.

Some patients may have myocardial swelling and chamber dilatation that prevent closure of the chest because of hemodynamic instability. In these circumstances it may be advantageous to leave the sternum open and cover the mediastinum with an impermeable sheet of Silastic sutured to the skin edges [132,133]. This procedure may be done in critically ill patients in the operating room at the initial closure or after the chest is opened in the cardiac surgical ICU for tamponade or low cardiac output. Once myocardial swelling has resolved and cardiac and pulmonary function have stabilized, the sternum may be electively closed in the ICU within 48–72 hours. In one series delayed sternal closure was a risk factor for Gram-negative mediastinitis [134].

Delayed cardiac tamponade from post-pericardiotomy syndrome can occur several days or weeks after the operation and manifests with low-grade fever and chest pain. Physical signs may include tachycardia, decreased pulse pressure, pericardial friction rub, and, in advanced cases, signs of low cardiac output. The extent of pericardial effusion is easily evaluated by echocardiography. We obtain a discharge echocardiogram and an anteroposterior and lateral chest radiograph in all patients before they leave the hospital to rule out post-pericardiotomy syndrome. Symptomatic treatment with nonsteroidal anti-inflammatory drugs or a short course of steroids is generally effective [135]. Sizable pericardial effusions may require subxiphoid needle aspiration. If this is unsuccessful, percutaneous insertion of a pigtail catheter may be needed. Otherwise open pericardial drainage may be necessary either by opening the lower portion of the sternum or through a left thoracotomy, creating a pericardial window.

Pulmonary Hypertensive Crises

Pulmonary hypertensive crisis describes a serious syndrome characterized by an acute rise in pulmonary artery pressure followed by a reduction in cardiac output and, in patients with residual intracardiac shunts, a fall in systemic oxygen saturation. Historically, pulmonary hypertensive crises were encountered in older infants and children who were recovering from repair of large left-to-right shunt lesions (e.g., truncus arteriosus, complete atrioventricular canal) or obstructed pulmonary venous return. Given that nearly all lesions with large left-to-right shunts at the ventricular or arterial level are now repaired in early infancy, pulmonary hypertensive crises are much less common, but may be life threatening in those patients in whom a crisis occurs. The pulmonary artery pressure may be essentially normal following the repair until an episode of pulmonary hypertension occurs. Pulmonary hypertensive crises may be precipitated by noxious stimuli (e.g., suctioning of the endotracheal tube), hypoxemia, hypothermia, or hypercarbia with resultant acidosis. Once the pulmonary hypertensive crisis begins it can be very difficult to break the vicious cycle of right ventricular dysfunction and low cardiac output. Treatment includes ventilation with 100% oxygen, hyperventilation, sedation with intravenous fentanyl or morphine, inhaled nitric oxide, and neuromuscular blockade. These crises may be fatal in spite of intensive therapy; therefore, their prevention is critically important. An important preventive measure in patients at risk is the initial maintenance of neuromuscular blockade and deep sedation for the first 24–48 hours following cardiac surgical intervention. This appears to minimize the incidence of pulmonary hypertensive crises. In infants and children at greatest risk of pulmonary hypertensive crisis, we also routinely use inhaled nitric oxide. In fact, inhaled nitric oxide has been the single most significant advance in the treatment of pulmonary hypertension [53,136]. It is a selective pulmonary vasodilator with essentially no systemic effects [137]. We have used nitric oxide in postoperative patients at doses of 5–20 ppm [138]. These patients must be monitored for methemoglobin toxicity (measured with arterial blood gases). In a randomized clinical trial, sildenafil, a selective phosphodiesterase type-V inhibitor, has been shown to facilitate weaning of children from inhaled nitric oxide [139]. Patients thought to need longer-term treatment also are transitioned to oral sildenafil [140]. Inhaled prostacyclin is an alternative pulmonary vasodilator that acts through cyclic adenosine monophosphate (cAMP)-mediated pulmonary vasodilatation. In children with inadequate response to nitric oxide, inhaled PGI_2 may be a useful alternative or adjunctive pulmonary vasodilator [141].

Cardiac Arrest

Cardiac arrest occurs in approximately 3% of all patients who are receiving care in pediatric cardiac ICU [142]. Common causes of cardiac arrest following pediatric cardiac surgery include progressive low cardiac output, severe pulmonary hypertension, arrhythmias, coronary ischemia, airway events, aortopulmonary shunt thrombosis, and cardiac tamponade. Many of these events are not sudden, and thoughtful and anticipatory circulatory and respiratory support as previously discussed likely prevents many evolving clinical situations from progressing to cardiac arrest. Although certain concepts in the management of cardiac arrest are based on pediatric advanced life support (PALS) guidelines issued by the American Heart Association, [143] special considerations are warranted for many patients recovering from cardiac surgery [142]. Resuscitative efforts should be directed by the most experienced team member, and this code leader should not become preoccupied with the performance of individual tasks. A patent airway and adequate ventilation is a priority. In nonintubated patients ventilation is started using a face mask and Ambu bag, followed by endotracheal intubation. If patients are already intubated, patency of the endotracheal tube must be ascertained. If obstructed, the tube should be replaced. The adequacy of ventilation is confirmed by end-tidal CO_2 detection, the quality of the (bilateral) breath sounds, and the inspiratory expansion of the chest. Note that in the absence of pulmonary blood flow, either because of an obstructed aortopulmonary shunt or cardiac arrest, end-tidal CO_2 will not be detectable even if the endotracheal tube is patent and its tip properly located in the mid-trachea. Care should be taken to avoid overventilation, which may increase intrathoracic pressure and impede pulmonary blood flow, particularly in patients with palliated single ventricle physiology.

Simultaneously attempts should be directed at restoring effective circulation. This is accomplished initially by external cardiac massage. In infants this is best done by placing both thumbs in front of the sternum and all other fingers on the patient's back. There should be no hesitation in performing closed cardiac massage in a patient who has had a recent sternotomy. The precordium should be compressed 100 times per minute (per PALS guidelines) while checking on the adequacy of massage by the quality of the femoral or carotid pulses, or by arterial pressure tracing when available. If an adequate cardiac output cannot be obtained with external cardiac compression, or if tamponade is suspected, the chest should be immediately opened and manual internal cardiac massage instituted. Epinephrine is the single most useful drug to assist in restoring cardiac action in a child who has experienced cardiac arrest. Epinephrine, 10 μg/kg, may be given either intravenously or by intracardiac injection via the left precordial or subxiphoid route. Injection directly into the heart is no longer practiced because of the possibility of injury to the coronary artery. For a patient without intravenous access, epinephrine may be given via the endotracheal tube at a dose of 100 μg/kg. Calcium chloride, 10–20 mg/kg, or calcium gluconate, 50–100 mg/kg, may be given as an inotropic agent. Sodium bicarbonate at a dose of 1 mEq/kg is administered to normalize arterial pH.

Concomitant with air exchange and restoration of circulation, evaluation must be made to ascertain the cause of cardiac arrest. If acute hypoxia preceded the cardiac arrest in patients with a Blalock–Taussig shunt, the possibility must be considered that it has thrombosed and the chest must be opened to "strip" the shunt. Cardiac rhythm is determined by electrocardiogram. Ventricular fibrillation is managed with defibrillation (1–2 J/kg), which must be repeated until an organized heart beat is restored. Ventricular arrhythmias should raise suspicion for coronary ischemia or hyperkalemia. Ventricular ectopy and ventricular tachycardia may necessitate lidocaine administration (1 mg/kg intravenously). For patients with heart block who are dependent on temporary pacing, it should be ensured that the wires have not become dislodged, the battery expired, or the ventricular capture threshold did not exceed the programmed voltage output.

Survival rates following in-hospital cardiac arrest in children with heart disease range from 40–66% [144,145]. It is noteworthy that infants and children seem to tolerate longer periods of hypotension from a cardiac arrest than do adult patients without neurologic or other organ system damage. In one report of pediatric cardiac patients who experienced an in-hospital cardiac arrest, 83% of survivors were grossly neurologically intact at hospital discharge [144]. Clinical trials have shown that mild hypothermia reduces mortality and neurologic outcomes in adult cardiac arrest victims and newborns with hypoxic–ischemic encephalopathy [146,147]. Ongoing clinical trials will determine whether therapeutic hypothermia reduces mortality and improves neurodevelopmental outcomes following pediatric cardiac arrest. A rapid-deployment system of ECMO support is life saving in some patients, particularly those with acute shunt thrombosis [110,148].

Pulmonary Dysfunction

Respiratory dysfunction after cardiac surgery is common, multifactorial in origin, and results in significant postoperative morbidity. Because of the nature of cardiorespiratory interactions, any alteration in cardiac performance can have a secondary effect on the lungs. Preoperative, long-standing modifications in respiratory function often exist as a consequence of the cardiac anomaly. Excess pulmonary blood flow is associated with increased airway resistance and decreased pulmonary compliance [149]. Restrictive lung disease may be present in patients with prior thoracotomy or sternotomy. Significant impairment of pulmonary mechanics can result from the systemic inflammatory response that occurs with CPB [150]. The exposure of blood to the CPB circuitry and other factors (bleeding, end-organ ischemia, changes in body temperature) have been shown

to trigger release of cytokines and cause complement activation [49,151]. The lungs are particularly susceptible to injury from this inflammatory cascade because they represent such a large vascular bed. Recent advances in perioperative ultrafiltration have shown promising results in attenuating these effects [152,153]. We have demonstrated an improvement in the postoperative alveolar-to-arterial O_2 gradient (A-aO_2) using a preoperative dose of intravenous dexamethasone [49].

Postoperative respiratory failure can result from endothelial dysfunction, left ventricular failure, pulmonary edema secondary to fluid overload, significant residual intracardiac left-to-right shunting, inadequate intraoperative left heart decompression, neuromuscular weakness, or a combination of these factors. Respiratory dysfunction can also be caused by retained tracheobronchial secretions, major atelectasis, phrenic nerve injury with diaphragmatic paralysis, sedatives and analgesics, and neuromuscular disorders affecting the respiratory muscles. When respiratory insufficiency is present, attempts at weaning the patient from the ventilator may result in tachypnea, labored breathing, cyanosis, arterial hypoxemia and hypercarbia, and respiratory acidosis. Under these circumstances, respiratory support should be continued until the underlying cause has been corrected and the patient can be safely weaned and extubated.

Tracheobronchial compression may be caused by vascular structures and, when suspected, bronchoscopy and/or computed tomography (CT) angiography are useful for evaluation. Diaphragmatic paralysis, if persistent for more than 1–2 weeks, can prevent weaning of an infant from the ventilator and should be managed with diaphragmatic plication, which often allows successful weaning from the ventilator [154]. In some patients who require extended respiratory support, tracheostomy must be considered to minimize complications associated with prolonged endotracheal intubation and facilitate rehabilitation. Patients who receive a tracheostomy after congenital heart surgery have few complications directly related to the tracheostomy and the majority are ultimately decannulated [155]. However, our experience shows that neonates and younger children can tolerate postoperative endotracheal intubation for several months with minimal complications. Over the past several years it has been very unusual for us to recommend a tracheostomy for a patient unless they are to be ventilator-dependent for an indeterminate period of time.

Renal Failure

Acute tubular necrosis after open heart surgery usually results from a period of inadequate renal perfusion pressure after cardiac surgery. Preexisting renal insufficiency, CPB-induced inflammation, and exposure to contrast or nephrotoxic agents may also be contributory. Markers of impending renal failure include persistent oliguria and elevation of blood urea nitrogen (BUN) and creatinine, whose levels should be carefully followed. Biochemical acute kidney failure may be defined as an increase in serum creatinine levels to twice or more the preoperative level [156]. The most important goal in patients with evolving renal failure is to maintain a normal renal perfusion pressure, which is calculated by subtracting the central venous pressure from the mean arterial pressure. Abdominal compartment syndrome, due to bowel wall edema and ascites, may compromise renal venous drainage. In patients with low cardiac output and a tense abdominal wall, we have seen dramatic improvement in renal function following placement of peritoneal drains, even in the presence of minimal ascites. Volume and electrolyte status must be carefully managed. To avoid fluid overload, intravenous intake must be limited to replacement of insensible losses, urinary output, gastric, and chest tube drainage. Serum electrolytes, BUN, and creatinine levels should be measured initially every 4–6 hours for early detection of excessive azotemia, hyponatremia or hypernatremia, and especially hyperkalemia. Hyperkalemia (>6mEq/L) may cause bradycardia, heart block, asystole, or ventricular fibrillation. Potassium must be removed from all intravenous fluids and from the diet. Acute treatment may require intravenous administration of calcium gluconate (30 mg/kg), sodium bicarbonate (1mEq/kg), insulin, and glucose. A sodium polystyrene sulfonate (Kayexalate; Sanofi Winthrop Pharmaceuticals, Morrisville, PA) retention enema (1g/kg) is frequently effective in temporarily lowering the serum potassium level. Persistent or increasing hyperkalemia demands peritoneal dialysis or hemodialysis. During the polyuric phase of recovery from acute renal failure, careful attention should be paid to urine output and serum electrolyte levels to avoid dehydration, hypovolemia, and electrolyte imbalance.

Infectious Complications

Moderate temperature elevation (37.9–38.5°C) is common during the first and second postoperative days and is usually related to surgical tissue injury or atelectasis. High fever (>39°C), however, should always raise the possibility of bacteremia or wound infection. Specimens of blood, tracheobronchial secretions, and urine should be obtained promptly for culture. Treatment with broad-spectrum antibiotics should be started early and modified later according to the results of bacteriologic and sensitivity studies. Positive blood culture results necessitate treatment with appropriate intravenous antibiotics for at least 10 days. Postoperative bacteremia is a catastrophic complication, because it can result in the development of infective endocarditis. Sternal wound infections occur in 2–5% of infants and children after median sternotomy [134,157]. Superficial wound infections occur in approximately 3–5% of patients and deep infection (mediastinitis) in 1–2% of patients [157]. Wound infections necessitate adequate drainage and intensive antibiotic treatment, especially in patients with intracardiac prosthetic patches or artificial valves. We previously treated deep sternal infections with muscle flaps [158], but since 2002 we have used vacuum-assisted closure (VAC) successfully in 16 of 19 patients with sternal infections. Central venous catheters are known to be associated with bloodstream infections. The prevention of central line-associated bloodstream infection can be reduced by a systematic, multidisciplinary initiative, as demonstrated by Costello *et al.* [82].

Septic shock can be caused by Gram-positive or Gram-negative bacterial infection. It is usually associated with arterial hypotension, peripheral vasodilation, splanchnic venous pooling, and oliguria. Septic shock is often complicated by disseminated intravascular clotting and consumptive coagulopathy. Initial empiric antibiotic therapy includes vancomycin (10–15 mg/kg/dose IV every 8 hours) and ceftazidime 100–150mg/kg/day until the results of bacteriologic and sensitivity studies determine the specific antimicrobial therapy. Respiratory syncytial viral (RSV) pneumonia can also cause the signs and symptoms of septic shock with respiratory compromise. Diagnosis is made with a nasopharyngeal swab. Currently, there are no clearly beneficial therapeutic interventions for RSV aside from supportive care [159]. Palivizumab is currently recommended as a preventive strategy in high-risk patients [160]. Other supportive measures include maintenance of an adequate blood volume and perfusion pressure as well as inotropic and ventilatory support.

Central Nervous System

It can be difficult to assess the neurologic status of a neonate or child in the immediate postoperative period because of the residual effects of anesthesia. The neurologic assessment includes vital signs, pupillary response to light, withdrawal from noxious stimuli, and symmetric movement in all extremities. Neurologic complications can result from cerebral ischemia, global hypoxia, electrolyte imbalance, acidosis, hypoglycemia, hypomagnesemia, and cerebral emboli. Evaluation of seizure activity includes an electroencephalographic (EEG) study and measurement of arterial blood gas and electrolyte levels. Hypocalcemia, hypoglycemia, hypomagnesemia, and fever can be causes of seizures in neonates. Because of the immature myelination of the neonatal brain, focal seizures may be caused by metabolic or structural abnormalities. Focal seizures require neurology consultation and evaluation including computerized tomography or magnetic resonance imaging (MRI) of the brain. Seizures should be controlled immediately to

avoid interference with adequate ventilation and the cardiovascular stress of increased metabolic activity. Hypoxemia, acidosis, and electrolyte imbalance should be
corrected. Fever should be controlled with antipyretics and
cooling blankets. Shum-Tim *et al.* found that postischemic
hyperthermia significantly exacerbates functional and
structural neurologic injury after deep hypothermic circulatory arrest and should be avoided [161]. Lorazepam
0.1 mg/dose IV is used initially to stop seizure activity.
Maintenance phenobarbital or phenytoin is then administered. The phenobarbital loading dose is 10–20 mg/kg followed by a maintenance dose of 5 mg/kg/day given every
12 hours. Phenobarbital can be a cardiac depressant and
should be given cautiously in a patient with borderline
cardiac output. Phenytoin loading dose is 15–20 mg/kg IV,
followed by a maintenance dose of 5–10 mg/kg/day given
every 8–12 hours. Phenytoin also has cardiac effects and is
contraindicated if the patient has heart block or bradycardia. Gaynor and coworkers have emphasized that routine
continuous EEG monitoring is necessary to rule out the
occurrence of subtle seizures [162]. They noted that
increased duration of deep hypothermic circulatory arrest
(DHCA) was identified as a predictor of seizures.

Choreoathetosis is a rare complication of deep hypothermia (<25 °C) and circulatory arrest [163]. This disorder
tends to develop 2–7 days after the operation and manifests
as seemingly purposeless continued movements of the
head, torso, and all extremities while awake but not while
asleep. Patients with the full-blown syndrome are unable
to swallow, support their head, or walk. The syndrome
tends to resolve over months to years. The cause of choreoathetosis remains undefined, but it appears related to
deep hypothermia (<25 °C), cooling with alpha-stat rather
than pH-stat, uneven brain cooling, and aortopulmonary
collaterals that "steal" blood flow from the cerebral circulation [164,165]. The incidence of this unusual complication
has dropped dramatically in the past 10 years, probably
related to more careful and even cooling/warming of the
brain and less frequent use of DHCA.

Conclusion

The perioperative care of children undergoing congenital
heart surgery can be complex and often is challenging.
There is no substitute for repeated physical examination
and vigilant serial observance of children in the postoperative period. The emphasis in the current era is on a team
concept of care for these children [166]. Dramatic improvements in ICU management, including ventilator care,
inotropic support, highly trained nurses, and improved
monitoring techniques, have helped to optimize the results
of congenital heart surgery procedures. Constant attention
to detail is essential, and anticipatory rather than reactive
care is the key to optimal postoperative outcomes.

References

1. Chang AC. (2005) Common problems and their solutions in paediatric cardiac intensive care. Cardiol Young 15(Suppl 1), 169–173.
2. Kane JM, Preze E. (2009) Nurses' perceptions of subspecializ-ation in pediatric cardiac intensive care unit: quality and patient safety implications. J Nurs Care Qual 24, 354–361.
3. Catchpole KR, de Leval MR, McEwan A, *et al.* (2007) Patient handover from surgery to intensive care: using Formula 1 pit-stop and aviation models to improve safety and quality. Paediatr Anaesth 17, 470–478.
4. Checchia PA, McCollegan J, Daher N, *et al.* (2005) The effect of surgical case volume on outcome after the Norwood procedure. J Thorac Cardiovasc Surg 129, 754–759.
5. Hannan EL, Racz M, Kavey RE, *et al.* (1998) Pediatric cardiac surgery: the effect of hospital and surgeon volume on in-hospital mortality. Pediatrics 101, 963–969.
6. Jenkins KJ, Newburger JW, Lock JE, *et al.* (1995) In-hospital mortality for surgical repair of congenital heart defects: preliminary observations of variation by hospital caseload. Pediatrics 95, 323–330.
7. Chang AC. (2002) How to start and sustain a successful pediatric cardiac intensive care program: a combined clini-cal and administrative strategy. Pediatr Crit Care Med 3, 107–111.
8. Khongphatthanayothin A, Wong PC, Samara Y, *et al.* (1999) Impact of respiratory syncytial virus infection on surgery for congenital heart disease: postoperative course and outcome. Crit Care Med 27, 1974–1981.
9. Heymann MA, Berman W Jr, Rudolph AM, *et al.* (1979) Dilatation of the ductus arteriosus by prostaglandin E1 in aortic arch abnormalities. Circulation 59, 169–173.
10. Meckler GD, Lowe C. (2009) To intubate or not to intubate? Transporting infants on prostaglandin E1. Pediatrics 123, e25–e30.
11. Lim DS, Kulik TJ, Kim DW, *et al.* (2003) Aminophylline for the prevention of apnea during prostaglandin E1 infusion. Pediatrics 112, e27–e29.
12. Backer CL, Baden HP, Costello JM, *et al.* (2003) Perioperative care. In: Mavroudis C, Backer CL, eds. *Pediatric Cardiac Surgery*, 3rd ed. Philadelphia, PA: Mosby, Inc.
13. Tabbutt S, Ramamoorthy C, Montenegro LM, *et al.* (2001) Impact of inspired gas mixtures on preoperative infants with hypoplastic left heart syndrome during controlled ventilation. Circulation 104, I159–I164.
14. McElhinney DB, Hedrick HL, Bush DM, *et al.* (2000) Necrotizing enterocolitis in neonates with congenital heart disease: risk factors and outcomes. Pediatrics 106, 1080–1087.
15. Neutze JM, Starling MB, Elliott RB, *et al.* (1977) Palliation of cyanotic congenital heart disease in infancy with E-type prostaglandins. Circulation 55, 238–241.
16. Rashkind WJ, Miller WW. (1966) Creation of an atrial septal defect without thoracotomy. A palliative approach to com-plete transposition of the great arteries. JAMA 196, 991–992.
17. Vida VL, Bacha EA, Larrazabal A, *et al.* (2007) Hypoplastic left heart syndrome with intact or highly restrictive atrial

septum: surgical experience from a single center. Ann Thorac Surg 84, 581–585; discussion 586.

18. Khoury MJ, Cordero JF, Mulinare J, et al. (1989) Selected midline defect associations: a population study. Pediatrics 84, 266–272.

19. Murugasu B, Yip WC, Tay JS, et al. (1990) Sonographic screening for renal tract anomalies associated with congenital heart disease. J Clin Ultrasound 18, 79–83.

20. Limperopoulos C, Majnemer A, Shevell MI, et al. (1999) Neurologic status of newborns with congenital heart defects before open heart surgery. Pediatrics 103, 402–408.

21. Licht DJ, Shera DM, Clancy RR, et al. (2009) Brain maturation is delayed in infants with complex congenital heart defects. J Thorac Cardiovasc Surg 137, 529–536; discussion 536–537.

22. Miller SP, McQuillen PS, Hamrick S, et al. (2007) Abnormal brain development in newborns with congenital heart disease. N Engl J Med 357, 1928–1938.

23. Licht DJ, Wang J, Silvestre DW, et al. (2004) Preoperative cerebral blood flow is diminished in neonates with severe congenital heart defects. J Thorac Cardiovasc Surg 128, 841–849.

24. Mahle WT, Tavani F, Zimmerman RA, et al. (2002) An MRI study of neurological injury before and after congenital heart surgery. Circulation 106, I109–I114.

25. Petit CJ, Rome JJ, Wernovsky G, et al. (2009) Preoperative brain injury in transposition of the great arteries is associated with oxygenation and time to surgery, not balloon atrial septostomy. Circulation 119, 709–716.

26. Graham EM, Bradley SM, Shirali GS, et al. (2004) Effectiveness of cardiac surgery in trisomies 13 and 18 (from the Pediatric Cardiac Care Consortium). Am J Cardiol 93, 801–803.

27. Costello JM, Polito A, Brown DW, et al. (2010) Birth before 39 weeks' gestation is associated with worse outcomes in neonates with heart disease. Pediatrics 126, e277–e284.

28. Chang AC, Hanley FL, Lock JE, et al. (1994) Management and outcome of low birth weight neonates with congenital heart disease. J Pediatr 124, 461–466.

29. Reddy VM, McElhinney DB, Sagrado T, et al. (1999) Results of 102 cases of complete repair of congenital heart defects in patients weighing 700 to 2500 grams. J Thorac Cardiovasc Surg 117, 324–331.

30. Kirklin JK, Kirklin JW. (1981) Management of the cardiovascular subsystem after cardiac surgery. Ann Thorac Surg 32, 311–319.

31. Nadas AS, Fyler DC, eds. (1972) *Pediatric Cardiology*, 3rd ed. Philadelphia, PA: WB Saunders.

32. Janke EL, Pilkington SN, Smith DC. (1996) Evaluation of two warming systems after cardiopulmonary bypass. Br J Anaesth 77, 268–270.

33. Cote CJ, Rolf N, Liu LM, et al. (1991) A single-blind study of combined pulse oximetry and capnography in children. Anesthesiology 74, 980–987.

34. Rudolph AM, Cayler GG. (1958) Cardiac catheterization in infants and children. Pediatr Clin North Am 5, 907–943.

35. Karakitsos D, Labropoulos N, De Groot E, et al. (2006) Real-time ultrasound-guided catheterisation of the internal jugular vein: a prospective comparison with the landmark technique in critical care patients. Crit Care 10, R162.

36. Tweddell JS, Hoffman GM, Mussatto KA, et al. (2002) Improved survival of patients undergoing palliation of hypoplastic left heart syndrome: lessons learned from 115 consecutive patients. Circulation 106, I82–I89.

37. Liakopoulos OJ, Ho JK, Yezbick A, et al. (2007) An experimental and clinical evaluation of a novel central venous catheter with integrated oximetry for pediatric patients undergoing cardiac surgery. Anesth Analg 105, 1598–1604.

38. Flori HR, Johnson LD, Hanley FL, et al. (2000) Transthoracic intracardiac catheters in pediatric patients recovering from congenital heart defect surgery: associated complications and outcomes. Crit Care Med 28, 2997–3001.

39. Gold JP, Jonas RA, Lang P, et al. (1986) Transthoracic intracardiac monitoring lines in pediatric surgical patients: a ten-year experience. Ann Thorac Surg 42, 185–191.

40. Santini F, Gatti G, Borghetti V, et al. (1999) Routine left atrial catheterization for the post-operative management of cardiac surgical patients: is the risk justified? Eur J Cardiothorac Surg 16, 218–221.

41. Ranucci M, Isgro G, de la Torre T, et al. (2008) Near-infrared spectroscopy correlates with continuous superior vena cava oxygen saturation in pediatric cardiac surgery patients. Paediatr Anaesth 18, 1163–1169.

42. Li J, Van Arsdell GS, Zhang G, et al. (2006) Assessment of the relationship between cerebral and splanchnic oxygen saturations measured by near-infrared spectroscopy and direct measurements of systemic haemodynamic variables and oxygen transport after the Norwood procedure. Heart 92, 1678–1685.

43. Kane JM, Steinhorn DM. (2009) Lack of irrefutable validation does not negate clinical utility of near-infrared spectroscopy monitoring: learning to trust new technology. J Crit Care 24, 472 e1–e7.

44. Carroll KC, Reeves LM, Andersen G, et al. (1998) Risks associated with removal of ventricular epicardial pacing wires after cardiac surgery. Am J Crit Care 7, 444–449.

45. Fishberger SB, Rossi AF, Bolivar JM, et al. (2008) Congenital cardiac surgery without routine placement of wires for temporary pacing. Cardiol Young 18, 96–99.

46. Batra AS, Balaji S. (2008) Post operative temporary epicardial pacing: When, how and why? Ann Pediatr Cardiol 1, 120–125.

47. Batra AS, Wells WJ, Hinoki KW, et al. (2003) Late recovery of atrioventricular conduction after pacemaker implantation for complete heart block associated with surgery for congenital heart disease. J Thorac Cardiovasc Surg 125, 1291–1293.

48. Agati S, Mignosa C, Gitto P, et al. (2006) A method for chest drainage after pediatric cardiac surgery: a prospective randomized trial. J Thorac Cardiovasc Surg 131, 1306–1309.

49. Bronicki RA, Backer CL, Baden HP, et al. (2000) Dexamethasone reduces the inflammatory response to cardiopulmonary bypass in children. Ann Thorac Surg 69, 1490–1495.

50. Checchia PA, Bronicki RA, Costello JM, et al. (2005) Steroid use before pediatric cardiac operations using cardiopulmonary bypass: an international survey of 36 centers. Pediatr Crit Care Med 6, 441–444.

51. Quasney MW, Goodman DM, Billow M, *et al.* (2001) Routine chest radiographs in pediatric intensive care units. Pediatrics 107, 241–248.

52. Robotham JL, Peters J, Takata M, *et al.* (1996) Cardiorespiratory interactions. In: Rogers MC, Nichols DG, eds. *Textbook of Pediatric Intensive Care*, 3rd ed. Baltimore, MD: Williams & Wilkins.

53. Wessel DL, Adatia I, Thompson JE, *et al.* (1994) Delivery and monitoring of inhaled nitric oxide in patients with pulmonary hypertension. Crit Care Med 22, 930–938.

54. Bradley SM, Simsic JM, Mulvihill DM. (1998) Hyperventilation impairs oxygenation after bidirectional superior cavopulmonary connection. Circulation 98, II372–II376; discussion II376–II377.

55. Bradley SM, Simsic JM, Mulvihill DM. (2003) Hypoventilation improves oxygenation after bidirectional superior cavopulmonary connection. J Thorac Cardiovasc Surg 126, 1033–1039.

56. Williams DB, Kiernan PD, Metke MP, *et al.* (1984) Hemodynamic response to positive end-expiratory pressure following right atrium-pulmonary artery bypass (Fontan procedure). J Thorac Cardiovasc Surg 87, 856–861.

57. Morales DL, Carberry KE, Heinle JS, *et al.* (2008) Extubation in the operating room after Fontan's procedure: effect on practice and outcomes. Ann Thorac Surg 86, 576–581; discussion 581–582.

58. Davis S, Worley S, Mee RB, *et al.* (2004) Factors associated with early extubation after cardiac surgery in young children. Pediatr Crit Care Med 5, 63–68.

59. Markovitz BP, Randolph AG. (2002) Corticosteroids for the prevention of reintubation and postextubation stridor in pediatric patients: a meta-analysis. Pediatr Crit Care Med 3, 223–236.

60. Treluyer JM, Tonnelier S, d'Athis P, *et al.* (2001) Antipyretic efficacy of an initial 30-mg/kg loading dose of acetaminophen versus a 15-mg/kg maintenance dose. Pediatrics 108, E73.

61. Booth KL, Roth SJ, Perry SB, *et al.* (2002) Cardiac catheterization of patients supported by extracorporeal membrane oxygenation. J Am Coll Cardiol 40, 1681–1686.

62. Zahn EM, Dobrolet NC, Nykanen DG, *et al.* (2004) Interventional catheterization performed in the early postoperative period after congenital heart surgery in children. J Am Coll Cardiol 43, 1264–1269.

63. Durward A, Tibby SM, Skellett S, *et al.* (2005) The strong ion gap predicts mortality in children following cardiopulmonary bypass surgery. Pediatr Crit Care Med 6, 281–285.

64. Murray DM, Olhsson V, Fraser JI. (2004) Defining acidosis in postoperative cardiac patients using Stewart's method of strong ion difference. Pediatr Crit Care Med 5, 240–245.

65. Patel HB, Yeh TF. (1985) Resuscitation. In: Yeh TF, ed. *Drug Therapy in the Neonate and Small Infant*. Chicago: Year Book.

66. Falcao G, Ulate K, Kouzekanani K, *et al.* (2008) Impact of postoperative hyperglycemia following surgical repair of congenital cardiac defects. Pediatr Cardiol 29, 628–636.

67. Polito A, Thiagarajan RR, Laussen PC, *et al.* (2008) Association between intraoperative and early postoperative glucose levels and adverse outcomes after complex congenital heart surgery. Circulation 118, 2235–2242.

68. Yates AR, Dyke PC 2nd, Taeed R, *et al.* (2006) Hyperglycemia is a marker for poor outcome in the postoperative pediatric cardiac patient. Pediatr Crit Care Med 7, 351–355.

69. Ballweg JA, Wernovsky G, Ittenbach RF, *et al.* (2007) Hyperglycemia after infant cardiac surgery does not adversely impact neurodevelopmental outcome. Ann Thorac Surg 84, 2052–2058.

70. Vlasselaers D, Milants I, Desmet L, *et al.* (2009) Intensive insulin therapy for patients in paediatric intensive care: a prospective, randomised controlled study. Lancet 373, 547–556.

71. Piper HG, Alexander JL, Shukla A, *et al.* (2006) Real-time continuous glucose monitoring in pediatric patients during and after cardiac surgery. Pediatrics 118, 1176–1184.

72. Mahesh B, Yim B, Robson D, *et al.* (2008) Does furosemide prevent renal dysfunction in high-risk cardiac surgical patients? Results of a double-blinded prospective randomised trial. Eur J Cardiothorac Surg 33, 370–376.

73. Costello JM, Thiagarajan RR, Dionne RE, *et al.* (2006) Initial experience with fenoldopam after cardiac surgery in neonates with an insufficient response to conventional diuretics. Pediatr Crit Care Med 7, 28–33.

74. Braudis NJ, Curley MA, Beaupre K, *et al.* (2009) Enteral feeding algorithm for infants with hypoplastic left heart syndrome poststage I palliation. Pediatr Crit Care Med 10, 460–466.

75. Mehta NM, Compher C. (2009) A.S.P.E.N. Clinical Guidelines: nutrition support of the critically ill child. JPEN J Parenter Enteral Nutr 33, 260–276.

76. Tiffany KF, Burke BL, Collins-Odoms C, *et al.* (2003) Current practice regarding the enteral feeding of high-risk newborns with umbilical catheters in situ. Pediatrics 112, 20–23.

77. Kanto WP Jr, Hunter JE, Stoll BJ. (1994) Recognition and medical management of necrotizing enterocolitis. Clin Perinatol 21, 335–346.

78. Costello JM, Graham DA, Morrow DF, *et al.* (2010) Risk factors for surgical site infection after cardiac surgery in children. Ann Thorac Surg 89, 1833–1841; discussion 1841–1842.

79. Anderson DJ, Kaye KS, Classen D, *et al.* (2008) Strategies to prevent surgical site infections in acute care hospitals. Infect Control Hosp Epidemiol 29(Suppl 1), S51–S61.

80. Alphonso N, Anagnostopoulos PV, Scarpace S, *et al.* (2007) Perioperative antibiotic prophylaxis in paediatric cardiac surgery. Cardiol Young 17, 12–25.

81. Costello JM, Graham DA, Morrow DF, *et al.* (2009) Risk factors for central line-associated bloodstream infection in a pediatric cardiac intensive care unit. Pediatr Crit Care Med 10, 453–459.

82. Costello JM, Morrow DF, Graham DA, *et al.* (2008) Systematic intervention to reduce central line-associated bloodstream infection rates in a pediatric cardiac intensive care unit. Pediatrics 121, 915–923.

83. Matlow AG, Wray RD, Cox PN. (2003) Nosocomial urinary tract infections in children in a pediatric intensive care unit: a follow-up after 10 years. Pediatr Crit Care Med 4, 74–77.

84. Wernovsky G, Wypij D, Jonas RA, *et al.* (1995) Postoperative course and hemodynamic profile after the arterial switch operation in neonates and infants. A comparison of

low-flow cardiopulmonary bypass and circulatory arrest. Circulation 92, 2226–2235.

85. Bryant RM, Shirley RL, Ott DA, et al. (1998) Left ventricular performance following the arterial switch operation: use of noninvasive wall stress analysis in the postoperative period. Crit Care Med 26, 926–932.

86. Romero T, Covell J, Friedman WF. (1972) A comparison of pressure-volume relations of the fetal, newborn, and adult heart. Am J Physiol 222, 1285–1290.

87. Friedman WF. (1972) The intrinsic physiologic properties of the developing heart. Prog Cardiovasc Dis 15, 87–111.

88. Zaritsky A, Chernow B. (1984) Use of catecholamines in pediatrics. J Pediatr 105, 341–350.

89. Friedman WF, George BL. (1985) Treatment of congestive heart failure by altering loading conditions of the heart. J Pediatr 106, 697–706.

90. Kouchoukos NT, Kirklin JW, Sheppard LC, et al. (1971) Effect of left atrial pressure by blood infusion on stroke volume early after cardiac operations. Surg Forum 22, 126–127.

91. Mavroudis C, Zales VR, Backer CL, et al. (1992) Fenestrated Fontan with delayed catheter closure. Effects of volume loading and baffle fenestration on cardiac index and oxygen delivery. Circulation. 86, II85–II92.

92. Lehot JJ, Villard J, Piriz H, et al. (1992) Hemodynamic and hormonal responses to hypothermic and normothermic cardiopulmonary bypass. J Cardiothorac Vasc Anesth 6, 132–139.

93. Chang AC, Atz AM, Wernovsky G, et al. (1995) Milrinone: systemic and pulmonary hemodynamic effects in neonates after cardiac surgery. Crit Care Med 23, 1907–1914.

94. Hoffman TM, Wernovsky G, Atz AM, et al. (2003) Efficacy and safety of milrinone in preventing low cardiac output syndrome in infants and children after corrective surgery for congenital heart disease. Circulation 107, 996–1002.

95. Kristof AS, Magder S. (1999) Low systemic vascular resistance state in patients undergoing cardiopulmonary bypass. Crit Care Med 27, 1121–1127.

96. Rosenzweig EB, Starc TJ, Chen JM, et al. (1999) Intravenous arginine-vasopressin in children with vasodilatory shock after cardiac surgery. Circulation 100, II182–II186.

97. Argenziano M, Chen JM, Choudhri AF, et al. (1998) Management of vasodilatory shock after cardiac surgery: identification of predisposing factors and use of a novel pressor agent. J Thorac Cardiovasc Surg 116, 973–980.

98. Davies MJ, Nguyen K, Gaynor JW, et al. (1998) Modified ultrafiltration improves left ventricular systolic function in infants after cardiopulmonary bypass. J Thorac Cardiovasc Surg 115, 361–369; discussion 369–370.

99. Burrows FA, Williams WG, Teoh KH, et al. (1988) Myocardial performance after repair of congenital cardiac defects in infants and children. Response to volume loading. J Thorac Cardiovasc Surg 96, 548–556.

100. Driscoll DJ, Gillette PC, Duff DF, McNamara DG. (1979) The hemodynamic effect of dopamine in children. J Thorac Cardiovasc Surg 78, 765–768.

101. Loeb HS, Bredakis J, Gunner RM. (1977) Superiority of dobutamine over dopamine for augmentation of cardiac output in patients with chronic low output cardiac failure. Circulation 55, 375–358.

102. Ando M, Park IS, Wada N, et al. (2005) Steroid supplementation: a legitimate pharmacotherapy after neonatal open heart surgery. Ann Thorac Surg 80, 1672–1628; discussion 1628.

103. Kilger E, Weis F, Briegel J, et al. (2003) Stress doses of hydrocortisone reduce severe systemic inflammatory response syndrome and improve early outcome in a risk group of patients after cardiac surgery. Crit Care Med 31, 1068–1074.

104. Suominen PK, Dickerson HA, Moffett BS, et al. (2005) Hemodynamic effects of rescue protocol hydrocortisone in neonates with low cardiac output syndrome after cardiac surgery. Pediatr Crit Care Med 6, 655–659.

105. Alsoufi B, Al-Radi OO, Gruenwald C, et al. (2009) Extracorporeal life support following cardiac surgery in children: analysis of risk factors and survival in a single institution. Eur J Cardiothorac Surg 35, 1004–1011; discussion 1011.

106. Cooper DS, Jacobs JP, Moore L, et al. (2007) Cardiac extracorporeal life support: state of the art in 2007. Cardiol Young 17(Suppl 2), 104–115.

107. Tissot C, Buckvold S, Phelps CM, et al. (2009) Outcome of extracorporeal membrane oxygenation for early primary graft failure after pediatric heart transplantation. J Am Coll Cardiol 54, 730–737.

108. Morris MC, Ittenbach RF, Godinez RI, et al. (2004) Risk factors for mortality in 137 pediatric cardiac intensive care unit patients managed with extracorporeal membrane oxygenation. Crit Care Med 32, 1061–1069.

109. Aharon AS, Drinkwater DC Jr, Churchwell KB, et al. (2001) Extracorporeal membrane oxygenation in children after repair of congenital cardiac lesions. Ann Thorac Surg 72, 2095–2101; discussion 2101–2102.

110. Chan T, Thiagarajan RR, Frank D, et al. (2008) Survival after extracorporeal cardiopulmonary resuscitation in infants and children with heart disease. J Thorac Cardiovasc Surg 136, 984–992.

111. del Nido PJ, Duncan BW, Mayer JE Jr, et al. (1999) Left ventricular assist device improves survival in children with left ventricular dysfunction after repair of anomalous origin of the left coronary artery from the pulmonary artery. Ann Thorac Surg 67, 169–172.

112. Karl TR, Horton SB, Brizard C. (2006) Postoperative support with the centrifugal pump ventricular assist device (VAD). Semin Thorac Cardiovasc Surg Pediatr Card Surg Annu 83–91.

113. Hetzer R, Alexi-Meskishvili V, Weng Y, et al. (2006) Mechanical cardiac support in the young with the Berlin Heart EXCOR pulsatile ventricular assist device: 15 years' experience. Semin Thorac Cardiovasc Surg Pediatr Card Surg Annu 99–108.

114. Hetzer R, Loebe M, Potapov EV, et al. (1998) Circulatory support with pneumatic paracorporeal ventricular assist device in infants and children. Ann Thorac Surg 66, 1498–1506.

115. Imamura M, Dossey AM, Prodhan P, et al. (2009) Bridge to cardiac transplant in children: Berlin Heart versus extracorporeal membrane oxygenation. Ann Thorac Surg 87, 1894–1901; discussion 1901.

116. Hoffman TM, Wernovsky G, Wieand TS, et al. (2002) The incidence of arrhythmias in a pediatric cardiac intensive care unit. Pediatr Cardiol 23, 598–604.

117. Hoffman TM, Bush DM, Wernovsky G, *et al.* (2002) Postoperative junctional ectopic tachycardia in children: incidence, risk factors, and treatment. Ann Thorac Surg 74, 1607–1611.

118. Dodge-Khatami A, Miller OI, Anderson RH, *et al.* (2002) Impact of junctional ectopic tachycardia on postoperative morbidity following repair of congenital heart defects. Eur J Cardiothorac Surg 21, 255–259.

119. Walsh EP, Saul JP, Sholler GF, *et al.* (1997) Evaluation of a staged treatment protocol for rapid automatic junctional tachycardia after operation for congenital heart disease. J Am Coll Cardiol 29, 1046–1053.

120. Laird WP, Snyder CS, Kertesz NJ, *et al.* (2003) Use of intravenous amiodarone for postoperative junctional ectopic tachycardia in children. Pediatr Cardiol 24, 133–137.

121. Saul JP, Scott WA, Brown S, *et al.* (2005) Intravenous amiodarone for incessant tachyarrhythmias in children: a randomized, double-blind, antiarrhythmic drug trial. Circulation 112, 3470–3477.

122. Dodge-Khatami A, Johnsrude CL, Backer CL, *et al.* (2000) A comparison of steroid-eluting epicardial versus transvenous pacing leads in children. J Card Surg 15, 323–329.

123. Gomes MM, McGoon DC. (1970) Bleeding patterns after open-heart surgery. J Thorac Cardiovasc Surg 60, 87–97.

124. Stark J, de Leval M. (1984) Experience with fibrin seal (Tisseel) in operations for congenital heart defects. Ann Thorac Surg 38, 411–413.

125. Gruenwald CE, McCrindle BW, Crawford-Lean L, *et al.* (2008) Reconstituted fresh whole blood improves clinical outcomes compared with stored component blood therapy for neonates undergoing cardiopulmonary bypass for cardiac surgery: a randomized controlled trial. J Thorac Cardiovasc Surg 136, 1442–1449.

126. Manno CS, Hedberg KW, Kim HC, *et al.* (1991) Comparison of the hemostatic effects of fresh whole blood, stored whole blood, and components after open heart surgery in children. Blood 77, 930–936.

127. Guay J, Rivard GE. (1996) Mediastinal bleeding after cardiopulmonary bypass in pediatric patients. Ann Thorac Surg 62, 1955–1960.

128. Costello JM, Backer CL, de Hoyos A, *et al.* (2003) Aprotinin reduces operative closure time and blood product use after pediatric bypass. Ann Thorac Surg 75, 1261–1266.

129. Fergusson DA, Hebert PC, Mazer CD, *et al.* (2008) A comparison of aprotinin and lysine analogues in high-risk cardiac surgery. N Engl J Med 358, 2319–2331.

130. Mangano DT, Tudor IC, Dietzel C. (2006) The risk associated with aprotinin in cardiac surgery. N Engl J Med 354, 353–365.

131. Greilich PE, Jessen ME, Satyanarayana N, *et al.* (2009) The effect of epsilon-aminocaproic acid and aprotinin on fibrinolysis and blood loss in patients undergoing primary, isolated coronary artery bypass surgery: a randomized, double-blind, placebo-controlled, noninferiority trial. Anesth Analg 109, 15–24.

132. McElhinney DB, Reddy VM, Parry AJ, *et al.* (2000) Management and outcomes of delayed sternal closure after cardiac surgery in neonates and infants. Crit Care Med 28, 1180–1184.

133. Tabbutt S, Duncan BW, McLaughlin D, *et al.* (1997) Delayed sternal closure after cardiac operations in a pediatric population. J Thorac Cardiovasc Surg 113, 886–893.

134. Long CB, Shah SS, Lautenbach E, *et al.* (2005) Postoperative mediastinitis in children: epidemiology, microbiology and risk factors for Gram-negative pathogens. Pediatr Infect Dis J 24, 315–319.

135. Horneffer PJ, Miller RH, Pearson TA, *et al.* (1990) The effective treatment of postpericardiotomy syndrome after cardiac operations. A randomized placebo-controlled trial. J Thorac Cardiovasc Surg 100, 292–296.

136. Miller OI, Tang SF, Keech A, *et al.* (2000) Inhaled nitric oxide and prevention of pulmonary hypertension after congenital heart surgery: a randomised double-blind study. Lancet 356, 1464–1469.

137. Frostell C, Fratacci MD, Wain JC, *et al.* (1991) Inhaled nitric oxide. A selective pulmonary vasodilator reversing hypoxic pulmonary vasoconstriction. Circulation 83, 2038–2047.

138. Curran RD, Mavroudis C, Backer CL, *et al.* (1995) Inhaled nitric oxide for children with congenital heart disease and pulmonary hypertension. Ann Thorac Surg 60, 1765–1771.

139. Namachivayam P, Theilen U, Butt WW, *et al.* (2006) Sildenafil prevents rebound pulmonary hypertension after withdrawal of nitric oxide in children. Am J Respir Crit Care Med 174, 1042–1047.

140. Huddleston AJ, Knoderer CA, Morris JL, *et al.* (2009) Sildenafil for the treatment of pulmonary hypertension in pediatric patients. Pediatr Cardiol 30, 871–882.

141. Carroll CL, Backer CL, Mavroudis C, *et al.* (2005) Inhaled prostacyclin following surgical repair of congenital heart disease – a pilot study. J Card Surg 20, 436–439.

142. Peddy SB, Hazinski MF, Laussen PC, *et al.* (2007) Cardiopulmonary resuscitation: special considerations for infants and children with cardiac disease. Cardiol Young 17(Suppl 2), 116–126.

143. American Heart Association. (2006) 2005 American Heart Association (AHA) guidelines for cardiopulmonary resuscitation (CPR) and emergency cardiovascular care (ECC) of pediatric and neonatal patients: pediatric basic life support. Pediatrics 117(5), e989–e1004.

144. Kane DA, Thiagarajan RR, Wypij D, *et al.* (2010) Rapid-response extracorporeal membrane oxygenation to support cardiopulmonary resuscitation in children with cardiac disease. Circulation. 122, S241–S248.

145. Rhodes JF, Blaufox AD, Seiden HS, *et al.* (1999) Cardiac arrest in infants after congenital heart surgery. Circulation 100, II194–II199.

146. Hypothermia after Cardiac Arrest Study Group. (2002) Mild therapeutic hypothermia to improve the neurologic outcome after cardiac arrest. N Engl J Med 346, 549–556.

147. Shankaran S, Laptook AR, Ehrenkranz RA, *et al.* (2005) Whole-body hypothermia for neonates with hypoxic-ischemic encephalopathy. N Engl J Med 353, 1574–1584.

148. Allan CK, Thiagarajan RR, del Nido PJ, *et al.* (2007) Indication for initiation of mechanical circulatory support impacts survival of infants with shunted single-ventricle circulation supported with extracorporeal membrane oxygenation. J Thorac Cardiovasc Surg 133, 660–667.

149. Bancalari E, Jesse MJ, Gelband H, *et al.* (1977) Lung mechanics in congenital heart disease with increased and decreased pulmonary blood flow. J Pediatr 90, 192–195.

150. DiCarlo JV, Steven JM. (1994) Respiratory failure in congenital heart disease. Pediatr Clin North Am 41, 525–542.

151. Wan S, LeClerc JL, Vincent JL. (1997) Inflammatory response to cardiopulmonary bypass: mechanisms involved and possible therapeutic strategies. Chest 112, 676–692.

152. Gaynor JW. (2003) The effect of modified ultrafiltration on the postoperative course in patients with congenital heart disease. Semin Thorac Cardiovasc Surg Pediatr Card Surg Annu 6, 128–139.

153. Naik SK, Knight A, Elliott M. (1991) A prospective randomized study of a modified technique of ultrafiltration during pediatric open-heart surgery. Circulation 84, III422–III431.

154. Baker CJ, Boulom V, Reemtsen BL, *et al.* (2008) Hemidiaphragm plication after repair of congenital heart defects in children: quantitative return of diaphragm function over time. J Thorac Cardiovasc Surg 135, 56–61.

155. Hoskote A, Cohen G, Goldman A, *et al.* (2005) Tracheostomy in infants and children after cardiothoracic surgery: indications, associated risk factors, and timing. J Thorac Cardiovasc Surg 130, 1086–1093.

156. Welke KF, Dearani JA, Ghanayem NS, *et al.* (2008) Renal complications associated with the treatment of patients with congenital cardiac disease: consensus definitions from the Multi-Societal Database Committee for Pediatric and Congenital Heart Disease. Cardiol Young 18(Suppl 2), 222–225.

157. Mehta PA, Cunningham CK, Colella CB, *et al.* (2000) Risk factors for sternal wound and other infections in pediatric cardiac surgery patients. Pediatr Infect Dis J 19, 1000–1004.

158. Backer CL, Pensler JM, Tobin GR, *et al.* (1994) Vascularized muscle flaps for life-threatening mediastinal wounds in children. Ann Thorac Surg 57, 797–801; discussion 802.

159. Davison C, Ventre KM, Luchetti M, *et al.* (2004) Efficacy of interventions for bronchiolitis in critically ill infants: a systematic review and meta-analysis. Pediatr Crit Care Med 5, 482–489.

160. American Academy of Pediatrics. (2006) Respiratory syncytial virus. In: Red book online. Available at: http://aapredbook.aappublications.org/content/dtl/2006/1/#SECTION___SUMMARIES_OF_INFECTIOUS_DISEASES. Accessed 4 April 2011.

161. Shum-Tim D, Nagashima M, Shinoka T, *et al.* (1998) Postischemic hyperthermia exacerbates neurologic injury after deep hypothermic circulatory arrest. J Thorac Cardiovasc Surg 116, 780–792.

162. Gaynor JW, Nicolson SC, Jarvik GP, *et al.* (2005) Increasing duration of deep hypothermic circulatory arrest is associated with an increased incidence of postoperative electroencephalographic seizures. J Thorac Cardiovasc Surg 130, 1278–1286.

163. Barratt-Boyes BG. (1990) Choreoathetosis as a complication of cardiopulmonary bypass. Ann Thorac Surg 50, 693–694.

164. DeLeon S, Ilbawi M, Arcilla R, *et al.* (1990) Choreoathetosis after deep hypothermia without circulatory arrest. Ann Thorac Surg 50, 714–719.

165. Wessel DL, du Plessis AJ. (1996) Choreoathetosis. In: Jonas RA, Newburger JW, Volpe JJ, eds. *Brain Injury and Pediatric Cardiac Surgery*. Boston, MA: Butterworth-Heinemann.

166. Bognar A, Barach P, Johnson JK, *et al.* (2008) Errors and the burden of errors: attitudes, perceptions, and the culture of safety in pediatric cardiac surgical teams. Ann Thorac Surg 85, 1374–1381.

CHAPTER 8

The Nurse Practitioner's Role in Patient Management

Nancy Benson, Denise Davis, Fejeania Hunter, Kim Teknipp, and Jamie Thomas

Center for Congenital Heart Surgery, Cleveland Clinic Children's Hospital, Cleveland, OH, USA

History of Nurse Practitioners in Cardiothoracic Surgery

Since surgeons began correcting congenital heart defects in the 1940s, this subspecialty has undergone formidable changes. Over the past seven decades, congenital heart surgery mortality rates have fallen from 80% to less than 5% as a result of improved technology, surgical techniques, and postoperative management [1]. With the institution of the intensive care unit came the development of critical care subspecialties and advanced practice nursing including the congenital heart surgery nurse practitioner (NP). The transition to incorporating NPs into the congenital heart surgery team came about by a decline in the number of residents and resident work hours, along with the acceptance of NPs to many medical institutions as integral members of the healthcare team.

Although the history of advanced practice nursing can be traced to the nineteenth century during the Civil War, the first pediatric NP program did not exist until the middle 1960s [2]. The most recent development in this field has been the inclusion of the acute care NP. Noticeable gaps in patient care lead to the creation of this role specifically for congenital heart disease (CHD) at Boston Children's Hospital in 1987 [3]. Since that time, NPs have become integral members of the congenital heart surgery team around the world [3].

Nurse practitioners specializing in pediatric and congenital heart surgery provide continual care for patients with CHD starting with the initial call to schedule surgery and continuing until hospital discharge and outpatient follow-up visits. Hravnak *et al.* described the core com-

petencies of the acute care NP as direct clinical practice including guidance, consultation, research skills, leadership, collaboration, and ethical decision-making [4]. The cardiothoracic surgery NP, as a member of a multidisciplinary team, must look at each of these competencies as an essential part of patient care and professional responsibility. The priority to provide high quality hospital-based care while maintaining a holistic approach to the patient and family is the foundation of the NP role within the team [5].

Diagnosis

Congenital heart disease continues to be the most common birth defect with an occurrence of 8 per 1000 births [6]. More than a third of infants who die from a congenital anomaly have a heart defect as part of the complex pathophysiology that lead to their demise [6]. Furthermore, the incidence of chromosome abnormalities in infants with CHD is estimated at 5–10% [7,8]. The frequency of fetuses with chromosomal anomalies and cardiac defects is actually higher than those found in live births [8,9]. In addition, extracardiac malformations occur in at least 25% of infants with CHD [8].

Etiologies of CHD include prematurity, low birth weight, advanced maternal age, and multiple gestation [10]. Risk factors for CHD have been studied by many and include infant sex, ethnicity, environmental exposure, and possibly maternal/paternal age [10]. Supplemental research and examination will broaden the ability to make consistent hypotheses regarding risk factors for CHD. Early diagnosis and analysis of infants with CHD allows for accurate monitoring and treatment at birth.

Pediatric Cardiac Surgery, Fourth Edition. Edited by Constantine Mavroudis and Carl L. Backer.
© 2013 Blackwell Publishing Ltd. Published 2013 by Blackwell Publishing Ltd.

Technological advances in fetal echocardiography allow pediatric cardiologists to diagnose CHD earlier in pregnancy and can be used at 12 weeks gestation [11]. Parents who have a child with a congenital heart defect are at an increased risk (3–4% or higher) of having another child with a defect [11]. These parents will want as much information as possible about the risks of having future children. Early fetal echocardiography can detect increased nuchal translucency, a thickened skin over the fetus' neck, which has been correlated with congenital heart abnormalities [11]. Early detection of a fetus with major structural cardiac anomalies permits the cardiologist to closely monitor the mother and fetus by reimaging during the second and third trimesters. Additionally, the cardiologist can implement a plan that ensures optimal delivery based on the severity of the cardiac defect.

With early diagnosis, the healthcare team has the best likelihood to prevent or minimize pathophysiology that may result from malformation [6]. Outcomes are improved for infants who are delivered at a tertiary center [6], and the infant benefits from prompt appropriate treatment, which is expedited by an expert medical team and can dictate whether there is a need for additional specialized care.

During the prenatal period, the NP establishes a relationship with the family, ensures effective communication, and acts as a liaison with the healthcare team. As part of the multidisciplinary team, the NP educates the parents concerning the diagnosis and preoperative management, identifies anticipatory needs, and arranges specialty service consults as warranted [12].

Preoperative Evaluation

The preoperative evaluation of the child with CHD begins with the initial contact with the family. This early communication may be in person or via telephone. Consideration of the family as a unit will ensure a smooth transition from preoperative evaluation through outpatient follow-up. The compilation of a thorough history ensures preoperative needs are addressed and fulfilled. Additionally, the NP becomes a resource to the family and maintains open communication with the healthcare team.

After preliminary communication about the need for surgery by their cardiologist, a preoperative encounter can be initiated to schedule surgery and obtain patient information. These details include past medical and surgical history, current or recent illnesses, hospitalizations, dental history, current medications, familial support, and financial means. The NP ensures proper identification of patient and family needs and referral to the proper individuals to meet those needs. The week before surgery, the family is contacted to discuss the child's present health, ensure no recent or current presence of viral illnesses, discuss discontinuing

certain medications before surgery, and reminders regarding the preoperative visit. Final consult recommendations (e.g., neurology, genetics, hematology, infectious disease) should be collected and comprehensively reviewed the week before surgery to ensure the child's medical needs are addressed throughout the hospital stay.

The next appointment is the preoperative visit. This office encounter includes chest radiograph, laboratory work, preoperative education, history and physical, and evaluation by the anesthesiologist. The NP reviews laboratory results and chest radiograph evaluation and conducts a thorough history and physical within 30 days before surgery. The NP discusses with the parents any current health and medical concerns, their readiness for the upcoming surgery, and any educational needs of the patient and/or family. The preoperative visit may include consultation with the on-service cardiologist, anesthesiologists, child-life personnel, and social workers.

Preoperative teaching is done in great detail including reinforcement of the child's heart defect, the surgical process, and postoperative expectations. The discussion may include computer-generated diagrams, pamphlets, and/or heart models. This concrete visualization and representation of the process needed to repair the heart defect allows families to understand and have realistic expectations. Proper evaluation of the child's developmental level is ascertained and appropriate educational material should be used. Child-life personnel have a positive impact on children and their siblings when discussing the surgical process. Identification of feelings and expression of these feelings is encouraged. Child-life personnel specialize in helping these children discuss their feelings, which drastically reduces the stress level of both child and family.

Perioperative Process

Intraoperative Phase

On the morning of surgery, the child is accompanied to the operating room by parent(s) or caregiver(s), and care is transferred to the operating room staff. This experience has proven to be stressful and emotional for families. Extended family support is encouraged and helpful. A location where caregivers and their support system can remain during the child's surgery is beneficial in decreasing the anxiety that is present throughout the process. The NP provides the family with necessary updates throughout the intraoperative phase, including the anesthetic, commencement of cardiopulmonary bypass, and the final outcome.

Emotional support is provided to the family if the surgical outcome will not be optimal, including cases of delayed chest closure, extracorporeal membrane oxygenation support, or surgical demise. Toward the end of the surgical case, the surgeon discusses the operative details with the family. In the case of poor outcome or death, the NP provides social and spiritual support as necessary.

Initial Postoperative Phase

Once the surgical procedure has been completed, the child is transferred to the intensive care unit. This transfer can be a physiologically stressful time for the child, where adequate assessment of hemodynamic support and pain management are vital. The NP communicates intraoperative concerns to the pediatric intensive care unit staff, writes postoperative orders, and assists with the admission of the child to the unit. Careful review of laboratory work, correction of electrolytes, treatment of coagulopathies, and blood administration is completed as indicated. Arterial blood gas measurements are reviewed to assure appropriate ventilation. Initial chest radiograph, after transfer, includes assessment of proper placement of lines and tubes. Pleural effusion, atelectasis, pulmonary vascular markings, heart size, and other abnormalities are noted, and appropriate treatments are started. The cardiac rhythm is assessed and a 12-lead electrocardiogram is obtained to rule out conduction abnormalities. Once this initial assessment is done, the parents are provided the opportunity to see their child.

Most parents require reintroduction to their surroundings, including the child's intravenous lines and tubes and their function to the child's recovery. Explanation of monitors will allow parents to understand what nurses and medical staff are doing to provide proper medical treatment to their child. The family should be introduced to the child's bedside nurse and be encouraged to ask questions. Nursing staff can promote family participation in their child's care by supporting them in simple tasks such as changing diapers, applying lotion, or even sponge bathing. This minimizes feelings of helplessness and allows a sense of accomplishment.

Subsequently, the NP monitors the child's progress and assesses potential problems by serial physical exams and attention to clinical signs. Common postoperative problems are managed and include low cardiac output, pulmonary edema, arrhythmias, and excessive bleeding. The NP confers with the surgeon, cardiologists, intensive care unit staff, and residents at daily rounds to develop a treatment plan for each child. The plan is communicated to the family at this time, and the NP provides emotional support as appropriate.

Postoperative Assessment and Complications

The NP must understand each patient's congenital heart defect, the preoperative clinical condition, the surgical procedure, and the potential postoperative sequela. The NP focuses on potential problems and proactively approaches preventing them.

Decreased Cardiac Output

The greatest concern of the postoperative period is maintaining adequate myocardial function and oxygen delivery to the tissues. The child with poor cardiac output will have cool extremities, decreased peripheral pulses, decreased capillary refill, lactate levels greater than 2 mmol/L, and poor urine output. Low cardiac output in the immediate postoperative period may result from hypovolemia, elevated systemic vascular resistance (SVR), arrhythmia, cardiac tamponade, and myocardial dysfunction. The management of low cardiac output requires replacement of intravascular volume, treating inappropriate SVR, and frequently supporting myocardial function with inotropic medications such as dopamine, milrinone, and dobutamine. It is also important that the child with decreased cardiac output be normothermic, well sedated, and maintain electrolytes in normal range, particularly calcium, magnesium, glucose, and potassium.

Arrhythmias

Hemodynamically significant arrhythmias occur frequently after congenital heart surgery in approximately 15% of patients [13,14]. Some examples of rhythm disturbances include heart block, junctional ectopic tachycardia (JET), premature ventricular contractions (PVCs), and supraventricular tachycardia (SVT). One study performed by Batra *et al.* [15], stated that surgical repairs with the highest risk for arrhythmia were Norwood procedure (90%), arterial switch operation (54%), and atrioventricular canal repair (37%). Among the group of 336 patients, PVCs (11%), JET (8%), nonsustained ventricular tachycardia (4%), and SVT (3%) were among the most common arrhythmias [15]. Close cardiac monitoring allows for frequent assessment of the child's rhythm and prompt intervention when necessary. Children who are at increased risk for arrhythmias may require pacing, and temporary pacing wires are used when available.

The most problematic and common arrhythmia that occurs in the immediate postoperative period, usually in infants after a complex repair, is JET. The loss of atrioventricular synchrony and decreased ventricular fill time can have a significant impact on cardiac output. Junctional ectopic tachycardia may not be obvious, so the NP must have a high index of suspicion in an infant with poor rate variability and decreased perfusion. A 12-lead electrocardiogram with atrial wire tracing is helpful when diagnosing JET. Treatment includes mild hypothermia, sedation, reduction of exogenous catecholamines, overdrive pacing and the use of antiarrhythmic medications, such as amiodarone [13].

Conduction defects can occur with procedures that relieve left ventricular outflow obstruction and where closure of a septal defect is involved. Patients may require temporary pacing until normal sinus rhythm returns or a permanent pacemaker is placed. The recommended acceptable waiting period for recovery is 7–10 days. Children who have surgical heart block are at risk for long-term conduction abnormalities [16].

Fluids/renal Function

Hypovolemia and interstitial fluid accumulation occur from capillary leak in the first 24–48 hours after cardiopulmonary bypass [17]. Fluid status needs to be carefully evaluated and appropriate treatment given. Intravascular volume needs to be replaced with colloid and/or blood products titrated to appropriate filling pressures to maintain cardiac output. Diuretics are usually started on the first postoperative day to encourage mobilization of interstitial fluid. During this active diuresis, the NP must monitor electrolytes and replace where warranted. The patient response to therapy, physical exam, daily weights, blood urea nitrogen, and creatinine needs to be followed to prevent over-diuresis and dehydration. Fluid loss from chest tubes, peritoneal drains, nasogastric tubes, and diarrhea must be accounted for and replaced as necessary.

Temporary oliguric renal dysfunction is common after long cardiopulmonary bypass times for complex CHD in infants. Acute renal injury after cardiac surgery is a serious adverse event, which can significantly impact patient morbidity and mortality [17]. Generally, this recovers as the systemic inflammatory response resolves and cardiac output improves, usually 24–48 hours postoperatively. If oliguria persists with electrolyte abnormalities and/or severe fluid overload occurs, peritoneal dialysis can be helpful. Children who recover from hemodynamic instability with improved cardiac output usually have good renal function recovery [18].

Potential Neurological Complications

Children with CHD are at increased risk for neurological impairment, particularly brain injury after open-heart surgery [19]. The brain may be at increased vulnerability to injuries due to hemodynamic, ventilatory, and oxygen disturbances [19]. The initial postoperative period focuses on the physiologic effects after cardiopulmonary bypass. Neurological complications after surgery include seizures, embolic stroke, intracerebral hemorrhage, choreoathetosis, quadriplegia, and long-term neurodevelopment deficits, which appear later in childhood.

Some children with CHD are at particularly greater risk for suboptimal outcomes including premature and low-birthweight infants, children with chromosomal anomalies or syndromes, and more complex heart defects [19–21]. Any of these complications can lead to learning and behavior disabilities. Adverse neurologic outcomes are multifactorial and relate to both patient-specific factors (genetic predisposition, in-utero central nervous system development, socioeconomic level) and potentially modifiable factors. Potentially modifiable factors include intraoperative variables, cardiopulmonary bypass, deep hypothermic circulatory arrest, and perioperative factors. Perioperative factors include low cardiac output, hypoxemia, hypotension, prolonged hospitalization, and sepsis [19–21].

Pulmonary Complications

A systematic pulmonary evaluation is done with each assessment, including notation of ventilator settings, lung auscultation, nature of secretions, and evaluation of arterial blood gas measurements. This detailed review will assist in assessment of the child's readiness for extubation.

Most children can be extubated within 72 hours after surgery. Inability to wean or separate from mechanical ventilation may be related to pleural effusion, phrenic nerve damage, recurrent nerve damage, airway edema, bronchomalacia, airway compression from vascular structures or conduits, or residual cardiac defects [22]. Frequently, the case is multifactorial in a small malnourished child with residual cardiac defects. Children who require prolonged intubation can be at increased risk for ventilator associated pneumonia (VAP) and increased length of stay [23]. Additionally, prolonged ventilation is associated with greater medical complications and mortality rates [24].

The NP monitors for appropriate fluid and electrolytes and ensures appropriate nutritional support. The surgeon can be alerted if drainage of pleural effusions is indicated. The NP can assist in determining the cause of respiratory failure by astute serial physical exam during weaning and extubation. Did the child fail because of tachypnea, stridor, inability to handle secretions, or poor cough? Was paradoxical breathing noted or did the child gradually become fatigued with poor inspiratory effort? Ultrasound of the diaphragm or a consult with an ear, nose, and throat physician may be indicated to rule out phrenic or vocal cord damage.

Causes for pleural effusion or excessive pleural drainage include fluid overload, pulmonary edema, and capillary leak from cardiopulmonary bypass and increased venous pressure as seen with patients after right ventriculotomy (e.g., tetralogy of Fallot), cavopulmonary shunts, and the Fontan procedure. Small to moderate pleural effusions can usually be handled medically with diuretics. However, a large effusion should be drained, especially if the patient is symptomatic. Serial physical exams and chest radiograph should be done to monitor effusions and response to therapy.

Chylothorax is the leakage of lymphatic fluid, a creamy white fluid called chyle, into the pleural space owing to injury of the thoracic duct or because of increased pressure within the intrathoracic lymph system [25]. Excessive chylous drainage can lead to hypoproteinemia, hypolipidemia, electrolyte loss, and immune dysfunction due to loss of T cells. Nutritional treatment consists of a diet low in long-chain triglycerides, and high in medium-chain triglycerides and protein. Electrolytes, serum protein, and albumin are followed and replaced as necessary. Some children require chemical or mechanical pleurodesis with parenteral nutrition. Octreotide, a somatostatin analogue, has been used in some institutions with some success in reducing chylous leakage [25].

Infection

Infections, particularly sepsis, can be a serious postoperative complication. Factors that increase the risk of infection include younger age, prolonged surgical procedure, prolonged intensive care unit course, prolonged mechanical ventilation, multiple lines and tubes, and delayed chest closure. Prevention and early treatment of line infections are particularly important for children who have intracardiac prosthesis or patches, as eradication of established infection on foreign material can be difficult.

A low-grade fever is common for 24 hours after surgery. However, if the fever is greater than $39\,^{\circ}C$, infection should be suspected and cultures sent. Other signs of infection include changes in white blood cell count, a drop in platelet count, hemodynamic instability, and/or change in mental status. All intravenous sites and the child's incision should be inspected daily for signs of infection. Good handwashing, meticulous line care, and early removal of lines and tubes are important in preventing infection. Other causes of fever could be atelectasis, pleural effusion, pneumonia, postcardiotomy syndrome, urinary tract infection, gastroenteritis, and otitis media. Respiratory syncytial virus (RSV) and other respiratory viruses should be suspected if the child has upper respiratory infection symptoms, chest radiograph changes, or low oxygen saturation.

Risk factors for wound infection include delayed chest closure, exploration for bleeding, and reoperation. The most common organisms are coagulase-negative *Staphylococcus* and *Staphylococcus aureus*. Severe infection requires incision and drainage, and healing is by second intention.

Vacuum-assisted closure (VAC) is a new therapy for children with mediastinitis that has shown promise in improving outcomes. However, studies in children have been limited. A VAC dressing consists of a piece of foam with an open cell structure placed loosely in the wound [26,27]. A wound drain with multiple lateral perforations is placed on top. The entire wound is then covered with a transparent dressing. The drain tube is then connected to a vacuum source, which is set between 25 and 125 mmHg. Fluid is drawn from the wound through the foam into a reservoir for disposal. The transparent dressing prevents air entry and allows a partial vacuum to form within the wound, which promotes debridement and decreases tissue bacterial levels, increases blood flow, and promotes healing [26,27].

Nutrition

Children with CHD are frequently malnourished and have failure to thrive before surgical intervention [28]. It is well known that patients who are malnourished are at increased risk for poor wound healing, infections, and an inability to wean from mechanical ventilation. Therefore, it is essential in the postoperative period when the child is in a hypermetabolic state that nutritional support be started early to prevent complications. Parenteral nutrition is indicated when hemodynamic instability and poor gastrointestinal function prevent using the gastrointestinal tract. The use of trophic feeds in conjunction with total parenteral nutrition can help prevent gastrointestinal complications, improve immune function, and lessen the risk of bacterial infection [24].

Neonates with complex repairs involving the aortic arch, and single-ventricle patients with an aorta pulmonary shunt are at increased risk for necrotizing enterocolitis [25]. The usual feeding regimen begins with continuous nasogastric feeds with breast milk or 20 kcal per ounce formula. Feeds are slowly increased over 3–5 days with serial abdominal examination. The calorie density of the breast milk or formula then is advanced until the infant is receiving at least 120 kcal/kg/day. Infants with two-ventricle repair typically are managed with a combination of oral and nasogastric feeding. Oral feeding is attempted for 15–20 minutes with nasogastric supplementation thereafter as necessary. This allows the infant to learn oral feeding skills while ensuring adequate calorie intake. Breast feeding should be encouraged and supported as long as the infant is able to gain weight. Lactation consultants can assist mother and baby to establish breast feeding. Infants may have feeding difficulties owing to congestive heart failure, poor cardiac output, vocal cord paresis, uncoordinated suck swallow or feeding aversion [29]. Infants with delayed gastric emptying, severe gastroesophageal reflux, or vocal cord dysfunction may require a transpyloric feeding tube to allow for enteral nutrition.

Parents of children who are poor feeders need a tremendous amount of support. Mothers often feel frustrated and stressed if their infant does not feed well, and that can negatively impact bonding and nurturing. Nasogastric feeding sometimes can help with the stress of feeding and allow for more relaxed bonding between mother and child. However, their families may feel the stress of learning nasogastric feeding and become overwhelmed. Children who have ongoing protein loss from chest tube drainage and chylothorax require a diet high in protein and low in long-chain triglycerides.

Pain Management

Every patient who has cardiac surgery will experience some degree of pain and anxiety. A pain assessment should be performed with every set of vital signs and with every physical examination. Poor pain management can lead to physical and psychologic stress, which can lead to increased morbidity and mortality. There are several self-reporting pain assessment tools now available for all ages of patients [30]:

OUCHER
- Facial photographs (3–4 years and up)
- Linear analogue scale (6–7 years and up)

Wong-Baker faces
- Cartoon faces (3–4 years and up)
- Word descriptors and numbers (6–7 years and up)

Visual analogue
Finger span scale or word anchors (6–7 years and up)

There are additionally, several behavioral and physiologic pain assessment tools currently being used by patients of all ages [30]:

CRIES (crying, requires oxygen, increased vital signs, expression, sleepless; infants)

FLACC (face, legs, activity, cry, consolability; 2 months to 7 years)

OPS (objective pain scale; <3 years)

CHEOPS (Children's Hospital of Eastern Ontario Pain Scale: cry, facial, verbal, torso, touch, legs; 1–7 years).

Scales that allow a child to self report pain are preferred whenever possible. Older children should be familiarized with an age-appropriate pain assessment tool and plans for postoperative pain management [30] discussed before surgery. Older children can be instructed in the use of the patient-controlled analgesia pump. Usually, the initial postoperative pain management regimen consists of continuous opioid infusion (morphine or fentanyl for the first 24–48 hours) (see Chapter 7, *Perioperative Care*). Other sedation, like benzodiazepines, may be used as needed to maintain comfort during mechanical ventilation. Most children can take medications by mouth by the third postoperative day and can be switched to acetaminophen and/or ibuprofen with codeine or oxycodone for breakthrough pain.

Critically ill infants and children after complex repairs are at risk for pulmonary hypertensive crisis, junctional tachycardia, or postoperative bleeding resulting from hypertension and are kept sedated with high-dose opioid infusion and scheduled benzodiazepines. As the child becomes hemodynamically stable, the sedation is weaned. Children who have received large doses of narcotics and benzodiazepines for longer than 5 days are at risk for withdrawal if medications are abruptly stopped. A slow wean by decreasing the narcotic or lorazepam dose by 10% and increasing the time between doses will usually prevent withdrawal symptoms [30]. Child-life personnel are significant members of the multidisciplinary team who provide nondrug strategies to children. For instance, watching television or listening to music can be helpful to relieve pain and anxiety associated with minor problems such as intravenous starts and lab draws. Painful procedures, such as chest tube removal, usually require treatment with both a narcotic and anxiolysis. The presence of a parent is a great source of comfort for the child, and he or she should be encouraged to be with the child and participate in care as much as possible [31].

Discharge Planning

Discharge teaching for patients undergoing congenital surgery is continuous and should begin at the time of admission [1,12]. As overall patient acuity and complexity of care has increased, so have the details of discharge planning for this patient population [32]. The patient's age, nutritional needs, home medical equipment needs, communication with the primary care physicians, as well as plans to return to work and school all require careful consideration. It has been said that the NP involved with these patients essentially becomes a patient care coordinator at this time. The experienced clinical judgment of the NP as well as his/her background in patient education and clinical research, comprises the best candidate for discharge planning [32].

Neonatal Discharge Planning

Organizing the discharge of neonates after congenital heart surgery requires a high degree of care coordination. It has been shown that a systematic discharge plan not only improves the neonate's recovery at home, but also increases parents' confidence in caring for their child [33]. It is of utmost importance to determine patient as well as parent readiness for discharge planning process [12]. The neonate with CHD is deemed ready for discharge once vital signs (including saturations) are stable, body temperature is maintained without warmers, and the infant is gaining weight steadily with oral or enteral tube feeding [12]. The best method of determining parent readiness is to have the parent or designated caregiver "room-in" with the infant [12]. While rooming in, the parent can assume all of their child's care with back-up help from the floor nurse or cardiothoracic NP. Also during this time, the NP can review with the parents wound care needs, medication dosing and administration, in addition to providing education regarding postoperative complications to watch for once at home.

One of the most common problems infants with CHD face is feeding difficulties and growth delay, particularly those who remain cyanotic after initial surgery [34]. Many of these infants will require assistance with feeding via nasogastric tube. Persistent postoperative congestive heart failure, stress of surgery, and wound healing can increase the metabolic rate of children with CHD, thus increasing their caloric needs. Most neonates are sent home on calorie-dense formula or fortified breast milk to provide proper nutritional requirements. Some of these patients require up to 160 kcal/kg/day to gain sufficient weight [35].

There are several other issues requiring attention before discharge including sending all pertinent neonatal screening tests (e.g., hearing screen, phenylketonuria testing). Other genetic anomalies may be present and certain testing can be done to address these issues. Hearing screens are routinely recommended for newborns before discharge and are especially recommended for those newborns with CHD. Various syndromes associated with CHD, as well as various medications these infants need before and after surgery can lead to hearing loss [12]. A brainstem evoked auditory response (BAER) exam can be performed at the bedside. Immunizations should be given as recommended for these infants a few days before discharge to allow time to observe for adverse reactions [12]. The hepatitis B series should be initiated and, depending on the child's age at discharge, the pneumococcal and rotavirus vaccines should be considered [36]. If discharge is occurring during the fall and winter months, all neonates with CHD should begin receiving monthly RSV prophylaxis until the season is over [37]. Palivizumab and RSV immune globulin can be given during the RSV season up to the age of 2 years [37].

Additional matters to be addressed include car seat safety and cardiopulmonary resuscitation (CPR) education for caregivers. Many institutions require a car seat challenge for premature or special needs infants going home for the first time. Car seat challenges ensure the infant can maintain adequate oxygen saturations while positioned in an infant car seat for up to an hour. The parents should be instructed on proper car seat positioning and demonstrate competence in securing their child.

Cardiopulmonary resuscitation training is essential for parents and caregivers of infants with CHD. In-hospital resources can be used for CPR training, or community resources are available for CPR training for these families and caregivers. Extensive teaching is done before discharge, including what to do in case of an emergency.

Discharge Planning Past the Neonatal Period

Central Nervous System Concerns

Pain management remains a primary concern for parents of children with CHD. For younger patients, giving acetaminophen (15 mg/kg) every 6 hours is usually sufficient.

Ibuprofen (10 mg/kg) can be alternated with acetaminophen dosing to give additional pain relief. Some children often require a mild narcotic regimen such as codeine (0.5–1 mg/kg/dose) every 6 hours or oxycodone (0.05–0.15 mg/kg/dose) every 4–6 hours. Older children and young adults may benefit from nonsteroidal anti-inflammatory agents such as ibuprofen or ketorolac provided they have normal renal function.

> **Education Point**
>
> Review expectations for pain management in an age-appropriate manner. Any increase in wound pain should be immediately reported to the surgical team.

Respiratory Concerns

Atelectasis is common postoperatively and usually resolves quickly in infants and younger children. Older children and adolescents should be encouraged to use bubbles, incentive spirometry, and other deep breathing exercises to assist in alveolar recovery. A repeat chest radiograph should be done at the postoperative visit to evaluate lung expansion and resolution of prior atelectasis. Some patients with increased pulmonary vascular resistance may require home oxygen therapy. Arrangements should be made before discharge from the hospital. Some institutions require home pulse oximetry, and parent education should be thorough regarding its use.

> **Education Point**
>
> Review signs and symptoms of pleural effusion. The surgical team should be notified immediately of increased work of breathing or retractions abnormal to the patient's baseline. Infants may develop poor feeding and tachypnea, both of which should be reported to the proper members of the healthcare team.

Cardiovascular Concerns

An overview of cardiovascular symptoms that may develop postoperatively should be reviewed with the family. This includes assessment of perfusion, presence of edema, irritability, and lethargy. Cardiovascular medications, administration guidelines, and review of medication interactions should be reviewed with patients and families before discharge. Postoperative complications should be communicated with the child's primary care physician so recurrence of these can be monitored appropriately. Families of children with complex CHD, including single-ventricle pathology, require staged palliative procedures. The need for appropriate follow-up and referral should be reinforced.

> **Education Point**
>
> Review the symptoms of worsening condition such as tachycardia, chest pain, or cyanotic episodes. Review side effects of cardiovascular medications and possible drug interactions.

Gastrointestinal Concerns

A nutritional plan should be made in collaboration with a dietitian before discharge and written instructions reviewed with caregivers. Dietary regimens may include both oral and nasogastric feedings while the child transitions to full oral feedings. Nasogastric tube insertion and verification of placement should be demonstrated by caregivers as appropriate. Additionally, constipation from narcotic regimen may become an issue postoperatively. Proper use of stool softeners is examined and dosage recommendations reviewed with families.

> **Education Point**
>
> Review plans for stool softeners and dietary changes until normal bowel movement pattern returns. Fluids should be encouraged and development of diarrhea, vomiting, or refusal of intake should be immediately reported.

Renal Concerns

Patients typically require diuretics during the immediate postoperative period, with some children requiring prolonged use. The administration timing of diuretics should be considered in older children to avoid disruption of the sleep cycle. Occasionally, viral illnesses will cause children with CHD to become dehydrated. Referral to the cardiologist and primary care physicians should be encouraged early in the course of the illness for proper medication adjustments.

> **Education Point**
>
> Review dosing, side effects, symptoms related to electrolyte imbalances, and dietary changes that can prevent hydration issues.

Hematologic/Infectious Disease Concerns

Anemia may be persistent postoperatively and iron supplementation initiated until adequate hemoglobin levels are achieved. Immunizations remain important and children over 6 months of age should be receiving yearly flu vaccination. Children over age 2 should receive the meningococcal vaccine as well [36]. Immunocompromised patients, such as those with asplenia, will require daily antibiotic prophylaxis. If wound infection occurs postoperatively, children may require long-term intravenous antibiotics. Home care nursing may be required and these arrangements should be made before discharge.

> **Education Point**
>
> Review with families the American Heart Association Guidelines for bacterial endocarditis prophylaxis. Parents are instructed to call for any fever over 38.3°C in all postoperative patients. Ensure the family has access to an appropriate thermometer and instruct prompt measurement when a fever is suspected.

Integumentary Concerns

Proper wound care is of vital importance in children who have undergone any invasive surgery. Thorough education and wound care procedures should be demonstrated by caregivers. Showering will be postponed until suture removal is performed at the postoperative visit. Soaking underneath water and swimming are discouraged until wounds are fully healed. If prolonged dressing changes are required for delayed incisional healing, extensive education and demonstration of technique should be performed. In some cases, home care nursing may be used.

> **Education Point**
>
> Education regarding signs and symptoms of wound infection are reviewed. If disruption of healing is suspected, the surgical team should be notified immediately.

Medication Concerns

The home medication regimen is examined before discharge and an administration schedule developed with the family. Rooming-in will allow for proper assessment of the caregiver's ability to draw up and administer any liquid medications [12]. Explanation of medication necessity should be thoroughly reviewed with adolescents and young adults to ensure compliance.

> **Education Point**
>
> A written list of medications, dosage, route, timing of administration, purpose of use, and side effects should be provided to the family. Prescriptions should be filled before discharge so proper measuring techniques can be demonstrated with liquid preparations.

Final Discharge Details

The transition from hospital to home consists of communication with the surgical team to primary care physician and cardiologist. Both should receive copies of the operative note and discharge for the child's medical record. Notification of discharge date and follow-up plans should be communicated to the primary care physician and cardiologist. Outstanding issues including laboratory or radiology testing can be addressed with this communication. This exchange of information enables primary care physicians the opportunity to ask specific questions regarding their patients.

Parenting methods and discipline are often a common topic of concern for parents following cardiac surgery. Parents of children with CHD commonly fear disciplining their child, as concern exists of a worsening heart condition. Early on, whether by a cardiologist or NP, the parents should be encouraged to treat their child as normal as possible to avoid "vulnerable child syndrome". This syndrome occurs as a result of a parent's perception of the child as weaker owing to life-threatening illness despite the child's recovery. This leads to disruption in the parent-child relationship, which eventually causes behavior disorders [38].

Another topic of concern for the older child and adolescent is return to school and/or work. There is limited information in the literature regarding timing of postoperative return to work or school. Individual recovery periods and variability in complications after surgery need to be accounted for when deciding the proper timing for return to school and work. Once the child has had their initial postoperative visit with their cardiologist, a return to work/school date can be identified. School-aged children are excused from physical education for 6–12 weeks and are encouraged to avoid heavy lifting (backpacks) for at least 6 weeks. It may be helpful for the school to provide the child with a second set of books during this recovery period. The primary cardiologist routinely gives adolescents clearance to return to the work environment. Depending on the adolescent's occupation, 2–4 weeks is usually sufficient time for recovery. High-intensity labor positions may require a further return to work date, especially if heavy lifting is involved. Cardiac rehabilitation is recommended for the adolescent population, and proper referral should be made before discharge.

Various details are needed in order to organize the child's discharge from the hospital after congenital heart surgery. A holistic approach should be used when planning for each patient's transition from hospital to home. The NP has an extensive opportunity to be engaged in the discharge process for these families from admission to the hospital through discharge. The NP ensures a comprehensive discharge plan for each patient based on their individual needs. However, the NP cannot complete the

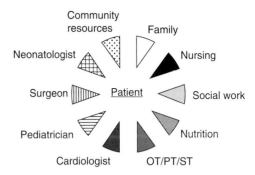

Figure 8.1 Multidisciplinary team. (Reproduced with permission from Dodds *et al.* [12].)

patient's discharge plan alone. A multidisciplinary team including physicians, nurses, and therapists is needed to ensure comprehensive care is delivered after hospital discharge (Figure 8.1) [12].

Patient and Family Satisfaction

The NP has a vital role in the assessment of patient and family satisfaction throughout the entire spectrum of care from preoperative diagnosis through postoperative follow up. Some quality improvement initiatives measure patient satisfaction data, including the Joint Commission on Accreditation of Healthcare Organizations (JCAHO). Collectively, institutions are required to comply with National Patient Safety Goals, and accreditation status can be affected by this data. Proper examination of the hospital experience for patient's with CHD permits a thorough evaluation of the surgical process and supports restructuring when satisfaction needs are unmet.

The NP continues to be at the forefront of delivering education and dissemination of information to families and patients. The literature suggests that some of the most important domains of satisfaction identified by parents are medical care, professional support in terms of communication and information, and the parents' own role in pediatric care [39]. Past research suggests that communication, staff courtesy, compassion and respect, information provided to the family, and level of healthcare received by the patient were predictors of overall family satisfaction [40]. The NP has the ability to witness, assess, and shape the hospital experience for patients and families and is essential to providing good patient satisfaction outcomes.

The child's perception and experience are both relevant to satisfaction, as well as parental insight and contentment with the perioperative process. The child's needs should be met from initial contact to hospital discharge, including age-appropriate education. Patient satisfaction scores may

Table 8.1 Hierarchy of needs used to assess patient and family satisfaction.

Physiologic needs	Medication, oxygenation, pain control, diet, bowel pattern, sleep
Safety	Secured side rails, availability of nursing
Love/belonging	Presence of caregivers, nursing, child-life personnel, NPs
Esteem	Confidence, respect of others, achievement of medical tasks
Self-actualization	Delivery of medical facts, prognosis

reflect suitable pain assessment and management, patient safety, building trustworthy relationships, age-appropriate communication and rationale for care, and family/nursing presence at the bedside. The caregiver level of satisfaction can be optimized by adequate delivery of medical information, developing empowering relationships, and decisive fulfillment of family centered care. Ensuring that these needs are met may be done in systematic fashion. For instance, an adaptation of a hierarchy of needs is demonstrated as a tool that could be used to ameliorate the assessment of patient and family satisfaction (Table 8.1) with the highest priority being physiologic needs.

Physiologic needs including medication, oxygen requirements, pain control, diet intake, bowel management, and adequate sleep are fundamental tasks that require careful assessment and adjustment as warranted. This element of the child's needs assessment highly impacts the other issues of concern.

Safety becomes an important and prioritized point for children during the hospital stay. Hospital safety is important to patients and families and has been shown to be a predictor of positive outcomes [40]. Physical safety should be guaranteed, along with the feeling of being safe while being hospitalized. This can be accomplished with locked patient care areas and secured bed side rails. Children may or may not have continued presence of a caregiver during their hospitalization. The NP is an advocate for the child and encourages caregiver presence whenever possible. If the caregiver or extended family is unable to be present, the nursing staff and NP compensate for this deficit until discharge is possible.

The ability of children and adolescents with CHD to feel love and belonging in the hospital environment is of great importance and should be maintained. Caregivers who are unable to be present because of work schedules or care requirements of other siblings need reinforcement of holistic hospital care and recovery in their absence. Nursing staff, child-life personnel, and the NP may need to compen-

sate for the absence of a consistent caregiver. Social work assessment is important in this situation.

The next phase of the needs assessment includes the child's self-esteem. This phase becomes a topic of interest in the older child. This age group has the ability to be active in their recovery process. Encouragement to be accountable for their nutritional and physical therapy needs can provide them with a sense of accomplishment and augment their healing time. Child-life personnel can be used when identifying the child's needs in collaboration with the NP. Providing rewards for accomplishing activities necessary for recovery (ambulation, bathing, medication intake, painful procedures) may be helpful.

The self-actualization phase includes assessment of child and caregiver, depending on the child's age and ability to understand and accept their medical diagnosis and prognosis. Delivery of information and discussion of medical facts with the family and child are common tasks needed for successful understanding of long-term outcomes.

A uniform way to evaluate parental or caregiver satisfaction can be done in addition to the child's assessment. The hierarchy of needs can be used and adapted for individual patients and families. The literature continues to have common themes for positive outcomes including delivery of medical information, building trustworthy relationships, and parental involvement in patient care. According to Dowling et al. [40], communication remains a powerful predictor of satisfaction and should be a key component of any initiative. The NP can modify and adapt a system that embodies the mission of their institution to ensure thorough needs assessment of their patient population. Evidenced-based research can allow for expanding on these processes and discovery of the best approach to ensure satisfaction.

Conclusion

Pediatric NPs bring their expertise in general pediatrics as well as in human development to specialty care in congenital heart surgery [3]. The NP role continues to evolve as new treatments become available, medical and surgical therapies progress, and the patient population lives longer. Judicious patient care assessment, coordination, and practice improvement enhance positive patient outcomes.

References

1. Allen AD, Driscoll DJ, Shaddy RE, et al. (2008) *Moss and Adams' Heart Disease in Infants, Children, and Adolescents: Including the Fetus and Young Adult*, 7th ed. Philadelphia, PA: Lippincott Williams & Wilkins.
2. Keeling AW. (2009) A brief history of advanced practice nursing in the United States. In: Hamric AB, Spross JA,

Hanson CM, eds. *Advanced Practice Nursing: An Integrative Approach*, 4th ed. St Louis, MO: Elsevier Saunders, pp. 3–32.

3. O'Brien P. (2007) The role of the nurse practitioner in congenital heart surgery. Pediatr Cardiol 28, 88–95.

4. Hravnak M, Kleinpell RM, Magdic KS, *et al.* (2009) The acute care nurse practitioner. In: Hamric AB, Spross JA, Hanson CM, eds. *Advanced Practice Nursing: An Integrative Approach*, 4th ed. St Louis, MO: Elsevier Saunders, pp. 403–436.

5. Cheek DJ, Harshaw-Ellis KS. (2005) Advanced practice nurses in non-primary care roles: the evolution of specialty and acute care practices. In: Stanley JM, ed. *Advanced Practice Nursing: Emphasizing Common Roles*. Philadelphia, PA: FA Davis Company, pp. 146–156.

6. McGrath JM. (2006) Early detection and immediate management of congenital heart disease is important to long-term outcomes. J Perinat Neonatal Nurs 20, 285–286.

7. Hook EB. (1982) Contribution of chromosome abnormalities to human morbidity and mortality. Cytogenet Cell Genet 33, 101–106.

8. Sivanandam S, Glickstein JS, Printz BF, *et al.* (2006) Prenatal diagnosis of conotruncal malformations: diagnostic accuracy, outcome, chromosomal abnormalities, and extracardiac anomalies. Am J Perinatol 23, 241–245.

9. Paladini D, Calabro R, Palmieri S, *et al.* (1993) Prenatal diagnosis of congenital heart disease and fetal karyotyping. Obstet Gynecol 81, 679–682.

10. Kornosky JL, Salihu HM. (2008) Getting to the heart of the matter: epidemiology of cyanotic heart defects. Pediatr Cardiol 29, 484–497.

11. Huhta JC. (2001) The first trimester cardiologist: one standard of care for all children. Curr Opin Pediatr 13, 453–455.

12. Dodds KM, Merle C. (2005) Discharging neonates with congenital heart disease after cardiac surgery: a practical approach. Clin Perinatol 32, 1031–1042.

13. Delaney JW, Moltedo JM, Dziura JD, *et al.* (2006) Early postoperative arrhythmias after pediatric cardiac surgery. J Thorac Cardiovasc Surg 131, 1296–1300.

14. Rekawek J, Kansy A, Miszczak-Knecht M, *et al.* (2007) Risk factors for cardiac arrhythmias in children with congenital heart disease after surgical intervention in the early postoperative period. J Thorac Cardiovasc Surg 133, 900–904.

15. Batra AS, Chun DS, Johnson TR, *et al.* (2006) A prospective analysis of the incidence and risk factors associated with junctional ectopic tachycardia following surgery for congenital heart disease. Pediatr Cardiol 27, 51–55.

16. Fischbach PS, Frias PA, Strieper MJ, *et al.* (2007) Natural history and current therapy for complete heart block in children and patients with congenital heart disease. Congenit Heart Dis 2, 224–234.

17. Welke KF, Dearani JA, Ghanayem NS, *et al.* (2008) Renal complications associated with the treatment of patients with congenital cardiac disease: consensus definitions from the Multi-Societal Database Committee for Pediatric and Congenital Heart Disease. Cardiol Young 18(Suppl 2), 222–225.

18. Moghal NE, Brocklebank JT, Meadow SR. (1998) A review of acute renal failure in children: incidence, etiology and outcome. Clin Nephrol 49, 91–95.

19. Ballweg JA, Wernovsky G, Gaynor JW. (2007) Neurodevelopmental outcomes following congenital heart surgery. Pediatr Cardiol 28, 126–133.

20. Hsia TY, Gruber PJ. (2006) Factors influencing neurologic outcome after neonatal cardiopulmonary bypass: what we can and cannot control. Ann Thorac Surg 81, S2381–S2388.

21. Trittenwein G, Nardi A, Pansi H, *et al.* (2003) Early postoperative prediction of cerebral damage after pediatric cardiac surgery. Ann Thorac Surg 76, 576–580.

22. Bandla HP, Hopkins RL, Beckerman RC, *et al.* (1999) Pulmonary risk factors compromising postoperative recovery after surgical repair for congenital heart disease. Chest 116, 740–747.

23. Davis S, Cox AC, Piedmonte M, *et al.* (2002) Prolonged mechanical ventilation after cardiac surgery in young children: incidence, etiology, and risk factors. J Intens Care Med 17, 302–307.

24. Kanter RK, Bove EL, Tobin JR, *et al.* (1986) Prolonged mechanical ventilation of infants after open heart surgery. Crit Care Med 14, 211–214.

25. Chan EH, Russell JL, Williams WG, *et al.* (2005) Postoperative chylothorax after cardiothoracic surgery in children. Ann Thorac Surg 80, 1864–1870.

26. Agarwal JP, Ogilvie M, Wu LC, *et al.* (2005) Vacuum-assisted closure for sternal wounds: a first-line therapeutic management approach. Plast Reconstr Surg 116, 1035–1040; discussion 1041–1043.

27. Salazard B, Niddam J, Ghez O, *et al.* (2008) Vacuum-assisted closure in the treatment of poststernotomy mediastinitis in the paediatric patient. J Plast Reconstr Aesthet Surg 61, 302–305.

28. Steltzer M, Rudd N, Pick B. (2005) Nutrition care for newborns with congenital heart disease. Clin Perinatol 32, 1017–1030.

29. Rosti L, De Battisti F, Butera G, *et al.* (2005) Octreotide in the management of postoperative chylothorax. Pediatr Cardiol 26, 440–443.

30. Diaz LK. (2006) Anesthesia and postoperative analgesia in pediatric patients undergoing cardiac surgery. Paediatr Drugs 8, 223–233.

31. Cunliffe M, McArthur L, Dooley F. (2004) Managing sedation withdrawal in children who undergo prolonged PICU admission after discharge to the ward. Paediatr Anaesth 14, 293–298.

32. Uzark K, LeRoy S, Callow L, *et al.* (1994) The pediatric nurse practitioner as case manager in the delivery of services to children with heart disease. J Pediatr Health Care 8, 74–78.

33. Yang HL, Chen YC, Mao HC, *et al.* (2004) Effect of a systematic discharge nursing plan on mothers' knowledge and confidence in caring for infants with congenital heart disease at home. J Formos Med Assoc 103, 47–52.

34. Davis D, Davis S, Cotman K, *et al.* (2008) Feeding difficulties and growth delay in children with hypoplastic left heart syndrome versus d-transposition of the great arteries. Pediatr Cardiol 29, 28–33.

35. Dooley KJ, Bishop L. (2002) Medical management of the cardiac infant and child after surgical discharge. Crit Care Nurs Q 25, 98–104.

36. Department of Health and Human Services Center for Disease Control and Prevention. The recommended immunization schedules for persons aged 0 through 18 years. Available at www.cdc.gov/vaccines/recs/acip and http://www.aap.org and http://www.aafp.org.

37. Cohen SA, Zanni R, Cohen A, *et al.* (2008) Palivizumab use in subjects with congenital heart disease: results from the 2000–2004 Palivizumab Outcomes Registry. Pediatr Cardiol 29, 382–387.

38. Lipstein EA. (2006) Helping "vulnerable" children – and their parents – lead normal lives. Contemp Pediatr 23, 26–37.

39. Lawoko S. (2007) Factors influencing satisfaction and well-being among parents of congenital heart disease children: development of a conceptual model based on the literature review. Scand J Caring Sci 21, 106–117.

40. Dowling J, Vender J, Guilianelli S, *et al.* (2005) A model of family-centered care and satisfaction predictors: the Critical Care Family Assistance Program. Chest 128, 81S–92S.

9

Palliative Operations

Carl L. Backer[1] and Constantine Mavroudis[2]

[1]Ann & Robert H. Lurie Children's Hospital of Chicago, formerly Children's Memorial Hospital, Chicago, IL, USA
[2]Florida Hospital for Children, Orlando, FL, USA

The word palliate originates from the Latin "palliare" (to cloak) and in medicine it is usually taken to mean the masking or lessening of an effect [1]. A palliative operation generally is one that provides symptomatic relief but leaves the main pathophysiology uncorrected. A palliative operation is one that affords relief (usually temporary) but is not a correction or a repair. In congenital heart surgery the two classic palliative procedures are the aortopulmonary shunt and the pulmonary artery band [2,3]. From a historical perspective, these were initially the only procedures available to treat many children with congenital heart disease. Over the past 50 years the advances in open-heart surgery, progressing to neonatal repair for many congenital heart lesions, have decreased markedly the indications for these palliative procedures. Although there are fewer and fewer indications for palliative procedures, there is a select, small group of patients for whom palliation is still (and may always be) necessary. The importance of the initial palliative procedure cannot be overemphasized. A poorly performed aortopulmonary shunt that destroys a pulmonary artery may prohibit the child from having a completion Fontan procedure. Hence, although these are older and seemingly less important procedures, they must be performed well to ensure a smooth eventual corrective procedure.

Some of the procedures reviewed in this chapter are now actually considered obsolete and are no longer performed. However, the surgeon must understand these procedures and their attendant complications because there are many surviving patients who have had these operations in the remote past but now require repeat surgical intervention. A thorough understanding of palliative procedures is necessary for appropriate staging and successful takedown at the time of correction.

In general, the goals of palliative procedures are to alter the hemodynamic physiology in such a manner as to make the cardiac malformation more tolerable, allow an improvement in the patient's condition, and allow continued growth until the child has complete correction. In the past, palliative procedures were performed on nearly all children and their complete "correction" was performed when they were older and larger. With improvements in cardiopulmonary bypass and in microsurgical techniques, the size of the patient is no longer as significant a consideration in deciding between palliation and complete repair [4]. Rather, it is the underlying cardiovascular physiology, in particular the normal high neonatal pulmonary vascular resistance, that usually mandates a palliative operation in the current era.

The two primary palliative procedures are the aortopulmonary shunts (Table 9.1) and the pulmonary artery band. Many of the aortopulmonary shunts noted in Table 9.1 are now obsolete and rarely used (Potts shunt, Waterston/Cooley shunt). Aortopulmonary shunts are designed to increase pulmonary blood flow in a cyanotic child with inadequate pulmonary blood flow. Pulmonary artery band is designed to limit pulmonary blood flow in a child with excessive pulmonary blood flow. A third palliative operation is the atrial septectomy, designed to increase mixing at the atrial level in patients with transposition of the great arteries or single ventricle and atrioventricular valve stenosis. The Blalock–Hanlon atrial septectomy was first reported in 1950 [5]. Interestingly, like many other "simple" congenital heart procedures, this is now most commonly performed using transcatheter techniques [6]. There are other more complex procedures that are considered palliative, such as the Norwood operation for hypoplastic left heart syndrome [7] and the Glenn procedure [8], but these are in general specific operative procedures for defined lesions

Table 9.1 Aortopulmonary shunts.

Shunt	Surgeon	Year
Blalock–Taussig shunt	Alfred Blalock	1944
Potts shunt	Willis Potts	1946
Waterston shunt	David Waterston	1962
Cooley shunt	Denton Cooley	1966
Modified Blalock–Taussig shunt	Marc de Leval	1976

and are discussed in detail in the chapters on those specific lesions. One palliative operation that has had a resurgence is pulmonary artery banding combined with a ductal stent for hypoplastic left heart syndrome, the so-called "hybrid" approach [9,10].

Pulmonary Artery band

Pulmonary artery banding was first reported by Muller and Dammann [3] in 1952 for children with a large left-to-right shunt or single ventricle and excessive pulmonary blood flow. For many years, pulmonary artery banding was the preferred initial palliation for any small child with a large left-to-right shunt and increased pulmonary blood flow. Examples of this would include ventricular septal defect, atrioventricular canal, and truncus arteriosus. However, as improvements in neonatal cardiac surgical techniques have taken place, pulmonary artery banding is now routinely used for only a very few specific lesions. These include (1) "Swiss-cheese" muscular ventricular septal defects; (2) multiple ventricular septal defects with coarctation; (3) single ventricle with increased pulmonary blood flow (i.e., tricuspid atresia type IIc) in preparation for eventual Fontan procedure [11,12]; (4) to prepare and retrain the left ventricle of a patient with transposition of the great arteries for the arterial switch procedure either (a) following late presentation after 6 weeks of age [13], or (b) following prior atrial repair [14]; and 5) to train the left ventricle in a patient with congenitally corrected transposition of the great arteries for a "double switch" [15,16]. Even these limited indications are controversial, and some surgeons recommend complete neonatal repair of coarctation of the aorta with multiple ventricular septal defects [17,18]. Others recommend a Damus–Stansel–Kaye procedure with aortopulmonary shunt instead of pulmonary artery band placement for single ventricle with increased pulmonary blood flow, especially when there is potential for subaortic obstruction [19].

Pulmonary artery banding in a child with normally related great vessels can be performed either through a left lateral thoracotomy or a median sternotomy incision. Although the left thoracotomy was historically the preferred approach, many surgeons now prefer the median sternotomy approach. The advantage of the left thoracotomy approach is that it frees the anterior mediastinum from

adhesions at the time of reoperation. The advantage of the median sternotomy is it allows a safe and usually quite easy approach to the pulmonary artery even with the frequently varied location of the pulmonary artery in complex defects (e.g., heterotaxy, situs inversus, etc.). In addition, as the band is tightened, the saturations reflect only the banding and not also the effect of the lung compression from a thoracotomy. The bands we have used are either Teflon-impregnated Dacron (infants) or a strip of polytetrafluoroethylene (PTFE) (older children). Figure 9.1 [20] shows the approach for pulmonary artery banding through a median sternotomy incision. If a left thoracotomy is used, the pericardium is opened anterior to the phrenic nerve. Stay sutures are placed to hold the pericardium open. The left atrial appendage generally sits just at the site where the band is to be applied and it can be retracted with a stay suture if needed. Directly encircling a dilated, thin-walled pulmonary artery can possibly lead to unwanted pulmonary artery entry and thus needs to be performed with great care. The safest way to encircle the pulmonary artery is by the subtraction technique. This is illustrated in Figure 9.1A [20]. The band is first placed around both the aorta and the main pulmonary artery proximally. This initial maneuver also avoids the complication of encircling only the left pulmonary artery, which can happen with the thoracotomy approach. A plane is then developed between the aorta and the pulmonary artery with a combination of sharp dissection and electrocautery. A right-angled clamp is then passed around the aorta (not the pulmonary artery) and the free end of the band is grasped (Figure 9.1A2) [20]. The band is pulled through the space between the aorta and pulmonary artery and (by subtraction technique) encircles the pulmonary artery. The band is then sequentially tightened by placing multiple interrupted sutures in the band, as illustrated in Figure 9.1B [20]. An alternative technique to tighten the band is with serial hemoclips, each placed below the prior clip, leading to a progressively tighter band. A catheter is placed in the distal pulmonary artery to monitor the distal pulmonary artery pressure in comparison with the aortic (radial) pressure as the band is being tightened (Figure 9.1C) [20]. Once the band has been tightened to the desired degree, the band is fixed to the proximal pulmonary artery with several interrupted prolene sutures to prevent distal migration of the band and encroachment on the right pulmonary artery (Figure 9.1C) [20].

Placement of the band should result in an elevation of the aortic systolic blood pressure by 10–20 mmHg. For a patient who will eventually have a two-ventricle repair, the distal main pulmonary artery systolic pressure should be reduced to less than 50% of the measured aortic systolic blood pressure. For a patient who is going to undergo an eventual Fontan procedure, the lowest possible distal main pulmonary artery pressure that can be achieved with acceptable oxygen saturations is desired. Oxygen

A1

A2

A3

B1

B2

B3

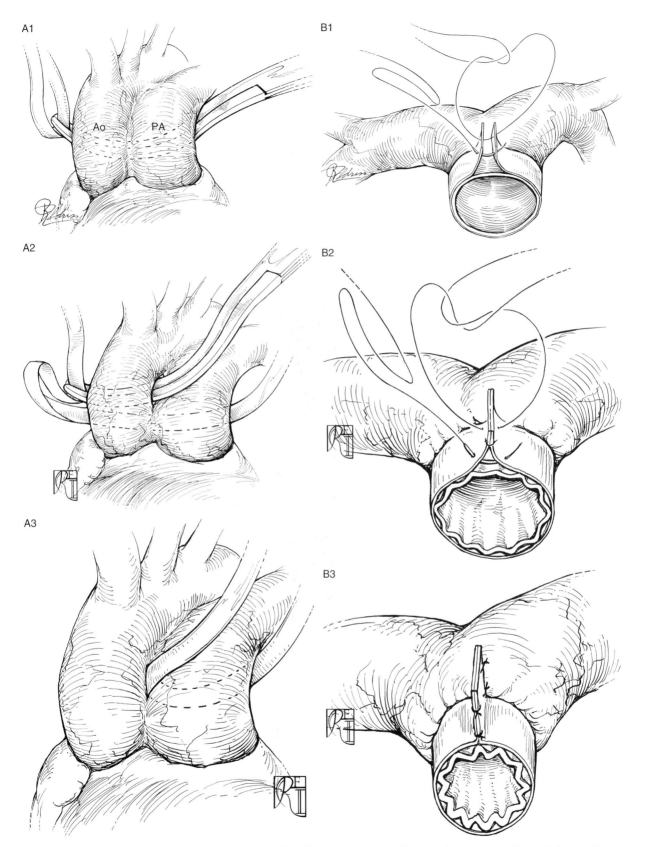

Figure 9.1 Placement of pulmonary artery band. **A,** Encircling the pulmonary artery by the subtraction technique. **B,** Suture placement to tighten the band. **C,** Pressure monitor in distal pulmonary artery to assess band tightness. (Ao, aorta; PA, pulmonary artery.)

C

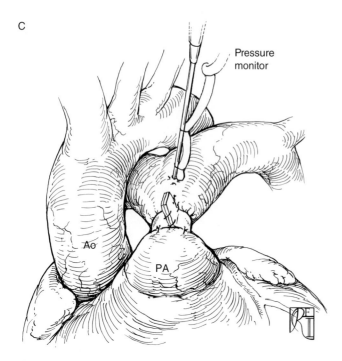

Pressure monitor

Ao

PA

Figure 9.1 (*Continued*)

saturations for a patient who is going to undergo biventricular repair should be left at 95%. For the patient who is going to undergo a Fontan operation, the oxygen saturation should preferably drop to between 80% and 85%. It should be kept in mind that as the child grows, the band will by default become "tighter" and further drop the distal pulmonary artery pressure (and saturations). One possible complication of band placement is the above-noted encroachment on the right pulmonary artery. The band can pinch off the right pulmonary artery while allowing excessive blood flow to the left pulmonary artery. This results in right pulmonary artery stenosis and left pulmonary artery hypertension. Once the band has been secured in place, the pericardium is irrigated with saline, so there is less chance of intrapericardial adhesions at the time of intracardiac repair. If performed through a left thoracotomy, the pericardium is approximated with several interrupted polypropylene sutures, with care being taken to avoid injury to the phrenic nerve.

Although the concept of an externally adjustable pulmonary artery band has been around for many years, it is only recently that several alternative techniques have been reported with considerable improvement in results. Cormo has reported the use of a patented device: FloWatch-R-PAB (EndoArt, S.A., Lausanne, Switzerland) [21]. This is a small clip-like device with a telemetric-controlled incorporated electric micrometer. The meter drives a piston that changes the area inside the clip. Because this band compresses the pulmonary artery in a noncircular fashion, pulmonary artery reconstruction may not be required when it is

removed [22]. Talwar reported a "double loop" of Ethibond suture passed around the pulmonary artery, through a pledget, and then up to the skin for external manual tightening [23]. In this series of 147 patients, the use of the adjustable pulmonary artery band was associated with a reduction in early multiple reoperations and band-related deaths. The total number of pulmonary artery band procedures reported in the Society of Thoracic Surgery (STS) congenital database was 739 for the period 2002–2005, corresponding to 1.9% of the total surgical procedures (739 of 38 431). The total number of pulmonary artery band procedures reported in the European Association of Cardiothoracic Surgery (EACTS) congenital database was 711, corresponding to 2.0% of the total surgical procedures (711 of 35 575). These figures contrast with the opinion that pulmonary artery band is an abandoned procedure [24]!

Another method of pulmonary artery band placement is the "intraluminal" technique. This technique is used only in patients who require cardiopulmonary bypass for other, simultaneous procedures. The technique utilizes a Gore-Tex patch with a calibrated precut hole in the center that is sutured as a patch in the main pulmonary artery. It results in a consistent and significant reduction in pulmonary artery pressure and flow. It essentially eliminates the problem of band "slipping" with resultant pinching of the right pulmonary artery. One of the advantages of this "band" is that it can be dilated with transcatheter techniques if the patient should become progressively cyanotic with growth. Pulmonary artery band takedown is performed by incising the pulmonary artery and resecting the Gore-Tex patch and then performing an end-to-end anastomosis. Many of the patients, however who have the intraluminal band go on to a bidirectional Glenn (Fontan strategy) in which case the pulmonary artery is transected at the site of the patch [25].

Pulmonary artery band takedown is performed at the time of intracardiac correction of the congenital cardiac lesion through a median sternotomy. Generally, the intracardiac repair is performed first, and the pulmonary artery reconstruction can be done while the patient is being warmed. All portions of the band should be removed because even a small portion of Dacron band left posteriorly can create scarring, which can cause late pulmonary artery stenosis. Removing the band completely, however, is not always adequate to prevent residual pulmonary stenosis at the band site because the pulmonary artery wall does not easily rebound open. If the band is left in place for only a period of weeks, simple removal is adequate. If the band is left in place for more than a few months, however, the area of banding must be either patched anteriorly or excised (Figure 9.2) [20]. The technique of excision of the scarred pulmonary artery banding site is shown in Figure 9.2A [20]. The area where the band was positioned is resected and then an end-to-end anastomosis is per-

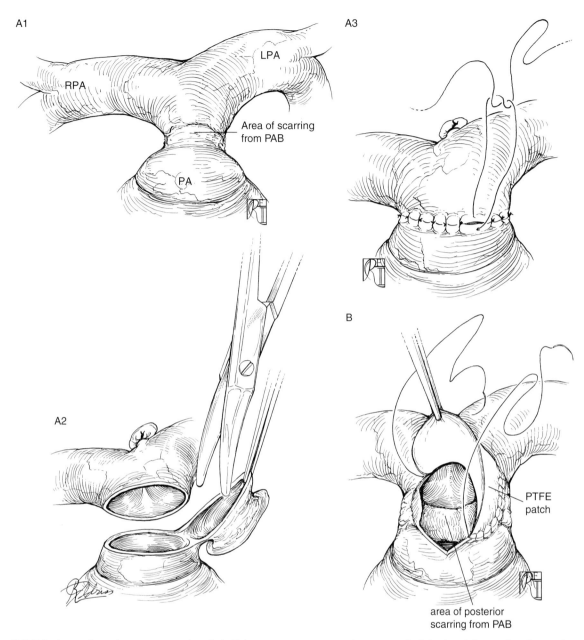

Figure 9.2 Takedown of a pulmonary artery band. **A,** Pulmonary artery transection, removal of the band site, and end-to-end reconstruction with interrupted absorbable suture. **B,** Takedown of a pulmonary artery band with anterior polytetrafluoroethylene (PTFE) patch placement. (LPA, RPA, left, right pulmonary artery; PA, pulmonary artery; PAB, pulmonary artery band.)

formed between the two remaining pulmonary arterial segments with interrupted, absorbable, fine monofilament suture. The distal right and left pulmonary arteries must be completely mobilized and the ligamentum arteriosum ligated and divided to provide a tension-free anastomosis. The patch technique is illustrated in Figure 9.2B [20]. A patch of either pericardium or PTFE is used to augment the pulmonary artery anteriorly over the posteriorly scarred area and allow flow into the right and left pulmonary arteries without hemodynamic obstruction to flow. This some-

times requires use of a "pantaloon" patch with extension into the right and left anterior sinuses of Valsalva. Although most surgeons have preferred to use a patch anteriorly, this usually still results in a mild main pulmonary artery stenosis and residual murmur. The use of transection of the site of the band and direct end-to-end anastomosis in most cases results in no gradient and no residual murmur. As mentioned previously, use of the newer adjustable bands may help prevent the need for pulmonary artery construction [22].

Aortopulmonary Shunts

Classic Blalock–Taussig Shunt

The Blalock–Taussig shunt was the first aortopulmonary shunt and was performed in 1944 by Alfred Blalock of the Johns Hopkins University Medical Center [2]. The classic Blalock–Taussig shunt is a direct end-to-side anastomosis of the transected subclavian artery to the pulmonary artery. Blalock had successfully created a left subclavian-to-pulmonary artery anastomosis while developing a canine model of pulmonary hypertension at Vanderbilt University. Helen Taussig suggested to Blalock that he apply his experimental procedure to patients who had cyanosis from insufficient pulmonary blood flow. The first operation was performed on 28 November 1944, on a 15-month-old girl with the diagnosis of tetralogy of Fallot and severe pulmonary stenosis. After that first successful case, hundreds of cyanotic children went to Baltimore for "the operation." In fact, between 1944 and 2006, 2016 patients had a Blalock–Taussig shunt at Johns Hopkins Medical Center [26].

The classic Blalock–Taussig shunt was typically constructed through a thoracotomy approach on the side opposite the aortic arch. When there is a left aortic arch, there is typically a right innominate artery, and using the subclavian artery on this side provides a gentle curve to the pulmonary artery. With a right aortic arch and mirror-image branching, the left innominate artery provides a similar gentle curve to the pulmonary artery. In contrast, the contralateral subclavian artery would require an angulation of the artery of nearly 180 degrees for the anastomosis. Figure 9.3 [20] illustrates the anatomy for exposure of the right subclavian and pulmonary arteries through a right thoracotomy. The branches of the right subclavian artery are ligated and divided along with the distal subclavian artery, and the subclavian artery is pulled through the loop formed by the right recurrent laryngeal nerve. The carotid artery is dissected out to provide more mobility. The azygos vein is doubly ligated and divided. The anastomosis is constructed to the main pulmonary artery with vascular clamps after 1 mg/kg of heparin is given intravenously. Care is taken to avoid the complication of performing the anastomosis to the right upper lobe branch. The subclavian artery will then lie in a groove just posterior to the superior vena cava and the phrenic nerve.

The classic Blalock–Taussig shunt does not require prosthetic material and provides a precise amount of pulmonary blood flow limited by the orifice of the subclavian artery. In addition, the shunt grows with the patient, providing more pulmonary blood flow as the child grows. However, the Blalock–Taussig shunt sacrifices the subclavian artery, which in a small number of cases can result in hand or arm ischemia [27]. The affected arm is usually shorter than the contralateral arm, is often somewhat cool

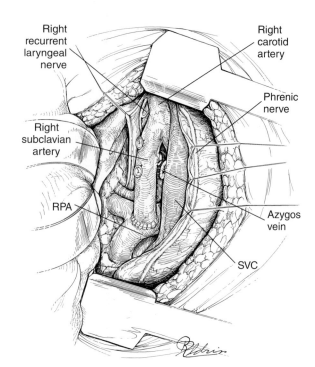

Figure 9.3 Classic Blalock–Taussig shunt (right thoracotomy). (RPA, right pulmonary artery; SVC, superior vena cava.)

to the touch, and will not have a palpable pulse. In addition, even with ample mobilization of the carotid artery and division of the inferior pulmonary ligament, the subclavian artery may still be so short as to cause the pulmonary artery to be "pulled" up and kink. Takedown of the classic right Blalock–Taussig shunt at the time of complete correction through a median sternotomy involves dissection posterior to the superior vena cava. The artery can then be encircled and double ligation performed. Because of the multiple disadvantages of the classic Blalock–Taussig shunt, we currently recommend the modified Blalock–Taussig shunt.

Modified Blalock–Taussig Shunt

The use of a PTFE tube for an aortopulmonary shunt was first reported by Gazzaniga and associates in 1976 [28]. Three infants with pulmonary atresia underwent aorta-to-pulmonary artery shunt using an interposed 4-mm PTFE tube. DeLeval [29] coined the term modified Blalock–Taussig shunt when he reported on 99 patients operated on between 1975 and 1979 having a prosthesis of Dacron (13) or PTFE (86) interposed between the subclavian and pulmonary arteries. Shunt failure rate was 6%, and operative mortality was 8%. The advantages of the modified Blalock–Taussig shunt, which has now become the shunt of choice at most congenital heart surgery centers [30], include 1) preservation of the circulation to the affected arm; 2) regulation of the shunt flow by the size of the systemic (subclavian or innominate) artery; 3) high early patency rate with expanded PTFE arterial prosthesis (Gore-Tex, W.L. Gore & Associates, Inc., Flagstaff, AZ); 4) guarantee of adequate shunt length; and 5) ease of shunt takedown. One disadvantage of the modified Blalock–Taussig shunt is the occasional leaking of serous fluid through the interstices of the fabric of the PTFE. This may result in excessive and prolonged chest tube drainage, localized seroma formation around the graft, or both [31]. This complication occurs in 3–5% of patients.

The modified Blalock–Taussig shunt can be performed through a right or left thoracotomy or a median sternotomy. The approach depends on the subclavian and pulmonary artery anatomy, the presence and location of a ductus arteriosus, the great vessel relationship, and surgeon preference. In the past several years, there has been a distinct trend toward performing the modified Blalock–Taussig shunt through a median sternotomy. This has been our approach of choice for the past 10 years. The sternotomy approach is technically less challenging and is associated with fewer shunt failures than the classic thoracotomy approach [32,33]. If necessary, the shunt can be performed with the use of cardiopulmonary bypass if the child has significant oxygen desaturation during the procedure. With a median sternotomy approach the side of the aortic arch is not a concern. The shunt can be placed to the main pulmonary artery if necessary. Access to the patent ductus arteriosus for ligation to remove a source of competitive flow is always possible. The potential theoretical disadvantage of increased adhesions at the time of sternal re-entry has not really been an issue [32].

For a thoracotomy approach, the latissimus dorsi muscle is divided; the serratus anterior is mobilized and spared. The thorax is entered through the fourth interspace. The lung is retracted anteriorly and inferiorly. The mediastinal pleura is opened posterior to the superior vena cava and phrenic nerve. The azygos vein is doubly ligated and divided. The subclavian artery is encircled with a vessel loop, with care being taken to avoid the right recurrent laryngeal nerve, which passes around the distal innominate artery at the takeoff of the subclavian and common carotid arteries. The right pulmonary artery is dissected free, with care being taken to identify the right upper lobe branch and main pulmonary artery continuation to the right lower and middle lobes. The right upper lobe and distal right pulmonary artery branches are encircled with vessel loops, which can then be occluded with small Rummel tourniquets. The patient is administered 1 mg/kg heparin intravenously.

The size of the PTFE graft selected is based on the size of the patient. Earlier series frequently used a 5-mm shunt. If the shunt is taken from the subclavian artery, this will

regulate the flow. However, if the shunt is from the innominate artery (which frequently is the case with a median sternotomy approach), consideration must be given to using a smaller shunt as then the shunt size will regulate the flow. We generally use a 4-mm graft for (3.5–5.0 kg) infants, and a 3.5-mm graft for babies weighing less than 3.5 kg. We have downsized the shunts because most of these children go on to complete repair at 6–9 months of age and the shunt flow is adequate and not excessive (even if the shunt comes from the innominate artery). The PTFE is cut to size before the clamps are placed; the clamps distort the relative distance between the subclavian and pulmonary arteries. The graft is usually cut to give it a gentle curve, which allows for patient growth. It should not kink or distort the pulmonary artery, which can easily happen if the length is not accurate. We prefer the "stretch" PTFE that is more forgiving vis-à-vis length estimates. The PTFE graft is beveled as illustrated in Figure 9.4A [20], and an arteriotomy is created in the inferior aspect of the subclavian artery after placement of a vascular clamp. The PTFE graft is anastomosed to the opening in the subclavian artery with 7-0 polypropylene suture (Figure 9.4B) [20]. The clamp on the subclavian artery is left in place until the pulmonary artery anastomosis is completed. Repositioning the clamp to the PTFE graft may increase the risk of blood stasis and shunt thrombosis. The pulmonary artery is controlled with another vascular clamp. Rummel tourniquets are snugged on the right upper and lower distal pulmonary arteries. A longitudinal arteriotomy is created in the superior aspect of the right pulmonary artery. Using a single 7-0 polypropylene suture, the PTFE graft is anastomosed to the pulmonary artery (Figure 9.4C) [20].

When the clamps are released and flow established through the shunt, there should be a nearly instantaneous rise of approximately 15–20% in the patient's oxygen saturation as monitored by pulse oximetry. A thrill should be palpable in the shunt and in the distal pulmonary artery. It is important to maintain adequate systemic perfusion pressure before, during, and after the operation to prevent early shunt thrombosis. This may require the use of inotropic support (dopamine, epinephrine). Bleeding is controlled with Gelfoam soaked with topical thrombin. The heparin is not routinely reversed with protamine unless there is excessive bleeding from the suture lines. The graft should lie in a groove posterior to the superior vena cava, where it is accessible at the time of takedown. We routinely sedate and ventilate the child for the first 24 hours postoperatively. We also routinely give an aspirin suppository (10 mg/kg) in the operating room when the shunt is completed and then 10 mg/kg PO daily until shunt takedown [34]. The Boston Children's group [33] reported 104 patients who underwent placement of a modified Blalock–Taussig shunt. The chosen approach was thoracotomy in 52 patients, and median sternotomy in 52. There were ten shunt failures

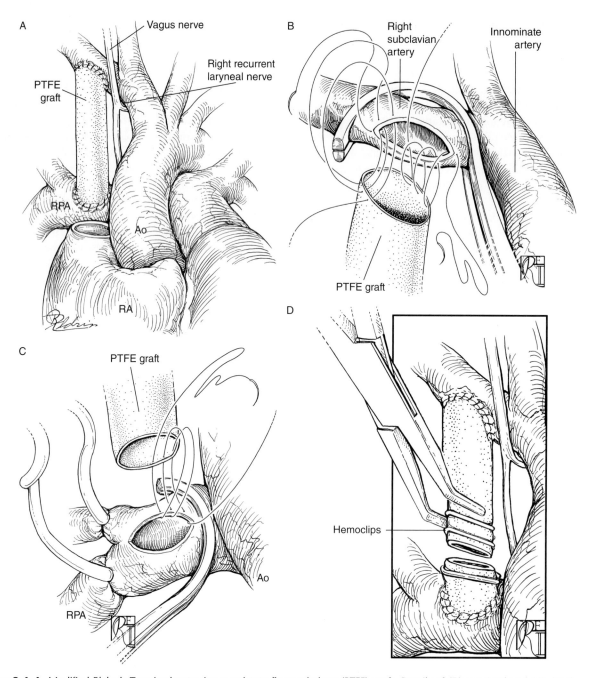

Figure 9.4 A, Modified Blalock–Taussig shunt using a polytetrafluoroethylene (PTFE) graft. Details of (**B**) proximal and (**C**) distal anastomosis for modified Blalock–Taussig shunt. **D,** Takedown of a modified Blalock–Taussig shunt with hemoclips and shunt division. (Ao, aorta; PTFE, polytetrafluoroethylene; RA, right atrium; RPA, right pulmonary artery.)

and three deaths in the thoracotomy group and four shunt failures and six deaths in the sternotomy group. They concluded that the median sternotomy approach was preferable. Alkhulaifi and colleagues [35] recently reported 79 neonates who had undergone modified Blalock–Taussig shunt placement. The shunts were placed via a right thoracotomy in 36 patients, through a left thoracotomy in six,

and through a median sternotomy in 33 patients. Indications for a shunt were pulmonary atresia with intact ventricular septum, pulmonary atresia with ventricular septal defect, severe tetralogy of Fallot, double-outlet right ventricle with pulmonary stenosis, transposition of the great arteries with pulmonary stenosis, and single-ventricle equivalent. Hospital mortality was 4% and there were seven shunt-related complications. Jahangiri and co-workers [36] reported 140 patients who had tetralogy of Fallot and had undergone a modified Blalock–Taussig shunt. All were done via thoracotomy. There were no hospital deaths and there was equal growth of the right and left pulmonary arteries, regardless of shunt location.

The takedown of a modified Blalock–Taussig shunt at the time of intracardiac repair through a median sternotomy is quite easily performed, particularly if the shunt was placed on the right side (Figure 9.4D) [20]. The shunt can be identified by dissecting the medial aspect of the superior vena cava posteriorly. Locating a shunt on the left side is more difficult, but it can be identified either by dissecting along the left pulmonary artery, along the aorta to the shunt, or by entering the pleural space and approaching the shunt laterally. A word of caution: the left-sided modified Blalock–Taussig shunt is often very close to the left phrenic nerve. The dissection will first encounter a thick fibrous "peel," which typically forms around the PTFE graft. Once the plane between the "peel" and the PTFE graft is entered, the dissection proceeds relatively quickly and enough graft length can be achieved for double hemoclip application proximally and single hemoclip distally. The graft should be divided between the hemoclips to prevent distortion of either the subclavian artery or the pulmonary artery as the patient grows and the distance between these two vessels naturally increases. No attempt is made to remove the proximal portion of the graft. In some patients the distal graft will require removal in order to facilitate performing a bidirectional Glenn anastomosis. However, if the operation involves repair at the site of the main pulmonary artery, the distal graft can be left in place and typically does not cause a residual peripheral pulmonary artery stenosis. Another word of caution regarding the takedown of these shunts. Preparation for cardiopulmonary bypass should be made prior to dissecting the shunt. For example, the aorta and right atrium should be accessible for cardiopulmonary bypass with purse strings placed and the pump primed. Sometimes dissection near the shunt dislodges the neointima causing acute desaturation, retrievable only by rapidly initiating cardiopulmonary bypass.

Waterston/Cooley Shunt

In 1962, David Waterston reported an aortopulmonary shunt that was an anastomosis between the posterior aspect of the ascending aorta and the anterior right pulmonary artery [37]. This procedure was performed through a right thoracotomy with the anastomosis posterior to the superior vena cava. Denton Cooley [38] reported the same technical shunt (right thoracotomy) but performed it in an intrapericardial fashion anterior to the superior vena cava. This shunt was initially widely used because of its ease of

construction, preservation of the subclavian artery, and lack of need for prosthetic material. However, because of the significant right pulmonary artery distortion it creates, the distinct possibilities of excessive or inadequate pulmonary blood flow, and the success of the modified Blalock–Taussig shunt, it is rarely applied in the current era.

The technique for construction of a Waterston/Cooley shunt through a right thoracotomy is shown in Figure 9.5

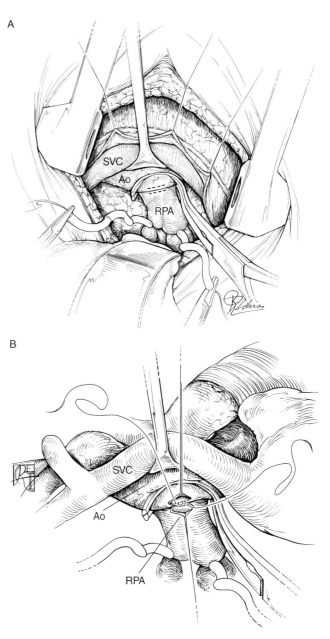

Figure 9.5 Waterston shunt. **A,** Clamps and Rummel tourniquets in place. **B,** Aorta-to-pulmonary artery anastomosis. (Ao, aorta; RPA, right pulmonary artery; SVC, superior vena cava.)

[20]. After mobilizing the right pulmonary artery, the distal pulmonary artery branches can be controlled with small Rummel tourniquets. Proximally, a Castaneda clamp is used to occlude both a portion of the ascending aorta and the entire right pulmonary artery. The aorta is rotated slightly anteriorly with a forceps so that a posterior rather than lateral portion of its wall is exteriorized by the clamp for the anastomosis. As illustrated in Figure 9.5 [20], matching incisions are made in the posterior aorta and anterior pulmonary artery. These incisions are between 3 mm and 4 mm in length, depending on the size of the patient. An anastomosis is then created with running polypropylene suture. The tourniquets are released and the clamp removed, and the oxygen saturation should increase appropriately.

A significant problem with the Waterston/Cooley shunt is that it is not as controlled a shunt as either the classic or modified Blalock–Taussig shunts. If the incisions in the aorta and pulmonary artery are too long and the anastomosis is too large, there will be excessive pulmonary blood flow with a risk of pulmonary vascular disease. If the incisions are too short and the opening is too small, there will be inadequate pulmonary blood flow and the patient will remain cyanotic. Another problem with the Waterston anastomosis is that as the patient grows and the aorta rotates, the anastomosis applies traction to the right pulmonary artery and kinks and distorts the right pulmonary artery. This may cause preferential flow to one lung and significant right pulmonary artery stenosis [39]. For this reason, almost all patients who have takedown of a Waterston shunt will require a major reconstruction of the right pulmonary artery.

The Waterston shunt is taken down at the time of intracardiac correction of the primary cardiac lesion through a median sternotomy (Figure 9.6) [20]. It is important to dissect the pulmonary arteries prior to cardiopulmonary bypass in order to occlude the pulmonary arteries on initiation of cardiopulmonary bypass to prevent pulmonary runoff with inadequate systemic perfusion. The repair is done with the patient on cardiopulmonary bypass with the aorta cross-clamped distal to the shunt. After cardioplegic solution has been administered (occluding the pulmonary arteries to prevent cardioplegic solution runoff), the aorta is separated from the right pulmonary artery with an incision made along the original anastomotic line. Typically, the aorta in these patients is large, and the opening in the aorta can be closed primarily with running suture. A PTFE or pericardial patch is then used to patch open the area of the right pulmonary artery where stenosis is usually created by the shunt. Another approach to the Waterston shunt at the time of takedown (originally described by Cooley) is to open the aorta anteriorly after the cross-clamp has been applied and close the opening from within the aorta itself. The aorta can also be completely transected to provide better exposure of the right pulmonary artery [40].

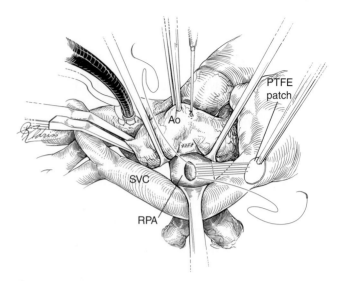

Figure 9.6 Takedown of a Waterston shunt with cardiopulmonary bypass and aortic cross-clamp, using a polytetrafluoroethylene (PTFE) patch to open the right pulmonary artery. The aortic opening has been closed primarily with a running suture. (Ao, aorta; RPA, right pulmonary artery; SVC, superior vena cava.)

The Waterston shunt has fallen out of favor because of the previously mentioned disadvantages and has been replaced in most centers by the modified Blalock–Taussig shunt. However, there are still a number of patients who have had this shunt who will require eventual takedown as described.

Potts Shunt

The Potts shunt (Figure 9.7) [20] is an anastomosis between the descending thoracic aorta and the left pulmonary artery performed through a left thoracotomy. It was first reported by Willis J Potts from Children's Memorial Hospital in Chicago [41]. This operation was first performed on 13 September 1946. The child was 21 months of age and weighed 8.3 kg. She had been cyanotic since 3 months after birth and had multiple hypercyanotic spells. She was intensely cyanotic and had severe clubbing. The Potts shunt was performed using a special clamp developed by Potts that only partially occluded the descending thoracic aorta to decrease the risk of paraplegia [42]. The proximal and distal left pulmonary artery were occluded. The anastomosis was performed between parallel 4-mm incisions made in the descending thoracic aorta and the posterior left main pulmonary artery. The completed shunt is shown in Figure 9.7A [20].

The Potts anastomosis was widely used at Children's Memorial Hospital; between 1946 and 1967, 659 such shunts were performed. The Potts shunt was technically easier than the classic Blalock–Taussig shunt and it pre-

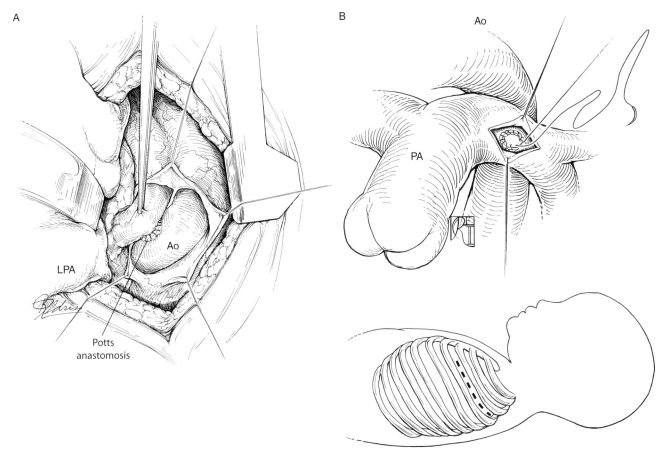

Figure 9.7 Potts shunts. **A,** Left thoracotomy showing spatial relationship of aorta to left pulmonary artery and completed anastomosis. Inset, Left thoracotomy. **B,** Takedown of a Potts anastomosis with placement of a polytetrafluoroethylene (PTFE) patch in the left pulmonary artery under circulatory arrest. (Ao, aorta; LPA, left pulmonary artery; PA, pulmonary artery.)

served the left subclavian artery. However, there were several serious complications that led to the abandonment of the Potts shunt. Many children developed large aneurysms of the left pulmonary artery that were very difficult to repair (Figure 9.8) [43]. Another complication was that the Potts shunt could be either too small and the patient remained cyanotic, or it was too large and caused congestive heart failure. The Potts shunt could not be used with a right arch (even with a right thoracotomy) because the right bronchus lies between the pulmonary artery and the aorta. The final and most significant problem with the Potts shunt was the difficulty in taking down the shunt at the time of complete correction of the intracardiac lesion [44]. Initial attempts at simply ligating the shunt resulted in uncontrollable hemorrhage in the operating room or in the immediate postoperative period. If the shunt was taken down with cardiopulmonary bypass and circulatory arrest, there was a risk of stroke from air embolism if the brachiocephalic vessels were not controlled. The preferred technique now is to use deep hypothermia and circulatory arrest, with adequate precautions taken to avoid

air embolism to the cerebral circulation with the descending thoracic aorta opened. After cardiopulmonary bypass is initiated through a median sternotomy, the aortic–pulmonary anastomosis is digitally occluded with a finger from outside the pulmonary artery to limit the left-to-right shunt and improve the efficiency of cooling. The brachiocephalic vessels are encircled with vessel loops. The aorta is cross-clamped and the heart arrested with cardioplegic perfusion. The brachiocephalic vessels are snared, and circulatory arrest is commenced once the target temperature (18 °C) is reached. Only then can the left pulmonary artery be safely opened. Under circulatory arrest, the communication between the pulmonary artery and the aorta can be visualized and closed with a PTFE patch (Figure 9.7B) [20]. All air is evacuated from the ascending aorta before the snares are released to the brachiocephalic vessels in order to prevent cerebral air embolism.

Because of the complications of left pulmonary artery aneurysm, frequent excessive pulmonary blood flow with resultant pulmonary hypertension, and the difficulties in taking down the Potts shunt, this procedure is essentially

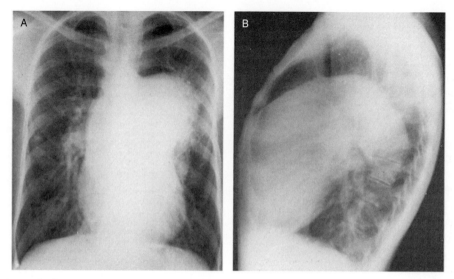

Figure 9.8 Chest radiographs (posteroanterior and lateral) of a 23-year old patient with tetralogy of Fallot 16 years after a Potts (descending aorta-to-pulmonary artery) anastomosis. The left pulmonary artery aneurysm projects from the mediastinum into the left chest (**A**) and fills the anterior compartment (**B**). (Reproduced with permission from de Hoyos *et al.* [43].)

no longer performed at congenital heart surgery centers. This has been true for many years, and there are very few patients alive with an intact Potts shunt.

Miscellaneous Palliative Procedures

A palliative procedure performed to improve mixing of blood at the atrial level in patients with transposition of the great arteries or single ventricle with atrioventricular valve stenosis/atresia is the atrial septectomy. The Blalock–Hanlon atrial septectomy was first performed in 1950 and was done through a right thoracotomy [5]. A portion of the right and left atria are occluded with a single clamp, occluding also the right pulmonary veins. The right atrium is then opened within the confines dictated by the clamp, and a portion of intra-atrial septum is grasped, pulled up, and excised from within the clamp. The clamp is then repositioned so that the atrial septum falls back into the atrial cavity and the clamp is only holding the cut edges of the atrium, and the atrial suture line is closed. This procedure is generally no longer performed, and most patients now who require an atrial septal defect undergo Rashkind balloon septostomy [6]. The Rashkind septostomy is typically performed in an infant with transposition of the great arteries and intact ventricular septum. A balloon-tipped catheter is passed up the femoral vein across the patent foramen ovale and into the left atrium. The balloon is initially inflated in the left atrium and then rapidly pulled across the septum into the right atrium, tearing the atrial septum. For patients with a thick atrial septum that is recalcitrant to Rashkind balloon septostomy, open atrial septec-

tomy with cardiopulmonary bypass is the safest procedure. The atrial septectomy can be performed either during a short period of aortic cross-clamping or with induced electrical fibrillation of the heart. The entire atrial septum within the fossa ovalis can be excised, with the surgeon taking care to avoid injury to the atrioventricular node or cutting outside the heart. Rashkind balloon septostomy in the cardiac catheterization laboratory now is the preferred approach for most cases.

Some patients with complex cyanotic congenital heart disease and suboptimal anatomy for complete correction undergo a Glenn operation (which is discussed in Chapters 28 and 31) or a Mustard procedure (Chapter 26) for palliation of their cyanotic heart disease. Ceresnak has described a palliative arterial switch procedure [45]. These patients will have an elevation in their oxygen saturations after these palliative procedures, but are not completely corrected. Other procedures that could be considered palliative procedures, that is, pulmonary and aortic valvotomy, modified Norwood, and bidirectional Glenn, are covered in other chapters. The hybrid procedure is probably the most notable recent "palliative" procedure and employs bilateral pulmonary artery bands and a ductal stent placed with transcatheter techniques in a "hybrid lab." This is discussed further in Chapter 31, *Hypoplastic Left Heart Syndrome*.

Conclusion

The primary palliative operations for children with congenital heart disease are aortopulmonary shunts and the pulmonary artery band. The aortopulmonary shunt of choice currently is the modified Blalock–Taussig shunt performed with a sternotomy approach. This provides a controlled source of pulmonary blood flow, does not sacrifice the subclavian artery, and is quite easy to take down at the time of intracardiac repair. Pulmonary artery banding is selected for very few patients now, but is still indicated for patients with Swiss-cheese muscular ventricular septal defects, for some infants with single ventricle and increased pulmonary blood flow, and to prepare the left ventricle in select patients. Advances in percutaneously adjustable bands has improved outcomes in these patients. Hybrid techniques have also led to a resurgent interest in pulmonary artery band techniques. Surgeons need to be aware of the Waterston/Cooley and Potts anastomosis, the associated complications, and the techniques required to safely take these shunts down at the time of complete repair.

References

1. Joffs C, Sade RM. (2000) Congenital Heart Surgery Nomenclature and Database Project. Palliation, correction, or repair? Ann Thorac Surg 69, S369–S372.
2. Blalock A, Taussig HB. (1945) The surgical treatment of malformations of the heart in which there is pulmonary stenosis or pulmonary atresia. JAMA 128, 189–202.
3. Muller WH Jr, Dammann JF Jr. (1952) The treatment of certain congenital malformations of the heart by creation of pulmonic stenosis to reduce pulmonary hypertension and excessive pulmonary blood flow: a preliminary report. Surg Gynecol Obstet 95, 213–219.
4. Rossi AF, Seiden HS, Sadeghi AM, et al. (1998) The outcome of cardiac operations in infants weighing two kilograms or less. J Thorac Cardiovasc Surg 116, 28–35.
5. Blalock A, Hanlon CR. (1950) Surgical treatment of complete transposition of the aorta and pulmonary artery. Surg Gynecol Obstet 90, 1–15.
6. Rashkind WJ, Miller WW. (1966) Creation of an atrial septal defect without thoracotomy. A palliative approach to complete transposition of the great arteries. JAMA 196, 991–992.
7. Norwood WI, Lang P, Hansen DD. (1983) Physiologic repair of aortic atresia-hypoplastic left heart syndrome. N Engl J Med 308, 23–26.
8. Glenn WWL. (1958) Circulatory bypass of the right side of the heart. IV. Shunt between superior vena cava and distal right pulmonary artery; report of a clinical application. N Engl J Med 259, 117–120.
9. Gibbs JL, Wren C, Watterson KG, et al. (1993) Stenting of the arterial duct combined with banding of the pulmonary arteries and atrial septectomy or septostomy: a new approach to palliation for the hypoplastic left heart syndrome. Br Heart J 69, 551–555.
10. Galantowicz M, Cheatham JP, Phillips A, et al. (2008) Hybrid approach for hypoplastic left heart syndrome: intermediate results after the learning curve. Ann Thorac Surg 85, 2063–2070.
11. Odim JN, Laks H, Drinkwater DC Jr, et al. (1999) Staged surgical approach to neonates with aortic obstruction and single-ventricle physiology. Ann Thorac Surg 68, 962–967.
12. Amin Z, Backer CL, Duffy CE, et al. (1998) Does banding the pulmonary artery affect pulmonary valve function after the Damus-Kaye-Stansel operation? Ann Thorac Surg 66, 836–841.
13. Boutin C, Jonas RA, Sanders SP, et al. (1994) Rapid two-stage arterial switch operation. Acquisition of left ventricular mass after pulmonary artery banding in infants with transposition of the great arteries. Circulation 90, 1304–1309.
14. Mavroudis C, Backer CL. (2000) Arterial switch after failed atrial baffle procedures for transposition of the great arteries. Ann Thorac Surg 69, 851–857.
15. Winlaw DS, McGuirk SP, Balmer C, et al. (2005) Intention-to-treat analysis of pulmonary artery banding in conditions with a morphological right ventricle in the systemic circulation with a view to anatomic biventricular repair. Circulation 111, 405–411.
16. Devaney EJ, Charpie JR, Ohye RG, et al. (2003) Combined arterial switch and Senning operation for congenitally corrected transposition of the great arteries: patient selection and intermediate results. J Thorac Cardiovasc Surg 125, 500–507.
17. Kitagawa T, Durham LA III, Mosca RS, et al. (1998) Techniques and results in the management of multiple ventricular septal defects. J Thorac Cardiovasc Surg 115, 848–855.
18. Seddio F, Reddy VM, McElhinney DB, et al. (1999) Multiple ventricular septal defects: how and when should they be repaired? J Thorac Cardiovasc Surg 117, 134–139.
19. Franklin RCG, Sullivan ID, Anderson RH, et al. (1990) Is banding of the pulmonary trunk obsolete for infants with tricuspid atresia and double inlet ventricle with a discordant ventriculoarterial connection? Role of aortic arch obstruction and subaortic stenosis. J Am Coll Cardiol 16, 1455–1464.
20. Backer CL, Mavroudis C. (2003) Palliative operations. In: Mavroudis C, Backer CL, eds. Pediatric Cardiac Surgery, 3rd ed. Philadelphia, PA: Mosby.
21. Corno AF, Bonnet D, Sekarski N, et al. (2003) Remote control of pulmonary blood flow: initial clinical experience. J Thorac Cardiovasc Surg 126, 1775–1780.
22. Corno AF, Prosi M, Fridez P, et al. (2006) The non-circular shape of FloWatch-PAB prevents the need for pulmonary artery reconstruction after banding. Computational fluid dynamics and clinical correlations. Eur J Cardiothorac Surg 29, 93–99.
23. Talwar S, Choudhary SK, Mathur A, et al. (2008) Changing outcomes of pulmonary artery banding with the percutaneously adjustable pulmonary artery band. Ann Thorac Surg 85, 593–598.
24. Corno AF. (2008) Invited commentary. Ann Thorac Surg 85, 598–599.
25. Piluiko VV, Poynter JA, Nemeh H, et al. (2005) Efficacy of intraluminal pulmonary artery banding. J Thorac Cardiovasc Surg 129, 544–550.
26. Williams JA, Bansal AK, Kim BJ, et al. (2007) Two thousand Blalock–Taussig shunts: a six-decade experience. Ann Thorac Surg 84, 2070–2075.

27. Geiss D, Williams WG, Lindsay WK, *et al.* (1980) Upper extremity gangrene: a complication of subclavian artery division. Ann Thorac Surg 30, 487–489.

28. Gazzaniga AB, Elliott MP, Sperling DR, *et al.* (1976) Microporous expanded polytetrafluoroethylene arterial prosthesis for construction of aortopulmonary shunts: experimental and clinical results. Ann Thorac Surg 21, 322–327.

29. DeLeval MR, McKay R, Jones M, *et al.* (1981) Modified Blalock-Taussig shunt. Use of subclavian artery orifice as flow regulator in prosthetic systemic-pulmonary artery shunts. J Thorac Cardiovasc Surg 81, 112–119.

30. Yuan SM, Shinfeld A, Raanani E. (2009) The Blalock-Taussig shunt. J Card Surg 24, 101–108.

31. LeBlanc J, Albus R, Williams WG, *et al.* (1984) Serous fluid leakage: a complication following modified Blalock-Taussig shunt. J Thorac Cardiovasc Surg 88, 259–262.

32. Morales D, Zafar F, Arrington K, *et al.* (2008) Repeat sternotomy in congenital heart surgery: no longer a risk factor. Ann Thorac Surg 86, 897–902.

33. Odim J, Portzky M, Zurakowski D, *et al.* (1995) Sternotomy approach for the modified Blalock–Taussig shunt. Circulation 92, II256–II261.

34. Al Jubair KA, Al Fagih MR, Al Jarallah AS, *et al.* (1998) Results of 546 Blalock–Taussig shunts performed in 478 patients. Cardiol Young 8, 486–490.

35. Alkhulaifi AM, Lacour-Gayet F, Serraf A, *et al.* (2000) Systemic pulmonary shunts in neonates: early clinical outcome and choice of surgical approach. Ann Thorac Surg 69, 1499–1504.

36. Jahangiri M, Lincoln C, Shinebourne EA. (1999) Does the modified Blalock–Taussig shunt cause growth of the contralateral pulmonary artery? Ann Thorac Surg 67, 1397–1399.

37. Waterston DJ. (1962) [Treatment of Fallot's tetralogy in infants under the age of 1 year.] Rozhl Chir 41, 181–183.

38. Cooley DA, Hallman GL. (1966) Intrapericardial aortic-right pulmonary arterial anastomosis. Surg Gynecol Obstet 122, 1084–1086.

39. Wilson JM, Mack JW, Turley K, *et al.* (1981) Persistent stenosis and deformity of the right pulmonary artery after correction of the Waterston anastomosis. J Thorac Cardiovasc Surg 82, 169–175.

40. Curran RD, Mavroudis C, Backer CL. (1997) Ascending aortic extension for right pulmonary artery stenosis associated with ventricular-to-pulmonary artery conduit replacement. J Card Surg 12, 372–379.

41. Potts WJ, Smith S, Gibson S. (1946) Anastomosis of aorta to pulmonary artery: certain types in congenital heart disease. JAMA 132, 627–631.

42. Baffes TG. (1987) Willis J. Potts: his contributions to cardiovascular surgery. Ann Thorac Surg 44, 92–96.

43. de Hoyos A, Dodge-Khatami A, Backer CL. (2009) Vascular masses of the mediastinum. In: Shields TW, Locicero J III, Reed CE, *et al.* eds. *General Thoracic Surgery*, 7th ed., vol. 2. Philadelphia, PA: Lippincott Williams & Wilkins/Wolters Kluwer, p. 2231

44. Kirklin JW, Devloo RA. (1961) Hypothermic perfusion and circulatory arrest for surgical correction of tetralogy of Fallot with previously constructed Potts' anastomosis. Dis Chest 39, 87–91.

45. Ceresnak SR. Quaegebeur JM, Pass RH, *et al.* (2008) The palliative arterial switch procedure for single ventricles: are these patients suitable Fontan candidates? Ann Thorac Surg 86, 583–587.

CHAPTER 10

Management of Pediatric Cardiopulmonary Bypass

Darryl H. Berkowitz[1] and J. William Gaynor[2]

[1]Pennsylvania Hospital, Philadelphia, PA, USA
[2]The Children's Hospital of Philadelphia, Philadelphia, PA, USA

History

In the early part of the twentieth century, at a time when technology did not exist to operate inside the heart, morbidity and mortality remained extremely high for children born with congenital heart defects such as atrial (ASD) and ventricular (VSD) septal defects. By 1950 surgeons were successfully operating on patients with patent ductus arteriosus and aortic coarctation. Battlefield experience from World War II, with descriptions of successful removal of intracardiac foreign bodies [1], as well as early experimentation with hypothermia, as described by Bigelow and colleagues in 1950, set the stage for technology to pump oxygenated blood to artificially support a patient whilst a surgeon delved into the heart to repair complex congenital malformations. Although a group led by F. John Lewis [2] successfully closed an ASD using deep hypothermic arrest in 1951 and Gross and Watkins [3] described an atrial well technique in 1953, other groups began to use early forms of cardiopulmonary bypass (CPB) apparatus. The initial pump was devised by DeBakey in 1934 and was a hand-driven roller type pump. The initial systems incorporated this pump with oxygenation via either bubble or film oxygenators. Early attempts from 1951 to 1954 were commonly failures, with 18 patients described by various groups and with only one survival. The first successful human intracardiac operation was performed by J.H. Gibbon on 18 May 1953. Although this first patient in his series did survive, he went on to record five deaths resulting in his abandonment of the technique [4]. Failures were attributable to incorrect preoperative diagnoses, ventricular dysfunction at termination of bypass, hypovolemia, surgical errors, and ventricular failure within the convalescence period (Table 10.1) [4–10].

Whilst efforts continued to develop a feasible technique for CPB, Lillehei and colleagues described controlled cross circulation, with the initial procedure in humans being performed in early 1954 [11]. In this technique Lillehei used another human, usually the patient's parent, as a pump/oxygenator. The "donor's" femoral vessels were cannulated, and oxygenated blood was pumped into the patient allowing the surgical team to perform intracardiac surgeries [11]. His initial series recorded 18 deaths in 45 patients. Mortality was attributed to pulmonary complications including atelectasis, pneumonitis, and underappreciated pulmonary vascular changes; incorrect diagnoses; and surgical complications. Although there was no donor mortality, there was morbidity from air embolism from a large-bore peripheral intravenous (IV) line and marked decrease in venous return through the exchange pump. The mortality rate of 40% was clearly still extremely high, but was nevertheless a great improvement from the almost 100% mortality of early CPB cases. Indeed some commentators suggested that further research into a bypass machine be abandoned [12]. Approximately 1 year later, in May 1955, Kirklin and colleagues at the Mayo Clinic described a series of eight patients (five with VSDs, two with atrioventricular canal defects and one with tetralogy of Fallot) who were operated on using a CPB machine similar to that previously used by Gibbon. In contrast to earlier series, this series had a 50% survival. This was attributable to a better understanding of the patient's pathology, improved diagnostic testing, and a perioperative team including physiologists, pathologists, anesthesiologists, and surgeons. In the conclusion of his landmark paper Kirklin declared, "Use of this system established excellent conditions for precise, unhurried intracardiac surgery" [13]. The modern age of cardiac surgery had begun.

Pediatric Cardiac Surgery, Fourth Edition. Edited by Constantine Mavroudis and Carl L. Backer.
© 2013 Blackwell Publishing Ltd. Published 2013 by Blackwell Publishing Ltd.

Table 10.1 Open-heart surgery with total cardiopulmonary bypass: results of all reported cases 1951 to 1954 (before cross-circulation on 26 March 1954).

Surgeon	No. patients	Oxygenator type	Year	Survivors	Deaths
Dennis *et al.* [5]	2	Film	1951	0	2
Helmsworth *et al.* [7]	1	Bubble	1952	0	1
Gibbon [4]	6	Film	1953	1 (ASD repair)	5
Dodrill *et al.* [8]	1	Autogenous	1953	0	1
Mustard *et al.* [9]	5	Monkey lungs	1951–1953	0	5
Clowes *et al.* [10]	3	Bubble	1953	0	3
Total	18			1 (5.5%)	17 (94.5%)

The Gibbons bypass machine incorporated three De-Bakey pumps and a screen type oxygenator [14] instead of the film type oxygenator used in his original animal experiments, as the film type would not support oxygenation in an animal larger than a cat. By the mid to late 1950s three types of oxygenators were in clinical use: 1) The Mayo–Gibbon pump oxygenator, although commercially available, was cumbersome, difficult to clean, and required a large prime volume; 2) the Kay-Cross disc oxygenator, which was also cumbersome despite the introduction of simpler commercial versions, was favored by many clinicians due to the perception that it caused less blood component trauma, particularly in longer procedures; and 3) the DeWall-Lillehei bubble oxygenator, which began clinical use in 1955 by Lillehei, gained widespread popularity, and by 1976 was being used in an estimated 90% of cardiac surgeries [15]. The advantage of this oxygenator was that it used a small volume prime, negating the need for donor blood, and, importantly, was disposable. The disadvantage, however, was that blood constituent trauma occurred, particularly with lengthy procedures.

Although conceptualized in the mid 1940s, membrane oxygenation only came into vogue in the late 1970s to early 1980s. The most important factor for this was that early materials were unsuitable with respect to permeability, strength, and how thinly they could be manufactured without defect allowing for blood-surface interaction. With the advent of microporous, hollow-fiber membranes, clinical usage began to shift toward membrane oxygenators. These oxygenators were made of bundles of hollow fibers within a hard plastic shell. They had a large surface area-to-volume ratio and were thus extremely efficient at gas exchange. Because of other advantages, such as being easy to produce in large numbers as well as in different sizes with noncompliant blood/gas compartments, they were well suited to pediatric cardiac surgery.

Thus the stage was set by the early 1980s for surgeons to successfully attempt to palliate and cure complex congenital cardiac disease. Looking forward, the question of functional survival into mid life, neurological outcomes, and such technical questions as blood conservation, further decreasing the inflammatory response to bypass, and circuit miniaturization will come to the forefront of research.

Cardiopulmonary Bypass in Infants versus Adults

Summarized in Table 10.2 are many of the important differences that occur in the management of the very young for CPB as compared with the adult patient [16]. The most important of these are the routine use of hypothermia with or without circulatory arrest, the use of low perfusion pressures, and, of great clinical importance, marked hemodilution. Thus pediatric patients will be exposed to the extremes of physiologic tolerance. These factors coupled with immature organ systems place pediatric patients at great risk during the period of CPB. In addition to the aforementioned factors that can be directly compared between the two age groups, there are additional issues that further complicate the management strategy (Table 10.3) [6].

From the surgical perspective, several technical challenges exist including placement of both venous and arterial cannulae (with their potential effect on hemodynamics); the effect of collateral vessels on both blood return to the heart (making visibility a challenge) and the phenomenon of stealing blood from vital organs (making organ preservation difficult) [17]; coronary anomalies (which accompany many of the congenital lesions); and multiple suture lines in patients with multifactorial coagulopathy.

Physiology of Cardiopulmonary Bypass

The safe conduct of CPB in the neonate and infant requires a comprehensive understanding of the physiologic associations that occur. These variables include circuit design, hemodilution, choice of cannulae, degree of hypothermia, acid–base strategies, and flow rates, which include the decision to use deep hypothermic circulatory arrest.

Hypothermia

The rationale for the use of hypothermia during CPB is myocardial and other vital organ protection. To this end

Table 10.2 Differences between adult and pediatric cardiopulmonary bypass. (Reproduced with permission from Dinardo [16].)

Parameter	Adult	Pediatrics
Hypothermic temperature	Rarely <25–32 °C	Commonly 15–20 °C
Circulatory arrest	Uncommon	Common
Pump prime		
Dilutional effect on blood volume	25–33%	200–300%
Additional additives	Blood, albumin	
Perfusion pressure	50–80 mmHg	20–50 mmHg
Influence of pH management	Minimal at moderate hypothermia	Marked at deep hypothermia
Measured PaCO$_2$ differences	30–45 mmHg	20–80 mmHg
Glucose regulation		
Hypoglycemia	Rare – requires liver injury	Common – ↓ glycogen stores
Hyperglycemia	Frequent – insulin bolus or infusion	Less common – rebound ↓↓ glucose

Table 10.3 Unique pediatric characteristics.

Smaller circulating blood volume
Higher oxygen consumption
Reactive pulmonary vascular bed
Intra- and extracardiac shunting
Altered thermoregulation
Poor tolerance for microemboli

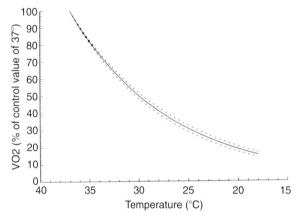

Figure 10.1 Whole body oxygen consumption (VO$_2$) as a function of body temperature.

three distinct methods are used: moderate hypothermia (25–32 °C), deep hypothermia (18–20 °C), and deep hypothermic circulatory arrest (DHCA) where circulation is shut down completely at 16–18 °C. There has been increasing interest in the use of normothermic CPB. Normothermia and moderate hypothermia are used on cases where the surgeon is able to safely cannulate both vena cavae to operate within the heart. This of course can be done even on the smallest of patients, bearing in mind that the cannulae may cause vena caval obstruction and impaired drainage that can adversely effect both the cerebral and abdominal perfusion independent of perfusion pressure. Deep hypothermia with reduced pump flow to as low as 25–50 mL/kg/min will allow the surgeon to perform corrective surgeries with only minimal return of blood to the surgical field whilst at the same time maintaining vital organ perfusion. DHCA is used for the repair of complex intracardiac lesions as well as reconstructions of the aorta. Once circulation has been stopped, the surgeon is able to remove all cannulae and work in a completely bloodless and unobstructed field. An alternative for aortic surgeries is DHCA with retrograde cerebral perfusion with an arterial cannula in the innominate artery and venous drainage either via pump suction in the open atrium or a cannula placed in the superior vena cava (SVC). Flow rates of 20–50 mL/kg/min to a perfusion pressure of 30–50 mmHg are used [18].

The principal clinical effect of hypothermia is the reduction in metabolic rate and molecular movement. As temperature is lowered, both basal and functional cellular metabolism is reduced, and the rate of adenosine triphosphate (ATP) consumption is decreased. Whole-body oxygen consumption decreases directly with body temperature (Figure 10.1) [6,19,20,21]. The cerebral metabolic rate (CMRO$_2$) has been found to exponentially decrease as temperature decreases throughout the clinically relevant temperature range of 37 °C to 18 °C [22,23]. The reduction in CMRO$_2$ has been calculated to be between 82% and 87% of baseline in the canine model and the pediatric population, respectively [22]. This relationship between temperature and metabolic rate can be quantified by calculating the Q10, which is a temperature coefficient defined as the ratio of metabolic rates at two temperatures separated by 10 °C. This has been calculated in adults to be 2.4–2.8; in the pediatric population, it has been shown to be 3.65. This indicates that there is a greater decrease in metabolic rate in neonates, infants, and children compared to adults as they become more hypothermic. In clinical terms this translates into better brain and organ protection with hypothermia in the pediatric population [22]. At deep hypothermia cellular metabolism is so low and membrane fluidity is reduced to such a large extent that cellular basal metabolic needs and cellular membrane integrity can be maintained for a relatively long period of time (Figure 10.2) [6,24]. Despite these beneficial effects cerebral blood flow (CBF) autoregulation is lost at deep hypothermia and becomes proportional to mean arterial pressure (Figure 10.3) [6,22]. In those patients who underwent deep hypothermia with low-flow bypass,

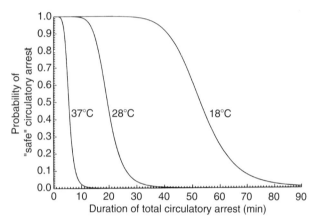

Figure 10.2 The probability of safe circulatory arrest is related to the duration of arrest and the temperature at which it occurs. (Reproduced with permission from Kirklin *et al.* [24].)

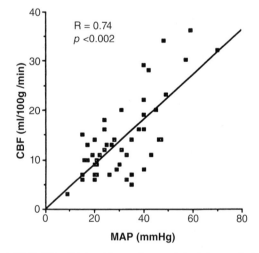

Figure 10.3 Data obtained from a human infant demonstrate that cerebral autoregulation is lost at deep hypothermic temperatures (<22°C) with cerebral blood flow (CBF) related in a linear manner to mean arterial pressure (MAP). (Reproduced with permission from Greeley *et al.* [22].)

CBF will return to normal with rewarming and may even exceed it in the post-bypass phase. Interestingly, in the group of patients who undergo DHCA it appears that CBF does not return to normal, remaining low into the post-bypass period. One study suggested that this may last for up to 40 hours post bypass despite adequate perfusion pressure [25]. Two apposing explanations exist for this phenomenon: the low CBF may be a function of a low metabolic demand seen post DHCA, or this prolonged low CBF is secondary to a pathologic no-reflow phenomenon as a result of a primary cerebral vascular abnormality secondary to DHCA [22,25,26].

In contrast to the role that hypothermia plays in cerebral protection, it is less important in protection of the myocardium; indeed it has been suggested that electrical quiescence accounts for ±90% of myocardial protection at normothermia [27]. It has been found that a decrease in perfusion temperature has a possible deleterious effect on the myocardium as it leads to abnormal calcium and sodium handling. As Na^+/K^+ ATPase inhibition occurs with a falling temperature it gives rise to an increase in intracellular sodium. This may then result in an increased activity of the Na^+/Ca^{2+} exchanger, with an increase in intracellular calcium [28]. This may play an important part in the development of an entity described as rapid cooling contracture, which is thought to play a role in post-bypass myocardial dysfunction. Experimental evidence suggests that rapid cooling of the myocardium, such as occurs with hypothermic CPB and cold cardioplegia, may result in an exacerbation of injury [29–31]. The increase in intracellular calcium will lead to an increase in ATP use, a decrease in ATP synthesis, activation of calcium-dependent degradative enzymes, and an increase in free-radical reactions [31]. Clinically this will be translated into an increase in contractility and a decrease in both systolic and diastolic function. Further evidence suggests that these changes in compliance of the myocardium will also increase resistance to coronary blood flow [32]. This effect of cooling on myocardial performance may be more pronounced in the neonatal and infant period, as the lower total body and cardiac mass make these patients susceptible to more rapid temperature changes [31].

The adverse effects of rapid cooling have been demonstrated experimentally in the kidneys, liver, and lungs as well. In clinical practice, however, many variables are involved and there does not seem to be readily apparent injury to the patient from rapid cooling [33–34]. It does appear that the neonate is able to tolerate the stress of profound hypothermia without difficulty. The reason for this may be the fact that neonates possess different ionic channel density or have different membrane function than do older patients. These theories remain speculative.

In summary hypothermia preserves organ function by maintaining cellular ATP stores despite reduced oxygen delivery, reducing excitatory neurotransmitter release and preventing calcium entry into the cell. In neonatal and infant congenital heart surgery, the use of some form of hypothermia remains commonplace. It aids in preservation of organ function during ischemia, allows the surgeon to operate in a potentially bloodless field, and increases the safety of CPB.

Pulsatile versus Nonpulsatile Flow

Whether pulsatile flow has improved outcomes over non-pulsatile flow remains an open question. The basis for this stems from the suggestion that nonpulsatile perfusion may be associated with microcirculatory dysfunction and, thus, may be important in the genesis of post-CPB myocardial, cerebral, and renal dysfunction [35]. The desirability of pulsatile perfusion has been contemplated and studied since the introduction of extracorporeal circulation in the 1950s.

The difference between these two modes of perfusion is not simply the generation of a pulse pressure. Pulsatile flow also depends on creation of an energy gradient; thus pump flow as well as arterial pressure must be included [36]. This relationship was described by Shepard in 1966 [37] and is known as the energy equivalent pressure (EEP) formula:

$$EEP = \left(\int fpdt \right) / \left(\int fdt \right)$$

Thus it is the ratio of the area under the hemodynamic power curve ($\int fpdt$) and the area under the pump flow curve ($\int fdt$) where f is the pump flow rate, p is the arterial pressure (in mmHg) and dt indicates that the integration is performed over time (t). Because EEP is measured in mmHg, a comparison can be made between it and mean arterial pressure (MAP). The difference between these two measurements is the energy generated by the bypass machine – be it a pulsatile or nonpulsatile device [36]. This difference must then be applied to the surplus hemodynamic energy (SHE) formula:

$$SHE = 1332(EEP - MAP)$$

The unit of measure of this formula (SHE) is the erg, which represents energy. Pulsatile flow is best represented by an energy gradient rather than a pressure gradient, and pulsatile perfusion produces more SHE units than nonpulsatile perfusion [38]. This improved generation of energy units may translate into improved regional and global blood flow to vital organs [39]. The converse is also true that when there is no difference in energy level generated between pulsatile and nonpulsatile flow then there is no difference in vital organ blood flow (Figure 10.4) [35–40].

As has been mentioned above, pulsatile flow appears to improve organ flow during CPB and function in the post-CPB period. In a pilot study of 50 patients Alkan and colleagues described improved myocardial function in the pulsatile group based on the observation that this group of patients required less inotropic support and at lower doses [41]. The same investigators found equivalent findings in a follow-up study of 215 patients [39]. This was similar to experimental findings of improved myocardial blood flow and function even after up to 60 minutes of DHCA [42].

Cerebral blood flow patterns have also been studied, and experimental animal models have been used to find differences in flow techniques. It is noted that both methods of perfusion show decreased flow when compared to pre-CPB cerebral blood flow. The findings showed that cerebral hemispheric, basal ganglia, brainstem, and cerebellar flows were better maintained in the pulsatile group. This was found at normothermic CPB, pre DHCA, post DHCA, and even post CPB. An important factor related to these findings is that cerebral vascular resistance is found to be lower under pulsatile perfusion during and after normothermic CPB [38]. Interestingly authors involved in this work have conducted other studies that do not agree with these findings; however, despite this they make a point of concluding that in their opinion pulsatile flow remains a better choice based on its ability to generate more hemodynamic energy, which in turn may maintain the microcirculation to a greater degree [40–43].

Postoperative ventilation and the effects of CPB on pulmonary function are important clinical markers in patients undergoing cardiac surgery. In their large clinical study, Alkan and colleagues found that time to extubation and length of intensive care unit (ICU) stay was significantly shorter in the pulsatile perfusion group, from which it can be concluded that pulmonary function was improved in this group [39]. Renal function was also a marker analyzed in this study, and it was found that, although the serum creatinine was similar in both groups, urine output was significantly improved in the pulsatile group. Indeed it has been shown that pulsatile perfusion increased renal and specifically renal cortical flow. Pulsatile perfusion also played a role in decreasing edema and ischemic changes found in renal tubules as compared to nonpulsatile flow [44].

One of the biggest problems faced by clinicians when patients are placed onto CPB is the inflammatory cascade that is initiated secondary to the exposure of patient's blood to the foreign surface of the bypass circuit, surgical trauma, ischemia/reperfusion hemodilution, hypothermia, and possibly changes related to the artificial nature of perfusion – the end result being organ dysfunction that affects the myocardial, pulmonary, hepatic, and renal systems. Damaged endothelium releases increased amounts of cytokines, including interleukin 8 (IL-8), and increased release of IL-8 is frequently used as a measure of inflammation. The use of pulsatile CPB has been associated with a lower concentration of IL-8, leading authors to speculate

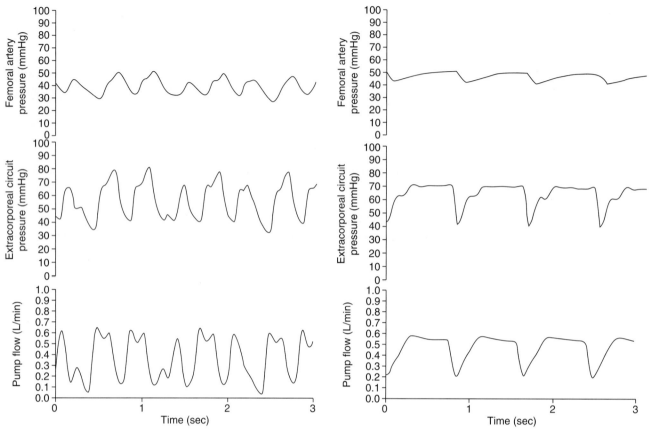

Figure 10.4 Femoral artery pressure, precannula extracorporeal circuit pressure, and pump flow during (left) pulsatile and (right) nonpulsatile cardiopulmonary bypass in a neonatal piglet. (Reproduced with permission from Undar *et al.* [35].)

that this may improve outcomes with regard to function and microcirculation of vital organs [32,36].

Despite encouraging experimental and clinical results with the use of pulsatile flow, this technique has not yet been brought into broad use. Multicenter trials have been called for but have not yet been reported. As such, nonpulsatile flow remains the perfusion technique most widely used in pediatric cardiac surgery.

Strategies for Blood Gas Management: alpha Stat and pH Stat

Another topic of considerable debate in pediatric CPB is the question of interpretation and management of pH, most specifically at deep hypothermia. In adult patients undergoing CPB, the most common cause of brain injury is related to the delivery of embolic material to the cerebral vasculature. The etiology of brain injury in children is thought to result from hypoperfusion during periods of low flow or DHCA [45]. As has been mentioned, many pediatric cardiac surgeries are performed under conditions of decreased flow rates with moderate to deep hypother-

mia in an effort to protect against vital organ injury. It would thus follow that strategies that result in the lowest $CMRO_2$ would offer the best protection.

The temperature at which the pH is reported is of fundamental importance. Within the body, maintenance of electrochemical neutrality is necessary to ensure that cellular protein and enzymes function optimally. This neutrality occurs when there are equal concentrations of positively and negatively charged ions within aqueous solutions. As the temperature begins to drop, the dissociation constant of aqueous systems will increase and thus the concentration of H^+ begins to decrease. As pH is the inverse log of H^+ and as electrochemical neutrality must be maintained, the pH of the solution will increase. Electrochemical neutrality is also maintained within cells; thus we can hypothesize that the pH within cells is a pH of neutrality. We would then assume that to maintain neutrality the intracellular pH would change with a change in temperature. Analysis of ectothermic animals shows that intracellular pH remains at or near this pH of neutrality even as body temperature drops. For this to occur, two additional processes must take place. The first is a buffer system with a pK value close to that of the intracellular pH and whose pK changes as temperature changes. The buffering capacity of the imidazole of the amino acid histidine has these characteristics. Histidine is found commonly within intracellular proteins and enzymes. The term "alpha" refers to the degree of dissociation of the imidazole, that is, the ratio of unprotonated to total imidazole; under normal conditions within the intracellular compartment this has a value of 0.55. This dissociation (and hence the alpha value) will remain constant over a range of temperatures as there is a proportional change of the neutral pH of water, the pKa of imidazole, and the tissue pH. The second necessary process is that the CO_2 content of the blood must remain constant as body temperature drops. This is the "alpha stat" condition. If, however, the pH remains constant during hypothermia, then the alpha number of the imidazole will change and thus there may be a change in protein structure or enzyme function. This is known as the "pH stat" condition. In this management technique, CO_2 is added so that the pH will remain constant through the range of hypothermic temperatures (Figure 10.5) [46].

Into the 1990s, based on adult studies and strategies, the alpha stat technique was thought to have a better neuroprotective outcome. Despite the lack of prospective data, it gained widespread use amongst institutions performing

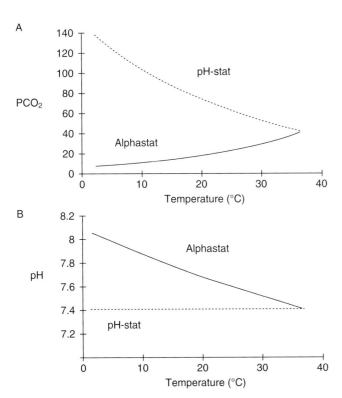

Figure 10.5 The effect of temperature on blood plasma pCO_2 (**A**) and pH (**B**) comparing the alphastat and pH-stat protocols of acid–base management. (Reproduced with permission from Tallman [46].)

cardiac surgeries on children [45]. In a neurodevelopmental follow-up of 16 patients who had undergone Senning operations, Jonas and colleagues reviewed perfusion techniques and pH strategy. They found that the use of alpha stat strategy before DHCA was associated with poorer developmental scores and postulated that the lower CBF associated with alpha stat may result in inadequate cooling. Despite the groups being of different ages at the time of assessment and despite the fact that it was underpowered, this study hinted at a possible need to change strategies in the pediatric population [47]. Another more devastating neurological complication of pediatric cardiac surgery is the development of choreoathetosis. In two studies, one from the above group, patients underwent DHCA and later went on to develop choreoathetosis. After analysis apart from the use of DHCA it was found that all of the affected patients were managed using alpha stat [48,49]. Laboratory studies with neonatal piglets and DHCA times varying from 60 to 90 minutes have demonstrated that the use of pH stat appears to offer better cerebral protection. In the studies referenced, the markers used to compare the two management strategies included microvascular diameter during cooling and rewarming, cerebral tissue oxygenation, brain cooling, and metabolic markers of ischemia (e.g., extrastriatal dopamine production) [50–52]. The effects on brain cooling include a faster rate of cooling that is uniform across all regions of the brain, especially the cortical white matter [53]. The results of these showed pH stat to be superior in all of the aforementioned categories in the cooling phases of DHCA as well as in the recovery phase.

In the first prospective trial into the use of pH stat management in the cooling phases of DHCA, du Plessis and colleagues found that there was a greater degree of cerebral cooling, as measured by tympanic membrane temperature, in the pH stat group. This they attributed to increased CBF that appeared to be equally distributed throughout the brain. In keeping with these data, this group also had recovery of electroencephalogram (EEG) activity more rapidly than those in whom alpha stat management had been used. EEG-confirmed seizures were also increased twofold in the alpha stat group [45]. Although a later section of this chapter will be dedicated to the discussion of near infrared spectroscopy (NIRS), in our current context it is important to note that monitoring studies have been undertaken in which there is evidence to suggest that the use of alpha stat is associated with lower signals during cooling. This indicates that this method results in insufficient CBF and oxygenation [54,55]. In 2003 Bellinger and colleagues from the group at Boston Children's Hospital presented 1-year follow-up data on a large group of patients who had been exposed to either alpha stat or pH stat management. These data showed that despite apparent advantages of pH early post-CPB, neurodevelopmentally there was no difference between the groups. Despite this the use of pH stat for cooling remains the management of choice.

The effects of pH/CO_2 on other organ systems have also been studied. Myocardial protection is also obviously of great concern to the entire care team. In a study performed by Nagy and colleagues in which troponin I was used as the marker of myocardial injury, it was found, across a spectrum of patients that included pulmonary hypertension and cyanotic congenital heart disease (CHD), that those in whom pH stat was used had better myocardial performance after CPB [56]. They postulated that pH stat may induce a more even myocardial temperature during cooling due to hypercapnia-induced vasodilation. Oxygen delivery may also be improved as the oxygen–hemoglobin dissociation curve shifts rightwards with the increase in CO_2. Lastly they suggested that the hypercapnia-induced inhibition of pyruvate dehydrogenase, which leads to a decrease in lactate production, may also be of great benefit. As a secondary outcome their study also suggested that postoperative ventilation and length of ICU stay may be shorter with pH stat. Improved myocardial performance had also been found in the du Plessis study where there appeared to be a higher cardiac index within the first 18 hours after CPB with lower inotropic use, less hypotension, and metabolic acidosis compared to the alpha stat group. These patients also had significantly less mechanical ventilation and ICU stays [45].

Despite these advantages there is concern that the use of pH stat may result in a change in the internal pH (pHi) of cells that would lead to a prolonged depletion of high-energy phosphates during rewarming, which in turn would lead to cellular damage. Experimental evidence, however, seems to suggest that the pHi of cells is regulated independently of the extracellular environment. Hiramatsu and colleagues showed that the pHi was alkalotic irrespective of the use of alpha stat or pH stat strategies during the cooling phase, but that it tended towards acidosis with the onset of DHCA [50]. The data then suggested that there was a quicker recovery of both pHi and ATP using the pH stat technique. As mentioned before, this was on the basis of a greater oxygen reserve secondary to increased blood flow and oxygen delivery in the cooling phase. In conclusion it would seem that the evidence presented here would undoubtedly indicate that a prudent approach would be for the use of pH stat management during the cooling phase of deep hypothermic CPB; indeed, there is also some evidence from these studies that this strategy should be employed in the rewarming phases as well. Many centers, including our own, use alpha stat during rewarming to good clinical effect.

Neurological Injury and Protection

As has been stressed throughout this chapter, protecting vital organs and especially the brain is of paramount importance. To this end investigators are continuously searching for ideal monitoring tools to ensure that there is minimal morbidity during all phases of CPB as well as into the recovery phase, as our perioperative management may directly correlate with long-term neurodevelopmental outcomes. Unlike in the adult population, where neurological injury commonly involves thromboembolic stroke, in the pediatric population the injury results in more subtle problems such as with attention, fine and gross motor control, visual motor integration, and executive functioning. The end result of these problems is school failure and low self-esteem. This "developmental signature" is similar to that seen in very low birthweight, premature infants [57].

It is quite alarming to note that long-term follow-up has found that neurodevelopmental impairment occurs in approximately 50% of children who have cardiac surgery as newborns or young infants [58]. Many studies of neurodevelopmental outcome after cardiac surgery in infancy have focused on injury during the intraoperative period as the likely cause of adverse outcomes. However, there is increasing evidence that brain development is abnormal in children with CHD, and injury often can be identified before surgery. Patient-specific factors such as genetic abnormalities, socioeconomic status, and maternal education are more important determinants of neurodevelopmental outcomes than are intraoperative management strategies [49]. From Table 10.4 it can be seen that a number of factors influence neurological outcome [59].

Table 10.4 Factors Influencing neurological injury. (Reproduced with permission from Hsai *et al.* [59].)

Fixed factors
Genetic syndromes
Structural CNS malformations
Socioeconomic status
Genetic predispositions
Modifiable factors
Preoperative
Hypotension
Glycemic control
Hyperthermia
Operative
Emboli – gaseous/particulate
CPB circuit/inflammation
Modified ultrafiltration
pH stat blood gas management
Cerebral ischemia
Steal
Hemodilution
Free radicals/reoxygenation

Preoperative Factors

Neonates with CHD have a higher incidence of cerebral dysgenesis than those in the general population [59]. The era of staged reconstruction of hypoplastic left heart syndrome (HLHS) began in the late 1970s, with this diagnosis being fatal prior to this time. In a series of postmortem examinations from the early to mid 1980s, the authors found 29% of the patients had either minor or major central nervous system (CNS) abnormalities. They also found that the absence of dysmorphic features did not preclude CNS abnormalities [60].

Periventricular leukomalacia (PVL) (Figure 10.6) is one of the most frequent and severe neuronal injuries specific to the neonatal brain [61]. It is caused by necrosis of deep white matter adjacent to the lateral ventricles. The mechanism is thought to be related to injury to immature oligodendrocytes. In early life the brain undergoes an intensive period of neuronal development and axonal growth. It is during this period that the brain is susceptible to ischemia–reperfusion injury due to its fragile vascularity, high metabolic activity, and immature autoregulation. At this time oligodendrocytes myelinate developing axons throughout the CNS, thus making the white matter particularly susceptible to oligodendrocytic injury [59]. PVL occurs not only in the period surrounding CPB but also in premature infants and after such insults as hypoxia, hypoglycemia, and meningitis. The incidence prior to CPB has been estimated to be between 16% and 25% [62,63] with this rate increasing to between 54% and 73% [61,63] post CPB based on magnetic resonance imaging (MRI) studies. The study subjects included a group of patients undergoing Norwood operation with regional low-flow cerebral perfusion, whilst the other cohort included patients with one or two ventricles with or without aortic arch obstruction. In this latter group, only 1 out of 23 (4%) of the older infants developed PVL [61]. In recent years MRI as well as prenatal ultrasound has been used to assess CBF. Fetal echocardiography has demonstrated that there are changes in the cerebral vascular resistance that vary according to the specific cardiac defect. Thus CBF and oxygen delivery may be impaired in fetuses with CHD, resulting in abnormal brain development [64]. Preoperative MRI has found similar anatomic findings to those already mentioned, with one study finding an incidence of >50% of neonates with a wide range of CHD having structural brain abnormalities, with PVL in 28% and microcephaly in 24%. The important point from this study, however, was that CBF was decreased from normal in the cohort and that, in some cases, flow was critically low at <10 mL/100 g/min [65]. Apart from abnormal intracardiac shunt these neonates have ductus arteriosus-dependent aortic or pulmonary blood flow, which leads to diastolic hypotension that may lead to compromised CBF. Other important preoperative factors may include the need for balloon atrial septostomy in those with transposition of the great vessels with resultant embolic events [66] and ongoing systemic inflammation secondary to endotoxin translocation from mesenteric hypoperfusion [58].

There are also genetic factors that play a role in the genesis of neurological damage. These include underlying congenital defects such as the presence of a VSD and aortopulmonary collaterals, abnormalities of cerebral vasculature, and genetic factors such as prothrombotic disorders and polymorphisms of apolipoprotein E (APOE). An important factor in neuronal repair, APOE also aids in regulation of cholesterol metabolism. There are three common isoforms of APOE (E2, E3, and E4) that are encoded by three alleles (ε2, ε3, and ε4). Research has shown that the APOE genotype has a strong association as a determinant of neurological recovery following CNS injury. In a study of 244 patients who had undergone repair of CHD ≤6 months of age with or without DHCA, Gaynor and colleagues found that in those who carried the APOE ε2 allele had significantly lower Psychomotor Developmental Index (PDI) than those who carried the other two alleles. It is important to note, however, that in this study all of the patients, irrespective of allele type, scored lower on PDI and Mental Developmental Index (MDI) than expected for their age [67]. A follow-up study by the same group at the Children's Hospital of Philadelphia enrolled a cohort of 550 patients all of whom had surgical procedures <105 days of age. The preoperative diagnoses included HLHS, tetralogy of Fallot, VSD with and without coarct, and transposition of the great arteries (TGA) with and without VSD. Of this original group 359 returned and participated in the study

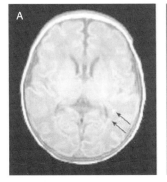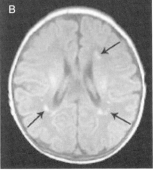

Figure 10.6 MRI evidence of periventricular leukomalacia. **(A)** Axial MRI image (T1-weighted) demonstrating two small areas of increased signal intensity in the periventricular white matter consistent with PVL, classified as mild (arrows). **(B)** Axial MRI image (T1-weighted) demonstrating multiple larger areas of increased signal density in the periventricular white matter consistent with PVL, classified as moderate (arrows).

at 1 year of age. Of the original cohort 49 patients had died (21 during the original hospitalization and 28 following discharge) and a further 142 did not return. Apart from motor and cognitive testing the patients also underwent genetic screening. The genetic evaluation was considered normal in 257 of the patients. As in the previous study the overall scores of the PDI and MDI were lower than the population norms. Risk factors for low scores amongst this cohort included confirmed genetic syndrome, lower birthweight, small head circumference at 1 year, preoperative intubation, longer hospital stay, use of extracorporeal membrane oxygenation (ECMO) or a ventricular assist device (VAD), and the presence of the APOE ε2 allele. Interestingly the investigators found that a higher hematocrit after hemodilution was associated with higher scores and the use or duration of DHCA was not associated with worse outcomes. Based on their findings the investigators advised preoperative genetic consultation that risk stratification be performed for those with positive genetic screens [59].

Intraoperative Factors

Despite the above-mentioned factors, the intraoperative period is still a time of great risk to the child. In two contrary sets of data, two apparently different neurological outcomes were found. In a study performed in patients undergoing ASD closure via surgical- versus catheter-based closure, there was a significant decrease in intelligence quotient [68]. In the other study, presented by Quartermain and colleagues as a scientific abstract at the 2008 American Heart Association's Scientific Sessions in New Orleans, a cohort of 41 patients from 5 to 18 years of age all of whom underwent CPB for closure of simple atrial or ventricular defects or simple valve surgeries showed no decrease in neurocognitive function [69]. The study group was compared with a similar group of patients undergoing noncardiac surgery.

Factors that will likely result in poorer outcomes include anesthetic-related issues encompassing a decrease in cardiac output with decreased oxygen delivery at the time of transition from negative- to positive-pressure ventilation and the negative inotropic effects of anesthetic agents. Hypoxia may worsen before establishment of CPB, particularly in those with ductal-dependent flow, as the surgeon dissects around the ductus, resulting in vasospasm. Once on CPB numerous factors may occur, including malposition of both the arterial and venous cannulae with resultant poor flow characteristics and venous drainage leading to cerebral hypoperfusion; embolic phenomena, including air and thrombus, may occur despite meticulous circuit check, adequate anticoagulation, and de-airing of the heart once repair is undertaken; the inflammatory response set up by CPB; the effects of DHCA with ischemia–reperfusion injury

and uneven cerebral cooling; hemodilution; pH management; and the effect of collateral steal of blood away from vital organs [58,59]. Once weaning from CPB has taken place, it is the effects of continued myocardial dysfunction with decreased oxygen delivery and hypoxia that may lead to ongoing brain injury. From 2–5% of patients require the use ECMO for postcardiotomy support [70], which itself has significant morbidity and mortality with up to 50% of survivors showing neurodevelopmental problems [71].

Postoperative Factors

In the postoperative period, ongoing low cardiac output and hypoxia result in continued neurological damage. Other factors that may play an important part in the genesis of damage during this period include hyperthermia, endocrine abnormalities, acid–base disturbance, and disruption of cerebral vasoregulation. In this latter etiologic factor autoregulation is disrupted after CPB; thus it is important to maintain adequate cerebral perfusion pressure. Longer postoperative length of stay has consistently been shown to be associated with worse neurodevelopmental outcomes, suggesting that events in the postoperative period modify the risk of an adverse outcome.

Neuromonitoring and Neuroprotection

As can be seen from the above discussion a multitude of factors can result in neurological injury either on their own or in combination. Neuroprotection should begin from birth. In the preoperative period clinicians should be aware that severe hypoxia, low perfusion pressure in the form of low diastolic pressure secondary to ductal runoff, low cardiac output states, respiratory alkalosis, and hyperthermia may be variables in neurological injury. In the transition to the operating room and controlled ventilation, clinicians should be attentive to changes that result in the aforementioned factors. How then can we protect the brain?

In recent years interest has been focused on neurological monitoring with NIRS, transcranial Doppler, electroencephalography, and jugular venous saturation alone or in combination as opposed to using surrogate markers of perfusion pressure, mixed venous saturation, and acid–base status [72]. NIRS provides a real-time, noninvasive assessment of regional cerebral oxygenation and has been validated with jugular venous saturation [72]. In this method a venous weighted approximation of tissue oxygen saturation is measured with a venous:arterial blood ratio of 85:15. This technology uses modifications of Beer's equation. Photons are injected through the skin, penetrate through tissue, and then return, whereupon the oxyhemoglobin saturation of tissues at a depth of 2 cm from the skin is measured. Subtraction of the shallow light path from the deep light path results in the approximation of brain oxygenation [72]. The INVOS 5100 (Somanetics, Inc, Troy, MI), which is approved by the United Stated Food and Drug Administration (US FDA) for use in adults and children, calculates a regional cerebral saturation index (rSO_2i) by computing the ratio of oxyhemoglobin to total hemoglobin. It has range of 15–95%. These monitors are best used as trend monitors, with a fall of 20% from baseline being significant [73]. Factors that affect cerebral oxyhemoglobin saturation include cerebral perfusion pressure, CBF, arterial oxyhemoglobin saturation, $PaCO_2$, and cerebral metabolic rate. The baseline values have been quantified with 70% being normal in adults. Normal and acyanotic children have similar values. In a study by Kurth *et al.* where cerebral oxygen saturation was measured preoperatively the mean saturation was found to be between 43% and 57% for a wide range of cyanotic heart disease [74]. The one group that fell outside this range comprised six patients with a diagnosis of pulmonary atresia and with an average saturation of 38% [74]. Studies looking at single-ventricle patients and from laboratory studies suggest that a saturation below 30% results in anaerobic metabolism [74,75]. It thus becomes obvious that many patients that we take care of must have saturations that fall below this anaerobic threshold. The question that would thus be answered by the use of this technology would be when does anaerobic metabolism occur, for how long, and what do our interventions do to either improve or worsen the situation? In this regard NIRS has been used to guide safe duration of DHCA, proper placement of cannulae, and also optimum flow during low-flow cerebral perfusion at deep hypothermia [76–78]. Some investigators have also suggested the use of concurrent cerebral NIRS and the placement of a probe over the anterior abdominal wall or renal bed to monitor the somatic bed [79,80]. Based on the assumption that the invasive technique of jugular venous bulb saturation (SjO_2) gives an extremely accurate measurement of cerebral oxygenation and metabolism, there are a few pitfalls in using NIRS. This includes a better correlation between SjO_2 and NIRS with patients <10 kg, which can be explained by an increased skin and skull thickness in larger children, the relatively small area of cerebral circulation, and the possible contribution of extracerebral tissue to the signal [81].

EEG monitoring is theoretically attractive for the detection of hypoperfusion or ischemia on the basis of altered signals. It is, however, not routinely feasible as the technology is bulky and the signals may be affected by the electrical interference of electrocautery, patient temperature, anesthetic agents used, and CPB itself. EEG is useful, however, for quantification of anesthetic depth, occurrence of electrical silence with DHCA, and of course the presence of epileptiform activity in the postoperative period, which may indicate neuronal damage [73]. The Bispectral Index

(Aspect Medical Systems, Newton, MA) uses processed EEG signals to compute a number in the range of 0 (complete EEG silence) to between 90 and 100, which is found in awake patients and thus has been used as a adjunct for anesthesiologists to predict the likelihood of recall under anesthesia. The monitor is easy to use in both the placement of the electrode and in the read-out display itself. An added advantage of this monitor is the ability to see an unprocessed EEG in real time, which can give an indication of burst suppression or electrical silence – an obvious advantage when patients are being cooled to deep hypothermia [82]. The BIS value is reported to decrease with hypothermia and thus decreasing anesthesia requirements. Conversely, upon rewarming BIS values increase, possibly reflecting a change in consciousness level [73].

Transcranial Doppler (TCD) provides a real-time monitor of CBF velocity and the occurrence of embolic phenomena during CPB. The instrument uses pulsed wave ultrasound, usually at 2 MHz frequency. The units display the frequency of the Doppler signals; peak systolic and mean flow velocities (cm/second); and the pulsatility index, which is the peak velocity minus the end-diastolic velocity divided by the mean velocity [82]. The added advantage of the device is the identification of microemboli via high-intensity transient signals that are displayed with an audible click for each event. The most consistent and reproducible technique is to monitor the middle cerebral artery through the temporal window, which is located superior to the zygoma and anterior to the tragus. The values reproduced are trended throughout the case; and a drop of 60% in the peak velocity is considered a moderate drop in perfusion whilst a drop of 80% is considered a severe drop. Clinically both an inflow arterial obstruction, which will be seen by a drop in the peak Doppler signal, or an outflow obstruction, which is diagnosed by a decrease in the diastolic flow signal, can be appreciated. The respective etiologies are malposition of the arterial cannula, arterial line obstruction, changes to perfusion pressure, and changes in the flow rates or, alternatively, obstruction to venous drainage from the head by superior vena caval cannula malposition, kinking of the venous line, or after the creation of a superior cavopulmonary anastomosis [72]. High-intensity transient signals at a rate of >1/minute are considered significant [72,82], but as has been mentioned previously with regard to the etiology of adverse neurological events in children being different to that in adult CPB, the embolic count has not been shown to correlate with early neurological outcome in infants and children [73].

Jugular venous bulb saturation (SjO_2), as its name implies, measures the saturation of the venous blood by the placement of a retrograde venous catheter into the jugular venous bulb located approximately just cephalad of the C1C2 disc. The jugular veins drain almost all blood from the brain, but it has been shown that up to 6.6% of this blood comes from extracranial sources, which include the emissary and frontal veins, and the facial vein, which contributes the most extracranial blood [83]. Another potential anatomic problem with this monitoring technology is that blood does not drain equally into the two jugular venous bulbs. Indeed mixing of blood from the cortical and deeper regions of the brain is incomplete. Autopsy studies have shown that blood draining from the subcortical areas draining via the straight sinus flow to the left lateral sinus whilst blood from the cortical areas drained mainly to the right lateral sinus. Despite this, sampling from normal individuals has shown that saturations at the level of the internal jugular vein are equal on both sides [83]. In the pediatric population the use of SjO_2 has been studied in the context of optimal cooling time in those undergoing DHCA. As the temperature drops the brain will extract less oxygen as its metabolic demands fall. Under optimal conditions as the temperature falls the SjO_2 rises until the difference between the arterial saturation and the jugular venous saturation becomes minimal [84]. At this point it can be concluded that the metabolic rate of the brain has reached a nadir where maximal protection is occurring. One acknowledged negative in the use of this technology is that it is invasive; thus investigators have performed comparative studies between SjO_2 and NIRS to assess whether the noninvasive infrared technology produces similar results. Studies demonstrate that although there appears to be a good correlation between the two modalities [85–88] certain limitations are evident: accuracy of NIRS at low SjO_2, difficulty in assessing whether cerebral metabolism has nearly ceased as NIRS values may not read >90%, and accuracy of NIRS at low flow rates. The best correlations between the modalities occur with patients who are less than 10 kg. Authors conclude that these patients have decreased skull and scalp thickness allowing for a larger area of deeper brain structures to be scanned [86,87].

From this discussion it can be understood why some centers use triple-modality neuromonitoring: NIRS, jugular venous oxygen, and EEG. The advantage of this is that the monitoring is noninvasive and relatively easy to apply. Once an abnormality is detected adjustments in patient positioning, cannula position, blood pressure, hemoglobin, $PaCO_2$ and depth of anesthesia may be all that is needed in the prevention of potential neurological injury [58,72,73,82]. In an early study, Austin and colleagues performed this triple monitoring on 250 patients. The initial phase was an attempt to validate this triple monitoring, so the investigators did not treat any changes that were observed as this phase. The findings were that 12 of 46 (26%) of these patients developed early postoperative neurological problems inclusive of seizures, coma, hemiparesis, and movement, vision, or speech disorders. In the group in which interventions were performed when a problem was found, the complication rate decreased to 7 out of 130 patients (6%). Of note in the study was that in the remaining 74 patients in whom no changes were detected 5 patients had adverse outcomes. Of the monitoring modalities EEG found 5% of the abnormalities whilst NIRS and TCD found 58% and 37%, respectively [89]. In a recent meta-analysis by Hirsch and colleagues studying NIRS alone, the authors concluded that although a useful adjunct it is of greater clinical relevance to combine modalities. Their study found that despite measuring regional cerebral saturation, there was a paucity of data to show improved neurological outcome based on these numbers alone. It appears therefore that this may give added support to the multimodal approach [90].

As discussed in prior sections of this chapter and alluded to in this section, neuroprotection does not involve a single strategy but rather is a multifactorial approach. Table 10.5 illustrates a comprehensive strategy.

Table 10.5 Comprehensive strategy for brain protection.

CPB factors

Adequate perfusion pressure

Adequate DO_2 as measured by SvO_2/ABG

Limit Inflammatory response – steroids/leukocyte depleting filters/ heparin coated circuitry

Use of filters to avoid air / particulate emboli

Ensure adequate anticoagulation

pH stat management for any temperature ≤normothermia

Hematocrit ≥30 (≤1 year of age) / ≥25 (≥1 year of age)

Hyperglycemia

Hypothermia

DHCA

Adequate cooling times of at least 20 minutes

Hyperoxygenation prior to arrest

Limit time to ≤40 minutes

Alternative perfusion strategies:

   Intermittent cerebral perfusion

   Low flow CPB

   Antegrade cerebral perfusion

Monitoring

Near infrared spectroscopy (NIRS)

Electroencephalography (EEG)

Transcranial Doppler (TCD)

Postoperative Factors

The prevention of neurological damage must be vigorously continued in the postoperative period. Cerebral autoregulation is not normal in the post-bypass period, and adequate perfusion pressure is reliant on systemic arterial blood pressure. In conjunction with this hypocarbia and alkalosis are best avoided as these may decrease CBF. Other important factors include the early treatment of hypoxia, hyperthermia, acid–base disturbance, and electrolyte abnormalities. NIRS monitoring is as useful in guiding therapy postoperatively as it is intraoperatively. Despite this the impact of postoperative NIRS on neurodevelopmental outcome remains unclear [58].

Myocardial Protection

In comparison to the adult heart, the pediatric heart undergoing surgery will suffer more complex interventions with greater temperature fluctuations. The ability of the myocardium, therefore, to withstand these perturbations and function adequately to deliver oxygen to the body will be directly related to the adequacy of myocardial protection. A large number of surgical interventions are carried out in the neonatal or early infant period when the myocardium may not be able to adequately deal with the stressors of CPB, hypothermia, and ischemia. An important factor in this is its immature metabolic capacity that in turn may affect the response to ischemia during the myocardial standstill that is frequently required during surgical repair of congenital defects.

Experimental evidence suggests that because of myocardial immaturity there is a more rapid accumulation of lactate, which results in earlier inhibition of glycolysis, which in turn results in a decrease in high-energy phosphates such as ATP. At a cellular level this results in an increased number of actin–myosin complexes that cannot dissociate. The decrease in ATP will also result in a decreased ability of the sarcoplasmic reticulum to take up calcium [91]. As the immature myocardium relies heavily on glucose as its major substrate and also has a greater reliance on extracellular calcium for calcium-mediated excitation coupling, the problems related to this metabolic immaturity are clear [92,93]. The end results are earlier ischemic injury compared with adults and possibly explain why certain pediatric patients have increased morbidity and mortality. Most of the laboratory data investigating this has been obtained on normal hearts and it is thus unclear what the ischemic tolerance is when there are pre-existing conditions such as cyanosis, hypertrophy, hypoxia, volume or pressure overload, and acidosis. Many of these conditions may be present and may compromise myocardial protection in neonates and infants who require surgical correction of their heart defects. Infants and children with chronic cyanosis as a result of inadequate pulmonary blood flow often have increased bronchial collateral flow. This increased blood return to the left heart can result in insufficient myocardial protection by warming the heart and washing out cardioplegia [94]. Hypertrophied ventricles also may have inadequate myocardial protection and subendocardial ischemia during prolonged arrest periods. It has been found that up to 90% of patients who do not survive the perioperative period show some form of myocardial necrosis that exists in the absence of coronary artery obstruction. This necrosis may effect the entire subendocardium and lead to endocardial fibrosis with late myocardial dysfunction [95].

As mentioned previously in this chapter electrical quiescence provides the cornerstone of myocardial protection. This coupled with the principles of hypothermia have been in practice since the 1960s in an attempt to protect the myocardium during periods of ischemia. Cold crystalloid cardioplegia was applied to pediatric surgery and remains in use today by many pediatric cardiac surgeons. Intraoperative myocardial protection can be viewed to have a number of components of which cardioplegia plays the most important part, with perfusion technique, surgical precision, and anesthetic management also playing important roles.

The principles that guide the composition of cardioplegia include: 1) the ability to produce rapid cardiac arrest; 2) hypothermia; 3) metabolic substrates; 4) appropriate pH; and 5) membrane stabilization (ie, low Ca^{2+}, Mg^{2+}, steroids, O_2 radical scavengers) [96]. The only monitor for the efficacy during CPB of the cardioplegia is electrical quiescence as we do not have a readily available test of myocardial metabolic status. The quality of cardioplegia can, however, be assessed in the immediate period after CPB by myocardial function, inotropic requirements, and troponin I level. Despite the theoretical efficacy of the troponin I level interpretation is difficult and influenced by type of cardiac defect, the myocardial incision, the assay system used, and the use of dexamethasone during CPB [97].

Historically crytalloid cardioplegia has been used. Examples of this include the del Nido solution, favored at Boston Children's Hospital and the Children's Hospital of Philadelphia, and St Thomas solution, which is used elsewhere. The del Nido solution contains Na^+ of 153 mmol/L, K^+ of 24 mmol/L, Cl^- of 132 mmol/L, Ca^{2+} of 0.4 mmol/L, Mg^{2+} of 6.2 mmol/L, lidocaine of 140 mg/L, and mannitol of 2.6 g/L. St Thomas's solution contains Na^+ of 129 mmol/L, K^+ of 16 mmol/L, Cl^- of 140 mmol/L, Ca^{2+} of 1.2 mmol/L, Mg^{2+} of 16 mmol/L, and no mannitol or lidocaine. A significant difference between these rwo solutions is the concentration of Ca^{2+}, although the St Thomas solution is still a normocalcemic value for ionized calcium. It has been found that high levels of intracellular Ca^{2+} during ischemia and reperfusion lead to increased cellular injury

[96]. The neonatal myocardium may be at increased risk for this effect as it possesses a diminished capacity to sequester calcium. Experimentally it has been found that in nonhypoxic hearts either normocalcemic or hypocalcemic cardioplegia results in preservation of myocardial and vascular function. In contrast to this in patients with hypoxic stress (i.e., cyanotic heart disease), hypocalcemic cardioplegia allows for repair of hypoxic myocardial damage, whereas normocalcemic cardioplegia is associated with increased cellular injury manifest as myocardial and endothelial dysfunction post-bypass. Another difference between these two solutions is the concentration of Mg^{2+}. At a myocardial level the increased Mg^{2+} will inhibit the entry of Ca^{2+} into the cell, offsetting the higher Ca^{2+} in the St Thomas solution. Another added benefit is that the higher Mg^{2+} cardioplegia has been associated with a decrease in post-bypass arrhythmia [96]. In early animal experimentation it was found that magnesium enrichment of hypocalcemic cardioplegia offered myocardial protection and functional preservation; however, when it was added to normocalcemic cardioplegia these positive effects did not occur [98].

There are three phases of cardioplegia described: induction, maintenance, and reperfusion. Induction of cardioplegia covers the initial dose that results in electrical silence given soon after initiation of CPB. All hearts receive noncoronary collateral blood flow via pericardial connections, and in some patients with aortopulmonary collaterals this may be more significant. The presence, size, and number of these vessels may be variable; thus the flow may be of sufficient volume to wash out the cardioplegia. This will result in an increase in myocardial temperature as the collateral flow will bring blood to the heart that is at the temperature of the systemic perfusate and also, importantly, a possible return of electrical activity. This is the rationale to give intermittent doses of cardioplegia every 10–30 minutes [95–97]. The periodic cardioplegia will result in: 1) maintenance of arrest; 2) restoring myocardial hypothermia; 3) buffering acidosis and washing away acidic metabolites; 4) replenishing high-energy phosphates; and 5) counteracting edema with hyperosmolarity [95]. This is therefore the maintenance phase of cardioplegia. The reperfusion phase is a critical time as the mode of reperfusion appears to be more important than the duration of ischemia. In a study performed on 103 patients with both cyanotic and acyanotic CHD, one group received intermittent boluses of cold cardioplegia whilst another group received the same cardioplegia strategy to which was added $300\,mL/m^2$ of the same cardioplegia solution at $35\,°C$ just prior to aortic cross-clamp removal. This is known as terminal warm blood cardioplegia (TWBCP) and is often used in adult cardiac surgery. The use of TWBCP was associated with higher numbers of patients resuming spontaneous sinus rhythm, decreased inotropic use to wean from CPB (although nearly all patients in the study required inotropic support postoperatively in the ICU), improved lactate extraction, and decreased troponin T and heart type fatty acid binding protein. The latter two markers are indicative of cellular damage and necrosis. It would thus appear that the use of TWBCP may provide additional protection by improving myocardial aerobic energy metabolism and decreasing cellular damage [99].

Three additional factors play an important role: adequate distribution of coronary flow, delivery pressure of the cardioplegia, and the question of crystalloid versus blood cardioplegia. To be effective the cardioplegia must be adequately distributed to the myocardium. Although pediatric coronary vessels do not suffer from occlusive disease there are certain pathologic conditions where retrograde perfusion may be a better choice: severe aortic insufficiency, arterial switch operation, and severe ventricular and septal hypertrophy. The delivery pressure of the cardioplegia may also influence myocardial damage. Despite the requirement that the cardioplegia be delivered at a certain pressure to ensure adequate distribution, care must be taken not to perfuse the myocardium at too high a pressure as this may itself lead to myocardial and vascular endothelial cell damage, increased edema, and decreased ATP levels. A pressure of 30–50 mmHg has been shown to be adequate [95]. The last factor of importance is the question of crystalloid versus blood cardioplegia. The use of blood cardioplegia results in myocardial arrest in an oxygenated state with no loss of ATP in the period of electrical activity prior to arrest. This is contrasted to the use of crystalloid where there is a high loss of ATP during this same period. In addition to this when warm blood cardioplegia is used as induction it can resuscitate injured myocardium, which allows it to better tolerate subsequent ischemia. Several authors and commentators have concluded that there appears to be a distinct advantage in the use of blood cardioplegia over crystalloid be it at cold or warm temperatures [95–97,100–103]. The investigators found improvements that included lower coronary sinus lactate, improved cardiac index, better echocardiographic evidence of left ventricular function, increased heat shock protein (produced in myocardial cells in response to stress), and decreased troponin I release, which may correlate with less myocardial injury.

In completion of this topic on myocardial protection perfusion technique, surgical and anesthesia factors must be mentioned. Although a more in-depth discussion will follow, the effect of appropriate perfusion is considerable. With respect to myocardial protection, the effect of perfusion is to maintain perfusion pressure to the coronary vessels, to adequately remove excess body water that may affect post-bypass myocardial performance, and to limit the inflammatory cascade triggered by the institution of

CPB. The surgeon is clearly in a unique position to directly affect the outcome of the attempts to preserve myocardial integrity. Surgical technique must be meticulous so as not to cause unnecessary trauma to myocardial tissue, which may result in global dysfunction, heart block, or coronary artery problems that include kinking, transaction, or air embolism owing to inadequate ventricular de-airing. Anesthesia factors that may aid myocardial protection include a thorough understanding of the underlying physiology both before and after surgical intervention, ventilator settings that will aid and not impede myocardial function (e.g., attempts to keep pulmonary artery pressures low so as to offload the right ventricle), and timely use of inotropic, inodilator, vasodilator, or antiarrhythmic therapies. In conclusion, as with protection of any organ system, a more multimodal approach will offer the best result.

Pulmonary Effects of Cardiopulmonary Bypass

The institution of CPB, as with other organ systems, has potential deleterious effects on the lungs. In the preoperative stages, particularly in those with increased pulmonary blood flow, the patient may suffer pulmonary edema that will require intense medical therapy before surgery. Indeed there is a group of patients who will present to the operating room owing to failed drug therapy thus placing them at a physiologic disadvantage before the impact of CPB. In another group of patients, because pulmonary blood flow has been unrestricted over time (e.g., trisomy 21 patients with uncorrected left to right shunts), the arterial media undergoes hypertrophy with resultant vascular reactivity and pulmonary hypertension. These changes may affect the management of patients at the termination of CPB. In some this may be severe enough that the patient may suffer acute right ventricular failure resulting in a failure to wean from CPB and necessitating the use of acute extracorporeal support. Other patients in whom vascular reactivity and pulmonary hypertension may be an issue in weaning from CPB include neonates, by virtue of their pulmonary vasoreactivity as a carryover from the fetal circulation, and those patients in whom there is an obstruction to pulmonary venous drainage, be it at the level of the pulmonary veins or because of restrictive atrial septa associated with left-sided obstructive lesions. The lungs may be a source as well as a target of the inflammatory response associated with CPB [104]. The result of this is capillary leak and extravasation of fluid into the alveolar spaces with resultant poor oxygen exchange and a detrimental effect on pulmonary mechanics. Etiologic factors associated with capillary leak include hemodilution with resultant decrease in oncotic pressure; ischemia-reperfusion injury; and the sequestration of activated neutrophils, cytokines, complement, and leukotrienes within the pulmonary vascular bed during the period of CPB. The institution of CPB decreases perfusion pressure through the pulmonary capillary bed. Under normal physiologic conditions continuous perfusion aids in alveolar stability; thus, when this ceases with CPB, changes occur in the architecture of the alveolar wall leading to a loss in its stability. It thus follows that there is a marked change in resting alveolar volume and with that gas exchange [105]. Clinical studies performed on children in the peribypass period have demonstrated that there will be an increase in the functional residual capacity (FRC) after median sternotomy. This could be explained by the decrease in the effect of chest wall recoil. As pulmonary flow ceases on CPB and the alveoli collapse there will be an associated decrease in FRC. This decrease is reversed with the reinstitution of flow but is decreased to below resting levels with chest closure. It was postulated that this is due to the effect of chest drains, inflammation, and the presence of extravasated fluid [105].

The use of modified ultrafiltration (MUF) at the termination of bypass has greatly improved pulmonary function and thus oxygenation/ventilation at this critical phase of congenital cardiac surgery. The effect of MUF that is directly related to pulmonary function is due to a reduction in total body water and an associated decrease in lung water. This will lead to improved lung compliance and decreased airway pressure [106]. In addition the use of MUF has been shown to decrease inflammatory markers and this may therefore affect the capillary leak that plagues the lung during CPB [107]. In addition the use of steroids has been shown to improve postoperative pulmonary function [104]. The clinical result is faster time to extubation, decreased mechanical ventilation, and decreased ICU time [106,108].

Although practices vary widely, it is our preference to attempt extubation soon after arrival to the ICU in a wide variety of patients from the early neonatal period up to adults presenting for revision of palliative repairs. The group of patients in whom every attempt is made for early extubation is the single-ventricle population presenting for cavopulmonary anastomosis and Fontan completion. It has been well established that physiologically these patients are at a distinct disadvantage with positive-pressure ventilation, as this will interfere with passive venous flow through the capillary bed and thus affect oxygenation and ultimately cardiac output. In a study in which 79% of patients were extubated in the operating room following cardiac surgery, increased bypass time, age <1 year, and high inotropic support were factors that were found in those not extubated [109]. Although performed on patients who underwent only ASD or VSD repair it was found that there did not appear to be any cardiovascular instability in those extubated within 6 hours of returning to the ICU [110].

Renal Function and Protection on Cardiopulmonary Bypass

The development of acute kidney injury (AKI) is multi-factorial and can be subdivided into preoperative, intraoperative, and postoperative causes. The etiologies of the preoperative injury are mainly associated with neonates and infants as their renal physiology is immature. Glomerular filtration rate (GFR) is lower in this age group due to lower MAP and high renovascular resistance, with GFR maintained by postglomerular efferent arteriolar vasoconstriction that is dependent on high levels of angiotensin II activity. It is for this reason that the angiotensin-converting enzyme inhibitors are used in these patients with extreme caution [111].

Preventive and treatment strategies aim to maintain systemic oxygen delivery, maintain perfusion pressure to vital organs, and prevent any further deterioration in function. Thus in the preoperative phase careful attention must be paid to balancing pulmonary and systemic perfusion (Qp:Qs). As is well described, soon after birth the pulmonary resistance begins to fall and thus, in patients with ductal-dependent systemic flow, pulmonary blood flow may increase. This potential increase in pulmonary blood flow results in a concomitant decrease in systemic flow with resultant decreased perfusion of vital organs. Management at this time will therefore include prostaglandin infusion to maintain ductal dependent flow, low fraction of inspired oxygen (FiO$_2$), support of cardiac function, and early corrective or palliative surgery. Intraoperative aims include many of the factors that are discussed elsewhere in this chapter including dampening the inflammatory response, decreasing DHCA time, the effects of nonpulsatile versus pulsatile CPB, decreasing circuit size, and limiting the exposure to blood products. After the completion of CPB the aims of preventative management include decreasing total body water and inflammatory mediators by means of modified ultrafiltration; ensuring that there are no residual lesions that may affect Qp:Qs or directly affect cardiac function; and ensuring appropriate and ongoing cardiac support in the form of inotropic drugs, vasopressors, vasodilators, and diuretics.

The incidence of AKI varies dependent on surgical procedure with a range of 0.7% for short, uncomplicated surgeries (e.g., ASD closure), increasing up to 59% for longer, more complicated operations (e.g., arterial switch). Across the entire spectrum of procedures the incidence is in the range of 6–17%; however, renal replacement therapy is required in 2.3–11.5% [112–114]. Mortality in this subgroup of patients may be as high as 79% [113]. Table 10.6 describes the risk factors associated with the development of AKI in the immediate post-CPB period. Although this has been collated from data collected over the last 10–15 years it seems that the incidence of acute post-CPB renal failure is

Table 10.6 Risk factors for the development of acute renal failure.

Age ≤1 year

Elevated Aristotle/RACHS-1 (categories 4–6) surgical complexity scores

Long bypass time

Long cross-clamp time

Deep hypothermic circulatory arrest

Increased use of blood products

Low post-CPB cardiac output

Inotropic support (especially epinephrine and isuprel)

Low trough blood pressure on POD 1

decreasing [113]. It is unknown whether this can be ascribed to improved perfusion techniques, improved surgical technique, improved drug therapies, or an improved understanding and management in the ICU. The development of AKI has been associated with a risk factor for mortality as well as prolonged hospital stay and associated increase in-hospital costs. Despite these alarming numbers the diagnosis may prove difficult as consensus as to the definition is not clear. In a small meta-analysis performed by Zappitelli and colleagues, definitions varied and included serum creatinine (SCr) doubling from baseline, SCr tripling from baseline, and the need for dialysis [114]. Another diagnostic marker is the use of the p-RIFLE (pediatric – risk, injury, failure, loss, and end-stage renal disease), which estimates the decrease in Cr clearance and thus renal dysfunction [115]. In a novel approach, investigators identified the gene for neutrophil gelatinase-associated lipocalin (NGAL) as one of the most up-regulated genes expressed in the kidney not only after ischemic injury but also during sepsis and post-transplantation. NGAL functions as a bacteriostatic by blocking the use of iron by microbial systems; more importantly in relation to renal injury it functions to limit renal damage, appearing rapidly in the urine and serum in response to injury [116]. Based on this, NGAL has been identified as an early predictor of AKI [117]. In the immediate post-CPB period it has been found that this marker increases in all patients, especially in those in whom prolonged CPB was necessary. In those patients in whom AKI occurred there was a marked sustained increase in NGAL. A grossly elevated level at 12 hours post-CPB correlated with mortality. Another biomarker that has been described is interleukin 18 (IL-18), which will rise between 4 and 6 hours after CPB, peaking at 12 hours and remaining elevated for 24–48 hours. It has been suggested that the combination of the two markers will identify patients who are at risk for AKI hours after CPB with treatment being instituted early rather than having to wait for 48–72 hours when SCr begins to rise [118]. By the time Cr begins to rise, as much as 50% of renal function has been lost.

Renal replacement therapy (RRT) is usually instituted in association with multiorgan failure, worsening renal function with increasing K$^+$, and total body fluid accumulation. Studies have shown that up to 20% of pediatric patients in multiorgan failure are associated with cardiac surgery and that the prevention of total body fluid accumulation is associated with improved survival [111]. Two forms of RRT are used, namely peritoneal dialysis (PD) and continuous renal replacement therapy (CRRT). PD is managed by placing a catheter into the peritoneal cavity, instilling solute into the cavity, and then removing it after a suitable length of time. It has advantages in that it requires no intravascular access, does not need heparinization, is well tolerated even during hemodynamically unstable periods, and may even remove proinflammatory mediators if used immediately after CPB [111]. Disadvantages of PD are the occurrence of peritonitis and that the removal of solution or electrolytes is a slow process. Advantages of CRRT include rapid removal of excess body fluid, treatment of life-threatening hyperkalemia, and ease in which the circuit can be placed in parallel with an ECMO circuit. In this setting CRRT is usually achieved by a venovenous circuit with the utilization of the internal jugular, subclavian, or femoral veins. In one study the results of this approach showed that in patients alive to discharge, up to 90% were discharged with normal renal function [112].

Endocrine Response to CPB

Patients undergoing cardiac surgery within the range of temperatures from normothermia all the way to deep hypothermia generate a significant hormonal stress response that involves both the sympathoadrenal pathway as well as the hypothalamic–pituitary–adrenal (HPA) axis. The interpretation of this release is problematic as there is considerable variability depending on age, nature of the surgery, and anesthetic technique [119]. In a study of 22 infants ranging in age from 2 days to 18 months with a mix of both cyanotic and acyanotic conditions who all underwent repair utilizing DHCA, the authors found that there was an increase in both epinephrine and norepinephrine. This increase persisted from the cooling phase through the warming phase and up to the end of the study, which unfortunately ended with chest closure. These findings led the authors to conclude that there is considerable sympathoadrenal stress associated with CPB and DHCA despite what appeared to be adequate anesthesia and analgesia. The nonlinear relationship between duration of arrest and the postarrest values possibly indicated that the tissues were beginning to become hypoxic, thus trending these values could suggest a safe time for DHCA [120].

Similar findings were found in both a clinical as well as an experimental study. In these investigations there was a small rise in levels with induction and surface cooling followed by a rise at the time of sternotomy. The levels had returned to near baseline at the time of DHCA with the same spike as seen in the aforementioned study with the onset of rewarming. The conclusions were also similar in that this rise could be related to either washout of products of metabolism indicating ongoing cellular metabolism or the onset of ischemia, or simply the washout of catecholamines produced during arrest [121,122]. It was found experimentally that epinephrine was released only from the adrenal whilst norepinephrine was released from the adrenal as well as from peripheral sources. Clinically, however, these elevations in catecholamines are of questionable significance.

The endpoint of the HPA axis (i.e., the secretion of glucocorticoids) is important in the setting of cardiac surgery as studies suggest that the effect of these glucocorticoids include: 1) enhanced vascular sensitivity to catecholamines; 2) increased myocardial β adrenergic receptors; 3) increased rennin substrate and calcium availability; and 4) inhibited vasodilation and catecholamine degradation. The end result of these factors may be that glucocorticoids enhance myocardial and vascular responsiveness to catecholamines. In studies performed on critically ill neonates, infants, and children with hypotension refractory to volume resuscitation as well as inotropic support, adrenal insufficiency was found with clinical improvement on administration of corticosteroids [123]. In an early study by Pollock and colleagues, the authors studied 20 acyanotic patients ranging in age from 1–16 years who presented for repair of lesions including ASD, VSD, canal defects, anomalous venous return, and aortic valve surgery. They divided the patients into two equal and comparative groups. The two groups were then exposed to either pulsatile or nonpulsatile flow, respectively, as the authors postulated that pulsatile flow would show a superior hormone response. However, this was shown not to be the case as both groups demonstrated normal corticosteroid responses. Although the initial focus of the study was on comparing the two forms of CPB and the effect on hormonal secretion, it could be concluded that despite the physiologic aberrancy of CPB the function of this axis remained intact [124]. In a recent study Gajarski and colleagues postulated that postcardiotomy infants with high vasopressor requirements would demonstrate adrenal insufficiency that would be proportional to CPB or DHCA times and vasopressors requirements. Although the results of the study did not demonstrate a difference between bypass techniques, a subgroup of patients was identified which demonstrated an apparent adrenal insufficiency. This subgroup, which was representative of both regular CPB and DHCA, demonstrated higher inotropic requirements, prolonged intubation, and prolonged ICU stay. The authors concluded that despite the effects of CPB with or without DHCA, including the surgical stress, hemodilution associated with CPB, and lastly the concentrating effects of ultrafiltration, it appeared that in the majority of cases the HPA axis was intact [123]. Similar findings have been shown in other studies [125,126]. It appears that, at least in a subset of patients, the use of perioperative steroids would be of clinical benefit; however, the use of steroids in pediatric CPB is not routine and has indeed been questioned [127]. The literature shows that the question in to the use of peri-CPB steroids remains unsolved as there does not appear to be a consensus amongst different institutions into dosing, timing, or even whether or not to use these drugs [128–131].

Thyroid hormone levels have been found to become suppressed after critical illness and surgical procedures. This has the potential to cause a number of problems in the post-CPB period including prolonged ventilation, increased inotropic requirements, and increased need for diuretic therapy [132]. Several mechanisms have been proposed for this decrease. The stress of surgery itself may lead to a suppression of hypothalamic–pituitary axis. The effects of CPB, which include hemodilution, hypothermia, and the use of inotropic support, also lead to a decline. The release of endogenous mediators inclusive of glucocorticoids, tumor necrosis factor, and IL-6 are released in response to CPB and lead to low postoperative tri-iodothyronine (T3). Interestingly there is an initial surge of free hormone after the institution of CPB followed by low total and free T3/ T4 levels. The nadir of this effect occurs between 12 and 48 hours after bypass and lasts up to 5 days [132,133]. At a cellular level the effect of thyroid hormone is to influence the entry and extrusion of calcium from the cardiac myocyte via the sarcoplasmic reticulum and cell membrane. Thus, the effect of low T3 is profound on myocardial function and may be manifest by both systolic and diastolic dysfunction and increased vascular resistance, which collectively are seen clinically as a low cardiac output state [133]. Treatment with T3 either as repeated bolus therapy or infusion in the immediate postoperative period has been shown to improve systolic, mean arterial blood pressure, and cardiac output, which in turn leads to improved renal perfusion and negative fluid balance [134,135].

The concentration of growth hormone (GH) has also been shown to increase secondary to CPB; however, there is no matching elevation in insulin-like growth factor 1 (IGF-1) or insulin-like growth factor binding protein 3 (IGFBP-3). The latter two proteins are the effector proteins for GH function. These findings indicate that, although GH secretion is appropriately elevated secondary to a stress response, the lack of effector protein elevation indicates an ongoing catabolic state that continues into the postoperative and recovery phases [136].

Hyperglycemia in the critically ill, adult patient is known to be associated with higher morbidity and mortality [137–139]. Hyperglycemia is a normal response to stress and with this is coupled the secretion of insulin, which aids the uptake of glucose into muscle where it is used for the ongoing production of energy. Surgery, with its associated stress response, results in an increase in counter-regulatory hormones (epinephrine, glucagon, growth hormone, and cortisol) as well as inflammatory cytokines (e.g., tumor necrosis factor and interleukins). The result is increased hepatic glucose mobilization, impaired peripheral glucose utilization, relative insulin deficiency, and, thus, hyperglycemia [139]. This is complicated by insulin resistance found in cardiac surgery patients. It has been found that during hypothermia glucose levels increase and insulin decreases. On rewarming glucose levels continue to rise with an associated rise in insulin as well as the previously described increase in catecholamine, cortisol, and growth hormone levels. These combined with increased inflammatory cytokines lead to the insulin resistance seen. In addition to these etiologic factors, the administration of corticosteroids and inotropes also plays a role. In three retrospective studies in the pediatric population, one of which was performed specifically in the cardiac population, the second in a general pediatric ICU (PICU), including postoperative cardiac patients, and the third in a large, tertiary care, general PICU, the conclusion appears to be similar to the adult studies – namely that hyperglycemia was associated with increased morbidity and mortality [140–142]. The differences, however, were that unlike in the adult experience where initial glucose level was associated with mortality, in the pediatric group it was the peak level as well as continued elevation that was associated with complications. The morbidities described in these studies included prolonged ventilation, prolonged ICU stay, and increased rates of infection. The unanswered question is what to do about the hyperglycemia, particularly in the immediate perioperative phase. The real concern amongst clinicians is for prolonged hypoglycemia and its effects on the brain. In an interesting study by Ballweg and colleagues, early postoperative hyperglycemia was not associated with worse neurodevelopmental outcomes at 1 year of age [143].

Systemic Inflammation

The perioperative period is a potentially deleterious time as the combination of anesthesia, the stress of surgery, and the immune-stimulating effects of the CPB circuit combine to result in a systemic inflammatory response. Indeed it has been found that certain patients, including those with single-ventricle physiology, may have an activated inflammatory response prior even to the commencement of CPB [144]. Possible etiologic factors responsible include: 1) cellular activation with contact of blood products with the surface of the bypass circuit; 2) mechanical shear stress as the blood passes through suction systems and filters; 3) tissue ischemia and reperfusion; 4) hypotension and hemodilution; 5) administration of blood products; and 6) hypothermia (mild, moderate, and deep hypothermia) [104]. These factors will result in the activation of both humoral and cellular immune responses, which generate the activation of the complement, coagulation, and fibrinolytic pathways. Collectively these pathways result in endothelial damage, capillary leak, and organ dysfunction. In the literature, up to 50% of children have pulmonary and cardiovascular dysfunction attributable to this proinflammatory response in the post-CPB period [145]. The pediatric population may be at increased risk compared with the adult population as the body surface area to circuit size is greater.

Figure 10.7 demonstrates the effects of surgical trauma and CPB [145]. Complement activation occurs by both the alternative (contact with foreign surfaces, i.e., bypass circuitry) and classical pathways (protamine related). These two pathways result in the elevation of C3a and C5a; and C4a with additional C3a respectively. Elevations of C3a and C5a lead to activation and degranulation of neutrophils, release of histamine from mast cells and basophils, and platelet aggregation. These elevations have been associated with poor outcomes with severe organ dysfunction, prolonged mechanical ventilation and poor outcome [104,146]. Contact activation of clotting factor XII results in the eventual activation of kallikrein and bradykinin. The

effect of increased kallikrein is the positive feedback on the activation of more factor XII whilst the increased bradykinin results in the stimulation of B1 and B2 receptors. The effects of their stimulation is the production of nitric oxide, free radicals, eicosanoids, and cytokines. This will result in vasodilation and increased capillary permeability which in turn may lead to organ dysfunction [144,147]. B2 receptors have also been found in the brain and this may play a role in the genesis of ischemia–reperfusion injury [104]. Cytokines are produced by a wide range of cells including monocytes, macrophages, lymphocytes, and endothelial cells. These factors are either proinflammatory in the form of IL-6, IL-8, and tumor necrosis factor α (TNFα) or anti-inflammatory in IL-10 and IL-1 receptor antagonist (IL-1ra). An increase in TNFα has been demonstrated to be associated with increased capillary leak [147]; however, other studies have failed to show any significant increase [145,148]. Elevations in IL-6 and IL-8 have been shown to correlate with compromised post-bypass cardiopulmonary function with increased inotropic requirements, severe capillary leak syndrome, and an increase in mortality [104,144,145,148]. The balance therefore between the proinflammatory and anti-inflammatory responses may thus be altered in those who demonstrate an aggressive systemic inflammatory response. In uncomplicated cases the systemic inflammatory response is self-limited and is only of a few days' duration [145].

The question that now begs answering therefore is what can be done to prevent initiation of this inflammatory process. Several therapeutic maneuvers have been proposed

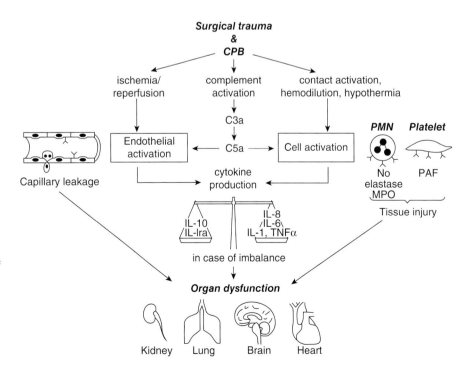

Figure 10.7 Illustration of effects of surgical trauma and CPB. Schematic representation of important mediators of the inflammatory response to surgical trauma and cardiopulmonary bypass (CPB). The different processes have a synergistic effect and may lead to organ dysfunction. (Reproduced with permission from Brix-Christensen [145].)

including the addition of steroids into the pump prime, the use of indomethacin, aprotinin, heparin-coated CPB circuitry, and the use of ultrafiltration [131]. The administration of steroids into the pump prime seems a logical therapeutic measure; however, data supporting this were derived from adult patients undergoing coronary artery bypass grafting [127]. Studies in the pediatric population have demonstrated variable results and indeed there does not appear to be agreement into timing or dosing of steroids, which may indicate the lack of data looking at dose, timing of dose, and clinically significant improvements after administration [129]. In one study there were measurable differences in the degree of inflammatory markers found between the 15 test subjects and the 14 controls. Although the age at the time of surgery, the CPB times, and the aortic cross-clamp times were similar in this study they did not reach statistical significance. The authors found that in the steroid group there was a decrease in the concentration of IL-6 and TNFα. They noted, however, that these decreases were after the initiation of bypass and before MUF in the TNFα group and after the removal of the cross-clamp in the IL-6 group. The concentration of C3a, however, was no different in both groups. In terms of clinical effect the steroid-treated group had lower alveolar arterial oxygen differences, lower temperatures (due to lower cytokine levels), required less supplemental fluid in the first 24 hours, had better renal function, and had less ICU time [149]. A further study looking into the effects of administration of preoperative steroids (methylprednisolone 30 mg/kg) 4 hours before surgery as well as intraoperatively compared with a cohort that received only intraoperative steroids found that the group who received two doses were at a laboratory (in the form of reduced levels of IL-6 and IL-10) as well as a clinical advantage as outlined in the first study [150]. Results of other studies have not, however, shown positive results. In a study that included patients ≥3 months of age but weighing ≤7 kg, 24 patients were given steroids while 26 were not. The strengths of this study included comparable age and surgical matching and the fact that all patients given steroids were operated on at one hospital while those who did not receive steroids were at another hospital. An obvious weakness of the study was that the dose and timing of the steroids were not mentioned in the study. Despite these factors the investigators found no differences in the inflammatory or clinical markers between the groups [127]. Possible explanations included that the patients had shorter CPB times, less surgical trauma, and dose and timing of the steroids. As has been indicated elsewhere in this discussion a large, randomized, prospective study is essential to properly elucidate this question.

Aprotinin, a serine protease inhibitor, was reported to be efficacious in the preservation of platelet function, to decrease bleeding diatheses associated not only with CPB but also other surgeries including spinal surgery, and also to have anti-inflammatory effects. Studies concluded that its use had beneficial effects on post-CPB organ function and improved hemodynamic stability. However, after published data in the adult literature suggested that there was a risk of thrombosis and renal failure with its use, the drug was voluntarily removed in November 2007 [151,152]. In the pediatric literature safety studies looking at these effects failed to concur with the adult studies [153,154]. As with many clinical questions in the literature some studies even questioned the drug's efficacy [155,156]. Aprotinin is, however, not available for clinical use.

As has been mentioned it is widely understood that the bypass circuit itself is probably the main culprit in inciting the inflammatory cascade. Following on this, two strategies have been used: miniaturization of bypass circuits (which will be discussed later) and the coating of the circuit in an attempt to make it more biocompatible. Other strategies that have been used by clinicians in an attempt to minimize the inflammatory effects include the use of aprotinin (which is no longer available for clinical use), ultrafiltration, the use of biocompatible circuits, and the use of smaller circuits. The latter three strategies will be discussed in greater detail in later sections. The conclusion that can be drawn from this discussion, however, is that it appears that a multimodal strategy is essential to decrease the deleterious effects of the multisystem inflammatory cascade that is incited during CPB.

Management of Cardiopulmonary Bypass

The trend in modern pediatric bypass equipment is to reduce the size of the extracorporeal circuit to reduce the prime volume. The priming volume may actually exceed the blood volume of the neonate by as much as 200–300%. This is in contrast to the adult CPB patient where the priming volume accounts for only 25–33% of the patient's blood volume. The effects of CPB have led surgeons to perform operations without the use of CPB and for interventional cardiologists to close ASDs and VSDs in the catheterization laboratory [157–162]. Indeed some undertake a hybrid approach for closure of VSDs, and other procedures such as stenting of the pulmonary arteries, in which the surgeon will obtain direct access to the heart and the procedure is performed using transcatheter techniques, often in conjunction with an interventional cardiologist [163].

Hemodilution

Research into the effects of CPB on the inflammatory cascade and organ dysfunction that occurs in the post-bypass period have also found that the use of blood products play a significant role in the inflammatory cascade.

These effects include an elevation in complement and inflammatory cytokines [164]. The use of blood in the pump prime, especially in neonates, infants and patients who will undergo DHCA and hypothermic low-flow bypass, is based on earlier published data that suggested that a hematocrit (HCT) of between 20 and 25 was associated with acute and long-term sequelae [165]. Acutely there appeared to be lower minimum cardiac index in the post-CPB phase, higher serum lactate levels at 60 minutes post-CPB, and a greater increase in total body water in the first postoperative day. At 1 year of age this same group tested lower in absolute number on the Psychomotor Development Index; a greater number of subjects also tested 2 standard deviations from the population mean. These authors concluded that an HCT diluted down to 20% was associated with the inferior results shown above; the optimal HCT above 25 could not be identified. In a further study of a cohort of patients undergoing two-ventricle and nonaortic arch surgery by the same group of researchers from Boston Children's Hospital, there appeared to be a point at an HCT of 23.5% where the 1-year psychomotor outcome was better than that below 23.5%. The authors noted that it was not possible to conclude, however, that there was an absolute safe HCT owing to the presence of confounding variables between subjects, for example age at operation, diagnosis, etc. [166]. A further study comparing HCT of 25% to HCT of 35% was also undertaken. Apart from a greater intraoperative fluid accumulation with lower HCT there were no reported differences between groups both in the early postoperative as well as at 1-year neurodevelopmental follow-up periods [167]. Thus, a conclusion that may be drawn is that an HCT of ≥25 may be adequate. At our institution we keep the HCT ≥30 in patients ≤1 year and ≥25 in those ≥1 year, irrespective of congenital abnormality. Based on this, blood is added into the prime volume so as to maintain the HCT at these levels that appear to be associated with improved outcomes.

Circuit Miniaturization

The desire to maintain HCT at these levels and also the previously mentioned discrepancy between patient size and circuit has lead researchers to attempt to miniaturize circuits, even for use in neonates. This has the advantage of not only decreasing the total surface area to which the patient will come into contact but also raising the possibility of bloodless prime. Methods that may be used to achieve this include using biocompatible coated circuitry and oxygenators, the use of vacuum-assisted venous drainage, the ability to decrease circuit length by bringing the pump as close to the patient as possible, and, finally, the exclusion of certain circuit components, for example arterial line filters and in-line cardioplegia [168].

Table 10.7 Properties of the ideal circuit. (Reproduced with permission from Janvier *et al.* [169].)

Inability to initiate thrombogenesis
Inability to initiate hemolysis
No complement activation
No toxicity of products extracted from the circuit by the blood
Chemical inertness so that no toxic metabolites generated

Biocompatible Circuits

As mentioned elsewhere the initiation of CPB will result in the activation of the five proteolytic plasma systems (coagulation, fibrinolysis, complement activation, kallikrein–kinin, and contact systems) and the cellular components (leukocytes, platelets, and endothelial cells). Thus, the theoretical ideal is to use surface modification of a circuit and thus dampen the response. Table 10.7 describes the ideal biocompatible circuit [169]. Surface modification can be achieved by four techniques: coating, chemical modification, attachment of macromolecules, and by blending of polymers [170].

The coating method will coat the surface of the circuit with another polymer thus attempting to reduce protein adsorption. The chemical modification technique uses a selected chemical group on the surface of the circuit to replace with another. In the blending method the surface polymers are altered to create hydrophilic/hydrophobic or natural/synthetic polymer combinations.

Polymethoxyethylacrylate (PMEA) (Terumo Medical Corporation, Somerset, NJ) consists of a hydrophobic polyethylene backbone with hydrophilic methoxyethyl pendant groups that have no chemically functioning attachments. Theoretically PMEA will not react with platelets and clotting factors, thus maintaining their number and function and reducing adsorption of proteins to the circuit surface, thus decreasing the inflammatory cascade. In two studies in the pediatric population there were some advantages to the PMEA-coated circuits with respect to a decreased activation of the inflammatory cascade as measured by neutrophil elastase activity and a decrease in the coagulation activation as measured by thrombin-antithrombin complexes [171]. Both of these studies interestingly found that there was no significant difference in the platelet number between the study and control group. This may indicate that these circuit alterations are ineffective with respect to platelet protection or that in the pediatric population factors other than contact activation are important. These factors may include platelet interactions with inflammatory mediators such as complement, leukotrienes, and collagenases. Limitations to these studies, however, included their small number of patients and that they tested the effects of these circuits alone and not in concert with antifibrinolytics, steroids, or modified ultrafiltration [171,172].

Phosphorycholine is used as a coating over the existing tubing material. It is marketed by Avant, Dideco, Mirandola, Italy, as Phisio and also incorporated into the SMART circuit, which is a combination of phosphorycholine coating and polycaprolactone–polydimethylsiloxilane additives to the base polymer resin of COBE (Cardiovascular, Inc., Arvada, Colorado). The mechanism of action of this coating is to mimic the surface of cell membranes within the vascular wall. The result is to attempt to decrease the thrombogenic and inflammatory responses as well as microbial adhesion to the surface of the circuit. An in vitro study performed by Hoel and colleagues comparing uncoated and Phisio-coated circuits showed no apparent differences in their effects on inflammation but there was a trend toward a lesser decrease on the platelet count in the coated group [173]. In another study the authors noted that the prime volume was large and that the hemodilution may have overshadowed any improvement in platelet number or function [172]. In this study the authors compared uncoated versus PMEA and phosphorylcholine circuits; they found no differences related to platelet count or function and also importantly no improvement in postoperative outcomes, suggesting that these circuits may not have had any effect on the inflammatory cascade either.

Heparin has been used as a component of the circuit in both adult and pediatric circuitry. Two examples of this are the biopassive surface from Medtronic, Minneapolis, Minnesota, and a heparin plus polymer coating from Gish Biomedical, Inc., Rancho Santa Margarita, California. The former consists of a polymer priming layer that is bonded to the surface of the circuit with the second polymer comprising a sulphate/sulphonate group and heparin. In the latter example a hydrophilic biopolymer binds to the circuit to which in turn heparin is bound. The use of this coating has been studied widely and appears to have some beneficial effect on the inflammatory response in children on CPB as measured by inflammatory markers directly as well as clinically by increased urine output and less time postoperatively requiring mechanical ventilation [174,175]. In both of these studies there was no mention of the use of any further methods to decrease the inflammatory response (i.e., antifibrinolytics, steroids, or the use of modified ultrafiltration). In a further study where heparin-coated circuits were compared with phosphorylcholine-coated circuits the results showed that there was a comparable decrease in inflammatory markers in both. In this study patients were divided into three groups. The first group had a 750-mL prime volume within a heparin-coated circuit whilst the other two groups used phosphorylcholine-coated circuits with 450-mL and 750-mL priming volumes, respectively. The authors noted that despite randomization the 750-mL phosphorylcholine group were a younger group of patients and displayed worse clinical outcome with respect to capillary leak, prolonged ventilation, and inotropic support.

Once again the care did not include antifibrinolytics or modified ultrafiltration [176]. Clearly future studies need to be directed at the use of small volume prime and anti-inflammatory adjuncts.

Circuit Design

The use of smaller circuit size and thus prime volume is aimed at decreasing hemodilution, which in theory will result in lower numbers of transfusions, decreased severity of the inflammatory response, and thus reduced hospital costs related to improved outcomes [177]. Techniques that investigators have used to create these smaller circuits have included: low prime volume oxygenators, reservoirs, and arterial filters; shorter extracorporeal circuitry, remote pump heads, use of venous vacuum (which can in turn result in the use of smaller venous tubing), and in certain configurations removal of parts of the classic circuit, most frequently the arterial line filter [164,177–182]. These investigators have demonstrated safety even in the neonatal population with priming volumes as low as 110 mL. In the descriptions of these configurations the bypass circuit is placed at the operating room table with the surgeon and assistants almost straddling the circuitry (Figure 10.8) [179]. The use of this technology clearly needs total team acceptance and understanding.

Surgeries performed in these case series range from relatively simple procedures (e.g., VSD or ASD closure) to cor-

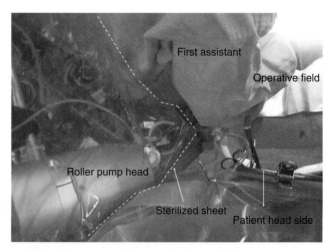

Figure 10.8 Operating field in cardiopulmonary bypass. Arrangement of the operating room and the sterilized polyvinyl chloride sheet is close to the first assistant's right elbow and functions as a protective barrier between the patient and the unsterilized CPB unit. The arterial, venous, and suction circuits are attached to the sheet. (Reproduced with permission from Miyaji *et al.* [179].)

rection of transposition of the great vessels, aortic arch hypoplasia, and even stage 1 Norwood procedures. In one of the studies there were descriptions of patients undergoing arterial switch, hypoplastic arch reconstructions, and interrupted aortic arch with VSD repairs without blood transfusions. Possibly the most startling fact of all was that one of the babies that underwent arterial switch operation weighed only 1.7 kg. These strategies clearly will lead to a degree of hemodilution, which is counter to what has been described earlier in this discussion. The patients were, however, monitored by using hemoglobin concentration, mixed venous saturation, regional cerebral oxygenation, and on-pump plasma lactate. Values of <7 g/dL, <70%, <50%, and >4 mmol/L, respectively, were used as transfusion triggers [179,181].

Laboratory experiments using neonatal piglets have demonstrated improved cardiopulmonary function post-deep hypothermia using miniaturized circuitry with asanguineous prime. The investigators found decreased TNFα, and the effect of primed neutrophils present in donor blood were of course absent. It has been found that these neutrophils are key factors in the genesis of the CPB-induced inflammatory cascade and capillary leak leading to organ dysfunction. Further analysis found improved right ventricular cardiac index, improved pulmonary vascular resistance index, and improved dynamic pulmonary compliance. The authors concluded that these could be attributed to a decrease in total lung water associated in turn with decreased inflammation [183]. In a separate study by the same group of investigators they were able to demonstrate improved CBF in a group of piglets that underwent CPB with the miniaturized circuit configuration. They demonstrated that the use of an asanguineous prime was associated with a decrease in the no-reflow phenomenon discussed earlier in the chapter. They further postulated that this may result in improved neurologic outcome [184].

Oxygenators

In the pediatric population, oxygenators must provide efficient gas exchange over a wide range of temperatures (10–40°C), pump flow rates (0–200 mL/kg/min), hematocrit as low as 15%, line pressures, and gas flow rates. Both bubble and membrane oxygenators can achieve effective gas exchange under these diverse conditions. Historically three different types of oxygenators have been used, namely the film type, bubble type, and membrane type. In the film type a thin blood film is created with gas exchange taking place on the surface of the film. In this method there is no mechanical introduction of gas into the blood and thus trauma to red blood cells is minimal; however, a large surface area is necessary with a large priming volume. The bubble oxygenator uses bubbles introduced directly into the blood. It has advantages in that the effective surface

area for gas exchange is large due to the surface area of the bubbles. The obvious disadvantage, however, is that the introduction of the bubbles causes red blood cell trauma. In addition to this the bubbles must clearly be removed from the circuit and this requires a settling chamber, which may in turn require added volume in the circuit. The final oxygenator is the one that is most widely used today. In this technique the blood is exposed to oxygen through a gas-permeable membrane and thus, because there is no direct contact between gas and blood, trauma is minimal [14]. Refinements in early membrane oxygenator design occurred in the 1980s with the introduction of microporous hollow fibers with blood flowing over the outside of the fiber and gas flowing down the fiber lumen. This increased the efficiency of gas exchange and at the same time decreased manufacturing costs in line with the cheaper bubble oxygenators [185].

Common to all CPB circuits are the presence of gaseous micro-emboli that have their genesis secondary to the following: pulsatile bypass, low venous reservoir levels, vacuum-assisted venous drainage, venous line air, field suckers, drug administration, and blood sampling. Perfusionists may use a number of methods to decrease this, ranging from filtration at the time of circuit set up, to ensuring adequate volumes within the venous reservoir and the placement of arterial line filters. Unfortunately, as has been mentioned before, the arterial line filter may add significant volume to the circuit. The use of arterial line filters has been reported in up to 96% of North American centers, whereas in Europe it has not been commonplace for a number of years [186]. The appropriate sizing of oxygenator for the pediatric population has been a focus in recent years as reducing the dimensions of this integral part of the CPB circuit will lead to significant reductions in prime volume. The first oxygenator designed specifically for the use in the neonatal population was the Dideco Kids D100 Neonatal Oxygenator (The Sorlin Group, Mirandola, Italy), which was initially evaluated in the USA at Duke University. The initial group of babies totaled six: two undergoing Norwood stage 1 palliations, two truncus arteriosus repairs, and two arterial switch operations. The investigators noted that the total priming volume for the oxygenator was only 31 mL and this enabled the priming volume of the circuit to be decreased by 12.5%. The change to this oxygenator did not compromise oxygenation and apart from the 1 unit of packed red blood cells (PRBC) and fresh frozen plasma (FFP) originally added as the prime no further blood products were used to maintain a hematocrit >35% [187]. As described above, the prime volume associated with the arterial line filter is significant adding between 20–40% in volume [186]. The Terumo Medical Corporation, Tokyo, Japan, have manufactured a miniature oxygenator, the CAPIOX® RX05 Baby RX™ Oxygenator, which has a prime volume of 43 mL with an added advantage of having an integrated arterial line filter. The group investigating it found that it was easy to use, decreased the number of gaseous emboli, and did not increase prime volume in their miniature circuit set up when compared to their regular oxygenator [186]. It can thus be appreciated that newer-generation neonatal oxygenators have an advantage in that they are specifically designed for this patient population, are easy to use, and have the benefit of small prime volumes that enable teams to attempt to achieve the goal of asanguineous prime.

Initiation of Cardiopulmonary Bypass

Before the initiation of surgery and CPB the entire team must plan strategy for the safe undertaking of the planned procedure. The surgical team ensures that the proper instrumentation is available, that the lines that will be used for the bypass are appropriately sized and that they are cut to appropriate length under the direction of the surgeon. In addition to this the surgical team assembles the appropriate mechanical or tissue valves and thaws homograft tissue patches that may be required by the surgeon for specific repairs (e.g., pulmonary artery patches or aortic augmentation). From the anesthetic perspective, apart from ensuring the patient transitions smoothly from spontaneous to controlled ventilation, the patient will be intubated for the procedure. The question of whether the patient is to be intubated orally or nasally is practitioner and institution dependent. In addition the anesthesia team will place peripheral intravenous lines, and invasive monitoring in the form of an arterial line with or without central venous line. Central venous catheters are also institution dependent with some groups avoiding them in favor of direct intracardiac lines being placed by the surgeon before termination of CPB. The reasoning is to avoid any thrombosis to the central veins, particularly in single-ventricle patients whose venous drainage from the head and neck is integral to survival. Other preparations include the placement of Foley catheters, the adjustment of the temperature of under body cooling blankets, the placement of topical cooling in the form of ice bags to the head (in those undergoing DHCA) and the placement of further monitoring (e.g., EEG, cerebral oximeters, or transcranial Doppler).

The surgeon must plan a strategy that will best enable repair of the given defect. Factors that need be considered include the potential for the use of DHCA, accessing defects through the right side of the heart, whether or not an aortic cross-clamp will be necessary, and if the size of the child being operated on will influence cannulation strategy. Options available to the surgeon include dual caval cannulation for patients having repairs of ASD, VSD, atrioventricular canal defects, tetralogy of Fallot, and transposition of the great vessels with VSD; single venous cannulation for mainly those cases in which DHCA will be employed

including augmentation of the aortic arch, Norwood stage 1 palliation, cavopulmonary anastomosis, and Fontan completion to name a few. In these cases CPB is used as a method to effectively decrease patient temperature. Once this has been achieved circulation is shut down and the cannulae are removed so that the repair may take place in a bloodless field. Importantly to this population group is meticulous de-airing of the circuit to avoid cerebral air embolus, keeping in mind that air may cross any of the intracardiac shunts.

As with the institution of CPB in the adult population, it is essential to check that the cannulae are appropriately positioned before going on to CPB. This will include the correlation of the pressure in the aorta with the invasive arterial line and that the venous cannulae are in the correct direction and that they are not potentially abutting the wall of either vena cava or right atrium. Once the patient is placed on to CPB, ventilation will cease and it is thus important to observe the oxygenation difference between the venous and the arterial cannulae as well as the SvO_2, which is measured from the bypass circuit. Table 10.8 lists both direct and indirect measures of adequate perfusion. Based on this list of measures there is a number of management strategies that may be employed should there be indicators of decreased perfusion. The perfusionist will ensure that the cardiac index is adequate based on the patient's weight or will increase MAP with the use of vasopressors agents. In the event that the cerebral saturations or SjO_2 decrease it is imperative that the surgeon check for correct placement of both arterial and venous cannulae. The arterial cannula may be directing blood away from the head vessels and the venous cannula may be positioned that it is causing obstruction to venous drainage from the head and thus decreasing cerebral perfusion pressure (CPP), which is calculated by CPP = MAP − ICP (or jugular venous pressure). Thus we see that alterations of either the arterial inflow or obstruction of outflow may result in a decrease in perfusion pressure. Other important factors that must be assessed are adequacy of hemoglobin concentration/hematocrit and oxygenation.

Table 10.8 Measures of adequate perfusion on CPB.

Direct measures
Cardiac index generated by pump
Mean arterial blood pressure generated by pump
Cerebral oximetry
Jugular bulb saturation
SvO_2

Indirect measures
Acid–base status
Plasma lactate
Urine output

Anticoagulation

At birth concentrations of the vitamin K-dependent clotting factors (II, VII, IX, X); contact factors (XI and XII); and the anticoagulant and inhibitory factors (antithrombin III, protein C, protein S, CI esterase inhibitor, and plasminogen) are all reduced. The mechanisms may include decreased hepatic synthesis or increased clearance secondary to increased metabolic rate [156,188]. Despite these apparent abnormalities normal neonates have preserved coagulation function. The same cannot be said, however, for patients with cyanotic heart disease. This patient group is known to have impaired coagulation before surgery on the basis of polycythemia, abnormal platelet count and function, decreased factor concentration (V, VII, and VIII), and increased fibrinolysis [188,189]. Table 10.9 lists factors that are associated with coagulopathy in neonates and infants presenting for surgery with CPB [188].

As has been mentioned, the institution of CPB will result in activation of the clotting cascade; thus therapeutic anticoagulation is vital to prevent the formation of clot within the circuit and the disastrous effects of possible thromboembolism into the arterial tree. The anticoagulant universally used in both adult and pediatric CPB is heparin. At the Children's Hospital of Philadelphia the patient is given 200 IU/kg either by the surgeon as a direct injection into the right atrium or by the anesthesiologist into a peripheral intravenous site. Other institutions use between 300 and 400 IU/kg. The goal activated clotting time (ACT) is ≥480 seconds. This is based on early work by Bull and colleagues who formulated a heparin-protamine dose-response curve in the attempt to avert the use of either excess heparin or protamine [190]. Heparin works by binding to antithrombin III (ATIII) resulting in a conformational change in the enzyme and enhancing its activity. Under normal conditions there is a continuous balance between coagulation and anticoagulation within the body.

ATIII functions to inactivate thrombin and other proteases, most notably Factor Xa, thus preventing ongoing propagation of the clotting cascade. The effect of heparin on ATIII is to increase its efficacy by a factor of a thousand. As mentioned earlier the level of ATIII is decreased in neonates and only will reach adult levels by 3–6 months. Patients in this age group may be at risk for inadequate anticoagulation. However, it has been found that there are two other thrombin inhibitors, namely heparin-cofactor II and α-2-macroglobulin, and indeed the concentration of α-2-macroglobulin in neonates and infants is twice as high as that of ATIII. Guzzetta and colleagues tested a group of patients with ages from the neonatal to more than 10 years of age. Interestingly they found that despite these concerns, statistically significant prolongation in the ACT and the heparin dose–response relationship occurred in the neonatal group. The authors postulated that this could be on the basis that either neonates generate less thrombin or that ACT is a poor indicator of anticoagulation in this age group. This could be explained by the fact that these neonates already have in place umbilical or central lines and many have had interventions performed in the cardiac catheterization laboratory that triggered hemostatic activation. It would thus seem unlikely that thrombin production is lower in this age group. The ACT as an indicator may play an important role for a number of reasons. Firstly the ACT value does not correlate with the heparin concentration on CPB, secondly hypothermia and hemodilution may cause inaccuracy, and thirdly the decreased levels of contact activation factors (factors XII and XI, prekallikrein, and high-molecular-weight kininogen) may complicate the interpretation of prolonged ACT [191]. Studies have shown that despite an adequate ACT and a lack of visible clot there may indeed be thrombin generation at a cellular level, which may lead to increased platelet binding and also decreased levels of factor VIII. Based on these factors investigators have suggested that a protocol based on heparin concentration may be more effective [192,193]. In a separate study Guzzetta and colleagues found that with the heparin concentration technique there was decreased thrombin generation as well as preserved factor VIII levels, suggesting improved anticoagulation. The authors did, however, indicate that this higher heparin concentration method lead to increased blood requirements [192].

A concern in patients who present for repeat cardiac surgery is the incidence of heparin-induced thrombocytopenia (HIT) in the pediatric population. There are two forms of HIT. HIT-1 is characterized by a transient early onset of a nonimmune-mediated decrease in platelet count that does not require the discontinuation of heparin. HIT-2 is characterized by an immune-mediated decrease in platelet count by >50% [194]. In the adult cardiac experience the quoted incidence of this phenomenon post CPB is 1–3% with a thrombotic morbidity of between 38% and 81% and

Table 10.9 Factors related to coagulopathic complications in neonates and infants. (Reproduced with permission from Jaggers et al. [188].)

Procedure-independent factors	Procedure-dependant factors
Ductal dependent flow	Hemodilution
Cyanosis	Hypothermia
Prematurity	DHCA
Low cardiac output	Redo surgery
Neurologic injury	Prolonged CPB
Sepsis	Use of prosthetic material
Malnutrition	Low cardiac output

a mortality of 28% [195]. The syndrome itself is an immune-mediated syndrome of platelet activation resulting in thrombocytopenia and diffuse venous and even arterial thrombosis. Thrombocytopenia will occur some days after the exposure to unfractionated heparin with platelet counts dropping to between 20 and $100 \times 10^9/L$. It is important, however, to be mindful of any drop in the platelet count as a drop in the count by 50%, even if the count is still in the normal range, is considered to be of significance. The antibodies are formed against platelet factor 4 (PF4) that is found on the surface of activated platelets as well as on endothelial cell surfaces secondary to heparin exposure. The presence of these antibodies occurs in up to 50% of adult cardiac surgery patients but only the quoted 1–3% will go onto develop the syndrome [195]. This seems to suggest that, although the platelet antibody is itself common after CPB, this in and of itself does not infer increased risk. It should, however, be noted that a positive antibody with thrombocytopenia places the patient at increased risk of developing HIT. In the adult population it seems that in those with a positive antibody the incidence of developing HIT is <10% [196]. The older pediatric population shows an incidence of a 50% positive antibody screen at the 10-day mark postoperatively [196]. In a case series of neonates, infants, and young children there were 10 cases of HIT with associated thrombotic complications [197]. These authors concluded that based on their experience, the incidence of HIT was equal to that in the adult population being 1.3%. In a separate study patients undergoing second surgeries were screened for presence of PF4 antibodies. The results once again echoed the prior studies in that there were 2/144 patients or 1.38% [198].

What are the alternatives to the use of heparin in a pediatric patient with a history of HIT or indeed HIT with associated thrombosis? In this regard three possible alternatives are available: 1) the use of an alternative anticoagulant with the complete avoidance of all heparin both intra- and postoperatively; 2) standard heparin anticoagulation with a platelet antagonist; and 3) waiting until the disappearance of HIT antibodies and proceeding with heparin anticoagulation [199]. A number of drugs are available for anticoagulation and are listed in Table 10.10. Of these aforementioned drugs it appears that only lepirudin and argatroban have been used to any degree. As they are both direct thrombin inhibitors they both work by directly and reversibly binding to the catalytic site of thrombin thus inhibiting the conversion of fibrinogen to fibrin. Successful use of both of these agents has been described in the literature in a wide range of procedures and ages. The advantage of the use of argatroban is that it is metabolized in the liver and can thus be used in patients with renal failure (lepirudin is renally excreted), can be monitored by ACT and has a half-life of <60 minutes. As HIT is a significant clinical problem but with a relatively low occurrence large clinical

Table 10.10 Alternative drugs to heparin for anticoagulation.

Glycoprotein IIb/IIIa inhibitors
Abciximab
Eptifibatide
Tirofiban

Direct Thrombin inhibitors
Hirudin
Lepirudin
Bivalirudin
Argatroban

Defibrinogenating enzymes
Ancrod

studies have not as yet been performed and thus dosing protocols are not standardized. Argatroban is used as an infusion with initial rates varying between 2 and 65 µg/kg/min. The use of an initial bolus was used inconsistently with a range of 35–750 µg/kg in divided doses. To maintain the ACT in the appropriate range further bolus doses of 20 µg/kg were used. The major adverse events related to these nonstandardized regimens were abnormally prolonged ACT and bleeding. There is no reversal drug as with heparin-protamine and thus the patient would require transfusions and even the use of factor VII [194,200,201]. Lepirudin has also been used for CPB although it may be more difficult to use based on its longer half life of 40–80 minutes, the need for ecarin clotting time (ECT) and renal excretion. It is also possible to monitor lepirudin with the activated partial thromboplastin time (aPTT) but this test would take too long in the setting of CPB. Just like with argatroban there is no reversal agent. Dosing of this agent follows the adult dosing of a bolus of 0.25 mg/kg and 0.2 mg/kg into the CPB circuit although a single group suggested increasing these doses due to a greater volume of distribution [198,202,203].

At the termination of CPB and as the cannulae are being removed protamine will be administered to reverse the anticoagulation owing to heparin. As with many areas in practice there is a range of dosing used in the clinical arena. As mentioned at the Children's Hospital of Philadelphia the heparin dosing is 200 IU/kg and for reversal the protamine dosing is 4 mg/kg with a maximum of 100 mg. This works out to be a ratio of protamine to heparin of 2:1 based on 1 mg of protamine to 100 IU (sometimes referred to as 1 mg) of heparin. In a survey of units within Great Britain and Ireland there was a reported ratio of 0.3:1 to 2:1 after a uniform heparin dose of 300 IU/kg. In adult cardiac surgery adverse reactions to the administration of protamine are well known and include anaphylactic and anaphylactoid reactions as well as pulmonary hypertensive events. The clinical result is a range from minor hypotensive events to fatal cardiovascular collapse. Although catastrophic events are rare, adverse events occur in up to 2.6% of adult patients [204]. Risk factors for adults include the use of protamine-containing insulin, previous drug reaction or exposure, vasectomy, rate of infusion, and allergy to protamine or fish. Pediatric patients, however, have different risks as they have less frequent or shorter exposures to cross-reacting antigens and lesser sensitivity to pulmonary intravascular macrophages to heparin–protamine complexes [205]. A study looking at the incidence in the pediatric population ≤16 years of age found that in a series of 1249 anesthetics the incidence of hypotension that persisted for >5 minutes was in the order of 1.76%. The authors noted that this might have included causes other than a protamine reaction due to the proximity to termination of CPB. Of interest in this study were the associated risk factors for hypotension namely: female sex, large dose of protamine, and a small heparin dose. The reason for the female sex being a risk could not be explained [205]. In a case report describing severe pulmonary hypertension, hypoxemia, and cardiovascular collapse after heparin reversal it appears that large protamine dosing of 10.7 mg/kg after an initial event and a subsequent 5.8 mg/kg after a second event were the etiological factors. Also of note was the female sex of the patient. This patient required inotropic support, jet ventilation, intravenous prostacyclin, and inhaled nitric oxide, but subsequently made a complete recovery [206]. In summary in relation to this reaction vigilance when giving any patient any drug cannot be overemphasized.

Termination of Bypass

In termination of CPB a number of important criteria need to be met. These will need to be identified and treated concomitantly at a time when the patient's clinical condition may be extremely tenuous.

General Principles

Before the termination of CPB an adequate cardiac rhythm must be established and if the native rhythm is inadequate either by rate or rhythm itself the heart will need external stimuli in the form of atrial and/or ventricular epicardial pacing. The use of inotropic support will obviously depend on the case, the presence of preexisting myocardial dysfunction, and the duration of CPB. In the pediatric setting this may take the form of dopamine, epinephrine, and milrinone but under certain circumstances vasopressin may be necessary. Concomitant with this will be the re-expansion of the lungs and resumption of ventilation. It is important that the lungs are fully re-expanded as atelectasis will lead to not only hypoxemia but also direct compression of the pulmonary bed. The combination of these two factors will lead to an increase in pulmonary artery pressure. In the neonate who already has an extremely reactive pulmonary

bed this may lead to a spiral of increasing hypoxia, worsening pulmonary artery pressure, and subsequent right ventricular failure, which may necessitate placing the patient back onto CPB or even ECMO. The principles of preventing this phenomenon include adequate ventilation as eluded to above, ensuring adequate oxygenation, avoiding hypothermia, avoiding acidosis, the use of the phosphodiesterase inhibitor milrinone, and, as a last resort, using inhaled nitric oxide as a direct pulmonary artery vasodilator.

Hypothermia

If the procedure was performed at anything but normothermia the patient needs to be rewarmed to normal. Hypothermia may result in a wide range of abnormalities. Experimental evidence suggests that hypothermia will result in a negative inotropic effect at the atrial level, an effect that may be detrimental at the termination of CPB as normal atrial function is an important contributor of ventricular preload [207]. Hypothermic effects on ventricular function include bradycardia, heart block, reduction of fibrillation threshold, and an increase in pacing threshold. These effects may occur even at moderate hypothermia [205]. Termination of CPB necessitates adequate heart rate that may require external pacing and thus normothermia is vital. Another important problem related to hypothermia in the cardiac surgery patient is the effect that it has on bleeding. It appears that hypothermia will affect both platelet function as well as the coagulation cascade. The defect in platelet function is related to an impaired release of thromboxane A2, which is necessary for the formation of the platelet plug. The coagulation is affected by a temperature-dependent decrease in enzyme function. These effects may occur at even 1–2 °C below normal [208,209]. Even if patients are normothermic on termination of CPB, for obvious reasons it is imperative to keep patients warm thereafter as temperature may drift downwards soon after resumption of spontaneous circulation placing them at risk once again.

Bleeding

The origins of the ongoing coagulopathy upon termination of bypass are multifactorial and include cascade activation due to CPB, therapeutic hypothermia as part of CPB, dilutional, consumptive, and due to ongoing bleeding from the surgical site. Obviously strategies at preventing blood loss must start at the beginning of CPB. These attempts focus on limiting hemodilution, the use of antifibrinolytic agents, and use of fresh whole blood in the prime volume. We have already discussed at length the effects of hemodilution and thus it will not be discussed again.

The antifibrinolytics in use are the serine protease inhibitor aprotinin and the lysine analogs ε-aminocaproic acid and tranexamic acid. Aprotinin inhibits kallikrein and plasmin with resultant decrease in hemostatic activation, inhibition of fibrinolysis, inhibition of the inflammatory cascade, and the preservation of platelet function. It is eliminated via the kidneys and then reabsorbed via the proximal tubule and then enzymatically broken down in phagolysosomes. Attempts have been made to establish the overall effects of the drug but this has been difficult as published studies have included small groups of patients, nonheterogeneous groups, and inconsistent dosing. It does appear that there were trends toward less bleeding, improved transpulmonary pressure gradients suggesting decreased inflammation and capillary leak, improved myocardial function, and decreased postoperative ventilation [156]. As mentioned prior problems were identified in the adult cardiac world with respect to postoperative renal failure and thrombosis risk in patients who received the drug and, despite these theoretical advantages, the drug is no longer used even in pediatric cardiac surgery, despite pediatric data, which may suggest that there is no statistically significant renal failure, need for dialysis, worsened neurological outcome or mortality (early or late) in the pediatric group [153,154,210–212]. At this time there is no plan to reintroduce the drug to market. The role of the lysine analogs has also long been studied. The mechanism of action is to interfere with the binding of plasminogen to fibrin, which is necessary for the activation of plasminogen to plasmin. Both drugs are eliminated via the kidneys with terminal half-life of 2 hours. The apparent advantages in comparison to aprotinin include the lack of an immunologic response, low cost, suggestion of platelet protection, and similar efficacy to aprotinin with respect to bleeding. In a meta-analysis containing more than 1000 patients it was found that in both cyanotic as well as acyanotic patients there was decreased bleeding, transfusion requirements, decreased sternal closure time, and improved re-exploration rates with the use of the lysine analogs. In two of the reviewed articles there was no improvement in postoperative ventilation time suggesting that these drugs have no anti-inflammatory effect [156]. In a further meta-analysis containing all three of the aforementioned drugs, the effect on bleeding was found to be similar comparing aprotinin to tranexamic acid with insufficient data to draw conclusions with the use of ε-aminocaproic acid [213]. In a further randomized study the two lysine analogs were compared in a cohort of patients ranging in age from 2 months to 14 years all with cyanotic heart disease. The results showed that both drugs had similar efficacy in decreasing postoperative blood loss as well as the use of blood products [214].

Introduced into the adult world in the late 1980s with investigations in pediatrics in the early 1990s, the use of fresh whole blood in the priming volume (between 24 hours and 48 hours old) carried a theoretical advantage over stored blood or reconstituted blood (made of packed red cells, FFP, and platelets) in that the coagulation factors

and platelets had little time to degrade due to cold storage thus improving post-bypass hemostasis. Other advantages sited by proponents are the decrease in systemic inflammation manifest as decreased edema and improved organ function [215]. An early study from the group at the Children's Hospital of Philadelphia followed three groups of patients all under 21 years of age and representing both cyanotic and acyanotic conditions. In this study one group received very fresh whole blood (<6 hours old), the second received fresh whole blood, whilst the third received reconstituted blood. All subjects who required blood in the prime solution received whole blood. Once the heparin was reversed any further bleeding and/or volume requirements were met with the assigned blood. It was found that patients who received the reconstituted blood had significantly more bleeding in comparison to the other two groups and that the most significant decrease in bleeding was in patients who were transfused fresh whole blood and were <2 years of age undergoing complex repairs. Another interesting finding from this was that despite theoretical advantages of the very fresh whole blood there was no significant difference in bleeding between the two whole blood groups [216]. Further study into the question of fresh whole blood has looked at comparing reconstituted fresh whole blood versus banked blood and also into reconstituted blood versus fresh whole blood [215,217]. A head-to-head comparison of fresh whole blood versus reconstituted blood (PRBC and FFP) in circuit prime had outcomes in favor of the reconstituted blood. Although there was no difference in chest tube output and requirements for transfusions between the two groups the fresh whole blood was associated with increased perioperative fluid overload, increased ventilation, and prolonged ICU stay. The authors concluded that, although the reconstituted blood group required more donor exposure by four donors as compared to 3.5 in the fresh whole blood group, in their opinion the clinical hazards of fresh whole blood outweighed the risk of increased exposure. Despite these findings there is ongoing debate and, as further research is performed into circuit size, this debate may be resolved by the use of asanguineous prime [217].

The question of ongoing bleeding despite the above strategies occurs in a multitude of cardiac surgeries including patients with cyanotic heart disease, patients having long bypass times, DHCA, and those with operations that involve multiple suture lines. In these patients it is useful to perform coagulation studies, platelet counts, and fibrinogen levels to better guide therapy. The problem, however, is that there are not many institutions that can perform these tests in a time period where the results are still clinically relevant. Ongoing bleeding is treated with packed red cells or fresh whole blood with component therapy transfused as needed in the form of cryoprecipitate, platelets, or even FFP. Desmopressin acetate (DDAVP) has been used due to the characteristic of the drug that it will decrease platelet dysfunction after CPB. DDAVP will increase the release of von Willebrand factor (vWF) multimers and factor VIII from endothelial storage sites. Factor VIII levels will increase immediately and that of vWF will peak in 30–60 minutes. The net effect of this is to augment platelet adhesion and aggregation [218]. Although the use of DDAVP has found success in adult cardiac surgery patients, the same results have not been found in pediatric patients, with studies finding no improvement in coagulation in patients who have been given the medication as a prophylactic measure [218,219].

In patients who continue to bleed despite the attempts to correct coagulopathy with blood products the use of recombinant factor VII has become a significant part of the armamentarium. The drug has been used clinically once coagulation factors, fibrinogen, and platelets have been administered and all attempts to correct surgical bleeding have failed; in some instances it has been used as a prophylactic measure in those surgeries which have seen long CPB times with a multitude of suture lines. Unfortunately, like with many drugs, pediatric dosing is extrapolated from adults. The dose thus is between 90 and 120 μg/kg, which is given every 2–3 hours. Studies have demonstrated that the half-life of fFactor VII in pediatrics may be half of that in the adult and that clearance is faster, possibly indicating a higher dose requirement [220]. It has also been suggested that transfusion of coagulation factors, fibrinogen, and platelets prior to the administration of factor VII may also affect the dosing regimen [220]. The pediatric experience thus far in the history of the drug has suggested it to be extremely efficacious but with some limitations and potential complications. The cost is extremely high with a 1- to 2-mg vial costing around $1000, with some patients obviously requiring more than just the one vial. The other concerns surround clot formation and thrombosis. Case reports have described mediastinal clot formation that in some cases has required emergency evacuation [221]. The drug has been used also in patients with intractable bleeding whilst on ECMO with success. In this subgroup of patients there is obviously concern for circuit thrombosis that would have catastrophic consequences and it has been suggested that the dosing be reduced to 30–50 μg/kg [221]. Yet another study has demonstrated no complications using the standard dose of 90–120 μg/kg in a group of ECMO patients [222]. Despite its very important place in the management of the post-CPB patient, there is still much investigation around the use of this drug with respect to optimal dosing as well as administration interval.

Anatomical Considerations and the Use of Transesophageal Echocardiography

Essential to the termination of CPB is an anatomically sound repair. This is true from a simple repair such as a secundum atrial septal defect to the complexities of a stage 1 Norwood reconstruction for the single ventricle. The effects of CPB on the myocardium are well proved and the longer the bypass time the worse these effects may become due to failure to establish electrical quiescence, unequal myocardial cooling, and the ongoing inflammatory cascade. It thus stands to reason a myocardium recovering from these insults will not function well should there be residual outflow tract obstruction, abnormal coronary flow, or abnormal flow through intracardiac baffles. Intraoperative transesophageal echocardiography (TEE) can thus be vital in diagnosing these problems in patients who are difficult to wean from CPB or who are possibly more cyanotic than expected. The problem in the early days of TEE was that probe size limited use in small patients and neonates – precisely the group of patients undergoing the most complex of procedures. Fortunately in recent years there has been development of probes that can be used in patients down to approximately 2.5 kg [223]. The incidence of post-CPB residual defects diagnosed by TEE, which will go on to require a second CPB run is approximately 7–9.6% across reported series [224–226]. This is clearly a significant number of patients who would possibly have required later reoperation or even postoperative emergent ECMO cannulation due to acute cardiac failure. Complications associated with passage of the TEE probe include failure to pass the probe, esophageal trauma that includes laceration or even perforation, airway compression, and hemodynamic compromise. The hemodynamic issues are related to compression of structures, which include the ascending and descending aorta, left atrium, pulmonary artery and veins, and superior vena cava [226]. Despite these possible complications they remain rare. In a study of 22 patients between 2 and 5 kg who underwent TEE examination before and after CPB no differences in lung function or arterial blood gas were found. In two patients the probe was removed because of concerns about ventilation unrelated to the TEE probe. The aforementioned parameters did not change before or after the removal of the probe [227]. In another study performed by the same authors looking this time at hemodynamic parameters, they found that there was an incidence of compromise in 1.7% of patients [226]. Despite the theoretical concerns in the very smallest of patients TEE examinations can be performed safely.

Modified Ultrafiltration

The institution of CPB will set up a proinflammatory state that is coupled with varying degrees of hemodilution. The net effect of this will be capillary leak that results in an increase in total body water and edema. This phenomenon, although affecting the entire body, will be especially problematic for the lungs, myocardium, and brain. Pulmonary compliance will decrease and the end result of myocardial edema is both systolic and diastolic dysfunction [108,228]. Strategies that have been employed include the use of steroids, coated CPB circuits, and miniaturized CPB circuits. First described in 1991 by Naik and colleagues, modified ultrafiltration (MUF) was formulated to improve the removal of this excess body fluid after the termination of CPB. These authors found that their new technique was better able to remove body water and elevate hematocrit when compared to conventional ultrafiltration that is employed whilst the patient is still on bypass [229]. The perfusionist employs a number of forms of filtration, all of which are aimed at limiting the inevitable increase in total body water, as well as removal of electrolytes and inflammatory mediators. Prime ultrafiltration (PUF) is used when packed red cells are added to the prime volume. The aim of this filtration technique is to remove any unfavorable electrolyte elevations associated with stored blood, increase the pH closer to physiological range, and also decrease the inflammatory response [230]. Conventional ultrafiltration (CUF) is employed throughout CPB with a common use being the removal of extra volume and electrolytes added to the circuit after the use of cardioplegia. In zero balance ultrafiltration (ZBUF) crystalloid is added to the circuit at the time of ultrafiltration. A complication of ultrafiltration is depletion of the venous reservoir volume and thus ZBUF is an attempt to counter this hypovolemia. Dilutional ultrafiltration is the last method of ultrafiltration used with the patient on CPB. The aim of this method is the dilution of a given electrolyte that is elevated. Dilution is achieved by the addition of hypotonic fluid (e.g., half normal saline) into the circuit at the time of the ultrafiltration. The common goal of these methods is removal of excess free water and inflammatory mediators and maintaining the hematocrit at a safe level whilst on CPB.

Studies have shown that MUF will improve both cardiac and pulmonary function, increase hematocrit, and remove inflammatory mediators and that these effects are improved over the other ultrafiltration techniques described. The technique of MUF includes the following modifications to the CPB circuit upon weaning from bypass. A clamp is applied which functionally disconnects the venous line from the venous reservoir. A line is then brought up to connect the ultrafilter directly onto the venous line (Figure 10.9) [228]. The direction of flow to the ultrafilter is then from the venous reservoir and from the arterial line. A roller pump is then interposed between the blood source and the filter to ensure blood moves toward the patient at a rate of approximately 200 mL/min. Suction is also applied to the filter at about -125 mmHg to achieve a filter rate of approximately 100–150 mL/min [228]. Saline is used to chase the blood still in the venous reservoir through the circuit and also to maintain right atrial filling pressure at the desired level. The endpoints are time of the MUF procedure (usually 15–20 minutes), the desired hematocrit of

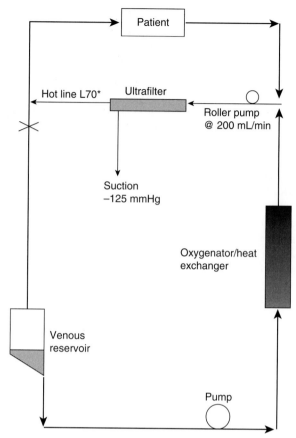

Figure 10.9 Set-up for modified ultrafiltration. (Reproduced with permission from Davies *et al.* [228].)

≥40, replacement of the venous reservoir with crystalloid, or the patient's inability to tolerate the procedure.

Table 10.11 shows the positive effects of MUF. The advantages of MUF with respect to cardiac function have been studied across the spectrum of patients [108,228,231,232]. The improvements in myocardial performance appear to be related to the decrease in myocardial edema that is seen after CPB. It has been shown that after MUF there is an increase in systolic function coupled with an increase in end-diastolic length and decrease in end-diastolic pressure. These improvements in diastolic function indicate improvement in left ventricular compliance [228]. In this study the myocardial dimensions were measured using intraoperative ultrasonic transducers. This was in agreement with earlier clinical observations made by Naik and his team in their original description. They observed that there was a universal rise in blood pressure and an apparent decrease in the myocardial dimension [230]. Overall MUF leads to improved left and right heart function. MUF has been shown to also improve pulmonary vascular resistance even in those patients who had elevated pulmonary pressure in the preoperative phase, an effect that lasts into the postoperative phase [108,231]. The patient

Table 10.11 Effects of modified ultrafiltration.

General effects
↓ Total body water
↓ Inflammatory markers

Cardiac effects
LV – improved systolic and diastolic function
RV – improved function secondary ↓ pulmonary arterial pressure

Pulmonary effects
↓ Interstitial water
↑ Compliance
↑ Ventilation/oxygenation
↓ Pulmonary artery pressure

Hematological effects
↑ Clotting factors/fibrinogen
↑ Plasma protein
↓ Transfusion requirements

with single-ventricle physiology is potentially at risk during the process of MUF because blood is being drawn away from the aorta, which is thus taking blood from the coronaries as well as the pulmonary flow (in those patients with a modified Blalock–Taussig shunt). In a study by Gaynor and colleagues, however, this was shown to be a safe procedure in this group with similar improvements in myocardial function as noted earlier [232].

Improving pulmonary function is important for not only myocardial function but for ventilation–oxygenation and the resulting decrease in the need for postoperative mechanical ventilation. Pulmonary dysfunction after CPB is manifest as lowered compliance, increased pulmonary vascular resistance, and a decrease in gas exchange. The mechanisms associated are related to hemodilution that decreases plasma oncotic pressure resulting in an increase in interstitial fluid. This is coupled with the atelectasis that occurs secondary to no ventilation on CPB. Furthermore the lung is obviously ischemic during bypass, which leads to the production of oxygen free radicals once the lung is reperfused. Lastly other factors such as hypothermia and foreign body contact of blood with the CPB circuit result in the release of inflammatory mediators that may further worsen pulmonary damage [231]. The effects of MUF are thus secondary to a decrease in interstitial fluid that in turn leads to increased pulmonary compliance, improved oxygenation, and a decrease in pulmonary artery pressure. All these positive factors will also lead to improvement of right ventricular function [108,231]. From the studies already referenced an added benefit to these pulmonary improvements is decreased postoperative ventilation and, in turn, ICU stay.

MUF has also been shown to improve the coagulopathy associated with CPB as well as decrease the transfusion requirements. CPB leads to a hemodilutional state which effects hematocrit and coagulation factors as well as a sepa-

rate effect on platelet number and function. The effect of MUF will lead to an increase in hematocrit (which in patients with single-ventricle physiology will improve oxygen saturation and oxygen-carrying capacity) and improvements in the level of coagulation factors by removing the aforementioned dilutional volume. This will in turn lead to improved coagulation, decreased bleeding, and decreased blood requirements. These effects have been shown in neonates and in those with prolonged CPB, two groups who are associated with increased bleeding. Despite these obvious advantages MUF has no effect on platelets [108,231,233,234].

Creation of a cavopulmonary anastomosis and Fontan completion will result in an increase in venous pressure. This is the primary etiologic association found in a subgroup of these patients who develop postoperative pulmonary or pericardial effusions. In an early study looking into the effect of MUF on associated morbidities it was found that there was a significant reduction in effusions. The difference was found to be most significant in the Fontan group where the incidence was 48.5% in the control group whereas in the MUF group this decreased to 10.5%. In those patients undergoing cavopulmonary anastomosis the control group showed 11.5% versus 4.9% [234]. The morbidity and mortality associated with ongoing effusions include chronic hypoxia and ongoing protein loss resulting in anasarca and immune suppression. These findings have been supported in other studies [108,235]. Clearly the use of MUF plays an important role in decreasing this morbidity and mortality. Recent advances have also included the creation of a fenestration in the Fontan baffle that serves as a pressure release from the now high pressure venous system into the atrial chamber.

The systemic inflammatory response that is generated with the onset of CPB can prove to be deleterious to organ function when attempts are made to wean from bypass. Inflammatory cytokines such as TNF, IL-6, IL-8, thromboxane B_2, and endothelin 1(ET-1) are released secondary to this inflammatory process. The first three of these are prominent in the systemic inflammatory response syndrome that occurs post CPB while the latter factors may contribute to the pulmonary vascular hyperactivity and pulmonary hypertension that occurs in certain individuals. As the use of MUF improves clinical outcomes, studies have attempted to show that it will lead to the decrease in these factors. Huang and colleagues showed that the use of continuous ultrafiltration and MUF will lead to a decrease in the concentration of IL-6 but had no effect on ET-1 [236]. Contrary to this study Bando and colleagues found that a combination of dilutional ultrafiltration with MUF will result in the decrease in ET-1, thus decreasing pulmonary/systemic pressure ratio and also lower ventilatory requirements [237]. In a third study the addition of a polysulfon ultrafilter to the MUF circuit for both conventional ultrafiltration and MUF improved the removal of IL-6 and TNF [107].

Despite all these positive effects of MUF there are important safety concerns. These include: inadvertent cooling during the procedure; hypotension if too much blood is drawn off via the arterial line; and varying technical difficulties with the circuit, for example air cavitating out of solution in the arterial line, clotted MUF circuit, and exsanguination owing to unclamping of the oxygenator circuit.

The effect of hypoperfusion/reperfusion has the potential to cause a breakdown in the normal gastrointestinal mucosal barrier. The translocation of endotoxins into the bloodstream may result in hypotension, fever, hypermetabolism, tissue damage, and coagulopathy, all factors that can cause problems as patients are being weaned from CPB. Yngaard and colleagues found that the endotoxin load significantly increased during CPB, peaking at the end of CPB. The use of MUF significantly decreased the load from 24.2 ng at the peak to 9 ng after MUF with the majority of the load found in the ultrafiltrate. In a separate study quoted by these authors it was found that an endotoxin load >4 ng/kg may depress myocardial function. The conclusion of the study was that despite not removing the load, MUF may aid in the modification of the inflammatory response seen [238].

The use of MUF has become standard in the performance of congenital cardiac surgery with the benefits as listed above. In most centers patients undergo continuous ultrafiltration in one form or another during CPB with MUF being performed on weaning from bypass. The disadvantages are mainly of a technical nature that can be overcome with experience. When combined with the other modalities already discussed in this chapter the use of MUF is an important adjuvant in combating the deleterious effects of CPB.

Treatment of Post Cardiotomy and Acute Cardiac Failure

In some patients there is an apparent period of hemodynamic and ventilatory stability that is followed by instability of varying degrees upon sternal closure. This may necessitate that the sternum remain open for a period ranging from a few hours up to 2–3 days. This is achieved by placing a tube strut between the two sternal edges (a rigid tube, e.g., a 4- to 5-mm endotracheal tube may suffice) and then closing the skin with a Gore-Tex patch. Concerns for this technique are obviously the risk of infection, tamponade due to inadequate drainage, and the inability to perform cardiopulmonary resuscitation (CPR) in the face of cardiopulmonary arrest. Sternal closure can then be achieved either in the ICU or in the operating room. At the Children's Hospital of Philadelphia this is routinely performed in the ICU with good results.

Table 10.12 Differences between ECMO and VAD.

	ECMO	VAD
Acute resuscitation	+	−
Bleeding at insertion	+	+++
Thromboembolic risk	+	+
Long-term support	−	++
Pulmonary support	+	−
Awake patient	−/+	+++
Able to ambulate	−	+++
Pulsatile flow	−	+

Cardiac failure may occur in a wide range of settings and may require immediate or planned intervention. The two modalities used are extracorporeal membrane oxygenation (ECMO) and ventricular assist devices (VAD). Table 10.12 lists some of the differences between these two modalities.

ECMO has been used in a number of settings that include mechanical cardiac failure or oxygenation failure upon weaning from CPB, ECMO-CPR (E-CPR) in a wide array of clinical settings, and emergent elective ECMO (e.g., severe myocarditis with impending cardiac failure secondary to nonperfusing rhythm or low cardiac output or even preoperative). In the majority of cases ECMO is established by cannulating either the neck or directly through the open chest at the time of cardiac surgery. The neck is cannulated by using the internal jugular vein to access the central venous circulation and the carotid artery to access the aorta. The advantage of ECMO is the speed at which it can be deployed and hence the concept of E-CPR has been widely promoted, with many institutions having ECMO teams on call on a 24 hours a day basis. An added advantage to this is that cannulation can be performed by noncardiac surgeons. This clearly requires a large institutional commitment of both manpower and resources. In a 2007 review from the Extracorporeal Life Support Organization it was found that in 73% of cases (499/682) E-CPR was used primarily for children with primary cardiac disease with the survival to discharge quoted as 38% [239]. Later series have quoted survival rates of 39–44% [240,241]. This is in comparison to a series of only cardiac patients who underwent ECMO placement both after cardiac surgery and as part of management for low cardiac output not associated with surgery [242]. In this series the survival to 24 hours post decannulation was 58%; however, the overall survival was only 39%. In 2005 the American Heart Association made the following recommendations regarding E-CPR: 1) E-CPR is considered if initial resuscitation attempts fail and the condition leading to the arrest is reversible or amenable to heart transplant; 2) CPR is started no more than a few minutes after no cardiac output; 3) ability to rapidly perform ECMO [243]. The survival rate in published series for patients treated only with CPR ranges from 16–34.5% [244–246]. These data include patients who underwent CPR for bradycardia with spontaneous but decreased perfusion. This group of patients will elevate the survival percentage; for patients who had an asystolic arrest the survival percentage was substantially less. At first glance this difference in survival does not appear to be that great but considering that a 10% difference between CPR and E-CPR translates to ten lives saved out of 100 this is undoubtedly a significant difference under the appropriate circumstances. Figure 10.10 shows a schematic representation of an ECMO circuit [247]. Although this drawing depicts cannulation through the chest, the same set-up is used for neck cannulation. In the group of patients who require cannulation as part of ongoing CPR or in the operating room where there is failure to wean from CPB either from a cardiac or pulmonary standpoint, the decision to proceed to ECMO cannulation is an obvious one. The decision, however, to "electively" cannulate a patient as part of ongoing management is a decision that is not taken lightly. The use of ECMO requires ongoing anticoagulation and just as with CPB an inflammatory cascade is started. The concerns with anticoagulation encompass both sides of the problem: undercoagulation with resultant circuit clot formation and the possibility of embolic phenomena to the brain, limbs or abdominal cavity; or overcoagulation with catastrophic cerebral hemorrhage as a devastating complication. Anticoagulation is achieved with the use of intravenous heparin with the

target ACT of 180–220 seconds. There are those patients who may even go on to develop heparin-induced thrombocytopenia that will necessitate anticoagulation with an alternative anticoagulant. Other concerns include the development of infection, renal failure, pulmonary hemorrhage, lack of improvement of the original etiological factor, and the inability to bridge the patient to transplant in the case of a primary cardiac etiology.

In a series of patients looking at the outcomes of patients placed on ECMO prior to corrective surgery the investigators had a number of interesting findings. This series of patients had a median age of 0.12 months with a range of 0–193 months with 17 patients being neonates and a further six being younger than 1 year. The patients in this series were representative of both single and biventricular repairs. Hypoxia was the predisposing factor in 65% and all patients were operated on whilst on ECMO. In all there were 16 patients who survived to hospital discharge. Failure to wean from ECMO/CPB at the end of corrective/palliative surgery was the most significant risk factor. Other associations were weight less than 2 kg and neonatal patients. Although the nature of the postoperative circulation was not found to be a significant risk factor, patients who underwent complex repairs of single-ventricle physiology had higher mortality [248].

The most devastating complication associated with either E-CPR or ECMO is neurological injury caused by hypoxia at the time of arrest or embolic and hemorrhagic events on ECMO. It has been found that in patients undergoing E-CPR those patients with cardiac causes for

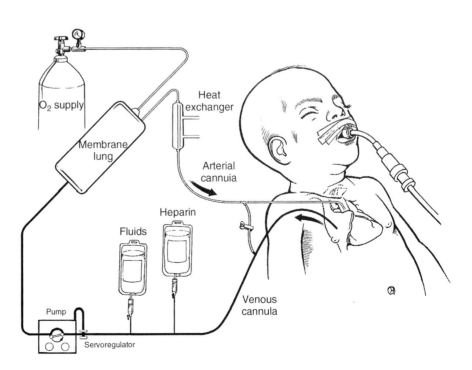

Figure 10.10 Schematic representation of ECMO circuit. (Reproduced with permission from Aharon *et al.* [247].)

requiring ECMO had improved neurological outcomes compared to those with pulmonary or metabolic etiologies. It has been postulated that this is due to the fact that post-operative cardiac patients are in ICU with continuous hemodynamic monitoring, vascular access, and, importantly, practitioners trained to rapidly deploy CPR and ECMO. Additionally patients who develop arrest secondary to respiratory causes are severely hypoxic at the time of arrest and thus are at increased risk of neurological damage [249]. The overall incidence of neurological complications was between 12% and 26%, which are indeed significant numbers [243,249,250]. Associated risk factors include severe metabolic acidosis at the time of going on ECMO, hypercarbia, venoarterial ECMO, ongoing inotrope and vasopressor requirement, and the need for further CPR whilst on ECMO. Location of cannulation was not found to be an independent risk factor for neurological outcome [249].

Assessing mortality risk factors is difficult in this patient subgroup. In the aforementioned cardiac ICU series the patients were divided into those post surgery and those not. In postoperative patients it appeared that age <1 month, male sex, and the development of renal and/or hepatic failure appeared to be risk factors. In the group who did not undergo surgery prior to going on ECMO there were no clearly significant factors, although male gender and renal/hepatic failure were nonstatistically significant associations. In this series the indication for ECMO (i.e., failure to separate from CPB or cardiac lesion such as single ventricle) was not found to be a predictor of mortality; similarly the duration of ECMO was no reason to withdraw support [242]. In an earlier series of 50 patients who required ECMO in the immediate post-CPB phase and ranging in age from 1 day to 11 years, it was found that those who had biventricular physiology had worse mortality than the single-ventricle patients in the same series. These findings were in contrast to earlier published data where it was found that patients undergoing the Norwood repair had the lowest survival rates amongst ECMO patients. These authors pointed to maintaining a balanced circulation for the single-ventricle patients as possible reasons for improved ECMO survival in this subgroup. Prolonged CPR and once again renal failure were associated with increased mortality; however, prolonged support worsened survival in this series [247].

In summary ECMO plays an important role in the management of patients with CHD and in those with acquired myocardial dysfunction due to myocarditis. It is used in the preoperative phase, as support in the immediate post-CPB period in those patients who cannot be weaned from CPB due to myocardial dysfunction or severe hypoxia, or in patients who undergo acute cardiopulmonary failure in the ICU after initially successful weaning from CPB. ECMO has also been used as support in patients who are being bridged to transplant or in those whose newly transplanted heart has failed. Although morbidity and mortality are high these figures would approach 100% without this life-saving modality.

The need for pediatric ventricular assist devices (VAD) has come about because of the increased rates of survival of patients with complex CHD but also because of improvements in medical therapy that has prolonged the life of patients with severe cardiomyopathy who may have otherwise succumbed to their disease years ago. Improvements in pediatric VAD therapy has lead to the development of miniaturized pumps and optimized cannulae appropriate for patients right down to neonatal size with stroke volumes of as little as 10 mL. In comparison to the adult population where VAD therapy is employed at the time of failed weaning from CPB this role is filled by ECMO in the pediatric population with VAD therapy being used in a patient where ongoing support is projected for weeks or months. In addition to this, advantages of VAD therapy include the ability to have the patient extubated, feeding enterally and, importantly, ambulating. The presence of respiratory failure, pulmonary hypertension, and residual intracardiac shunts are possible contraindications [251]. VAD therapy can be divided into paracorporeal (devices where the assist device is outside of the body) and intracorporeal (where the device is implantable within the patient). The paracorporeal systems include the Thoratec ventricular assist device (Thoratec Laboratories, Pleasanton, CA, USA), Abiomed BVS 5000 and Abiomed AB 5000 (Abiomed, Danvers, MA, USA), Berlin Heart EXCOR VAD (Berlin Heart AG, Berlin, Germany), and MEDOS HIA VAD (MEDOS, Medizintechnik AG, Stolberg, Germany). Intracorporeal (implantable) devices include the Micromed Debakey VAD (Micromed Technologies, Houston, Texas, USA), Jarvik 2000 Flowmaker (Jarvik Heart, Inc., New York, NY, USA), the Berlin Incor (Berlin Heart AG, Berlin, Germany), and the Thoratec Heartmate II VAD (Thoratec Laboratories, Pleasanton, California, USA). Of these VAD systems the following four are the most widely used: The Berlin Excor, MEDOS HIA VAD, and the Thoratec VAD are pulsatile paracorporeal systems whilst the Micromed DeBakey VAD is an intracorporeal axial flow device. The Berlin Heart Excor Pediatric VAD was the first system that was commercially available designed especially for the pediatric patient. It is paracorporeally placed and air driven with pumps of 10-, 12-, 15-, 25-, 30-, 50-, 60-, and 80-mL stroke volume. This will translate to the possibility of supporting a patient down to 2.5 kg. Figure 10.11 demonstrates a size comparison between pediatric and adult size as well as how the unit works [252]. The support configuration can be as LVAD, RVAD, or BiVAD. Overall survival is between 40% and 60%, and these statistics include patients who have been successfully weaned from support and those bridged to transplant [251,253]. The MEDOS HIA VAD is

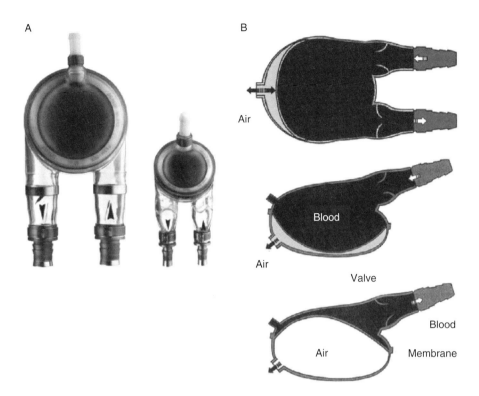

Figure 10.11 Adult versus pediatric Berlin heart chamber and pumping mechanism. **(A)** Adult (left) and pediatric (right) Berlin Excor® VADs. The adult pump has a stroke volume of 80 mL and tilting disc valves. The pediatric-sized pump is suitable for children with body weight of 3–9 kg. This pump has a stroke volume of 10 mL and polyurethane trileaflet valves. Pumps of all sizes are now available with polyurethane valves. **(B)** Cross-section of the Berlin heart pump with polyurethane valves. (Reproduced with permission from Potapov *et al.* [252].)

available in Europe in three sizes for the left ventricle (10, 25, and 60 mL) and three sizes for the right ventricle of (9, 22.5, and 54 mL). It can thus be used in RVAD, LVAD, or BiVAD formation. The Thoratec VAD has been used successfully worldwide in the pediatric population with a body surface area of 0.7–2.1 m². Multicenter experience has shown 60% survival to transplantation. Patients who required support for cardiomyopathy/myocarditis showed better survival than those presenting with CHD [254]. The Micromed DeBakey intracorporeal axial flow VAD is FDA approved for use in children 5–16 years of age with body surface areas between 0.7 and 1.5 m². Figure 10.12 shows the working parts of this system and its placement within the body [251]. Initially designed for use in adult patients by researchers at Baylor College of Medicine in Houston, Texas, and engineers at NASA, the first patient in the USA into whom this device was placed was a 10-year-old girl with a body surface area of 1.2 m² who presented with a dilated cardiomyopathy. She was successfully bridged to transplant after 84 days [255]. Disadvantages of this system include its availability only as an LVAD system, its size that precludes its use in patients with body surface area <0.7 m² and the requirement for normal pulmonary function.

Factors associated with morbidity and mortality in patients managed with VAD therapy are similar to the ECMO population. These include bleeding at the time of insertion and explantation, thrombosis with devastating embolic phenomena, infection, and organ failure. The bleeding experienced on insertion and explantation are secondary to the dissection that takes place with a large area of surgical trauma, the suture lines created in the major vessels and within the ventricular wall, and the coagulation cascade abnormalities associated with the blood–circuit interface. Although the major concern will be thrombosis in the circuit, later on this coagulopathy must be aggressively treated so as not to compromise VAD function due to hypovolemia. Therapy is similar to treatment of bleeding which accompanies separation from bypass including platelets, FFP, cryoprecipitate, blood or fresh whole blood, and the use of factor VII preparations. Keeping the use of indwelling catheters to a minimum and maintaining the skin area around the cannulae insertion clean can control infection. Long-term anticoagulation is one of those continuously evolving topics. It has been established that in these patients even viral infections that are otherwise well tolerated in healthy children are dangerous in this

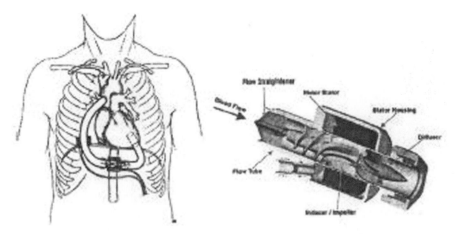

Figure 10.12 Mechanism of MicroMed DeBakey VAD. (Reproduced with permission from Fynn-Thompson *et al.* [251].)

population as the endogenous reactions to these infections may further activate the coagulation cascade and hence adjustments may be necessary at these times [253]. The strategy that is employed involves heparin-coated circuitry, frequent checks of the circuit by trained personnel, the use of heparin which is monitored by means of aPTT (60–80 seconds) and thromboelastography, monitoring anti-thrombin III with replacement if the level drops below 70%, and the use of antiplatelet drugs to prevent aggregation and adhesion. These drugs include aspirin and dipyridi-mole [253,255]. Platelet aggregation tests should be performed with target activation of 30%. Another possible improvement in the coagulation strategy has been the placement of the drainage cannula at the ventricular apex as apposed to the atrium. This may improve flow through the ventricle and outflow from the device [255].

This discussion would not be complete without comparison of survival between ECMO and VAD although this may be a case of comparing apples to oranges as ECMO plays a vital role in acute resuscitation, a role that VAD cannot. Despite the previously quoted studies a multi-center review by Blume and colleagues showed that in the current era the rate of patients successfully bridged to transplant was as high as 86% in the VAD population. Also of note was that the post-transplant survival in the VAD group was similar to those status 1 transplant patients not requiring support. This is in contrast to ECMO patients where 47–57% of patients survived to transplant [256]. Improvements in survival of VAD patients over earlier experience is related to improved surgical techniques; better timing of VAD placement (i.e., placement as function shows signs of deterioration versus waiting for end-organ damage); improved postoperative management with respect to myocardial support, earlier nutrition, earlier extubation, and better understanding of coagulation therapy; and improved patient selection [256]. Neurological

outcome is a major morbidity in both groups. Early experi-ence showed that in-hospital neurological complications occurred in 30% of ECMO patients and 10% of VAD patients [257]. The authors did however note that these patients, representative of both systems, improved with time with only 5 of 31 demonstrating ongoing severe disability. Despite the improved management outlined above there remains a 20% risk of stroke in VAD patients of which >50% prove fatal [254]. The worse outcome in the ECMO group may be associated with younger age at the time of support, this group has more complex disease, more cyanotic heart disease, that a large part of the ECMO group were neonates, and that greater anticoagulation was needed in the ECMO group. This higher anticoagulation translated into ACT of between 180 and 220 seconds that puts these neonates at higher risk for intracranial hemorrhage. In addition to these factors the ECMO circuit is more complex with the oxygenator and long tubing lengths increasing throm-boembolic risk [257].

What then is the future of pediatric mechanical support? At this time only the MicroMed DeBakey VAD has FDA approval for use in the pediatric population with the afore-mentioned systems being given permission by the FDA on a case-by-case basis on compassionate grounds. In the spring of 2004 the National Heart, Lung and Blood Institute (NHLBI) awarded five companies sponsorship for basic and applied research into new circulatory assist devices and other systems exclusively for infants and children with congenital and acquired heart disease. The objective is to provide circulatory support for infants and children while minimizing the risks of bleeding, infection, and throm-boembolism [252,258]. Unfortunately none of these devices has yet undergone clinical testing.

In conclusion the use of mechanical support in the pediatric population has improved vastly over the last two decades from a scaled-down adult machine to therapy dedicated and researched exclusively for children. As outlined there is still a long way forward and we await the NHLBI projects.

Conclusions

The use of CPB has progressed greatly in the last 60–70 years with clinicians and researchers overcoming a large number of obstacles; for example giving surgeons, anesthesiologists, perfusionists, and critical care cardiologists the ability to palliate single-ventricle patients into their third and even fourth decade of life as opposed to the nearly 100% mortality this diagnosis carried as little as 30 years ago. One of our greatest challenges moving forward will be limiting the neurological damage that occurs in some of our patients and, failing that, giving us the ability to help these patients with the challenges that they will face in their lives.

As can be seen this is a field of medicine where a team approach is of extreme importance as each group of practitioners has a vital role in patient care. The management is multimodal with no single therapy outweighing the others in importance. This concept cannot be stressed enough. Many questions remain unanswered, but the most important principle to remember is that these patients require care specific to them and not anything that is simply made smaller from adult principles.

References

1. Harken D. (1946) Foreign bodies in, and in relation to, the thoracic blood vessels and heart, I: techniques for approaching and removing foreign bodies from chambers of the heart. Surg Gynecol Obstet 83, 117–125.
2. Lewis FJ, Taufic M. (1953) Closure of atrial septal defects with the aid of hypothermia: experimental accomplishments and the report of one successful case. Surgery 33, 52–59.
3. Gross RE, Watkins E. (1953) Surgical closure of atrial septal defects. AMA Arch Surg 67, 670–685.
4. Gibbon JH. (1954) Application of a mechanical heart and lung apparatus to cardiac surgery. Minn Med 37, 171–185.
5. Dennis C, Spreng DS Jr, Nelson GE, et al. (1951) Development of a pump-oxygenator to replace the heart and lungs; an apparatus applicable to human patients, and application to one case. Ann Surg 134, 709–721.
6. Jaggers J, Ungerleider RM. (2003) Cardiopulmonary bypass in infants and children. In: Mavroudis C, Backer CL, eds. Pediatric Cardiac Surgery, 3rd ed. Philadelphia, PA: Mosby.
7. Helmsworth JA, Clark LC Jr, Kaplan S, et al. (1953) An oxygenator-pump for use in total by-pass of heart and lungs; laboratory evaluation and clinical use. J Thor Surg 26, 617–631; discussion 631–632.
8. Dodrill FD, Hill E, Gerisch RA, et al. (1953) Pulmonary valvuloplasty under direct vision using the mechanical heart for a complete by-pass of the right heart in a patient

with congenital pulmonary stenosis. J Thor Surg 26, 584–594; discussion 595–597.
9. Mustard WT, Thomson JA. (1957) Clinical experience with the artificial heart lung preparation. Can Med Assoc J 76, 265–269.
10. Clowes GH Jr, Neville WE, Hopkins A, et al. (1954) Factors contributing to success or failure in the use of a pump oxygenator for complete by-pass of the heart and lung, experimental and clinical. Surgery 36, 557–579.
11. Lillehei CW. (1955) Controlled cross circulation for direct-vision intracardiac surgery. Correction of ventricular septal defects, atrioventricularis communis, and tetralogy of Fallot. Postgrad Med 17, 388–396.
12. Daly RC, Dearani JA, Mcgregor CGA, et al. (2005) Fifty years of open heart surgery at the Mayo Clinic. Mayo Clin Proc 80, 636–640.
13. Kirklin JW, DuShane JW, Patrick RT, et al. (1955) Intracardiac surgery with the aid of a mechanical pump-oxygenator system (Gibbon type): report of eight cases. Proc Staff Meet Mayo Clin 10, 201–206.
14. Iwahashi H, Yuri K, Nose Y. (2004) Developement of the oxygenator. J Artif Organs 7, 111–120.
15. Lillehei CW. (1993) History of the development of extracorporeal circulation In: Arensman RM, Cornish JD, eds. Extracorporeal Life Support. Boston, MA: Blackewell Scientific Publication, pp. 9–30.
16. Dinardo JA. (2005) Physiology and techniques of extracorporeal circulation in the pediatric patient. In: Lake CL, Booker PD, eds. Pediatric Cardiac Anesthesia. Philadelphia, PA: Lippincott Williams & Wilkins, p. 229.
17. Davies LK. (1999) Cardipulmonary bypass in infants and children: how is it different? J Cardiothor Vasc Anes 13, 330–345.
18. Liu J, Feng Z, Li C, et al. (2007) Application of modified perfusion technique on one stage repair of interrupted aortic arch in infants: a case series and literature review. ASAIO Journal 53, 666–669.
19. Bigelow WG, Callaghan JC, Hopps JA. (1950) General hypothermia for experimental intracardiac surgery; the use of electrophrenic respirations, an artificial pacemaker for cardiac standstill and radio-frequency rewarming in general hypothermia. Ann Surg 132, 531–539.
20. Penrod KE. (1949) Oxygen consumption and cooling rates in immersion hypothermia in the dog. Am J Physiol 157, 436.
21. Ross DN. (1954) Hypothermia: part 2. Physiological observations during hypothermia. Guys Hosp Rep 103, 116.
22. Greeley WJ, Kern FH, Ungerleider RM, et al. (1991) The effect of hypothermic CPB and total circulatory arrest on cerebral metabolism in neonates, infants, and children. J Thorac Cardiovasc Surg 101, 783.
23. Arrica M, Bissonnette B. (2007) Therapeutic hypothermia. Sem Cardiothorac Vasc Anes 11, 6–15.
24. Kirklin JW, Barratt-Boyes BG. (1993) Cardiac Surgery, 2nd ed. New York: Churchill Livingstone.
25. Pua HL, Bissonnette B. (1998) Cerebral physiology in pediatric cardiopulmonary bypass. Can J Anaesth 45, 960–978.
26. Greeley WJ, Kern FH, Meliones JN, et al. (1993) Effect of deep hpothermia and circulatory arrest on cerebral blood flow and metabolism. Ann Thorac Surg 56, 1464–1466.

27. Buckberg GD, Brazier JR, Nelson RL, *et al.* (1977) Studies on the effects of hypothermia on regional myocardial blood flow and metabolism during cardiopulmonary bypass. I. The adequately perfused beating, fibrillating and arrested heart. J Thorac Cardiovasc Surg 73, 87–94.

28. Kondratiev TV, Wold RM, Aasum E, *et al.* (2007) Myocardial mechanical dysfunction and calcium overload following rewarming from experimental hypothermia *in vivo*. Cryobiology 56, 15–21.

29. Tveita T, Skandfer M, Refsum H, *et al.* (1996) Experimental hypothermia and rewarming: changes in mechanical function and metabolism of rat hearts. J Applied Physiol 80, 291–297.

30. Navas JP, Anderson W, Marsh JD. (1990) Hypothermia increases calcium content of hypoxic myocytes. Am J Physiol 259, H333–H339.

31. Rebeyka IM, Hanan SA, Borges MR, *et al.* (1990) Rapid cooling contracture of the myocardium. J Thorac Cardiovasc Surg 100, 240–249.

32. Lahorra JA, Torchiana DF, Tolis G, *et al.* (1997) Rapid cooling contracture with cold cardioplegia. Ann Thorac Surg 63, 1353–1360.

33. Compagnoni G, Bottura C, Cavallaro G, *et al.* (2007) Safety of deep hypothermia in treating neonatal asphyxia. Neonatology 93, 230–235.

34. Azzopardi D, Edwards AD. (2007) Hypothermia. Sem Fetal Neonatal Med 12, 303–310.

35. Undar A, Masai T, Yang S-Q, *et al.* (1999) Effects of perfusion mode on regional and global organ blood flow in a neonatal piglet model. Ann Thorac Surg 68, 1336–1346.

36. Ji B, Undar A. (2006) An evaluation of the benefits of pulsatile versus nonpulsatile perfusion during cardiopulmonary bypass procedures in pediatric and adult cardiac patients. ASAIO J 52, 357–361.

37. Shepard RB, Simpson DC, Sharp JF. (1996) Energy equivalent pressure. Arch Surg 93, 730–740.

38. Rider AR, Schreiner RS, Undar A. (2007) Pulsatile perfusion during cardiopulmonary bypass procedures in neonates, infants, and small children. ASAIO J 73, 706–709.

39. Alkan T, Akcevin A, Turkoglu H, *et al.* (2007) Benefits of pulsatile perfusion on vital organ recovery during and after pediatric open heart surgery. ASAIO J 53, 651–654.

40. Undar A, Eichstaedt HC, Bigley JE, *et al.* (2002) Effects of pulsatile and nonpulsatile perfusion on cerebral hemodynamics investigated with a new pediatric pump. J Thorac Cardiovasc Surg 124, 413–416.

41. Alkan T, Akcevin A, Undar A, *et al.* (2007) Effects of pulsatile and nonpulsatile perfusion on vital organ recovery in pediatric heart surgery: a pilot clinical study. ASAIO J 52, 530–535.

42. Undar A, Masai T, Yang S-Q, *et al.* (2002) Pulsatile perfusion improves regional myocardial blood flow during and after hypothermic cardiopulmonary bypass in a neonatal piglet model. ASAIO J 48, 90–95.

43. Lodge AJ, Undar A, Daggett WM, *et al.* (1997) Regional blood flow during pulsatile cardiopulmonary bypass and after circulatory arrest in an infant model. Ann Thorac Surg 63, 1243–1250.

44. Sezai A, Shiono M, Orime Y, *et al.* (1997) Renal circulation and cellular metabolism during left ventrucular assisted circulation: comparison study pulsatile and nonpulsatile assists. Artificial Organs 21, 830–835.

45. du Plessis AJ, Jonas RA, Wypij D, *et al.* (1997) Perioperative effects of alpha-stat versus pH-stat strategies for deep hypothermic cardiopulmonary bypass in infants. J Thorac Cardiovasc Surg 114, 991–1001.

46. Tallman RD Jr (1997) Acid-base regulation, alpha-stat, and the emperor's new clothes. J Cardiothorac Vasc Anesth 11, 282–288.

47. Jonas RA, Bellinger DC, Rappaport LA. (1993) Relation of pH strategy and developemental outcome after hypothermic circulatory arrest. J Thorac Cardiovasc Surg 106, 362–368.

48. Wong PC, Barlow CF, Hickey PR, *et al.* (1992) Factors associated with choreoathetosis after cardiopulmonary bypass in chikdren with congenital heart disease. Circulation 86, 118–126.

49. Levin DA, Seay AR, Fullerton DA, *et al.* (2005) Profound hypothermia with alpha-stat pY management during open-heart surgery is associated with choreoathetosis. Pediatr Cardiol 26, 34–38.

50. Hiramatsu T, Miura T, Forbess JM, *et al.* (1995) pH strategies and cerebral energetics before and after circulatory arrest. J Thorac Cardiovasc Surg 109, 948–958.

51. Markowitz SD, Mendoza-Peredes A, Liu H, *et al.* (2007) Response of brain oxygenation and metabolism to deep hypothermic circulatory arrest in newborn piglets: comparison of pH-stat and alpha stat strategies. Ann Thorac Surg 84, 170–176.

52. Duebener LF, Hagino I, Sakamoto T, *et al.* (2002) Effects of pH management duting deep hypothermic bypass on cerebral microcirculation: alpha-stat versus pH-stat. Circulation 106(suppl 1), 103–108.

53. Kurth CD, O'Rourke MM, O'Hara IB, *et al.* (1997) Brain cooling efficiency with pH-stat and alpha-stat cardiopulmonary bypass in newborn pigs. Circulation 96, 385–363.

54. Sakamoto T, Zurakowski D, Duebener LF, *et al.* (2002) Combination of alpha-stat strategy and hemodilution exacerbates neurologic injury in a survival piglet model with deep hypothermic circulatory arrest. Ann Thorac Surg 73, 180–190.

55. Sakamoto T, Zurakowski D, Duebener LF, *et al.* (2004) Interaction of temperature with hematocrit level and pH determines safe duration of hypothermic circulatory arrest J Thorac Cardiovasc Surg 128, 220–232.

56. Nagy ZL, Collins M, Sharpe T, *et al.* (2003) Effect or two different techiniques on the serum troponin-T levels in newborns and children. Does pH-stat provide better protection? Circulation 108, 577–582.

57. Wernovsky G, Shillingford AJ, Gaynor JW. (2005) Central nervous system outcomes in children with complex congenital heart disease. Curr Opin Cardiol 20, 94–99.

58. Nelson DP, Andropoulos DB, Fraser CD. (2008) Perioperative neuroprotective strategies. Semin Thorac Cardiovasc Surg Pediatr Card Surg Ann 11, 49–56.

59. Hsia T-Y, Gruber PJ. (2006) Factors influencing neurologic outcome after neonatal cardiopulmonary bypass: what we can and cannot control. Ann Thorac Surg 81, S2381–S2388.

60. Glauser TA, Rorke LB, Weinberg PM, et al. (1990) Congenital brain anomalies associated with the hypoplastic left heart syndrome. Pediatr 1990, 984–990.

61. Galli KK, Zimmerman RA, Jarvik GP, et al. (2004) Periventricular leukomalacia is common after neonatal cardiac surgery. J Thorac Cardiovasc Surg 127, 692–704.

62. Mahle WT, Tavani F, Zimmerman RA, et al. (2002) An MRI study of neurological injury before and after congenital heart surgery. Circulation 106, 109–114.

63. Dent CL, Spaeth JP, Jones BV, et al. (2006) Brain magnetic resonance imaging abnormalities after the Norwood procedure using regional cerebral perfusion. J Thorac Cardiovasc Surg 131, 190–197.

64. Kaltman JR, Di H, Tian Z, et al. (2005) Impact of congenital heart disease on cerebrovascular blood flow dynamics in the fetus. Ultrasound Obstet Gynecol 25, 32–36.

65. Licht DJ, Wang J, Silvestre DW, et al. (2004) Preoperative cerebral blood flow is diminished in neonates with severe congenital heart defects. J Thorac Cardiovasc Surg 128, 841–849.

66. McQuillen PS, Hamrick SEG, Perez MJ, et al. (2006) Balloon atrial septostomy is associated with preoperative stroke in neonates with transposition of the great arteries. Circulation 113, 280–285.

67. Gaynor JW, Gerdes M, Zackai EH, et al. (2003) Apolipoprotein E genotype and neurodevelopmental sequelae of infant cardiac surgery. J Thorac Cardiovasc Surg 126, 1736–1745.

68. Ballweg JA, Wernovsky G, Gaynor JW. (2007) Neurodevelopmental outcomes following congenital heart surgery. Pediatr Cardiol 28, 126–133.

69. Quartermain MD, Ittenbach RF, Flynn TB, et al. (2010) Neuropsychological status in children after repair of acyanotic congenital heart disease. Pediatrics 126, e351–e359.

70. Salvin JW, Laussen PC, Thiagarajan RR. (2008) Extracorporeal membrane oxygenation for postcardiotomy mechanical cardiovascular support in children with congenital heart disease. Paediatr Anaesth 18, 1157–1162.

71. Hamrick SEG, Gremmels DB, Keet CA, et al. (2003) Neurodevelopmental outcome of infants supported with extracorporeal membrane oxygenation after cardiac surgery. Pediatr 111, e672–675.

72. Ghanayem NS, Mitchell ME, Tweddell JS, et al. (2006) Monitoring the brain before, during, and after cardiac surgery to improve long-term neurodevelopmental outcomes. Cardiol Young 16(Suppl 3), 103–109.

73. Williams GD, Ramamoorthy C. (2007) Brain monitoring and protection during pediatric cardiac surgery. Semin Cardiothorac Vas Anesth 11, 23–33.

74. Kurth CD, Steven JM, Montenegro LM, et al. (2001) Cerebral oxygen saturation before congenital heart surgery. Ann Thorac Surg 72, 187–192.

75. Hoffman GM, Ghanayem NS, Kampine JM, et al. (2000) Venous saturation and the anaerobic threshold in neonates after the Norwood procedure for hypoplastic left heart syndrome. Ann Thorac Surg 70, 1515–1521.

76. Andropoulos DB, Stayer SA, McKenzie ED, et al. (2003) Novel cerebral physiologic monitoring to guide low-flow cerebral perfusion during neonatal aortic arch reconstruction. J Thorac Cardiovasc Surg 125, 491–499.

77. Gottlieb EA, Fraser CD, Andropoulos DB, et al. (2006) Bilateral monitoring of cerebral oxygen saturation results in recognition of aortic cannula malposition during p ediatric congenital heart surgery. Pediatr Anaesth 16, 787–789.

78. Sakamoto T, Hatsuoka S, Stock UA, et al. (2001) Prediction of safe duration of hypothermic circulatory arrest by near-infrared spectroscopy. J Thorac Cardiovasc Surg 122, 339–350.

79. Kaufman J, Almodovar MC, Zuk J, et al. (2008) Correlation of abdominal site near-infrared spectroscopy with gastric tonometry in infants following surgery for congenital heart disease. Pediatr Crit Care Med 9, 62–68.

80. Berens RJ, Stuth EA, Robertson FA, et al. (2006) Near infrared spectroscopy monitoring during pediatric aortic coarctation repair. Pediatr Anaesth 16, 777–781.

81. Fagdyman N, Fleck T, Schubert S, et al. (2005) Comparison between cerebral tissue oxygenation index measured by near-infrared spectroscopy and venous jugular bulb saturation in children. Intensive Care Med 31, 846–850.

82. Andropoulos DB, Stayer SA, Diaz LK, et al. (2004) Neurological monitoring for congenital heart surgery Anesth Analg 99, 1368–1375.

83. Macmillan CSA, Andrews PJD. (2000) Cerebrovenous oxygen saturaiton monitoring: practical considerations and clinical relevance. Intensive Care Med 26, 1028–1036.

84. Kern FH, Ungerleider RM, Schulman SR, et al. (1995) Comparing two strategies of cardiopulmonary bypass cooling on jugular venous oxygen saturation in neonates and infants. Ann Thorac Surg 60, 1198–1202.

85. Ranucci M, Isgro G, De La Torre T, et al. (2008) Near-infrared spectroscopy correlates with continuous superior vena cava oxygen saturation in pediatric cardiac surgery patients. Pediatr Anaesth 18, 1163–1169.

86. Nagdyman N, Fleck T, Schubert S, et al. (2005) Near-infrared spectroscopy correlates with continuous superior vena cava oxygen saturation in pediatric cardiac surgery patients. Intensive Care Med 31, 846–850.

87. Daubeney PEF, Pilkington SN, Janke E, et al. (1996) Cerebral oxygenation measured by near-infrared spectroscopy: comparison with jugular bulb oximetry. Ann Thorac Surg 61, 930–934.

88. Tortoriello TA, Stayer SA, Mott AR, et al. (2005) A noninvasive estimation of mixed venous oxygen saturation using near-infrared spectroscopy by cerebral oximetry in pediatric cardiac surgery patients. Pediatr Anaesth 15, 495–503.

89. Austin EH, Edmonds HL, Auden SM, et al. (1997) Benefit of neurophysiological monitoring for pediatric cardiac surgery. J Thorac Cardiovasc Surg 114, 707–717.

90. Hirsch JC, Charpie JR, Ohye RG, et al. (2009) Near-infrared spectroscopy: what we know and what we need to know–a systematic review of the congenital heart disease literature. J Thorac Cardiovasc Surg 137, 154–159.

91. Wittnich C, Belanger MP, Bandali KS. (2007) Newborn hearts are at greater "metabolic risk" during global ischemia – advantages of continous coronary washout. Can J Cardiol 23, 195–200.

92. Boucek RJJ, Citak M, Graham TPJ, *et al.* (1984) Postnatal development of calcium release from cardiac sarcoplasmic reticulum Pediatr Res 18, 119.

93. Rolph TP, Jones CT. (1983) Regulation of glycolytic flux in the heart of fetal guinea pig. J Dev Physiol 5, 31–49.

94. Hetzer R, Warnecke H, Wittock H. (1980) Extracoronary collateral myocardial flow during cardioplegic arrest. J Thorac Cardiovasc Surg 28, 191.

95. Allen BS, Barth MJ, Ilbawi MN. (2001) Pediatric myocardial protecion: an overview. Semin Thorac Cardiovasc Surg 13, 56–72.

96. Allen BS. (2004) Pediatric myocardial protection: a cardioplegic strategy is the "solution". Semin Thorac Cardiovasc Surg: Ped Card Surg Ann 7, 141–154.

97. Durandy Y. (2008) Pediatric myocardial protection. Curr Opin Cardiol 23, 85–90.

98. Kronon MT, Allen BS, Hernan J, *et al.* (1999) Superiority of magnesium cardioplegia in neonatal myocardial protection. Ann Thorac Surg 68, 2285–2291; discussion 2291–2292.

99. Toyoda Y, Yamaguchi M, Yoshimura N, *et al.* (2003) Cardioprotective effects and the mechanisms of terminal warm blood cardioplegia in pediatric cardiac surgery. J Thorac Cardiovasc Surg 125, 1242–1251.

100. Guru V, Omura J, Alghamdi AA, *et al.* (2006) Is blood superior to crystalloid?: a meta-analysis of randomized clinical trials. Circulation 114, 331–338.

101. Jacob S, Kallikourdis A, Sellke F, *et al.* (2008) Is blood cardioplegia superior to crystalloid cardioplegia? Interact CadioVasc Thorac Surg 7, 491–498.

102. Amark K, Berggren H, Bjork K, *et al.* (2005) Blood cardioplegia provides superior protection in infant cardiac surgery. Ann Thorac Surg 80, 989–994.

103. Caputo M, Modi P, Imura H, *et al.* (2002) Cold blood versus cold crystalloid cadioplegia for repair of ventricular septal defects in pediatric heart surgery: a randomized controlled trial. Ann Thorac Surg 74, 530–535.

104. Kozik DJ, Tweddell JS. (2006) Characterizing the inflammatory response to cardiopulmonary bypass in children. Ann Thorac Surg 81, S2347–S2354.

105. von Ungern-Sternberg BS, Petak F, Saudan S, *et al.* (2007) Effect of cardiopulmonary bypass and aortic clamping on functional residual capacity and ventilation distribution in children. J Thorac Cardiovasc Surg 134, 1193–1198.

106. Montenegro LM, Greeley WJ. (1998) Pro: the use of modified ultrafiltration during pediatric cardiac surgery is a benefit. J Cadiothorac Vasc Anesth 12, 480–482.

107. Berdat PA, Eichenberger E, Ebell J, *et al.* (2004) Elimination of proinflammatory cytokines in pediatric cardiac surgery: analysis of ultrafiltration method and filter type. J Thorac Cardiovasc Surg 127, 1688–1696.

108. Bando K, Turrentine MW, Vijay P, *et al.* Effect of modified ultrafiltration in high-risk patients undergoing operations for congenital heart disease. Ann Thorac Surg 66, 821–827; discussion 828.

109. Mittnacht AJC, Thanjan M, Srivastava S, *et al.* (2008) Extubation in the operating room after congenital heart surgery in children. J Thorac Cardiovasc Surg 136, 88–93.

110. Meibner U, Scharf J, Dotsch J, *et al.* (2008) Very early extubation after open-heart surgery in children does not influence cardiac function. Pediatr Cardiol 29, 317–320.

111. Picca S, Ricci Z, Picardo S. (2008) Acute kidney injury in an infant after cardiopulmonary bypass. Semin Nephrol 28, 470–476.

112. Kist-van Hothe tot Echten JE, Goedvolk CA, Doornaar MBME, *et al.* (2001) Acute renal insufficiency and renal replacement therapy after pediatric cardiopulmonary bypass surgery. Pediatr Cardiol 22, 321–326.

113. Pedersen KR, Povlsen JV, Christensen S, *et al.* (2007) Risk factors for acute renal failure requiring dialysis after surgery for congenital heart disease in children. Acta Anaesthesiol Scand 51, 1344–1349.

114. Zappitelli M, Bernier P-L, Saczkowski RS, *et al.* (2009) A small post-operative rise in serum creatinine predicts acute kidney injury in children undergoing cardiac surgery. Kidney Int 29, 1–8.

115. Plotz FB, Bouma AB, van Wijk JAE, *et al.* (2008) Pediatric acute kidney injury in the ICU: an independant evaluation of pRIFLE criteria. Intensive Care Med 34, 1713–1717.

116. Mishra J, Ma Q, Prada A, *et al.* (2003) Identification of neutrophil gelatinase-associated lipocalin as a novel early urinary biomarker for ischemic renal injury J Am Soc Nephrol 14, 2534–2543.

117. Schimdt -Ott KM, Mori K, Yi Li J, *et al.* (2007) Dual action of neutrophil gelatinase-associated lipocalin. J Am Soc Nephrol 18, 407–413.

118. Parikh CR, Mishra J, Thiessen-Philbrook H, *et al.* (2006) Urinary IL-18 is an early predictive biomarker of acute kidney injury after cardiac surgery. Kidney Int 70, 199–203.

119. Gruber E, Laussen PC, Casta A, *et al.* (2001) Stress response in infants undergoing cardiac urgery: a randomized study of fentanyl bolus, fentanyl infusion, and fentanyl-midazolam infusion. Anesth Analg 92, 882–890.

120. Firmin RK, Boulox P, Allen P, *et al.* (1985) Sympathoadrenal function during cardiac operations in infants with the technique of surface cooling, limited cardiopulmonary bypass, and circulatory arrest. J Thorac Cardiovasc Surg 90, 729–735.

121. Turley K, Roizen M, Vlahakes GJ, *et al.* (1980) Catecholamine response to deep hypothermia and total circulatory arrest in the infant lamb. Circulation 62(suppl 1), I175–I179.

122. Wood M, Shand DG, Wood AJJ. (1980) The sympathetic response to profound hypothermia and circulatory arrest in infants. Canad Anaesth Soc J 27, 125–131.

123. Gajarski RJ, Stefanelli CB, Graziano JN, *et al.* (2010) Adrenocortical response in infants undergoing cardiac surgery with cardiopulmonary bypass and circulatory arrest. Pediatr Crit Care Med 11, 44–51.

124. Pollock EMM, Pollock JCS, Jamieson MPG, *et al.* (1988) Adrenocortical hormone concentrations in children during cardiopulmonary bypass with and without pulsatile flow. Br J Anaesth, 60 536–541.

125. Makoto A, Park I-S, Wada N, *et al.* (2005) Steroid supplementation: a legitimate pharmacotherapy after neonatal open heart surgery. Ann Thorac Surg 80, 1672–1678.

126. Suominem PK, Dickerson HA, Moffett BS, *et al.* (2005) Hemodynamic effects of rescue protocol hydrocortisone in neonates with low cardiac output syndrome after cardiac surgery. Pediatr Crit Care Med 6, 655–659.

127. Gessler P, Hohl V, Carrel T, *et al.* (2005) Administration of steroids in pediatric cardiac surgery: impact on clinical outcome and systemic inflammatory response. Pediatr Cardiol 26, 595–600.

128. Allen M, Sundararajan S, Pathan N, *et al.* (2009) Anti-inflammatory modalities: the current use in pediatric cardiac surgery in the United Kingdom and Ireland. Pediatr Crit Care Med 10, 341–345.

129. Checchia PA, Bronicki RA, Costello JM, *et al.* (2005) Steroid use before pediatric cardiac operations using cardiopulmonary bypass: an international survey of 36 centers. Pediatr Crit Care Med 6, 441–444.

130. Robertson-Malt S, Afrane B, Elbarbary M. (2007) Prophylactic steroids for pediatric open heart surgery (Review). The Cochrane Collaboration 4, 1–24.

131. Varan B, Tokel K, Mercan S, *et al.* (2002) Systemic inflammatory response related to cardiopulmonary bypass and its modification by methyl prednisolone: high dose versus low dose. Pediatr Cardiol 23, 437–441.

132. Dimmick S, Badawi N, Randell T. (2004) Thyroid hormone supplementation for the prevention of morbidity and mortality in infants undergoing cardiac surgery. Cochrane Database Syst Rev 3 (CD004220).

133. Ross OC, Petros A. (2001) The sick euthyroid syndrome in paediatric cardiac surgery patients. Intensive Care Med 27, 1124–1132.

134. Mackie AS, Booth KL, Newburger JW, *et al.* (2005) A randomized, double-blind, placebo controlled pilot trial of triiodothyronine in neonatal heart surgery. J Thorac Cardiovasc Surg 130, 810–816.

135. Bettendorf M, Schmidt KG, Grulich-Henn J, *et al.* (2000) Tri-iodothyronine treatment in children after cardiac surgery: a double-blind, randomised, placebo-controlled study. Lancet 356, 529–534.

136. Balcells J, Moreno A, Audi L, *et al.* (2001) Growth hormone/insulin-like growth factors axis in children undergoing cardiac surgery. Crit Care Med 29, 1234–1238.

137. McAlister FA, Man J, Bistritz L, *et al.* (2003) Diabetes and coronary artery bypass surgery. An examination of perioperative glycemic control and outcomes. Diabetes Care 26, 1518–1524.

138. Knapik P, Nadziakiewicz P, Urbanska E, *et al.* (2009) Cardiopulmonary bypass increases postoperative glycemia and insulin consumption after coronary surgery. Ann Thorac Surg 87, 859–865.

139. Shine TSJ, Uchikado M, Crawford CC, *et al.* (2007) Importance of perioperative blood glucose management in cardiac surgical patients. Asian Cardiovasc Thorac Annals 15, 534–538.

140. Faustino EV, Apkon M. (2005) Persistent hyperglycemia in critically ill children. J Pediatr 146, 30–34.

141. Yates AR, Dyke PC, Taeed R, *et al.* (2006) Hyperglycemia is a marker for poor outcome in the postoperative pediatric cardiac patient. Pediatr Crit Care Med 7, 351–355.

142. Srinivasan V, Spinella PC, Drott HR, *et al.* (2004) Association of timing, duration, and intensity of hyperglycemia with intensive care unit mortality in critically ill children. Pediatr Crit Care Med 5, 329–336.

143. Ballweg JA, Wernovsky G, Ittenbach RF, *et al.* (2007) Hyperglycemia after infant cardiac surgery does not adversely impact neurodevelopmental outcome. Ann Thorac Surg 84, 2052–2058.

144. Appachi E, Mossad E, Mee RBB, *et al.* (2007) Perioperative serum interleukins in neonates with hypoplastic left-heart syndrome and transposition of the great arteries. J Cardiothorac Vasc Anesth 21, 184–190.

145. Brix-Christensen V. (2001) The systemic inflammatory response after cardiac surgery with cardiopulmonary bypass in children. Acta Anaesthesiol Scand 45, 671–679.

146. Seghaye MC, Duchateau J, Grabitz RG, *et al.* (1993) Complement activation during cardiopulmonary bypass in infants and children. Relation to postoperative multiple system organ failure. J Thorac Cardiovasc Surg 106, 978–987.

147. Seghaye MC, Grabitz RG, Duchateau J, *et al.* (1996) Inflammatory reaction and capillary leak syndrome related to cardiopulmonary bypass in neonates undergoing cardiac operations. J Thorac Cardiovasc Surg 112, 687–697.

148. Madhok AB, Ojamaa K, Haridas V, *et al.* (2006) Cytokine response in children undergoing surgery for congenital heart disease. Pediatr Cardiol 27, 408–413.

149. Bronicki RA, Backer CL, Baden HP, *et al.* (2000) Dexamethasone reduces the imflammatory response to cardiopulmonary bypass in children. Ann Thorac Surg 69, 1490–1495.

150. Schroeder VA, Pearl JM, Schwartz SM, *et al.* (2003) Combined steroid treatment for congenital heart surgery improves oxygen delivery and reduces postbypass inflammatory mediator expression. Circulation 107, 2823–2328.

151. Mangano DT, Tudor IC, Ditzel C. (2006) The risk with aprotinin in cardiac surgery. New Engl J Med 354, 353–365.

152. Karkouti K, Beattie WS, Dattilo KM, *et al.* (2006) A propensity score case-control comparison of aprotinin and tranexamic acid in high-transfusion-risk cardiac surgery. Transfusion 46, 327–338.

153. Guzzetta NA, Evans FM, Rosengerg ES, *et al.* (2009) The impact of aprotinin on postoperative renal dysfunction in neonates undergoing cardiopulmonary bypass: a retrospective analysis. Anesth Analg 108, 448–455.

154. Szekely A, Sapi E, Breuer T, *et al.* (2008) Aprotinin and renal dysfunction after pediatric cardiac surgery. Pediatr Anesth 18, 151–159.

155. Williams GD, Ramamoorthy C, Pentcheva K, *et al.* (2008) A randomized, controlled trial of aprotinin in neonates undergoing open-heart surgery. Pediatr Anesth 18, 812–819.

156. Eaton MP. (2008) Antifibrinolytic therapy in surgery for congenital heart disease. Anesth Analg 106, 1087–1100.

157. Tireli E, Ugurlucan M, Kafali E, *et al.* (2006) Extracardiac Fontan operation without cardiopulmonary bypass. J Cardiovasc Surg 47, 699–704.

158. Kawahira Y, Uemura H, Yagihara T. (2006) Impact of the off-pump Fontan procedure on complement activation and cytokine generation. Ann Thorac Surg 81, 685–689.

159. Petrossian E, Reddy VM, Collins KK, *et al.* (2006) The extracardiac conduit Fontan operation using minimal approach extracorporeal circulation: Early and midterm outcomes. J Thorac Cardiovasc Surg 132, 1054–1063.

160. Waight DJ, Hijazi ZM. (2001) Pediatric interventional cardiology: the cardiologist's role and relationship with pediatric cardiothoracic surery. Adv Card Surg 13, 143–167.

161. Huang TC, Hsieh K-S, Lin C-C. (2008) Clinical results of percutaneous closure of large secundum atrial septal defects in children using the Amplatzer septal occluder. Heart Vessels 23, 187–192.

162. Carminati M, Butera G, Chessa M, *et al.* (2007) Transcatheter closure of congenital ventricular septal defects: results of the European Registry. Europ Heart J 28, 2361–2368.

163. Bacha EA, Hijazi ZM, Cao Q-L, *et al.* (2005) Hybrid pediatric heart surgery. Pediatr Cardiol 26, 315–322.

164. Hickey E, Karamlou T, You J, *et al.* (2006) Effects of circuit miniaturization in reducing inflammatory response to infant cardiopulmonary bypass by elimination of allogeneic blood products. Ann Thorac Surg 81, S2367–S2372.

165. Jonas RA, Wypij D, Roth SJ, *et al.* (2003) The influence of hemodilution on outcome after hypothermic cardiopulmonary bypass: results of a randomized trial in infants. J Thorac Cardiovasc Surg 126, 1765–1774.

166. Wypij D, Jonas RA, Bellinger DC, *et al.* (2008) The effect of hematocrit during hypothermic cardiopulmonary bypass in infant heart surgery: results from the combined Boston hematocrit trials. J Thorac Cardiovasc Surg 135, 355–360.

167. Newburger JW, Jonas RA, Soul J, *et al.* (2008) Randomized trial of hematocrit 25% versus 35% during hypothermic cardiopulmonary bypass in infant heart surgery. J Thorac Cardiovasc Surg 135, 347–354.

168. Shen I, Giacomuzzi C, Ungerleider RM. (2003) Current strategies for optimizing the use of cardiopulmonary bypass in neonates and infants. Ann Thorac Surg 75, S729–734.

169. Janvier G, Baquey C, Roth C, *et al.* (1996) Extracorporeal circulation, hemocompatibility, and biomaterials. Ann Thorac Surg 62, 1926–1934.

170. Gunaydin S. (2004) Emerging technologies in biocompatible surface modifying additives: quest for physiologic cardiopulmonary bypass. Curr Med Chem 2, 295–302.

171. Suzuki Y, Daitoku K, Minakawa M, *et al.* (2008) Poly-2-methoxyethylacrylate-coated bypass circuits reduce activation of coagulation system and inflammatory response in congenital cardiac surgery. J Artif Organs 11, 111–116.

172. Kirshbom PM, Miller BE, Spitzer K, *et al.* (2006) Failure of surface-modified bypass circuits to improve platelet function during pediatric cardiac surgery. J Thorac Cardiovasc Surg 132, 675–680.

173. Hoel TN, Thiara AS, Videm V, *et al.* (2009) In vitro evaluation of PHISIO-coated sets for pediatric cardiac surgery. Scand Cardiovasc J 43, 129–135.

174. Miyaji K, Hannan RL, Ojito J, *et al.* (2000) Heparin-coated cardiopulmonary bypass circuit: clinical effects in pediatric cardiac surgery. J Cardiac Surg 15, 194–198.

175. Olsson C, Siegbahn A, Henze A, *et al.* (2000) Heparin-coated cardiopulmonary bypass circuits reduce circulating complement factors and interleukin-6 in paediatric heart surgery. Scand Cardiovasc J 34, 33–40.

176. Boning A, Scheewe J, Ivers T, *et al.* (2004) Phosphorylcholine or heparin coating for pediatric extracorporeal circulation causes similar biologic effects in neonates and infants. J Thorac Cardiovasc Surg 127, 1458–1465.

177. Charette K, Hirata Y, Bograd A, *et al.* (2007) 180 ml and less: cardiopulmonary bypass techniques to minimize hemodilution for neonates and small infants. Perfusion 22, 327–331.

178. Miyaji K, Miyamoto T, Kohira S, *et al.* (2008) Miniaturized cardiopulmonary bypass system in neonates and small infants. Interact Cardiovasc Thorac Surg 7, 75–78.

179. Miyaji K, Kohira S, Miyamoto T, *et al.* (2007) Pediatric cardiac surgery without homologous blood transfusion, using a miniaturized bypass system in infants with lower body weight. J Thorac Cardiovasc Surg 134, 284–289.

180. Ando M, Takahashi Y, Suzuki N. (2004) Open heart surgery for small children without homologous blood transfusion by using remote pump head system. Ann Thorac Surg 78, 1717–1722.

181. Koster A, Huebler M, Boettcher W, *et al.* (2009) A new miniaturized cardiopulmonary bypass system reduces transfusion requirements during neonatal cardiac surgery: initial experience in 13 consecutive patients. J Thorac Cardiovasc Surg 137, 1565–1568.

182. Nakanishi K, Shichijo T, Shinkawa Y, *et al.* (2001) Usefulness of vacuum-assisted cardiopulmonary bypass circuit for pediatric open-heart surgery in reducing homologous blood transfusion. Eur J Cardiothorac Surg 20, 233–238.

183. Karamlou T, Schultz JM, Silliman C, *et al.* (2005) Using a miniaturized circuit and an asanguineous prime to reduce neutrophil-mediated organ dysfunction following infant cardiopulmonary bypass. Ann Thorac Surg 80, 6–13; discussion 614.

184. Karamlou T, Hickey E, Silliman CC, *et al.* (2005) Reducing risk in infant cardiopulmonary bypass: the use of a miniaturized circuit and a crystalloid prime improves cardiopulmonary function and increases cerebral blood flow. Semin Thorac Cardiovasc Surg Pediatr Card Surg Annu 3–11.

185. Haworth WS. (2003) The development of the modern oxygenator. Ann Thorac Surg 76, S2216–S2219.

186. Gomez D, Preston TJ, Olshove VF, *et al.* (2009) Evaluation of air handling in a new generation neonatal oxygenator with integral arterial filter. Perfusion 24, 107–112.

187. Lawson DS, Smigla GR, McRobb CM, *et al.* (2008) A clinical evaluation of the Dideco Kids D100 neonatal oxygenator. Perfusion 23, 39–42.

188. Jaggers J, Lawson JH. (2006) Coagulopathy and inflammation in neonatal heart surgery: mechanisms and strategies. Ann Thorac Surg 81, S2360–S2366.

189. Tempe DK, Virmani S. (2002) Coagulation abnormalities in patients with cyanotic congenital heart disease. J Cardiothorac Vasc Anesth 16, 752–765.

190. Bull BS, Huse WM, Brauer FS, *et al.* (1975) Heparin therapy during extracorporeal circulation. II. The use of a dose-

response curve to individualize heparin and protamine dosage. J Thorac Cardiovasc Surg 69, 685–689.

191. Guzzetta NA, Miller BE, Todd K, *et al.* (2006) Clinical measures of heparin's effect and thrombin inhibitor levels in pediatric patients with congenital heart disease. Anesth Analg 103, 1131–1138.

192. Guzzetta NA, Bajaj T, Fazlollah T, *et al.* (2008) A comparison of heparin management strategies in infants undergoing cardiopulmonary bypass. Anesth Analg 106, 419–425.

193. Codispoti M, Ludlam CA, Simpson D, *et al.* (2001) Individualized heparin and protamine management in infants and children undergoing cardiac operations. Ann Thorac Surg 71, 922–927; discussion 927–928.

194. Dyke PC 2nd, Russo P, Mureebe L, *et al.* (2005) Argatroban for anticoagulation during cardiopulmonary bypass in an infant. Paediatr Anaesth 15, 328–333.

195. Boshkov LK, Kirby A, Shen I, *et al.* (2006) Recognition and management of heparin-induced thrombocytopenia in pediatric cardiopulmonary bypass patients. Ann Thorac Surg 81, S2355–S2359.

196. Mullen MP, Wessel DL, Thomas KC, *et al.* (2008) The incidence and implications of anti-heparin-platelet factor 4 antibody formation in a pediatric cardiac surgical population. Anesth Analg 107, 371–378.

197. Alsoufi B, Boshkov LK, Kirby A, *et al.* (2004) Heparin-induced thrombocytopenia (HIT) in pediatric cardiac surgery: an emerging cause of morbidity and mortality. Sem Thorac Cardiovasc Surg 7, 155–171.

198. Boning A, Morschheuser T, Blase U, *et al.* (2005) Incidence of heparin-induced thrombocytopenia and therapeutic strategies in pediatric cardiac surgery. Ann Thorac Surg 79, 62–65.

199. Schreiber C, Dietrich W, Braun S, *et al.* (2006) Use of heparin upon reoperation in a pediatric patient with heparin-induced thrombocytopenia after disappearance of antibodies. Clin Res Cardiol 95, 379–382.

200. Hursting MJ, Dubb J, Verme-Gibboney CN. (2006) Argatroban anticoagulation in pediatric patients: a literature analysis. J Pediatr Hematol Oncol 28, 4–10.

201. Malherbe S, Tsui BC, Stobart K, *et al.* (2004) Argatroban as anticoagulant in cardiopulmonary bypass in an infant and attempted reversal with recombinant activated factor VII. Anesthesiology 100, 443–445.

202. Knoderer CA, Knoderer HM, Turrentine MW, *et al.* (2006) Lepirudin anticoagulation for heparin-induced thrombocytopenia after cardiac surgery in a pediatric patient. Pharmacotherapy 26, 709–712.

203. Iannoli ED, Eaton MP, Shapiro JR. (2005) Bidirectional Glenn shunt surgery using lepirudin anticoagulation in an infant with heparin-induced thrombocytopenia with thrombosis. Anesth Analg 101, 74–76.

204. Welsby IJ, Newman MF, Phillips-Bute B, *et al.* (2005) Hemodynamic changes after protamine administration: association with mortality after coronary artery bypass surgery. Anesthesiology 102, 308–314.

205. Seifert HA, Jobes DR, Ten Have T, *et al.* (2003) Adverse events after protamine administration following cardiopulmonary bypass in infants and children. Anesth Analg 97, 383–389.

206. Boigner H, Lechner E, Brock H, *et al.* (2001) Life threatening cardiopulmonary failure in an infant following protamine reversal of heparin after cardiopulmonary bypass. Paediatr Anaesth 11, 729–732.

207. Goetzenich A, Schroth SC, Emmig U, *et al.* (2009) Hypothermia exerts negative inotropy in human atrial preparations: in vitro-comparison to rabbit myocardium. J Cardiovasc Surg 50, 239–245.

208. Rajagopalan S, Mascha E, Na J, *et al.* (2008) The effects of mild perioperative hypothermia on blood loss and transfusion requirement. Anesthesiology 108, 71–77.

209. Rundgren M, Engstrom M. (2008) A thromboelastometric evaluation of the effects of hypothermia on the coagulation system. Anesth Analg 107, 1465–1468.

210. Twite MD, Hammer GB. (2008) The use of aprotinin in pediatric cardiac surgery: should we bid "good riddance" or are we throwing out the baby with the bath water? Paediatr Anaesth 18, 809–811.

211. Manrique A, Jooste EH, Kuch BA, *et al.* (2009) The association of renal dysfunction and the use of aprotinin in patients undergoing congenital cardiac surgery requiring cardiopulmonary bypass. Anesth Analg 109, 45–52.

212. Backer CL, Kelle AM, Stewart RD, *et al.* (2007) Aprotinin is safe in pediatric patients undergoing cardiac surgery. J Thorac Cardiovasc Surg 134, 1421–1426; discussion 1426–1428.

213. Schouten ES, van de Pol AC, Schouten AN, *et al.* (2009) The effect of aprotinin, tranexamic acid, and aminocaproic acid on blood loss and use of blood products in major pediatric surgery: a meta-analysis. Pediatr Crit Care Med 10, 182–190.

214. Chauhan S, Das SN, Bisoi A, *et al.* (2004) Comparison of epsilon aminocaproic acid and tranexamic acid in pediatric cardiac surgery. J Cardiothorac Vasc Anesth 18, 141–143.

215. Mou SS, Giroir BP, Molitor-Kirsch EA, *et al.* (2004) Fresh whole blood versus reconstituted blood for pump priming in heart surgery in infants. New Engl J Med 351, 1635–1644.

216. Manno CS, Hedberg KW, Kim HC, *et al.* (1991) Comparison of the hemostatic effects of fresh whole blood, stored whole blood, and components after open heart surgery in children. Blood 77, 930–936.

217. Gruenwald CE, McCrindle BW, Crawford-Lean L, *et al.* (2008) Reconstituted fresh whole blood improves clinical outcomes compared with stored component blood therapy for neonates undergoing cardiopulmonary bypass for cardiac surgery: a randomized controlled trial. J Thorac Cardiovasc Surg 136, 1442–1449.

218. Oliver WC Jr, Santrach PJ, Danielson GK, *et al.* (2000) Desmopressin does not reduce bleeding and transfusion requirements in congenital heart operations. Ann Thorac Surg 70, 1923–1930.

219. Reynolds LM, Nicolson SC, Jobes DR, *et al.* (1993) Desmopressin does not decrease bleeding after cardiac operation in young children. J Thorac Cardiovasc Surg 106, 954–958.

220. Warren OJ, Rogers PL, Watret AL, *et al.* (2009) Defining the role of recombinant activated factor VII in pediatric cardiac surgery: where should we go from here? Pediatr Crit Care Med 10, 572–582.

221. Agarwal HS, Bennett JE, Churchwell KB, *et al.* (2007) Recombinant factor seven therapy for postoperative bleeding in neonatal and pediatric cardiac surgery. Ann Thorac Surg 84, 161–168.

222. Wittenstein B, Ng C, Ravn H, *et al.* (2005) Recombinant factor VII for severe bleeding during extracorporeal membrane oxygenation following open heart surgery. Pediatr Crit Care Med 6, 473–476.

223. Scohy TV, Gommers D, Jan ten Harkel AD, *et al.* (2007) Intraoperative evaluation of micromultiplane transesophageal echocardiographic probe in surgery for congenital heart disease. Eur J Echocardiogr 8, 241–246.

224. Bettex DA, Pretre R, Jenni R, *et al.* (2005) Cost-effectiveness of routine intraoperative transesophageal echocardiography in pediatric cardiac surgery: a 10-year experience. Anesth Analg 100, 1271–1275.

225. Bettex DA, Schmidlin D, Bernath MA, *et al.* (2000) Intraoperative transesophageal echocardiography in pediatric congenital cardiac surgery: a two-center observational study. Anesth Analg 97, 1275–1282.

226. Andropoulos DB, Stayer SA, Bent ST, *et al.* (2000) The effects of transesophageal echocardiography on hemodynamic variables in small infants undergoing cardiac surgery. J Cardiothorac Vasc Anesth 14, 133–135.

227. Andropoulos DB, Ayres NA, Stayer SA, *et al.* (2000) The effect of transesophageal echocardiography on ventilation in small infants undergoing cardiac surgery. Anesth Analg 90, 47–49.

228. Davies MJ, Nguyen K, Gaynor JW, *et al.* (1998) Modified ultrafiltration improves left ventricular systolic function in infants after cardiopulmonary bypass. J Thorac Cardiovasc Surg 115, 361–369; discussion 369–370.

229. Naik SK, Knight A, Elliott MJ. (1991) A successful modification of ultrafiltration for cardiopulmonary bypass in children. Perfusion 6, 41–50.

230. Shimpo H, Shimamoto A, Sawamura Y, *et al.* (2001) Ultrafiltration of the priming blood before cardiopulmonary bypass attenuates inflammatory response and improves postoperative clinical course in pediatric patients. Shock 16, 51–54.

231. Raja SG, Yousufuddin S, Rasool F, *et al.* (2006) Impact of modified ultrafiltration on morbidity after pediatric cardiac surgery. Asian Cardiovasc Thorac Ann 14, 341–350.

232. Gaynor JW, Kuypers M, van Rossem M, *et al.* (2005) Haemodynamic changes during modified ultrafiltration immediately following the first stage of the Norwood reconstruction. Cardiol Young 15, 4–7.

233. Friesen RH, Campbell DN, Clarke DR, *et al.* (1997) Modified ultrafiltration attenuates dilutional coagulopathy in pediatric open heart operations. Ann Thorac Surg 64, 1787–1789.

234. Koutlas TC, Gaynor JW, Nicolson SC, *et al.* (1997) Modified ultrafiltration reduces postoperative morbidity after cavopulmonary connection. Ann Thorac Surg 64, 37–42; discussion 43.

235. Gaynor JW, Bridges ND, Cohen MI, *et al.* (2002) Predictors of outcome after the Fontan operation: is hypoplastic left heart syndrome still a risk factor? J Thorac Cardiovasc Surg 123, 237–245.

236. Huang H, Yao T, Wang W, *et al.* (2003) Continuous ultrafiltration attenuates the pulmonary injury that follows open heart surgery with cardiopulmonary bypass. Ann Thorac Surg 76, 136–140.

237. Bando K, Vijay P, Turrentine MW, *et al.* (1998) Dilutional and modified ultrafiltration reduces pulmonary hypertension after operations for congenital heart disease: a prospective randomized study. J Thorac Cardiovasc Surg 115, 517–525; discussion 525–527.

238. Yndgaard S, Andersen LW, Andersen C, *et al.* (2000) The effect of modified ultrafiltration on the amount of circulating endotoxins in children undergoing cardiopulmonary bypass. J Cardiothorac Vasc Anesth 14, 399–401.

239. Thiagarajan RR, Laussen PC, Rycus PT, *et al.* (2007) Extracorporeal membrane oxygenation to aid cardiopulmonary resuscitation in infants and children. Circulation 116, 1693–1700.

240. Raymond TT, Cunnyngham CB, Thompson MT, *et al.* (2010) Outcomes among neonates, infants, and children after extracorporeal cardiopulmonary resuscitation for refractory inhospital pediatric cardiac arrest: a report from the National Registry of Cardiopulmonary Resuscitation. Pediatr Crit Care Med 11, 362–371.

241. Tajik M, Cardarelli MG. (2008) Extracorporeal membrane oxygenation after cardiac arrest in children: what do we know? Eur J Cardiothorac Surg 33, 409–417.

242. Morris MC, Ittenbach RF, Godinez RI, *et al.* (2004) Risk factors for mortality in 137 pediatric cardiac intensive care unit patients managed with extracorporeal membrane oxygenation. Crit Care Med 32, 1061–1069.

243. Fiser RT, Morris MC. (2008) Extracorporeal cardiopulmonary resuscitation in refractory pediatric cardiac arrest. Pediatr Clin N Am 55, 929–941, x.

244. Rodriguez-Nunez A, Lopez-Herce J, Garcia C, *et al.* (2006) Effectiveness and long-term outcome of cardiopulmonary resuscitation in paediatric intensive care units in Spain. Resuscitation 71, 301–309.

245. Nadkarni VM, Larkin GL, Peberdy MA, *et al.* (2006) First documented rhythm and clinical outcome from in-hospital cardiac arrest among children and adults. JAMA 295, 50–57.

246. Donoghue A, Berg RA, Hazinski MF, *et al.* (2009) Cardiopulmonary resuscitation for bradycardia with poor perfusion versus pulseless cardiac arrest. Pediatrics 124, 1541–1548.

247. Aharon AS, Drinkwater DC Jr, Churchwell KB, *et al.* (2001) Extracorporeal membrane oxygenation in children after repair of congenital cardiac lesions. Ann Thorac Surg 72, 2095–2101; discussion 2101–2102.

248. Bautista-Hernandez V, Thiagarajan RR, Fynn-Thompson F, *et al.* (2009) Preoperative extracorporeal membrane oxygenation as a bridge to cardiac surgery in children with congenital heart disease. Ann Thorac Surg 88, 1306–1311.

249. Barrett CS, Bratton SL, Salvin JW, *et al.* (2009) Neurological injury after extracorporeal membrane oxygenation use to aid pediatric cardiopulmonary resuscitation. Pediatr Crit Care Med 10, 445–451.

250. Cengiz P, Seidel K, Rycus PT, *et al.* (2005) Central nervous system complications during pediatric extracorporeal life

support: incidence and risk factors. Crit Care Med 33, 2817–2824.

251. Fynn-Thompson F, Almond C. (2007) Pediatric ventricular assist devices. Pediatr Cardiol 28, 149–155.

252. Potapov EV, Stiller B, Hetzer R. (2007) Ventricular assist devices in children: current achievements and future perspectives. Pediatr Transplant 11, 241–255.

253. Hetzer R, Stiller B. (2006) Technology insight: Use of ventricular assist devices in children. Nature Clin Pract 3, 377–386.

254. Padalino MA, Ohye RG, Chang AC, *et al*. (2006) Bridge to transplant using the MicroMed DeBakey ventricular assist device in a child with idiopathic dilated cardiomyopathy. Ann Thorac Surg 81, 1118–1121.

255. Arabia FA, Tsau PH, Smith RG, *et al*. (2006) Pediatric bridge to heart transplantation: application of the Berlin Heart, Medos and Thoratec ventricular assist devices. J Heart Lung Transplant 25, 16–21.

256. Blume ED, Naftel DC, Bastardi HJ, *et al*. (2006) Outcomes of children bridged to heart transplantation with ventricular assist devices: a multi-institutional study. Circulation 113, 2313–2319.

257. Duncan BW, Hraska V, Jonas RA, *et al*. (1999) Mechanical circulatory support in children with cardiac disease. J Thorac Cardiovasc Surg 117, 529–542.

258. Duncan BW. (2005) Pediatric mechanical circulatory support. ASAIO J 51, ix–xiv.

CHAPTER 11

Intraoperative Myocardial Protection

Paul J. Chai

All Children's Hospital, Saint Petersburg, FL, USA

Myocardial protection is a critical component of cardiac surgery. Without the use of myocardial protection techniques, permanent ischemic damage begins to occur in the heart after 20 minutes [1,2]. A complete understanding of the principles of myocardial protection is essential for the cardiac surgeon. A variety of myocardial protection techniques exists, and cardioplegia protocols can vary significantly from one center to another. Despite this variation in technique, these key principles of myocardial protection remain constant: the reduction of metabolic activity by hypothermia and the cessation of contractile and electrical activity of the heart. These principles remain important in the special circumstances of cardiac surgery in the neonate and infant.

Considerations for myocardial protection in pediatric cardiac surgery differ from those for adult cardiac surgery in a number of significant ways. The coronary arteries and myocardium are generally nondiseased in patients with congenital heart disease; therefore, in most cases the congenital heart surgeon does not need to worry about the uniform delivery of cardioplegia or deal with significantly scarred or impaired regional or global ventricular function. The congenital heart surgeon needs to deal with a heart in varying stages of maturity. This variation is significant because, as the myocardium matures, fundamental changes occur that directly influence the ability of the heart to withstand periods of ischemia and injury. The point of transition is not well known but likely occurs in the first year of life and potentially within the first 3 months of life.

It is generally believed that normal neonatal myocardium is more resistant to ischemia and reperfusion injury than mature adult myocardium [3,4]. It is important that this added resistance does not seem to be present in the hearts of cyanotic neonates and children or those with acute or chronic heart failure. These differences must be taken into account when considering the optimal strategy for myocardial protection during cardiac surgery of the neonate and infant. Myocardial protection techniques must be tailored to the age of the patient and complexity of the procedure in order to ensure the best outcomes.

Physiologic Differences Between Immature and Mature Myocardium

There are a number of specific physiologic differences between the immature myocardium of the infant and the mature myocardium of the adult that are important to understanding the greater tolerance to ischemia of the pediatric heart. These differences include a disparity in preferred substrate for metabolism, dissimilar levels of glycogen content, and differences in calcium and catecholamine sensitivities (Table 11.1) [5].

Substrate for Energy Production

Myocardium derives its energy production (adenosine triphosphate [ATP]) from the oxidation of fatty acids, glucose, lactate, ketone bodies, and amino acids. Additional energy production is also used from endogenous substrates such as glycogen and triglycerides. In the adult heart, long chain fatty acids are the main substrate for myocardial energy production. The adult myocardium gains as much as 90% of its ATP production from the oxidation of these fatty acids [6]. In contrast, the neonatal heart uses glucose as its main substrate. Energy production is supplemented by the use of fatty acids, ketones, and amino acids [7]. This shift in substrate preference from glucose to fatty acids occurs within the first few weeks of life and is caused by upregulation of 5'-adenosine monophosphate-activated protein kinase [8]. During this period of development, the neonatal myocardium has a diminished sensitivity to insulin [9] as well as a much greater capacity to store glycogen [10]. It is

Pediatric Cardiac Surgery, Fourth Edition. Edited by Constantine Mavroudis and Carl L. Backer.
© 2013 Blackwell Publishing Ltd. Published 2013 by Blackwell Publishing Ltd.

Table 11.1 Physiologic differences between pediatric and adult myocardium and potential effect of these differences on ischemia tolerance of the pediatric heart. (Reproduced with permission from Doenst *et al.* [5].)

	Pediatric	Adult	Potential effect on ischemia tolerance in the pediatric heart
Preferred substrate for adenosine triphosphate production	Glucose	Fatty acids	Increase
Glycogen content	High	Low	Increase
Insulin sensitivity	Impaired	Normal	?
Calcium handling (intracellular)	Impaired	Normal	?
Calcium sensitivity	Increased	Normal	Decrease?
Antioxidant defense	Low	High	Decrease
5′-nucleotidase	Low	High	Increase
Catecholamine sensitivity	Low	Normal	?
Ischemic preconditioning	Absent	Present	?

? indicates potential effect unknown.

generally accepted that the immature myocardium has a greater ability to use anaerobic metabolism.

The relevance of these physiologic differences between the neonatal and adult myocardium is not completely understood at this time. There may be some correlation between the neonatal heart's increased use of glucose with its increased tolerance to ischemia. For instance, Liu *et al.* found that after a period of ischemia in the adult heart, fatty acid oxidation rapidly normalized while glucose oxidation, as well as contractile function, remained depressed [11]. A positive correlation between return of contractile function and enhanced glucose uptake was demonstrated in patients undergoing coronary artery bypass operations [12]. In different experimental settings, activation of glucose oxidation enhanced functional recovery of cardiac muscle during or after ischemia [13,14].

Doenst proposed several explanations for these findings [5]. First, glucose is a more efficient substrate because it carries more of its own oxygen [6]. Second, more protons generated during ischemia are consumed when glucose is oxidized at the pyruvate dehydrogenase step [11,14]. Third, ATP generated from glycolysis supports the function of key ion pumps and calcium homeostasis [15]. Fourth, metabolism of glycogen may help with the maintenance of function of sarcoplasmic reticulum [16]. It is possible that some or all of the mechanisms responsible for these findings may be already present in hearts using glucose as a primary substrate (such as pediatric hearts) and may explain its prolonged tolerance to ischemia.

Calcium Metabolism

Pediatric myocardium is significantly more sensitive to extracellular calcium compared to adult myocardium. This may be because of the underdevelopment of the sarcoplasmic reticulum in pediatric myocardium, resulting in a reduction in storage capacity of calcium. The adult heart gets most of the calcium required for contraction from the sarcoplasmic reticulum [17,18]. In pediatric hearts, the reduced storage capacity of the sarcoplasmic reticulum forces much of the calcium to be provided by influx of calcium from the extracellular space [19]. The activity of sarcoplasmic Ca-ATPase (the enzyme necessary for calcium reuptake into the sarcoplasmic reticulum) is reduced in the pediatric heart. This reduction of sarcoplasmic Ca-ATPase activity results in a decreased ability to release calcium on stimulation of the ryanodine receptor, as well as a reduction in calcium reuptake into the sarcoplasmic reticulum. This biochemical variation found in the pediatric heart may explain why postischemic calcium overload may easily occur with the use of a perfusion medium containing high or normal levels of calcium. Several studies have described adverse effects using cardioplegic solutions containing high or normal concentrations of calcium during pediatric cardiac surgery and have recommended the use of subphysiologic levels of calcium in cardioplegia solutions [20–22]. As a result, most cardioplegic solutions in use today contain very low levels of calcium [23–25].

Enzyme Systems

Two enzyme systems seem to be relevant to the protection of the heart during periods of ischemia. The first of these systems is the antioxidant system, which includes the enzymes superoxide dismutase, catalase, and glutathione reductase. The activity of this enzyme system, which is important in the protection of the heart from free radicals, is reduced in immature myocardium [26]. Free radical generation is markedly elevated during reperfusion after a period of ischemia, and so a decreased defense mechanism would render the heart more susceptible to free radical injury. Children with tetralogy of Fallot are known to have a significant reduction in the activity of glutathione reductase [26–28] and may be at even greater risk from free radical damage than others. Some groups have incorporated the use of leukocyte filtration in the cardiopulmonary bypass circuit in an attempt to reduce the amount of free radical generation. Studies have so far yielded mixed results [29–31].

The enzyme 5'-nucleotidase, which catalyzes the conversion of adenosine monophosphate (AMP) to adenosine, is the second enzyme system of potential importance. While AMP is unable to pass through the plasma membrane, adenosine easily passes through the plasma membrane and is subsequently lost. The adenine nucleotide pool can become depleted with the production of adenosine. The size of this adenine nucleotide pool is important for postischemic recovery of the heart [32–34]. If the pool is depleted more than 50%, immediate full recovery of contractile function is impossible. Some groups have demonstrated improved ischemic tolerance by inhibition of this enzyme system [35–37]. This enzyme system is also reduced in immature myocardium and may be an additional reason why immature myocardium is more tolerant to ischemia [24,35].

Catecholamine Sensitivity

The sensitivity to catecholamines is decreased in immature hearts. In vitro studies suggest that a decreased coupling of myocardial beta-adrenergic receptors to adenylate cyclase at birth is the cause [38]. In contrast, the kinetics of cyclic adenosine monophosphate hydrolysis and the inhibitory potential of phosphodiesterase inhibitors such as milrinone are not affected by age. This explains the wide use of phosphodiesterase inhibitors in the postoperative care of neonates and infants. The question of whether this decreased sensitivity in the immature heart contributes to its increased tolerance to ischemia is difficult to answer at this time.

Summary

The preference of the immature heart for the use of glucose, the large stores of glycogen, and the low activity of 5'-nucleotidase may contribute to the neonatal and infant heart's extended tolerance to ischemia. In contrast, however, the reduced activity of the free radical scavenger system, the increased sensitivity to calcium, and unknown factors related to the unique environment of the cyanotic heart may serve to reduce the heart's ischemia tolerance. These findings, in addition to the observation that the immature heart is less sensitive to the effects of catecholamines postoperatively, suggest an even more important need for optimal myocardial protection in patients with congenital heart disease. The most important strategies for pediatric myocardial protection compared with adult myocardial

protection should include consideration of all of these findings.

Clinical Strategies for Myocardial Protection

There is no clear consensus concerning the optimal strategy for myocardial protection in the neonate and infant. Strategies vary significantly from center to center, as does the composition of cardioplegia used. Published studies often demonstrate conflicting results, which makes it difficult to recommend a "best" method of myocardial protection. Some of the mechanisms and principles behind myocardial protection strategies are discussed below.

Hypothermia

Hypothermia alone can provide a significant amount of myocardial protection and may be the single most important factor concerning myocardial protection in the neonate and infant. Some authors have suggested that under specific conditions, cardioplegia may in fact even be unnecessary [5,39]. This is demonstrated by a number of studies that have shown equivalent or better myocardial protection using hypothermia alone compared with the use of hypothermia with the addition of cardioplegia [40–43]. It should be noted, however, that these studies were performed at very low systemic temperatures of 15 °C or less. Studies at higher temperatures consistently demonstrate an advantage with the addition of cardioplegia [44–46].

Cooling of the human body to 32 °C reduces whole-body oxygen consumption by 45% [47]. At temperatures below 12 °C, oxygen consumption of the heart is below 1% of normal, and contractile function ceases [48]. In one study conducted in Siberia, because of the constraints of equipment availability, various forms of congenital heart disease were repaired using hypothermic circulatory arrest *without* cardiopulmonary bypass. Patients were packed in ice to achieve temperatures of 24–26 °C, and the repair was completed within 70 minutes. Results were remarkable, with mortality below 10% and neurologic complications at 13% [49].

Cardioplegia

Cardioplegia provides an additional level of protection during cardiac surgery. The essential use of cardioplegia is for cessation of all contractile and electrical activity of the heart. This results in a significant reduction of energy consumption, even at normothermia [24]. Almost all cardioplegic solutions exert their protective effects via depolarization or hyperpolarization of the membrane and mechanical arrest of the heart. The actual composition and method of delivery can vary significantly from institution to institution because there is currently no consensus on the type of cardioplegia that should be used. This variation is reflected in the fact that more than 150 cardioplegia solutions are used clinically for cardiac transplantation in the United States [50]. Many studies attempt to address this issue; however, these studies are fairly contradictory in their conclusions [21,46,51–54]. The primary differences in the composition of cardioplegia solution seek to address the mechanisms involved in ischemia-reperfusion injury. These can include elevated osmotic pressure to prevent edema formation, addition of buffering agents to reduce acidosis, addition of free radical scavengers, or supplementation with substrates to improve energy production during rewarming and reperfusion [20,23,55–57]. Indeed, the neonatal heart may be more prone to problematic myocardial edema, which may lead to decreased ventricular compliance, increased ventricular stiffness, and diastolic dysfunction; therefore, cardioplegia with normal and possibly slightly elevated osmotic pressure may be beneficial.

Many studies have examined the efficacy of cardioplegia (Table 11.2) [5,21,39–46,49,51–54,58–67]. All of the studies demonstrate some protective benefit of using either hypothermia or cardioplegia or both. There is no clear conclusion as to whether the use of hypothermia or cardioplegia alone is superior. There is benefit from cardioplegia over the establishment of the same temperature by a noncardioplegic method (i.e., topical cooling, blood perfusion, etc) as a function of myocardial temperature during ischemia (Figure 11.1) [5]. The benefit of cardioplegia in the neonatal period appears to be directly related to myocardial temperature. Baker demonstrated in rabbits that the importance of cardioplegia in addition to hypothermia increases with age [58]. The maintenance of deep myocardial hypothermia, therefore, is of critical importance in the clinical setting. This can be difficult to maintain in the pediatric setting, considering the small size of neonatal and infant hearts. Multiple strategies, such as systemic hypothermia, cold ambient temperatures in the operating room, and the periodic reinfusion of cold cardioplegia, are therefore necessary. Since the main purpose of reinfusion of cold cardioplegia is to cool the heart, the potassium concentration is often lowered to avoid excessive hyperkalemia [20].

Blood Versus Crystalloid Cardioplegia

The relative advantage of blood cardioplegia compared with crystalloid cardioplegia is still the subject of debate. Blood cardioplegia offers several theoretical advantages over crystalloid cardioplegia, such as the ability to carry oxygen and an excellent buffering capacity. Other theoretical advantages include a more similar electrolyte and osmotic composition and the potential to scavenge free radicals and minimize oxidative damage to the heart. In spite of these advantages, it has been difficult to demonstrate a clinical

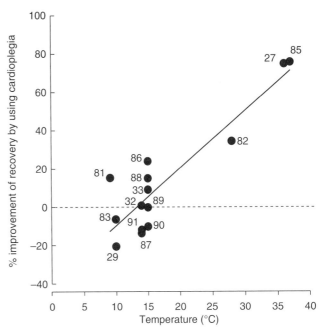

Figure 11.1 Benefit of cardioplegia over establishment of the same temperature by a noncardioplegic method (i.e., topical cooling, blood perfusion, perfusion with crystalloid buffer) as a function of myocardial temperature during ischemia. A positive value indicates that cardioplegia was better than the noncardioplegic method; a negative value indicates that the noncardioplegic method was better. (Reproduced with permission from Doenst *et al.* [5].)

superiority of blood cardioplegia over crystalloid cardioplegia. The research literature remains inconclusive, and crystalloid cardioplegia remains in use at numerous centers.

In the field of pediatric heart surgery, only a few clinical investigations comparing blood and crystalloid cardioplegia have been reported [54,68–70]. One recent study demonstrated better preservation of myocardial metabolism and ventricular function in infants receiving blood cardioplegia [68]. In another study, no significant differences in clinical outcomes were demonstrated between the two cardioplegic methods; however, in cyanotic patients, cold blood cardioplegia followed by terminal warm blood cardioplegic reperfusion ("hot shot") significantly reduced the decrease in adenosine triphosphate, indicating better myocardial protection [70]. Researchers concluded that, for cyanotic patients, cold blood cardioplegia with a hot shot is the best method of myocardial protection.

Potassium Depolarization Arrest Versus Hyperpolarization Arrest

Potassium depolarization arrest via hyperkalemia has become a fundamental component of cardioplegia solutions

Table 11.2 Synopsis of comparative studies on protection of the pediatric heart during ischemia. BCP, blood cardioplegia; CCP, crystalloid/cardioplegia; CP, cardioplegia; CPB, cardiopulmonary bypass; Hypo, hypothermia alone; ND, no data available. (Reproduced with permission from Doenst et al. [5].)

Year	Authors	Species	Age	Cardioplegia versus hypothermia alone, comments	Evidence-based medicine[a] score
1984	Bull et al. [39]	Children	ND	CCP better than fibrillation	3
1986	Bove et al. [51]	Rabbits	1, 4, 18 wk	Neonatal hearts show greater ischemia tolerance than adults	4
1987	Corno et al. [60]	Pigs	1–5 d	Hypo better than CCP; BCP better than CCP	4
1987	Bove et al. [45]	Rabbits	1 wk	CCP better than hypo	4
1988	Litasova et al. [49]	Children and adults	15 mo–44 y	Congenital heart surgery without CPB	3
1988	Ganzel et al. [63]	Pigs	Neonatal	CCP slightly better than hypo	4
1988	Magovern et al. [43]	Pigs	4, 24 wk	Hypo better than CCP	4
1988	Lynch et al. [67]	Rabbits	Neonatal	CP effective at normothermia	3
1989	Avkiran et al. [44]	Rats	3–5 d; 3–4 mo	Hypo better than CCP	4
1989	Konishi et al. [66]	Rabbits	Neonatal	CP better than hypo	4
1990	Baker et al. [40]	Rabbits	1 wk	Hypo better than CP	4
1990	Diaco et al. [61]	Rabbits	Neonatal	CP better than hypo	4
1991	Julia et al. [46]	Dogs	6–8 wk	Metabolic support with amino acids effective	4
1988	Fujiwara et al. [62]	Lambs	Neonatal	CCP slightly better than BCP	4
1991	Kofsky et al. [65]	Dogs	6–8 wk	Adult CP works well in children	4
1992	Hosseinzadeh et al. [42]	Pigs	1 wk	Hypo better than CCP; rapid cooling best	4
1993	Baker et al. [41]	Rabbits	1 wk	pH 6.8 better than hypo; hypo better than CCP	4
1993	Pearl et al. [53]	Pigs	1–2 d	CCP equal to BCP; normal Ca^{2+} better than low Ca^{2+}	4
1995	Baker et al. [58]	Rabbits	1–8 wk	Hypoxic hearts more ischemia tolerant. CP-protective effect increases with age	4
1996	Karck et al. [52]	Rats	4 wk	Hypo better than CP	4
1996	Bolling et al. [21]	Pigs	5–18 d	Normal Ca^{2+} detrimental in hypoxic hearts only	4
1997	Bolling et al. [59]	Pigs	Neonatal	BCP better than CCP in hypoxic states	4
1997	Young et al. [54]	Children	1–15 y	No difference between CCP and BCP	2
2001	Imura et al. [64]	Children	1 mo; 10 y	Hypoxic heart less ischemia tolerant	3

[a]Evidence-based medicine score is the modified American Heart Association/American College of Cardiology score.

today [71]. Depolarization arrest significantly reduces the metabolic energy demands of the myocyte. Studies indicate that normothermic arrest at 37°C decreases the oxygen demands of the heart by 90% to 1 mL O_2 × 100 g per minute [72]. Although depolarization arrest has become a fundamental component of cardioplegia, the merits of hyperpolarization arrest deserve some consideration. Certain energy-dependant processes, such as the sarcolemmal and sarcoplasmic reticular Ca2+-ATPases and Na-K-ATPase pumps, remain active during depolarization arrest. Some groups have argued that the energy requirements of these pumps may contribute to ischemic injury during potassium depolarization arrest through continued energy depletion and ionic imbalances [73]. A comparison of hyperpolarized cardioplegic arrest with a potassium ATP channel agent versus depolarization arrest with a traditional agent in rabbits found improved functional outcome in the hyperpolarized group [64]. These results are intriguing and merit further exploration into possible improvements to the traditional cardioplegic solutions in use today.

Warm Induction

A small subset of patients with left-ventricular dysfunction was found to have a reduced tolerance to aortic clamping. This poor tolerance to myocardial ischemia was thought to be because of depletion of myocardial energy stores. Rosenkranz et al. tested this hypothesis by depleting myocardial energy stores in dogs using 45 minutes of ischemia [33]. The dogs were then treated with either cold or warm induction of cardioplegia before receiving 2 hours of aortic cross-clamping with intermittent doses of cold cardioplegia. This group found that the dogs that had received warm induction had improved ventricular function and improved aerobic metabolism. Other groups have further demonstrated this finding as well [74].

Warm blood induction is felt to be beneficial in dysfunctional hearts because arrest at 37°C without ischemia enhances metabolic repair by channeling aerobic ATP production to reparative processes. The use of a warm induction dose of cardioplegia may therefore add a further level of myocardial protection by replenishing energy stores of previously abnormal hearts during cardiac surgery. This technique may deserve serious consideration in patients who come to the operating room with energy-depleted hearts, such as patients with severe cyanosis, hemodynamic instability, or heart failure.

Substrate Enhancement

Further enhancements to cardioplegia solution include the addition of substrates such as aspartate and glutamate. Studies investigating amino acid use through anaerobic pathways found that infusion of three amino acids – aspartate, glutamate, and ornithine – during ischemia augmented recovery of contractile function in isolated rabbit hearts [75]. Glutamate directly enters the tricarboxylic acid cycle as alpha-ketoglutarate and provides for nonglycolytic generation of ATP. Aspartate use is via the malate-aspartate shuttle. Aspartate is converted to oxaloacetate and then to malate. Malate enters the mitochondria where it is converted back to oxaloacetate, which liberates the reducing equivalents needed for ATP synthesis.

Lazar et al. demonstrated the benefit of using glutamate-enriched cardioplegia solution [76]. That group found increased rates of contraction and relaxation, improved stroke work index, and improved recovery of ATP using glutamate-enriched cardioplegia. Engelman et al. found that the use of a glutamate and aspartate enriched solution during reperfusion resulted in a reduction in infarct size and improved levels of ATP and acetyl coenzyme A in swine model of ischemia-reperfusion injury [77]. Other experimental studies have also suggested that including glutamate and aspartate in the warm induction of cardioplegia and also in the reperfusate provides an additional level of myocardial protection and recovery [20,46,62,65,78].

Clinical Techniques

The clinical techniques used among institutions today vary widely. Cardiac surgery in the neonate and infant is a team approach, which makes it difficult to assess clinical outcomes of any one specific technique of myocardial protection from another. Differences in operative techniques, operative times, and quality of postoperative care can significantly camouflage any possible differences in myocardial protection. What may work well for one surgeon in a particular center may not work for another.

The lack of clear and consistent data makes it difficult to recommend a single strategy of myocardial protection, especially because primary myocardial failure after cardiac surgery is a rare cause of death today [79,80]. Although myocardial failure as a cause of death remains rare, a decrease in cardiac output after pediatric cardiac surgery is fairly common. This decrease in cardiac output is especially apparent between 6 and 18 hours postoperatively, as documented by multiple studies from Children's Hospital Boston [81–84]. This phenomenon would suggest that areas of improvement pertaining to myocardial management techniques remain. Still, it is unclear whether this decrease in cardiac output would be obviated by improved strategies of myocardial protection; in fact, this phenomenon may be independent of myocardial protective strategies and instead be related to any of a variety of alternative etiologies including a generalized post-cardiopulmonary bypass inflammatory response, cytokine activity, enzymatic activity, and hormonal variations [85,86].

The Boston group found that a residual volume or pressure load on the heart (i.e., an imperfect repair) was the most important cause of an excessive drop in postoperative cardiac output [79]. Other important factors included ventricular distention during surgery (from failure to vent the heart adequately), retraction and stretch injury to the myocardium (from excessive retraction on tissues for exposure), coronary artery injury, ventriculotomy, edema, perfusion factors, and reperfusion conditions [87].

Cardiac Distention

In contrast to the findings that the immature myocardium is significantly more resistant to ischemia compared with the adult heart, there is a general feeling among surgeons that immature myocardium is significantly more vulnerable to stretch injury. Stretch injury occurs mainly from overdistention of the left heart and excessive retraction on myocardial tissues. Overdistention of the left heart can have many detrimental consequences other than primary myocardial contractile dysfunction. Overdistention of the left ventricle also leads to distention of the left atrium and pulmonary veins, which eventually results in a high transcapillary pressure in the lungs. This elevated pulmonary transcapillary pressure eventually leads to significant pulmonary edema and pulmonary dysfunction.

The cardiac surgeon needs to be acutely aware of instances when distention of the left heart is occurring. Palpation of the left ventricle, or even the main pulmonary artery, should alert the surgeon when overdistention is present. Left-heart venting should be performed either through the right superior pulmonary vein or through an atrial septal defect to keep left-ventricular pressures low. The safest time to insert a left atrial vent is after the aortic cross-clamp is applied, to negate any chance that air could be introduced to the left side and embolize to the brain. Instant measures to reduce left-ventricular overdistention include having the perfusionist immediately drop the flow rate and/or temporarily releasing the aortic cross-clamp until the issue is resolved.

Cardioplegia Protocols

Clinical techniques vary from groups who advocate the use of single-dose cold cardioplegia in neonates and infants to groups who favor a more conventional approach adapted from use in adult cardiac surgery. The group at Children's Hospital Boston is one group that advocates the use of a single dose of cold cardioplegia in specific circumstances. Their practice is to use a single dose of cardioplegia infusion (20 mL/kg) combined with systemic deep hypothermia for neonatal procedures. In patients older than 2–3 months of age, periodic doses of cold cardioplegia are repeated at 20- to 30-minute intervals. Beyond 1 year of age, repeat doses of cardioplegia are administered every 20 minutes using an initial dose of 20 mL/kg followed by subsequent doses of 10 mL/kg [87].

Another cardioplegia protocol from Boston uses an innovative single-dose cardioplegia protocol for all patients, with usually no repeat doses. The formulation was based on animal studies done by McGowan et al. and Takeuchi et al. [56,88]. Occasionally, a repeat dose is given in larger patients with sick myocardium. Cardioplegia is a custom mix crystalloid cardioplegia with 1 part oxygenated pump blood and 4 parts crystalloid. Blood is added for its buffering capability. Components of the crystalloid solution include Plasmalyte A, sodium bicarbonate, mannitol (decreases myocardial edema and acts as a free radical scavenger), potassium (depolarization), lidocaine (maintains arrest in a hyperpolarized state), and magnesium (Table 11.3) [89].

The group at the Congenital Heart Institute of Florida currently uses a cardioplegia protocol that involves the administration of up to four distinct cardioplegia solutions, depending on the particular procedure being performed (Table 11.4).

For standard cases at mild to moderate levels of hypothermia, a warm-induction dose is given initially (10–20 mL/kg), followed immediately by a high K cold-induction dose (20–30 mL/kg). Total induction volume is 40 mL/kg. Subsequent maintenance cardioplegia doses are given at roughly 20-minute intervals using the low K maintenance solution at half-induction doses (10–20 mL/kg). Before removal of the cross-clamp, a hot-shot dose of physiologic K warm perfusion is administered (10–20 mL/kg), followed by warm oxygenated blood reperfusion for 2 minutes.

Patients undergoing procedures that require a period of circulatory arrest are cooled to systemic temperatures of 18 °C. For myocardial protection, only the high K cold-induction dose is given (40 mL/kg). The warm-induction dose is not administered for circulatory arrest cases.

For cardiac transplant patients, initial reperfusion of the recipient heart with an aspartate- and glutamate-enriched leukocyte-filtered solution is used [90].

Table 11.3 Custom mix cardioplegia, Children's Hospital Boston. (Reproduced from Talwar [89].)

Plasmalyte A	1000 mL
Mannitol 20%	16.30 mL
Magnesium sulfate 50%	4.0 mL
Sodium bicarbonate 1 mEq/mL	13.0 mL
Lidocaine 1%	13.0 mL
Potassium chloride 2 mEq/mL	13.0 mL

Table 11.4 Neonatal/pediatric cardioplegia composition at the Congenital Heart Institute of Florida. (D5W, 5% dextrose; NaCl, sodium chloride; THAM, tromeThamine.)

	High K+ cold induction	Low K+ maintenance	Warm induction	Physiologic K+ warm reperfusion
D5W/0.22 NaCl	165 mL	165 mL	165 mL	165 mL
THAM 0.3 M	60 mL	60 mL	60 mL	60 mL
Potassium chloride	15 mEq	6 mEq	15 mEq	1.5 mEq
Magnesium sulfate	5.6 mEq	5.2 mEq	15.6 mEq	14.3 mEq
Aspartate 3.92%/Glutamate 4.28%			75 mL	75 mL
Volume dispensed	233.9 mL	229.3 mL	311.4 mL	304.4 mL

Retrograde Cardioplegia

Retrograde cardioplegia is an effective technique for administering cardioplegia in selective cases. Retrograde cardioplegia is routinely used for cases involving an open aortic root and coronary artery transfers such as the arterial switch procedure and Ross procedure. Retrograde cardioplegia is also particularly helpful in cases where the ability to arrest the heart because of severe aortic insufficiency is in question.

The retrograde cardioplegia cannula is placed under direct vision into the coronary sinus and secured by either balloon insufflation or placement of a purse-string suture (6-0 Prolene) around the coronary sinus. For larger patients, the retrograde cannula can be placed "blindly" by feel through a small stab incision in the right atrium. A 6-Fr retrograde cannula (DLP®; Medtronic) is the preferred cannula for neonatal surgery. During infusion of retrograde cardioplegia, flow through the retrograde cannula is adjusted to result in a cardioplegia perfusion pressure no higher than 50 mmHg.

Disadvantages for the use of retrograde cardioplegia include the potential nonuniform distribution of cardioplegia away from portions of the right ventricle and right atrium. Using retrograde cardioplegia in patients with a left-sided superior vena cava draining into the coronary sinus may also cause problems. Placement of the retrograde cannula can be difficult in the neonate and may require a carefully placed purse-string suture around the coronary sinus to prevent dislodgement. Care must be taken in placement of the purse-string suture to avoid the conduction system and prevent complete heart block. Direct coronary ostial administration of cardioplegia is an alternative technique when retrograde cardioplegia is difficult or impossible.

Conclusion

Pediatric cardiac surgery is a unique process, with many differences from adult cardiac surgery. Techniques for myocardial protection must take into account a myriad of factors including the physical size of the heart and operating field as well as the physiologic differences of the immature heart.

Many different techniques and forms of cardioplegia are successfully used by multiple centers with excellent results. In 2004, Ungerleider published a review of practice patterns of congenital heart surgeons collected from surveys of the Congenital Heart Surgeon's Society and from audience response at the American Association for Thoracic Surgery (May 2003) and the Society of Thoracic Surgeons (January 2004) [91]. This review demonstrated that numerous practice patterns exist, with unanimity only in the recommended use of cardioplegia, although the delivery, type, and timing of doses varied.

It is difficult to effectively compare techniques used at one institution with another because multiple variables exist, including surgical technique, operative times, anesthetic management, and perfusion methods. What may give excellent results at one institution may truly be surgeon or center specific and may not translate well for use at another institution.

The fact that multiple protocols for cardioplegia exist suggests that we still have much to learn about the optimal methods for myocardial protection. Further investigations, specifically in the field of pediatric myocardial protection, will increase our understanding and continue to improve outcomes.

References

1. Reimer KA, Jennings RB, Tatum AH. (1983) Pathobiology of acute myocardial ischemia: metabolic, functional and ultrastructural studies. Am J Cardiol 52, 72A–81A.
2. Spieckermann PG, Braun U, Hellberg K, et al. (1970) [Survival and resuscitation time of the heart during ketamine, barbiturates and halothane anesthesia]. Z Prakt Anasth 5, 365–372.
3. Bove EL, Gallagher KP, Drake DH, et al. (1988) The effect of hypothermic ischemia on recovery of left ventricular

function and preload reserve in the neonatal heart. J Thorac Cardiovasc Surg 95, 814–818.

4. Grice WN, Konishi T, Apstein CS. (1987) Resistance of neonatal myocardium to injury during normothermic and hypothermic ischemic arrest and reperfusion. Circulation 76, V150–V155.

5. Doenst T, Schlensak C, Beyersdorf F. (2003) Cardioplegia in pediatric cardiac surgery: do we believe in magic? Ann Thorac Surg 75, 1668–1677.

6. Goodwin GW, Ahmad F, Doenst T, et al. (1998) Energy provision from glycogen, glucose, and fatty acids on adrenergic stimulation of isolated working rat hearts. Am J Physiol 274, H1239–H1247.

7. Lopaschuk GD, Spafford MA, Marsh DR. (1991) Glycolysis is predominant source of myocardial ATP production immediately after birth. Am J Physiol 261, H1698–H1705.

8. Makinde AO, Gamble J, Lopaschuk GD. (1997) Upregulation of 5'-AMP-activated protein kinase is responsible for the increase in myocardial fatty acid oxidation rates following birth in the newborn rabbit. Circ Res 80, 482–489.

9. Clark CM, Jr. (1973) Characterization of glucose metabolism in the isolated rat heart during fetal and early neonatal development. Diabetes 22, 41–49.

10. Johnson B, Everitt B. (1988) The high concentration of glycogen in fetal cardiac muscle probably explains why the heart can maintain its contractile activity in the face of severe hypoxia. In: *Essential Reproduction*, 3rd ed. Oxford: Blackwell Publishing, p. 275.

11. Liu B, Clanachan AS, Schulz R, et al. (1996) Cardiac efficiency is improved after ischemia by altering both the source and fate of protons. Circ Res 79, 940–948.

12. Depre C, Vanoverschelde JL, Melin JA, et al. (1995) Structural and metabolic correlates of the reversibility of chronic left ventricular ischemic dysfunction in humans. Am J Physiol 268, H1265–H1275.

13. Lopaschuk GD, Wambolt RB, Barr RL. (1993) An imbalance between glycolysis and glucose oxidation is a possible explanation for the detrimental effects of high levels of fatty acids during aerobic reperfusion of ischemic hearts. J Pharmacol Exp Ther 264, 135–144.

14. Mallet RT. (2000) Pyruvate: metabolic protector of cardiac performance. Proc Soc Exp Biol Med 223, 136–148.

15. Weiss JN, Lamp ST. (1987) Glycolysis preferentially inhibits ATP-sensitive K+ channels in isolated guinea pig cardiac myocytes. Science 238, 67–69.

16. Xu KY, Zweier JL, Becker LC. (1995) Functional coupling between glycolysis and sarcoplasmic reticulum Ca2+ transport. Circ Res 77, 88–97.

17. Klitzner TS. (1991) Maturational changes in excitation-contraction coupling in mammalian myocardium. J Am Coll Cardiol 17, 218–225.

18. Pieske B, Schlotthauer K, Schattmann J, et al. (1997) Ca(2+)-dependent and Ca(2+)-independent regulation of contractility in isolated human myocardium. Basic Res Cardiol 92(suppl) 1, 75–86.

19. Boland R, Martonosi A, Tillack TW. (1974) Developmental changes in the composition and function of sarcoplasmic reticulum. J Biol Chem 249, 612–623.

20. Allen BS, Barth MJ, Ilbawi MN. (2001) Pediatric myocardial protection: an overview. Semin Thorac Cardiovasc Surg 13, 56–72.

21. Bolling K, Kronon M, Allen BS, et al. (1996) Myocardial protection in normal and hypoxically stressed neonatal hearts: the superiority of hypocalcemic versus normocalcemic blood cardioplegia. J Thorac Cardiovasc Surg 112, 1193–1200; discussion 1200–1201.

22. Kronon MT, Allen BS, Hernan J, et al. (1999) Superiority of magnesium cardioplegia in neonatal myocardial protection. Ann Thorac Surg 68, 2285–2291; discussion 2291–2292.

23. Bilfinger TV, Moeller JT, Kurusz M, et al. (1992) Pediatric myocardial protection in the United States: a survey of current clinical practice. Thorac Cardiovasc Surg 40, 214–218.

24. Buckberg GD. (1995) Update on current techniques of myocardial protection. Ann Thorac Surg 60, 805–814.

25. Rebeyka IM, Diaz RJ, Augustine JM, et al. (1991) Effect of rapid cooling contracture on ischemic tolerance in immature myocardium. Circulation 84, III389–III393.

26. Teoh KH, Mickle DA, Weisel RD, et al. (1992) Effect of oxygen tension and cardiovascular operations on the myocardial antioxidant enzyme activities in patients with tetralogy of Fallot and aorta-coronary bypass. J Thorac Cardiovasc Surg 104, 159–164.

27. del Nido PJ, Mickle DA, Wilson GJ, et al. (1987) Evidence of myocardial free radical injury during elective repair of tetralogy of Fallot. Circulation 76, V174–V179.

28. del Nido PJ, Mickle DA, Wilson GJ, et al. (1988) Inadequate myocardial protection with cold cardioplegic arrest during repair of tetralogy of Fallot. J Thorac Cardiovasc Surg 95, 223–229.

29. Englander R, Cardarelli MG. (1995) Efficacy of leukocyte filters in the bypass circuit for infants undergoing cardiac operations. Ann Thorac Surg 60, S533–S535.

30. Hayashi Y, Sawa Y, Nishimura M, et al. (2000) Clinical evaluation of leukocyte-depleted blood cardioplegia for pediatric open heart operation. Ann Thorac Surg 69, 1914–1919.

31. Kawata H, Sawatari K, Mayer JE Jr. (1992) Evidence for the role of neutrophils in reperfusion injury after cold cardioplegic ischemia in neonatal lambs. J Thorac Cardiovasc Surg 103, 908–917; discussion 917–918.

32. Rosenkranz ER, Okamoto F, Buckberg GD, et al. (1986) Biochemical studies: failure of tissue adenosine triphosphate levels to predict recovery of contractile function after controlled reperfusion. J Thorac Cardiovasc Surg 92, 488–501.

33. Rosenkranz ER, Vinten-Johansen J, Buckberg GD, et al. (1982) Benefits of normothermic induction of blood cardioplegia in energy-depleted hearts, with maintenance of arrest by multidose cold blood cardioplegic infusions. J Thorac Cardiovasc Surg 84, 667–677.

34. Taegtmeyer H, Goodwin GW, Doenst T, et al. (1997) Substrate metabolism as a determinant for postischemic functional recovery of the heart. Am J Cardiol 80, 3A–10A.

35. Bolling SF, Olszanski DA, Bove EL, et al. (1992) Enhanced myocardial protection during global ischemia with 5'-nucleotidase inhibitors. J Thorac Cardiovasc Surg 103, 73–77.

36. Kitakaze M, Weisfeldt ML, Marban E. (1988) Acidosis during early reperfusion prevents myocardial stunning in perfused ferret hearts. J Clin Invest 82, 920–927.

37. Pridjian AK, Bove EL, Bolling SF, *et al.* (1994) Developmental differences in myocardial protection in response to 5'-nucleotidase inhibition. J Thorac Cardiovasc Surg 107, 520–526.

38. Artman M, Kithas PA, Wike JS, *et al.* (1989) Inotropic responses to cyclic nucleotide phosphodiesterase inhibitors in immature and adult rabbit myocardium. J Cardiovasc Pharmacol 13, 146–154.

39. Bull C, Cooper J, Stark J. (1984) Cardioplegic protection of the child's heart. J Thorac Cardiovasc Surg 88, 287–293.

40. Baker JE, Boerboom LE, Olinger GN. (1990) Cardioplegia-induced damage to ischemic immature myocardium is independent of oxygen availability. Ann Thorac Surg 50, 934–939.

41. Baker JE, Boerboom LE, Olinger GN. (1993) Age and protection of the ischemic myocardium: is alkaline cardioplegia appropriate? Ann Thorac Surg 55, 747–755.

42. Hosseinzadeh T, Tchervenkov CI, Quantz M, *et al.* (1992) Adverse effect of prearrest hypothermia in immature hearts: rate versus duration of cooling. Ann Thorac Surg 53, 464–471.

43. Magovern JA, Pae WE Jr, Waldhausen JA. (1988) Protection of the immature myocardium. An experimental evaluation of topical cooling, single-dose, and multiple-dose administration of St. Thomas' Hospital cardioplegic solution. J Thorac Cardiovasc Surg 96, 408–413.

44. Avkiran M, Hearse DJ. (1989) Protection of the myocardium during global ischemia. Is crystalloid cardioplegia effective in the immature myocardium? J Thorac Cardiovasc Surg 97, 220–228.

45. Bove EL, Stammers AH, Gallagher KP. (1987) Protection of the neonatal myocardium during hypothermic ischemia. Effect of cardioplegia on left ventricular function in the rabbit. J Thorac Cardiovasc Surg 94, 115–123.

46. Julia P, Young HH, Buckberg GD, *et al.* (1991) Studies of myocardial protection in the immature heart. IV. Improved tolerance of immature myocardium to hypoxia and ischemia by intravenous metabolic support. J Thorac Cardiovasc Surg 101, 23–32.

47. Bigelow WG, Callaghan JC, Hopps JA. (1950) General hypothermia for experimental intracardiac surgery; the use of electrophrenic respirations, an artificial pacemaker for cardiac standstill and radio-frequency rewarming in general hypothermia. Ann Surg 132, 531–539.

48. Niazi SA, Lewis FJ. (1955) The effect of carbon dioxide on ventricular fibrillation and heart block during hypothermia in rats and dogs. Surg Forum 5, 106–109.

49. Litasova EE, Lomivorotov VN. (1988) Hypothermic protection (26–25 degrees C) without perfusion cooling for surgery of congenital cardiac defects using prolonged occlusion. Thorax 43, 206–211.

50. Demmy TL, Biddle JS, Bennett LE, *et al.* (1997) Organ preservation solutions in heart transplantation–patterns of usage and related survival. Transplantation 63, 262–269.

51. Bove EL, Stammers AH. (1986) Recovery of left ventricular function after hypothermic global ischemia. Age-related differences in the isolated working rabbit heart. J Thorac Cardiovasc Surg 91, 115–122.

52. Karck M, Ziemer G, Haverich A. (1996) Myocardial protection in chronic volume-overload hypertrophy of immature rat hearts. Eur J Cardiothorac Surg 10, 690–698.

53. Pearl JM, Laks H, Drinkwater DC, *et al.* (1993) Normocalcemic blood or crystalloid cardioplegia provides better neonatal myocardial protection than does low-calcium cardioplegia. J Thorac Cardiovasc Surg 105, 201–206.

54. Young JN, Choy IO, Silva NK, *et al.* (1997) Antegrade cold blood cardioplegia is not demonstrably advantageous over cold crystalloid cardioplegia in surgery for congenital heart disease. J Thorac Cardiovasc Surg 114, 1002–1008; discussion 1008–1009.

55. Beyersdorf F, Kirsh M, Buckberg GD, *et al.* (1992) Warm glutamate/aspartate-enriched blood cardioplegic solution for perioperative sudden death. J Thorac Cardiovasc Surg 104, 1141–1147.

56. McGowan FX Jr., Cao-Danh H, Takeuchi K, *et al.* (1994) Prolonged neonatal myocardial preservation with a highly buffered low-calcium solution. J Thorac Cardiovasc Surg 108, 772–779.

57. Pearl JM, Hiramoto J, Laks H, *et al.* (1994) Fumarate-enriched blood cardioplegia results in complete functional recovery of immature myocardium. Ann Thorac Surg 57, 1636–1641.

58. Baker EJ, Boerboom LE, Olinger GN, *et al.* (1995) Tolerance of the developing heart to ischemia: impact of hypoxemia from birth. Am J Physiol 268, H1165–H1173.

59. Bolling K, Kronon M, Allen BS, *et al.* (1997) Myocardial protection in normal and hypoxically stressed neonatal hearts: the superiority of blood versus crystalloid cardioplegia. J Thorac Cardiovasc Surg 113, 994–1003; discussion 1003–1005.

60. Corno AF, Bethencourt DM, Laks H, *et al.* (1987) Myocardial protection in the neonatal heart. A comparison of topical hypothermia and crystalloid and blood cardioplegic solutions. J Thorac Cardiovasc Surg 93, 163–172.

61. Diaco M, DiSesa VJ, Sun SC, *et al.* (1990) Cardioplegia for the immature myocardium. A comparative study in the neonatal rabbit. J Thorac Cardiovasc Surg 100, 910–913.

62. Fujiwara T, Kurtts T, Anderson W, *et al.* (1988) Myocardial protection in cyanotic neonatal lambs. J Thorac Cardiovasc Surg 96, 700–710.

63. Ganzel BL, Katzmark SL, Mavroudis C. (1988) Myocardial preservation in the neonate. Beneficial effects of cardioplegia and systemic hypothermia on piglets undergoing cardiopulmonary bypass and myocardial ischemia. J Thorac Cardiovasc Surg 96, 414–422.

64. Imura H, Caputo M, Parry A, *et al.* (2001) Age-dependent and hypoxia-related differences in myocardial protection during pediatric open heart surgery. Circulation 103, 1551–1556.

65. Kofsky E, Julia P, Buckberg GD, *et al.* (1991) Studies of myocardial protection in the immature heart. V. Safety of prolonged aortic clamping with hypocalcemic glutamate/aspartate blood cardioplegia. J Thorac Cardiovasc Surg 101, 33–43.

66. Konishi T, Apstein CS. (1989) Comparison of three cardioplegic solutions during hypothermic ischemic arrest in neonatal blood-perfused rabbit hearts. J Thorac Cardiovasc Surg 98, 1132–1137.

67. Lynch MJ, Bove EL, Zweng TN, et al. (1988) Protection of the neonatal heart following normothermic ischemia: a comparison of oxygenated saline and oxygenated versus nonoxygenated cardioplegia. Ann Thorac Surg 45, 650–655.

68. Amark K, Berggren H, Bjork K, et al. (2005) Blood cardioplegia provides superior protection in infant cardiac surgery. Ann Thorac Surg 80, 989–994.

69. Caputo M, Modi P, Imura H, et al. (2002) Cold blood versus cold crystalloid cardioplegia for repair of ventricular septal defects in pediatric heart surgery: a randomized controlled trial. Ann Thorac Surg 74, 530–534; discussion 535.

70. Modi P, Suleiman MS, Reeves B, et al. (2004) Myocardial metabolic changes during pediatric cardiac surgery: a randomized study of 3 cardioplegic techniques. J Thorac Cardiovasc Surg 128, 67–75.

71. Conti VR, Bertranou EG, Blackstone EH, et al. (1978) Cold cardioplegia versus hypothermia for myocardial protection. Randomized clinical study. J Thorac Cardiovasc Surg 76, 577–589.

72. Buckberg GD, Brazier JR, Nelson RL, et al. (1977) Studies of the effects of hypothermia on regional myocardial blood flow and metabolism during cardiopulmonary bypass. I. The adequately perfused beating, fibrillating, and arrested heart. J Thorac Cardiovasc Surg 73, 87–94.

73. Cohen NM, Wise RM, Wechsler AS, et al. (1993) Elective cardiac arrest with a hyperpolarizing adenosine triphosphate-sensitive potassium channel opener. A novel form of myocardial protection? J Thorac Cardiovasc Surg 106, 317–328.

74. Tixier D, Matheis G, Buckberg GD, et al. (1991) Donor hearts with impaired hemodynamics. Benefit of warm substrate-enriched blood cardioplegic solution for induction of cardioplegia during cardiac harvesting. J Thorac Cardiovasc Surg 102, 207–213; discussion 213–214.

75. Rau EE, Shine KI, Gervais A, et al. (1979) Enhanced mechanical recovery of anoxic and ischemic myocardium by amino acid perfusion. Am J Physiol 236, H873–H879.

76. Lazar HL, Buckberg GD, Manganaro AM, et al. (1980) Myocardial energy replenishment and reversal of ischemic damage by substrate enhancement of secondary blood cardioplegia with amino acids during reperfusion. J Thorac Cardiovasc Surg 80, 350–359.

77. Engelman RM, Rousou JA, Flack JE 3rd, et al. (1991) Reduction of infarct size by systemic amino acid supplementation during reperfusion. J Thorac Cardiovasc Surg 101, 855–859.

78. Kronon MT, Allen BS, Rahman S, et al. (2000) Reducing postischemic reperfusion damage in neonates using a terminal warm substrate-enriched blood cardioplegic reperfusate. Ann Thorac Surg 70, 765–770.

79. Jonas R, Krasna M, Sell J, et al. (1991) Myocardial failure is a rare cause of death after pediatric cardiac surgery (abstr). J Am Coll Cardiol 17, 110A.

80. Jonas RA. (1998) Myocardial protection for neonates and infants. Thorac Cardiovasc Surg 46(suppl 2), 288–291.

81. du Plessis AJ, Jonas RA, Wypij D, et al. (1997) Perioperative effects of alpha-stat versus pH-stat strategies for deep hypothermic cardiopulmonary bypass in infants. J Thorac Cardiovasc Surg 114, 991–1000; discussion 1000–1001.

82. Jonas RA, Wypij D, Roth SJ, et al. (2003) The influence of hemodilution on outcome after hypothermic cardiopulmonary bypass: results of a randomized trial in infants. J Thorac Cardiovasc Surg 126, 1765–1774.

83. Newburger JW, Jonas RA, Wernovsky G, et al. (1993) A comparison of the perioperative neurologic effects of hypothermic circulatory arrest versus low-flow cardiopulmonary bypass in infant heart surgery. N Engl J Med 329, 1057–1064.

84. Wernovsky G, Wypij D, Jonas RA, et al. (1995) Postoperative course and hemodynamic profile after the arterial switch operation in neonates and infants. A comparison of low-flow cardiopulmonary bypass and circulatory arrest. Circulation 92, 2226–2235.

85. Saatvedt K, Lindberg H. (1996) Depressed thyroid function following paediatric cardiopulmonary bypass: association with interleukin-6 release? Scand J Thorac Cardiovasc Surg 30, 61–64.

86. Saatvedt K, Lindberg H, Geiran OR, et al. (1998) Thyroid function during and after cardiopulmonary bypass in children. Acta Anaesthesiol Scand 42, 1100–1103.

87. Jonas RA. (2004) Myocardial protection. In: Jonas RA, ed. *Comprehensive Surgical Management of Congenital Heart Disease*. London: Arnold, pp. 175–184.

88. Takeuchi K, Takashima K, Kawai A, et al. (1995) [Prolonged preservation due to acceleration of anaerobic glycolysis with histidine buffered cardioplegia in canine heart]. Nippon Kyobu Geka Gakkai Zasshi 43, 1895–1901.

89. Talwar S. (2010) Controversies in managing cardiopulmonary bypass in neonates and infants. Ind J Extra Corpor Technol 20, 12–18.

90. Jacobs JP, Quintessenza JA, Boucek RJ, et al. (2004) Pediatric cardiac transplantation in children with high panel reactive antibody. Ann Thorac Surg 78, 1703–1709.

91. Ungerleider RM. (2005) Practice patterns in neonatal cardiopulmonary bypass. Asaio J 51, 813–815.

CHAPTER 12

Patent Ductus Arteriosus

Muhammad Ali Mumtaz,[1] Athar Qureshi,[2] Constantine Mavroudis,[3] and Carl L. Backer[4]

[1]Children's Hospital of the King's Daughters, Norfolk, VA, USA
[2]Cleveland Clinic Children's Hospital, Cleveland, OH, USA
[3]Florida Hospital for Children, Orlando, FL, USA
[4]Ann & Robert H. Lurie Children's Hospital of Chicago, formerly Children's Memorial Hospital, Chicago, IL, USA

Introduction

The ductus arteriosus is an arterial connection between the pulmonary artery and the aorta. It is normally present in the fetus to direct the pulmonary arterial blood to the aorta. The ductus arteriosus closes shortly after birth, and the term *patent ductus arteriosus* (PDA) refers to the pathologic persistence of the ductal lumen after birth.

Patent ductus arteriosus was first ligated by Strieder [1] in Boston in 1937 in a patient with infective endocarditis. Although he achieved technical success, the patient died from aspiration in the postoperative period. The first successful ligation to a PDA is credited to Gross [2] in a 7-year-old girl in 1938. This ushered in a new era of cardiac surgery. Interestingly, treatment of PDA is also the lesion that was the substrate for closure by interventional cardiology methods when Porstmann [3] closed a PDA with a foam plug placed with a catheter. Furthermore, PDA happens to be the first anatomic lesion treated with pharmacologic manipulation [4]. This chapter discusses PDA occurring as an isolated lesion and not in association with other cardiac malformations.

Anatomy

The ductus arteriosus is a normal fetal structure connecting the pulmonary artery to the aorta. During the fourth week of embryonic development, the pharyngeal arches develop. Each arch has its own artery and nerve. The arteries join in the front with the truncus arteriosus and in the back with the dorsal aorta. The sixth aortic arch gives rise to the ductus and proximal branch pulmonary arteries. On the right side, the proximal aortic arch gives a branch toward the lung bud. The distal connection to the dorsal aorta disappears, and the proximal portion remains connected to the right lung and forms the right pulmonary artery. On the left side, the distal connection to the dorsal aorta persists as ductus arteriosus, and the proximal portion connects to the lung bud forming the left pulmonary artery. This results in the interesting relation between the recurrent laryngeal nerve and the ductus. The recurrent laryngeal nerve is the branch to the sixth pharyngeal arch. As the heart and great vessels descend into the thorax, the nerves are pulled into the thorax. Since on the right side the distal sixth arch disappears, the recurrent laryngeal nerve hooks around the derivative of the right fourth aortic arch (proximal subclavian artery), because there is no fifth aortic arch in humans. On the left side, the nerve hooks around the ductus because it is the persisting derivative of the sixth left aortic arch.

The pulmonic origin of the duct is typically at the pulmonary artery bifurcation, somewhat closer to the left pulmonary artery. It then gently curves posteriorly and inferiorly to be inserted into the descending aorta beyond the origin of the left subclavian artery. The angle between the superior edge of the ductus and the underside of the aorta is acute. It is occasionally "reversed" when this angle is greater than 90 degrees. Reversed ductus is commonly associated with pulmonary atresia and right ventricular outflow obstruction [5]. Ductus is occasionally inserted at the base of the subclavian artery. In the case of right aortic arch, it frequently inserts at the base of the left-sided innominate artery. It is typically absent in truncus arteriosus, pulmonary atresia/ventricular septal defect (VSD) with absent central pulmonary arteries, and in tetralogy of Fallot with absent pulmonary valve. It may occasionally be absent in tetralogy of Fallot. It is rarely bilateral or just right sided. The media of the ductus arteriosus is composed of longitudinally and spirally arranged layers of smooth muscle fibers within loose, concentric layers of elastic tissue. The intima of the ductus arteriosus is thickened and irregular, with abundant mucoid material, sometimes referred to as intimal cushions. This is in contrast to the media of aorta and pulmonary artery, which have circumferentially arranged layers of elastic fibers [6].

Etiologic Factors

Prostaglandins

During fetal life, as the lungs are collapsed and fluid-filled, pulmonary vascular resistance is high, and ductal flow is right to left. The patency is maintained by low oxygen saturation and circulating prostaglandins. In mice, this effect appears to be mediated by cyclooxygenase-2 (COX-2) isoform. In a mouse fetus, ductal constriction can be achieved by selective COX-2 inhibitors but not selective COX-1 inhibitors [4]. The role of prostaglandins constitutes the rationale for the administration of nonsteroidal anti-inflammatory drugs in the treatment of PDA [7]. After birth, the increase in arterial oxygen results in inhibition of the prostaglandin synthase followed by a fall in the circulating prostaglandin level. This may be mediated via an oxygen-sensitive potassium channel [8]. This leads to ductal constriction and eventual closure.

Prematurity

A number of factors are responsible for the patency of the duct in the premature infant. Hypoxia and respiratory distress accompanying the lung disease of prematurity are the major factors. In neonatal lambs, respiratory distress results in elevation of prostaglandin levels that may lead to persistence of the PDA [9]. Similarly, cortisone increases the sensitivity of the ductal tissue to circulating prostaglandins, leading to earlier or premature closure [10].

Drugs

Various drugs, including angiotensin-converting enzyme (ACE) inhibitors, have been implicated in ductal patency.

Genetic Factors

Genetic factors also seem to play a role in persistence of PDA. Patients with trisomy-21 seem to have a higher incidence of PDA [11]. Siblings of patients with PDA had an increased incidence of up to 2–4% [12]. Char syndrome is an autosomal dominant trait characterized by PDA, facial dysmorphism, and hand anomalies. The mutation related to Char syndrome has been mapped to chromosome 6. Similarly, other mutations have been linked to PDA [13]. Others have found increased incidence in cases of parental consanguinity. Mutations on chromosome 12 have been linked to high incidence of PDA in children of consanguineous Iranian parents [14].

Congenital Infections

Infections such as rubella are associated with PDA. In addition, sepsis in premature babies frequently results in reopening of the PDA [15].

Pathophysiology

After birth, with the drop in pulmonary vascular resistance, there is increased blood flow from the aorta to the pulmonary artery through the PDA during both phases of the cardiac cycle. As a result, size-for-size, a PDA results in more pulmonary overcirculation than a VSD or an atrial septal defect (ASD). The resulting pulmonary congestion results in typical symptoms of congestive heart failure. Pulmonary hypertension from a persistent patent duct can develop earlier as well. The diastolic steal of systemic blood flow into the pulmonary circulation in neonates and premature babies is thought to be the mechanism for development of renal and gastrointestinal dysfunction. Because of velocity acceleration in a small or restrictive PDA, endothelial damage can occur. This may be a contributing factor for development of infective endocarditis.

Natural History

Recent studies have documented PDA to be present in 0.9% of full-term live births at 1 month of age [16]. One study reports an incidence of 4.5% in full-term normal babies at 2–6 months of age [17]. The incidence had previously been reported as much lower (1 in 2000) [18]. This discrepancy is probably related to the occurrence of "silent PDA" picked up by echocardiography. The incidence of PDA is around 30% in very low birthweight premature infants (<1500 g) [19] and decreases with age after birth. However, a very small percentage of PDAs close after 6 months of age. The mortality from untreated PDA is high, and 30% of patients born with an isolated PDA die within the first year. The most common mode of death is heart failure. Pulmonary hypertension, pulmonary hemorrhage, and infective endocarditis are other modes of death. Infective endocarditis has been reported in all age groups, including neonates [20]. Although the incidence of infective endocarditis in a patient with PDA has been debated, it is probably underreported [21,22].

Clinical Features

Clinical features of patients with PDAs vary depending on the resistances of the systemic and pulmonary circulations, the age of the patient, and the anatomy of the PDA. Preterm infants with PDAs may initially need their PDA as an obligatory shunt because of initial high pulmonary vascular resistance. With severe pulmonary hypertension, the PDA serves as a mechanism to maintain cardiac output and prevent right heart failure. However, despite prematurity, many of these babies have significant left-to-right shunts through a PDA very early on in life and sometimes within hours of birth [23]. As pulmonary vascular resistance falls, if the PDA is significant, these babies develop signs of congestive heart failure, or "pulmonary overcirculation." This often manifests as an inability to wean from the ventilator or as an increase in ventilatory requirements. In extreme situations, poor systemic cardiac output may be seen with signs of poor peripheral perfusion and multiorgan failure. Although controversy still exists, the presence and hemodynamic consequence of a PDA may lead to chronic lung disease (bronchopulmonary dysplasia), necrotizing enterocolitis, intraventricular hemorrhage, and renal failure [24]. An uncommon and not often thought of consequence of a PDA is pulmonary hemorrhage, which can be catastrophic in some cases. Kluckow *et al.* found an incidence of 9.5% of pulmonary hemorrhage in premature newborns in a study where a ductus with a hemodynamically significant left-to-right shunt was seen in 92% of patients [25]. Left untreated, PDAs in premature babies are associated with increased mortality [26].

Infants with a significant left-to-right shunt present with signs of congestive heart failure (i.e., tachypnea, poor feeding, and poor growth). Children may present with symptoms of a left-to-right shunt, such as poor growth and fatigue, particularly with exertion, if the PDA is large. Infants and children can develop episodes of frequent upper respiratory tract infections or pneumonias. However, many children and adults are asymptomatic. Patients with large PDAs that are not treated have features of pulmonary hypertension and, in fact, may develop Eisenmenger syndrome [27,28]. Although rarely seen in the developed world, this is unfortunately still seen in developing nations.

Diagnosis

In patients with a significant left-to-right shunt through the ductus, a wide pulse pressure is present because of diastolic run off. The precordium is hyperactive, and a continuous, "machinery" murmur is audible in the left infraclavicular area and throughout the precordium (in small babies). In clinical practice, however, the diastolic component of this murmur is not always heard in premature babies. A diastolic rumble because of increased flow across the mitral valve is heard when the shunt is very large. Hepatomegaly is also present. Rales are not usually heard in congestive heart failure in babies and children. In patients who have significant pulmonary hypertension, the oxygen saturation in the lower extremities may be lower than in the upper extremities because of the predominant right-to-left shunt. An increased right ventricular impulse

may be felt. A loud pulmonary component of the second heart sound is present. Often, no murmur is heard because of the elevated pulmonary vascular resistance. If, however, significant tricuspid regurgitation is present, a systolic regurgitant murmur is heard.

Elevations in plasma B-type natriuretic peptide levels have been found in preterm babies with symptomatic PDAs [29]. The electrocardiogram may support pulmonary hypertension (right-ventricular hypertrophy) or left-ventricular volume load depending on the presenting physiology. Chest roentograms show a normal-sized heart if pulmonary hypertension is present (may be enlarged if pulmonary hypertension is longstanding), and cardiomegaly with increased flow to the lungs is present if the left ventricle is volume loaded. Transthoracic echocardiography is the standard for diagnosis and defines the anatomy and hemodynamic significance of the shunt. In premature babies, defining a hemodynamically significant PDA on the basis of clinical grounds alone may be fraught with difficulty in the presence of other comorbidities. In these patients, echocardiographic parameters such as left-ventricular dilation, a left atrial to aortic root ratio of more than 1.3:1 or more than 1.5:1 (depending on hydration status), and diastolic flow reversal in the descending aorta are all indicators of a hemodynamically significant left-to-right shunt [30]. The left atrium may, however, not be significantly dilated in the presence of a significant atrial level shunt, which decompresses the left atrium. In preterm infants weighing less than 1500 g, an absolute PDA diameter of more than 1.5 mm at a mean age of 19 hours has been found to predict a hemodynamically significant PDA that would require treatment [31]. Details of the anatomy of the PDA, aortic arch, and brachiocephalic vessel branching pattern are extremely important, with obvious surgical implications. Transverse arch hypoplasia and typical juxtaductal coarctation should be ruled out (by careful ductal arch imaging and evaluation of the aortic isthmus). Cardiac catheterization is no longer used for diagnosis. However, in rare cases where pulmonary hypertension is present, diagnostic catheterization may be needed for hemodynamic purposes and to test the reactivity of the pulmonary vascular bed with pulmonary vasoactive agents.

Management

Medical treatment in children and adults who present with hemodynamically significant PDAs includes diuretics, digoxin, and afterload-reducing agents such as ACE inhibitors. Definitive treatment via interventional catheterization or surgery is relatively easily performed, and, in practice, few patients remain on medical therapy for congestive heart failure for prolonged periods of time. Antibiotic prophylaxis before potentially bacteremic procedures is no longer recommended per the recently revised American

Heart Association guidelines [32]. The management of a silent ductus is controversial, because there have been only few reports of silent PDAs as a source of endarteritis [33,34].

Management in Premature Infants

In the premature infant, PDAs can be challenging to manage and are a source of significant hemodynamic compromise. Medical and supportive treatment should target the hemodynamic effects of the left-to-right shunt. Optimizing the hematocrit, fluid restriction, and diuresis are all advantageous. Other measures include instituting intravenous inotropes (or oral digoxin) and ACE inhibitors.

Definitive treatment is either achieved by pharmacologic means or by surgery. In two separate reports in 1976, Friedman *et al.* and Heymann *et al.* reported the initial experience of closure of the ductus with indomethacin [4,35]. Indomethacin is a nonsteroidal anti-inflammatory agent (NSAID) that inhibits cyclo-oxygenase and, thus, prostaglandin synthesis [36]. Traditionally, intravenous indomethacin has been administered, and a variety of dosing regimens have been proposed. At our institution, we administer intravenous indomethacin at a dose of 0.2 mg/kg followed by 0.1 mg/kg for two additional doses at 12-hour intervals. If needed, this course is repeated at a dose of 0.2 mg/kg for three doses at 12-hour intervals. It is important to note, however, that indomethacin can effect platelet function (which can lead to necrotizing enterocolitis and intraventricular hemorrhage) and cause oliguria and renal toxicity. Recently, the use of intravenous ibuprofen has been shown to have similar closure rates (70% initial closure rate), with significantly decreased renal toxicity [37]. Moreover, oral ibuprofen has been shown to be as effective as intravenous ibuprofen with fewer adverse effects in very low birthweight infants [38].

If a hemodynamically significant PDA does not close or get significantly smaller despite medical therapy, surgical ligation is performed. Surgical ligation is also performed in these babies if there are contraindications to pharmacologic treatment with NSAIDs. Although there are reports of coil occlusion of the ductus in select preterm babies [39], we currently recommend surgical ligation in this group of patients. Prophylactic treatment of PDAs in preterm babies is controversial. It has been shown that it is possible to predict PDAs that are likely to become hemodynamically significant on the basis of early echocardiographic parameters [31]. Although this is advocated by some centers, in general this has not been our routine practice.

Surgical Repair of PDA

Isolated PDA can be repaired via thoracotomy or sternotomy or minimally invasive procedures.

Left Thoracotomy

Left thoracotomy is the more common approach for isolated PDA repair. Although anterolateral thoracotomy was used in the initial cases [1,2], muscle-sparing posterolateral thoracotomy is the more common approach at present. This can be done in any size patient. The alternate approach of transaxillary thoracotomy, which is really a modification of lateral thoracotomy, can also be used with good cosmetic results. The patient is placed in the right lateral position. An axillary roll of cushioned material is placed, and the left arm is secured appropriately. It is important to avoid pressure on skin and nerves while in this position (peroneal nerve, ankle, etc.). We prefer to use a rather small incision that is posterior to the midaxillary line and is about 1 cm or less below the tip of the scapula and to use a muscle-sparing approach to preserve the periosteum of the ribs. Entry is typically through the third or fourth intercostal space. Others have used an extrapleural approach [40], although transpleural is equally safe. The lung is gently retracted anteriorly using a small gauze sponge or a retractor.

Before dissection is begun, it is important to identify the complete anatomy, including the left recurrent and phrenic nerves, the left subclavian artery, the distal aortic arch, the descending aorta, and the PDA. It is important to stay as posterior as possible to the recurrent nerve. We typically do not identify the left pulmonary artery from this approach. We believe it is unnecessary and potentially hazardous to the recurrent laryngeal nerve. If the steps as noted above are followed, especially in that particular order, the anatomy can easily be understood, and ligation of the inappropriate vessel will not occur. The PDA is dissected at 1 or 2 mm from its aortic end, taking care not to injure it, especially in the window between its superior edge and the aortic arch. The duct can then be ligated or clipped. The technique of double ligation and excision ensures complete interruption and is the most reliable technique. It is our preferred technique in older children; however, it may be difficult in very small babies. Double ligation or double clipping is also used to ensure complete occlusion of the duct. A single chest tube is placed and can be removed after closure of the chest or 24 hours later as clinically indicated.

Median Sternotomy

Median sternotomy is rarely used for isolated PDA ligation. However, it is an option in cases where left lung compression is not possible (e.g., unilateral right lung diseases such as interstitial emphysema or bilobar right-sided pneumonia). Another situation requiring an anterior approach is for the window-like duct, which is short and wide. This may require cardiopulmonary bypass. In adults with a calcified ductus, the anterior approach is preferred. A lower partial sternotomy or ministernotomy may be used if appropriate. The pericardium is incised longitudinally, and pericardial stays are applied. The PDA is dissected close to the pulmonary arterial location because the recurrent nerve is closer to the aorta. Furthermore, use of electrocautery should be very limited in dissection of the PDA, especially laterally to avoid thermal injury to the recurrent laryngeal nerve. It is critical to identify the right and left pulmonary arteries, especially in a small baby. Dissection can be facilitated using a fine-tipped clamp. The PDA can then be ligated with silk or braided polyester or clipped using metal clips. Alternatively, ligation and division ensures interruption of the PDA. A single pericardial or pleuropericardial drain is placed, while ensuring that it is not compressing the heart.

Minimally Invasive Techniques

Patent ductus arteriosus ligation has been accomplished using video-assisted techniques as well as robotic surgery [41–43]. Video-assisted surgery has gained more popularity, and some centers use this technique exclusively. Incidence of conversion to open technique is low, and in experienced hands, the surgical time is comparable. With the availability of 3 mm ports and camera, video-assisted techniques are feasible even in premature babies [42,44]. Lung retraction instead of lung collapse can be used. Costs and early morbidity of video-assisted techniques compared with the open technique are similar [45]; however, the long-term sequelae of thoracotomy are avoided. Robotic surgery is currently limited to children more than 12–15 kg. Operative times are long, and it is difficult to show any benefit over video-assisted technique at this time [46].

Special Considerations in Premature Infants

A premature baby presents significant challenges. The PDA may not be necessarily more fragile, but the small size of the baby creates technical issues. Airway and intravenous access are critically important. The endotracheal tube can easily be dislodged during positioning. Careful temperature management of the baby to avoid hypothermia is imperative. We perform the surgery in the neonatal intensive care unit. Our usual approach is a muscle sparing posterolateral left thoracotomy through the third intercostal space. The basic surgical steps are similar to those described earlier. The PDA can be singly ligated or clipped. It is important to identify the anatomy to avoid ligation of the incorrect vessel. We typically leave a single chest tube overnight, although others have been removed at the end of the case.

Special Consideration in Infants and Children

Children and infants can be in significant congestive heart failure because of a PDA. Whereas most of these patients will have PDA occlusion via percutaneous technique, those coming to surgery typically have a large and possibly shorter duct. They may come to surgery after a failed attempt at percutaneous occlusion, in which case the device or coil may still be deployed. If no device or coil is in place, left posterolateral thoracotomy is safe. A muscle sparing approach via the fourth intercostal space is our preferred approach. The duct should be doubly ligated and preferably divided to avoid any chance of residual shunt. In cases where the duct is very short and wide, it may best be addressed via median sternotomy with options for cardiopulmonary bypass. This situation is rather rare. If a PDA closure is required in a child with a failed device and the device is still in place, it is usually best to address this from the front with a full or partial median sternotomy because the device can be extracted from the pulmonary artery with or without the use of cardiopulmonary bypass [47].

Special Considerations in Adults

Surgical closure of PDA in adults is rarely required because of advances in percutaneous techniques. Patients requiring surgery are best addressed via a median sternotomy and preparation for cardiopulmonary bypass. This is because of frequent calcification of the duct. A calcified duct can be closed under circulatory arrest or regional cerebral perfusion. It is common to use a patch or primary closure through the pulmonary artery. Another excellent option avoids or limits the use of circulatory arrest by using a balloon-tipped catheter to occlude the duct [48,49]. This then allows the surgeon to sew a patch on the pulmonary arterial end from the inside of the pulmonary artery.

Surgical Outcomes

Excellent outcomes have been reported after surgical ligation of PDA with little or no surgical mortality and a low morbidity [45]. Recurrent laryngeal nerve injury has been reported, with a low incidence except for one study with 52% incidence [32]. Cases of chylous leaks are rare. Incidence of scoliosis after thoracotomy has been noted in 19–31% of patients [50–52]. By preserving the periosteum of the ribs and performing a posterolateral muscle sparing thoracotomy, there is potential to avoid some of the sequelae of thoracotomy. Video-assisted techniques further decrease the trauma of thoracotomy and its long-term sequelae. The incidence of residual PDA is low in some studies (3.1%); however, with ligation and division, the incidence is zero [53].

Percutaneous Closure of PDA

In 1967, Portsmann performed the first transcatheter PDA closure, which was a landmark event in the field of interventional cardiology [54]. His initial technique, however, required a large sheath and arterial cutdown [54,55]. Since his pioneering work, numerous devices have been used [56–58]. Over the years, modifications of the technique and devices used have resulted in smaller delivery systems and the ability to occlude even large PDAs safely in small patients.

Currently, the two most widely used methods of closing PDAs in the catheterization laboratory employ the use of coils or the Amplatzer® Duct Occluder (AGA Medical Corporation; Plymouth, Minnesota). Generally, coil occlusion is performed in PDAs less than 3 mm in diameter. There are numerous types of coils that can be used. The coils that are most often used are 0.038-inch Gianturco stainless steel coils (Cook, Inc; Bloomington, Indiana). Dacron fibers are present on the coils to promote thrombus formation and closure of the PDA. Coils can be deployed antegrade (from the venous side; Figure 12.1) or retrograde (from the arterial side). The diameter of coil chosen is about twice the size of the smallest dimension of the duct, with 1.5 loops or less of the coil deployed on the pulmonary artery side and the majority of loops deployed in the ampulla on the aortic side of the duct. Coils are advantageous in that they are cheaper than Amplatzer Duct Occluders. Coil occlusion in very small infants is often not feasible, particularly in large PDAs with little constriction at the pulmonary end. In a large cohort of patients from the European Coil Registry, 5% of patients had a residual leak 1 year after coil implant [59]. In our experience however, the vast majority of residual leaks are clinically insignificant.

The Amplatzer Duct Occluder has helped overcome many of the shortcomings of coils (i.e., occurrence of residual leaks and limitations in occlusion of large ducts). They are mainly used to occlude PDAs larger than 3 mm and are approved for use in infants more than 6 months of age and weighing more than 6 kg. The device consists of a pulmonary end and a larger aortic end with a retention disc. The device has memory and is made of nitinol, which is easily collapsed into the appropriate-sized delivery sheath. Polyester fabric is added to the device to promote thrombus formation. The size of the device chosen should have

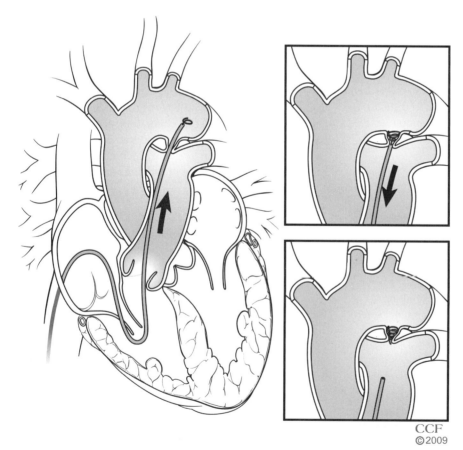

CCF
©2009

Figure 12.1 A coil being deployed antegrade (from the venous side) in a patent ductus arteriosus. Note that most of the loops of the coil are on the aortic side of the ductus (i.e., in the ampulla). (Reproduced with permission from the Cleveland Clinic Center for Medical Art & Photography. Copyright © 2009–2012. All rights reserved.)

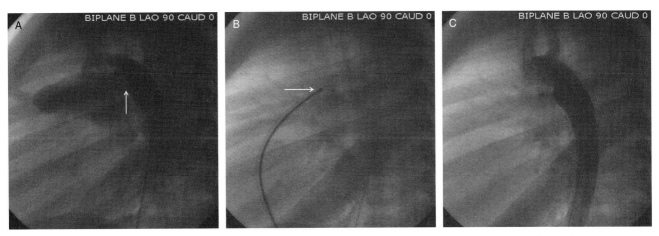

Figure 12.2 A, This straight lateral aortogram in a 2-year-old boy shows a moderate-sized PDA (arrow). **B,** An 8/6 Amplatzer Duct Occluder is advanced antegrade (from the venous side). The device has been deployed and the retension disc is seen opposing the aortic side of the ampulla, while the delivery cable (arrow) is still attached to the pulmonary end of the device. **C,** After release of the device, no residual shunt through the PDA is seen.

a pulmonary end diameter that is 1–2 mm larger than the narrowest dimension of the duct. These devices are available in sizes up to 14 mm in diameter (pulmonary end of the device). The device is always deployed antegrade to allow for the retention disc to appose the aortic side of the ampulla (Figure 12.2). An advantage of this device is that it can be fully retrieved before complete release into the delivery sheath (while still being attached to the delivery cable on the pulmonary end) if the device is not deemed appropriate or is in improper position. The experience with this device thus far has been promising, and the results of a multicenter trial using the Amplatzer Duct Occluder device showed complete closure rate of 98% up to 1 year after implantation [60]. Numerous other techniques, such as simultaneous deployment of multiple coils, have also been described for large PDAs [55,56,58].

The recent availability of a variety of coils and devices in the catheterization laboratory has limited suboptimal results and complications related to transcatheter closure of the ductus. A suboptimal outcome of transcatheter closure of PDAs was seen in patients from the European Coil Registry, which was defined as coil embolization, an abandoned procedure; persistent hemolysis; residual leak requiring a further procedure; flow impairment in adjacent structures (obstruction to left pulmonary artery or aortic flow); and duct recanalization [59]. Large PDAs and tubular PDAs were risk factors for a suboptimal outcome, and for those PDAs, the Amplatzer Duct Occluder is probably better suited. Serious and minor complication rates have been seen in 7.1% of patients undergoing closure with the Amplatzer Duct Occluder [60].

Many of the inadvertently embolized coils/devices can be safely retrieved in the catheterization laboratory, and important hemolysis can be treated by device/coil removal

in the catheterization laboratory or by placement of another coil if needed. With newer technologies and smaller delivery sheaths, femoral arterial complications are now seen much less than in prior years. Infection is rare, but all patients undergoing PDA occlusion in the catheterization laboratory receive prophylactic antibiotics for 24 hours and should receive prophylactic antibiotics before potentially bacteremic procedures up to 6 months after the implant. Antibiotic prophylaxis is also recommended if residual shunts are present.

The overwhelming majority of PDAs (except those in very small infants) can be closed safely in the catheterization laboratory. In addition, catheter-based closure is as effective as and cheaper than surgical closure [61]. Surgical closure is generally performed in small infants with large ducts (less than 6 months of age or weighing less than 6 kg). Preterm babies whose ducts do not constrict after the administration of NSAIDs (or if there are contraindications to NSAID therapy) should also undergo surgical closure of their PDAs. Surgical closure of PDA is rarely performed in the older child or adult unless a concomitant surgical procedure is being performed.

Conclusion

We recommend occluding all hemodynamically significant or audible PDAs. For premature infants or symptomatic children weighing less than 6 kg, surgical PDA ligation via muscle sparing posterolateral thoracotomy is offered, though video-assisted PDA ligation may be a better long-term solution. For older children and adults, a percutaneous route is favored and surgery is reserved for cases where the percutaneous approach fails.

References

1. Graybiel A, Strieder JW, Boyer NH. (1938) An attempt to obliterate the patent ductus arteriosus in a patient with subacute bacterial endarteritis. Am Heart J 15, 621.

2. Gross RE, Hubbard JP. (1939) Surgical ligation of a patent ductus arteriosus. Report of first successful case. JAMA 112, 729–731.

3. Porstmann W, Wierny L, Warnke H. (1967) Closure of persistent ductus arteriosus without thoracotomy. Ger Med Mon 12, 259–261.

4. Heymann MA, Rudolph AM, Silverman NH. (1976) Closure of the ductus arteriosus in premature infants by inhibition of prostaglandin synthesis. N Engl J Med 295, 530–533.

5. Hinton R, Michelfelder E. (2006) Significance of reverse orientation of the ductus arteriosus in neonates with pulmonary outflow tract obstruction for early intervention. Am J Cardiol 97, 716–719.

6. Silver MM, Freedom RM, Silver MD, et al. (1981) The morphology of the human newborn ductus arteriosus: a reappraisal of its structure and closure with special reference to prostaglandin E1 therapy. Hum Pathol 12, 1123–1136.

7. Loftin CD, Trivedi DB, Langenbach R. (2002) Cyclooxygenase-1-selective inhibition prolongs gestation in mice without adverse effects on the ductus arteriosus. J Clin Invest 110, 549–557.

8. Thebaud B, Michelakis ED, Wu XC, et al. (2004) Oxygen-sensitive Kv channel gene transfer confers oxygen responsiveness to preterm rabbit and remodeled human ductus arteriosus: implications for infants with patent ductus arteriosus. Circulation 110, 1372–1379.

9. Clyman RI, Mauray F, Roman C, et al. (1980) Circulating prostaglandin E2 concentrations and patent ductus arteriosus in fetal and neonatal lambs. J Pediatr 97, 455–461.

10. Clyman RI, Mauray F, Roman C, et al. (1981) Effects of antenatal glucocorticoid administration on ductus arteriosus of preterm lambs. Am J Physiol 241, H415–H420.

11. Vida VL, Barnoya J, Larrazabal LA, et al. (2005) Congenital cardiac disease in children with Down's syndrome in Guatemala. Cardiol Young 15, 286–290.

12. Nora JJ. (1968) Multifactorial inheritance hypothesis for the etiology of congenital heart diseases. The genetic-environmental interaction. Circulation 38, 604–617.

13. Zhu L, Bonnet D, Boussion M, et al. (2007) Investigation of the MYH11 gene in sporadic patients with an isolated persistently patent arterial duct. Cardiol Young 17, 666–672.

14. Mani A, Meraji SM, Houshyar R, et al. (2002) Finding genetic contributions to sporadic disease: a recessive locus at 12q24 commonly contributes to patent ductus arteriosus. Proc Natl Acad Sci U S A 99, 15054–15059.

15. Gonzalez A, Sosenko IR, Chandar J, et al. (1996) Influence of infection on patent ductus arteriosus and chronic lung disease in premature infants weighing 1000 grams or less. J Pediatr 128, 470–478.

16. Jan SL, Hwang B, Fu YC, et al. (2004) Prediction of ductus arteriosus closure by neonatal screening echocardiography. Int J Cardiovasc Imaging 20, 349–356.

17. Hoffman JI, Kaplan S. (2002) The incidence of congenital heart disease. J Am Coll Cardiol 39, 1890–1900.

18. Mitchell SC, Korones SB, Berendes HW. (1971) Congenital heart disease in 56,109 births. Incidence and natural history. Circulation 43, 323–332.

19. Lemons JA, Bauer CR, Oh W, et al. (2001) Very low birth weight outcomes of the National Institute of Child health and human development neonatal research network, January 1995 through December 1996. NICHD Neonatal Research Network. Pediatrics 107.

20. Grover A, Barnes N, Chadwick C, et al. (2008) Neonatal infective endarteritis complicating patent ductus arteriosus. Acta Paediatr 97, 663–665.

21. Huggon IC, Qureshi SA. (1997) Is the prevention of infective endarteritis a valid reason for closure of the patent arterial duct? Eur Heart J 18, 364–366.

22. Sadiq M, Latif F, Ur-Rehman A. (2004) Analysis of infective endarteritis in patent ductus arteriosus. Am J Cardiol 93, 513–515.

23. Kluckow M, Evans N. (2001) Low systemic blood flow in the preterm infant. Semin Neonatol 6, 75–84.

24. Knight DB. (2001) The treatment of patent ductus arteriosus in preterm infants. A review and overview of randomized trials. Semin Neonatol 6, 63–73.

25. Kluckow M, Evans N. (2000) Ductal shunting, high pulmonary blood flow, and pulmonary hemorrhage. J Pediatr 137, 68–72.

26. Noori S, McCoy M, Friedlich P, et al. (2009) Failure of ductus arteriosus closure is associated with increased mortality in preterm infants. Pediatrics 123, e138–e144.

27. Brickner ME, Hillis LD, Lange RA. (2000) Congenital heart disease in adults. Second of two parts. N Engl J Med 342, 334–342.

28. Brickner ME, Hillis LD, Lange RA. (2000) Congenital heart disease in adults. First of two parts. N Engl J Med 342, 256–263.

29. Choi BM, Lee KH, Eun BL, et al. (2005) Utility of rapid B-type natriuretic peptide assay for diagnosis of symptomatic patent ductus arteriosus in preterm infants. Pediatrics 115, e255–e261.

30. Skinner J. (2001) Diagnosis of patent ductus arteriosus. Semin Neonatol 6, 49–61.

31. Kluckow M, Evans N. (1995) Early echocardiographic prediction of symptomatic patent ductus arteriosus in preterm infants undergoing mechanical ventilation. J Pediatr 127, 774–779.

32. Wilson W, Taubert KA, Gewitz M, et al. (2007) Prevention of infective endocarditis: guidelines from the American Heart Association: a guideline from the American Heart Association Rheumatic Fever, Endocarditis, and Kawasaki Disease Committee, Council on Cardiovascular Disease in the Young, and the Council on Clinical Cardiology, Council on Cardiovascular Surgery and Anesthesia, and the Quality of Care and Outcomes Research Interdisciplinary Working Group. Circulation 116, 1736–1754.

33. Balzer DT, Spray TL, McMullin D, et al. (1993) Endarteritis associated with a clinically silent patent ductus arteriosus. Am Heart J 125, 1192–1193.

34. Parthenakis FI, Kanakaraki MK, Vardas PE. (2000) Images in cardiology: silent patent ductus arteriosus endarteritis. Heart 84, 619.

35. Friedman WF, Hirschklau MJ, Printz MP, *et al.* (1976) Pharmacologic closure of patent ductus arteriosus in the premature infant. N Engl J Med 295, 526–529.

36. Hammerman C, Kaplan M. (1999) Patent ductus arteriousus in the premature neonate: current concepts in pharmacological management. Paediatr Drugs 1, 81–92.

37. Van Overmeire B, Smets K, Lecoutere D, *et al.* (2000) A comparison of ibuprofen and indomethacin for closure of patent ductus arteriosus. N Engl J Med 343, 674–681.

38. Cherif A, Khrouf N, Jabnoun S, *et al.* (2008) Randomized pilot study comparing oral ibuprofen with intravenous ibuprofen in very low birth weight infants with patent ductus arteriosus. Pediatrics 122, e1256–e1261.

39. Roberts P, Adwani S, Archer N, *et al.* (2007) Catheter closure of the arterial duct in preterm infants. Arch Dis Child Fetal Neonatal Ed 92, F248–F250.

40. Leon-Wyss J, Vida VL, Veras O, *et al.* (2005) Modified extrapleural ligation of patent ductus arteriosus: a convenient surgical approach in a developing country. Ann Thorac Surg 79, 632–635.

41. Le Bret E, Folliguet TA, Laborde F. (1997) Videothoracoscopic surgical interruption of patent ductus arteriosus. Ann Thorac Surg 64, 1492–1494.

42. Le Bret E, Papadatos S, Folliguet T, *et al.* (2002) Interruption of patent ductus arteriosus in children: robotically assisted versus videothoracoscopic surgery. J Thorac Cardiovasc Surg 123, 973–976.

43. Suematsu Y, Mora BN, Mihaljevic T, *et al.* (2005) Totally endoscopic robotic-assisted repair of patent ductus arteriosus and vascular ring in children. Ann Thorac Surg 80, 2309–2313.

44. Burke RP, Jacobs JP, Cheng W, *et al.* (1999) Video-assisted thoracoscopic surgery for patent ductus arteriosus in low birth weight neonates and infants. Pediatrics 104, 227–230.

45. Kennedy AP Jr, Snyder CL, Ashcraft KW, *et al.* (1998) Comparison of muscle-sparing thoracotomy and thoracoscopic ligation for the treatment of patent ductus arteriosus. J Pediatr Surg 33, 259–261.

46. Mavroudis C. (2005) Invited commentary. Ann Thorac Surg 80, 2313.

47. Shahabuddin S, Atiq M, Hamid M, *et al.* (2007) Surgical removal of an embolised patent ductus arteriosus amplatzer occluding device in a 4-year-old girl. Interact Cardiovasc Thorac Surg 6, 572–573.

48. Tekin Y, Ozer S, Murat B, *et al.* (2007) Closure of adult patent ductus arteriosus under cardiopulmonary bypass by using foley balloon catheter. J Card Surg 22, 219–220.

49. Thilen U, Astrom-Olsson K. (1997) Does the risk of infective endarteritis justify routine patent ductus arteriosus closure? Eur Heart J 18, 503–506.

50. Bal S, Elshershari H, Celiker R, *et al.* (2003) Thoracic sequels after thoracotomies in children with congenital cardiac disease. Cardiol Young 13, 264–267.

51. Seghaye MC, Grabitz R, Alzen G, *et al.* (1997) Thoracic sequelae after surgical closure of the patent ductus arteriosus in premature infants. Acta Paediatr 86, 213–216.

52. Shelton JE, Julian R, Walburgh E, *et al.* (1986) Functional scoliosis as a long-term complication of surgical ligation for patent ductus arteriosus in premature infants. J Pediatr Surg 21, 855–857.

53. Mavroudis C, Backer CL, Gevitz M. (1994) Forty-six years of patent ductus arteriosus division at Children's Memorial Hospital of Chicago. Standards for comparison. Ann Surg 220, 402–409; discussion 409–410.

54. Portsmann W, Wierny L, Warnke H. (1967) The closure of the patent ductus arteriosus without thoractomy (preliminary report). Thoraxchir Vask Chir 15, 199–203.

55. Portsmann W, Wierny L, Warnke H, *et al.* (1971) Catheter closure of patent ductus arteriosus. 62 cases treated without thoracotomy. Radiol Clin North Am 9, 203–218.

56. Grifka RG. (2004) Transcatheter closure of the patent ductus arteriosus. Catheter Cardiovasc Interv 61, 554–570.

57. Mullins CE. Transcatheter occlusion of the patent ductus arteriosus (PDA). *Cardiac Catheterization in Congenital Heart Disease: Pediatric and Adult.* Malden, MA: Blackwell Futura 2006, pp. 693–727.

58. Rome JJ, Perry SB. Defect closure – coil embolization (technology, methodology in aorto pulmonary venous collaterals; PDA; coronary arteriovenous fistulae; shunts, other). In: Lock JE, Keane JF, Perry SB, eds. *Diagnostic and Interventional Catheterization in Congential Heart Disease.* 2nd edn. Norwell, MA: Kluwer Academic Publishers 2000, pp. 199–220.

59. Magee AG, Huggon IC, Seed PT, *et al.* (2001) Transcatheter coil occlusion of the arterial duct; results of the European Registry. Eur Heart J 22, 1817–1821.

60. Pass RH, Hijazi Z, Hsu DT, *et al.* (2004) Multicenter USA Amplatzer patent ductus arteriosus occlusion device trial: initial and one-year results. J Am Coll Cardiol 44, 513–519.

61. Prieto LR, DeCamillo DM, Konrad DJ, *et al.* (1998) Comparison of cost and clinical outcome between transcatheter coil occlusion and surgical closure of isolated patent ductus arteriosus. Pediatrics 101, 1020–1024.

CHAPTER 13

Vascular Rings and Pulmonary Artery Sling

Carl L. Backer[1] and Constantine Mavroudis[2]

[1]Ann & Robert H. Lurie Children's Hospital of Chicago, formerly Children's Memorial Hospital, Chicago, IL, USA
[2]Florida Hospital for Children, Orlando, FL, USA

Classification

The term "vascular ring" is used to describe vascular anomalies that result from abnormal development of the aortic arch complex and cause compression of the trachea, esophagus, or both. The first vascular ring described was a double aortic arch by Hommel in 1737 [1]. The phrase "vascular ring" was introduced to the surgical literature by Robert E Gross in 1945 [2]. At that time he reported the first successful division of a double aortic arch causing tracheal obstruction in a 1-year-old infant. "A ring of blood vessels was found encircling the intrathoracic portion of the esophagus and trachea." Most children with vascular rings present with symptoms in the first few months of life and require surgery within the first year of life [3]. Some of these anomalies are anatomically complete rings, or true vascular rings; others are anatomically incomplete, or partial vascular rings, but present similar symptoms because of the tracheoesophageal compression. In particular, a pulmonary artery sling is a rare vascular anomaly in which the left pulmonary artery originates from the right pulmonary artery and encircles the right mainstem bronchus and distal trachea before entering the hilum of the left lung. This anomaly was first reported by Glaevecke and Doehle in 1897 as a postmortem finding in a 7-month-old infant with severe respiratory distress [4]. The classification of vascular rings we have used at Children's Memorial Hospital in Chicago is based on anatomic and clinical features, particularly the location of the aortic arch(es). This classification scheme was recently endorsed by the Congenital Heart Surgery International Nomenclature and Database Project for the Society of Thoracic Surgeons database [5].

The history of vascular ring surgery began with the division of a double aortic arch by Gross at Boston Children's Hospital on 9 June 1945 [2]. Gross was also the first to suspend the innominate artery to the posterior sternum for innominate artery compression syndrome in 1948 [6]. The first repair of a pulmonary artery sling was by Willis J Potts at Children's Memorial Hospital in 1953 [7]. More recently, for the complex subset of patients with pulmonary artery sling who also have tracheal stenosis from complete tracheal rings, the pericardial patch tracheoplasty technique was first performed by Farouk S Idriss in 1982 [8]. The first tracheal autograft for tracheal stenosis also was performed at Children's Memorial Hospital [9]. Since Potts' first operation on an infant with double aortic arch at our institution on 27 July 1946 [10] we have operated on over 400 patients at the Children's Memorial Hospital with different types of vascular tracheoesophageal compression syndromes and this experience forms the basis for this chapter (Table 13.1).

Embryology and Pathology

In 1922 Congdon [11] reported his extensive experience with the study of the embryonic development of the human aortic arch system. Edwards [12] proposed a schematic model with a double aortic arch system and bilateral ductus arteriosus. More recently, Stewart and associates [13] summarized the pathologic, embryologic, and roentgenographic correlations of these lesions. In embryonic vascular development six pairs of aortic arches connect the two primitive ventral and dorsal aortae (Figure 13.1) [14]. The formation of a vascular ring depends on preservation or deletion of specific segments of the rudimentary embryonic aortic arch complex. Most portions of the first, second, and fifth arches regress. The third arches become the carotid arteries. A branch from the ventral bud of the sixth arch

Pediatric Cardiac Surgery, Fourth Edition. Edited by Constantine Mavroudis and Carl L. Backer.
© 2013 Blackwell Publishing Ltd. Published 2013 by Blackwell Publishing Ltd.

Table 13.1 Vascular ring patients operated on at Children's Memorial Hospital: 1946–2009.

Complete vascular rings	
Double aortic arch	139
Right arch dominant	
Left arch dominant	
Balanced arches	
Right aortic arch with left ligamentum arteriosum	140
Retroesophageal left subclavian artery	
Mirror-image branching	
Partial vascular rings	
Innominate artery compression syndrome	87
Pulmonary artery sling	40
Left aortic arch, aberrant right subclavian artery	6
Total	**412**

meets the lung bud to form the pulmonary artery. On the right side the dorsal contribution to the sixth arch disappears; on the left it persists as the ductus arteriosus. The seventh intersegmental arteries arise from the dorsal aorta and form the subclavian arteries. Normally a portion of the right fourth arch involutes at 36–38 days in the 16 mm embryo, leaving the usual left aortic arch configuration (Figure 13.1) [14]. The apex of the aortic arch in this (normal) situation is to the left of the trachea.

Double Aortic Arch

If the right and left fourth arches both persist, a double aortic arch is formed (Figure 13.1) [14]. Two arches arise from the ascending aorta and pass on both sides of the trachea and esophagus, joining the descending aorta, producing a true ring. The right (posterior) arch gives origin to the right carotid and subclavian arteries. The left carotid and subclavian arteries arise from the usually smaller left (anterior) arch. In 70% of these infants, the right-sided arch is dominant, in 20% the left arch is dominant, and in 5% the arches are equal in size. The trachea and esophagus are encircled and compressed by the two arches.

Right Aortic Arch

If the left fourth arch involutes, a right aortic arch system is created (Figure 13.1) [14]. The apex of the aortic arch in these patients is to the right of the trachea. Depending on the exact site(s) of interruption of the left arch and the branching pattern to the left subclavian artery, left carotid artery, and ductus arteriosus, different configurations of right aortic arch are possible (Figure 13.2) [14]. The two common variations are retroesophageal left subclavian artery (65%) and mirror-image branching (35%) [15]. The right aortic arch with a retroesophageal left subclavian artery results from persistence of the right fourth arch and

deletion of the left arch between the left carotid and subclavian arteries. The subclavian artery originates from the descending aorta and courses to the left behind the esophagus. The ligamentum extends from the descending aorta to the left pulmonary artery, completing the vascular ring (Figure 13.2A).

A right aortic arch with mirror-image branching and left ligamentum arteriosum results from persistence of the right fourth aortic arch and disappearance of the left arch between the subclavian artery and the dorsal descending aorta. When the ligamentum originates from the descending aorta, a complete vascular ring is formed (Figure 13.2B). If the ligamentum originates from the innominate artery, which is more common in this group, a vascular ring is not formed and the child is asymptomatic (Figure 13.2C). Although one third of patients with tetralogy of Fallot and truncus arteriosus have a right aortic arch [16], we did not find a reverse association with a specific cardiac defect when a vascular ring was formed by a right arch.

Pulmonary Artery Sling

The embryonic origin of pulmonary artery sling occurs when the developing left lung captures its arterial supply from derivatives of the right sixth arch through capillaries caudad rather than cephalad to the developing tracheobronchial tree [17]. The left pulmonary artery originates from the right pulmonary artery instead of the main pulmonary artery. The left pulmonary artery passes around the right main bronchus and courses between the trachea and esophagus, forming a "sling" that compresses the tracheobronchial tree (Figure 13.3) [14]. The airway may also be compromised by associated complete cartilage tracheal rings, the so-called "ring-sling" complex where the membranous portion of the trachea is absent and the tracheal cartilages are circumferential (Figure 13.3) [14,18].

Innominate Artery Compression

Innominate artery compression syndrome results from anterior compression of the trachea by the innominate artery. Why an innominate artery, which normally crosses in front of the trachea, should compress the trachea in some cases and not others is not well understood. The innominate artery appears to originate somewhat more posteriorly and leftward on the aortic arch than usual. As the artery courses to the right, upward, and posterior to reach the right thoracic outlet, it compresses the trachea anteriorly (Figure 13.4) [14,19].

Aberrant Right Subclavian Artery

A left aortic arch with aberrant right subclavian artery develops when the right fourth arch between the subclavian and carotid arteries regresses. The right subclavian artery (originating from the intersegmental artery) traverses

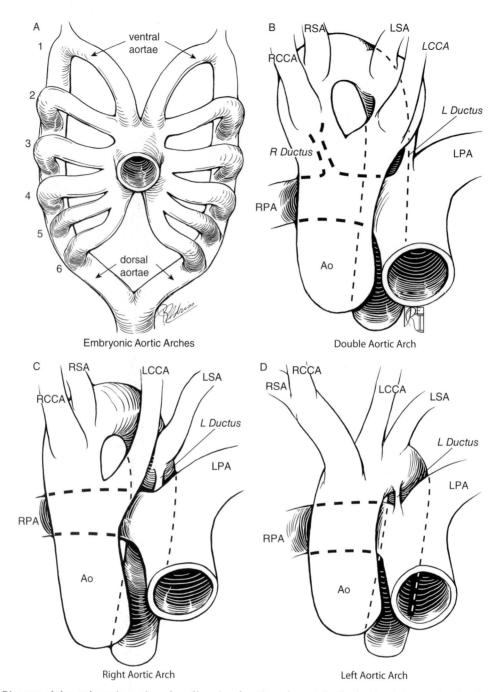

Figure 13.1 (A), Diagram of the embryonic aortic arches. Six pairs of aortic arches originally develop between the dorsal and ventral aorta. The first, second, and fifth arches regress. Preservation or deletion of different segments of the rudimentary arches results in either a double aortic arch **(B)**, a right aortic arch **(C)**, or the "normal" left aortic arch **(D)**. (Ao, aorta; CCA, common carotid artery; L, left; PA, pulmonary artery; R, right; SA, subclavian artery.)

the mediastinum and inserts on the descending aorta. The right subclavian artery then becomes a branch off the descending aorta and courses to the right, posterior to the esophagus. This produces an indentation of the esophagus, but does not form a complete vascular ring (Figure 13.5) [14]. In fact, this is the most common vascular anomaly of the aortic arch system (0.5% of humans) [20]. Because it is so common, it has been blamed in the past, mistakenly, for vague swallowing symptoms, earning the label "dysphagia lusoria," [21] or "difficulty in swallowing due to a trick of nature." The aberrant right subclavian is actually nearly always a "red herring," and not the true etiology of the child's symptoms [22]. We have not operated on a child with this diagnosis since 1973, although we are aware of some very rare cases where the aberrant right subclavian artery does compress the trachea causing symptoms.

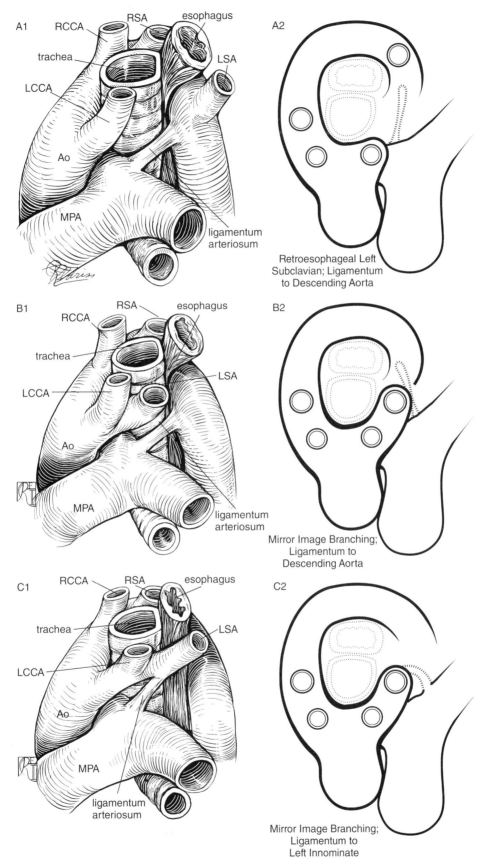

Figure 13.2 Right aortic arch types. **A,** Retroesophageal left subclavian artery, ligamentum to descending aorta. **B,** Mirror image branching, ligamentum to descending aorta. **C,** Mirror image branching, ligamentum to left innominate artery. (Ao, aorta; CCA, common carotid artery; L, left; PA, pulmonary artery; R, right; SA, subclavian artery.)

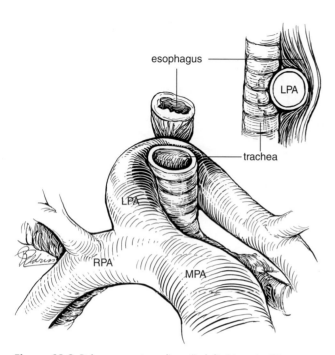

Figure 13.3 Pulmonary artery sling. (L, left; M, main; PA, pulmonary artery; R, right.)
Inset: Left lateral view of anterior compression of the esophagus and posterior compression of the trachea.

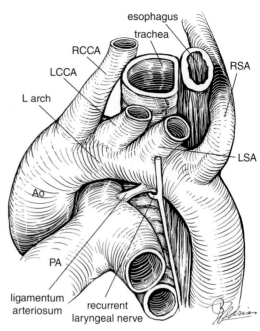

Figure 13.5 Left aortic arch with aberrant right subclavian artery causing posterior compression of the esophagus. (Ao, aorta; L, left; LCCA, RCCA, left, right carotid artery; LSA, RSA, left, right subclavian artery; PA, pulmonary artery.)

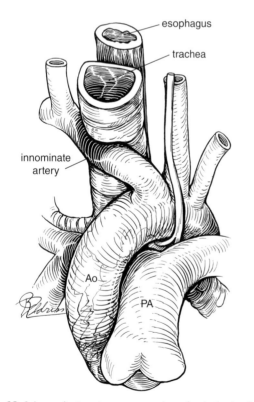

Figure 13.4 Innominate artery compression of anterior trachea. (Ao, aorta; PA, pulmonary artery.)

Rare Vascular Rings

In the unusual combination of left aortic arch and right descending aorta, if there is a right patent ductus arteriosus or ligamentum arteriosum, a vascular ring is formed [23]. The left aortic arch in these cases is often a cervical arch, resulting from persistence of the third rather than the fourth embryonic aortic arch [24]. A large sweeping cervical arch may independently compress the trachea anteriorly, even in the absence of a right ductus. This combination is one of the very few vascular rings that are best approached with a right thoracotomy rather than a left thoracotomy [25]. These patients are very rare and often have associated cardiac anomalies [26]. Because we now obtain a computed tomographic (CT) or magnetic resonance image (MRI) on all vascular ring patients prior to an operation the exact anatomy and decision about the approach has become less of an "art" [27].

A single case report has described a ductus arteriosus traveling from the right pulmonary artery to the descending aorta between the trachea and esophagus with an aberrant right subclavian artery (ductus arteriosus sling) [28]. The ductus was compressing the trachea and right bronchus in a manner analogous to pulmonary artery sling. We reported a 5-month-old infant with a right aortic arch, right ligamentum, and absent left pulmonary artery who required division of the right ligamentum to relieve respiratory failure [29]. Robotin and colleagues [30] reported three groups of unusual forms of tracheobronchial compression in a series of over 500 patients with vascular rings. Three patients had an encircling right aortic arch with a left-sided descending aorta and ligamentum ("circumflex aorta"), two patients had airway compression from a pincer effect between a malposed and enlarged ascending aorta and the descending aorta, and three patients had airway compression after an arterial switch. Van Son [31] recently reviewed two patients with a right cervical aortic arch and McElhinney [32] reviewed six patients with a cervical aortic arch. Another rare vascular ring occurs when a patient has situs inversus and has a left aortic arch with an aberrant right subclavian artery, with a right ligamentum. These patients (we have had one) require a right thoracotomy and ligation/division of the right ligamentum.

Clinical Presentation and Diagnosis

Most children with vascular rings present with symptoms within the first several weeks to months of life. The symptoms typically include some combination of the following: respiratory distress, stridor, the classic "seal bark" cough, apnea, dysphagia, and recurrent respiratory tract infections. (Table 13.2) [27]. Some older children will present only with symptoms of dysphagia or slow feeding where they tend to be the last child to leave the table because they have to chew their food carefully as a learned procedure. Infants may hold their head hyperextended to splint the trachea and lessen the obstruction, improving their breathing. Apnea or cyanosis may be precipitated by swallowing a bolus of solid food that presses on the soft posterior trachea within the restrictive confines of a ring. Most infants are well nourished, however, because they tolerate liquid formula well. When they are advanced to solid food, symptoms become more evident. The diagnosis of vascular rings requires a high index of suspicion because of the relative infrequency of this diagnosis compared with other conditions that cause respiratory distress in children such as asthma, reflux, and upper respiratory tract infection. Symptoms appear earlier and tend to be more severe in cases with a double aortic arch. A simple "cold" may precipitate severe respiratory difficulty. Children with innominate artery compression syndrome present with symptoms of tracheal compression, and nearly one half have had apneic episodes. It is of importance in these infants to rule out other causes of apneic spells. This includes a complete neurologic evaluation, investigation for gastroesophageal reflux, and sleep studies. Physical examination may reveal stridor, wheezing, tachypnea, a brassy cough, or noisy breathing. If the obstruction is severe, there may be obvious subcostal retractions, and nasal flaring. The number of patients presenting with various symptoms in our series of vascular ring patients is shown in Table 13.1.

The diagnosis of a vascular ring starts with the plain chest radiograph. There is a myriad of other diagnostic procedures that may be employed. These include barium esophagogram, bronchoscopy, tracheograms, computed tomography, magnetic resonance imaging, echocardiography, and cardiac catheterization. The emphasis should be to arrive at a diagnosis with the most efficient use of the multiple tests available. Once the diagnosis has been made, further studies are not required and the clinician should resist the tendency to obtain more studies that simply continue to confirm the diagnosis in a slightly different way.

Table 13.2 Symptoms leading to clinical presentation in patients with vascular rings*. (Reproduced with permission from Backer *et al.* [27].)

	Double aortic arch (n = 80)†	Right aortic arch (n = 78)†
Stridor	46 (57%)	18 (23%)
Recurrent upper respiratory tract infections	22 (27%)	18 (23%)
Cough	17 (21%)	8 (10%)
Dysphagia	12 (15%)	12 (15%)
Respiratory distress	8 (10%)	13 (17%)
Ventilator preoperatively	7 (9%)	3 (4%)

*More than one symptom occurred in many patients.
†Our records did not provide symptoms for the earlier patients in the series.

Chest Radiograph

The evaluation of a child with a possible vascular ring begins with anteroposterior and lateral chest radiography [33]. The mediastinum should be evaluated for a left aortic arch, right aortic arch, or double aortic arch as determined by the location of the aortic arch in relation to the trachea. When the location of the arch is not clear, a double aortic arch should be suspected. The lateral chest radiograph should be carefully evaluated for tracheal narrowing at the level of the aortic arch. High kilovoltage magnification technique is very helpful. If a right aortic arch or double aortic arch is suspected or narrowing of the trachea is seen on lateral images, further investigation for a vascular ring should be initiated. Unilateral hyperinflation of the right lung suggests a pulmonary artery sling. A completely normal chest radiograph is strong evidence against the presence of a vascular ring.

Barium Esophagogram

The barium esophagogram was historically the most widely used study for the diagnosis of vascular rings [34]. This is no longer the case and barium swallow has been supplanted by CT and MRI [27,35,36]. The impressions produced in the barium-filled esophagus by the anomalous aortic arch and/or branches often are quite characteristic for each lesion and may allow strong suspicion of the specific ring type present. A double aortic arch or right aortic arch with left ligamentum will appear as a deep persistent extrinsic indentation on the posterior aspect of the esophagus (Figure 13.6) [14]. Bilateral persistent compressions of the esophagus on the anteroposterior views are usually present with a double aortic arch (Figure 13.7) [3]. The dominant arch is usually on the right, higher, and more posterior than the lesser arch. A right aortic arch and retroesophageal left subclavian artery will produce an oblique indentation angled toward the left shoulder. A high posterior oblique indentation directed from left to right on the esophagogram is indicative of an aberrant right subclavian artery. A pulmonary artery sling is suggested by an anterior indentation of the esophagus (Figure 13.8) [14]. The diagnosis of a complete vascular ring can usually be established with some level of certainty with a barium esophagogram. However, determining the specific type of ring with a chest radiograph and esophagogram alone is not usually possible. Although historically surgeons would operate on these patients with only a barium swallow and a chest X-ray, we currently recommend CT or MRI on all vascular ring patients prior to surgical intervention [27].

Computed Tomography (CT)

CT scanning is very accurate in the identification of vascular anomalies of the aortic arch and great vessels and is our diagnostic method of choice [27,35]. A double aortic arch is diagnosed with certainty when both limbs are patent and enhanced with the intravenous administration of contrast material. However, in some cases the vascular ring may be completed by a nonenhanced segment, either the ligamentum arteriosum or an atretic portion of the lesser arch. In these cases the diagnosis of a complete ring depends on recognizing the arterial branching pattern, the side of the aortic arch, and focal narrowing of the airway. Three-dimensional reconstruction of the vascular structures establishes a very clear "road map" for the surgeon (Figure 13.9) [37].

One clue to an arch anomaly is the "four artery sign," which can be seen on sections obtained cephalad to the

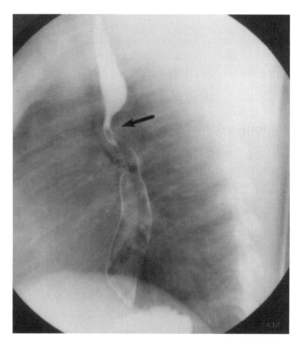

Figure 13.6 Lateral esophagogram of an 11-month-old boy with a double aortic arch, right arch dominant. Arrow points to the deep posterior indentation in the esophagus caused by the right arch.

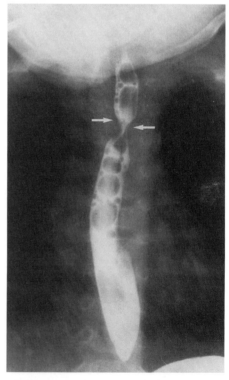

Figure 13.7 Anteroposterior esophagogram of a 4-month-old boy who presented with stridor and was found to have a double aortic arch. (Reproduced with permission from Backer *et al.* [3].)

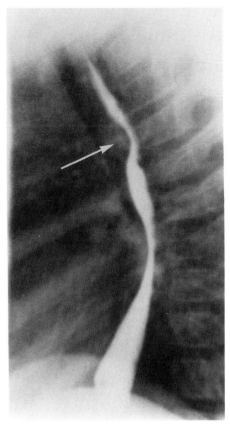

Figure 13.8 Lateral esophagogram of a 1½ -year-old girl with repeated episodes of stridor and respiratory tract infections. Arrow points to anterior indentation of esophagus caused by the anomalous left pulmonary artery.

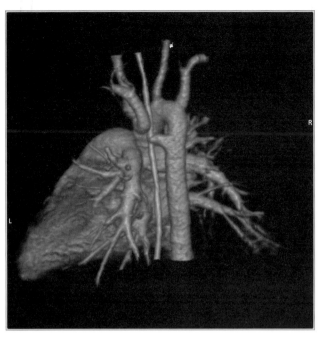

Figure 13.9 Three-dimensional (3D) reconstruction of CT scan. A 5-month-old child with a double aortic arch, right arch dominant. The distal left arch can be clearly seen projecting like a thumb from the descending aorta. The vertical structure inside the "ring" is the nasogastric tube. The anterior portion of this left arch is atretic just distal to the left subclavian artery. The left aortic arch had eroded into the esophagus. (Reproduced with permission from Backer et al. [37].)

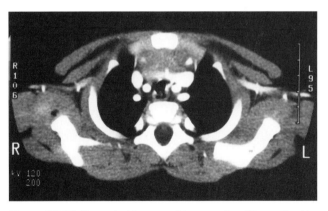

Figure 13.10 Computed tomographic scan of an 11-month-old boy with a right dominant double aortic arch. Note the four brachiocephalic vessels grouped symmetrically around the trachea.

aortic arch and consists of two dorsal subclavian arteries and two ventral carotid arteries evenly spaced around the trachea [38]. The sign is present when the two dorsal subclavian arteries arise directly from the aortic arch and not from a brachiocephalic artery. This occurs with double aortic arches and configurations with aberrant subclavian arteries (Figure 13.10) [14].

In patients with innominate artery compression syndrome, CT scan with contrast will show the anterior compression of the trachea by the innominate artery and helps to confirm the visual impression at the time of bronchoscopy (Figure 13.11) [14]. In children with a pulmonary artery sling, CT demonstrates the left pulmonary artery originating from the right pulmonary artery, encircling the trachea and coursing to the hilum of the left lung anterior to the esophagus and aorta (Figure 13.12) [37]. In addition, the presence of associated complete tracheal rings can be seen, and the extent of the tracheal narrowing can be used to plan the surgical approach.

Magnetic Resonance Imaging (MRI)

MRI is well suited for imaging vascular structures of the mediastinum (Figures 13.13 and 13.14) [3,39–42]. Axial images provide the same information as CT without ionizing radiation or the need for intravenously administered

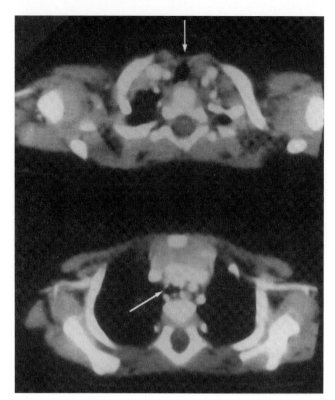

Figure 13.11 Computed tomographic scan with contrast of an infant with innominate artery compression syndrome. The superior cut shows a normal size trachea (arrow). The inferior cut shows the trachea (arrow) compressed by the innominate artery.

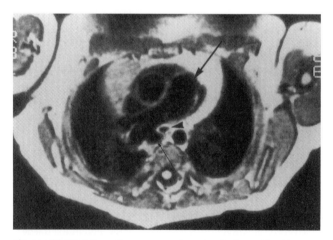

Figure 13.13 Magnetic resonance imaging in 7-month-old female infant with pulmonary artery sling and tracheal stenosis. Large arrow points to main pulmonary artery. Small arrow points to left pulmonary artery, which is curling around trachea. Trachea forms a complete ring easily visible on this study (arrowhead). (Reproduced with permission from Backer *et al.* [42].)

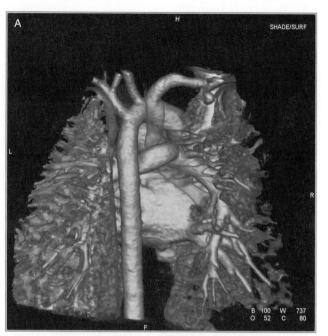

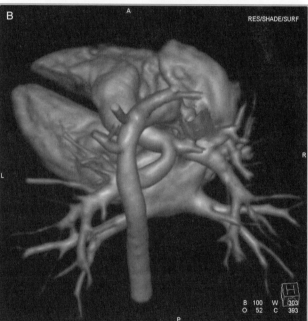

Figure 13.12 Three-dimensional (3D) reconstruction (pulmonary artery sling). **A,** This is a 3D reconstruction of a 2-month-old boy who had several apneic episodes requiring CPR. The child had a pulmonary artery sling causing significant tracheal compression. This posterior view shows the left pulmonary artery wrapping around and compressing the distal trachea and right bronchus. **B,** More cranial view of the same patient with the trachea removed to show the origin of the left pulmonary artery from the right pulmonary artery. The child had no further apneic spells after sling repair. (Reproduced with permission from Backer *et al.* [37].)

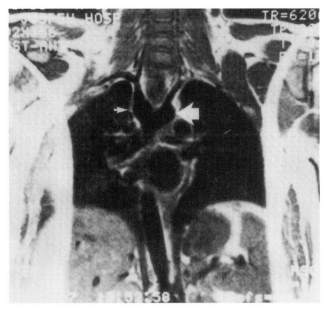

Figure 13.14 A 17-year-old patient with dysphagia. Magnetic resonance imaging shows a right aortic arch (small arrow) and a Kommerell diverticulum (large arrow) at the origin of the left subclavian artery. (Reproduced with permission from Backer *et al.* [3].)

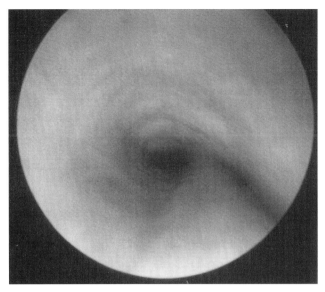

Figure 13.15 Bronchoscopic view of a 5-month-old boy with severe progressive stridor from innominate artery compression. Bronchoscopy shows the classic pulsatile anterior compression of the trachea extending from left to right.

contrast material. In addition, coronal and sagittal sections or images can be helpful in confusing cases. As with CT, the diagnosis of a vascular ring is based on the vascular branching pattern, the side of the aortic arch or arches, and narrowing of the airway. Unfortunately, like CT, MRI cannot reveal a small ligamentum or atretic segment. A disadvantage to MRI is the length of time required for the study necessitating sedation. When there is significant respiratory distress, sedation may not be safe. It seems that more often than not, the quality of MRI studies is poorer than CT scans because of patient movement. Sedation is not always necessary with CT since in a restrained infant dynamic scanning can be performed quickly. Because of these issues CT remains our imaging modality of choice. Both CT and MRI also can be helpful by revealing unsuspected mediastinal or tracheobronchial abnormalities.

Bronchoscopy

Bronchoscopy is often employed in children with respiratory distress who do not have a definite diagnosis [43]. External compression of the trachea just above the carina suggests either a double aortic arch or a right aortic arch with left ligamentum. The initial diagnosis of innominate artery compression is nearly always made with bronchoscopy. In these patients, bronchoscopy classically shows a pulsatile anterior compression of the trachea extending from left to right at a location closer to the vocal cords than

true vascular rings (Figure 13.15) [14]. Indication of significant innominate artery compression occurs only when the extent of the compression is more than 70–80% of the lumen of the trachea. Anterior compression of this area with the tip of the bronchoscope while monitoring the right radial pulse is a useful diagnostic maneuver with resultant obliteration or weakening of the pulse. Bronchoscopy can also be used to rule out other causes of respiratory distress such as aspiration of a foreign body or subglottic stenosis. In cases of pulmonary artery sling, bronchoscopy is required to assess for associated complete tracheal rings. In all cases an extreme degree of caution is necessary during and after bronchoscopy as the tracheal lumen, already narrowed by the vascular compression, may be compromised further by edema from bronchoscopic manipulation We now obtain bronchoscopy in all patients with a vascular ring prior to surgical repair because of the 3–5% incidence of unsuspected tracheal pathology [27].

Tracheograms

Although tracheograms were used frequently in the era before CT/MRI studies, they are much less commonly performed currently. They should be obtained only with the utmost caution to avoid further ventilatory compromise. If excess contrast is used, the lung may be permanently damaged by the barium. CT scanning and MRI are proving to be good noninvasive alternatives to tracheograms for evaluating the tracheal anatomy. There are still occasional difficult diagnostic cases, however, where a tracheogram can be quite useful [29].

Cardiac Catheterization

Cardiac catheterization formerly was used extensively to diagnose vascular rings in some institutions [44]. Because of the precision and noninvasive nature of CT and MRI, these tests have replaced angiography [42]. The only children for whom we now recommend cardiac catheterization are those with associated congenital cardiac anomalies. In particular, patients with a left aortic arch with right descending aorta and right ligamentum arteriosum often have associated cardiac disease and the diagnosis is often made by angiogram [28].

Echocardiography

Although echocardiography can detect aortic arch anomalies such as vascular rings, because of the limited windows it has not become a dominant diagnostic tool. The addition of Doppler color flow imaging is helpful in assessing for a ductus arteriosus and arch patency. Vascular ring segments without lumens cannot be displayed [45]. However, many patients with a vascular ring also have associated congenital heart disease. In our series of patients this occurred in 12% of the cases [27]. In Ruzmetov's series from Indiana, this occurred in 30% of the cases [46]. In our practice, if a child receives a diagnosis of complete tracheal rings, we use echocardiography as the procedure of choice to rule out an associated pulmonary artery sling if the child is too unstable for a CT scan [47].

Surgical Management

An operation is indicated in all symptomatic patients who have a vascular ring [48]. On close and pertinent questioning, nearly all patients with an anatomic vascular ring will be found to have significant airway symptoms. Initiation of early and appropriate surgical treatment is important to avoid serious complications that may arise after hypoxic or apneic spells. Delayed treatment may result in either sudden death or further tracheobronchial damage. Diagnostic errors may also lead to improper management of the respiratory obstruction with prolonged endotracheal intubation and occasional catastrophic erosion of the aortic arch into the trachea or esophagus [49–51]. Other reported complications of unrepaired vascular ring include aortic dissection and aneurysm formation [52]. The surgical approach varies depending on the specific vascular ring diagnosed (Table 13.3). A left posterolateral thoracotomy provides excellent exposure in almost all cases of the true vascular rings, i.e., double aortic arch and right aortic arch

Table 13.3 Surgical management of vascular rings.

Double aortic arch
1. Left thoracotomy (muscle sparing – 4th interspace)
2. Divide lesser of two arches at insertion with descending aorta
3. Preserve blood flow to carotid/radial arteries
4. Ligate and divide ligamentum arteriosum
5. Leave pleura open

Right aortic arch/left ligamentum
1. Left thoracotomy (muscle sparing – 4th interspace)
2. Ligate and divide ligamentum arteriosum
3. Resect Kommerell's diverticulum (if present) and transfer left subclavian artery to left carotid artery
4. Leave pleura open

Innominate artery compression syndrome
1. Right anterolateral thoracotomy (3rd interspace)
2. Resect right lobe of thymus
3. Suspend innominate artery to posterior sternum
4. Postoperative bronchoscopy

Pulmonary artery sling
1. Median sternotomy/extracorporeal circulation
2. Ligate/divide left pulmonary artery (PA)
3. Implant left PA into main PA anterior to the trachea
4. Slide Tracheoplasty for associated tracheal rings

with left ligamentum. We use a right thoracotomy for the innominate artery compression syndrome, and a median sternotomy for pulmonary artery sling with or without complete tracheal rings.

Double Aortic Arch

Nearly all of these patients are best approached through a left thoracotomy. The exception is the patient with a dominanent left arch where the approach is best with a right thoracotomy. The left thoracotomy can be performed with a muscle-sparing technique, elevating the serratus and latissimus muscles and entering the thorax through the fourth intercostal space. The mediastinal pleura is widely opened. Careful dissection in the posterior mediastinum should be performed to clearly delineate the anatomic configuration of the vascular ring. In particular, the left subclavian artery, ligamentum arteriosum, and descending aorta should be identified (Figure 13.16A) [14]. Typically, the left (anterior) arch is the smaller of the two arches, and it may be atretic where it inserts into the descending aorta. In our series of patients the right arch (posterior arch) was dominant in 75% of the patients, the left arch (anterior arch) was dominant in 18%, and the arches were of equal size in 7%. With a dominant right arch segments of the left arch were atretic in 34% of the patients. With a dominant left arch segments of the right arch were atretic in 25% of the patients. The atretic area occurred most frequently at the posterior or distal end of

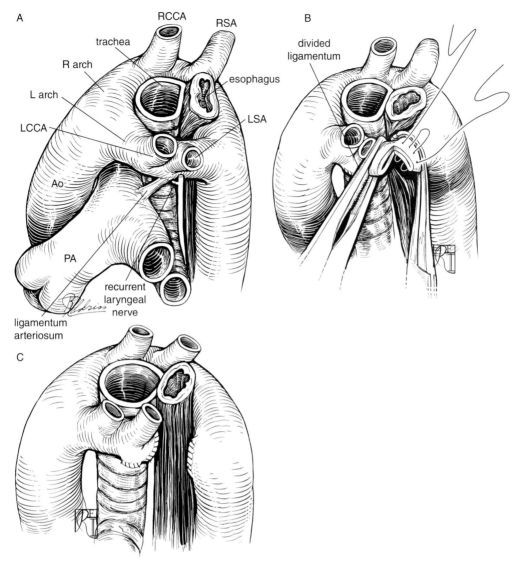

Figure 13.16 Double aortic arch division. **A,** Double aortic arch, right arch dominant. **B,** Dividing left aortic arch. **C,** Arch divided. (Ao, aorta; CA, carotid artery; L, left; LCCA, RCCA, left, right carotid artery; PA, pulmonary artery; R, right; SA, subclavian artery.)

the lesser arch. The vascular ring caused by the double aortic arch is released by dividing the lesser of the two arches, usually at the posterior insertion site into the descending aorta. The lesser arch is divided between clamps at a site selected to preserve brachiocephalic blood flow (Figure 13.16B) [14]. After applying the vascular clamps the anesthesiologist carefully checks the carotid and radial pulses on both the left and right sides. This ensures that the blood flow to these vessels is not interrupted. We place a pulse oximeter on both upper extremities and one lower extremity and that trace is also useful to watch for signs of vessel occlusion. Then the ring is divided and the two stumps are oversewn, each with a double layer of running polypropylene suture (Figure 13.16C) [14]. In addition, the ligamentum arteriosum is

always ligated and divided and careful dissection performed around the esophagus and the trachea to lyse any residual adhesive bands. The recurrent laryngeal nerve and phrenic nerve are identified and protected throughout the case. The mediastinal pleura is left widely open to decrease the chance of recurrent stenosis in the area of ring division. This is quite important; I have noted that many of the patients with recurrent symptoms referred to our center from other institutions have had their pleura closed at the initial operation. The resultant scar tissue from this pleural closure can be quite dense.

Results of Double Aortic Arch Repair

Since the first case reported by Potts at Children's Memorial Hospital in 1946, 139 patients have had repair of a double aortic arch at Children's Memorial Hospital. There has been no operative mortality from repair of an isolated double aortic arch since 1952. Two patients required reoperation for persistent symptoms arising from scar tissue at the divided posterior left arch. Nearly all patients were extubated in the operating room. We did not do routine postoperative bronchoscopy. In the past 15 years, we have only rarely used a tube thoracostomy [27]. The patients are monitored overnight in the cardiac intensive care unit, and discharged home on the second or third postoperative day. In most cases, it takes weeks to months for the barky cough to completely disappear, although it is nearly always significantly improved immediately postoperatively.

Right Aortic Arch with Left Ligamentum

For the patient with a right aortic arch and a left ligamentum, the same left thoracotomy muscle-sparing approach is used. After careful dissection and identification of the configuration of the aortic arch, the ligamentum arteriosum is identified. The ligamentum is either doubly ligated and divided or doubly clamped and divided with the two stumps oversewn (Figure 13.17) [14]. Any adhesive bands are lysed and the recurrent laryngeal nerve and phrenic nerve are carefully identified and protected. Patients with a right aortic arch and a left ligamentum may have a Kommerell's diverticulum at the origin of the left subclavian artery from the descending aorta [53]. This diverticulum is embryologically a remnant of the left fourth aortic arch. This diverticulum may enlarge to proportions that can independently compress the esophagus or trachea. Rupture of this aneurysm has also been reported [54]. We have become concerned about the size of this diverticulum when it is more than 1.5–2.0 times the diameter of the left subclavian artery. In this instance, the diverticulum or aneurysmal dilatation should be resected and the left subclavian artery transferred to the left carotid artery to prevent its independent compression of the trachea and esophagus (Figure 13.18) [55].

An unusual group of patients with a right aortic arch and left ligamentum have a left-sided descending aorta, the so-called "circumflex aorta." Robotin and associates [30] have described an aortic "uncrossing" operation for these rare patients (3 of 468 patients). This procedure is performed through a median sternotomy with cardiopulmonary bypass and hypothermic circulatory arrest. The aortic arch is mobilized, divided, and brought in front of the tracheobronchial tree, then reanastomosed end-to-side to the lateral aspect of the ascending aorta. All three patients described by Robotin had prior ligamentum division via left thoracotomy. We have performed this operation in two patients, one of whom had a dramatic improvement, the other a marginal improvement.

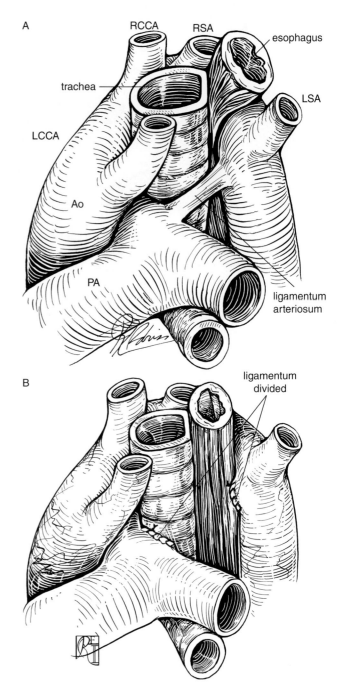

Figure 13.17 Right aortic arch – division and oversewing **(B)** of ligamentum arteriosum **(A)**. (Ao, aorta; CCA, common carotid artery; L, left; MPA, main pulmonary artery; R, right; SA, subclavian artery.)

Results of Right Aortic Arch with Left Ligamentum Division

One hundred and forty patients at Children's Memorial Hospital have had division of the ligamentum for a diagnosis of right aortic arch, retroesophageal left subclavian artery, and left ligamentum. There has been no operative mortality since 1959. No patient in our series has required

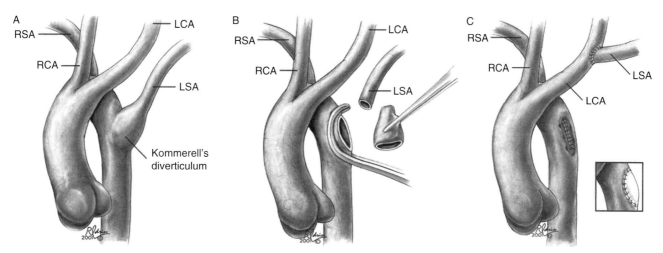

Figure 13.18 A, The typical anatomy of a patient with a right aortic arch, retroesophageal left subclavian artery, and large Kommerell's diverticulum. The Kommerell's diverticulum is an embryologic remnant of the left fourth aortic arch. (LCA/RCA, left/right carotid artery; LSA/RSA, left/right subclavian artery.) **B,** A schematic illustration of the resection of a Kommerell's diverticulum through a left thoracotomy. There is a vascular clamp partially occluding the descending thoracic aorta at the origin of the Kommerell's diverticulum. The Kommerell's diverticulum has been completely resected. The clamp on the distal left subclavian artery is not illustrated. **C,** The completed repair. The orifice where the Kommerell's diverticulum was resected is usually closed primarily, or, as shown in the inset, the orifice can be patched with polytetrafluoroethylene if necessary. The left subclavian artery has been implanted into the side of the left common carotid artery with fine running polypropylene suture. (Reproduced with permission from Backer et al. [55].)

a reoperation. In 66% of the patients a retroesophageal left subclavian artery was present. In 34% of patients there was a mirror image left innominate artery. In the past 10 years, 10 children who had recurrent symptoms after ligamentum division elsewhere underwent reoperation at our center. All had a large Kommerell's diverticulum compressing their esophagus and/or trachea that required resection. In these patients we resected the Kommerell's diverticulum and reimplanted the left subclavian artery into the left carotid artery, to relieve a sling-like effect of the right arch and left subclavian artery on the trachea. Eight patients have had diverticulum resection and left subclavian transfer done as a primary procedure. These 18 patients have all had dramatic relief of their symptoms, with no neurologic complications and all left subclavian arteries patent.

Innominate Artery Compression Syndrome

The management of compression of the trachea by the innominate artery has classically been with suspension of the innominate artery to the posterior aspect of the sternum [56]. This technique as originally described by Gross was performed through a left anterolateral thoracotomy [6], and at Boston Children's Hospital the left thoracotomy is still the approach of choice [57]. However, at our institution we have preferred a small right submammary anterolateral thoracotomy for these infants (Figure 13.19) [58]. The right lobe of the thymus is excised, taking care not to injure the right phrenic nerve. The innominate artery is secured with

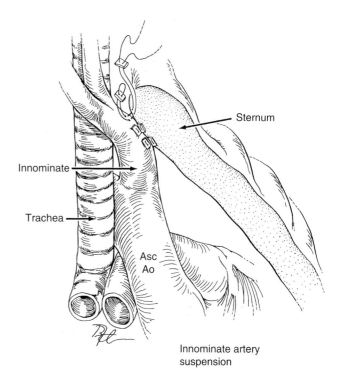

Figure 13.19 Innominate artery suspension. Exposure is through a right submammary thoracotomy. Fixing the adventitia of the innominate artery to the posterior table of the sternum with pledgeted sutures pulls the innominate artery anteriorly and actively pulls the tracheal wall forward and opens it. (Asc. Ao, ascending aorta.) (Reproduced with permission from Backer et al. [58].)

pledget-supported sutures to the posterior periosteum of the sternum to lift the innominate artery away from the trachea, simultaneously pulling the anterior tracheal wall open. Typically, three separate mattress sutures are used. The first is on the anterior surface of the aortic arch in line with the origin of the innominate artery, the second at the junction between the innominate artery and the aorta, and the third 0.5 cm distal to the origin of the innominate artery. Bronchoscopy is then performed after the suspension to confirm relief of the tracheal compression. Pre- and postoperative CT scans of a patient having innominate artery suspension are shown in Figure 13.20 [59]. Other authors have described using a median sternotomy with division of the innominate artery and reimplantation into the

ascending aorta at a site more to the right and anterior to the native site [60]. This technique would seem to sacrifice the active suspending mechanism on the tracheal wall provided by the classical innominate artery suspension. In addition, there is some risk of cerebrovascular accident with the technique of division and reimplantation [59]. We and others [61] continue to recommend innominate artery suspension to the sternum through a right thoracotomy.

Results of Innominate Artery Compression Syndrome Repair

Eighty-seven patients have had innominate arteriopexy at Children's Memorial Hospital. There have been no operative mortalities for isolated innominate artery suspension. Two patients have required reoperation for resuspension. The cessation of apneic spells is very reassuring to parents! However, it is our suspicion that this diagnosis was previously made too often, and the number of patients we have operated on for this diagnosis has decreased dramatically in the past 20 years (Figure 13.21) [62].

Pulmonary Artery Sling

The management of the infant with pulmonary artery sling has changed considerably since the original procedure by Potts at Children's Memorial Hospital in 1953 [7]. Potts operated on a patient without a precise preoperative diagnosis through a right thoracotomy. He doubly clamped and transected the left pulmonary artery, translocated it anterior to the trachea, and then reimplanted it into the original division site on the right pulmonary artery. The child survived the operation but on long-term follow-up has an occluded left pulmonary artery [63]. The next step in the evolution of surgical technique for this condition was to approach through a left thoracotomy with implantation of

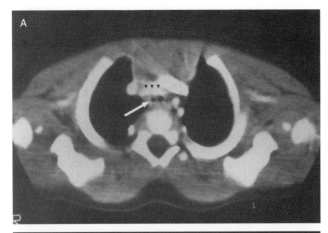
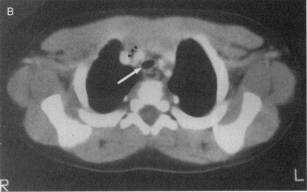

Figure 13.20 Computed tomographic scan before and after innominate artery suspension. **A,** Computed tomographic scan with contrast material preoperatively shows severe anterior compression of the trachea (large arrow) by the innominate artery (small arrowheads). In this instance the trachea is septated into two lumina by the severe compression. **B,** Computed tomographic scan with contrast material of the same child after innominate artery suspension shows a dramatic increase in the size of the tracheal lumen (large arrow). The innominate artery (small arrowheads) has been shifted anteriorly and to the right by the sutures fixed to the sternum. (Reproduced with permission from Backer et al. [59].)

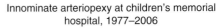
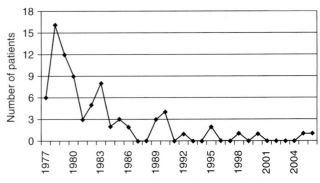

Figure 13.21 Innominate arteriopexy: Changing incidence of operative procedures at Children's Memorial Hospital from 1977 to 2006. (Reproduced with permission from Backer et al. [62].)

the left pulmonary artery into the main pulmonary artery at a site that approximated its normal origin from the main pulmonary artery [64]. This procedure initially had a high incidence of left pulmonary artery stenosis or occlusion, along with a high mortality [17]. Because between 50% and 65% of patients with pulmonary artery sling will have associated complete tracheal rings, the "ring-sling" complex [18], we have advocated an approach with median sternotomy and the use of extracorporeal circulation [42,65]. This allows accurate transection of the left pulmonary artery with implantation into the main pulmonary artery anterior to the trachea (Figure 13.22) [14]. The operation can be performed without respiratory compromise (patient is on cardiopulmonary bypass), and enough time and care can be taken to ensure patency of the left pulmonary artery. An alternative technique for pulmonary artery sling relief is to translocate the left pulmonary artery at the time of distal tracheal resection for tracheal stenosis [66]. We have only used this when the right pulmonary artery was severely hypoplastic or absent. Van Son and colleagues [67] compared the two techniques and demonstrated that the translocation technique had a higher incidence of residual left pulmonary artery stenosis.

Results of Pulmonary Artery Sling Repair

Between 1953 and 2008, 40 infants underwent repair of pulmonary artery sling at Children's Memorial Hospital, Chicago. Median age at repair was 4 months. One patient (the first) was approached through a right thoracotomy. Six patients were approached through a left thoracotomy (1972–1979). Thirty-three patients were repaired through a median sternotomy (1970, 1985–2008), and of these, 32 were repaired with the use of cardiopulmonary bypass. There has been no operative mortality. There were four late deaths, all from respiratory complications of simultaneous tracheoplasty. All left pulmonary arteries in patients repaired with the use of cardiopulmonary bypass are patent and blood flow to the left lung by nuclear scan ranges from 24% to 46% (mean $35 \pm 9\%$). If there are associated complete tracheal rings, we previously used the pericardial tracheoplasty technique simultaneous with the pulmonary artery sling repair [8,68]. From 1996–2004 we used the tracheal autograft technique [9,69,70], and since 2004 we have used the slide tracheoplasty [71,72]. These techniques are discussed in depth in the next section.

Tracheal Stenosis

Infants born with complete cartilage tracheal rings often present with life-threatening respiratory distress in infancy [73]. There is absence of the normal membranous trachea, and at the site of the complete rings the tracheal lumen is often only 2–3 mm (Figure 13.23A) [14]. Medical management is associated with at least a 40% mortality [74].

Pericardial patch tracheoplasty as a surgical solution was first performed by Farouk S Idriss at Children's Memorial Hospital in 1982 [8]. These patients were operated on using cardiopulmonary bypass through a median sternotomy. The trachea was exposed and incised anteriorly through the extent of the complete tracheal rings. An autologous pericardial patch was sutured in place with interrupted polyglactin 910 (Vicryl™, Ethicon, Inc., Somerville, NJ) or polydioxanone (PDS™, Ethicon, Inc., Somerville, NJ) sutures (Figure 13.23B) [14]. The endotracheal tube was used to stent the trachea and patch for 1–2 weeks postoperatively. These patients survived, which was a major achievement, but had a high incidence of recurrent stenosis from patch tracheomalacia and granulation tissue [75].

The slide tracheoplasty is currently our procedure of choice for the patient with tracheal stenosis secondary to complete tracheal rings (Figure 13.24) [71,72,76–79]. The slide tracheoplasty is performed through a median sternotomy with extracorporeal circulation. We have used a collar incision in the neck like a "T" (at the top of the sternotomy incision) to adequately visualize the cervical portion of the trachea. If a pulmonary artery sling or cardiac anomaly is present, they are repaired first. After initiating cardiopulmonary bypass with an aortic and single atrial venous cannula, the trachea is divided in the midportion of the tracheal stenosis. This location is determined either by external visual inspection or fiberoptic bronchoscopy. The inferior portion of the trachea is incised anteriorly and the superior portion of the trachea is incised posteriorly. The corners of the tracheal openings are trimmed. An anastomosis is performed with running 5-0 or 6-0 PDS suture starting at the superior aspect and finishing by the carina. The patient then undergoes bronchoscopy to aspirate secretions and to ensure the stenosis has been relieved. The repair is stented with an endotracheal tube for 3–5 days, and the child is kept on a ventilator. Follow-up bronchoscopy is performed to remove granulation tissue, clear secretions, and identify residual stenosis. The child is then weaned from the ventilator and extubated.

Between 1996 and 2004, we developed and used the tracheal autograft technique in 20 patients. The use of this method was sparked by successful reports using tracheal homograft [80], and our own initial marginal results with the slide tracheoplasty [76]. The autograft technique employs excision of the midportion of the stenotic trachea (this piece becomes the autograft), performance of an end-to-end anastomosis posteriorly, and then patching the trachea anteriorly with the autograft [9,69,70]. We have essentially abandoned this approach and now use the slide tracheoplasty. The other surgical alternative for complete tracheal rings is simple resection with end-to-end anastomosis for shorter segments [66,81–83]. We used this technique if the length of stenosis is less than 30% of the total tracheal length, usually less than seven rings.

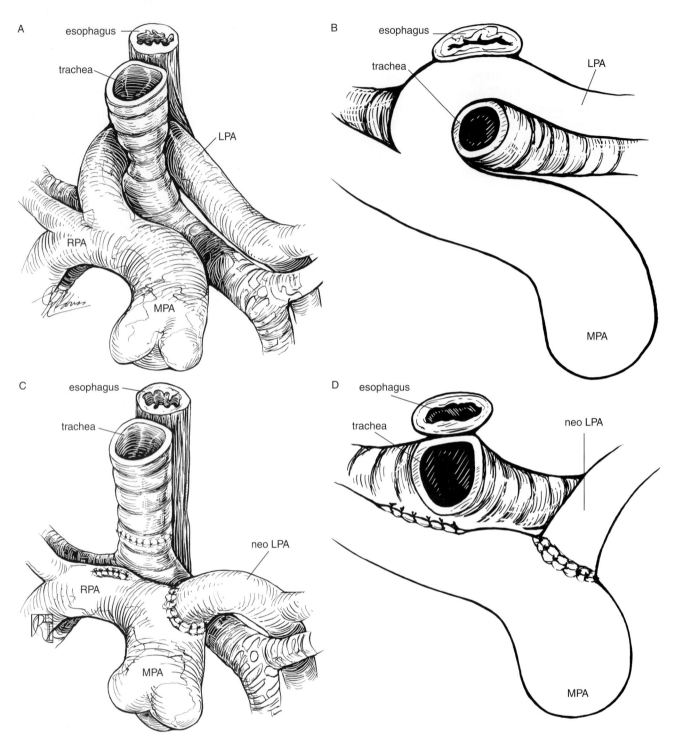

Figure 13.22 Illustration of operative technique for pulmonary artery sling repair with tracheal resection (performed with cardiopulmonary bypass). **A,** LPA encircles and compresses distal area of trachea and right main stem bronchus. **B,** Relationship of LPA to trachea and esophagus. **C,** Repair is by transecting LPA at its origin from RPA and anastomosing the LPA to the MPA at a site that approximates usual anatomic configuration. The tracheal stenosis has also been resected, and an end-to-end tracheal anastomosis is shown. **D,** Postoperative relationship of neo-LPA to MPA anastomosis shows the relatively long distance from the original LPA takeoff from the RPA. (LPA, left pulmonary artery; MPA, main pulmonary artery; RPA, right pulmonary artery.)

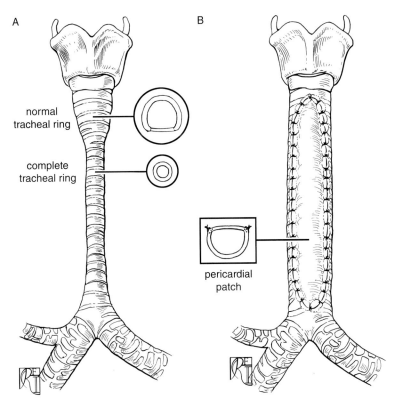

Figure 13.23 Pericardial patch tracheoplasty technique. **A,** Long segment tracheal stenosis with complete tracheal rings. The trachea is incised anteriorly through the extent of the complete tracheal rings. **B,** Completed repair with trachea patched anteriorly with autologous pericardial patch.

Results of Tracheal Stenosis Repair

Between 1982 and 2009, 75 patients have had repair of congenital tracheal stenosis at Children's Memorial Hospital. Median age at repair was 4 months. Techniques included pericardial patch tracheoplasty (n = 28), tracheal autograft (n = 20), tracheal resection (n = 13), and slide tracheoplasty (n = 14). Twenty-five of these patients (33%) had an associated pulmonary artery sling and 17 (23%) had an associated intracardiac anomaly. Twelve patients had unilateral lung agenesis or severe hypoplasia. Despite the increased severity of the pathology and more critical presentation, outcomes in patients with one lung physiology were not different from patients with two lungs [79]. There were seven early deaths (9%) and five late deaths (7%). Our current procedures of choice for infants with congenital tracheal stenosis are resection with end-to-end anastomosis for short-segment stenosis (up to six rings) and the slide tracheoplasty for long-segment stenosis. Associated pulmonary artery sling and intracardiac anomalies should be repaired simultaneously.

Postoperative Care

The postoperative care of all infants with vascular rings includes high humidity to loosen secretions, oxygen therapy when needed as monitored with pulse oximetry, and careful nasopharyngeal suctioning and chest physiotherapy. Early extubation is attempted for all patients except for those following tracheoplasty. Other helpful postoperative modalities include inhaled corticosteroids, albuteral treatments, and heliox. Most patients have a relatively uncomplicated course if no additional trauma is inflicted in the trachea and upper part of the airway. Antibiotic treatment of any associated pneumonitis is also indicated. Complete relief of symptoms may not be noted immediately after surgery, but most patients are generally significantly improved. A period of months to 1 year may be required before disappearance of the noisy respirations caused by tracheomalacia. This fact should be clearly explained to the parents preoperatively and also to the nurses to allay their fears regarding the residual noisy breathing.

Video-Assisted Thoracoscopic Surgery

An alternative to an open thoracotomy is video-assisted thoracoscopic surgery (VATS) for the division of vascular rings [84]. This has occurred as an extension of VATS use for patent ductus arteriosus ligation [85]. Burke [86] reported VATS use for eight patients with vascular rings. Anatomy of the rings included double aortic arch with an

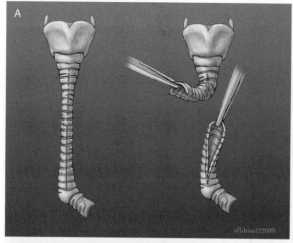

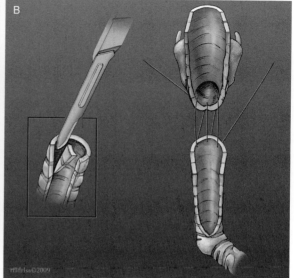

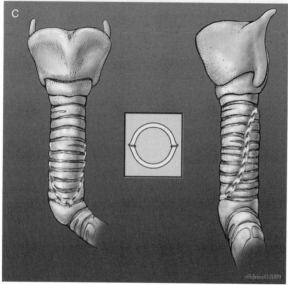

Figure 13.24 Slide tracheoplasty; absent right lung. **A,** The patient has been placed on cardiopulmonary bypass with mild hypothermia to 32 °C. The trachea is transected in the midportion of the tracheal stenosis. This site is determined by either external examination or by internal bronchoscopic findings. The inferior portion of the trachea is incised anteriorly and the superior portion of the trachea is incised posteriorly. **B,** The ends of the trachea are beveled as shown in the small inset. The anastomosis is performed with running 6.0 polydioxanone suture. The suture line is started superiorly (parachute technique) and finished inferiorly just above the carina. **C,** Completed slide tracheoplasty. The everting running suture line helps to avoid the "figure of 8" configuration problem after the completed repair. (Reproduced with permission from Backer *et al.* [79].)

atretic left arch (three patients) and right aortic arch, left ligamentum arteriosum (five patients). Three patients (37.5%) required a thoracotomy to complete the procedure. The median operating time was 4 hours; median hospital stay was 3 days. It is interesting to note there were no patients with a patent arch. A concern for the patient with a patent arch is that once the clips are applied and the ring divided, the two stumps retract because of the tension on the ring. The posterior stump often retracts into the mediastinum, and if the clip should slip off, the risk of hemorrhage is great. We are aware of anecdotal reports of this severe complication. It is not always possible to tell exter-

nally whether a segment of the ring is atretic or patent. Even quite recent series have yet to demonstrate a significant advantage to VATS over open repair [87].

Conclusion

The diagnosis of a vascular ring should be suspected in any infant or child who presents with symptoms of respiratory distress. The diagnosis is best established by CT or MRI which accurately delineate the anatomy of the ring. Echocardiography should be obtained in all patients to assess for congenital heart disease. Bronchoscopy should be performed in all cases to assess for additional tracheal pathology and provide an assessment of tracheobronchomalacia. The surgical approach for both double aortic arch and right aortic arch is usually a left thoracotomy (muscle-sparing approach). Some rare vascular rings are best approached through a right thoracotomy. We have used a right thoracotomy for innominate artery suspension. A median sternotomy and the use of extracorporeal circulation is recommended for the repair of pulmonary artery sling and patients who have associated complete tracheal rings. Our current procedure of choice for long-segment tracheal stenosis is the slide tracheoplasty. Surgical intervention successfully provides relief of tracheoesophageal compression from vascular structures in over 95% of infants and children.

References

1. Hommel, cited by Turner W. (1962) On irregularities of the pulmonary artery, arch of the aorta and the primary branches of the arch with an attempt to illustrate their mode of origin by a reference to development. Br Foreign Med Chir Rev 30, 173, 461.
2. Gross RE. (1945) Surgical relief for tracheal obstruction from a vascular ring. N Engl J Med 233, 586–590.
3. Backer CL, Ilbawi MN, Idriss FS, *et al.* (1989) Vascular anomalies causing tracheoesophageal compression. Review of experience in children. J Thorac Cardiovasc Surg 97, 725–731.
4. Glaevecke H, Doehle W. (1897) Ueber eine seltene angeborene anomalie der pulmonalarterie. Munch Med Wochenschr 44, 950.
5. Backer CL, Mavroudis C. (2000) Congenital heart surgery nomenclature and database project: vascular rings, tracheal stenosis, pectus excavatum. Ann Thorac Surg 69(4 Suppl), S308–S318.
6. Gross RE, Neuhauser EBD. (1948) Compression of the trachea by an anomalous innominate artery: an operation for its relief. Am J Dis Child 75, 570–574.
7. Potts WJ, Holinger PH, Rosenblum AH. (1954) Anomalous left pulmonary artery causing obstruction to right main bronchus: report of a case. JAMA 155, 1409–1411.
8. Idriss FS, DeLeon SY, Ilbawi MN, *et al.* (1984) Tracheoplasty with pericardial patch for extensive tracheal stenosis in infants and children. J Thorac Cardiovasc Surg 88, 527–536.
9. Backer CL, Mavroudis C, Dunham ME, *et al.* (1998) Repair of congenital tracheal stenosis with a free tracheal autograft. J Thorac Cardiovasc Surg 115, 869–874.
10. Potts WJ, Gibson S, Rothwell R. (1948) Double aortic arch: report of two cases. Arch Surg 57, 227–233.
11. Congdon ED. (1922) Transformation of the aortic arch system during the development of the human embryo. Contrib Embryol 14, 47.
12. Edwards JE. (1948). Anomalies of the derivatives of the aortic arch system. Med Clin North Am 32, 925–949.
13. Stewart JR, Kincaid OW, Edwards JE. (1964) *An Atlas of Vascular Rings and Related Malformations of the Aortic Arch System.* Springfield, Ill: Charles C Thomas Publisher.
14. Backer CL, Mavroudis C. Vascular rings and pulmonary artery sling. In: Mavroudis C, Backer CL, eds. *Pediatric Cardiac Surgery*, 3rd ed. Philadelphia, PA: Mosby, 2003.
15. Felson B, Palayew MJ. (1963) The two types of right aortic arch. Radiology 81, 745–759.
16. Hastreiter AR, D'Cruz IA, Cantez T, *et al.* (1966) Right-sided aorta. I. Occurrence of right aortic arch in various types of congenital heart disease. II. Right aortic arch, right descending aorta, and associated anomalies. Br Heart J 28, 722–739.
17. Sade RM, Rosenthal A, Fellows K, *et al.* (1975) Pulmonary artery sling. J Thorac Cardiovasc Surg 69, 333–346.
18. Berdon WE, Baker DH, Wung JT, *et al.* (1984) Complete cartilage-ring tracheal stenosis associated with anomalous left pulmonary artery: the ring-sling complex. Radiology 152, 57–64.
19. Ardito JM, Ossoff RH, Tucker GF Jr, *et al.* (1980) Innominate artery compression of the trachea in infants with reflex apnea. Ann Otol Rhinol Laryngol 89, 401–405.
20. Abbott ME. (1936) *Atlas of Congenital Cardiac Disease.* New York: American Heart Association.
21. Bayford D. (1794) Account of singular case of obstructed deglutition. Mem Med Soc London 2, 275.
22. Beabout JW, Stewart JR, Kincaid OW. (1964) Aberrant right subclavian artery, dispute of commonly accepted concepts. Am J Roentgen 92, 855.
23. Murthy K, Mattioli L, Diehl AM. (1970) Vascular ring due to left aortic arch, right descending aorta, and right patent ductus arteriosus. J Pediatr Surg 5, 550–554.
24. Whitman G, Stephenson LW, Weinberg P (1982). Vascular ring: left cervical aortic arch, right descending aorta, and right ligamentum arteriosum. J Thorac Cardiovasc Surg 83, 311–315.
25. McFaul R, Millard P, Nowicki E. (1981) Vascular rings necessitating right thoracotomy. J Thorac Cardiovasc Surg 82, 306–309.
26. Park SC, Siewers RD, Neches WH, *et al.* (1976) Left aortic arch with right descending aorta and right ligamentum arteriosum. A rare form of vascular ring. J Thorac Cardiovasc Surg 71, 779–784.
27. Backer CL, Mavroudis C, Rigsby CK, *et al.* (2005) Trends in vascular ring surgery. J Thorac Cardiovasc Surg 129, 1339–1347.
28. Binet JP, Conso JF, Losay J, (1978) Ductus arteriosus sling: report of a newly recognized anomaly and its surgical correction. Thorax 33, 72–75.
29. Dodge-Khatami A, Backer CL, Dunham ME, *et al.* (1999) Right aortic arch, right ligamentum, absent left pulmonary artery: a rare vascular ring. Ann Thorac Surg 67, 1472–1474.
30. Robotin MC, Bruniaux J, Serraf A, *et al.* (1996) Unusual forms of tracheobronchial compression in infants with congenital heart disease. J Thorac Cardiovasc Surg 112, 415–423.
31. van Son JAM, Bossert T, Mohr FW. (1999) Surgical treatment of vascular ring including right cervical aortic arch. J Card Surg 14, 98–102.
32. McElhinney DB, Thompson LD, Weinberg PM, *et al.* (2000) Surgical approach to complicated cervical aortic arch: anatomic, developmental, and surgical considerations. Cardiol Young 10, 212–219.

33. Pickhardt PJ, Siegel MJ, Gutierrez FR. (1997) Vascular rings in symptomatic children: frequency of chest radiographic findings. Radiology 203, 423–426.

34. Stark J, Roesler M, Chrispin A, et al. (1985) The diagnosis of airway obstruction in children. J Pediatr Surg 20, 113–117.

35. Lambert V, Sigal-Cinqualbre A, Belli E, et al. (2005) Preoperative and postoperative evaluation of airways compression in pediatric patients with 3-dimensional multislice computed tomographic scanning: effect on surgical management. J Thorac Cardiovasc Surg 129, 1111–1118.

36. Malik TH, Bruce IA, Kaushik V, et al. (2006) The role of magnetic resonance imaging in the assessment of suspected extrinsic tracheobronchial compression due to vascular anomalies. Arch Dis Child 91, 52–55.

37. Backer CL (2009) Compression of the trachea by vascular rings. In: Shields TW, Locicero J III, Reed CE, Feins RH, eds. General Thoracic Surgery, 7th ed., vol. 1. Philadelphia, PA: Wolters Kluwer/Lippincott Williams & Wilkins.

38. Lowe GM, Donaldson JS, Backer CL. (1991) Vascular rings: 10-year review of imaging. RadioGraphics 11, 637–646.

39. Bisset GS 3rd, Strife JL, Kirks DR, et al. (1987) Vascular rings: MR imaging. AJR Am J Roentgenol 149, 251–256.

40. Kensting-Sommerhoff BA, Sechtem UP, Fisher MR, et al. (1987) MR imaging of congenital anomalies of the aortic arch. AJR Am J Roentgenol 149, 9–13.

41. van Son JAM, Julsrud PR, Hagler DJ, et al. (1994) Imaging strategies for vascular rings. Ann Thorac Surg 57, 604–610.

42. Backer CL, Idriss FS, Holinger LD, et al. (1992) Pulmonary artery sling. Results of surgical repair in infancy. J Thorac Cardiovasc Surg 103, 683–691.

43. Holinger LD. (1989) Diagnostic endoscopy of the pediatric airway. Laryngoscope 99, 346–348.

44. Azarow KS, Pearl RH, Hoffman MA, et al. (1992) Vascular ring: does magnetic resonance imaging replace angiography? Ann Thorac Surg 53, 882–885.

45. Lillehei CW, Colan S. (1992) Echocardiography in the preoperative evaluation of vascular rings. J Pediatr Surg 27, 1118–1120.

46. Ruzmetov M, Vijay P, Rodefeld MD, et al. (2009) Follow-up of surgical correction of aortic arch anomalies causing tracheoesophageal compression: a 38-year single institution experience. J Pediatr Surg 44, 1328–1332.

47. Alboliras ET, Backer CL, Holinger LD, et al. (1996) Pulmonary artery sling: diagnostic and management strategy. Pediatrics 98, 530A.

48. van Son JA, Julsrud PR, Hagler DJ, et al. (1993) Surgical treatment of vascular rings: the Mayo Clinic experience. Mayo Clin Proc 68, 1056–1063.

49. Othersen HB Jr, Khalil B, Zellner J, et al. (1996) Aortoesophageal fistula and double aortic arch: two important points in management. J Pediatr Surg 31, 594–595.

50. Heck HA Jr, Moore HV, Lutin WA, et al. (1993) Esophageal-aortic erosion associated with double aortic arch and tracheomalacia. Experience with 2 infants. Tex Heart Inst J 20, 126–129.

51. Angelini A, Dimopoulos K, Frescura C, et al. (2002) Fatal aortoesophageal fistula in two cases of tight vascular ring. Cardiol Young 12, 172–176.

52. Midulla PS, Dapunt OE, Sadeghi AM, et al. (1994) Aortic dissection involving a double aortic arch with a right descending aorta. Ann Thorac Surg 58, 874–875.

53. Kommerell B. (1936) Verlagerung des osophagus durch eine abnorm verlaufende arteria subclavia dextra (arteria lusoria). Fortschr Geb Rontgenstr 54, 590.

54. Fisher RG, Whigham CJ, Trinh C. (2005) Diverticula of Kommerell and aberrant subclavian arteries complicated by aneurysms. Cardiovasc Intervent Radiol 28, 553–560.

55. Backer CL, Hillman N, Mavroudis C, et al. (2002) Resection of Kommerell's diverticulum and left subclavian artery transfer for recurrent symptoms after vascular ring division. Eur J Cardiothorac Surg 22, 64–69.

56. Moes CAF, Izukawa T, Trusler GA. (1975) Innominate artery compression of the trachea. Arch Otolaryngol 101, 733–738.

57. Jones DT, Jonas RA, Healy GB. (1994) Innominate artery compression of the trachea in infants. Ann Otol Rhinol Laryngol 103, 347–350.

58. Backer CL, Mavroudis C. (1997) Surgical approach to vascular rings. In: Karp R, et al., eds. Advances in Cardiac Surgery, Vol. 9. St. Louis, MO: Mosby-Year Book.

59. Backer CL, Holinger LD, Mavroudis C. (1992) Invited letter: Innominate artery compression – division and reimplantation versus suspension. J Thorac Cardiovasc Surg 103, 817–820.

60. Hawkins JA, Bailey WW, Clark SM. (1992) Innominate artery compression of the trachea. Treatment by reimplantation of the innominate artery. J Thorac Cardiovasc Surg 103, 678–682.

61. Adler SC, Isaacson G, Balsara RK. (1995) Innominate artery compression of the trachea: diagnosis and treatment by anterior suspension. A 25-year experience. Ann Otol Rhinol Laryngol 104, 924–927.

62. Backer CL, Mavroudis C, Stewart RD, et al. (2006) Congenital anomalies: vascular rings. In: Patterson GA, ed. Pearson's Thoracic and Esophageal Surgery. Philadelphia, PA: Elsevier.

63. Campbell CD, Wernly JA, Koltip PC, et al. (1980) Aberrant left pulmonary artery (pulmonary artery sling): successful repair and 24 year follow-up report. Am J Cardiol 45, 316–320.

64. Koopot R, Nikaidoh H, Idriss FS. (1975) Surgical management of anomalous left pulmonary artery causing tracheobronchial obstruction. Pulmonary artery sling. J Thorac Cardiovasc Surg 69, 239–246.

65. Backer CL, Mavroudis C, Dunham ME, et al. (1999) Pulmonary artery sling: results with median sternotomy, cardiopulmonary bypass, and reimplantation. Ann Thorac Surg 67, 1738–1745.

66. Jonas RA, Spevak PJ, McGill T, et al. (1989) Pulmonary artery sling: primary repair by tracheal resection in infancy. J Thorac Cardiovasc Surg 97, 548–550.

67. van Son JAM, Hambsch J, Haas, GS, et al. (1999) Pulmonary artery sling: reimplantation versus antetracheal translocation. Ann Thorac Surg 68, 989–994.

68. Heimansohn DA, Kesler KA, Turrentine MW, et al. (1991) Anterior pericardial tracheoplasty for congenital tracheal stenosis. J Thorac Cardiovasc Surg 102, 710–716.

69. Backer CL, Mavroudis C, Dunham ME, et al. (2000) Intermediate-term results of the free tracheal autograft for

long segment congenital tracheal stenosis. J Pediatr Surg 35, 813–819.

70. Backer CL, Holinger LD, Mavroudis C. (2007) Congenital tracheal stenosis: tracheal autograft technique. Op Tech Thorac Cardiovasc Surg 12, 178–183.

71. Tsang V, Murday A, Gillbe C, *et al.* (1989) Slide tracheoplasty for congenital funnel-shaped tracheal stenosis. Ann Thorac Surg 48, 632–635.

72. Grillo HC. (1994) Slide tracheoplasty for long-segment congenital tracheal stenosis. Ann Thorac Surg 58, 613–621.

73. Janik JS, Nagaraj HS, Yacoub U, *et al.* (1982) Congenital funnel-shaped tracheal stenosis: an asymptomatic lethal anomaly of early infancy. J Thorac Cardiovasc Surg 83, 761–766.

74. Benjamin B, Pitkin J, Cohen D. (1981) Congenital tracheal stenosis. Ann Otol Rhinol Laryngol 90, 364–371.

75. Backer CL, Mavroudis C, Dunham ME, *et al.* (1997) Reoperation after pericardial patch tracheoplasty. J Pediatr Surg 32, 1108–1112.

76. Dayan SH, Dunham ME, Backer CL, *et al.* (1997) Slide tracheoplasty in the management of congenital tracheal stenosis. Ann Otol Rhinol Laryngol 106, 914–919.

77. Kocyildirim E, Kanani M, Roebuck D, *et al.* (2004) Long-segment tracheal stenosis: slide tracheoplasty and a multidisciplinary approach improve outcomes and reduce costs. J Thorac Cardiovasc Surg 128;876–882.

78. Manning PB, Rutter MJ, Border WL. (2008) Slide tracheoplasty in infants and children: risk factors for prolonged postoperative ventilatory support. Ann Thorac Surg 85;1187–1192.

79. Backer CL, Kelle AM, Mavroudis C, *et al.* (2009) Tracheal reconstruction in children with unilateral lung agenesis or severe hypoplasia. Ann Thorac Surg 88, 624–631.

80. Jacobs JP, Elliott MJ, Haw MP, *et al.* (1996) Pediatric tracheal homograft reconstruction: a novel approach to complex tracheal stenoses in children. J Thorac Cardiovasc Surg 112, 1549–1560.

81. Backer CL, Mavroudis C, Gerber ME, *et al.* (2001) Tracheal surgery in children: an 18-year review of four techniques. Eur J Cardiothorac Surg 19, 777–784.

82. Cotter CS, Jones DT, Nuss RC, *et al.* (1999) Management of distal tracheal stenosis. Arch Otolaryngol Head Neck Surg 125, 325–328.

83. Wright CD, Graham BB, Grillo HC, *et al.* (2002) Pediatric tracheal surgery. Ann Thorac Surg 74, 308–313.

84. Burke RP, Chang AC. (1993) Video-assisted thoracoscopic division of a vascular ring in an infant: a new operative technique. J Card Surg 8, 537–540.

85. Laborde F, Noirhomme P, Karam J, *et al.* (1993) A new video-assisted thoracoscopic surgical technique for interruption of patent ductus arteriosus in infants and children. J Thorac Cardiovasc Surg 105, 278–280.

86. Burke RP, Wernovsky G, van der Velde M, *et al.* (1995) Video-assisted thoracoscopic surgery for congenital heart disease. J Thorac Cardiovasc Surg 109, 499–508.

87. Kogon BE, Forbess JM, Wulkan M, *et al.* (2007) Video-assisted thoracoscopic surgery: is it a superior technique for the division of vascular rings in children? Congenit Heart Dis 2, 130–133.

CHAPTER 14

Coarctation of the Aorta

Carl L. Backer,[1] Sunjay Kaushal,[2] and Constantine Mavroudis[3]

[1]Ann & Robert H. Lurie Children's Hospital of Chicago, formerly Children's Memorial Hospital, Chicago, IL, USA
[2]University of Maryland, Baltimore, MD, USA
[3]Florida Hospital for Children, Orlando, FL, USA

The word coarctation originates from the Latin *coarctere*, to contract. A coarctation of the aorta is a congenital narrowing of the descending thoracic aorta usually (but not always) occurring just distal to the left subclavian artery adjacent to the site of insertion of the ductus arteriosus (ligamentum arteriosum). The occurrence rate is 0.2–0.6 per 1000 live births and coarctation of the aorta represents 5–8% of all cases of congenital heart disease [1,2]. Coarctation of the aorta is the eighth most common congenital heart defect. Coarctation is often associated with other congenital heart defects including patent ductus arteriosus, bicuspid aortic valve, ventricular septal defect, and mitral valve abnormalities [3]. The clinical presentation of coarctation varies from cardiovascular collapse in infancy after ductal closure to asymptomatic hypertension in an adult.

Robert Gross [4] experimented with repair of coarctation in animals in 1938, and documented the possible complications of severe hemorrhage and paraplegia. The first successful repair of coarctation of the aorta in a human was performed in Stockholm, Sweden in 1944 by Clarence Crafoord [5]. He resected a coarctation and performed an end-to-end anastomosis in a 12-year-old boy with severe hypertension. Crafoord's patient had relief of hypertension and normalization of lower extremity blood pressure. The surgical management of coarctation of the aorta has evolved over the years mainly in attempts to prevent recoarctation. Other techniques described, in historical order, include prosthetic patch aortoplasty [6], subclavian flap aortoplasty [7], and resection with *extended* end-to-end anastomosis [8,9]. There are many other techniques with subtle variations described for coarctation repair, including: subclavian flap aortoplasty with preservation of arterial blood flow to the left arm [10], subclavian free flap [11], subclavian flap

with resection of ductal tissue [12], coarctation resection with radically extended end-to-end anastomosis [13], end-to-side anastomosis of the descending aorta to the proximal aortic arch [14], and pulmonary homograft patch aortoplasty [15]. This chapter will review the embryology, anatomy, pathophysiology, natural history, diagnostic techniques, surgical alternatives, and postoperative considerations for coarctation of the aorta.

Embryology and Anatomy

Coarctation of the aorta was first noted as an autopsy finding by Morgagni in 1760 [16]. He described a localized constriction of the descending aorta. In 1903, Bonnet [17] suggested dividing patients with coarctation of the aorta into two groups, infantile and adult. "Infantile" later became known as preductal, and "adult" as postductal. In the infantile group, the ductus arteriosus is open and there is a tubular narrowing of the isthmus of the aorta proximal to the ductus. The ductus supplies the blood flow to the descending aorta (Figure 14.1A) [18]. In the adult type of coarctation the ductus is closed and there is a shelf-like narrowing within the lumen of the aorta (Figure 14.1B) [18]. The key difference between these two types is the patent ductus arteriosus provides blood flow to the lower extremity in the preductal (infantile) group and the ductus arteriosus is closed in the postductal (adult) coarctation. The critical factors that determine the hemodynamic burden to the patient are whether the ductus is patent, the size of the transverse arch, and the degree of narrowing at the coarctation site. In surgical series, particularly for evaluating outcome, a classification system of three groups of coarctation patients has been widely used: group I, patients with

Pediatric Cardiac Surgery, Fourth Edition. Edited by Constantine Mavroudis and Carl L. Backer.

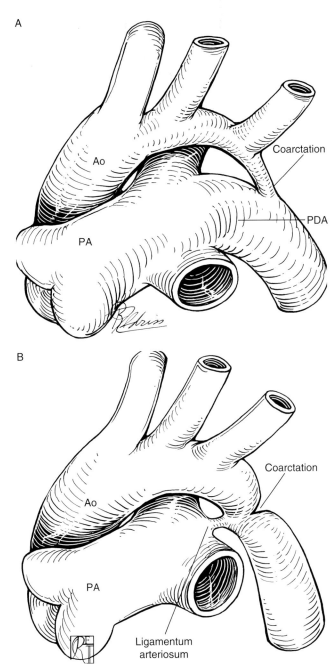

Figure 14.1 A, Infantile or "preductal" coarctation of the aorta. The patent ductus arteriosus (PDA) provides the majority of blood flow to the descending aorta. There is tubular narrowing of the transverse arch and a small aortic isthmus. **B,** Adult or "postductal" coarctation of the aorta. The area of narrowing is actually juxtaductal and consists of a prominent posterior ridge projecting into the lumen. The ductus arteriosus has closed and is now a ligamentum arteriosum. (Ao, aorta; PA, pulmonary artery.)

isolated coarctation; group II, patients with coarctation and ventricular septal defect; and group III, patients with coarctation and complex intracardiac anomalies other than isolated ventricular septal defect [19–21]. The classification system proposed by the International Nomenclature and Database Conferences for Pediatric Cardiac Surgery [22] is as follows: coarctation of the aorta, isolated; coarctation of the aorta, with ventricular septal defect; and coarctation of the aorta, with complex intracardiac anomaly. Other modifiers are isthmus hypoplasia and/or arch hypoplasia. The aortic arch can be divided into three parts, the proximal transverse arch (arch between the innominate and left carotid arteries), the distal transverse arch (arch between the left carotid and left subclavian arteries), and the aortic isthmus (arch between the left subclavian and insertion of the patent ductus arteriosus). Isthmus hypoplasia is defined as present if the isthmus is less than 40% of the diameter of the ascending aorta [23]. Arch hypoplasia is defined as present if the proximal or distal transverse arch are less than 60% or 50% respectively of the diameter of the ascending aorta [24]. We have also used a relatively simple clinical definition of hypoplastic transverse aortic arch as occurring when the transverse aortic arch dimension measured in mm is less than the weight of the patient in kgs plus one [25].

Embryology

There are two complementary theories explaining the embryology of coarctation of the aorta: 1) the flow theory and 2) the ductal sling theory. The flow theory is based on the hypothesis that blood flow through the cardiac chambers and great arteries during fetal life often determines their size at birth [26]. In a normal fetus, the left and right ventricles have approximately equal stroke volumes, although they function in parallel rather than in series. If there is an increase in blood flow through the right heart because of an intracardiac septal defect (VSD), then there is a decrease in flow through the left heart and hence the aortic isthmus. If there is an upstream left-sided obstructive lesion (i.e., mitral or aortic stenosis), again, there will be less flow through the ascending aorta and the isthmus. This theory holds that coarctation of the aorta forms because of a lack of fetal blood flow across the aortic isthmus. The intracardiac defects that would cause coarctation on the basis of the flow theory are in fact clinically commonly associated with patients with coarctation of the aorta. These include ventricular septal defect, bicuspid aortic valve, congenital aortic stenosis, and congenital mitral valve stenosis [3]. The hemodynamic disturbances in embryonic circulatory pathways that lead to reduced aortic arch flow need not be dramatic [27]. The role of the limbus of the foramen ovale is to deflect the appropriate proportion of the inferior vena caval blood to the ascending aorta. Prenatal narrowing of the foramen ovale or an improper angulation of its limbus can lead to variable degrees of hypoplasia of the left-sided structures. This may explain Shone's syndrome [28] (coarctation of the aorta, parachute mitral valve, supravalvar mitral ring of the left atrium, and subaortic stenosis). Corroborating evidence is the corollary that lesions that reduce right heart output such as tetralogy of Fallot, pulmonary stenosis, and tricuspid atresia are almost never associated with coarctation of the aorta [26].

The flow theory, however, is not very convincing for patients with no obvious intracardiac defects. For these patients the ductal sling theory is more appealing. More than 100 years ago Skoda [29] postulated that abnormal extension of contractile ductal tissue into the aorta is a significant factor in the pathogenesis of coarctation of the aorta. More recently it has been microscopically shown that the obstructing shelf of coarctation can be composed of cells similar to that found in the ductus arteriosus [30]. Careful histological examination of resected coarctation specimens has demonstrated extension of ductal tissue in a circumferential sling extending from the ductus arteriosus and into the adjacent aorta [31]. Contraction and fibrosis of this "ductal sling" at the time of ductal closure would lead to constriction of the aorta and a primary coarctation

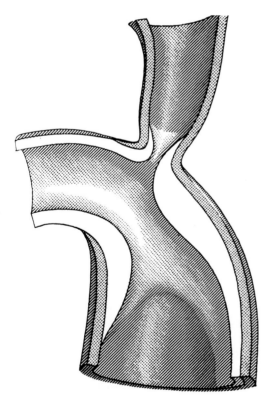

Figure 14.2 Illustration of the extent of ductal tissue present in a coarctation of the aorta specimen. The white areas show the coarctation shelf, circumferential ductal sling, and the prolongations of ductal tissue distally in the aorta. (Reproduced with permission from Russell *et al.* [31].)

(Figure 14.2) [31]. There is confirmatory echocardiographic evidence for this theory [32]. This may explain the origin of coarctation of the aorta when there is no associated intracardiac lesion.

Other investigators have advanced ideas that may also play some role in the embryology of coarctation of the aorta. Kappetein and colleagues [33] believe that an abnormality of neural crest development plays a role in the pathogenesis of coarctation of the aorta. There may also be genetic factors given the increased incidence of coarctation of the aorta in females with Turner's syndrome [34]. This syndrome was originally described in adult karyotype XO female patients having sexual infantilism, webbed neck, and cubitus valgus; 15–36% of these patients have associated coarctation of the aorta.

Anatomy

The anatomic features of coarctation depend on the age of the patient, whether there is an associated patent ductus arteriosus, and the degree of hypoplasia of the transverse aortic arch and isthmus. In a typical infant with coarctation of the aorta and patent ductus arteriosus, there is often a diffuse narrowing of the aorta distal to the left common carotid artery. A large patent ductus arteriosus the size of the descending aorta connects the descending aorta to the pulmonary artery. The opened aorta reveals a coarctation membrane proximal to the entrance of the ductus. There is minimal post-stenotic dilatation of the descending aorta and only minor enlargement of the intercostal arteries. In an older child with a juxtaductal coarctation, there is often a visible external narrowing of the descending aorta at the level of the ligamentum. The degree of external narrowing, however, does not necessarily correlate with the inner lumen of the aorta, which will contain a shelf-like concentric narrowing that may result in a pinpoint lumen (Figure 14.3). Rarely, there is complete occlusion of the lumen, and all flow to the descending aorta is from collateral arteries. The aorta proximal and distal to the coarctation is often dilated with enlargement of the proximal subclavian artery. The aortic wall may be very thin in the region of post-stenotic dilatation. The intercostal vessels entering the descending aorta are large, thin-walled, and may even become aneurysmal.

When a coarctation is present, there is progressive enlargement of collateral blood vessels around the coarctation. This collateral flow is predominantly from the subclavian artery and its branches; the internal thoracic, intercostal, scapular, cervical, vertebral, epigastric, and spinal arteries. These vessels enlarge steadily, and in older children (more than 4 years of age) and adults the chest radiograph may show the characteristic "rib notching" of the inferior aspect of the ribs due to the presence of dilated and tortuous collaterals. These large collateral vessels

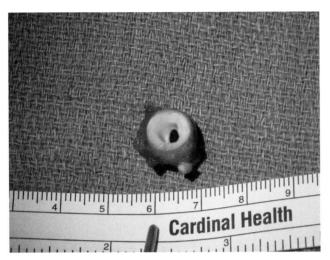

Figure 14.3 Coarctation lumen in a 14-year-old child who underwent coarctation resection and placement of an 18-mm interposition graft. Lumen measures 3 mm.

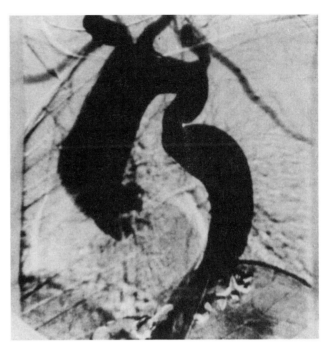

Figure 14.4 Pseudocoarctation. Aortogram showing a dilated ascending aorta, elongation of the arch, and kinking of the descending thoracic aorta in the region of the ligamentum. There was only a 20 mmHg systolic pressure gradient across the pseudocoarctation, but marked post-stenotic dilatation of the descending thoracic aorta. Resection with interposition graft was performed to relieve dysphagia. (Reproduced with permission from Kessler *et al.* [36].)

provide enough flow to the lower body to maintain organ function and growth.

Pseudocoarctation of the aorta is a rare condition presumably resulting from a congenital elongation of the aortic arch [35]. The elongation leads to redundancy and kinking of the aorta, which may appear similar to a coarctation of the aorta but has no actual obstruction to blood flow (Figure 14.4) [36]. There is usually little or no demonstrable pressure gradient present in pseudocoarctation [36]. Because of the tortuous nature of the aorta, however, there is a tendency for dilatation and aneurysm formation presumably related to turbulent flow beyond the kink [37]. These patients should be followed closely and surgical intervention may be required if dilatation compresses surrounding structures (i.e., esophagus) or aneurysm formation is discovered [38].

Coarctation of the abdominal aorta occurs in only 0.5–2% of all coarctations [1]. The embryology of abdominal coarctation may be congenital or related to congenital rubella, Takayasu's arteritis, or von Recklinghausen's disease [39]. In two-thirds of cases the narrowing is circumscribed, and in one-third there is a long diffuse hypoplasia. Diagnosis is confirmed by angiography. It is important to establish the status of the renal arteries in these patients. Effective surgical therapy has included patch aortoplasty and bypass grafts [40–42].

Natural History and Pathophysiology

The presentation of patients with coarctation of the aorta occurs in a bimodal distribution. There is a group that presents in the first week of life whose blood flow to the lower body is dependent on a patent ductus arteriosus. If they are not diagnosed before ductal closure, they present in cardiovascular shock. Collateral flow is inadequate in

infancy and ischemia of organs distal to the coarctation results in renal failure and acidosis. At the same time the sudden increased afterload on the left ventricle results in acute congestive heart failure. The management of these neonates was greatly improved by the introduction of prostaglandin E1 (PGE_1), which opens and maintains the patency of the ductus arteriosus. PGE_1 was initially used (1975) successfully for infants with cyanotic heart disease (pulmonary atresia, transposition of the great arteries) [43], and later (1979) applied to infants with aortic arch interruption and coarctation of the aorta [44]. Intravenous infusion of PGE_1 dilates and maintains the patency of the ductus arteriosus, which normalizes perfusion to the lower body and unloads the left ventricle. In some patients PGE_1 may not open the patent ductus arteriosus, but it does improve flow through the coarctation site by acting on the "ductal sling" tissue [32]. This slight increase in coarctation orifice diameter is often enough to help stabilize the patient prior to elective surgical repair. The use of PGE_1 combined with intubation and ventilation, intravenous inotropic support (dopamine and dobutamine), and intravenous sodium bicarbonate acts to correct the low output state and reverse metabolic acidosis and renal failure. Surgical intervention can then be planned on a semielective basis at a time when the function of the various organ systems has been optimized.

The other arm of this bimodal presentation is a group of patients who are "asymptomatic" but present with hypertension on a routine physical examination. The main cause of symptoms in these patients is the proximal systemic hypertension, which may cause headaches or epistaxis. They may also have claudication from inadequate lower extremity perfusion with exercise. Alterations in renal, adrenal, and baroreceptor function all contribute to the development of this proximal systemic hypertension. This may lead to circle of Willis aneurysms, aortic aneurysm proximal or distal to the coarctation, aortic dissection, and increased coronary atherosclerotic heart disease with associated myocardial infarction [45]. The following diagnoses are the causes of death in patients with unrepaired coarctation: congestive heart failure (26%), bacterial endocarditis (25%), spontaneous rupture of the aorta (21%), and intracranial hemorrhage (13%) [46]. The frequency of intracranial aneurysms among adult patients with coarctation (mean age 42 years) is 10% as compared to 2% in the general population [47]. The survival curve of patients with an unoperated coarctation of the aorta is shown in Figure 14.5 [48]. In a review of 200 autopsies in patients with coarctation of the aorta, Abbott found the average age at death was 33.5 years [49]. Reifenstein and associates [46] in a similar study of 104 autopsies quoted a figure of 35.0 years. In these patients pregnancy increases the risk of associated complications. There is essentially no medical therapy for coarctation and these patients should be referred at the time of diagnosis for surgical intervention.

Diagnosis

The newborn infant with critical coarctation and ductus closure will present in shock. On physical examination the child will be tachypneic and tachycardic, and will appear pale. Lower extremity pulses are absent, and upper extremity pulses may be thready. The child may be hypotensive, even in the arms, and the liver will be enlarged. Chest radiograph will demonstrate cardiomegaly and evidence of congestive heart failure. Electrocardiogram shows a left ventricular strain pattern. Two-dimensional echocardiography with color Doppler interrogation is diagnostic in most instances [50–52]. The echocardiogram will demonstrate lack of pulsatile flow in the descending aorta, the anatomic coarctation site, the size of the transverse arch, and any other associated intracardiac anomalies. In many instances, for newborn infants a comprehensive echocardiogram is all that is required to prepare a patient for surgical intervention after stabilization of organ systems. However, if there are complex associated cardiac anomalies cardiac catheterization can safely be performed in a stable baby who is being maintained on prostaglandin infusion. This will reveal the precise great vessel morphology, significant hemodynamic parameters, and intracardiac anatomy [27]. For the child that does not need a cardiac catheterization for the intracardiac anatomy, but has an arch that is difficult to image, computed tomography (CT) scan is our current procedure of choice. Ultrafast scan with 3D reconstruction reveals the anatomy beautifully and gives the surgeon a very clear "road map" (Figure 14.6) [53].

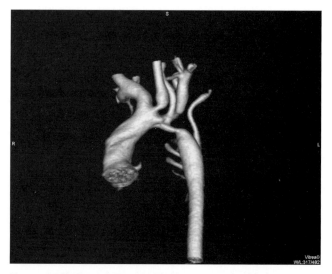

Figure 14.6 Three-dimensional computed tomographic reconstruction of a newborn with coarctation of the aorta. By echocardiographic analysis adequate visualization of the transverse arch could not be obtained. Because of the CT angiogram showing complex hypoplasia of the transverse aortic arch and stenosis of the origin of the left carotid and left subclavian artery, repair was electively performed through a sternotomy with modified cerebral perfusion. (Reproduced with permission from Kaushal et al. [53].)

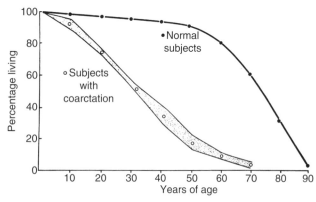

Figure 14.5 Survival curve of patients with coarctation of the aorta surviving the first year of life as compared with normal subjects. (Reproduced with permission from Campbell [48].)

Physical examination of an older child (often with no symptoms) reveals upper extremity hypertension and absent or greatly diminished femoral pulses. Electrocardiogram demonstrates left ventricular hypertrophy and left ventricular strain. Chest radiograph will often demonstrate "notching" of the ribs if the patient is over 4 years of age. In addition, the classic "3" sign on chest radiograph is caused by dilatation of the left subclavian artery, the narrowing of the coarctation site, and poststenotic dilatation of the descending aorta. The echocardiogram in most instances of simple coarctation in older children, adolescents, and adults will provide the diagnosis without requiring cardiac catheterization. Cardiac catheterization is required for these patients only if there are associated intracardiac anomalies, a question with regard to the size of the collateral vessels, or poor visualization by echocardiography. In all older patients who do not have a catheterization we also obtain either a CT or magnetic resonance imaging (MRI) image to fully delineate the anatomy (Figure 14.7) [18,54,55]. The presence or absence of collaterals is noted to help in predicting the need for left heart bypass. In summary, assessment of aortic coarctation can be accomplished accurately and comprehensively in many instances by using the combined methodologies of two-dimensional and Doppler echocardiography. Computed tomography is useful for infants and MRI and CT are used for older children and adults to precisely define the arch anatomy [56]. In all cases a complete two-dimensional and Doppler echocardiographic examination of intracardiac anatomy is necessary to reach appropriate therapeutic and surgical recommendations.

Surgical Techniques

General Considerations

The surgical approach to coarctation in most instances is through a left posterolateral thoracotomy incision entering the thorax through the third or fourth intercostal space. The exception to this is a median sternotomy approach for patients with associated cardiac anomalies that are to be repaired simultaneously or the patient with a hypoplastic transverse aortic arch. The arterial blood pressure is monitored in the right radial artery. Should the right subclavian artery arise anomalously below the coarctation the temporal artery provides a useful site for monitoring the proximal aortic pressure. One must be very careful with this site, however, as there is a chance of injecting air or debris to the cerebral circulation. In some cases like this we have done the repair with only near infrared spectroscopy (NIRS) monitoring of the brain. Using the left thoracotomy approach, we divide the latissimus dorsi muscle, but spare the serratus anterior by retracting it anteriorly. In older children the multiple chest wall collateral vessels should be individually ligated and divided to prevent hemorrhage either during the operation or postoperatively. The lung is retracted anteriorly and the mediastinal pleura overlying the coarctation site is incised. Any large lymphatic channels are either preserved or ligated and divided. The vagus nerve and recurrent laryngeal nerve are carefully preserved by retracting and dissecting these structures with the mediastinal pleura anteriorly. The descending aorta, left subclavian artery, isthmus of the aorta, ductus arteriosus (or ligamentum), and transverse aortic arch distal to the left carotid artery are mobilized. An anomalous artery originally described by Abbott is an occasionally encountered collateral vessel originating from the posterior wall of the aortic arch or left subclavian artery [57]. This vessel is not found in normal subjects or described in standard anatomy textbooks (Figure 14.8) [58]. If present it should be ligated and divided to facilitate the repair. In older children there are often large collateral intercostal vessels entering the descending aorta distal to the coarctation. These should be carefully mobilized and either encircled with vessel loops or ligated and divided in order to fully mobilize the area of the coarctation.

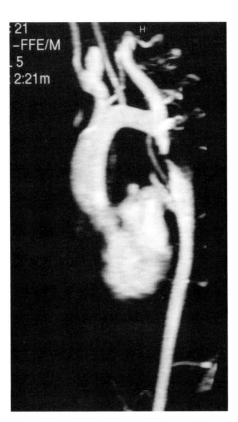

Figure 14.7 Magnetic resonance image of a severe coarctation of the aorta in a 24-year-old. The anatomy is very clearly demonstrated.

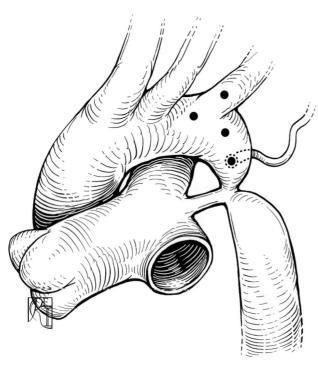

Figure 14.8 Abbott's artery. Drawing outlines the area on the posterior wall of the aortic arch or subclavian artery from which a blood vessel, which Gross chose to call Abbott's artery, may take its origin. X = possible sites of origin. (Reproduced with permission from Schuster *et al.* [58].)

Table 14.1 Surgical milestones.

Surgical procedure	Author	Year	Country
Resection with end-to-end anastomosis	Crafoord [5]	1944	Sweden
Prosthetic interposition graft	Gross [64]	1951	USA
Prosthetic patch augmentation	Vossschulte [6]	1957	Germany
Subclavian flap aortoplasty	Waldhausen and Nahrwold [7]	1966	USA
Resection with extended end-to-end anastomosis	Amato [8]	1986	USA

It is very important that the proximal aortic pressure be allowed to stay quite high (100–120 mmHg for infants, 160–200 mmHg for older children and adults) during the time of the aortic cross-clamp to provide adequate mean aortic arterial blood pressure distal to the clamp to help prevent the complication of paraplegia. Sodium nitroprusside should never be used during the time of cross-clamping for coarctation repair. The use of nipride while the aorta is clamped has actually been shown to increase the incidence of paraplegia postoperatively [59]. A distal aortic pressure monitoring line should be placed in older children in the femoral artery. In these older children the mean distal aortic pressure should be maintained above 45 mmHg during the period of aortic cross-clamp [60,61]. During the first 10 minutes of cross-clamping the mean distal aortic pressure usually increases 5 mmHg. Maintaining the distal aortic pressure can be done by the administration of volume expanders, use of inotropes such as dopamine or dobutamine, or reduced anesthetic during the time period of the cross-clamp. Other useful maneuvers are to readjust the proximal clamp (if anatomically feasible) to allow flow in the left subclavian artery or to allow more intercostal arteries to remain open. Should the mean pressure drop below 45 mmHg, alternative techniques such as the use of partial left heart cardiopulmonary bypass with left atrial and descending aortic cannulation should be used [61–63]. We are very proactive in using left heart bypass should there by any question regarding the distal perfusion pressure during the coarctation repair. Hypoperfusion of the spinal cord can lead to the dreaded complication of paraplegia which will be discussed in detail later in this chapter. The various techniques of repair are now reviewed separately (Table 14.1) [5–8,64].

Resection and End-to-End Anastomosis

Crafoord and Nylin [5] reported the first successful resection of coarctation of the aorta with end-to-end anastomosis. Their two patients were a 12-year-old boy and a 27-year-old man operated on in October 1944. Kirklin and associates [65] described the successful surgical treatment of coarctation of the aorta in an infant when they operated on a 10-week-old child performing successful coarctation resection with end-to-end anastomosis (and ligation of the left subclavian artery) in 1951. The technique of resection and end-to-end anastomosis is shown in Figure 14.9 [18]. The obviously narrowed coarctation segment is excised with a direct end-to-end circumferential anastomosis of the aorta. Early repairs utilized silk suture in a continuous fashion posteriorly and interrupted everting horizontal mattress sutures anteriorly. The mortality and recoarctation rates using resection and end-to-end anastomosis in several series are shown in Table 14.2 [13,66–72]. Although the mortality rate was very acceptable in large series [73] several institutions reported a relatively high recoarctation rate (20–86%) particularly in the age group <1 year [13,66,69,71]. This high rate of stenosis in retrospect is attributed to: 1) the use of silk sutures instead of the currently available fine monofilament suture [58]; 2) inadequate resection of all ductal tissue, which may extend into

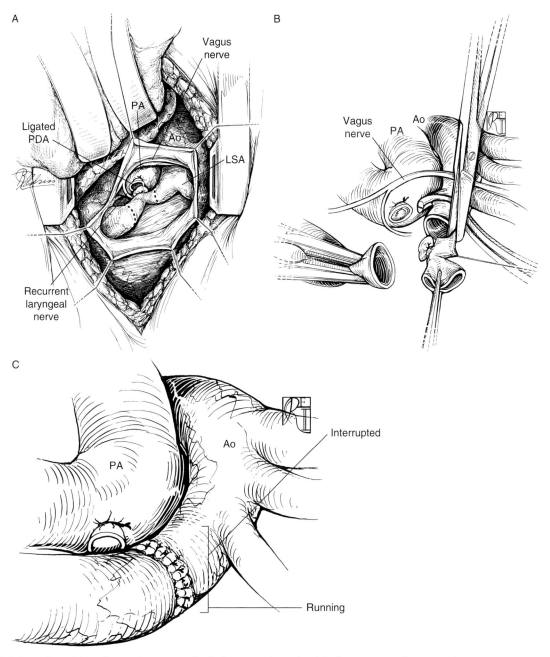

A

Vagus
nerve

PA

Ligated
PDA

Ao

LSA

Recurrent
laryngeal
nerve

B

Vagus
nerve

PA

Ao

C

PA

Ao

Interrupted

Running

Figure 14.9 Resection with end-to-end anastomosis. **A,** Exposure through a left thoracotomy. The patent ductus arteriosus (PDA) has been ligated and divided. Dotted lines show area to be resected. **B,** Clamps have been applied and the coarctation segment is being resected. **C,** Anastomosis has been constructed with running suture for the back wall and interrupted suture anteriorly. (Ao, aorta; LSA, left subclavian artery; PA, pulmonary artery.)

areas of normal-appearing aorta [69]; 3) lack of growth at a circumferential suture line [74]; and 4) lack of growth of a hypoplastic transverse arch. More recent series [70,72] tend to indicate that with modern sutures and microvascular techniques, the recoarctation rate is reduced. However, this technique does not address the issue of a hypoplastic transverse arch, which is present in many infants. This

technique is not easily applicable to older children in whom the location of the arch and descending aorta is more "fixed" than in infants and is difficult to mobilize for a safe tension-free anastomosis. Simple resection with end-to-end anastomosis has been essentially abandoned at most centers because of new, superior techniques that prevent recoarctation.

Table 14.2 Results of resection with end-to-end anastomosis.

Author	Age	Year	Patients	Mortality	Recoarctation
Williams [66]	<1 yr	1980	176	66 (38%)	39 (33%)
Cobanoglu [67]	<3 mo	1985	55	16 (29%)	3 (8%)
Körfer [68]	<4 mo	1985	55	2 (4%)	3 (6%)
Ziemer [69]	<1 mo	1986	24	8 (33%)	4 (25%)
Brouwer [70]	<2 yr	1991	32	2 (6%)	4 (13%)
Kappetein [71]	<3 yr	1994	48	5 (10%)	41 (86%)[a]
Van Heurn [13]	<3 mo	1994	42	5 (10%)	11 (30%)
Quaegebeur [72][b]	<1 mo	1994	139	20 (14%)	6 (4%)
TOTALS			571	124 (21%)	111 (19%)

[a]Kaplan-Meier estimate at 30 years.
[b]Congenital Heart Surgeon's Society.

Prosthetic Patch Aortoplasty

Chiefly because of the high rate of recoarctation with the classic end-to-end anastomosis technique, the technique of prosthetic patch aortoplasty was introduced. Vossschulte [6] in 1957 described an "isthmusplastic" procedure that developed into the prosthetic patch aortoplasty. For many years this was our procedure of choice for older children (1–16 years of age). However, as will be seen in this section, the potential for aneurysm formation has led us to now only rarely use this technique [75–77]. As discussed earlier under general considerations, this operation is performed through a left thoracotomy and fourth intercostal space incision. After vessel dissection and ductus ligation, the aorta is occluded proximal and distal to the coarctation with vascular clamps. The aorta is then incised longitudinally through the site of the coarctation with the incision being extended well beyond the level of the coarctation both distally and proximally. Proximally this means that the patch often extends up onto the left subclavian artery. If the isthmus is hypoplastic with stenosis between the left subclavian and left carotid artery, the patch may be extended up into this area by placing the proximal clamp proximal to the left carotid artery. In the initial descriptions of this procedure, the posterior coarctation membrane or fibrous shelf was excised. This maneuver, however, can cause disruption of the intima and predispose to aortic aneurysm formation and is no longer recommended [78]. A circular prosthetic patch (slightly elliptical) made of polytetrafluoroethylene is sutured in place longitudinally along the aortotomy edge. An effort is made to use the largest patch feasible and place the widest portion of the patch at the level of the aortic constriction (Figure 14.10) [18]. The pleura should be closed as completely as possible over the patch.

The prosthetic patch technique offers several advantages over simple resection with end-to-end anastomosis,

1) the collateral vessels are all preserved and do not require ligation and division; 2) the technique allows simultaneous enlargement of isthmic hypoplasia if necessary; 3) the anastomosis is tension free; 4) the posterior aortic wall and even a hypoplastic aortic arch will grow after prosthetic patch repair [79]. The primary worrisome late complication of this technique is aneurysm formation of the posterior aortic wall opposite the patch [75–77]. This may be explained by several different factors. Most reported aneurysm formation occurred after resection of the coarctation membrane with violation of the intimal layer [80,81]. The patch causes altered hemodynamics arising from the different tensile strengths of the prosthetic patch and the posterior aortic wall, the pulsatile waveform being completely directed to the posterior aortic wall by the inflexible anterior patch [82]. Resection of the coarctation ridge (which is no longer performed) significantly predisposes to this complication. Another theory to explain aneurysm formation is a congenital abnormality of the aortic wall at the coarctation site [83]. Mortality, recoarctation rates, and incidence of aneurysm formation in several series [79–82,84–87] of patch aortoplasty are shown in Table 14.3. In a collected series of 815 patients, 9% had recoarctation and 4% had aneurysm formation. The issue of aneurysm formation is addressed in greater detail in the section on postoperative complications.

For many years the patch aortoplasty was our operation of choice for children older than 1 year and less than 16 years of age. The potential for late aneurysm formation however has now led us to use this procedure only in rare cases. In our experience the younger children (<5 years of age) are frequently candidates for a resection with an extended end-to-end anastomosis (to be discussed later in the chapter). The older children and certainly those over 10 years of age are now in our opinion better served by an interposition graft with essentially no risk for aneurysm formation or disruption of the anastomosis because of

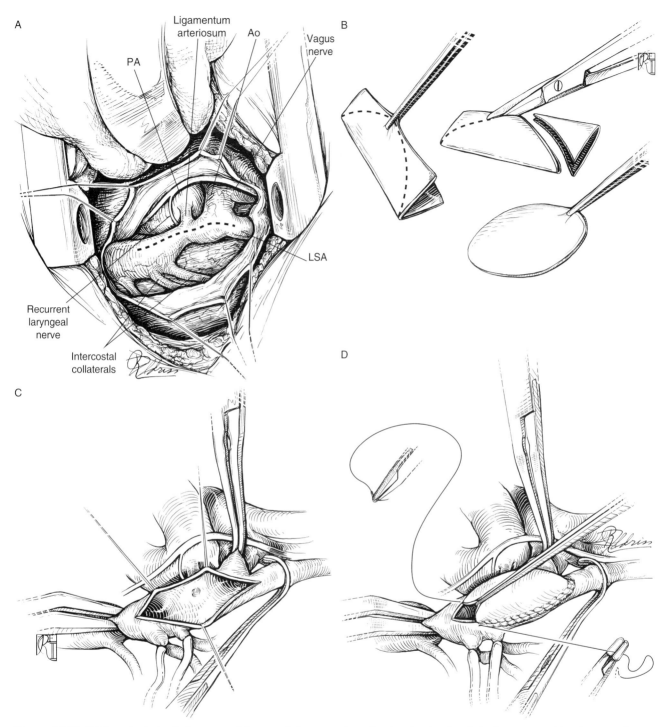

A — Ligamentum arteriosum
PA
Ao
Vagus nerve
LSA
Recurrent laryngeal nerve
Intercostal collaterals

B

C

D

Figure 14.10 Patch aortoplasty. **A,** Exposure of the coarctation through a left thoracotomy. Note juxtaductal coarctation and enlarged intercostal collateral arteries. **B,** An elliptical polytetrafluoroethylene (PTFE) patch is fashioned prior to clamp placement. **C,** Clamps have been applied and the aorta opened laterally opposite the site of the ligamentum. Note intercostal arteries are controlled with small Rumel tourniquets. The coarctation ridge is *not* excised. **D,** The patch is sutured in place in such a manner that the PTFE creates a "roof" over the coarctation ridge. (Ao, aorta; LSA, left subclavian artery; PA, pulmonary artery.)

Table 14.3 Results of patch aortoplasty. (NS, not specified; PTFE, polytetrafluoroethylene,)

Author	Age	Year	Patients	Operative mortality	Recoarctation	Aneurysm	Patch
Yee [84]	<1yr	1984	100	0	10 (12%)	0	PTFE
Clarkson [82]	>15yr	1985	38	NS	6 (16%)	5 (13%)	Dacron
Hehrlein [80]	2d–64yr	1986	317	16 (5%)	4 (1.3%)	18 (6%)	Dacron
Del Nido [85]	3d–32yr	1986	63	1(2%)	8 (13%)	3 (5%)	Dacron
Ungerleider [86]	NS	1991	54	0	2 (5%)	0	PTFE
Backer [87]	5.1yr (mean)	1994	125	4 (3%)	10 (8%)	0	PTFE
Walhout [81]	1.8yr (mean)	2003	118	4 (3%)	30 (25%)	8 (7%)	PTFE
TOTALS			815	25 (3%)	70 (9%)	34 (4%)	

tension. We last used a patch aortoplasty for a primary coarctation repair in 2002. We reported our results with this procedure in 1995 [87]. Between 1979 and 1993, 125 infants and children underwent polytetrafluoroethylene patch aortoplasty. The posterior coarctation ridge was *not* excised in any patient. There were 111 primary repairs and 14 reoperations. The mean age at the time of surgery was 5.1 years. There were no cases of intraoperative mortality or postoperative paraplegia. There were four deaths (3% mortality) at 10–40 days postoperatively all neonates having additional intracardiac procedures for complex lesions. We have had only one patient develop an aneurysm and this was a false aneurysm detected 4 months after the surgery. One of the lessons that we did learn from this series was that infants who have this approach at less than 1 month of age had a high incidence of residual or recurrent coarctation. That experience has been confirmed by others [81,88]. Because of these experiences we do not recommend the patch aortoplasty for infants who are less than 1 year of age. We also do not use patch aortoplasty in patients older than 16 years of age because of the increased risk of aneurysm formation in older patients [75]. In summary, we currently believe that the patch aortoplasty should only be used in the rare patient who is too small for an interposition graft and whose anatomy precludes resection with extended end-to-end anastomosis, and for recoarctation. All patients having patch aortoplasty should be carefully followed for aneurysm formation.

Prosthetic Interposition Graft

The use of a prosthetic interposition graft was first described by Robert Gross [64] in 1951 when he used an aortic homograft as a replacement for a coarctation in a child with a long narrowed coarctation segment. In 1960 Morris, Cooley, DeBakey, and Crawford [89] described the use of a Dacron prosthetic interposition graft in 3% of 171 patients undergoing coarctation repair. Currently we recommend prosthetic interposition grafts (Figure 14.11) [18] for patients over 10 years of age, patients with an associated aneurysm,

patients with complex long-segment coarctation, and selected patients with recurrent coarctation. It is also a useful technique if during a planned resection and end-to-end anastomosis it appears that the anastomosis will be under tension or the aorta requires further resection because of a thinned aortic wall secondary to post-stenotic dilatation. Aris and colleagues [90] reported successful use of this technique in eight patients over 50 years of age, using 16- or 18-mm Dacron tube grafts. We have used Hemashield or Gelweave (Vascutek-Terumo, Renfrewshire, Scotland) grafts for these patients to minimize bleeding, especially if partial cardiopulmonary bypass is used (Plate 14.1, see plate section opposite p.594). The obvious disadvantage of the interposition graft is the developmental size discrepancy in the growing child, making the operation more applicable for older patients. Another consideration is the longer aortic cross-clamp time taken to perform two circular anastomoses. This is now our procedure of choice for patients over 10 years of age where an adult sized graft can be inserted. We have used this technique in 24 patients in the past 20 years.

Subclavian Flap Aortoplasty

The subclavian flap aortoplasty technique was introduced by Waldhausen and Nahrwold [7] in 1966. Successful coarctation repair was reported in three patients aged 4 months, 6 months, and 3 years (Figure 14.12) [18]. The operation is performed through the left fourth intercostal space as described earlier under general considerations. The ligamentum or ductus arteriosus is ligated. The aorta is clamped proximal to the left subclavian artery as well as distal to the coarctation. The left subclavian artery is ligated distally (near the origin of the vertebral artery), which may or may not be included in the ligature. The subclavian artery is then opened along its lateral margin and divided near the ligature. The incision is extended through the isthmus across the coarctation site into the area of poststenotic dilatation. The subclavian artery is folded down onto the incision in the aorta and then the

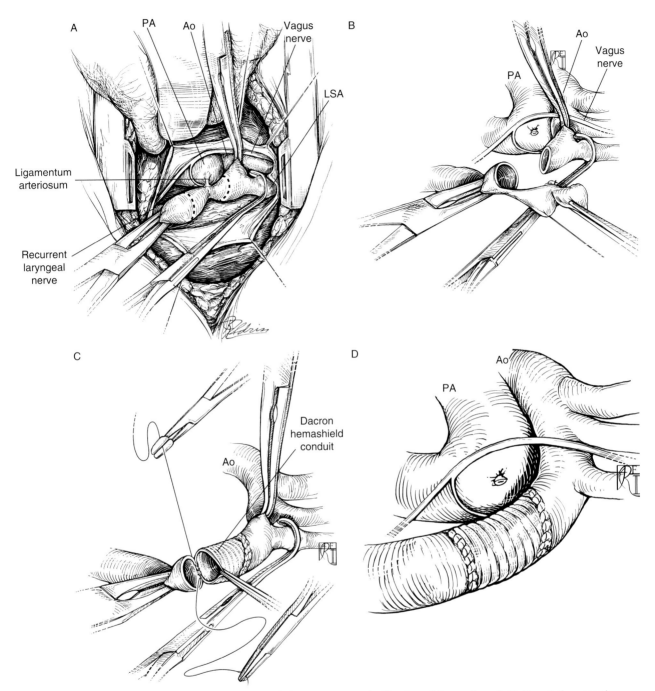

Figure 14.11 Interposition graft. **A,** Exposure through a left thoracotomy. Clamps are in place and the ligamentum has been ligated. The area to be resected is shown by the dotted lines. Frequently, in long-standing coarctation there is pre- and post-stenotic dilatation of the aortic wall. **B,** Coarctation resection. **C,** Proximal oblique anastomosis has been completed and the distal anastomosis is being performed. **D,** Completed interposition graft. (Ao, aorta; LSA, left subclavian artery; PA, pulmonary artery.)

subclavian "flap" is sutured in place with continuous fine polypropylene suture. The clamps are released and the appearance is of the subclavian patch creating a "roof" over the area of the previous coarctation. The issue of ligation of the vertebral artery is decided on a case-by-case basis. Leaving it intact provides collateral circulation to the arm but may possibly cause subclavian steal syndrome as the child grows. If possible, the internal mammary artery and the thyrocervical trunk are left intact to provide collateral circulation to the left arm. Occasionally more length

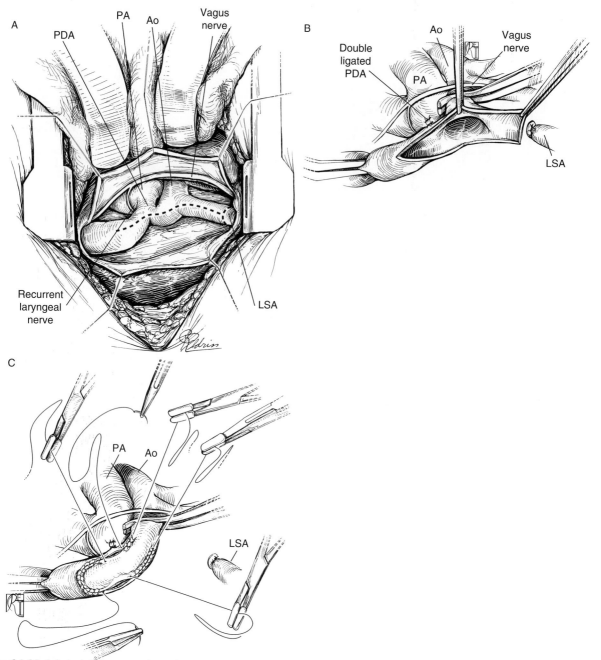

Figure 14.12 Subclavian flap aortoplasty. **A,** Exposure through a left thoracotomy. **B,** Clamps are applied, the left subclavian artery (LSA) is ligated, opened, and divided. **C,** The LSA is then turned down as a flap over the coarctation site, carrying the flap as far distal as is possible. Three polypropylene sutures are then used to create the anastomosis. (Ao, aorta; PA, pulmonary artery; PDA, patent ductus arteriosus.)

is required to span the coarctation site and sacrifice of these vessels is required. Failure to extend the incision far enough downstream across the coarctation and onto the area of post-stenotic dilatation may contribute to restenosis at a later date. Several variations of this technique have been described for complex coarctations. In 1983 Hart and Waldhausen [91] described the reversed subclavian flap

technique for repair of a coarctation proximal to the left subclavian artery. Meier and colleagues [10] also described a technique for subclavian reimplantation in 1986 to preserve the arterial blood flow to the left arm. Dietl and associates [92] used a combined technique of coarctation resection and subclavian flap aortoplasty. Allen and coworkers [93] recently described a modification of the subclavian flap adding a side-to-side transverse aortic anastomosis at the level of the coarctation. Kanter [94] has described using a reverse subclavian flap for repair of a hypoplastic transverse arch.

The advantages of the subclavian flap technique include its simplicity, short cross-clamp time, avoidance of prosthetic material, easy anastomotic hemostatic control, and increased anastomotic growth owing to the use of an autogenous noncircumferential flap [95]. Until the late 1980s the subclavian flap repair was widely utilized as the method of choice for repair of coarctation of the aorta in infants and children under 1 year of age [96,97]. However, there are some significant disadvantages of this technique which have led to many centers abandoning it in the current era. We do not perform this procedure in older children because of the fear of left arm ischemia following ligation of the subclavian artery [98–100]. We are aware of a patient who actually required amputation of a gangrenous arm after subclavian flap aortoplasty [101]. In addition, sacrifice of the left subclavian artery may affect long-term growth and function in the left upper limb [102]. Aneurysm occurrence has been described after subclavian flap aortoplasty [103] and in our institution we had one child who developed a false aneurysm following a subclavian flap aortoplasty utilizing absorbable suture. Subclavian flap aortoplasty was widely used from the mid-1970s to the late-1980s [104]. As the long-term follow-up was continued it appeared that the incidence of recoarctation, initially thought to be low, was higher than expected ranging up to 42% in some series [13,69,72,93,97,105,106,107–110]. In a collected series from 10 authors, 1181 patients had subclavian flap aortoplasty with a 13% recoarctation rate (Table 14.4) [13,69,72,93,97, 105,106,107–110]. It was particularly in the smaller infant less than 2 months in age that the subclavian flap aortoplasty appeared to have a high recurrence rate [106]. Because of this, surgeons became interested again in the

resection with end-to-end anastomosis technique, this time, however, with an "extended" anastomosis. Some surgeons continue to feel that subclavian flap aortoplasty is the procedure of choice for neonatal coarctation of the aorta, although they appear to be in the minority [105,109,110].

Resection with Extended End-to-End Anastomosis

In 1977, Amato [8] reported four infants with hypoplasia of the distal transverse arch who underwent a new technique of resecting the coarctation and performing an extended anastomosis under the left carotid artery. In 1986 Lansman and associates [9] reported a series of 17 infants operated on between 1977 and 1985 having resection with extended end-to-end anastomosis. Forty-seven percent of these patients had a hypoplastic distal aortic arch and isthmus. Brown and colleagues [111] described an "isthmus flap" aortoplasty in 1985 as an alternative to subclavian flap for long-segment coarctation of the aorta in infants. This procedure is essentially a resection with extended end-to-end anastomosis.

Resection with extended end-to-end anastomosis can be performed via a left thoracotomy or through a median sternotomy. We have used a thoracotomy approach for 80% of our coarctation repairs [53]. We use a sternotomy approach if there is an associated intracardiac lesion or a hypoplastic transverse aortic arch. We also favor a sternotomy approach if there is an aberrant right subclavian artery or a common brachiocephalic trunk. Our current frequent use of CT imaging for these issues has been extremely helpful. The illustrations show the approach via a left thoracotomy (Figure 14.13) [18]. The initial exposure is as described earlier for the other techniques. The ductus arteriosus is ligated. The descending aorta is extensively mobilized – usually the first two or three sets of intercostal

Table 14.4 Results of subclavian flap aortoplasty. (NS, not specified.)

Author	Age	Year	Patients	Mortality	Recoarctation
Metzdorff [106]	<2 mo	1985	60	11 (18%)	10 (17%)
Ziemer [69]	<1 mo	1986	70	8 (11.4%)	9 (15%)
Ehrhardt [108]	<1 mo	1989	45	14 (31%)	7 (23%)
Milliken [97]	<1 mo	1990	123	11 (9%)	20 (16%)
Van Heurn [13]	<3 mo	1994	15	1 (7%)	6 (42%)
Quaegebeur [72][a]	<1 mo	1994	112	9 (8%)	12 (12%)
Allen [93]	<3 mo	2000	53	0	2 (4%)
Jahangiri [109]	<1 yr	2000	185	6 (3%)	11 (6%)
Pandey [105]	< 4 yr	2006	399	51 (12.8%)	61 (15.3%)
Barreiro [110]	<1 yr	2007	119	5 (4%)	12 (11%)
TOTALS			1181	116 (10%)	150 (13%)

[a]Congenital Heart Surgeon's Society.

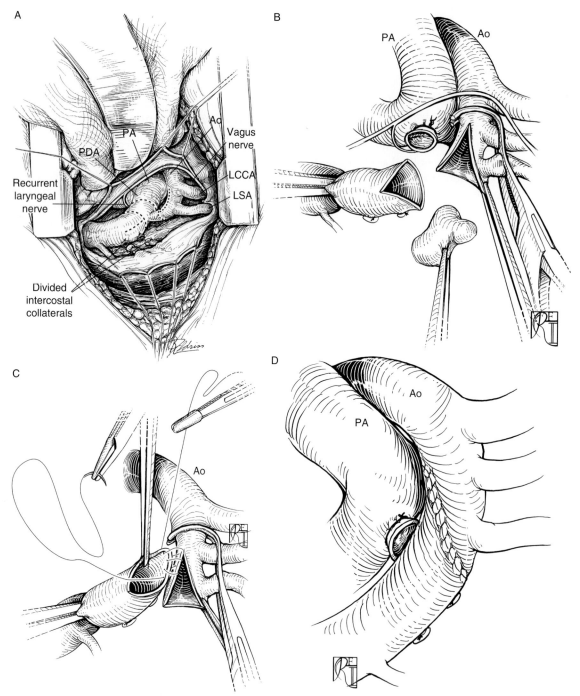

Figure 14.13 Resection with extended end-to-end anastomosis. **A,** Exposure through a left thoracotomy. Two sets of intercostal collaterals have been ligated and divided. The dotted lines show the area to be resected and the incisions to be made in the undersurface of the transverse arch and in the lateral descending aorta. **B,** The coarctation has been resected and the ductus ligated and divided. **C,** Running polypropylene is used to create the anastomosis. **D,** Completed oblique anastomosis extends to a point opposite the left carotid artery, nicely addressing arch hypoplasia. (Ao, aorta; LCC, left common carotid artery; LSA, left subclavian artery; PA, pulmonary artery; PDA, patent ductus arteriosus.)

Table 14.5 Results of resection with "extended" end-to-end anastomosis.

Author	Age	Year	Patients	Operative mortality	Recoarctation
Lansman [9]	6 mo	1986	17	1 (6%)	2 (12%)
Vouhé [19]	3 mo	1988	80	21 (26%)	6 (10%)
Zannini [112]	3 mo	1993	21	4 (19%)	4 (23%)
Van Heurn [13]	3 mo	1994	77	5 (6%)	8 (11%)
Kappetein [71]	3 yr	1994	26	4 (15%)	0%
Conte [21]	<1 mo	1995	307	23 (7%)	24 (9%)
Van Son [116]	<1 mo	1997	25	0	1 (4%)
Wood [118]	<1 yr	2004	181	1	4 (2.2%)
Wright [117]	<1 yr	2005	83	2 (2%)	4 (6%)
Thomson [119]	<1 yr	2006	191	9 (5%)	7 (4.2%)
Kaushal [53]	1 yr	2009	201	4 (2%)	8 (4%)
TOTALS			1209	74 (6%)	68 (6%)

vessels are ligated and divided. The left subclavian and left carotid arteries are dissected and encircled with vessel loops. The proximal aortic clamp is positioned between the innominate artery and the left carotid artery. The distal vascular clamp is placed well below the coarctation. The entire coarctation segment and ductus are excised. Proximally, an incision is made on the inferior surface of the transverse arch up to the proximal clamp. Distally the descending aorta is incised laterally in a "mirror" fashion to the other incision and the anastomosis is then performed with running polypropylene suture. We have used 7-0 prolene for neonates, 6-0 prolene for infants (30 days – 1 year) and 8-0 prolene for babies less than 1.5 kg. In our series from Children's Memorial Hospital (n = 201) mean clamp time was 18 minutes, operative mortality was 2% and reintervention for recoarctation was 4% [53]. Zannini and colleagues [112] described a similar technique in the Italian literature. Elliott [113] modified the technique to address transverse arch hypoplasia utilizing a clamp proximally to occlude the left subclavian artery, the left carotid artery, and even part of the right innominate artery. This allowed extension of the aortic arch incision more proximally than the "radically extended end-to-end anastomosis." Zannini and colleagues described another modification of this technique using a median sternotomy approach and cardiopulmonary bypass, with ligation of the isthmus and end-to-side anastomosis of the descending to the ascending thoracic aorta [114]. Although an interrupted suture technique would be theoretically attractive to promote growth of the anastomosis, Lansman proposed a running suture technique to decrease cross-clamp time. Growth of the anastomosis will occur because of eventual disruption of the suture line as the anastomotic site matures. This appears to be substantiated by indirect evidence of growth of a circumferential suture line following the arterial switch procedure [115]. Results of resection with extended end-to-end anastomosis are shown in Table 14.5 [9,13,19,21,71,110, 112,115,119]. In 1209 patients, operative mortality was 6% and the recoarctation rate was also 6%.

Many surgeons now feel that this is the procedure of choice for the infant with coarctation. There are several advantages of this technique. All coarctation tissue with uncertain potential for future growth is completely resected. The left subclavian artery is preserved, avoiding potential left arm ischemia or growth disorders. The procedure addresses and corrects hypoplasia of the transverse arch, the distal aortic arch, and the aortic isthmus. The technique avoids prosthetic material, limits the potential for aneurysm formation, and preserves normal vascular anatomy. Paraplegia has not been reported as a complication of resection with extended end-to-end anastomosis, despite the ligation of multiple collaterals in 1209 patients (Table 14.5) [9,13,19,21,71,110,112,115,119]. When applied to the infant with complex associated cardiac lesions, one-stage total repair with this technique through a median sternotomy is quite successful [120]. Surgeons have demonstrated that a hypoplastic arch will grow with increased flow across a standard end-to-end anastomosis [121] or subclavian flap aortoplasty [122]. Extended arch repair is particularly useful for the small group of infants with transverse aortic arch-to-ascending aorta diameter ratios of less than 0.25 [123]. Resection with extended end-to-end anastomosis is currently our procedure of choice for all infants under 1 year of age and many children over one year of age.

Balloon Dilation Angioplasty

In 1979 Sos and associates [124] demonstrated that a surgically resected neonatal aortic coarctation could be successfully enlarged with a balloon dilation catheter. Lock and colleagues [125] performed dilatation on seven resected coarctation segments and showed that eight atmospheres of pressure produced considerable increase in internal aortic diameter as a result of linear intimal tearing with medial extension. Lababidi and coworkers [126] reported successful balloon angioplasty in 27 patients with native coarctation in 1984. In 1986 Marvin and colleagues [127] first reported the development of aortic aneurysms near the site of balloon dilation angioplasty for native coarctation. Four of 11 patients undergoing dilation had aneurysm formation at the previously dilated site within 1 year. Surgical excision of the coarctation segments revealed an absence of muscle and elastic lamella in the area of the aneurysms [128]. This report led to an immediate suspension of the technique in patients with native coarctation of the aorta at all but a few centers. Cooper and associates [129] reported aneurysm formation in three of seven patients. Microscopy revealed disruption of the intima and elastic media, which resulted in thinning of the intact adventitial wall of the vessel. In 1989 the Valvuloplasty and Angioplasty of Congenital Anomalies (VACA) Registry reported data from 140 patients for native coarctation of the aorta. A residual gradient of more than 20 mmHg was detected in 23 patients (16%) and late aneurysms were detected in six patients (4%) [130]. The study group concluded that although balloon angioplasty reduced the pressure gradient and increased the coarctation diameter, concerns about femoral artery injury and the late appearance of aneurysms called into question inclusion of the technique in the armamentarium of the interventional cardiologist [131]. Controversy continues to exist regarding the safety and efficacy of balloon angioplasty in the management of native coarctation of the aorta [132]. One of the few comparison studies (surgery vs. balloon) was reported by Fiore from St. Louis University [133]. Between 1994 and 2004, 17 patients had balloon angioplasty and 15 had surgery. Fifty-seven percent of the balloon angioplasty patients went on to require surgical intervention. Based on our experience we limit the use of balloon angioplasty for native coarctation of the aorta to patients with major systemic illnesses that significantly increase the risk of surgical intervention, and to older patients with mild discrete coarctation of the aorta and poorly developed collaterals. Some centers are still investigating balloon angioplasty for native coarctations [134,135]. Outcomes in these patients may be improved by the use of balloon-expandable stents [136]. However, stents are not a panacea for transcatheter therapy. There are multiple case reports of aortic rupture with stents [137,138]. In addition, younger age (9.8 vs. 18.6 years) and lower weight (37 kg vs. 59 kg) at the time of the initial procedure was associated with the development of in-stent stenosis [139]. Finally, Forbes recently reported a 31% incidence of complications in stents placed in patients over 40 years of age, "making this a high risk group" [140]. We recently operated on a patient who had unsuccessful dilation of a coarctation with a stent (Plate 14.2A, see plate section opposite p. 594). The coarctation and stent were excised (Plate 14.2B, see plate section opposite p. 594) and replaced with a 24-mm Gelweave Interposition graft.

In contrast to the above described results with balloon dilation for native coarctation the results of dilation for *recurrent* coarctation (Figure 14.14) [132] have been consistently more successful with a much lower incidence of aneurysm formation [141,142]. Saul and colleagues [143] reported a 90% success rate in a large series of patients with recurrent coarctation. The fibrous perivascular postsurgical scar appears to allow safe use of this technique for recoarctation in contrast to the danger of aneurysm formation when balloon dilation is used for native coarctation of the aorta. A multicenter prospective study [144] of balloon angioplasty for recurrent coarctation of the aorta reported 200 patients from 26 institutions. The prior method of surgical repair did not affect the postangioplasty gradient relief or diameter. A residual gradient of more than 21 mmHg was present in only 41 patients (20%). There were five deaths (2.5%) from aortic rupture (1), unexplained sudden death (2), cerebrovascular accident (1), and left heart failure (1). One patient had a cerebrovascular accident, another aortic dissection requiring urgent surgical intervention. There were no late aneurysms. Hijazi and associates [142] reported 27 patients undergoing balloon angioplasty for recurrent coarctation of the aorta. One patient was undilatable, one patient developed a stable aneurysm, and two patients developed restenosis. Yetman [145] reported 90 patients having balloon dilation of recurrent coarctation, with one death and one aortic tear requiring urgent surgical intervention. Good early results were obtained in 88% of the patients and at long-term follow-up (12 years) 72% of these patients remained free of intervention. Reich reported 99 patients with a 93% success rate of balloon angioplasty for recurrent coarctation [146]. We feel that balloon angioplasty is the procedure of choice for recurrent coarctation of the aorta following surgical repair.

Complications

The list of possible complications both during and following coarctation repair is extensive and their prevention requires careful attention to all details of the technique (Table 14.6).

Hemorrhage

During the time period that the aortic clamps are in place and following their removal, the anesthesiologist should have blood available and prepared for administration so that it is immediately accessible in the event of excessive suture line hemorrhage after clamp release. Even though none of the techniques utilized requires intravenous heparin (except if cardiopulmonary bypass is used) the suture lines nearly always have an initial moderate degree of bleeding until clots form within the needle holes. At the

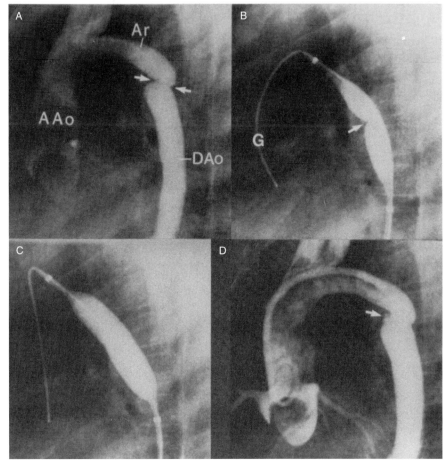

Figure 14.14 Balloon angioplasty of recoarctation after surgical repair with subclavian flap. **A,** Predilation aortogram demonstrating the narrowed recoarcted segment (arrows). **B,** Initial balloon inflation with creation of waist from obstructive shelf. **C,** Upon full inflation, waist is relieved. **D,** Postangioplasty aortogram shows successful dilation of recoarcted segment. Note irregularity of vessel wall in the dilated area (arrow). (AAo, ascending aorta; Ar, aortic arch; G, guideline; DAo, descending aorta.) (Reproduced with permission from Zales et al. [132].)

Table 14.6 Potential complications of surgery.

Recoarctation
Paradoxical hypertension
Paraplegia
Recurrent laryngeal nerve injury
Left arm ischemia
Hemorrhage
Aneurysm formation
Chylothorax
Horner's syndrome
Phrenic nerve injury
Cerebral-vascular accident

---

termination of the procedure, chest tubes (or Blake drains) should be left in position to monitor and evacuate postoperative blood loss. Any sudden increase in the amount of bleeding from the chest tube should result in the patient's immediate return to the operating room for control of bleeding.

Paradoxical Postoperative Hypertension

That the correction of a coarctation of the aorta, an apparently straightforward cause of hypertension, can provoke a postoperative increase in blood pressure is unexpected and illogical, hence the name paradoxical hypertension [147]. The etiology of the postoperative hypertension is felt to occur secondary to two hypertensive responses [148]. The first response occurs immediately and subsides in most patients within 24 hours and is due to the release of the stretch on the baroreceptors in the carotid arteries and aortic arch after removal of the aortic obstruction. This increase in blood pressure occurs until the baroreceptors are set at a lower level. The best evidence for this is the marked increase in sympathetic activity indicated by elevations in norepinephrine level after operation [149]. This occurs in slightly over half of patients and in most cases subsides within 24 hours [150]. The second phase (which is more pronounced in diastole) appears within 48–72 hours and occurs in about one-third of those experiencing the first phase of hypertension. It is associated with elevated levels of renin and angiotensin, which may be stimulated by the first phase of paradoxical hypertension [151,152]. This second response may be the adaptation gone awry that ensures adequate flow to exercising muscles below the coarctation, above and beyond that delivered by increasing the systolic pressure.

Unchecked hypertension in either postoperative phase can have disastrous results. Because the mesenteric arteries have been accustomed to a very low blood pressure, the sudden increase of arterial pressure in these arterioles may lead to severe reactive acute inflammatory changes. This may result in mesenteric arteritis and subsequent evolution to mesenteric ischemia [153,154]. The child then develops severe abdominal pain, distension, and tenderness. On occasion this will cause gastrointestinal bleeding and may require laparotomy with bowel resection. Thus postoperative hypertension must be very carefully monitored and managed. In the immediate postoperative period the administration of esmolol or nicardipine intravenously can be used to titrate the blood pressure [155]. We have also found it useful to use intravenous enalapril (angiotensin converting enzyme inhibitor) beginning shortly after the procedure with eventual conversion to oral captopril or vasotec after several days. Oral propranolol is also quite useful in blunting the sympathetic response and managing the hypertensive response [156]. Gidding and coworkers [157] showed that *preoperative* administration of propranolol helped prevent the postoperative hypertensive response. Because of the risk of mesenteric arteritis, we usually keep our patients NPO for the first 24–36 hours following coarctation repair. We have only had one (mild) case of mesenteric arteritis in the past 20 years with careful postoperative management of hypertension.

The tendency to have persistence of the hypertension late after coarctation repair is proportional to the age of the child at the time of the operative repair [158]. Seirafi and colleagues [159] reported only 2 of 48 infants (<12 months of age) operated on for coarctation having late hypertension (4%) versus 16 of 59 (27%) patients operated on after 1 year of age (Figure 14.15) [159]. Sigurdardottir [160] confirmed these findings in exercise studies. Of course persistent hypertension following repair of coarctation of the aorta despite medical intervention merits investigation to rule out a recurrent coarctation. All patients with coarctation should have life-time follow-up by a cardiologist. Warnes and colleagues have made the point that coarctation should be regarded not as a localized abnormality but as a diffuse arteriopathy deserving long-term follow-up [161,162].

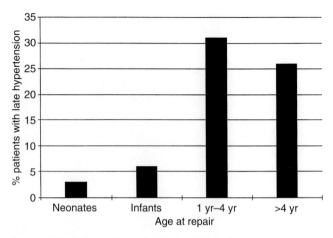

Figure 14.15 Percentage of patients with persistent or late hypertension listed according to age at operation. The percentage of patients with late hypertension was significantly less in the neonatal and infant groups (n = 48, 4.2%) than in toddlers and older children (n = 59, 27.1%; $p < 0.002$). YR, years. (Reproduced with permission from the Society of Thoracic Surgeons from Seirafi *et al.* [159].)

Paraplegia

Paraplegia was first reported by Gross and Hufnagel [4] as a possible complication in animals following coarctation repair and to this day remains a serious and feared complication. Bing and colleagues [163] reported the first human to develop paraplegia after coarctation repair in 1948. In a landmark review from 1972, Brewer and coworkers [164] surveyed 12 532 cases of coarctation of the aorta repair and found an incidence of 0.41% spinal cord complications (1 in 250 patients). They were unable to correlate these complications with any specific factor such as number of intercostals divided or length of cross-clamp time. Lerberg and associates [165] more recently reported an incidence of paraplegia of 1.5% (5/334). Paraplegia correlated with the length of aortic cross-clamping (mean cross-clamp time in those patients with paraplegia was 49 minutes) and the presence of an aberrant origin of the right subclavian artery below the coarctation (one of eight patients). Crawford and Sade [166] reported three patients in whom intraoperative hyperthermia appeared (temperature maximum 38.7°C, 39.8°C, 40°C) to play a significant role in the development of postoperative spinal cord injury. As previously discussed under operative technique, the distal aortic pressure during clamp placement is very important and this pressure should be kept over 45 mmHg [60]. To effect this the proximal aortic pressure must be kept high (120–200 mmHg, depending on the age of the patient) during the clamp time. Acidosis should be avoided during the time of the aortic cross-clamp as this may contribute to low cardiac output and hypotension [63]. Somatosensory evoked potentials (SSEP) are a possible method of assessing reversible spinal cord ischemia [167].

In summary, to avoid paraplegia we recommend: 1) aortic cross-clamp time as short as possible, 2) careful technical anastomosis so reapplication of clamps is not necessary, 3) moderate hypothermia (34–35 °C), 4) high proximal blood pressure, 5) no acidosis, and 6) adequate distal mean blood pressure (>45 mmHg). The key among these is perhaps the distal mean blood pressure. In patients over 1 year of age we monitor both the radial artery pressure and the distal femoral pressure. At the time of test clamp if the pressure drops below 45 mmHg we perform the case with partial left heart bypass [61]. Left heart bypass is performed with systemic heparinization and a venous cannula placed in the left atrial appendage by opening the pericardium. The descending thoracic aorta is cannulated with an appropriately sized aortic cannula. Typical left heart bypass flows are 50–60% calculated total flow, all of which goes to the lower extremities. Our mean cardiopulmonary bypass time was 27 minutes, the mean aortic clamp time was 21 minutes. The mean hospital stay in the patients where cardiopulmonary bypass was used was not different from the mean hospital stay in the patients where cardiopulmonary bypass was not used. There were no complications related to the cardiopulmonary bypass (bleeding, recurrent laryngeal nerve injury, recurrent coarctation, or neurologic injury). We have now used left heart bypass for coarctation repair in 22 patients without complications.

Aneurysm Formation

Both true and false aneurysms have been reported as complications after all types of coarctation of the aorta repair [168]. Aneurysms are also known to occur in patients with coarctation *not* undergoing surgical treatment [77]. However, there have been more reports of true aneurysm formation following prosthetic patch aortoplasty than any other technique. In 1980 Bergdahl [76] reported four adult patients with aneurysm formation in the aortic wall opposite a Dacron patch. Two of the patients had the patch placed at the time of reoperation after prior resection with end-to-end anastomosis. Microscopy revealed degenerative changes in the aortic wall opposite the patch. They postulated that the reason for the aneurysm formation was that part of the circumference of the aorta was replaced by a material with tensile characteristics differing from those of the aorta itself. In 1986 Rheuban and associates [169] reported eight aneurysms in a follow-up of 45 patients who had Dacron patch aortoplasty at a mean age of 8.5 years. In this series if a significant coarctation ridge was noted it was excised, even though the authors state this did not increase the incidence of aneurysm formation. Clarkson and colleagues [82] reported "aneurysm" formation in 5 of 38 patients (13%) in whom a Dacron patch aortoplasty was performed. In 20 of these patients the

intimal ridge was excised. Only one patient had a true aneurysm after primary coarctation repair without excision of the intima, four patients had false aneurysms. Del Nido and associates [85] reported a 5% incidence of aneurysm formation after 63 patch aortoplasties. Two of the three patients developing an aneurysm had the patch placed as a repair of recoarctation following primary resection of coarctation with end-to-end anastomosis during infancy.

In one of the largest series reported, starting with the patients originally operated on by Vossschulte, Hehrlein and coworkers [80] reported 18 aneurysms occurring in 317 patients (6%). Of the 14 patients for whom detailed information was available, 12 of 14 had an extensive resection of the fibrous coarctation membrane. Hehrlein and associates concluded that resection of a fibrous membrane of the aortic isthmus at the first intervention seemed to be an essential predisposing factor for development of aneurysms and the posterior ridge should not be excised. Experimental evidence confirming this observation was provided by DeSanto and colleagues [78] who studied Dacron and PTFE patches in dogs with and without concomitant intimal excision opposite the patch. Aneurysms formed in 8 of 12 dogs undergoing intimal excision and none of the control animals. Heikkinen and associates [83] reported histopathological studies of aneurysms and found medionecrosis in 13 of 14 patients and foreign body reaction in 11 patients. They concluded that these patients have an inherent weakness of the segment of the aortic wall owing to medial cystic degeneration. The same group reported successful management of such patients with aneurysm resection and insertion of a tubular prosthesis using femorofemoral or left atriofemoral bypass [75]. This group, which has the highest reported incidence of aneurysm formation (33%), speculated that this might reflect the fact that most of the patients were adults when the primary repair was done. Prolonged hemodynamic stress may have weakened the aortic wall of these patients. Bogaert and colleagues [170] reported that transverse arch hypoplasia also predisposes to aneurysm formation. The risk of aneurysm formation would appear to be higher for patients having a patch at >16 years of age or operated on as a recoarctation following resection with end-to-end anastomosis. The incidence of aneurysm formation also appears to be significantly higher after Dacron patch as compared to PTFE patch use [171]. Bertolini and associates [172] performed MRIs on 26 patients at a mean of 7 years after PTFE patch placement and found no aneurysms.

The risk of aneurysm formation is what has led us to significantly reduce the number of patients undergoing patch aortoplasty at our institution. We essentially now reserve that operation for patients who are having transverse arch repair or recoarctation repair and the child is not large enough for an interposition graft.

Recoarctation and Reoperation

Recurrent or residual coarctation has been reported after every type of coarctation repair. Numerous factors have been shown to increase the risk of recoarctation including age less than 2 to 3 months [71,106,107], weight less than 2 kg [173], silk suture material instead of polypropylene [58], and residual ductal tissue [174]. Recoarctation is defined as a postoperative arm-to-leg peak systolic pressure gradient exceeding 20 mmHg across the repaired area [175]. The resting gradient is not necessarily sensitive enough to "rule out" significant hypertension seen with exercise. Simultaneous arm/leg pressure measurements after exercise are the best way to exclude the possibility of residual obstruction at the coarctation repair site [176]. Magnetic resonance imaging, digital subtraction angiography, and bicycle exercise testing may also be useful in detecting residual coarctation of the aorta [177]. The most "cost-effective" approach may be to combine physical examination with MRI [178].

It seems clear that the initial reports of resection and end-to-end anastomosis had a high recoarctation rate (19%) [66]. This was probably secondary to the use of silk sutures instead of the currently available fine monofilament suture, inadequate resection of all ductal tissue that may extend into areas of normal-appearing aorta, lack of growth at a circumferential suture line, and lack of growth of a hypoplastic transverse arch. Recent reports of resection and end-to-end anastomosis using microvascular technique appear to have a much lower recoarctation rate [53]. The subclavian flap aortoplasty, although originally felt to nearly eliminate recoarctation, definitely has a rate of recoarctation higher than initially thought (13%) [66]. The patch aortoplasty should not be used in infants because of the high recoarctation rate. Resection with extended end-to-end anastomosis appears to have the lowest recoarctation rate (6%) [53]. Our current approach is to use resection with extended end-to-end anastomosis for all neonates and infants and some older children. For children over 10 years of age we use an interposition graft.

As discussed in the section on balloon angioplasty, this procedure is now considered the initial procedure of choice for most children with recurrent coarctation of the aorta [130,144]. The initial success rate is high with a low incidence of complications. If balloon dilation is not successful or not indicated, reoperation may be required. In most cases reoperation is considerably more difficult owing to dense scarring in the region of the previous repair. The gradient is usually not high, decreasing the impetus for collateral formation and possibly increasing the risk of spinal cord complications [179]. The previously discussed indications for partial left atriofemoral bypass to maintain adequate distal aortic perfusion pressure should be seriously considered for every reoperation. No single technique of reoperation is applicable to all patients but the majority of patients can be managed by either patch graft angioplasty, resection and interposition graft, or a local bypass graft technique [180,181]. Resection and primary end-to-end anastomosis may be difficult secondary to adhesions and the amount of mobilization required to avoid tension on the suture line of what is usually a very friable aorta.

Sweeney and associates [180] reported 53 patients who underwent reoperation for aortic coarctation. Interestingly, no temporary shunts or left heart bypass was used, all patients survived, and there were no instances of paraplegia. Twenty-six patients had Dacron patch angioplasty, 16 had bypass grafts around the coarctation, 8 had resection and interposition grafting, and 3 had resection and end-to-end anastomosis. Only three patients had a postoperative gradient more than 10 mmHg and none more than 20 mmHg. Kron and colleagues [182] reported 24 reinterventions in 23 patients with recoarctation with one death and no paraplegia. Techniques employed included patch aortoplasty (13), balloon dilation (6), end-to-end anastomosis (2), interposition graft (2), and subclavian flap (1). They recommended balloon dilation as primary therapy for restenosis. Sakapoulos and colleagues [183] reported reoperation for recurrent coarctation in 56 patients, the vast majority of repairs using a prosthetic patch technique. There were no deaths or major complications and a 96% success rate. For patients with a long segment recoarctation, very dense adhesions, or requiring a cardiac operation, Jacob and coworkers [184] reported success in 10 patients using an ascending aorta-to-descending aorta bypass graft placed with a combined left thoracotomy, median sternotomy approach. Kanter [185] also reports successful extra-anatomic bypass for complex recurrent coarctation. Moderate-to-severe hemodynamic abnormalities may persist during exercise after reoperation for coarctation of the aorta [186]. Diligent efforts to repair all hemodynamically significant residual and recurrent coarctations are necessary if the natural fate of premature death is to be avoided for patients with these lesions.

Conclusion

The management of the infant and child with coarctation of the aorta has become fairly standardized. Echocardiography is the primary diagnostic tool. Computed tomographic imaging is very useful if the echocardiogram is not fully diagnostic. PGE₁ has dramatically improved the outcome for neonates with critical coarctation. Coarctation should be repaired at the time of diagnosis to minimize the incidence of late hypertension. We recommend resection with extended end-to-end anastomosis for neonates, infants, and young children. For complex coarctation of the aorta (associated intracardiac lesions), we recommend transmediastinal repair of the cardiac defect and resection with extended end-to-end anastomosis. We recommend resection with interposition graft placement for older children. In older children femoral artery pressure should be monitored and strong consideration should be given to partial left heart bypass to avoid paraplegia. Balloon dilatation is the initial procedure of choice for recoarctation. If this is unsuccessful, reoperation with patch aortoplasty or graft interposition has excellent results.

References

1. Keith JD. (1978) Coarctation of the aorta. In: Keith JD, Rowe RD, VIad P, eds. *Heart Disease in Infancy and Childhood*, 3rd ed. New York: Macmillan, pp. 736–760.
2. Rudolph AM. (1974) *Congenital Diseases of the Heart*. Chicago, IL: Year Book Medical Publishers.
3. Tawes RL Jr, Aberdeen E, Waterston DJ, et al. (1969) Coarctation of the aorta in infants and children. A review of 333 operative cases, including 179 infants. Circulation 39, I173–I184.
4. Gross RE, Hufnagel CA. (1945) Coarctation of the aorta. Experimental studies regarding its surgical correction. N Engl J Med 233, 287–293.
5. Crafoord C, Nylin G. (1945) Congenital coarctation of the aorta and its surgical treatment. J Thorac Surg 14, 347–361.
6. Vossschulte K. (1961) Surgical correction of coarctation of the aorta by an "isthmusplastic" operation. Thorax 16, 338–345.
7. Waldhausen JA, Nahrwold DL. (1966) Repair of coarctation of the aorta with a subclavian flap. J Thorac Cardiovasc Surg 51, 532–533.
8. Amato JJ, Rheinlander HF, Cleveland CJ. (1977) A method of enlarging the distal transverse arch in infants with hypoplasia and coarctation of the aorta. Ann Thorac Surg 23, 261–263.
9. Lansman S, Shapiro AJ, Schiller MS, et al. (1986) Extended aortic arch anastomosis for repair of coarctation in infancy. Circulation 74, I37–I41.
10. Meier MA, Lucchese FA, Jazbik W, et al. (1986) A new technique for repair of aortic coarctation. Subclavian flap aortoplasty with preservation of arterial blood flow to the left arm. J Thorac Cardiovasc Surg 92, 1005–1012.
11. Kubota H, Camilleri L, Legault B, et al. (1998) Surgical correction of the hypoplastic aortic arch by the subclavian free flap method in the neonate. J Thorac Cardiovasc Surg 116, 519–521.
12. Asano M, Mishima A, Yamamoto S, et al. (1998) Modified subclavian flap aortoplasty for coarctation repair in patients less than three months of age. Ann Thorac Surg 66, 588–589.
13. van Heurn LWE, Wong CM, Spiegelhalter OJ, et al. (1994) Surgical treatment of aortic coarctation in infants younger than 3 months: 1985 to 1990. Success of extended end-to-end arch aortoplasty. J Thorac Cardiovasc Surg 107, 74–85.
14. Rajasinghe HA, Reddy VM, van Son JAM, et al. (1996) Coarctation repair using end-to-side anastomosis of descending aorta to proximal aortic arch. Ann Thorac Surg 61, 840–844.
15. Tchervenkov CI, Tahta SA, Jutras L, et al. (1998) Single-stage repair of aortic arch obstruction and associated intracardiac defects with pulmonary homograft patch aortoplasty. J Thorac Cardiovasc Surg 116, 897–904.
16. Morgagni JB. (1760) De sedibus et causis morborum. Epist XVIII, Article 6.
17. Bonnet LM. (1903) Stenose congenitale de l'aorte. Rev Med Paris 23, 108–225.
18. Backer CL, Mavroudis C. (2003) Coarctation of the aorta. In: Mavroudis C, Backer CL, eds. *Pediatric Cardiac Surgery*, 3rd ed. Philadelphia, PA: Mosby.
19. Vouhé PR, Trinquet F, Lecompte Y, et al. (1988) Aortic coarctation with hypoplastic aortic arch. Results of extended end-to-end aortic arch anastomosis. J Thorac Cardiovasc Surg 96, 557–563.
20. Backer CL, Mavroudis C, Zias EA, et al. (1998) Repair of coarctation with resection and extended end-to-end anastomosis. Ann Thorac Surg 66, 1365–1370.
21. Conte S, Lacour-Gayet F, Serraf A, et al. (1995) Surgical management of neonatal coarctation. J Thorac Cardiovasc Surg 109, 663–674.
22. Backer CL, Mavroudis C. (2000) Congenital Heart Surgery Nomenclature and Database Project: patent ductus arteriosus, coarctation of the aorta, interrupted aortic arch. Ann Thorac Surg 69, S298–S307.
23. Moulaert AJ, Bruins CC, Oppenheimer-Dekker A. (1976) Anomalies of the aortic arch and ventricular septal defects. Circulation 53, 1011–1015.
24. Machii M, Becker AE. (1997) Hypoplastic aortic arch morphology pertinent to growth after surgical correction of aortic coarctation. Ann Thorac Surg 64, 516–520.
25. Karl TR, Sano S, Brawn W, et al. (1992) Repair of hypoplastic or interrupted aortic arch via sternotomy. J Thorac Cardiovasc Surg 104, 688–695.
26. Rudolph AM, Heymann MA, Spitznas U. (1972) Hemodynamic considerations in the development of narrowing of the aorta. Am J Cardiol 30, 514–525.
27. Muster AJ. (1993) Angiographic anatomy of aortic coarctation: A classification based on the associated morphology of the aortic arch. In: Mavroudis C, Backer CL, eds. *Coarctation and Interrupted Aortic Arch*. Philadelphia, PA: Hanley & Belfus; Cardiac Surgery: State of the Art Reviews 7, 23–31.
28. Shone JD, Sellers RD, Anderson RC, et al. (1963) The developmental complex of "parachute mitral valve," supravalvular ring of left atrium, subaortic stenosis, and coarctation of aorta. Am J Cardiol 11, 714–720.
29. Skoda J. (1855) Demonstration eines Falles von Obliteration der Aorta. Wochenblatt der Zeitschrift der Kaiserlichen-Königliche Gesellschaft der Aertze zur Wein 1, 710.
30. Elzenga NJ, Gittenberger-de Groot AC, Oppenheimer-Dekker A. (1986) Coarctation and other obstructive aortic arch anomalies: their relationship to the ductus arteriosus. Int J Cardiol 13, 289–308.
31. Russell GA, Berry PJ, Watterson K, et al. (1991) Patterns of ductal tissue in coarctation in the first three months of life. J Thorac Cardiovasc Surg 102, 596–601.

32. Callahan PF, Quivers ES, Bradley LM, *et al.* (1998) Echocardiographic evidence for a ductal tissue sling causing discrete coarctation of the aorta in the neonate: case report. Pediatr Cardiol 19, 182–184.

33. Kappetein AP, Gittenberger-de Groot AC, Zwinderman AH. (1991) The neural crest as a possible pathogenic factor in coarctation of the aorta and bicuspid aortic valve. J Thorac Cardiovasc Surg 102, 830–836.

34. Sybert VP. (1998) Cardiovascular malformations and complications in Turner syndrome. Pediatrics 101, E11–E18.

35. Hoeffel JC, Henry M, Mentre B, *et al.* (1975) Pseudocoarctation or congenital kinking of the aorta: radiologic considerations. Am Heart J 89, 428–436.

36. Kessler RM, Miller KB, Pett S, *et al.* (1993) Pseudocoarctation of the aorta presenting as a mediastinal mass with dysphagia. Ann Thorac Surg 55, 1003–1005.

37. Gay WA Jr, Young WG Jr. (1969) Pseudocoarctation of the aorta. A reappraisal. J Thorac Cardiovasc Surg 58, 739–745.

38. Bahabozorgui S, Bernstein RG, Frater RWM. (1971) Pseudocoarctation of the aorta associated with aneurysm formation. Chest 60, 616–617.

39. Riemenschneider TA, Emmanouilides GC, Hirose F, *et al.* (1969) Coarctation of the abdominal aorta in children: report of three cases and review of the literature. Pediatrics 44, 716–726.

40. Scott HW Jr, Dean RH, Boerth R, *et al.* (1979) Coarctation of the abdominal aorta: pathophysiologic and therapeutic considerations. Ann Surg 189, 746–757.

41. Pierce WS, Vincent WR, Fitzgerald E, *et al.* (1975) Coarctation of the abdominal aorta with multiple aneurysms. Operative correction. Ann Thorac Surg 20, 687–693.

42. Bergamini TM, Bernard JD, Mavroudis C, *et al.* (1995) Coarctation of the abdominal aorta. Ann Vasc Surg 9, 352–356.

43. Elliott RB, Starling MB, Neutze JM. (1975) Medical manipulation of the ductus arteriosus. Lancet 1, 140–142.

44. Heymann MA, Berman W Jr, Rudolph AM, *et al.* (1979) Dilatation of the ductus arteriosus by prostaglandin E1 in aortic arch abnormalities. Circulation 59, 169–173.

45. Cokkinos DV, Leachman RD, Cooley DA. (1979) Increased mortality rate from coronary artery disease following operation for coarctation of the aorta at a late age. J Thorac Cardiovasc Surg 77, 314–318.

46. Reifenstein GH, Levine SA, Gross RE. (1947) Coarctation of the aorta. A review of 104 autopsied cases of the "adult type," 2 years of age or older. Am Heart J 33, 146–168.

47. Connolly HM, Huston J III, Brown RD Jr, *et al.* (2003) Intracranial aneurysms in patients with coarctation of the aorta: a prospective magnetic resonance angiographic study of 100 patients. Mayo Clin Proc 78, 1491–1499.

48. Campbell M. (1970) Natural history of coarctation of the aorta. Br Heart J 32, 633–640.

49. Abbott ME. (1928) Coarctation of the aorta of the adult type; statistical study and historical retrospect of 200 recorded cases with autopsy, of stenosis or obliteration of descending arch in subjects above age of 2 years. Am Heart J 3, 574–615.

50. Weyman AE, Caldwell RL, Hurwitz RA, *et al.* (1978) Cross-sectional echocardiographic detection of aortic obstruction. 2. Coarctation of the aorta. Circulation 57, 498–502.

51. Shaddy RE, Snider AR, Silverman NH, *et al.* (1986) Pulsed Doppler findings in patients with coarctation of the aorta. Circulation 73, 82–88.

52. Simpson IA, Sahn DJ, Valdes-Cruz LM, *et al.* (1988) Color Doppler flow mapping in patients with coarctation of the aorta: new observations and improved evaluation with color flow diameter and proximal acceleration as predictors of severity. Circulation 77, 736–744.

53. Kaushal S, Backer CL, Patel JN, *et al.* (2009) Coarctation of the aorta: midterm outcomes of resection with extended end-to-end anastomosis. Ann Thorac Surg 88, 1932–1938.

54. Stern HC, Locher D, Wallnofer K, *et al.* (1991) Noninvasive assessment of coarctation of the aorta: comparative measurements by two-dimensional echocardiography, magnetic resonance, and angiography. Pediatr Cardiol 12, 1–5.

55. Simpson IA, Chung KJ, Glass RF, *et al.* (1988) Cine magnetic resonance imaging for evaluation of anatomy and flow relations in infants and children with coarctation of the aorta. Circulation 78, 142–148.

56. Riquelme C, Laissy P, Menegazzo D, *et al.* (1999) MR imaging of coarctation of the aorta and its postoperative complications in adults: assessment with spin-echo and cine-MR imaging. Magn Reson Imaging 17, 37–46.

57. Lerberg DB. (1982) Abbott's artery. Ann Thorac Surg 33, 414–418.

58. Schuster SR, Gross RE. (1962) Surgery for coarctation of the aorta. A review of 500 cases. J Thorac Cardiovasc Surg 43, 54–70.

59. Marini CP, Grubbs PE, Toporoff B, *et al.* (1989) Effect of sodium nitroprusside on spinal cord perfusion and paraplegia during aortic cross-clamping. Ann Thorac Surg 47, 379–383.

60. Watterson KG, Dhasmana JP, O'Higgins JW, *et al.* (1990) Distal aortic pressure during coarctation operation. Ann Thorac Surg 49, 987–990.

61. Backer CL, Stewart RD, Kelle AM, *et al.* (2006) Use of partial cardiopulmonary bypass for coarctation repair through a left thoracotomy in children without collaterals. Ann Thorac Surg 82, 964–972.

62. Wong CH, Watson B, Smith JR, Hamilton AH. (2001) The use of left heart bypass in adult and recurrent coarctation repair. Eur J Cardiothorac Surg 20, 1199–1201.

63. Christenson JT, Sierra J, Didier D, *et al.* (2004) Repair of aortic coarctation using temporary ascending to descending aortic bypass in children with poor colateral circulation. Cardiol Young 14, 39–45.

64. Gross RE. (1951) Treatment of certain aortic coarctations by homologous grafts; report of 19 cases. Ann Surg 134, 753–768.

65. Kirklin JW, Burchell HB, Pugh DG, *et al.* (1952) Surgical treatment of coarctation of the aorta in a ten week old infant: report of a case. Circulation 6, 411–414.

66. Williams WG, Shindo G, Trusler GA, *et al.* (1980) Results of repair of coarctation of the aorta during infancy. J Thorac Cardiovasc Surg 79, 603–608.

67. Cobanoglu A, Teply JF, Grunkemeier GL, *et al.* (1985) Coarctation of the aorta in patients younger than three months. A critique of the subclavian flap operation. J Thorac Cardiovasc Surg 89, 128–135.

68. Körfer R, Meyer H, Kleikamp G, *et al.* (1985) Early and late results after resection and end-to-end anastomosis of coarctation of the thoracic aorta in early infancy. J Thorac Cardiovasc Surg 89, 616–622.

69. Ziemer G, Jonas RA, Perry SB, *et al.* (1986) Surgery for coarctation of the aorta in the neonate. Circulation 74, I25–I31.

70. Brouwer MHJ, Kuntze CEE, Ebels T, *et al.* (1991) Repair of aortic coarctation in infants. J Thorac Cardiovasc Surg 101, 1093–1098.

71. Kappetein AP, Zwinderman AH, Bogers AJJC, *et al.* (1994) More than thirty-five years of coarctation repair. An unexpected high relapse rate. J Thorac Cardiovasc Surg 107, 87–95.

72. Quaegebeur JM, Jonas RA, Weinberg AD, *et al.* (1994) Congenital Heart Surgeons Society: Outcomes in seriously ill neonates with coarctation of the aorta. A multiinstitutional study. J Thorac Cardiovasc Surg 108, 841–851.

73. Harlan JL, Doty DB, Brandt B III, *et al.* (1984) Coarctation of the aorta in infants. J Thorac Cardiovasc Surg 88, 1012–1019.

74. Hartmann AF Jr, Goldring D, Hernandez A, *et al.* (1970) Recurrent coarctation of the aorta after successful repair in infancy. Am J Cardiol 25, 405–410.

75. Ala-Kulju K, Heikkinen L. (1989) Aneurysms after patch graft aortoplasty for coarctation of the aorta: long-term results of surgical management. Ann Thorac Surg 47, 853–856.

76. Bergdahl L, Ljungqvist A. (1980) Long-term results after repair of coarctation of the aorta by patch grafting. J Thorac Cardiovasc Surg 80, 177–181.

77. Roth M, Lemke P, Schönburg M, *et al.* (2002) Aneurysm formation after patch aortoplasty repair (Vossschulte): reoperation in adults with and without hypothermic circulatory arrest Ann Thorac Surg 74, 2047–2050.

78. DeSanto A, Bills RG, King H, *et al.* (1987) Pathogenesis of aneurysm formation opposite prosthetic patches used for coarctation repair. An experimental study. J Thorac Cardiovasc Surg 94, 720–723.

79. Sade RM, Crawford FA, Hohn AR, *et al.* (1984) Growth of the aorta after prosthetic patch aortoplasty for coarctation in infants. Ann Thorac Surg 38, 21–25.

80. Hehrlein FW, Mulch J, Rautenburg HW, *et al.* (1986) Incidence and pathogenesis of late aneurysm after patch graft aortoplasty for coarctation. J Thorac Cardiovasc Surg 92, 226–230.

81. Walhout RJ, Lekkerkerker JC, Oron GH, *et al.* (2003). Comparison of polytetrafluoroethylene patch aortoplasty and end-to-end anastomosis for coarctation of the aorta. J Thorac Cardiovasc Surg 126, 521–528.

82. Clarkson PM, Brandt PWT, Barratt-Boyes BG, *et al.* (1985) Prosthetic repair of coarctation of the aorta with particular reference to Dacron onlay patch grafts and late aneurysm formation. Am J Cardiol 56, 342–346.

83. Heikkinen L, Sariola H, Sala J, *et al.* (1990) Morphological and histopathological aspects of aneurysms after patch aortoplasty for coarctation. Ann Thorac Surg 50, 946–948.

84. Yee ES, Soifer SJ, Turley K, *et al.* (1986) Infant coarctation: a spectrum in clinical presentation and treatment. Ann Thorac Surg 42, 488–493.

85. Del Nido PJ, Williams WG, Wilson GJ, *et al.* (1986) Synthetic patch angioplasty for repair of coarctation of the aorta: experience with aneurysm formation. Circulation 74, I32–I36.

86. Ungerleider RM. (1991) Commentary: Is there a role for prosthetic patch aortoplasty in the repair of coarctation? Ann Thorac Surg 52, 601.

87. Backer CL, Paape K, Zales VR, *et al.* (1995) Coarctation of the aorta. Repair with polytetrafluoroethylene patch aortoplasty. Circulation 92(9 Suppl), II132–II136.

88. Messmer BJ, Minale C, Mühler E, *et al.* (1991) Surgical correction of coarctation in early infancy: does surgical technique influence the result? Ann Thorac Surg 52, 594–600.

89. Morris GC Jr, Cooley DA, DeBakey ME, *et al.* (1960) Coarctation of the aorta with particular emphasis upon improved techniques of surgical repair. J Thorac Cardiovasc Surg 40, 705–722.

90. Aris A, Subirana T, Ferrés P, *et al.* (1999) Repair of aortic coarctation in patients more than 50 years of age. Ann Thorac Surg 67, 1376–1379.

91. Hart JC, Waldhausen JA. (1983) Reversed subclavian flap for arch coarctation of the aorta. Ann Thorac Surg 36, 714–717.

92. Dietl CA, Torres AR, Favaloro RG, *et al.* (1992) Risk of recoarctation in neonates and infants after repair with patch aortoplasty, subclavian flap, and the combined resection-flap procedure. J Thorac Cardiovasc Surg 103, 724–732.

93. Allen BS, Halldorsson AO, Barth MJ, *et al.* (2000) Modification of the subclavian patch aortoplasty for repair of aortic coarctation in neonates and infants. Ann Thorac Surg 69, 877–881.

94. Kanter KR, Vincent RN, Fyfe DA. (2001) Reverse subclavian flap repair of hypoplastic transverse aorta in infancy. Ann Thorac Surg 71, 539–536.

95. Moulton AL, Brenner JI, Roberts G, *et al.* (1984) Subclavian flap repair of coarctation of the aorta in neonates. Realization of growth potential? J Thorac Cardiovasc Surg 87, 220–235.

96. Bergdahl LAL, Blackstone EH, Kirklin JW, *et al.* (1982) Determinants of early success in repair of aortic coarctation in infants. J Thorac Cardiovasc Surg 83, 736–742.

97. Milliken JC, Brawn WJ, Mee RB. (1990) Neonatal coarctation: clinical spectrum and improved results. J Am Coll Cardiol 15, 78A.

98. Geiss D, Williams WG, Lindsay WK, *et al.* (1980) Upper extremity gangrene: a complication of subclavian artery division. Ann Thorac Surg 30, 487–489.

99. Wells WJ, Castro LJ. (2000) Arm ischemia after subclavian flap angioplasty: repair by carotid–subclavian bypass. Ann Thorac Surg 69, 1574–1576.

100. Diemont FF, Chemla ES, Julia PL, *et al.* (2000) Upper limb ischemia after subclavian flap aortoplasty: unusual long-term complication. Ann Thorac Surg 69, 1576–1578.

101. Mellgren G, Friberg LG, Erikson BO, *et al.* (1987) Neonatal surgery for coarctation of the aorta. The Gothenburg experience. Scand J Thorac Cardiovasc Surg 21, 193–197.

102. Todd PJ, Dangerfield PH, Hamilton DI, *et al.* (1983) Late effects on the left upper limb of subclavian flap aortoplasty. J Thorac Cardiovasc Surg 85, 678–681.

103. Martin MM, Beekman RH, Rocchini AP, *et al.* (1988) Aortic aneurysms after subclavian angioplasty repair of coarctation of the aorta. Am J Cardiol 61, 951–953.

104. Penkoske PA, Williams WG, Olley PM, *et al.* (1984) Subclavian arterioplasty. Repair of coarctation of the aorta in the first year of life. J Thorac Cardiovasc Surg 87, 894–900.

105. Pandey R, Jackson M, Ajab S, *et al.* (2006) Subclavian flap repair: review of 399 patients at median follow-up of fourteen years. Ann Thorac Surg 81, 1420–1428.

106. Metzdorff MT, Cobanoglu A, Grunkemeier GL, *et al.* (1985) Influence of age at operation on late results with subclavian flap aortoplasty. J Thorac Cardiovasc Surg 89, 235–241.

107. Sanchez GR, Balsara RK, Dunn JM, *et al.* (1986) Recurrent obstruction after subclavian flap repair of coarctation of the aorta in infants. Can it be predicted or prevented? J Thorac Cardiovasc Surg 91, 738–746.

108. Ehrhardt P, Walker DR. (1989) Coarctation of the aorta corrected during the first month of life. Arch Dis Child 64, 330–332.

109. Jahangiri M, Shinebourne EA, Zurakowski D, *et al.* (2000) Subclavian flap angioplasty: does the arch look after itself? J Thorac Cardiovasc Surg 120, 224–229.

110. Barreiro CJ, Ellison TA, Williams JA, *et al.* (2007) Subclavian flap aortoplasty: still a safe, reproducible, and effective treatment for infant coarctation. Eur J Cardiothorac Surg 31, 649–653.

111. Brown JW, Fiore AC, King H. (1985) Isthmus flap aortoplasty: an alternative to subclavian flap aortoplasty for long-segment coarctation of the aorta in infants. Ann Thorac Surg 40, 274–279.

112. Zannini L, Lecompte Y, Galli R, *et al.* (1985) [Aortic coarctation with hypoplasia of the arch: description of a new surgical technique.] G Ital Cardiol 15, 1045–1048.

113. Elliott MJ. (1987) Coarctation of the aorta with arch hypoplasia: improvements on a new technique. Ann Thorac Surg 44, 321–323.

114. Zannini L, Gargiulo G, Albanese SB, *et al.* (1993) Aortic coarctation with hypoplastic arch in neonates: a spectrum of anatomic lesions requiring different surgical options. Ann Thorac Surg 56, 288–294.

115. Jonas RA. (1991) Coarctation: do we need to resect ductal tissue? Ann Thorac Surg 52, 604–607.

116. van Son JAM, Falk V, Schneider P, *et al.* (1997) Repair of coarctation of the aorta in neonates and young infants. J Card Surg 12, 139–146.

117. Wright GE, Nowak CA, Goldberg CS, *et al.* (2005) Extended resection and end-to-end anastomosis for aortic coarctation in infants: results of a tailored surgical approach. Ann Thorac Surg 80, 1453–1459.

118. Wood AE, Javadpour H, Duff D, *et al.* (2004) Is extended arch aortoplasty the operation of choice for infant aortic coarctation? Results of 15 years' experience in 181 patients. Ann Thorac Surg 77, 1353–1357.

119. Thomson JD, Mulpur A, Guerrero R, *et al.* (2006) Outcome after extended arch repair for aortic coarctation. Heart 92, 90–94.

120. Lacour-Gayet F, Bruniaux J, Serraf A, *et al.* (1990) Hypoplastic transverse arch and coarctation in neonates. Surgical reconstruction of the aortic arch: a study of sixty-six patients. J Thorac Cardiovasc Surg 100, 808–816.

121. Brouwer MHJ, Cromme-Dijkhuis AH, Ebels T, *et al.* (1992) Growth of the hypoplastic aortic arch after simple coarctation resection and end-to-end anastomosis. J Thorac Cardiovasc Surg 104, 426–433.

122. Myers JL, McConnell BA, Waldhausen JA. (1992) Coarctation of the aorta in infants: does the aortic arch grow after repair? Ann Thorac Surg 54, 869–875.

123. Siewers RD, Ettedgui J, Pahl E, *et al.* (1991) Coarctation and hypoplasia of the aortic arch: will the arch grow? Ann Thorac Surg 52, 608–614.

124. Sos T, Sniderman KW, Rettek-Sos B, *et al.* (1979) Percutaneous transluminal dilatation of coarctation of thoracic aorta post mortem. Lancet 2, 970–971.

125. Lock JE, Castaneda-Zuniga WR, Bass JL, *et al.* (1982) Balloon dilation of excised aortic coarctations. Radiology 143, 689–691.

126. Lababidi ZA, Daskalopoulos DA, Stoeckle H Jr. (1984) Transluminal balloon coarctation angioplasty: experience with 27 patients. Am J Cardiol 54, 1288–1291.

127. Marvin WJ, Mahoney LT, Rose EF. (1986) Pathologic sequelae of balloon dilation angioplasty for unoperated coarctation of the aorta in children. J Am Coll Cardiol 7, 117A.

128. Brandt B 3rd, Marvin WJ Jr, Rose EF, *et al.* (1987) Surgical treatment of coarctation of the aorta after balloon angioplasty. J Thorac Cardiovasc Surg 94, 714–719.

129. Cooper RS, Ritter SB, Rothe WB, *et al.* (1987) Angioplasty for coarctation of the aorta: long-term results. Circulation 75, 600–604.

130. Tynan M, Finley JP, Fontes V, *et al.* (1990) Balloon angioplasty for the treatment of native coarctation: results of Valvuloplasty and Angioplasty of Congenital Anomalies Registry. Am J Cardiol 65, 790–792.

131. Lock JE. (1984) Now that we can dilate, should we? Am J Cardiol 54, 1360.

132. Zales VR, Muster AJ. (1993) Balloon dilation angioplasty for the management of aortic coarctation. In: Mavroudis C, Backer CL, eds. Coarctation and interrupted aortic arch. *Cardiac Surgery: State of the Art Reviews.* Philadelphia, PA: Hanley & Belfus, 7, 133–146.

133. Fiore AC, Fischer LK, Schwartz T, *et al.* (2005) Comparison of angioplasty and surgery for neonatal aortic coarctation. Ann Thorac Surg 80, 1659–1665.

134. Ovaert C, McCrindle BW, Nykanen D, *et al.* (2000) Balloon angioplasty of native coarctation: clinical outcomes and predictors of success. J Am Coll Cardiol 35, 988–996.

135. Fletcher SE, Nihill MR, Grifka RG, *et al.* (1995) Balloon angioplasty of native coarctation of the aorta: midterm follow-up and prognostic factors. J Am Coll Cardiol 25, 730–734.

136. Ebeid MR, Prieto LR, Latson LA. (1997) Use of balloon-expandable stents for coarctation of the aorta: initial results and intermediate-term follow-up. J Am Coll Cardiol 30, 1847–1852.

137. Varma C, Benson LN, Butany J, *et al.* (2003) Aortic dissection after stent dilatation for coarctation of the aorta: a case

report and literature review. Catheter Cardiovasc Interv 59, 528–535.

138. Korkola SJ, Tchervenkov CI, Shum-Tim D, *et al.* (2003) Aortic rupture after stenting of a native coarctation in an adult. Ann Thorac Surg 74, 936.

139. Forbest TJ, Moore P, Pedra CA, *et al.* (2007) Intermediate follow-up following intravascular stenting for treatment of coarctation of the aorta. Catheter Cardiovasc Interv 70, 569–577.

140. Forbest TJ, Garekar S, Amin Z, *et al.* (2007) Procedural results and acute complications in stenting native and recurrent coarctation of the aorta in patients over 4 years of age: a multi-institutional study. Catheter Cardiovasc Interv 70, 276–285.

141. Hess J, Mooyaart EL, Busch HJ, *et al.* (1986) Percutaneous transluminal balloon angioplasty in restenosis of coarctation of the aorta. Br Heart J 55, 459–461.

142. Hijazi ZM, Fahey JT, Kleinman CS, *et al.* (1991) Balloon angioplasty for recurrent coarctation of the aorta. Immediate and long-term results. Circulation 84, 1150–1156.

143. Saul JP, Keane JF, Fellows KE, *et al.* (1987) Balloon dilation angioplasty of postoperative aortic obstructions. Am J Cardiol 59, 943–948.

144. Hellenbrand WE, Allen HD, Golinko RJ, *et al.* (1990) Balloon angioplasty for aortic recoarctation: results of Valvuloplasty and Angioplasty of Congenital Anomalies Registry. Am J Cardiol 65, 793–797.

145. Yetman AT, Nykanen D, McCrindle BW, *et al.* (1997) Balloon angioplasty of recurrent coarctation: a 12-year review. J Am Coll Cardiol 30, 811–816.

146. Reich O, Tax P, Bartáková H, *et al.* (2008). Long-term (up to 20 years) results of percutaneous balloon angioplasty of recurrent aortic coarctation without use of stents. Eur Heart J 29, 2042–2048.

147. Sealy WC, Harris JS, Young WG Jr, *et al.* (1957) Paradoxical hypertension following resection of coarctation of aorta. Surgery 42, 135–147.

148. Sealy WC. (1990) Paradoxical hypertension after repair of coarctation of the aorta: a review of its causes. Ann Thorac Surg 50, 323–329.

149. Goodall MC, Sealy WC. (1969) Increased sympathetic nerve activity following resection of coarctation of the thoracic aorta. Circulation 39, 345–351.

150. Sealy WC. (1967) Coarctation of the aorta and hypertension. Ann Thorac Surg 3, 14–28.

151. Rocchini AP, Rosenthal A, Barger AC, *et al.* (1976) Pathogenesis of paradoxical hypertension after coarctation resection. Circulation 54, 382–387.

152. Fox S, Pierce WS, Waldhausen JA. (1980) Pathogenesis of paradoxical hypertension after coarctation repair. Ann Thorac Surg 29, 135–141.

153. Lober PH, Lillehei CW. (1954) Necrotizing panarteritis following repair of coarctation of aorta: report of two cases. Surgery 35, 950–956.

154. Benson WR, Sealy WC. (1956) Arterial necrosis following resection of coarctation of the aorta. Lab Invest 5, 359–376.

155. Tabbutt S, Nicolson SC, Adamson PC, *et al.* (2008) The safety, efficacy, and pharmacokinetics of esmolol for blood pressure control immediately after repair of coarctation of the aorta in infants and children: a multicenter, double-blind, randomized trial. J Thorac Cardiovasc Surg 136, 321–328.

156. Leenen FHH, Balfe JA, Pelech AN, *et al.* (1987) Postoperative hypertension after repair of coarctation of aorta in children: protective effect of propranolol? Am Heart J 113, 1164–1173.

157. Gidding SS, Rocchini AP, Beekman R, *et al.* (1985) Therapeutic effect of propranolol on paradoxical hypertension after repair of coarctation of the aorta. N Engl J Med 312, 1224–1228.

158. Presbitero P, Demarie D, Villani M, *et al.* (1987) Long term results (14.30 years) of surgical repair of aortic coarctation. Br Heart J 57, 462–469.

159. Seirafi PA, Warner KG, Geggel RL, *et al.* (1998) Repair of coarctation of the aorta during infancy minimizes the risk of late hypertension. Ann Thorac Surg 66, 1378–1382.

160. Sigurdardottir LY, Helgason H. (1996) Exercise-induced hypertension after corrective surgery for coarctation of the aorta. Pediatr Cardiol 17, 301–307.

161. Warnes CA. (2003) Bicuspid aortic valve and coarctation: two villains part of a diffuse problem. Heart 89, 965–966.

162. Cohen M, Fuster V, Steele PM, *et al.* (1989) Coarctation of the aorta: long-term follow-up and prediction of outcome after surgical correction. Circulation 80, 840–845.

163. Bing RJ, Handelsman JC, Campbell JA, *et al.* (1948) The surgical treatment and physiopathology of coarctation of the aorta. Ann Surg 128, 803–824.

164. Brewer LA 3rd, Fosburg RG, Mulder GA, *et al.* (1972) Spinal cord complications following surgery for coarctation of the aorta. A study of 66 cases. J Thorac Cardiovasc Surg 64, 368–381.

165. Lerberg DB, Hardesty RL, Siewers RD, *et al.* (1982) Coarctation of the aorta in infants and children: 25 years of experience. Ann Thorac Surg 33, 159–170.

166. Crawford FA Jr, Sade RM. (1984) Spinal cord injury associated with hyperthermia during aortic coarctation repair. J Thorac Cardiovasc Surg 87, 616–618.

167. Pollock JC, Jamieson MP, McWilliam R. (1986) Somatosensory evoked potentials in the detection of spinal cord ischemia in aortic coarctation repair. Ann Thorac Surg 41, 251–254.

168. Nguyen DM, Tsang J, Tchervenkov CI. (1999) Aneurysm after subclavian flap angioplasty repair of coarctation of the aorta. Ann Thorac Surg 68, 1392–1394.

169. Rheuban KS, Gutgesell HP, Carpenter MA, *et al.* (1986) Aortic aneurysm after patch angioplasty for aortic isthmic coarctation in childhood. Am J Cardiol 58, 178–180.

170. Bogaert J, Gewillig M, Rademakers F, *et al.* (1995) Transverse arch hypoplasia predisposes to aneurysm formation at the repair site after patch angioplasty for coarctation of the aorta. J Am Coll Cardiol 26, 521–527.

171. Aebert H, Laas J, Bednarski P, *et al.* (1993) High incidence of aneurysm formation following patch plasty repair of coarctation. Eur J Cardiothorac Surg 7, 200–205.

172. Bertolini A, Dalmonte P, Toma P, *et al.* (1992) Gore-Tex patch aortoplasty for coarctation in children: nuclear magnetic resonance assessment at 7 years. J Cardiovasc Surg (Torino) 33, 223–228.

173. Sudarshan CD, Cochrane AD, Jun ZH, *et al.* (2006) Repair of coarctation of the aorta in infants weighing less than 2 kilograms. Ann Thorac Surg 82, 158–163.

174. Goldman S, Hernandez J, Pappas G. (1986) Results of surgical treatment of coarctation of the aorta in the critically ill neonate. Including the influence of pulmonary artery banding. J Thorac Cardiovasc Surg 91, 732–737.

175. Kirklin JW, Barratt-Boyes BG. (1986) *Cardiac Surgery*. New York: John Wiley Inc.

176. Freed MD, Rocchini A, Rosenthal A, *et al.* (1979) Exercise-induced hypertension after surgical repair of coarctation of the aorta. Am J Cardiol 43, 253–258.

177. Kappetein PA, Guit GL, Bogers AJJC, *et al.* (1993) Noninvasive long-term follow-up after coarctation repair. Ann Thorac Surg 55, 1153–1159.

178. Therrien J, Thorne SA, Wright A, *et al.* (2000) Repaired coarctation: a "cost-effective" approach to identify complications in adults. J Am Coll Cardiol 35, 997–1002.

179. Foster ED. (1984) Reoperation for aortic coarctation. Ann Thorac Surg 38, 81–89.

180. Sweeney MS, Walker WE, Duncan JM, *et al.* (1985) Reoperation for aortic coarctation: techniques, results, and indications for various approaches. Ann Thorac Surg 40, 46–49.

181. Connolly HM, Schaff HV, Izhar U, *et al.* (2001) Posterior pericardial ascending-to-descending aortic bypass: an alternative surgical approach for complex coarctation of the aorta. Circulation 104, I133–I137.

182. Kron IL, Flanagan TL, Rheuban KS, *et al.* (1990) Incidence and risk of reintervention after coarctation repair. Ann Thorac Surg 49, 920–926.

183. Sakopoulos AG, Hahn TL, Turrentine M, *et al.* (1998) Recurrent aortic coarctation: is surgical repair still the gold standard? J Thorac Cardiovasc Surg 116, 560–565.

184. Jacob T, Cobanoglu A, Starr A. (1988) Late results of ascending aorta-descending aorta bypass grafts for recurrent coarctation of the aorta. J Thorac Cardiovasc Surg 95, 782–787.

185. Kanter KR, Erez E, Williams WH, *et al.* (2000) Extra-anatomic aortic bypass via sternotomy for complex aortic arch stenosis. J Thorac Cardiovasc Surg 120, 885–890.

186. Beekman RH, Rocchini AP, Behrendt DM, *et al.* (1981) Reoperation for coarctation of the aorta. Am J Cardiol 48, 1108–1114.

CHAPTER 15

Interrupted Aortic Arch

Richard A. Jonas

Children's National Medical Center, Washington, DC, USA

Introduction

Interrupted aortic arch (IAA) is a rare abnormality that accounts for approximately 1.5% of all congenital heart anomalies [1]. It is a fascinating example of the role that apoptosis plays in both normal and abnormal development. Apoptosis is usually responsible for resorption of most of the original six branchial arches in the embryo. However, when it occurs in excess, apoptosis can interrupt the aortic arch [2,3]. Although early mortality for primary one-stage surgical repair is now relatively low in centers managing large volumes of neonates, there is a frequent association with underdevelopment of left-sided structures that can result in the need for late reintervention, particularly for subaortic stenosis. Previous controversy regarding one-stage versus two-stage repair and the role of direct anastomosis versus interposition graft have largely subsided in favor of one-stage, direct anastomotic repair. However, new controversy has emerged regarding the role of selective cerebral perfusion in protecting the brain during repair. Developmental studies to resolve this controversy will be complicated by the important association of IAA with microdeletion of chromosome 22, which has important implications for cognitive development.

Pathologic Anatomy of the Aortic Arch

The arch of the aorta has a proximal component, the proximal aortic arch, and extends from the takeoff of the innominate artery to the left common carotid artery. The distal component, the distal aortic arch, extends from the left common carotid artery to the takeoff of the left subclavian artery. The segment of aorta that connects the distal aortic arch to the juxtaductal region of the descending aorta is termed the *isthmus* (Figure 15.1) [4]. In the embryo, these different segments are derived from different components: the proximal arch is derived from the *aortic sac*, the distal arch from the *fourth embryonic arch*, and the isthmus from the junction of the *sixth embryonic arch* (ductus) with the left dorsal aorta and fourth embryonic arch.

A useful classification of IAA was introduced by Celoria and Patton in 1959 (Figure 15.2) [5,6]. Type A interruption occurs at the level of the isthmus. It is often seen in a milder form in which a short fibrous chord connects across the interruption even though there is no luminal continuity. This has been termed aortic arch *atresia* and generally represents less of a surgical challenge than a long segment complete discontinuity.

Type B interruption occurs between the left common carotid artery and the left subclavian artery. It is the most common type seen. In a review of the experience at Children's Hospital Boston between 1974 and 1987 by Sell *et al.*, 69% of the 71 patients had type B interruption [7]. In a more recent multi-institutional study by the Congenital Heart Surgeon's Society (CHSS) [8], updated in 2005 [9], 70% of 468 neonates with IAA and associated ventricular septal defect (VSD) had type B interruption. Type B interruption is often associated with an aberrant origin of the right subclavian artery from the descending aorta. This is important because in this subtype, more flow must pass through the ductus arteriosus during fetal development and less flow through the left ventricular outflow tract and ascending aorta than with the standard type B interruption, with normal origin of the right subclavian from the innominate artery. Thus, it is not surprising to find that the risk of subaortic stenosis is increased when the right subclavian artery arises aberrantly.

Type C interruption occurs between the innominate artery takeoff and left common carotid. It is extremely rare, having been described in less than 4% of most large clinical

Pediatric Cardiac Surgery, Fourth Edition. Edited by Constantine Mavroudis and Carl L. Backer.
© 2013 Blackwell Publishing Ltd. Published 2013 by Blackwell Publishing Ltd.

and pathologic series. There were seven cases among the 468 patients with IAA reviewed by the CHSS [9].

Associated Anomalies

Isolated IAA is exceedingly rare. Apart from patent ductus arteriosus (PDA), a single VSD is the most common associ-

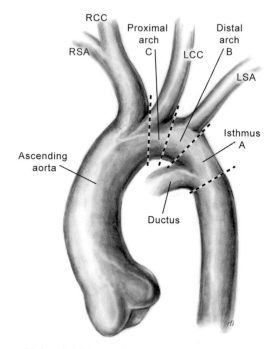

Figure 15.1 Helpful terminology for the segments of the aortic arch include *proximal arch* for the segment between the innominate artery and left common carotid artery (C), *distal arch* for the segment between the left common carotid and left subclavian arteries (B), and *isthmus* for the segment between the left subclavian artery and the ductus arteriosus (A). (LCC, left common carotid artery; LSA, left subclavian artery; RCC, right common carotid artery; RSA, right subclavian artery.)

ated anomaly. In a CHSS study, 72% of 472 patients had an isolated VSD as the only associated anomaly [9]. There is frequently posterior malalignment of the conal septum relative to the ventricular septum, which contributes to left ventricular outflow tract obstruction (LVOTO) [10]. Other anatomic features that may contribute to LVOTO include the aortic annulus itself, which is usually at least moderately hypoplastic. The aortic valve is frequently bicuspid, and there may be commissural fusion. Opposite the septum, there may be a prominent muscle bundle on the left ventricular free wall that projects into the outflow tract, the so-called "muscle of Moulaert" (Kreutzer J and Jonas R, unpublished observations). A fibrous subaortic membrane is almost never seen in the neonate with IAA but sometimes develops within a year or two of repair.

An atrial septal defect is frequently seen in conjunction with IAA. This is usually in the form of a stretched patent foramen ovale but can be quite large and therefore hemodynamically important. Perhaps this is caused by the left-to-right shunt that occurs during *in utero* development because of the left-sided obstruction that results from the interruption itself as well as associated LVOTO.

There are other anomalies seen in association with IAA (Table 15.1) [9]. Various forms of single ventricle are seen in 3% of patients with IAA and truncus arteriosus is seen in 11%.

Pathophysiology and Clinical Features

Prenatal diagnosis by ultrasound is becoming increasingly common. Prostaglandin E1 (PGE$_1$) is started immediately after birth, and an acidotic insult is avoided. For the patient who is not diagnosed prenatally with the most common form of IAA (an associated PDA and posterior malalignment VSD) there may be little suspicion of serious heart disease during the early neonatal period until ductal closure begins. If that should occur abruptly or is not recognized rapidly, the child will soon become profoundly

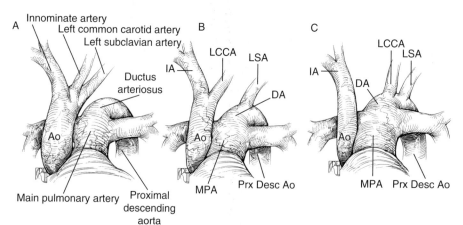

Figure 15.2 Anatomic types of interrupted aortic arch. **A,** Type A, interruption distal to the left subclavian artery. **B,** Type B, interruption between the left subclavian and left carotid arteries. **C,** Type C, interruption between the left carotid and innominate artery. (Ao, aorta; DA, ductus arteriosus, IA, innominate artery; LCCA, left common carotid artery; LSA, left subclavian artery; MPA, main pulmonary artery; Prx Desc Ao, proximal descending aorta.)

Table 15.1 Major cardiac anomalies associated with interrupted aortic arch in the most recent report from the Congenital Heart Surgeons Society. (VSD, ventricular septal defect.) (Reproduced with permission from McCrindle *et al.* [9].)

Variable	No.	Missing	Value	Deaths (n = 186)
None – isolated VSD	472	0	341 (72%)	121 (35%)
None – intact ventricular septum	472	0	7 (1%)	2 (29%)
Aortopulmonary window	472	0	20 (4%)	3 (15%)
Complete atrioventricular septal defect	472	0	3 (<1%)	3 (100%)
Atrioventricular discordance	472	0	2 (<1%)	1 (50%)
Double-outlet right ventricle	472	0	8 (2%)	4 (50%)
Partial anomalous pulmonary venous return	472	0	1 (<1%)	1 (100%)
Single ventricle	472	0	13 (3%)	9 (69%)
Transposition of great arteries with VSD	472	0	26 (6%)	9 (35%)
Truncus arteriosus	472	0	51 (11%)	34 (67%)
Bicuspid aortic valve	229	243	149 (65%)	57 (38%)
Anomalous right subclavian artery	427	45	108 (25%)	45 (42%)
Left superior vena cava	440	32	35 (8%)	19 (54%)
Large patent ductus arteriosus	281	191	251 (89%)	94 (37%)
Large VSD	392	80	322 (82%)	123 (38%)
Multiple VSDs	383	89	31 (8%)	14 (45%)
Malalignment of VSD	472	0	165 (35%)	74 (32%)

acidotic and anuric as perfusion of the lower body becomes entirely dependent on collateral communications between the two separate aortic systems. The distribution of palpable pulses will depend on the anatomical subtype. For example, with the common type B IAA, the right arm pulse will be palpable when the left arm pulse and femoral pulses become impalpable secondary to ductal closure. Ischemic injury to the liver will be reflected in a marked elevation of hepatic enzymes (serum glutamic oxaloacetic transaminase [SGOT] and lactic acid dehydrogenase [LDH]), and ischemic injury to the gut may be followed by evidence of necrotizing enterocolitis, such as bloody stools. Renal injury can be quantitated to some extent by the elevation observed in serum creatinine.

A very severe degree of systemic acidosis (prolonged pH < 7.0) will ultimately result in injury to all tissues of the body, including the brain and the heart itself. The child may have seizures and become flaccid and poorly responsive. Myocardial injury will be apparent in the form of a low cardiac output state despite normalization of parameters. Since pulmonary blood flow is preserved during ductal closure, it is rare to see evidence of pulmonary insufficiency.

Occasionally the ductus will not close during the neonatal period, and diagnosis may be delayed for several weeks. As pulmonary resistance falls, there will be an increasing left-to-right shunt, and the child will present with evidence of congestive heart failure, including failure to thrive.

Historical Perspective

Interrupted aortic arch was first described by Steidele in 1778 [11]. Celoria and Patton reported their anatomical classification in 1959 [5]. Successful surgical repair was first described by Merrill *et al.* in 1955 in a patient with short segment type A IAA [12]. A direct anastomosis was possible; however, the associated VSDs were not closed at the time of the arch repair. One-stage repair was first accomplished by Barratt-Boyes [13]. In the procedure he described, arch continuity was established using a synthetic conduit. One-stage repair, including direct arch anastomosis, was first described by Trusler in 1975 [14]. Interrupted aortic arch carried an extremely high mortality risk until the introduction of PGE$_1$ by Elliott *et al.* in 1976 [15]. Over the next 5–10 years, it became apparent that careful resuscitation of the neonate, often over a time span of days, before proceeding to surgery was associated with a dramatic improvement in surgical outcome (Figure 15.3) [6,7]. The concept of selective cerebral perfusion to minimize or eliminate the use of circulatory arrest has been described by many authors including Sakurada *et al.* and Asou *et al.* in 1996 [16,17].

Diagnosis of Interrupted Aortic Arch

Anatomy

Accurate anatomic diagnosis can currently be made using echocardiography alone. This is an important advantage to

A

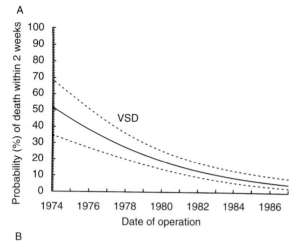

B

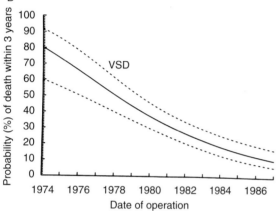

Figure 15.3 Results of surgery for interrupted aortic arch with ventricular septal defect according to year of operation at Children's Hospital, Boston, illustrating the remarkable effect of the introduction of prostaglandin E1 in the late 1970s. **A,** Probability of death within 2 weeks. **B,** Probability of death within 3 years. (VSD, ventricular septal defect.) (Reproduced with permission from Sell *et al.* [7].)

the neonate who presents in extremis and in whom invasive cardiac catheterization may be a serious additional insult. In addition to localizing the site of the interruption, the echocardiographer should provide the following information. The length of the discontinuity should be measured. The narrowest dimension of the left ventricular outflow tract (generally secondary to posterior displacement of the conal septum), the diameter of the aortic annulus, and the diameter of the ascending aorta should also be measured. It is unusual for segments of the arch that are present to be so hypoplastic that they cause hemodynamic compromise. The features of associated anomalies must be carefully defined. For example, the location of an associated VSD should be defined in relation to its margins. The conal septum is often severely hypoplastic, rendering approach to the superior margin of the defect through the

tricuspid valve particularly difficult. Additional VSDs are very rare. The presence or absence of the thymus can usually be ascertained by echocardiography. An absent thymus has important implications because of its association with microdeletion of chromosome 22 and DiGeorge syndrome.

Magnetic resonance angiography is emerging as a useful adjunct to echocardiography [18]. For uncomplicated cases of IAA with VSD, it would appear to have little advantage in the unrepaired neonate over echocardiography alone [19]. However, if there are important associated anomalies or unusual features (e.g., aortic atresia with hypoplastic ascending aorta and retrograde flow through the carotid arteries to the coronary circulation from the circle of Willis), it can be helpful [20].

Hemodynamic Assessment

Because diagnosis will generally be made when ductal patency has been re-established using PGE_1, pressure data will be of little use in formulating a plan for surgical management. The question that most commonly arises is the adequacy of the left ventricular outflow tract. Attempts to quantitate the degree of obstruction by measuring a pressure gradient are hampered by lack of information regarding the amount of flow passing through this area. The VSD will usually be nonrestrictive. There is no evidence that multiple VSDs are more accurately identified by angiography than by color flow Doppler echocardiography [21].

Management of Interrupted Aortic Arch

Medical and Interventional

The introduction of PGE_1 in 1976 revolutionized the management of IAA. Before this time, which also predated the introduction of two-dimensional echocardiography, it was necessary to manage acidotic neonates symptomatically as they underwent emergency cardiac catheterization and were then rushed from the catheterization laboratory to the operating room. Not surprisingly, few actually survived this sequence.

Prostaglandin E1 must be infused through a secure intravenous line. If ductal patency does not become apparent in any neonate younger than 1 week of age within 1 hour, it should be assumed until proven otherwise that there is a technical problem with delivery of the medication into the central bloodstream. Establishing ductal patency represents just the first step in medically resuscitating the neonate with IAA. Because the lower half of the body is dependent on perfusion through the ductus, and because blood in the ductus also has the choice of passing into the pulmonary circulation, it is important that pulmonary resistance be maximized. This can be achieved by avoiding a high level of inspired oxygen (usually room air is appropriate), as well as avoiding respiratory alkalosis caused by hyperventilation. In fact, control of ventilation is best achieved by intubating the neonate as well as sedating the child and inducing paralysis. A peak inspiratory pressure and ventilatory rate should be selected that will achieve a pCO_2 level of 40–50 mm. Metabolic acidosis should be aggressively treated with boluses of sodium bicarbonate, although care must be taken to avoid producing an overall alkalotic pH. Because myocardial function is likely to be depressed somewhat at the time of presentation, and it may be necessary for the heart to handle a moderate volume load (depending on the success with which pulmonary resistance is maximized), an inotropic agent such as dopamine is almost routinely employed. Dopamine has the added advantage of maximizing renal perfusion in this context of an ischemic renal insult. It is not uncommon to persist with medical resuscitation in the manner described for 1–2 days before surgery is undertaken. It should be very unusual that a child is taken to the operating room with any abnormalities of acid-base, renal, or hepatic indices [7].

Surgical Techniques: Interrupted Arch and Ventricular Septal Defect

The ideal method of surgical management has become less controversial over the last decade. There is now fairly widespread agreement that primary one-stage repair in the neonatal period is optimal management, although minor controversy persists regarding some of the details. Palliative options were commonly used in the past but are less frequently employed now as more units have become familiar with corrective neonatal surgery [22]. Noncorrective procedures include application of a pulmonary artery band during the neonatal period, with closure of the associated VSD at some time beyond infancy and usually before 5 years of age. Rather than a corrective direct anastomosis, arch continuity can be achieved by insertion of a synthetic conduit [23]. Both of these palliative options are generally undertaken working through a left thoracotomy, although some surgeons prefer to use a combined thoracotomy and sternotomy approach for placement of an ascending to descending aortic conduit. Our current preference is to undertake one-stage repair during the neonatal period including a direct aortic arch anastomosis [8].

During transport to the operating room and while preparing and positioning the child, it is important to maintain scrupulously the management principles that have been employed during the resuscitation of the child over the previous few days in the intensive care unit. In particular, a high level of inspired oxygen and hyperventilation must be avoided. In addition to the usual monitoring equipment, careful consideration must be given to monitoring arterial pressure. It is preferable to be able to measure blood pressure both above and below the forthcoming arch anastomosis. Often this is achieved by placing a right radial arterial line in addition to an umbilical arterial line. Not only does this allow one to immediately assess any pressure gradient across the anastomosis, but also the adequacy of perfusion of the separate upper and lower body circulation can be assessed during the cooling phase on cardiopulmonary bypass. Near infrared spectroscopy is also emerging as a useful technique, particularly with the application of two sensors, one for the brain and one for the lower body, either thigh or flank [24].

Approach is via a median sternotomy alone. If a thymus is present, it is largely excised. Pericardium is not usually harvested. Accurate arterial cannulation is an essential key to the success of the procedure. Although a single arterial cannula will usually ultimately achieve complete cooling, cannulation of both the ascending aorta and pulmonary artery optimize tissue perfusion, particularly of the brain and heart in the critical early phase of cooling when all organs are still warm. Generally an 8 or 6-Fr thin-walled wire-wrapped (e.g., Bio-Medicus®; Medtronic) arterial cannula is used for the ascending aorta. This cannula should be inserted on the right lateral aspect of the ascending aorta exactly opposite the anticipated location of the arch anastomosis (Figure 15.4) [4]. The tip of the cannula should not extend more than 1.5–2 mm into the lumen of the ascending aorta. This will decrease the chance that either retrograde flow to the coronary arteries or antegrade flow to the brain will be compromised. This is also an advantage of the 6-Fr cannula, although this cannula is too small to accommodate full flow in larger neonates (e.g., >3 kg) during the rewarming phase. The second arterial cannula is connected to the arterial tubing by a Y connector and is inserted in the anterior surface of the distal ductus. Because of the larger size of the main pulmonary artery relative to the ascending aorta (often 10–12 mm vs. 5–6 mm), a larger cannula (e.g., 8 Fr) can be employed. Immediately after beginning bypass, it is necessary to tie a suture ligature of 5/0 Prolene around the proximal ductus, as is done for the Norwood operation for hypoplastic left heart syndrome. Venous cannulation is routine, with a single straight cannula in the right atrium.

During cooling, the ascending aorta and its branches are thoroughly mobilized. The ductus and descending aorta are also mobilized to minimize tension on the arch anastomosis. If an aberrant right subclavian artery is present, it should be ligated and divided at its origin from the descending aorta. It is also often useful to divide the left subclavian artery in a type B interruption to further minimize anastomotic tension as well as simplifying the anastomosis, thereby decreasing the risk of bleeding and stenosis. When both rectal and tympanic temperatures are less than 18 °C, bypass is discontinued. Tourniquets are no

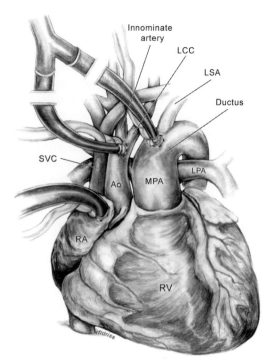

Figure 15.4 Arterial cannulation is a critically important component of the repair of interrupted aortic arch in the neonate. For type B interruption, two arterial cannulae are employed connected by a Y. Generally an 8-Fr thin-walled cannula is inserted into the small ascending aorta. The cannula should be positioned on the right side of the ascending aorta opposite the intended site of aortic anastomosis. A single venous cannula is placed in the right atrium. Either the branch pulmonary arteries are controlled with separate tourniquets or, alternatively, the second arterial cannula can be placed in the ductus and a ligature tightened around the proximal ductus immediately after commencing bypass. (Ao, aorta; LCC, left common carotid artery; LPA, left pulmonary artery; LSA, left subclavian artery; MPA, main pulmonary artery; RA, right atrium; RV, right ventricle; SVC, superior vena cava.)

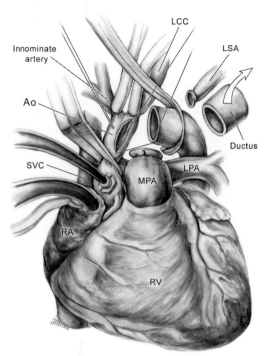

Figure 15.5 After the onset of hypothermic circulatory arrest, both arterial cannulae are removed. A cardioplegic cannula is noted with an aortic cross-clamp. The ductus is ligated proximally. Ductal tissue is excised up to the level of the descending aorta opposite the left subclavian artery. It may be helpful to divide the left subclavian artery to reduce tension on the arch anastomosis. The intended site of the anastomosis on the ascending aorta is indicated. A "C" clamp applied across the descending aorta is helpful in minimizing tension on the anastomosis as it is performed. (Ao, aorta; LCC, left common carotid artery; LPA, left pulmonary artery; LSA, left subclavian artery; MPA, main pulmonary artery; RA, right atrium; RV, right ventricle; SVC, superior vena cava.)

longer placed around the right and left common carotid arteries, as has become standard practice in adult aortic arch surgery where clamps and tourniquets are no longer used. Cardioplegia is infused through a sidearm on the ascending arterial connector, with temporary occlusion of the distal ascending aorta with forceps. Both arterial cannulae are then removed together with the venous cannula.

The ductus is ligated and divided at its junction with the descending aorta. Any residual ductal tissue is excised from the descending aorta. A C-clamp applied across the descending aorta helps to draw the ascending aorta to the level of the anastomosis, which can be performed with the opposing tissues under no tension (Figure 15.5) [4]. The anastomosis should be sited on the ascending aorta where tension will be minimized. Although many surgeons believe that this requires siting the anastomosis partially

on the left common carotid artery, some generally prefer to site the anastomosis completely on the ascending aorta. The anastomosis will be exactly opposite the ascending aortic cannulation site (Figure 15.6) [4]. Continuous absorbable polydioxanone 6-0 suture may be used, although there is no evidence that use of this suture results in a lower incidence of anastomotic stenosis. Many surgeons continue to prefer polypropylene suture, either 6/0 or 7/0. Its lesser tissue drag distributes tension more evenly through the suture line, which appears to enhance hemostasis. Data from the CHSS study supports not supplementing the anastomosis with a patch of pericardium or arterial allograft tissue when associated left heart obstruction is present, although this is practiced by some. One arterial cannula (the 6 or 8-Fr cannula, depending on the child's size) is carefully reinserted in the ascending aorta only before tying the anastomotic suture line. Aortic cross-clamped brachiocephalic vessel snuggers are preferred by

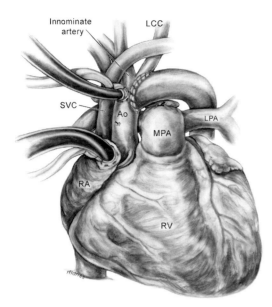

Figure 15.6 The ascending aortic cannula has been reinserted after carefully de-airing the aorta and arch vessels. A period of cold reperfusion of 5 minutes may be employed if a second period of hypothermic circulatory arrest is necessary for transatrial approach to the ventricular septal defect. However, commonly, the ventricular septal defect is approached through the main pulmonary artery, and bypass can be continued. (Ao, aorta; LCC, left common carotid artery; LPA, left pulmonary artery; MPA, main pulmonary artery; RA, right atrium; RV, right ventricle; SVC, superior vena cava.)

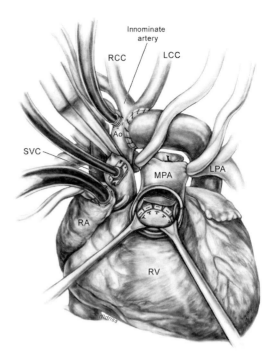

Figure 15.7 Because there is frequently severe hypoplasia of the conal septum the best approach for ventricular septal defect closure for interrupted aortic arch is often through a transverse incision in the main pulmonary artery. This can usually be performed with hypothermic bypass continuing. An aortic cross-clamp is usually applied to the ascending aorta during this period as illustrated. Vessel loops are placed to control bleeding from the left and right pulmonary arteries. (Ao, aorta; LCC, left common carotid artery; LPA, left pulmonary artery; MPA, main pulmonary artery; RA, right atrium; RV, right ventricle; SVC, superior vena cava.)

some authors (Figure 15.5) [4]. The author generally does not apply the cross-clamp on snuggers, preferring to perform the anastomosis without the instruments in the field. Trickle flow allows air to be displaced from the arch before the suture is tied. Bypass is recommenced at a flow rate of 50 mL/kg/min. Deep hypothermia is maintained.

The approach to the VSD will depend on the preoperative echocardiographic assessment that must be carefully viewed by the surgeon preoperatively. Frequently, there will be marked hypoplasia of the conal septum. In such cases, the optimal approach for VSD closure is via a transverse incision in the proximal main pulmonary artery immediately distal to the pulmonary valve (Figure 15.7) [4]. This approach has the advantage that bypass can be maintained with a single venous cannula in the right atrium. The VSD is closed in the routine fashion for a subpulmonary VSD [25]. At the superior margin, sutures are passed through the pulmonary annulus, with the pledgets lying above the pulmonary valve leaflets. Although this has the potential to distort the pulmonary valve, thereby excluding its use for a Ross procedure, there is at least one report of a successful Ross procedure after transpulmonary approach to the VSD [26].

A preoperative decision should be made regarding the need to close an atrial septal defect, which will be present in most patients. Because of the poor left-sided compliance that is often present with IAA with VSD, even a small atrial septal defect can result in a large left-to-right shunt postoperatively. The atrial septal defect can usually be closed by direct suture, working through a short low right atriotomy during a brief second period of circulatory arrest.

Routine monitoring lines (i.e., a left atrial and right atrial line) are placed during rewarming. Separating from bypass and early postoperative management should be uncomplicated because a biventricular repair has been achieved. If problems are encountered, a residual VSD or anastomotic stenosis must be excluded. It is unusual for LVOTO to result in hemodynamic compromise early after surgery.

Selective Cerebral Perfusion

It is usually possible to complete the dissection, mobilization, and anastomosis with a circulatory arrest time of little more than 20 minutes. With modern methods of circulatory arrest (i.e., hematocrit of at least 25, pH stat strategy, and a cooling time of at least 15–20 minutes), this is unlikely to lead to any detectable neurologic consequences. Nevertheless, many surgeons feel more comfortable and under less time pressure if they maintain flow to the brain using the technique of selective cerebral perfusion. Many different methods have been described, although probably the most popular involves direct cannulation of the innominate artery with tourniquet occlusion of the head vessels, including the innominate artery. A clamp is also required for the distal descending aorta to prevent a steal of flow from the head. One of the unresolved issues with this technique is how to decide on the optimal flow rate. Various formulas have been empirically applied, some of which include near infrared monitoring [27–29]. The only prospective randomized trial of selective cerebral perfusion failed to demonstrate any advantage over circulatory arrest, with a trend toward a worse outcome [30].

Interrupted Aortic Arch with VSD and LVOTO

Occasionally, LVOTO in the neonatal period may be sufficiently severe to justify a radical alternative primary procedure that has come to be known as the "Yasui procedure" [31]. The principle employed is analogous to the Damus-Kaye-Stansel procedure described for transposition (Figure 15.8) [6,8,31]. Left ventricular output is directed through the VSD by a baffle patch to the pulmonary artery. The main pulmonary artery is divided proximal to its bifurcation. The proximal divided main pulmonary artery is anastomosed to the side of the ascending aorta. A tube graft

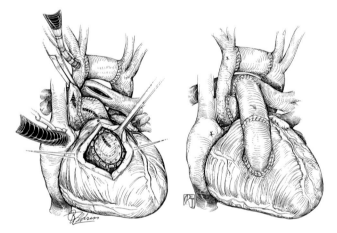

Figure 15.8 Modification of the Damus-Kaye-Stansel procedure described by Yasui *et al.* [31] for interrupted aortic arch with ventricular septal defect and very severe subaortic stenosis. This procedure carries a high mortality in the Congenital Heart Surgeons Society reports [8] and is rarely indicated.

bridges the arch interruption itself [31]. A conduit, preferably an aortic or pulmonary homograft or, more recently, a valved cryopreserved femoral vein, is placed between the right ventricle and the distal divided main pulmonary artery. Another variation of this theme is to supply pulmonary blood flow with a shunt following the pulmonary to aortic anastomosis and arch repair [32]. This is essentially a Norwood procedure with the addition of arch repair [33]. However, since two ventricles are present, it is difficult to recommend such a palliative procedure, although satisfactory results have been reported with this approach from centers very familiar with the Norwood procedure.

Interrupted Arch with Other Anomalies

The general principle should be applied that if two ventricles are present, a biventricular repair incorporating growth potential should be undertaken during the neonatal period. For example, the child with transposition of the great arteries, VSD and interrupted arch should undergo an arterial switch procedure with VSD closure and direct arch anastomosis. Although this complex procedure requires a long cross-clamp time, it is generally well tolerated so long as an accurate repair is achieved [34]. Transfer of the aorta posteriorly as part of the arterial switch in fact helps to reduce tension on the arch anastomosis. Various technical modifications have been proposed [35]. Similarly, with truncus arteriosus and interrupted arch, the large size of the truncus decreases the difficulty with which aortic cannulation is achieved relative to the child with simple interrupted arch where the ascending aorta is often very hypoplastic. An analysis of the results of surgery at Children's Hospital Boston suggests that IAA is no longer a risk factor for early death after repair of truncus with IAA in the current era [36].

Management of the child with a single functional ventricle and interrupted arch remains a significant challenge, presenting many of the same problems experienced with management of hypoplastic left heart syndrome, particularly when arch interruption is combined with aortic atresia and severe hypoplasia of the ascending aorta. There is frequently important obstruction present within the single ventricle when it is associated with IAA, often in the form of an obstructive bulboventricular foramen. This must either be bypassed using a pulmonary to aortic anastomosis (Damus-Kaye-Stansel; Norwood) or must be relieved by resection of the bulboventricular foramen. Residual arch obstruction is very poorly tolerated with either a shunt dependent circulation (after a pulmonary-aortic anastomosis) or a pulmonary artery band if bulboventricular foramen enlargement is undertaken. Such obstruction will result in excessive pulmonary blood flow unless the band itself is very tight. This creates a highly unstable situation.

Postoperative Management of Interrupted Aortic Arch

After biventricular repair of simple IAA with VSD, postoperative management should be routine. Failure to progress appropriately (e.g., minimal inotropic requirement within 24–48 hours and satisfactory progress toward extubation within 2–3 days, depending largely on preoperative status) should stimulate an aggressive search for residual hemodynamic lesions. A residual VSD should be excluded by oxygen saturation data collected from the pulmonary artery line on the first postoperative morning. An anastomotic gradient should have been excluded both intraoperatively and in the early postoperative period by appropriate blood pressure determination. Echocardiography, including intraoperative transesophageal echocardiography and, if there is any doubt, cardiac catheterization, can exclude important LVOTO. A left-to-right shunt at atrial level should also be excluded. If an important residual hemodynamic lesion is identified, the child should be expeditiously returned to the operating room for correction of the problem.

Results of Surgery

Dramatic improvement in both early and late results of surgery for IAA with VSD occurred at Children's Hospital Boston between 1974 and 1987 (Figure 15.3) [6,7]. The risk of death within 2 weeks of surgery in 1974 was greater than 50%, and by 1987, the risk was less than 10%. There were many changes in the management of neonates during this timeframe that may have contributed to this improvement. Our analysis in 1988 did not conclusively demonstrate that one-stage repair during the neonatal period or that direct arch anastomosis rather than placement of a conduit contributed to the reduction in mortality. This was also the case in the analysis by the CHSS in 1994 [8], as well as a more recent report by Brown et al. [22]. Nevertheless, current results and recent reports from large neonatal centers have encouraged an approach of one-stage direct anastomotic repair because of the multiple psychosocial, economic, and logistical advantages [37–39]. Furthermore, the most recent analysis by the CHSS demonstrated that techniques other than direct anastomosis are associated with a higher risk of reintervention [9].

Complications of Surgery

Early

Potential technical complications have been enumerated above. In addition, bleeding can be troublesome. Bleeding is more likely if the arch anastomosis is performed under excessive tension, which will usually be the result of inad- equate mobilization of the ascending and descending aorta. Extreme friability of tissue also contributes to the risk of bleeding. Friability can be associated with prematurity and can result from severe preoperative acidosis but is also apparent if ductal tissue is incorporated in the anastomosis. Including ductal tissue presumably also increases the risk of late anastomotic stenosis. As with all neonatal surgery, hemostasis must be accelerated by appropriate use of blood replacement, with fresh blood representing the optimal choice. In the absence of fresh blood, judicious but nevertheless aggressive transfusion of concentrated factors, including cryoprecipitate as well as platelet concentrates, is indicated. The selection of an appropriate perfusion hematocrit is also an important factor in achieving rapid hemostasis. Crystalloid hemodilution to 20% can result in inadequate levels of fibrinogen and other coagulation factors. Both conventional and modified ultrafiltration have roles to play in maintaining an ideal hematocrit. Aprotinin has been widely and effectively used to optimize hemostasis. However, the possibility of renal failure in adults raised the concern of the manufacturer and hospitals that this might be duplicated in neonates. New drugs are being developed to simulate the beneficial properties of aprotinin without the significant side effects. Lysine analogues, such as tranexamic acid, are less effective than aprotinin.

Both the left recurrent laryngeal and phrenic nerves are at risk during repair of IAA. Phrenic nerve injury is particularly common after placement of an ascending to descending aortic conduit, despite meticulous care of the nerve itself. It is speculated that direct compression of the nerve by the synthetic material may be the cause of this problem. Phrenic nerve palsy has been rare after direct arch anastomosis.

Late

Pressure Gradient Across Arch

Ultimately all patients who have a tube graft inserted during the neonatal period will develop obstruction (defined as a pressure gradient >30 mmHg) across the graft secondary to somatic growth alone. In addition, synthetic grafts have a variable rate of accumulation of a pseudointima that may accelerate the rate of obstruction. The actuarial freedom from tube graft obstruction in our early experience was 55% by 5 years [7]. In contrast, patients who had a direct arch anastomosis were more likely to have obstruction, with only 40% having less than a 30 mm gradient within 18 months of surgery [7]. However, balloon dilation can successfully relieve such gradients in most children who have had a direct arch anastomosis, and conduit replacement is inevitable for those with conduits. In the earlier analysis by the CHSS, the freedom from reintervention for arch obstruction was approximately

86% at 3 years for patients who had undergone a direct anastomosis, with a trend to a higher rate of reintervention for those patients who had undergone some form of arch reconstruction, including placement of a tube graft ($p = 0.15$) [8]. This also held true in the more recent analysis [9]. It is likely that the lower rate of reintervention in the more recent timeframe reflects increasing familiarity with wide mobilization of the ascending aorta, arch vessels, and the descending aorta.

LVOTO

The large CHSS experience suggested that performance of conal septal resection or performance of a pulmonary to aortic (Damus-Kaye-Stansel) anastomosis during the neonatal period carries a greater risk of early death than simple repair [8]. This is true by multivariate analysis of either the entire group or by analysis of just the subgroup with important left heart hypoplasia in addition to IAA. It is important to remember, however, that this report describes a multi-institutional experience in which there was a very wide range of patient volume and outcomes. Reports by Jacobs *et al.* [40] and Suzuki *et al.* [41] suggest that the Norwood procedure or conal septal resection can be performed with an acceptable mortality but probably should not be attempted at centers unfamiliar with these approaches. Another approach described by Luciani *et al.* [42] involves anchoring VSD sutures on the left side of the conal septum, thereby resulting in a rightward shift of the posteriorly displaced septum when the left ventricle is pressurized (Figure 15.9) [6]. There is no evidence, however, that this approach has any advantage from this perspective than the usual placement of sutures on the right side of the conal septum.

Although LVOTO is rarely sufficiently severe to justify an alteration in surgical strategy during the neonatal reparative procedure, it is by contrast not uncommon for surgical intervention to be required for LVOTO late postoperatively [10]. Among 33 patients reviewed by Sell *et al.* who underwent repair of a conoventricular VSD as the only associated anomaly with IAA, only 58% were free of evident LVOTO (defined as a gradient of greater than 40 mm) by 3 years postoperatively [7]. In the initial CHSS report, 77% were free from reintervention at 3 years. Since the morphology of LVOTO with IAA is variable, surgical management for LVOTO beyond the neonatal period will vary according to the specific circumstances. In some cases, it is possible to resect the posteriorly deviated conal septum working through the aortic valve. An aortic valvotomy may also be required if there is valvar stenosis. If there is tunnel subaortic stenosis, we perform a modified Konno procedure (i.e., ventricular septoplasty) [43]. Working through a right ventricular infundibular incision, an incision is made in the ventricular septum into the left ventricular outflow tract. The incision is carried up to the aortic

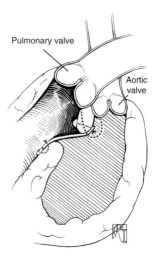

Figure 15.9 Technique of one-stage repair of interrupted aortic arch with ventricular septal defect and posteriorly malaligned conal septum. The technique involves (1) tailoring the patch to the shape of the ventricular septal defect but downsizing its area to avoid bulging toward the left ventricular outflow tract, and (2) positioning the stitches relative to the apical portion of the ventricular septal defect patch on the left side of the conal septum to promote deflection of the displaced septum (dashed line) away from the left ventricular outflow tract.

valve. A patch is placed on the right ventricular aspect of the surgically created VSD. If there is also aortic annular hypoplasia as well as tunnel subaortic stenosis, our current approach is to perform a Ross/Konno procedure (i.e., placement of a pulmonary autograft in the aortic position with an anterior incision into the ventricular septum). Alternative procedures used in the past include the Konno procedure and left ventricular apical to descending aortic conduit [44]. There is little place for the latter procedure today.

DiGeorge Syndrome

Absence or severe hypoplasia of the thymus was commonly seen in the Children's Hospital Boston series with IAA but was limited to patients with type B interruption [7]. Comprehensive testing of lymphocyte function was undertaken in only a small number of patients so that no concrete inferences can be drawn regarding the incidence of the complete syndrome. Although a large calcium requirement is often seen during the early postoperative period, it is rarely necessary for children to leave the hospital receiving oral calcium supplements (fortunately, because these are often poorly tolerated). Occasionally vitamin D supplements are useful to maintain serum calcium levels during the first few postoperative weeks. We are not aware that serious problems with immune function have been encountered among long-term survivors of IAA surgery. The association of IAA with microdeletion of chromosome 22 should be tested by fluorescence in situ hybridization (FISH) analysis. There are important implications for the developmental potential with respect to both cognitive and motor abilities of affected children [45].

Left Bronchial Obstruction

The left main bronchus usually passes under the arch of the aorta. If a direct anastomosis is performed without adequate mobilization, a bowstring effect over the left main bronchus may result. This will cause air trapping in the left lung with hyperexpansion seen on plain chest X-ray. The diagnosis can be confirmed by bronchoscopy together with computed tomography scan or magnetic resonance imaging. Surgical management may entail placement of an ascending to descending aortic conduit after division of the arch. With adequate initial mobilization of the ascending and descending aorta, this should almost never be necessary.

Conclusion

Prostaglandin E1 revolutionized the management of IAA in the late 1970s. Complete resuscitation should proceed over several days, if necessary, before surgery is undertaken. One-stage primary neonatal repair with direct arch anastomosis and VSD closure is the preferred surgical approach. Selective cerebral perfusion with near infrared monitoring is being used with increasing frequency. Although repair of interrupted arch is physiologically corrective, it should not be viewed as fully corrective because of the high incidence of important LVOTO. This may respond to a simple surgical reintervention such as subaortic resection, but in some cases an extensive procedure to enlarge the left ventricular outflow tract will be necessary. However, procedures directed against subaortic stenosis should rarely, if ever, be employed as part of the initial surgical management during the neonatal period.

References

1. Collins-Nakai RL, Dick M, Parisi-Buckley L, *et al.* (1976) Interrupted aortic arch in infancy. J Pediatr 88, 959–962.
2. Molin DG, DeRuiter MC, Wisse LJ, *et al.* (2002) Altered apoptosis pattern during pharyngeal arch artery remodelling is associated with aortic arch malformations in Tgfbeta2 knock-out mice. Cardiovasc Res 56, 312–322.
3. Poelmann RE, Gittenberger-de Groot AC. (2005) Apoptosis as an instrument in cardiovascular development. Birth Defects Res C Embryo Today 75, 305–313.
4. Jonas RA. (2004) *Comprehensive Surgical Management of Congenital Heart Disease.* London: Hodder Arnold, An Hachette UK Company.
5. Celoria GC, Patton RB. (1959) Congenital absence of the aortic arch. Am Heart J 58, 407–413.
6. Jonas RA. (2003) Interrupted aortic arch. In: Mavroudis C, Backer CL, eds. *Pediatric Cardiac Surgery*, 3rd ed. Philadelphia, PA: Mosby Inc.
7. Sell JE, Jonas RA, Mayer JE, *et al.* (1988) The results of a surgical program for interrupted aortic arch. J Thorac Cardiovasc Surg 96, 864–877.
8. Jonas RA, Quaegebeur JM, Kirklin JW, *et al.* (1994) Outcomes in patients with interrupted aortic arch and ventricular septal defect. A multiinstitutional study. Congenital Heart Surgeons Society. J Thorac Cardiovasc Surg 107, 1099–1109; discussion 1109–1113.
9. McCrindle BW, Tchervenkov CI, Konstantinov IE, *et al.* (2005) Risk factors associated with mortality and interventions in 472 neonates with interrupted aortic arch: a Congenital Heart Surgeons Society study. J Thorac Cardiovasc Surg 129, 343–350.
10. Jonas RA, Sell JE, Van Praagh R. (1989) Left ventricular outflow obstruction associated with interrupted aortic arch and ventricular septal defect. In: Crupi G, Parenzan L, Anderson RH, eds. *Perspectives in Pediatric Cardiology*, Vol 2. Pediatric Cardiac Surgery. Part 2. New York: Futura.
11. Steidele RJ. (1778) Samml Chir u Med Beob (Vienna). 2, 114.
12. Merrill DL, Webster CA, Samson PC. (1957) Congenital absence of the aortic isthmus; report of a case with successful surgical repair. J Thorac Surg 33, 311–320.
13. Barratt-Boyes BG, Nicholls TT, Brandt PW, *et al.* (1972) Aortic arch interruption associated with patent ductus arteriosus, ventricular septal defect, and total anomalous pulmonary venous connection. Total correction in an 8-day-old infant by means of profound hypothermia and limited cardiopulmonary bypass. J Thorac Cardiovasc Surg 63, 367–373.
14. Trusler GA, Izukawa T. (1975) Interrupted aortic arch and ventricular septal defect. Direct repair through a median sternotomy incision in a 13-day-old infant. J Thorac Cardiovasc Surg 69, 126–131.
15. Elliott RB, Starling MB, Neutze JM. (1975) Medical manipulation of the ductus arteriosus. Lancet 1, 140–142.
16. Asou T, Kado H, Imoto Y, *et al.* (1996) Selective cerebral perfusion technique during aortic arch repair in neonates. Ann Thorac Surg 61, 1546–1548.
17. Sakurada T, Kazui T, Tanaka H, *et al.* (1996) Comparative experimental study of cerebral protection during aortic arch reconstruction. Ann Thorac Surg 61, 1348–1354.
18. Dillman JR, Yarram SG, D'Amico AR, *et al.* (2008) Interrupted aortic arch: spectrum of MRI findings. AJR Am J Roentgenol 190, 1467–1474.
19. Roche KJ, Krinsky G, Lee VS, *et al.* (1999) Interrupted aortic arch: diagnosis with gadolinium-enhanced 3D MRA. J Comput Assist Tomogr 23, 197–202.
20. Tannous HJ, Moulick AN, Jonas RA. (2006) Interrupted aortic arch and aortic atresia with circle of Willis-dependent coronary perfusion. Ann Thorac Surg 82, e11–e13.
21. Spevak PJ, Mandell VS, Colan SD, *et al.* (1993) Reliability of Doppler color flow mapping in the identification and localization of multiple ventricular septal defects. Echocardiography 10, 573–581.
22. Brown JW, Ruzmetov M, Okada Y, *et al.* (2006) Outcomes in patients with interrupted aortic arch and associated

anomalies: a 20-year experience. Eur J Cardiothorac Surg 29, 666–673; discussion 673–674.

23. Mainwaring RD, Lamberti JJ. (1997) Mid- to long-term results of the two-stage approach for type B interrupted aortic arch and ventricular septal defect. Ann Thorac Surg 64, 1782–1785; discussion 1785-1786.

24. Berens RJ, Stuth EA, Robertson FA, *et al.* (2006) Near infrared spectroscopy monitoring during pediatric aortic coarctation repair. Paediatr Anaesth 16, 777–781.

25. Castaneda AR, Jonas RA, Mayer JE, *et al.* (1994) *Cardiac Surgery of the Neonate and Infant.* Philadelphia, PA: Saunders.

26. Luciani GB, Starnes VA. (1998) Pulmonary autograft after repair of interrupted aortic arch, ventricular septal defect, and subaortic stenosis. J Thorac Cardiovasc Surg 115, 266–267.

27. Dahlbacka S, Alaoja H, Makela J, *et al.* (2007) Effects of pH management during selective antegrade cerebral perfusion on cerebral microcirculation and metabolism: alpha-stat versus pH-stat. Ann Thorac Surg 84, 847–855.

28. Minatoya K, Ogino H, Matsuda H, *et al.* (2008) Evolving selective cerebral perfusion for aortic arch replacement: high flow rate with moderate hypothermic circulatory arrest. Ann Thorac Surg 86, 1827–1831.

29. Takeda Y, Asou T, Yamamoto N, *et al.* (2005) Arch reconstruction without circulatory arrest in neonates. Asian Cardiovasc Thorac Ann 13, 337–340.

30. Goldberg CS, Bove EL, Devaney EJ, *et al.* (2007) A randomized clinical trial of regional cerebral perfusion versus deep hypothermic circulatory arrest: outcomes for infants with functional single ventricle. J Thorac Cardiovasc Surg 133, 880–887.

31. Yasui H, Kado H, Nakano E, *et al.* (1987) Primary repair of interrupted aortic arch and severe aortic stenosis in neonates. J Thorac Cardiovasc Surg 93, 539–545.

32. Sinha P, Talwar S, Moulick A, *et al.* (2010) Right ventricular outflow tract reconstruction using a valved femoral vein homograft. J Thorac Cardiovasc Surg 139, 226–228.

33. Ilbawi MN, Idriss FS, DeLeon SY, *et al.* (1988) Surgical management of patients with interrupted aortic arch and severe subaortic stenosis. Ann Thorac Surg 45, 174–180.

34. Wernovsky G, Mayer JE Jr, Jonas RA, *et al.* (1995) Factors influencing early and late outcome of the arterial switch operation for transposition of the great arteries. J Thorac Cardiovasc Surg 109, 289–301; discussion 302.

35. Liddicoat JR, Reddy VM, Hanley FL. (1994) New approach to great-vessel reconstruction in transposition complexes with interrupted aortic arch. Ann Thorac Surg 58, 1146–1150.

36. Jahangiri M, Zurakowski D, Mayer JE, *et al.* (2000) Repair of the truncal valve and associated interrupted arch in neonates with truncus arteriosus. J Thorac Cardiovasc Surg 119, 508–514.

37. Kobayashi M, Ando M, Wada N, *et al.* (2009) Outcomes following surgical repair of arotic arch obstructions with associated cardiac anomalies. Eur J Cardiothorac Surg 35, 565–568.

38. Oosterhof T, Azakie A, Freedom RM, *et al.* (2004) Associated factors and trends in outcomes of interrupted aortic arch. Ann Thorac Surg 78, 1696–1702.

39. Schreiber C, Eicken A, Vogt M, *et al.* (2000) Repair of interrupted aortic arch: results after more than 20 years. Ann Thorac Surg 70, 1896–1899; discussion 1899–1900.

40. Jacobs ML, Chin AJ, Rychik J, *et al.* (1995) Interrupted aortic arch. Impact of subaortic stenosis on management and outcome. Circulation 92, II128–II131.

41. Suzuki T, Ohye RG, Devaney EJ, *et al.* (2006) Selective management of the left ventricular outflow tract for repair of interrupted aortic arch with ventricular septal defect: management of left ventricular outflow tract obstruction. J Thorac Cardiovasc Surg 131, 779–784.

42. Luciani GB, Ackerman RJ, Chang AC, *et al.* (1996) One-stage repair of interrupted aortic arch, ventricular septal defect, and subaortic obstruction in the neonate: a novel approach. J Thorac Cardiovasc Surg 111, 348–358.

43. Jahangiri M, Nicholson IA, del Nido PJ, *et al.* (2000) Surgical management of complex and tunnel-like subaortic stenosis. Eur J Cardiothorac Surg 17, 637–642.

44. Konno S, Imai Y, Iida Y, *et al.* (1975) A new method for prosthetic valve replacement in congenital aortic stenosis associated with hypoplasia of the aortic valve ring. J Thorac Cardiovasc Surg 70, 909–917.

45. Rauch A, Hofbeck M, Leipold G, *et al.* (1998) Incidence and significance of 22q11.2 hemizygosity in patients with interrupted aortic arch. Am J Med Genet 78, 322–331.

CHAPTER 16

Atrial Septal Defect, Partial Anomalous Pulmonary Venous Connection, and Scimitar Syndrome

Carl L. Backer[1] and Constantine Mavroudis[2]

[1]Ann & Robert H. Lurie Children's Hospital of Chicago, formerly Children's Memorial Hospital, Chicago, IL, USA
[2]Florida Hospital for Children, Orlando, FL, USA

An atrial septal defect (ASD) is defined as an opening, or hole, in the interatrial septum. Ostium secundum ASD is one of the most common congenital heart defects to occur as an isolated lesion. ASD occurs in 1 in every 1500 births and represents 6–10% of all congenital heart defects. ASD is more frequent in females, by a 2:1 ratio. Surgical closure of an ASD was first performed in 1952 by F. John Lewis [1,2] at the University of Minnesota using hypothermia and inflow occlusion. Atrial septal defect was also the first congenital cardiac defect to be repaired using cardiopulmonary bypass. On May 6, 1953 John Gibbon [3] used the pump oxygenator that he had developed in his laboratory to close an atrial septal defect. Atrial septal defect was also the first intracardiac lesion to be successfully treated using percutaneous transcatheter techniques [4]. In fact, with advances in technology and the evolution of transcatheter techniques, the majority of ostium secundum ASDs are now closed in the catheterization laboratory rather than in the operating room.

Anatomy and Pathology

The normal intraatrial anatomy as viewed through the opened right atrium is illustrated in Figure 16.1 [5]. The normal atrial septum is made up of two components, the septum secundum and the septum primum. The septum secundum is the thick, rounded superior portion derived from the infolded atrial roof. The septum primum is the lower portion of the atrial septum and is usually a relatively thin flap. The septum primum extends superiorly and to the left of the limbus of the septum secundum, so that it will close the foramen ovale as a flap valve. Normally, the left atrial pressure exceeds right atrial (RA) pressure and causes physiologic closure of this opening over time. The foramen ovale, of course, is necessary for the shunting of blood *in utero* from the right to the left atrium when the lungs are not functioning. The other significant anatomic structures within the right atrium are the orifice of the coronary sinus and the eustachian valve, guarding the orifice of the inferior vena cava. The crista terminalis is a thickened portion of infolding of the lateral right atrial wall running from superior to inferior.

There are three main types of ASDs, the ostium secundum (80%), sinus venosus (10%), and ostium primum (10%) type defects. Because it is a phenotypic variation of an atrioventricular septal defect (AVSD), the label "ostium primum" should probably be replaced by "partial AVSD" or "partial AV canal." In the Congenital Heart Surgery Nomenclature and Database Project [6], three other types of ASDs were identified. These included the common atrium (single atrium), coronary sinus type (unroofed coronary sinus), and patent foramen ovale. An atrial septal defect can coexist with multiple other anomalies, both simple and complex.

Ostium Secundum Atrial Septal Defect

As illustrated in Figure 16.2 [5], this is an ASD confined to the region of the fossa ovalis. The etiology is a deficiency of the septum primum. The resulting defect varies in size from a small pinhole to a large opening with essentially no inferior rim.

Pediatric Cardiac Surgery, Fourth Edition. Edited by Constantine Mavroudis and Carl L. Backer.
© 2013 Blackwell Publishing Ltd. Published 2013 by Blackwell Publishing Ltd.

Sinus Venosus Atrial Septal Defect

Sinus venosus defects occur most commonly at the junction between the superior vena cava and the right atrium (Figure 16.3) [5]. They are posterior in the atrial septum and cranial to the superior limbic band. They are almost always associated with anomalous drainage of the right superior pulmonary vein. This vein (veins) tends to enter at the junction of the superior vena cava and right atrium, along the rightward margin of the ASD, as illustrated in Figure 16.3B [5]. Sometimes these veins drain directly into the superior vena cava, adjacent to the entrance of the azygos vein (Figure 16.3A) [5]. Rarely, sinus venosus defects occur adjacent to the inferior vena cava orifice, and the anomalous vein is the right inferior pulmonary vein. This defect is an anomalous venoatrial communication rather than an actual atrial septal defect, but results in a left-to-right shunt of blood at the atrial level. The defect is produced by anomalous pulmonary venous connections to the inferior vena cava with retention of the pulmonary venous connection

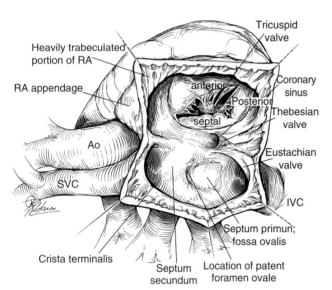

Figure 16.1 Normal intraatrial anatomy as viewed through the opened right atrium. (Ao, aorta; IVC, SVC, inferior, superior vena cava; RA, right atrium.)

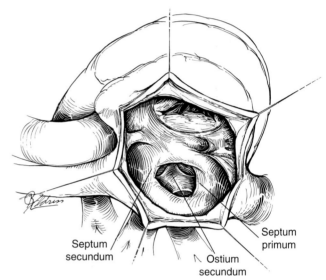

Figure 16.2 Ostium secundum atrial septal defect. This is the most common type of atrial septal defect, created by a deficiency in the septum primum.

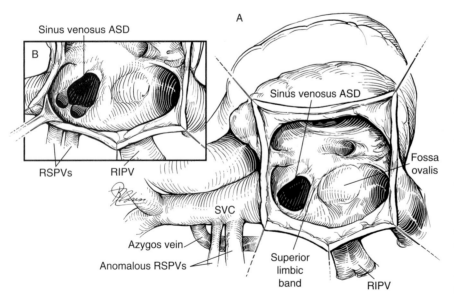

Figure 16.3 Sinus venosus ASD. **A,** The opening between the superior vena cava orifice and the superior limbic band is illustrated, with anomalous drainage of the right superior pulmonary veins directly to the superior vena cava, adjacent to the azygos vein. **B,** Another variant of sinus venosus defect is illustrated, showing the right superior pulmonary veins draining to the confluence of the superior vena cava and right atrium. (ASD, atrial septal defect; RIPV, right inferior pulmonary vein; RSPV, right superior pulmonary vein; SVC, superior vena cava.)

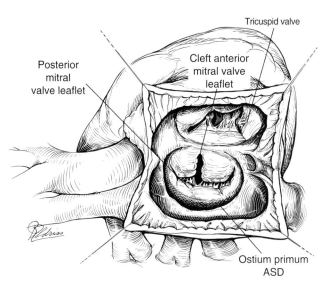

Figure 16.4 Partial atrioventricular canal defect or partial atrioventricular septal defect. These patients commonly have a cleft in the anterior leaflet of the mitral valve, as illustrated. (ASD, atrial septal defect.)

to the left atrium [7]. Anomalous drainage of the pulmonary veins to the right atrium can occur *without* an ASD.

Partial Atrioventricular Septal Defect

A partial atrioventricular septal defect (AVSD) defect is a crescent-shaped defect in the inferior portion of the atrial septum immediately adjacent to the atrioventricular valves (Figure 16.4) [5]. This was previously called an ostium primum ASD which is somewhat of a misnomer as it has nothing to do with the septum primum. Patients with a partial AVSD frequently have a cleft in the anterior leaflet of the mitral valve that may cause mitral valve insufficiency.

Common Atrium

Occasionally, the entire atrial septum will fail to develop and this will result in a "common atrium," or "single atrium." This is frequently found in patients with heterotaxy syndromes.

Patent Foramen Ovale

A patent foramen ovale is a small interatrial communication between the septum secundum and septum primum that is characterized by no deficiency of the septum primum and a normal limbus with no deficiency of the septum secundum. The flap of the patent foramen ovale is normally kept closed by the higher left atrial pressure. A true patent foramen ovale opens only when the right-sided pressure increases above that of the left, i.e., during coughing or Valsalva maneuver.

Unroofed Coronary Sinus

The coronary sinus is the confluence of the coronary veins draining the heart itself. A communication directly between the tube-like structure of the coronary sinus and the left atrium is called a coronary sinus ASD. This allows blood to shunt in an indirect fashion from the left atrium through the coronary sinus defect out of the actual coronary sinus and into the right atrium. Although there is no opening in the interatrial septum per se, the coronary sinus defect allows blood at the atrial level to shunt from left to right, physiologically exactly like an ASD that is a true opening in the atrial septum. These patients frequently have a left superior vena cava draining to the coronary sinus and that finding should be used as a "tip-off" to look for this defect. In some instances, the left superior vena cava may drain directly to the left atrium, which then causes an obligatory right-to-left shunt and cyanosis.

Pathophysiology and Natural History

The degree of left-to-right shunting at the atrial level is determined by the size of the ASD and the right and left ventricular compliance. Normally, the compliance of the left ventricle is less than that of the right ventricle, therefore there is a left-to-right shunt. This leads to right ventricular dilatation and excessive pulmonary blood flow. Patients with a large ASD can have a Qp/Qs ratio of greater than 4:1. There are very rare anatomic variations reported where a large persistent eustachian valve actually directs inferior vena caval blood flow through the ASD into the left atrium. These patients would then present with cyanosis. Patients with an unroofed coronary sinus and a left superior vena cava may also present with cyanosis. Finally, patients with a common atrium may have enough interatrial mixing of pulmonary and systemic venous return to cause a mild degree of cyanosis.

The natural history of an ASD has been determined by retrospective studies on patients who were not surgically repaired prior to the availability of surgical closure of ASDs. These patients are known to be at risk of atrial arrhythmias (most commonly, atrial flutter and atrial fibrillation), right ventricular dysfunction, pulmonary hypertension, paradoxical emboli, and eventual congestive heart failure. Without surgical intervention, the mean age of death in patients with a significant ASD is 36 years of age [8]. In young children, atrial septal defects larger than 8–10 mm in diameter are very unlikely to undergo spontaneous closure; defects smaller than 4–5 mm are reported to commonly undergo spontaneous closure [9,10]. Spontaneous closure occurring after the age of 4 years is very rare [11]. Bacterial endocarditis does not occur in patients with ostium secundum ASD unless they have an associated cardiovascular lesion. Of note, the existence of an isolated ASD is not an indication for prophylaxis of endocarditis, as per the American Heart Association guidelines [12].

Patients with an uncomplicated ASD typically do not have symptoms and present only with an audible murmur. The murmur typically has two components, a fixed split second heart sound related to the prolonged time period for flow of blood through the right side of the heart and delay of the pulmonary valve closure, and a systolic murmur of relative (physiologic) pulmonary stenosis. Patients with a large ASD may have a diastolic rumble secondary to relative (physiologic) tricuspid stenosis. The volume overload of the right ventricle and the pulmonary vascular bed is usually well tolerated for many years. There are only rare infants who develop congestive heart failure secondary to an uncomplicated atrial septal defect. The chance of developing obstructive pulmonary vascular disease is much less than for patients with ventricular septal defects or atrioventricular septal defects, however, it can occur in ASD patients. In a review of 169 adult patients with an ASD, pulmonary hypertension (defined as mean pulmonary artery pressure >30 mmHg) occurred in 10–25% of adults with an ASD and elevated pulmonary vascular resistance occurred in 5–15% of adults with an ASD [13]. Pulmonary hypertension was more common in adults with a sinus venosus ASD (16% of 31 patients) as compared to an ostium secundum ASD (4% of 138 patients). In these patients, the pulmonary vascular resistance may increase to a point where it is greater than the systemic vascular resistance. The intracardiac shunt will reverse (instead of left-to-right, right-to-left shunting occurs), and at that time surgical closure will be contraindicated [14]. The most common cause of late mortality in ASD patients is congestive heart failure and arrhythmias, which increase in frequency as the patient ages and in rough proportion to the shunt magnitude. In Murphy's review [15] of 123 patients undergoing repair of an ASD at the Mayo Clinic, the incidence of late atrial fibrillation was 4% if the ASD was closed before the age of 11, versus 55% if the ASD was closed after the age of 41.

Because of the known eventual complications of atrial arrhythmias, right ventricular dysfunction, and pulmonary hypertension, resulting in a dramatic reduction in life expectancy from congestive heart failure, closure of ASD is recommended. This can now be accomplished either with surgical or transcatheter techniques. Closure of an uncomplicated ASD is recommended in any patient with physical signs of an ASD or catheterization or echocardiographic evidence of a left-to-right shunt exceeding 1.5:1. In general,

patients with a significant ASD do not have a shunt less than 1.5:1 if they have physical findings of a significant systolic murmur and a fixed split second heart sound. In our series of 271 patients operated on between 1990 and 2009 at Children's Memorial Hospital for an ostium secundum defect, the median age at ASD closure was 3.3 years. Most centers prefer to electively close an ostium secundum ASD before a child starts school.

Diagnosis

Physical examination of a patient with an ASD typically reveals a fixed split second heart sound and a systolic murmur of relative physiologic pulmonary stenosis. There may also be a diastolic murmur or rumble of relative (physiologic) tricuspid stenosis. Chest X-ray evaluation will show cardiomegaly. When there is significantly increased pulmonary blood flow, there may be a bulging pulmonary artery at the upper left cardiac border. Electrocardiogram will demonstrate right ventricular hypertrophy. Typically, there is an rSr' or rsR' pattern in lead V_1 and right axis deviation. Of note, the appearance of left axis deviation on the electrocardiogram should alert the surgeon to the possible presence of a partial AVSD type of defect.

The most common and widely used diagnostic technique to definitively arrive at the diagnosis of ASD is two-dimensional echocardiography with color Doppler interrogation. The echocardiogram will visualize the defect in the atrial septum, estimate its size, and determine the location of the pulmonary veins. For patients with a partial AVSD, the degree of mitral insufficiency and evaluation of the mitral valve cleft can be obtained with color Doppler examination. In our series of patients with an ASD, less than 10% of the patients underwent cardiac catheterization and this percentage has dropped as the accuracy of echocardiographic techniques has improved. Cardiac catheterization is now only indicated when the diagnosis is uncertain or associated anomalies are suspected. Cardiac catheterization will reveal, on blood gas analysis, an oxygen step-up from the right atrium onward with a pulmonary blood flow typically two to four times the systemic flow. Quite commonly, there can be a gradient of 10–30 mmHg across the pulmonary valve because of the increased flow of blood through the right side. Pulmonary artery pressures are frequently normal unless pulmonary vascular obstructive disease has developed, usually only in older patients (over 20 years of age). Cardiac catheterization, computed tomographic (CT) scan, and magnetic resonance imaging (MRI) can be used to localize the pulmonary veins and rule out partial anomalous pulmonary venous connection if the veins are unable to be visualized with echocardiography. A left superior vena cava will be present in approximately 2% of patients with an ASD.

Transcatheter Closure

In the current era, transcatheter closure has evolved [4,16] and is now commonly used for many patients with ostium secundum ASDs that have an adequate rim for anchoring the device. There are currently two different FDA-approved devices available: the Amplatzer® device (AGA Medical Corp., Golden Valley, MN) [17–19] and the HELEX device (W.L..Gore and Associates, Flagstaff, AZ) [20]. These devices are currently used only for ostium secundum ASDs. These devices are not indicated for closure of a sinus venosus defect with anomalous drainage of the right superior pulmonary vein because of the potential for creation of superior vena caval or right superior pulmonary vein stenosis; or for partial AVSDs where the device would interfere with mitral and tricuspid valve function. As experience with these devices has been obtained, the incidence of complete closure has improved and the incidence of complications, such as device malposition or migration, has decreased significantly. Currently at Children's Memorial Hospital over 90% of ostium secundum ASDs are closed with the Amplatzer® device (Figure 16.5) [21]. The most common reason for referral of a patient with an ostium secundum ASD for surgery is that there is no inferior rim to anchor the device. Fischer reported that in 236 patients with an ostium secundum ASD 18 patients (8%) were not suitable for device closure because of anatomic issues determined in the catheterization lab [18]. At Children's Memorial Hospital, out of 143 patients undergoing attempted device closure, 11 (8%) were referred for surgery because a device could not be safely positioned.

Surgical Technique

Our preferred surgical technique for ASD closure is through a median sternotomy approach. Over the years, the length of the median sternotomy incision for ASD has steadily shortened, and many centers now close ASDs without opening the entire sternum [22–24]. This allows for a cosmetic closure, especially for females. An alternative technique is the right thoracotomy [25]. We have not used this approach because of the increased risk of air embolus and reports of right phrenic nerve injury [26]. The median sternotomy incision in particular permits repair of associated intracardiac lesions should they be discovered at the time of surgery. We currently use transesophageal echocardiography (TEE) in all ASD cases to confirm the diagnosis, to assess the pulmonary veins, and to confirm complete closure at the end of the case. In most cases, the thymus can be divided in the midline and resection of the thymus is not necessary. Our preferred closure technique has been to use an autologous pericardial patch. This patch is harvested at the beginning of the operation with stay sutures to retract the corners and placed in a sterile Petri dish filled

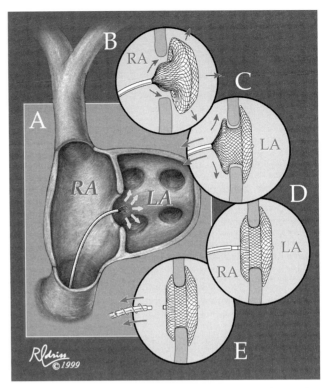

Figure 16.5 Implantation of the Amplatzer ASD occluder. **A,** The delivery catheter is positioned across the atrial defect. **B,** The left atrial disc with the self-centering connecting stalk is delivered. **C,** The device is withdrawn so that the connecting stalk is within the ASD and the left disc is firm against the atrial septum. **D,** The right atrial disc is delivered. **E,** The delivery cable is disconnected from the device. Until the delivery cable is disconnected, the device can be withdrawn back into the catheter and removed from the body. (LA, RA, left, right atrium.) (Reproduced with permission from Wax [21].)

with saline. We do not "tan" this patch with glutaraldehyde. Cardiopulmonary bypass is initiated with an aortic cannula and two venous cannulas. For an ostium secundum defect, the right atrial appendage can be cannulated first. This cannula is later advanced into the superior vena cava. The inferior vena cava should be cannulated at the junction with the right atrium, low enough so that if there is no inferior rim to the ASD adequate exposure in this area can still be obtained. A different cannulation strategy is used for sinus venosus ASD. The superior vena cava should be cannulated directly with a right-angled cannula superior to the azygous vein. Our preference for ASD closure has been to cool to 32 °C. We do not use a vent for ostium secundum or sinus venosus ASDs. In both defects, the left side is effectively decompressed through the ASD. We do use a vent for patients with a partial AVSD.

Following the initiation of cardiopulmonary bypass and the placement of caval tapes around the superior and inferior venae cavae, cold blood cardioplegia is administered

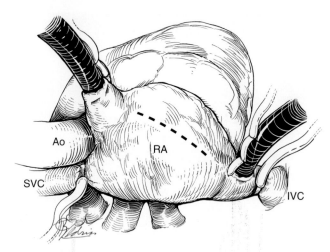

Figure 16.6 Operative closure of an ostium secundum ASD. This patient has been placed on cardiopulmonary bypass with bicaval cannulation. Dotted line indicates incision site in the right atrium. Aortic cannula is not shown. (Ao, aorta; IVC, SVC, inferior, superior vena cava; RA, right atrium.)

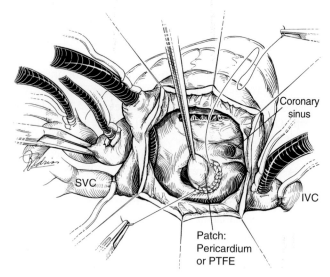

Figure 16.7 Closure of an ostium secundum atrial septal defect with a patch. Cardioplegia has been delivered and the heart arrested. The right atrium has been opened. The ASD is being closed with a patch – usually of autologous pericardium, although PTFE (polytetrafluoroethylene) may also be used. (IVC, SVC, inferior, superior vena cava.)

through the ascending aorta. Once the cardioplegia is begun, the caval tapes are deployed and the right atrium is opened. Our incision for an ostium secundum ASD is an oblique incision that is carried from the right atrial appendage in the direction of the inferior vena caval cannula (Figure 16.6) [5]. An attempt is made not to cross the crista terminalis, to preserve all possible conduction fibers from the sinoatrial node to the atrioventricular node. For sinus venosus ASDs, the incision in the right atrium is different, and is carried from the tip of the right atrial appendage in the direction of the superior vena cava–right atrial junction. The incision stops short of the crista terminalis and we do not cut across the cavoatrial junction. Superior retraction on the atrial wall nicely exposes the superior vena cava–right atrial junction.

For closure of an ostium secundum defect, the opening in the atrial septum is easily visualized through the opened right atrium (Figure 16.7) [5]. The cardiotomy sucker is used to control the blood coming up through the opening of the atrial septal defect from the left atrium. Excessive amounts of blood coming up from the left atrium should make the surgeon consider the possibility of a patent ductus arteriosus or relatively high cardiopulmonary bypass pump flow. Care is taken not to suction the left atrium empty; this prevents air from going across the mitral valve into the left ventricle. In cases where there is a question about pulmonary venous drainage, of course the atrium can be emptied of blood, but additional care must be taken at the conclusion of the operation to remove the air from the left side. The autologous pericardial patch is brought onto the field. In most cases, a 5-0 polypropylene

suture is sufficient to anchor this patch to the edges of the ASD. This suture is started at the inferior aspect of the defect, adjacent to the inferior vena cava. At this point, care must be taken to assure that the eustachian valve is not mistaken for the edge of the ASD. Suturing the eustachian valve to the septum secundum would create an obligatory shunt of the inferior vena cava blood into the left atrium; the patient would be cyanotic following the procedure [27]. The suturing of the patch is carried superiorly along the edge of the ASD, first adjacent to the crista terminalis and then adjacent to the coronary sinus. In the area of the coronary sinus some care must be taken not to take deep bites or grasp the area with pickups to avoid injury to the atrioventricular node. The suturing is completed superiorly, which is the "highest" point of the left and right atrial junction. When the suturing has been completed, but prior to tying the knot, an opening is created at the junction between the patch and the ASD and a Valsalva maneuver is performed by the anesthesiologist. This effectively pushes blood and air from the left atrium and pulmonary veins up through the opening in the patch. Usually there is an initial bubbling of air as the left side is de-aired, then followed solely by blood with no air. During the Valsalva maneuver, the suture is pulled tight and the knot is tied. The initial Valsalva maneuver is then relaxed, and then a second Valsalva maneuver is performed to test the suture line for leaks. Leaks will be seen as blood from the left atrium being forced out between the edges of the patch and the ASD. At this point the left side of the heart can be decompressed by venting through the cardioplegia needle site. Care must be taken not to vent too strongly and pull air into the left side of the system. The right atrial incision is then closed. The right side is also de-aired prior to releasing the cross clamp. During the suturing of the right atrium, the patient can be rewarmed.

Air embolism is one of the most feared possible complications of ASD closure. The left side of the heart has been open to air and the atmosphere during the repair period. Besides the maneuvers mentioned above, de-airing is performed by aspirating the cardioplegia needle site while gently massaging the left ventricle and left atrium, after the right atrial incision is closed. In addition, another Valsalva maneuver can be performed to push blood through the left side and out of the cardioplegia needle, along with any residual air. The aortic cross-clamp is then removed, applying suction to the ascending aorta at the time the cross-clamp is removed. Transesophageal echocardiography can be used to assess for air in the cardiac chambers during the weaning process from cardiopulmonary bypass. A vent tubing can be attached to the cardioplegia needle site to aspirate any air that might come up from the pulmonary veins or left atrium during the weaning from cardiopulmonary bypass. Warming is completed and the patient is ventilated and weaned from cardiopulmonary bypass. In most cases at Children's Memorial Hospital ASD patients are weaned from cardiopulmonary bypass with intravenous milrinone and low-dose dopamine. The venous cannulas are removed and we perform modified ultrafiltration (MUF) for 10 minutes. The use of MUF has been shown to decrease the need for blood transfusion in patients undergoing ASD closure [28]. The heparin is reversed with protamine, the aortic cannula is removed, and the patient is closed in the usual fashion. We do not place pacemaker wires at the conclusion of an ostium secundum defect repair. These patients are frequently able to be extubated in the operating room or shortly thereafter and usually spend only 24 hours in the intensive care unit.

Alternative techniques of closure for an ostium secundum ASD include direct suturing of the edges of the defect and the use of a polytetrafluoroethylene patch. We have preferred not to use a Dacron patch because the Dacron in some cases does not become completely endotheliazed. If there should be any mitral valve insufficiency, the jet of mitral insufficiency striking the patch can place the patient at risk for hemolysis. In our series of patients, we have previously used direct suturing in approximately 50% of the patients. In the current era, however, we use a patch in nearly all cases because the only referrals for ASD closure are those with large holes not amenable to device closure. The direct suture closure of an atrial septal defect is done with two layers of running 5-0 polypropylene suture.

Several reviews [29,30] have shown that the incidence of ASD recurrence may be reduced when a patch is employed, presumably because there is less tension on the suture line. However, if there is adequate useful septum primum tissue, we feel that successful suture closure can nearly always be accomplished.

Sinus venosus defects always require closure with a patch because of their location at the junction between the superior vena cava and the right atrium. Direct suture closure can lead to right superior pulmonary vein or superior vena caval stenosis (or both). We use transesophageal echocardiography for all sinus venosus defects. The preoperative study is useful for assessing the drainage point of the right pulmonary veins. At the conclusion of the procedure one can look for residual atrial level shunting, pulmonary vein stenosis, and superior vena cava stenosis. Another goal is to preserve sinus rhythm, which is complicated by the close proximity of the sinoatrial node. Another anatomic structure at risk is the right phrenic nerve, located on the other side of the pericardium immediately adjacent to the right lateral aspect of the superior vena cava. Great care in dissection of the superior vena cava is required in this area to prevent phrenic nerve injury with resultant diaphragm paralysis.

Between 20% and 45% of sinus venosus ASDs can be closed by a simple autologous intracardiac pericardial patch (Figure 16.8) [5, 31,32]. The suture line is started between the orifice of the right superior pulmonary vein and the orifice of the superior vena cava. Once the suturing has been completed in the superior aspect, it simply is carried around the remaining orifice of the ASD. At the posterior aspect of the junction of the superior vena cava and the right atrium, suturing should be relatively superficial to avoid injuring the sinoatrial node by deep bites into the atrial septum and junction with the superior vena cava. If the atrial septal defect requires enlargement to allow an adequate channel to the left atrium for the anomalous pulmonary veins, this is performed by making an incision towards the fossa ovalis and resecting a portion of the limbus of the septum secundum. Very rarely, partial anomalous pulmonary venous return of the right upper lobe or the right upper and middle lobes will occur to the superior vena cava–right atrial junction without an ASD. In these patients, an opening must be created in the atrial septum so that the pulmonary veins can be diverted into the left atrium underneath the pericardial baffle.

When the anomalous pulmonary veins enter the high superior vena cava, an alternative technique to the single patch must be used. In the past we used a "two-patch" technique where the cavoatrial junction was incised and a second pericardial patch was placed to augment the superior vena cava. Because of a high incidence of sinus node dysfunction with that technique, we have abandoned it and now use the "Warden" procedure for these patients

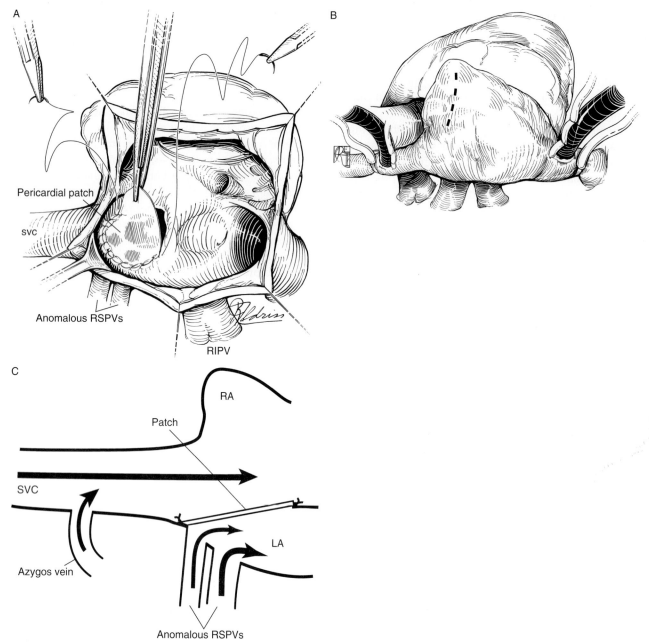

Figure 16.8 Single-patch closure of sinus venosus atrial septal defect. **A,** Pericardial patch closure of sinus venosus atrial septal defect where the anomalous veins drain to the superior vena cava-right atrial junction. **B,** Dotted line indicating incision for sinus venosus ASD closure. **C** shows in cross-section the relationship of the completed patch to the superior vena cava, right atrium, left atrium, and anomalous pulmonary veins. The postoperative blood flow in the superior vena cava and anomalous pulmonary veins is unobstructed. (LA, RA, left, right atrium; RIPV, right inferior pulmonary veins; SVC, superior vena cava.)

[31]. Warden first described this technique in 15 patients with partial anomalous pulmonary venous connection to the superior vena cava [33]. The Warden technique is illustrated in Figure 16.9 [31]. Important details of our technique include high cannulation of the superior vena cava (right-angle cannula) with division of the superior vena cava immediately above the partial anomalous pulmonary venous connection to save proximal superior vena cava length (Figure 16.9A) [31]. A pericardial patch is used to patch the cardiac stump of the superior vena cava to prevent stenosis or obstruction of the pulmonary venous return. The right atrial appendage is opened with an incision in the tip and care is taken to excise all trabeculations to avoid late stenosis (Figure 16.9B) [31]. The superior vena

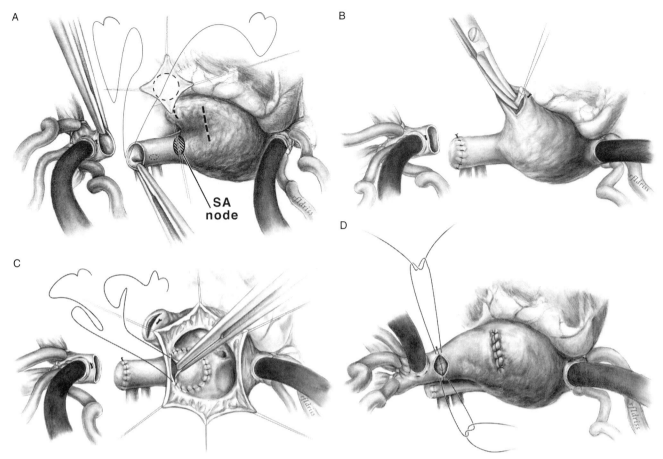

Figure 16.9 A, Details of the Warden technique. High cannulation of the superior vena cava (SVC) is performed with a right-angle cannula with division of the SVC immediately above the partial anomalous pulmonary venous connections to save proximal SVC length. A pericardial patch is used to patch the cardiac orifice of the SVC to prevent stenosis or obstruction of the pulmonary venous return (SA, sinoatrial). **B,** The right atrial appendage is opened with an incision in the tip, and care is taken to excise all trabeculations to avoid late stenosis. The completed pericardial patch on the superior vena cava is shown. **C,** The sinus venosus atrial septal defect is not "closed" but is used as an orifice through which the superior vena cava is baffled to the left atrium. The partial anomalous pulmonary venous connection blood flow goes through the remnant of superior vena cava through the sinus venosus atrial septal defect to the left atrium. **D,** The cut superior vena cava is anastomosed to the right atrial appendage using interrupted absorbable sutures to prevent purse-stringing and to allow growth. (Reproduced with permission from Stewart *et al.* [31].)

cava orifice in the right atrium is baffled to the left atrium through the sinus venosus atrial septal defect with a fresh autologous pericardial patch (Figure 16.9C) [31]. Finally, the cut superior vena cava is anastomosed to the right atrial appendage using absorbable interrupted sutures to prevent purse-stringing and to allow growth (Figure 16.9D) [31]. The azygos vein is preserved in case there is superior vena cava stenosis.

Partial atrioventricular septal defects are also closed with a pericardial patch (Figure 16.10) [5]. We use transesophageal echocardiography in all these cases. We use a vent placed through the right superior pulmonary vein. After cardioplegia has been administered and the right atrium opened, the vent is removed from the orifice of the

mitral valve and left ventricle and placed in the posterior left atrium. The mitral valve can then be irrigated with cold saline to assess the patient for mitral insufficiency and to assess the area of the cleft in the mitral valve. The cleft in the mitral valve leaflet is closed with simple interrupted polypropylene sutures. This repair is facilitated by placing the first suture at the leading edge of the mitral valve at the junction of the chordae tendineae with the edge of the mitral valve on either side. This then splays out the cleft and it can be closed with simple interrupted polypropylene sutures. We do not like to use a running suture technique because of the risk of foreshortening the valve when the suture is tied. Some surgeons have elected not to repair this cleft in those patients who do not have mitral regurgitation.

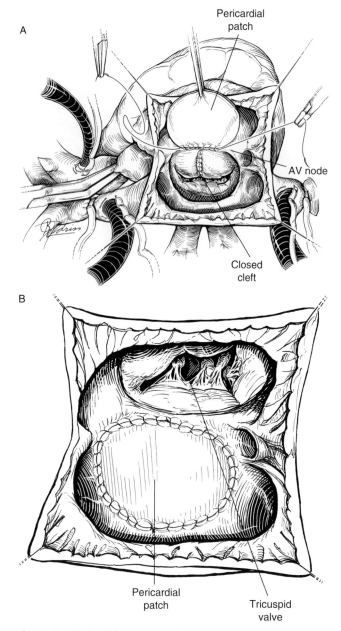

A

Pericardial patch

AV node

Closed cleft

B

Pericardial patch

Tricuspid valve

Figure 16.10 Partial atrioventricular septal defect closure. **Inset A:** Pericardial patch placement between the tricuspid and mitral valves has started and the cleft in anterior mitral valve leaflet has been closed. Vent in the right superior pulmonary vein is not illustrated. **B** shows completed ASD closure. (AV, atrioventricular.)

In our experience, we have had several patients with this type of repair performed elsewhere; these patients have then been referred with moderate or severe mitral insufficiency and sometimes with elevated pulmonary artery pressures. It is our opinion that all patients with a partial atrioventricular septal defect and a mitral valve cleft should have the cleft closed at the time of ASD closure. The pericardial patch is then brought onto the field and secured to the leaflet tissue that bridges the crest of the ventricular

septum between the mitral and tricuspid valves. As the surgeon progresses with the suturing in a clockwise fashion and gets close to the coronary sinus, superficial bites must be taken to avoid the atrioventricular node. Injury to the atrioventricular node can be minimized by carrying this suture line almost into the left ventricle, very close to the mitral valve. Once one passes the area of the coronary sinus, firmer bites can be taken. The suture line is completed by bringing a second suture line counterclockwise, again along the area of bridging leaflet tissue and up to the edge of the ASD. The remainder of the closure and de-airing are similar to that for an ostium secundum defect. Some surgeons prefer to carry the suture line on the right side of the coronary sinus, allowing the coronary sinus to drain to the left side to the left atrium. We have not found this necessary to prevent creation of atrioventricular heart block. After completing the cleft repair, the vent can be replaced across the mitral valve and into the left ventricle. The vent can then be used as part of the deairing process.

Postoperative Care

Following ASD closure, most patients can be extubated in the operating room or shortly thereafter. Our policy has been to monitor them in the intensive care unit for arrhythmias, postoperative bleeding, and potential airway problems for the first 24 hours postoperatively. They are then transferred to the regular ward. Chest tubes are removed usually on postoperative day 2 and the patients are discharged home on postoperative day 3 or 4. Most patients following ASD repair require only minimal short-term inotropic support and oxygen is usually only necessary while the patient is sedated. Price and colleagues [34] have confirmed that the use of critical pathways can reduce the length of hospitalization for ASD closure to a mean of 3.1 days. Most patients can be discharged with only medications for pain. After being seen by their cardiac surgeon at 1 week postoperatively, patients follow-up with their pediatric cardiologist. Nearly all of these patients will have no residual hemodynamic abnormalities.

Technical Pitfalls

As mentioned, the lower edge of a large ostium secundum defect may be difficult to visualize, especially if the inferior vena cava cannula has been placed too high. This is particularly true for the patient who has no inferior rim and who has been declined for device closure. Another pitfall in this area is a large, prominent eustachian valve that can be mistaken for the lower edge of the ASD. Suturing the edge of the ASD to the eustachian valve would cause an obligatory right-to-left shunt from the inferior vena cava to the left atrium. This would become immediately obvious due to severe oxygen desaturation of the patient following the procedure [27]. Proper cannulation of the inferior vena

Table 16.1 Results of surgical repair of ostium secundum ASD.

Institution	Years	Number of patients	Mortality	Significant morbidity
Hasbro Childrens [40]	1988–2002	176	0	3%*
CMH	1990–2009	271	0	0
UC-San Francisco [37]	1992–1997	115	0	0
Halifax [39]	1994–2001	100	0	3%*
Bambino Gesù [38]	1996–1998	122	0	2%*
Boston Children's [24]	1996–1998	135	0	0
University of Leipzig [41]	1996–2005	297	0	0
TOTAL		1217	0	1–2%

*post-pericardiotomy syndrome

cava, adequate sized atriotomy, and careful placement of the initial sutures in the inferior area where the visualization is most critical, should prevent these complications. Small fenestrations in the interatrial septum primum are a potential cause of residual shunting. These defects can be closed, often primarily, with interrupted 5-0 polypropylene simple or mattress sutures, depending on the size of the fenestration. Another unusual cause of persistent postoperative interatrial shunting is a partially unroofed coronary sinus [35]. This allows left atrial blood to enter into the right atrium through the coronary sinus ostium. This entity should be suspected when no atrial septal defect or anomalous pulmonary vein can be found in the right atrium in a patient with a documented oxygen step-up. To expose the defect in the roof of the coronary sinus, an incision should be made in the interatrial septum. A right-angle clamp can then be passed into the orifice of the coronary sinus and the opening into the left atrium visualized. This opening can be closed with a pericardial patch or primarily if the coronary sinus is dilated. Frequently these patients have a left superior vena cava that makes the coronary sinus quite large. In some cases, the left superior vena cava will drain directly into the left atrium with complete absence of the coronary sinus [36]. In these cases, the left superior vena cava must be ligated (if small) or in some fashion connected to the right side of the circulation. Our current preference for these patients is to do a left superior cavopulmonary anastomosis (Glenn procedure), anastomosing the left superior vena cava to the left pulmonary artery. An alternative technique that has been reported is an intra-atrial baffle of pericardium, however, this is complicated by the location of the pulmonary veins.

Results of Operation

At the Children's Memorial Hospital between 1990 and 2009, 271 patients underwent surgical closure of an ostium secundum ASD. The median age at ASD closure was 3.3 years. All of these patients were approached through a median sternotomy with the use of cardiopulmonary bypass, aortic cross-clamping, and cold blood cardioplegia.

In 50% of the cases, the defect was closed with a pericardial patch and in the other 50% direct suture closure was performed. However, since the advent of device closure, essentially all patients referred for surgery have required a patch. In this series, there were no deaths and no recurrences of the ASD. The mean hospital stay was 3.5 days. There have been multiple other series demonstrating outstanding surgical results of ASD closure in children (Table 16.1) [24,37–41]. In a large population-based study from Finland [42], the survival of children with a surgically closed ASD (812 patients) was comparable to that of the general population. In Murphy's [15] review from the Mayo Clinic, if the ASD was closed before the age of 25 years, there was no difference in actuarial survival at 27 years postoperatively from age-matched controls.

The results with sinus venosus defect are also very good. We have had no mortality from sinus venosus defect closure in 86 patients operated on between 1990 and 2009. In 54 patients that we recently reviewed [31], partial anomalous pulmonary venous connection was present in all but two patients; drainage was to the right atrium in eight patients (15%), the right atrial–superior vena cava junction in 17 patients (33%), and directly to the SVC in 27 patients (52%). Techniques utilized were single patch repair (24), two-patch repair (25), and Warden repair (5). The incidence of low atrial or junctional rhythm was 55% in the two-patch group, and 0 in the Warden group. Because of that finding we now use the Warden technique in all patients where a single patch repair is not achievable. Several other centers have reported no mortality and a very low incidence of sinoatrial node dysfunction using the Warden technique [43–46]. Superior vena cava stenosis and right pulmonary vein stenosis are also very rare with this technique. In the Mayo Clinic review, long-term survival of patients with a sinus venosus ASD was not different from age- and sex-matched populations [47].

Partial atrioventricular septal defect repair has a different set of possible complications than ostium secundum and sinus venosus repair. This is because though lacking a ventricular level communication, partial AVSDs share the same anatomic features of the scooped-out ventricular septum, elongated left ventricular outflow tract (LVOT), and trifoliate left AV valve configuration characteristic of complete atrioventricular septal defects [48]. These include mitral valve insufficiency, atrioventricular block requiring pacemaker placement, and left ventricular outflow tract obstruction. Najm and colleagues [49] at the Hospital for Sick Children reported their results with 180 patients having repair of an ostium primum ASD. Mean age at repair was 4.6 years. Early mortality occurred in three patients (1.6%), two of whom were less than 1 year of age at time of repair. Actuarial survival was 98% at 10 years, with no late deaths. Reoperation was required in 17 of the 180 patients (9%), five of whom were in the infant group. Indications for reoperation were subaortic obstruction in five patients (3%), and left atrioventricular valve regurgitation in 12 patients (7%). Eleven patients underwent valve repair, one patient required valve replacement.

At Children's Memorial Hospital, we have operated on 66 patients with partial AVSD from 1990 to 2007. Median age at repair was 16 months, mean age was 2.3 years. There was no operative mortality. Two patients required a reoperation for mitral valve insufficiency, two patients required reoperation for subaortic stenosis, and one patient required a permanent pacemaker for third-degree AV block. Nunn reported 126 patients having partial AVSD repair, from 1983 to 2005. Median age at operation was 2.9 years. Two patients required reoperation on the mitral valve and eight patients required reoperation for subaortic stenosis [50].

Results of Transcatheter Closure

In the past 30 years, several percutaneous transcatheter techniques have been explored for closure of ASDs. Excellent initial results were described with the Clamshell occluder device (USCI Division of CR Bard Inc, Billerica, MA) [16]. On late follow-up, however, the device was taken off the market because of fractures of the struts of the device. More recently, the Amplatzer® device [16–18], a self-expanding wire mesh double-mushroom device, has been successfully employed. The HELEX device is a double disc occluder composed of an expanded PTFE membrane bonded to a single nitinol wire frame [20]. The Amplatzer® device and the HELEX® are now FDA-approved. With ongoing improvements in device construction and placement, they have become the technique of choice for closure of most small-to-medium size ostium secundum ASDs in older children.

Chan and colleagues [51] from the United Kingdom reported 100 ASD closures with the Amplatzer® device in a multicenter study. There were seven failures and one embolization requiring surgical removal. Occlusion rate at 3 months was 98.9%. Berger and associates [52] reported 200 patients undergoing placement of the Amplatzer® device with trivial residual shunts in only 1.9% of the patients. In a separate study, Berger and coworkers [53] compared Amplatzer® and surgical closure. Closure rates were identical, but the duration of hospital stay was less and there was less morbidity with the device. These conclusions are somewhat biased in that the surgical candidates had larger ASDs not suitable for the device. There are possible complications of device closure that the surgeon should be familiar with [41,54]. DiBardino reported 223 adverse events in an estimated 18 333 implants (1.2%), resulting in 17 deaths (8%) and 152 surgical rescue operations (68%) [54]. Walther reported 15 reoperations on patients with an Amplatzer device – five for dislocation, five for neurologic events, and four for residual defect [41]. The most commonly reported complications are device malposition, dislocation, or embolization [41,54–56]. Another more serious complication is device erosion into the ascending aorta or the dome of the left atrium [41,54,57]. This tends to occur when the device is "oversized" because the ASD has deficient "rims" [58]. One of the ways to avoid this complication with the Amplatzer device is to not "oversize" the device to "make up for" a deficient aortic and/or superior rim. This complication occurred in 0.1% of patients tracked in the United States. We have had to operate on three patients at Children's Memorial Hospital after device closure. Two were for embolization (left atrium and mitral valve), and one for erosion into the dome of the left atrium causing a bloody pericardial effusion. Other reported complications include atrioventricular block [59], endocarditis [60], and anterior mitral valve perforation [61]. Another issue in the debate between surgical and device closure of ASD is cost. In developing countries, percutaneous occlusion costs were higher than those for surgical closure [62].

Results in Older Patients

The value of surgical closure of an ASD in an adult was previously controversial because of the higher operative risk in adults with multiple medical problems and questions regarding improvement in quality of life. Comparisons of medical therapy versus surgical therapy initially had mixed conclusions; however, recent series have found that surgical therapy has a better outcome [63]. Two studies [64,65] in the early 1990s suggested that surgical treatment is not of benefit to older patients with an ASD. Konstantinides and colleagues [66] evaluated patients diagnosed with ASD when they were more than 40 years of age. The surgical treatment group was comprised of 84 patients, and 95 patients were medically treated. Multivariate analysis revealed that surgical closure of the ASD significantly reduced mortality from all causes. The adjusted 10-year survival rate of surgically treated patients was 95% as compared with 84% for the medically treated patients. In addition, surgical treatment prevented functional deterioration as measured by the New York Heart Association class. Both Vogel [67] and Gatzoulis [68] and their associates showed that surgical closure of an ASD in adults had a very low operative mortality, and was associated with an improved quality of life and a significant reduction in arrhythmia occurrences. Patients with ASD and atrial fibrillation should have a Cox-maze III procedure at the time of ASD closure [69,70]. Older patients require anticoagulation following ASD repair. Hawe and coworkers [71] observed postoperative embolism in 35 of 546 adults undergoing ASD closure. Coronary embolism has also been reported in adults following ASD repair [72]. We recommend anticoagulation with warfarin in all patients over the age of 35 who undergo ASD closure. This is then continued for 6 months following the procedure.

Scimitar Syndrome

Scimitar syndrome consists of a rare constellation of anomalies, the constant being total or partial anomalous pulmonary venous connection of the right lung to the inferior vena cava. On a chest radiograph, the gently curved vertical shape of this vein resembles a curved Turkish sword, or scimitar [73]. The other frequently associated anomalies include dextroposition of the heart, hypoplasia of the right lung and right pulmonary artery, and an anomalous systemic artery to the right lung from the abdominal aorta that penetrates the diaphragm. Up to 70% of patients with scimitar syndrome also have associated intracardiac defects, most commonly ASD [74].

Symptoms are related to the amount of left-to-right shunting from the anomalous vein, the degree of pulmonary hypertension, parenchymal lung disease, and associated intracardiac lesions. Patients tend to present with two distinct clinical profiles [75]. In the "adult" form the patient is usually only mildly symptomatic with exertional dyspnea and recurrent respiratory infections [76]. In the "infantile" form, patients present in the first few months of life with failure to thrive, cyanosis, respiratory distress, and congestive heart failure. Infants often have severe pulmonary hypertension. Chest radiograph shows a small right lung, displacement of the heart to the right, and the shadow of the anomalous vein. Electrocardiogram reveals right ventricular hypertrophy. Echocardiography should be able to establish the diagnosis, identify intracardiac lesions, and visualize the location of the anomalous vein [74]. Cardiac catheterization and angiography are diagnostic and identify the anomalous systemic artery from the descending aorta that penetrates the diaphragm and supplies blood to the right lower lobe (Figure 16.11) [5]. Cardiac catheterization is now also part of the therapeutic strategy for these patients. They can have the anomalous systemic artery embolized at the time of the catheterization [77].

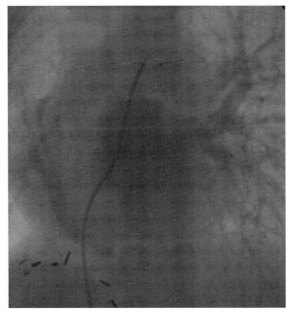

Figure 16.11 Scimitar syndrome. Levo-phase of a pulmonary angiogram. The left pulmonary veins drain normally to the left atrium. The right pulmonary veins drain to a vertical confluence that is directed toward the right diaphragm and enters the inferior vena cava. It is this vein that looks like a "scimitar."

Operative intervention is individualized and based on the degree of symptoms and findings at cardiac catheterization. In all instances, the systemic arterial supply to the lung is divided, if it was not occluded at the time of cardiac catheterization. Kirklin and colleagues [78] reported that the anomalous vein can either be anastomosed directly to the left atrium or an intracardiac patch can be used as a baffle to direct the flow from the anomalous vein to the left atrium through an atrial septal defect. Najm and coworkers [79] in Toronto reported 32 patients with scimitar syndrome seen over a 20-year time period. Nineteen were diagnosed in the first year of life. In 17 patients, the anomalous vein was baffled to the left atrium. Eight patients had postoperative evidence of pulmonary vein stenosis. Brown and colleagues [80] recently reported nine patients undergoing right thoracotomy with direct anastomosis of the scimitar vein to the left atrium without the use of cardiopulmonary bypass. All nine patients (mean age, 11.5 years) survived. That series was recently updated to 12 patients [81].

If inflammatory parenchymal changes are extensive, if the patient has persistent hemoptysis, or if there is marked hypoplasia of the right lung, pulmonary resection or pneumonectomy should be considered. Resection eliminates the left-to-right shunt as well as the lung infection. Huddleston and associates [82] reported 12 infants with scimitar syndrome. Primary pneumonectomy was performed in two patients, and three patients had a pneumonectomy after a baffle procedure became occluded. Overall mortality in this critically ill infant group was 30%.

In general, results depend primarily on the degree of preoperative pulmonary hypertension and associated cardiac lesions. Older patients with minimal symptoms have an excellent prognosis, however, infants with cyanosis, failure to thrive, and severe pulmonary hypertension have a high mortality.

Conclusion

Atrial septal defect was the first congenital cardiac defect closed with an operation. It was the first congenital cardiac defect closed with cardiopulmonary bypass, and it was the first intracardiac lesion closed with a device in the catheterization laboratory. The history of ASD closure has exemplified the progress made in congenital heart surgery over the past 50 years. Ostium secundum defects are now primarily closed with transcatheter devices in the catheterization lab. Large ostium secundum defects are closed in the operating room with a pericardial patch with essentially no mortality or morbidity with a 50 year follow-up. Sinus venosus defects require attention to the associated partial anomalous pulmonary veins and are repaired with either a pericardial patch or with the Warden procedure. Partial atrioventricular septal defect is addressed with a pericardial patch and attention to the cleft in the left AV valve. The outcome with both surgery and transcatheter techniques is extraordinarily good and the vast majority of these patients have no residual hemodynamic sequelae and a normal life expectancy. Optimal outcomes depend on proper selection of surgical and transcatheter techniques tailored to the individual patient anatomy.

References

1. Lewis FJ, Taufic M. (1953) Closure of atrial septal defects with the aid of hypothermia: experimental accomplishments and report of one successful case. Surgery 33, 52–59.
2. Shumway NE. (1996) F. John Lewis, MD: 1916–1993. Ann Thorac Surg 61, 250–251.
3. Gibbon JH Jr. (1954) Application of a mechanical heart and lung apparatus to cardiac surgery. Minnesota Med 37, 171–185.
4. King TD, Mills NL. (1976) Secundum atrial septal defects: nonoperative closure during cardiac catheterization. JAMA 235, 2506–2509.
5. Backer CL, Mavroudis C. (2003) Atrial septal defect, partial anomalous pulmonary venous connection, and scimitar syndrome. In: Mavroudis C, Backer CL, eds. *Pediatric Cardiac Surgery*, 3rd ed. Philadelphia, PA: Mosby.
6. Jacobs JP, Burke RP, Quintessenza JA, *et al.* (2000) Atrial septal defect. Ann Thorac Surg 69(suppl), S18–S24.
7. Crystal MA, Al Najashi K, Williams WG, *et al.* (2009) Inferior sinus venosus defect: echocardiographic diagnosis and surgical approach. J Thorac Cardiovasc Surg 137, 1349–1355.
8. Campbell M. (1970) Natural history of atrial septal defect. Br Heart J 32, 820–826.
9. Helgason H, Jonsdottir G. (1999) Spontaneous closure of atrial septal defects. Pediatr Cardiol 20, 195–199.
10. Hanslik A, Pospisil U, Salzer-Muhar U, *et al.* (2006) Predictors of spontaneous closure of isolated secundum atrial septal defect in children: a longitudinal study. Pediatrics 118, 1560–1565.
11. Cockerham JT, Martin TC, Gutierrez FR, *et al.* (1983) Spontaneous closure of secundum atrial septal defect in infants and young children. Am J Cardiol 52, 1267–1271.
12. Wilson W, Taubert KA, Gewitz M, *et al.* (2007) Prevention of infective endocarditis: guidelines from the American Heart Association: a guideline from the American Heart Association Rheumatic Fever, Endocarditis, and Kawasaki Disease Committee, Council on Cardiovascular Disease in the Young, and the Council on Clinical Cardiology, Council on Cardiovascular Surgery and Anesthesia, and the Quality of Care and Outcomes Research Interdisciplinary Working Group. Circulation 116, 1736–1754.
13. Vogel M, Berger F, Kramer A, *et al.* (1999) Incidence of secondary pulmonary hypertension in adults with atrial septal or sinus venosus defects. Heart 82, 30–33.
14. Steele PM, Fuster V, Cohen M, *et al.* (1987) Isolated atrial septal defect with pulmonary vascular obstructive disease – long-term follow-up and prediction of outcome after surgical correction. Circulation 76, 1037–1042.
15. Murphy JG, Gersh BJ, McGoon MD, *et al.* (1990) Long-term outcome after surgical repair of isolated atrial septal defect: follow-up at 27 to 32 years. N Engl J Med 323, 1645–1650.
16. Rome JJ, Keane JF, Perry SB, *et al.* (1990) Double-umbrella closure of atrial defects: initial clinical applications. Circulation 82, 751–758.
17. Yew G, Wilson NJ. (2005) Transcatheter atrial septal defect closure with the Amplatzer septal occluder: five-year follow-up. Catheter Cardiovasc Interv 64, 193–196.
18. Fischer G, Stieh J, Uebing A, *et al.* (2003) Experience with transcatheter closure of secundum atrial septal defects using the Amplatzer septal occluder: a single centre study in 236 consecutive patients. Heart 89, 199–204.
19. Du ZD, Hijazi ZM, Kleinman CS, *et al.* (2002) Comparison between transcatheter and surgical closure of secundum atrial septal defect in children and adults: results of a multicenter nonrandomized trial. J Am Coll Cardiol 39, 1836–1844.
20. Jones TK, Latson LA, Zahn E, *et al.* (2007) Results of the U.S. multicenter pivotal study of the HELEX septal occluder for percutaneous closure of secundum atrial septal defects. J Am Coll Cardiol 49, 2215–2221.
21. Wax DF. (1999) Therapeutic cardiac catheterization in children. The Child's Doctor, Fall, 15.
22. Cremer JT, Böning A, Anssar MB, *et al.* (1999) Different approaches for minimally invasive closure of atrial septal defects. Ann Thorac Surg 67, 1648–1652.
23. Khan JH, McElhinney DB, Reddy VM, *et al.* (1998) Repair of secundum atrial septal defect: limiting the incision without sacrificing exposure. Ann Thorac Surg 66, 1433–1435.

24. Bichell DP, Geva T, Bacha EA, *et al.* (2000) Minimal access approach for the repair of atrial septal defect: the initial 135 patients. Ann Thorac Surg 70, 115–118.

25. Rosengart TK, Stark JF. (1993) Repair of atrial septal defect through a right thoracotomy. Ann Thorac Surg 55, 1138–1140.

26. Helps BA, Ross-Russell RI, Dicks-Mireaux C, *et al.* (1993) Phrenic nerve damage via a right thoracotomy in older children with secundum ASD. Ann Thorac Surg 56, 328–330.

27. Desnick SJ, Neal WA, Nicoloff DM, *et al.* (1976) Residual right-to-left shunt following repair of atrial septal defect. Ann Thorac Surg 21, 291–295.

28. Gurbuz AT, Novick WM, Pierce CA, *et al.* (1998) Impact of ultrafiltration on blood use for atrial septal defect closure in infants and children. Ann Thorac Surg 65, 1105–1108.

29. Cohn LH, Morrow AG, Braunwald E. (1967) Operative treatment of atrial septal defect: clinical and haemodynamic assessments in 175 patients. Br Heart J 29, 725–734.

30. Fagan S, Veinot JP, Chan K-L. (2001) Residual sinus venosus atrial septal defect after surgical closure of atrial septal defects. J Am Soc Echocardiogr 14, 738–741.

31. Stewart RD, Bailliard F, Kelle AM, *et al.* (2007) Evolving surgical strategy for sinus venosus atrial septal defect: effect on sinus node function and late venous obstruction. Ann Thorac Surg 84, 1651–1655.

32. Gustafson RA, Warden HE, Murray GF, *et al.* (1989) Partial anomalous pulmonary venous connection to the right side of the heart. J Thorac Cardiovasc Surg 98, 861–868.

33. Warden HE, Gustafson RA, Tarnay TJ, *et al.* (1984) An alternative method for repair of partial anomalous pulmonary venous connection to the superior vena cava. Ann Thorac Surg 38, 601–605.

34. Price MB, Jones A, Hawkins JA, *et al.* (1999) Critical pathways for postoperative care after simple congenital heart surgery. Am J Manag Care 5, 185–192.

35. Lee ME, Sade RM. (1979) Coronary sinus septal defect: surgical considerations. J Thorac Cardiovasc Surg 78, 563–569.

36. Foster ED, Baeza OR, Farina MF, *et al.* (1978) Atrial septal defect associated with drainage of left superior vena cava to left atrium and absence of the coronary sinus. J Thorac Cardiovasc Surg 76, 718–720.

37. Khan JH, McElhinney DB, Reddy VM, *et al.* (1999) A 5-year experience with surgical repair of atrial septal defect employing limited exposure. Cardiol Young 9, 572–576.

38. Formigari R, DiDonato RM, Mazzera E, *et al.* (2001) Minimally invasive or interventional repair of atrial septal defects in children: experience in 171 cases and comparison with conventional strategies. J Am Coll Cardiol 37, 1707–1712.

39. Baskett RJ, Tancock E, Ross DB. (2003) The gold standard for atrial septal defect closure: current surgical results, with an emphasis on morbidity. Pediatr Cardiol 24, 444–447.

40. Hopkins RA, Bert AA, Buchholz B, *et al.* (2004) Surgical patch closure of atrial septal defects. Ann Thorac Surg 77, 2144–2150.

41. Walther T, Binner C, Rastan A, *et al.* (2007) Surgical atrial septal defect closure after interventional occluder placement: incidence and outcome. J Thorac Cardiovasc Surg 134, 731–737.

42. Nieminen HP, Jokinen EV, Sairanen HI. (2001) Late results of pediatric cardiac surgery in Finland: a population-based study with 96% follow-up. Circulation 104, 570–575.

43. Gustafson RA, Warden HE, Murray GF. (1995) Partial anomalous pulmonary venous connection to the superior vena cava. Ann Thorac Surg 60(6 Suppl), S614–S616.

44. Shahriari A, Rodefeld MD, Turrentine MW, *et al.* (2006) Caval division technique for sinus venosus atrial septal defect with partial anomalous pulmonary venous connection. Ann Thorac Surg 81, 224–230

45. Gaynor JW, Burch M, Dollery C, *et al.* (1995) Repair of anomalous pulmonary venous connection to the superior vena cava. Ann Thorac Surg 59, 1471–1475.

46. DiBardino DJ, McKenzie ED, Heinle JS, *et al.* (2004) The Warden procedure for partially anomalous pulmonary venous connection to the superior caval vein. Cardiol Young 14, 64–67.

47. Jost CH, Connolly HM, Danielson GK, *et al.* (2005) Sinus venosus atrial septal defect: long-term postoperative outcome for 115 patients. Circulation 112, 1953–1958.

48. Manning PB. (2007) Partial atrioventricular canal: pitfalls in technique. Semin Thorac Cardiovasc Surg Pediatr Card Surg Ann 10, 42–46

49. Najm HK, Williams WG, Chuaratanaphong S, *et al.* (1998) Primum atrial septal defect in children: early results, risk factors, and freedom from reoperation. Ann Thorac Surg 66, 829–835.

50. Nunn GR. (2007) Atrioventricular canal: modified single patch technique. Semin Thorac Cardiovasc Surg Pediatr Card Surg Annu 10, 28–31.

51. Chan KC, Godman MJ, Walsh K, *et al.* (1999) Transcatheter closure of atrial septal defect and interatrial communications with a new self expanding nitinol double disc device (Amplatzer septal occluder): multicentre UK experience. Heart 82, 300–306.

52. Berger F, Ewert P, Bjornstad PG, *et al.* (1999) Transcatheter closure as standard treatment for most interatrial defects: experience in 200 patients treated with the Amplatzer Septal Occluder. Cardiol Young 9, 468–473.

53. Berger F, Vogel M, Alexi-Meskishvili V, *et al.* (1999) Comparison of results and complications of surgical and Amplatzer device closure of atrial septal defect. J Thorac Cardiovasc Surg 118, 674–678.

54. DiBardino DJ, McElhinney DB, Kaza AK, *et al.* (2009) Analysis of the US Food and Drug Administration Manufacturer and User Facility Device Experience database for adverse events involving Amplatzer septal occluder devices and comparison with the Society of Thoracic Surgery congenital cardiac surgery database. J Thorac Cardiovasc Surg 137, 1334–1341.

55. Hekmat K, Mehlhorn U, de Vivie ER. (1997) Surgical repair of a large residual atrial septal defect after transcatheter closure. Ann Thorac Surg 63, 1456–1458.

56. Berdat PA, Chatterjee T, Pfammatter JP, *et al.* (2000) Surgical management of complications after transcatheter closure of an atrial septal defect or patent foramen ovale. J Thorac Cardiovasc Surg 120, 1034–1039.

57. Divekar A, Gaamangwe T, Shaikh N, *et al.* (2005) Cardiac perforation after device closure of atrial septal defects with the Amplatzer septal occluder. J Am Coll Cardiol 45, 1213–1218.

58. Amin Z, Hijazi ZM, Bass JL, *et al.* (2004) Erosion of Amplatzer septal occluder device after closure of secundum atrial septal defects: review of registry of complications and recommendations to minimize future risk. Catheter Cardiovasc Interv 63, 496–502

59. Suda K, Raboisson M-J, Piette E, *et al.* (2004) Reversible atrioventricular block associated with closure of atrial septal defects using the Amplatzer device. J Am Coll Cardiol 43, 1677–1682.

60. Balasundaram RP, Anandaraja S, Juneja R, *et al.* (2005) Infective endocarditis following implantation of amplatzer atrial septal occluder. Indian Heart J 57, 167–169.

61. Dialetto G, Covino FE, Scognamiglio G, *et al.* (2006) A rare complication of atrial septal occluders: diagnosis by transthoracic echocardiography. J Am soc Echocardiogr 19, 836, e5–8.

62. Vida VL, Barnoya J, O'Connell M, *et al.* (2006) Surgical versus percutaneous occlusion of ostium secundum atrial septal defects. J Am Coll Cardiol 47, 326–331.

63. Moodie DS, Sterba R. (2000) Long-term outcomes excellent for atrial septal defect repair in adults. Cleve Clin J 67, 591–597.

64. Shah D, Azhar M, Oakley CM, *et al.* (1994) Natural history of secundum atrial septal defect in adults after medical or surgical treatment: a historical prospective study. Br Heart J 71, 224–227.

65. Ward C. (1994) Secundum atrial septal defect: routine surgical treatment is not of proven benefit. Br Heart J 71, 219–223.

66. Konstantinides S, Geibel A, Olschewski M, *et al.* (1995) A comparison of surgical and medical therapy for atrial septal defect in adults. N Engl J Med 333, 469–473.

67. Vogel M, Berger F, Kramer A, *et al.* (1999) [Diagnosis and surgical treatment of atrial septal defects in adults]. Dtsch Med Wochenschr 124, 35–38.

68. Gatzoulis MA, Redington AN, Somerville J, *et al.* (1996) Should atrial septal defects in adults be closed? Ann Thorac Surg 61, 657–659.

69. Berger F, Vogel M, Kramer A, *et al.* (1999) Incidence of atrial flutter/fibrillation in adults with atrial septal defect before and after surgery. Ann Thorac Surg 68, 75–78.

70. Kobayashi J, Yamamoto F, Nakano K, *et al.* (1998) Maze procedure for atrial fibrillation associated with atrial septal defect. Circulation 98(19 Suppl), II399–II402.

71. Hawe A, Rastelli GC, Brandenburg RO, *et al.* (1969) Embolic complications following repair of atrial septal defects. Circulation 39, I185–I191.

72. Backer CL, Hartz RS, Meyers SN, *et al.* (1988) Coronary embolism following atrial septal defect repair. Ann Thorac Surg 45, 561–563.

73. Neill CA, Ferencz C, Sabiston DC, *et al.* (1960) The familial occurrence of hypoplastic right lung with systemic arterial supply and venous drainage: "scimitar syndrome". Bull Johns Hopkins Hosp 107, 1–21.

74. Shibuya K, Smallhorn JE, McCrindle BW. (1996) Echocardiographic clues and accuracy in the diagnosis of scimitar syndrome. J Am Soc Echocardiogr 9, 174–181.

75. Pelletier GJ, Spray TL. (2001) Repair of scimitar syndrome. Oper Tech Thorac Cardiovasc Surg 6, 32–49.

76. Kiely B, Filler J, Stone S, *et al.* (1967) Syndrome of anomalous venous drainage of the right lung to the inferior vena cava: a review of 67 reported cases and three new cases in children. Am J Cardiol 20, 102–116.

77. Dickinson DF, Galloway RW, Massey R, *et al.* (1982) Scimitar syndrome in infancy: role of embolisation of systemic arterial supply to right lung. Br Heart J 47, 468–472.

78. Kirklin JW, Ellis FH Jr, Wood EH. (1956) Treatment of anomalous venous connection in association with interatrial communications. Surgery 39, 389–398.

79. Najm HK, Williams WG, Coles JG, *et al.* (1996) Scimitar syndrome: twenty years' experience and results of repair. J Thorac Cardiovasc Surg 112, 1161–1168.

80. Brown JW, Edwards C, Fiore AC, *et al.* (2003) Surgical management of the scimitar syndrome: an alternative approach. J Thorac Cardiovasc Surg 125, 238–245.

81. Gudjonsson U, Brown JW. (2006) Scimitar syndrome. Semin Thorac Cardiovasc Surg Pediatr Card Surg Ann 9, 56–62.

82. Huddleston CB, Exil V, Canter CE, *et al.* (1999) Scimitar syndrome presenting in infancy. Ann Thorac Surg 67, 154–160.

Ventricular Septal Defect

Constantine Mavroudis,[1] Carl L. Backer,[2] Jeffrey P. Jacobs,[3] and Robert H. Anderson[4,5]

[1]Florida Hospital for Children, Orlando, FL, USA
[2]Ann & Robert H. Lurie Children's Hospital of Chicago, formerly Children's Memorial Hospital, Chicago, IL, USA
[3]All Children's Hospital, Saint Petersburg, FL, USA
[4]University of Newcastle, Newcastle, UK
[5]Medical University of South Carolina, Charleston, SC, USA

Definition and Prevalence

A ventricular septal defect (VSD) is a hole between the ventricles. Such holes can be located anywhere in the normal ventricular septum but can also exist at sites where, in the normal heart, there are no septal structures, such as directly beneath the leaflets of the pulmonary valve. They are characterized into anatomic types based on their location relative to the components of the right ventricle and their anatomic borders. The holes may vary in size, may be single or multiple, and may be associated with a number of other intracardiac and extracardiac anomalies. In this chapter, we discuss the management of isolated VSDs and those associated with persistent patency of the arterial duct (PDA), coarctation of the aorta, and acquired aortic insufficiency. Other associated major anomalies involving the ventricular outflow tracts, such as the defects seen in the setting of tetralogy of Fallot, double-outlet right ventricle, common arterial trunk (truncus arteriosus), and transposition, are discussed elsewhere in the appropriate chapters. Also in other chapters are discussions of those defects associated with atrioventricular anomalies and those with discordant atrioventricular connections.

Isolated VSD is the most commonly recognized congenital heart defect [1], excluding the aortic valve with two leaflets [2]. Ventricular septal defects occur in isolation at a rate of about 2 per 1000 live births, and account for about one-fifth of all forms of congenital heart disease [3]. When considered together, isolated VSDs and those associated with other major defects account for over half of the patients with congenitally malformed hearts.

Historical Perspectives

The clinical manifestations attributed to VSD were first described by Roger in 1879 [4]. Eisenmenger (1897) [5], when studying the heart of a 32-year-old cyanotic patient, noted the presence of a large VSD with an overriding aorta but in the absence of subpulmonary stenosis. It was much later that Abbott [6] and Selzer [7] formulated the pathophysiologic features of the VSD.

The era of surgical intervention began in 1952, when Muller and Dammann placed a band on the pulmonary trunk to limit the flow of blood to the lungs in a patient with a VSD [8]. The first operative repair was performed by Lillehei and associates in 1954 [9]. They used controlled cross-circulation with an adult acting as the pump oxygenator. The development of the heart–lung machine and cardiopulmonary bypass led rapidly to more widespread successful clinical results. DuShane and associates [10] had already shown, by 1956, that transventricular repair could be performed with an acceptable mortality rate, while Stirling and coworkers [11] showed that closure could be accomplished transatrially, thereby avoiding a ventriculotomy. In 1961, Kirklin and associates [12], and later Sigmann and associates [13], reported on the successful repair in infants, an approach which in the majority of cases obviated the need for palliative banding. Later reports by Okamoto (1969) [14] and Barratt-Boyes and colleagues (1976) [15] established the feasibility of repair in infants using deep hypothermia and circulatory arrest. Since that time, multiple refinements in methods of cardiopulmonary bypass and myocardial protection have allowed surgeons

Pediatric Cardiac Surgery, Fourth Edition. Edited by Constantine Mavroudis and Carl L. Backer.
© 2013 Blackwell Publishing Ltd. Published 2013 by Blackwell Publishing Ltd.

the time to perform accurate closure without incremental risk to the patient [16]. These advances have resulted in excellent short- and long-term clinical results.

Embryology and Pathologic Anatomy

An interventricular communication is part of the circulatory pattern during the first 8 weeks of fetal life; the hole is bound by the atrioventricular endocardial cushions, the developing muscular ventricular septum, and the proximal ends of the endocardial cushions, or ridges, the latter structures separating the flow pathways in the developing ventricular outflow tract. Failure to close this embryonic communication is the reason for persistence of the most common type of VSD requiring surgical correction, the perimembranous variant. But VSDs due to inappropriate compaction of the muscular septum can result in defects in any part of the septum, while failure to muscularize the outflow ridges produces doubly committed defects. There are chromosomal, familial, and geographic influences on normal closure of the embryonic interventricular communication and normal formations of the ventricular septum and the subpulmonary infundibulum. There is variation in incidence for certain years, different seasons, and different geographic areas [17,18]. It is well known that Asian populations have a higher incidence of the defects that exist because of failure of formation of the subpulmonary infundibulum [19,20]. Children of patients with VSDs have a higher incidence of congenital heart disease [21], although not necessarily specifically for VSD [22]. There is also a higher incidence of VSDs in premature infants [23] although there is no correlation with birth order or maternal age.

As an isolated lesion, a VSD can occur in one of three main locations, albeit that subtypes of such defects have been defined and interpreted in different fashion by many authors [24–29]. Systems for naming the VSDs have developed based on varied embryologic and anatomic principles, and differences of opinion persist, although there is a move toward consensus. In this respect, nonetheless, it is important to agree on the locus of space identified as representing the defect. Consider, for example, the situation in which the aortic valvar orifice overrides the crest of the muscular ventricular septum (Figure 17.1). There are at least three loci that could reasonably be defined as the VSD. The direct cranial continuation of the long axis of the ventricular septum marks the plane of the anatomic interventricular communication, but this plane is limited cranially during ventricular diastole by the undersurface of the closed leaflets of the aortic valve. The surgeon would never place a patch to close this plane. A second plane represents the outflow tract from the left ventricle, and the surgeon would take great pains to ensure that this hole was unobstructed at the completion of the repair. It is, in fact, the entrance to the overriding aortic root that is the locus around which the surgeon places the patch to close the hole between the ven-

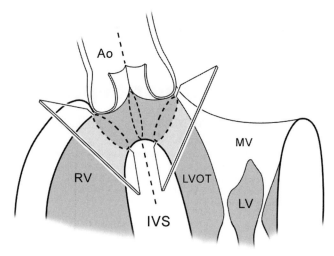

Figure 17.1 There are at least three potential loci that could reasonably be defined as the VSD. The direct cranial continuation of the long axis of the ventricular septum marks the plane of the anatomic interventricular communication, but this plane is limited cranially during ventricular diastole by the undersurface of the closed leaflets of the aortic valve. The surgeon would never place a patch to close this plane. A second plane represents the outflow tract from the left ventricle, and the surgeon would take great pains to ensure that this hole was unobstructed at the completion of the repair. It is, in fact, the entrance to the overriding aortic root that is the locus around which the surgeon places the patch to close the hole between the ventricles. It is, therefore, this view of the hole as seen from the right ventricle that we take to represent the VSD. (Ao, aorta; IVS, interventricular septum; MV, mitral valve; LV, left ventricle; LVOT, left ventricular outflow tract; RV, right ventricle.

tricles. It is, therefore, this view of the hole as seen from the right ventricle that we take to represent the VSD.

When considering anatomic variants for the VSD, the initial, time-honored, surgical classification accounted for four types of defects (Figure 17.2) [3,30]. The type I defect, also referred to as doubly committed and juxta-arterial, conal, supracristal, infundibular, and subarterial, is the consequence of failure of formation of the muscular subpulmonary infundibulum. The phenotypic feature of the defect is the presence of fibrous continuity between the leaflets of the aortic and pulmonary valves in its cranial margin. In consequence of this feature, the superior rim has a direct relationship with the right coronary aortic sinus and the corresponding leaflet of the aortic valve. The inferior margin of the defect is usually muscular with the bar formed by fusion of the caudal limb of the septal band fusing with the musculature of the inner heart curve serving to protect the atrioventricular conduction axis. Defects of this type, however, can also extend to become adjacent to the remnant of the membranous septum and could then also be classified as the type II defect. Defects opening directly into the subpulmonary infundibulum can also, on occasion have exclusively muscular borders. While some authors might still identify such defects as being type

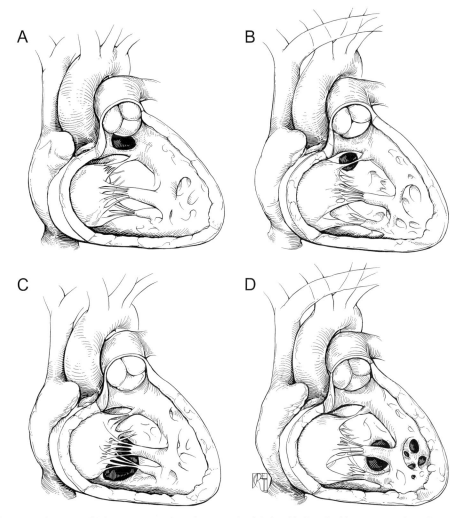

Figure 17.2 Classic anatomic types of VSD. **A,** Type I (conal, supracristal, infundibular, doubly committed, and juxta-arterial) VSD; **B,** Type II or perimembranous VSD; **C,** Type III VSD (atrioventricular canal type or inlet septum type); and **D,** Type IV VSD (single or multiple), also called muscular VSDs.

I in that they lack the phenotypic feature of fibrous continuity between the leaflets of the arterial valves, they are better defined as muscular outlet or muscular conal defects. In these defects also, the leaflets of the aortic valve can prolapse through the VSD and cause aortic insufficiency. In the presence of the muscular posteroinferior margin, the atrioventricular conduction axis is not in direct surgical proximity to the margins. Defects of this type account for less than one-tenth of isolated defects in Caucasian populations [16,31]. In contrast, reports from Asian countries show that the defects opening directly beneath the pulmonary valve are more frequent, accounting for up to one-third of all VSDs requiring surgical closure [32,33].

It is the type II VSD that is most frequently encountered at surgery [31]. It is the term perimembranous, in our opinion, that best describes this kind of defect, as the area of the defect is directly adjacent to the atrioventricular part of the membranous septum. This fibrous area, therefore,

forms part of the perimeter of the VSD. These VSDs used to be described as being membranous. They exist because of failure to close the embryonic interventricular communication by appropriate formation of the membranous septum. A remnant of the interventricular part of the membranous septum, nonetheless, known as the membranous flap, is frequently found in the inferior and caudad margin of the defect. The defect, therefore, existing because of deficiency of the muscular margins of the defect, can open into various parts of the right ventricle according to the precise areas of the muscular deficiency [34]. Despite arguments as to the appropriateness of the term "perimembranous," common use trumps the best interpretations of ancient Greek and Latin. Current database assessments show that most surgeons now closing these VSDs describe them as being perimembranous. The VSDs are usually bordered cranially by the muscular subpulmonary infundibulum, often with malalignment of the muscular outlet septum, so that they are directly related to the right and noncoronary leaflets of the aortic valve. The phenotypic feature of the defect, nonetheless, is fibrous continuity in the inferocaudad margin between the leaflets of the aortic and tricuspid valves (TVs), this area incorporating the atrioventricular component of the membranous septum. Because of this feature, the atrioventricular conduction axis penetrates directly through this border of the defect and is always at risk of damage during surgical closure.

The type III defects are also known as atrioventricular canal types, although this term is controversial. The feature of these defects is that they open to the inlet of the right ventricle, but they can take various anatomic forms (Figure 17.3). The true atrioventricular canal defect, as the name implies, has a common atrioventricular junction. These defects are atrioventricular rather than ventricular but with the bridging leaflets of the common atrioventricular valve attached to the underside of the atrial septum so that shunting is possible only at the ventricular level (Figure 17.3A). These VSDs, the rarest variant of atrioventricular septal defect with common atrioventricular junction, are associated with trifoliate left atrioventricular valves. They have the conduction axis arising from a posteroinferior atrioventricular node, as in all atrioventricular canal malformations. The more common defect described as being a type III VSD is no more than a perimembranous defect that opens predominantly to the inlet of the right ventricle (Figure 17.3B). These defects are shielded by the septal leaflet of the TV but retain fibrous continuity with both the noncoronary leaflet of the aortic valve and the leaflets of the mitral valve. They do not, however, possess a common atrioventricular canal. A third variant has also been described as being an atrioventricular canal defect. This is the defect associated with straddling of the leaflets of the TV and overriding of the right atrioventricular junction (Figure 17.3C). Such defects can also be considered perimembranous, in that they show fibrous continuity between the leaflets of the aortic, tricuspid, and mitral valves, but their phenotypic feature is malalignment between the atrial and muscular ventricular septal structures. Because of this, the atrioventricular node is deviated posteroinferiorly, being formed at the point of union between the muscular septum and the right atrioventricular junction. The node is no longer at the apex of the triangle of Koch and is at major risk during surgical closure of the defect. These VSDs again are not associated with a common atrioventricular canal. Some also include muscular defects opening to the inlet of the right ventricle in this group but on the basis of their phenotypic features, such VSDs with exclusively muscular borders should be considered as type IV defects (Figure 17.3D).

The various defects making up the type III VSDs have different embryologic origins. The perimembranous defects are the consequence of failure of proper formation of the muscular septum normally interposed between the ventricular inlets. The true atrioventricular canal defects, in contrast, reflect the failure to divide the atrioventricular canal into its right and left components, with the attachment of the bridging leaflets of the common valve serving to confine shunting at the ventricular level. The VSD associated with a straddling TV reflects inappropriate transfer of the developing right atrioventricular junction to the right ventricle. This defect is part of a spectrum leading to double-inlet left ventricle with right-sided incomplete right ventricle.

The phenotypic feature of the final type of defect, the type IV defect, is that, when viewed from the right ventricular aspect, it has exclusively muscular borders. Hence, they are also called muscular VSDs. They can be located in any part of the muscular ventricular septum and can be single or multiple. Some of the type I and type III defects, having exclusively muscular rims, should properly be defined as type IV defects. The muscular defects can be difficult to visualize and repair surgically, in part because their borders are often formed on different planes and take various shapes. When opening to the apical part of the right ventricle, they can also be difficult to reach. A particular subtype of muscular VSDs is the "Swiss-cheese" VSD. This defect can involve all components of the muscular septum, the morphologic characteristics suggesting failure of compaction during embryologic development [35,36]. Multiple, well formed muscular defects should be differentiated from the "Swiss-cheese" variant, as patients with the former type can undergo primary closure as opposed to banding of the pulmonary trunk, while those with the Swiss-cheese septum are better treated by banding.

A defect not included in the time-honored classification is the Gerbode defect. This is a direct communication between the left ventricle and the right atrium [37]. The first pathologic description was provided by Buhl in 1857 [38], and it was Kirby who performed the first surgical correction in 1956 [39]. Despite these antecedent reports, it was the report by Frank Gerbode and his associates in 1958 [40] that placed the moniker on this defect (Figure 17.4) [37,40].

In their description of five patients, four had a perimembranous VSD with an associated deficiency of the septal leaflet of the TV, thus permitting a shunt from left ventricle to right atrium (Figure 17.5) [37,40]. Their fifth patient, in contrast, exhibited a congenital deficiency of the atrioventricular component of the membranous septum (Figures 17.6, 17.7) [37,40]. It is this variant that is generally thought to represent the true Gerbode defect. Such true defects have been considered very rare, but at Children's Memorial Hospital over a period of 18 years, we encountered six patients with the true defect [37]. The patients had several diagnostic and therapeutic features in common,

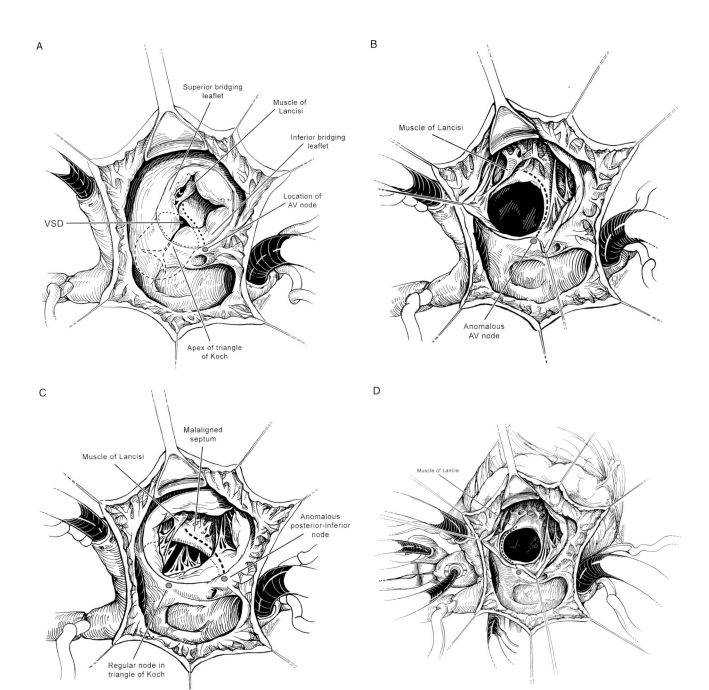

Figure 17.3 Composite representation of the various forms of inlet types of VSD, which have been identified historically as type III, atrioventricular canal type, and inlet VSDs. **A** shows an artists' view of a true atrioventricular canal defect. There is a common atrioventricular junction. These defects are basically atrioventricular rather than ventricular but with bridging leaflets of the common atrioventricular valve attached to the underside of the elongated atrial septum. The shunting therefore is possible only at the ventricular level. Note the location of the atrioventricular node, which conforms with the anatomy of complete atrioventricular septal defect and is not located within the triangle of Koch. **B** shows the more common inlet type of VSD, which is no more than a perimembranous defect that opens predominantly into the inlet of the right ventricle. The atrioventricular node and the conduction system is shown. **C** shows the lesion previously described as an "atrioventricular canal defect", but which has separate right and left atrioventricular junctions, and hence does not have an atrioventricular canal. The phenotypic feature of this defect is malalignment between the atrial septum and the muscular

ventricular septum, associated with straddling and overriding of the tricuspid valve. Because of the septal malalignment, the ventricular septum inserts postero-inferiorly away from the crux of the heart. The feature underscores the grossly abnormal arrangement of the atrioventricular conduction axis, which arises from an anomalous atrioventricular node formed at the point where the muscular ventricular septum meets the atrioventricular junction. The regular atrioventricular node is present at the apex of the triangles of Koch, but because of the septal malalignment, is unable to make contact with the ventricular conduction tissues. **D** shows the defect with exclusively muscular borders that opens to the inlet of the right ventricle. This defect would correctly be classified as being muscular, but because of its position, and its exclusively muscular borders, it has a different relationship to the atrioventricular conduction axis when compared to the perimembranous defect that opens to the right ventricular inlet (B). Of great importance is the location of the conduction system, which proceeds superiorly around the defect as noted.

A

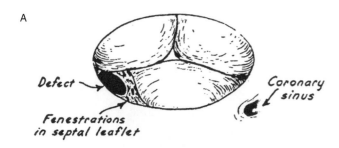

B

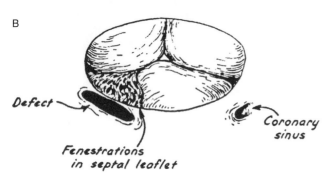

Figure 17.4 A, Indirect left ventricular to right atrial shunt through defect in tricuspid valve. **B**, The true or direct left ventricular to right atrial shunt. (Reproduced with permission from Gerbode *et al.* [40].)

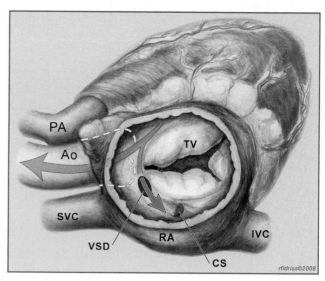

Figure 17.6 The anatomy of the Gerbode defect, the direct left ventricular to right atrial communication. (Ao, aorta; CS, coronary sinus; IVC, inferior vena cava; PA, pulmonary artery; RA, right atrium; SVC, superior vena cava; TV, tricuspid valve; VSD, ventricular septal defect.) (Reproduced with permission from Kelle *et al.* [37].)

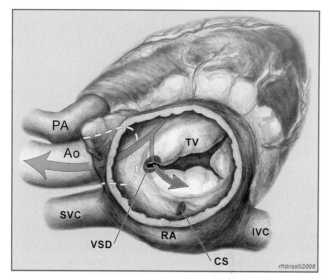

Figure 17.5 The more common, indirect type of communication where the flow of blood is from the left ventricle through a ventricular septal defect and then through a defect in the tricuspid valve into the right atrium. (Ao, aorta; CS, coronary sinus; IVC, inferior vena cava; PA, pulmonary artery; RA, right atrium; SVC, superior vena cava; TV, tricuspid valve; VSD, ventricular septal defect.) (Reproduced with permission from Kelle *et al.* [37].)

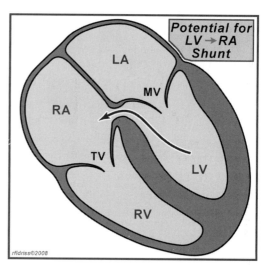

Figure 17.7 The blood in the left ventricle goes through the small area of the membranous septum where there is the potential for a left ventricular to right atrial shunt as shown in lateral view. (LA, left atrium; LV, left ventricle; MV, mitral valve; RA, right atrium; RV, right ventricle; TV, tricuspid valve.) (Reproduced with permission from Kelle *et al.* [37].)

which enhanced their clinical management. The defect is usually diagnosed by echocardiography, which shows a high Doppler gradient from left ventricle to right atrium in association with an unusually dilated right atrium. The absence of tricuspid regurgitation distinguishes the true defect from the indirect forms. Spontaneous closure is very rare, so surgical closure is recommended and is associated with excellent results [37,41,42].

New Concepts of Nomenclature

Nowadays, many surgeons classify VSDs on the basis of the borders of the defect rather than the area they occupy relative to the components of the right ventricle, as it is recognition of the borders that provides the crucial information concerning the location of the atrioventricular conduction axis (Figure 17.8) [29,30,35,43]. According to the nature of the borders, all defects can then be placed into three rather than four groups. Perimembranous defects are bordered directly by fibrous continuity between the leaflets of the atrioventricular and arterial valves. Muscular defects are completely embedded in the septal musculature and have exclusively muscular rims when viewed from the right ventricle. Doubly committed and juxta-arterial defects are bordered directly by fibrous continuity between the

leaflets of the aortic and pulmonary valves. The perimembranous and muscular defects are then subdivided into three additional subgroups, based on whether they mainly open into the inlet, apical trabecular, or outlet portions of the right ventricle.

Van Praagh and colleagues advocate a third system for nomenclature [34,44]. This system again includes four main types of VSDs, albeit with subtle differences from the time-honored groupings (Figure 17.9) [30,34,44]. In this system, VSDs are classified as being of atrioventricular canal, muscular, conoventricular, or conal types. Atrioventricular canal-type VSDs are those in the alleged atrioventricular canal portion of the muscular ventricular septum, being located beneath the TV and limited by the TV annulus. These defects, however, do not have a common atrioventricular junction but do have overriding of the orifice of the TV. Muscular VSDs have a rim totally made up of muscle and may occur anywhere in the muscular septum. Such muscular VSDs may be subdivided into anterior, midventricular, posterior, and apical types depending on their location in the muscular septum. Conoventricular defects can include defects of the membranous septum alone, but most involve more than just the membranous septum and are, therefore, termed paramembranous. Van Praagh *et al.* [34] use the term paramembranous and not perimembranous, arguing that these defects are beside the membranous septum and confluent with it. Such conoventricular defects include those with anterior malalignment of the conal septum, as seen in tetralogy of Fallot, and those

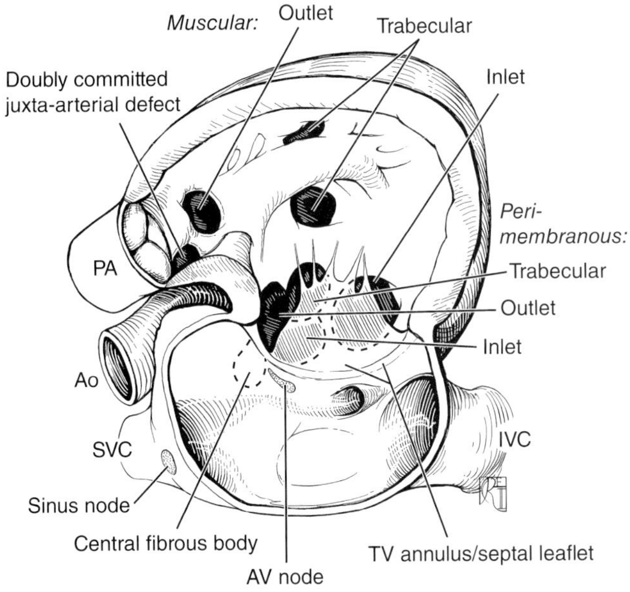

Figure 17.8 This drawing depicts the VSD nomenclature system advocated by the European school. VSDs are subdivided into three main types: perimembranous defects, muscular defects, and doubly committed juxta-arterial defects. (Ao, aorta; IVC, inferior vena cava; PA, pulmonary artery; SVC, superior vena cava.)

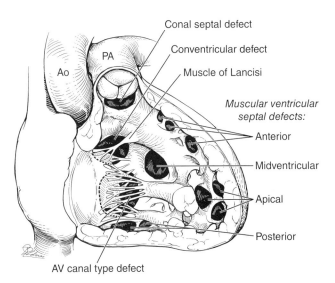

Figure 17.9 This diagram depicts the VSD nomenclature system advocated by Van Praagh. Ventricular septal defects are subdivided into four main types: conal, conoventricular, atrioventricular canal type, and muscular defects. (Ao, aorta; PA, pulmonary artery.)

with posterior malalignment, as seen in interrupted aortic arch. The conal septal defects result from a defect within the conal septum, being limited upstream by the muscular subpulmonary infundibulum and being surrounded by conal musculature.

Steps are currently in place to unify these various systems of nomenclature. Computer-generated images can now be used to demonstrate how the various previously described nomenclature systems can all coexist and be interrelated, providing that accurate phenotypes are provided for the defects as defined within the various systems [45].

Such a system that attempts to unify all the classifications may seem overly complex, but in reality, it is based on the existence of three types of interventricular communications: subarterial, perimembranous, and muscular. The myriad of other more detailed choices for coding is then manageable with the use of computer-generated coding and the hierarchical scheme as described by Jacobs and associates [45,46].

Thus, the basic hierarchy accounts simply for a VSD. The second level of the hierarchy divides the VSDs into the aforementioned main types. In the third level, each type of defect is modified according to its location relative to the components of the right ventricle. The fourth and fifth levels then provide further definitive descriptions for each subtype. These descriptors, which include malalignment between the atrial and ventricular septal structures, posterior or anterior malalignment of the muscular outlet septum, multiple VSDs, and so forth, thus account for multiple synonyms and appropriate systemic associations. Modern-day computer graphics, therefore, simplify the process of naming, as the more important issues are the location of the hole and the nature of its borders as seen from the right ventricle, rather than what it is called. The modern-day surgeon must be conversant with all classifications in order to describe, understand, and close the defects.

Pathophysiology

It is the size of the VSD, along with the pulmonary vascular resistance, which determines the magnitude of the left-to-right shunt. Other factors include ventricular compliance and obstructions to pulmonary or aortic outflows. The physiologic effects are age-dependent, being related early in life to pulmonary vascular resistance and later in life to the degree of narrowing and eventual closure of the VSD. For example, at birth pulmonary vascular resistance is predictably high and usually blunts the potential left-to-right shunt to the extent that the diagnosis often may go unrecognized. Within weeks to months, the pulmonary vascular resistance falls, resulting in an increasing left-to-right shunt and audible murmur. When shunting is excessive, congestive heart failure develops manifested by dyspnea, poor

feeding, frequent upper respiratory infections, and failure to thrive. In these patients, pulmonary vascular changes may begin to develop as early as the first months of life with pulmonary arteriolar thickening [47]. Typically, after 2–3 years, these changes may progress resulting in irreversible pulmonary vascular obstructive disease. In later stages, pulmonary vascular resistance may exceed systemic vascular resistance resulting in reversal of the shunt, cyanosis, and eventual death.

Children with restrictive defects and decreased left-to-right shunting usually remain asymptomatic with little or no medical therapy. They may improve symptomatically as the relative size of the VSD decreases. This leads to a clinical dilemma concerning the most prudent time for reference for surgical closure. Although the progression of pulmonary vascular disease is variable, it is generally agreed that irreversible pulmonary vascular disease will not occur before 1–2 years of age.

Natural History

The clinical course of patients born with a VSD is quite variable, depending to a large degree on the size of the defect, the magnitude of the left-to-right shunt, and the pulmonary vascular resistance. Most VSDs are restrictive, being less than 0.5 cm diameter. They frequently become smaller or undergo spontaneous closure during the first year of life, obviating the need for surgical closure in the majority of cases [48–51]. The mechanisms of spontaneous closure include fibrosis of the margins induced by hemodynamic changes; adherence of the septal leaflet of the TV to the defect, often forming a tricuspid tissue pouch; and muscular hypertrophy, which occurs most commonly with muscular defects [52]. The incidence of spontaneous closure is highest during the first year of life but continues to a lesser degree up to about 5 years, after which spontaneous closure is rare. An undesirable mechanism of spontaneous occlusion is prolapse of an aortic valvar leaflet into the defect, oftentimes causing aortic insufficiency. This is an indication for prompt surgical repair, albeit that it is preferable to identify the defects associated with this potential complication and close them before its development.

In patients with larger VSDs, symptoms develop soon after birth concomitant with the fall in the elevated neonatal pulmonary vascular resistance. Congestive heart failure, manifested by dyspnea, repeated pulmonary infections, hepatomegaly, sweating, and failure to thrive, usually responds to medical therapy but may persist. Increased pulmonary vascular resistance secondary to hypertensive pulmonary vascular disease worsens with increasing age [53–55]. Patients are at risk of developing irreversible pulmonary vascular disease after 1–2 years of age. This process may lead to the Eisenmenger syndrome, which is characterized by greater pulmonary than systemic vascular resistance, reversal of the ventricular shunt with resultant cyanosis, and eventual right ventricular failure. Although some patients show increased pulmonary vascular tone in the first year of life, the Eisenmenger syndrome typically takes much longer to develop, appearing most frequently in the second and third decade of life and typically leading to death by the age of 40 [56].

Some children with isolated defects develop subpulmonic stenosis due to right ventricular infundibular hypertrophy, producing physiology similar to tetralogy of Fallot. Because the pulmonary arteriolar beds have been protected from the high ventricular pressures, these patients are not at risk for pulmonary vascular destructive disease, in much the same way as if the patient had undergone palliative banding of the pulmonary trunk.

Bacterial endocarditis is a rare complication and occurs at a rate of approximately 0.3% per year for each patient with a VSD [57–61]. Its development is indicated by fever, bacteremia, and recurrent pulmonary infections. The locus of infection is usually the septal leaflet of the TV, which may result in an altered systolic murmur and localized vegetations identifiable by echocardiography. Antibiotic treatment is usually effective in controlling the active infection. After such an episode, closure of the VSD, regardless of its size, and TV repair are indicated. Prophylactic closure of restrictive VSDs in the absence of traditional indications for closure remains controversial. This is because of the small incidence of endocarditis compared with the small, but nevertheless present, risk of morbidity and mortality from surgical closure, as well as emotional and cosmetic considerations.

Ventricular septal defects are often associated with other lesions that develop because of their anatomic and hemodynamic characteristics. Prolapse of the leaflets of the aortic valve occurs most frequently with the defects opening directly into the outlet of the right ventricle, be these defects doubly committed and juxta-arterial, muscular outlet, or perimembranous defects opening to the right ventricular outlet with malalignment of the muscular outlet septum. Either the right or noncoronary leaflets of the aortic valve can be involved. With advancing age, untreated prolapse of the aortic valvar leaflets results, first, in a decreased left-to-right shunt because the involved leaflet often prolapses into the defect and reduces the shunt and, second, worsening aortic insufficiency. Early surgical closure may prevent the development of aortic insufficiency in those patients who initially had prolapse without insufficiency. If aortic insufficiency is present, repair can be performed at the time of surgical closure. Chronic turbulence through the VSD can also lead to bacterial endocarditis, which most often affects the septal leaflet of the TV [58].

Diagnosis

Patients with restrictive VSDs are generally diagnosed by the discovery of a loud holosystolic murmur heard best at the left sternal border, rarely accompanied by a hyperactive precordium and a ventricular bulge. The intensity of the murmur may vary significantly and can be inversely related to the size of the defect. The smaller its size, the louder the murmur. As the pulmonary vascular resistance rises, the murmur becomes shorter, softer, and limited to the early part of systole. It may disappear entirely, leaving a loud second heart sound due to closure of the pulmonary valve and indicative of severe pulmonary hypertension. The liver may be enlarged, and the neck veins can be distended.

Changes in chest X-ray are relative to the size of the left-to-right shunt. They include varying degrees of increased pulmonary vascularity and cardiomegaly with biventricular enlargement (Figure 17.10) [30]. The electrocardiogram may be normal or may show right, left, or combined ventricular hypertrophy.

Cross-sectional echocardiography, coupled with Doppler interrogation, now permits cardiologists not only to diagnose the presence of VSDs, but also to establish their phenotype. Multiple views help determine the location and size of the VSD, its borders, the morphology of the ventricular outflow tracts, the involvement of the aortic valve, and the proximity to the tension apparatus of the atrioventricular valves (Figure 17.11) [30]. This technique, however,

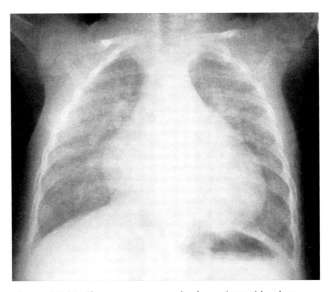

Figure 17.10 Chest roentgenograph of a patient with a large VSD showing cardiomegaly and increased pulmonary vascularity due to the large left-to-right shunt.

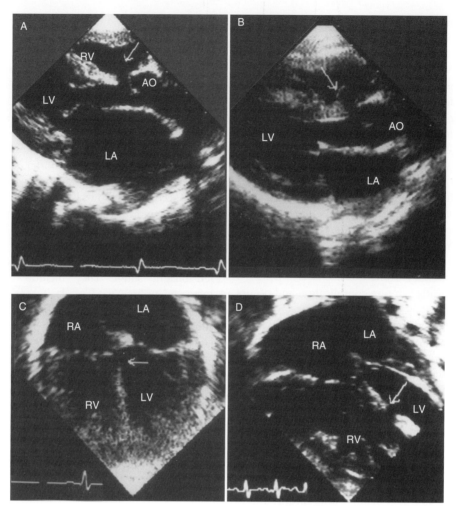

Figure 17.11 Echocardiographic views showing examples of the various types of VSDs. **A,** Parasternal long-axis view showing a doubly committed and juxta-arterial VSD. Arrow indicates the VSD with the right coronary leaflet of the aortic valve prolapsing into the defect. **B,** Parasternal long-axis view showing a perimembranous VSD. Arrow indicates tricuspid pouch (accessory tricuspid tissue). **C,** Apical four-chamber view showing a so-called atrioventricular canal type VSD (inlet VSD). Arrow indicates the position of the VSD in relation to the mitral and tricuspid valves at the inlet portion of the right ventricle. Note that the patient does not have a common atrioventricular canal. **D,** Apical four-chamber view showing a midmuscular VSD. Arrow indicates the position of the VSD. (AO, aorta; LA, left atrium; LV, left ventricle; RA, right atrium; RV, right ventricle.)

does not provide other important information that is determined by cardiac catheterization, such as quantification of ratio of systemic and pulmonary flows, the pulmonary arterial pressure, and accurate identification of multiple defects (Figure 17.12) [30] (see Chapter 4, *Preoperative Diagnostic Evaluation*). The current diagnostic trend, nonetheless, is away from cardiac catheterization, with greater reliance on echocardiographic and Doppler interrogation. The reason for this change is based on surgical trends toward earlier closure. For instance, a 3–6-month-old infant with a demonstrated large VSD and related symptoms almost assuredly has elevated pulmonary arterial pressures and a large left-to-right shunt. Moreover, the chance

of irreversible pulmonary vascular disease approaches zero. Consequently, cardiac catheterization, while technically informative, does not impact on the decision to advocate surgical closure in light of the current advances in echocardiographic techniques. On the other hand, a child or young adult with a large VSD may have increased pulmonary vascular resistance, which cannot accurately be determined by echocardiography. In these circumstances cardiac catheterization is required to measure pulmonary arterial pressure, to calculate pulmonary vascular resistance, and to determine the response of the pulmonary arteries to vasodilators, all of which will influence the decision regarding surgical closure.

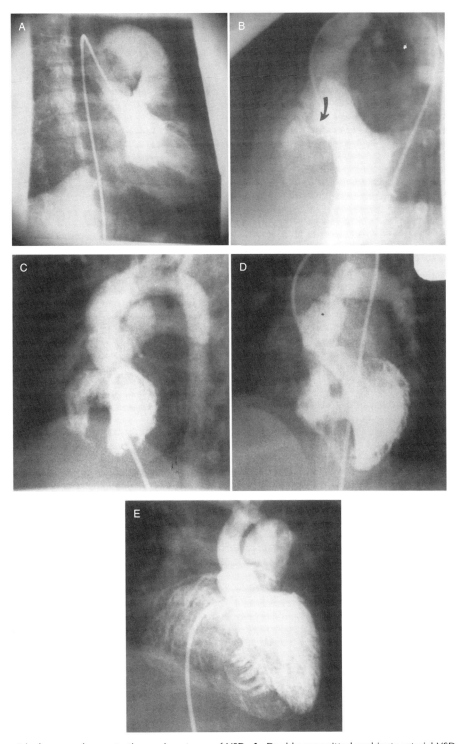

Figure 17.12 Left ventriculograms demonstrating various types of VSD. **A,** Doubly committed and juxta-arterial VSD (conal, supercristal, subarterial). **B,** Perimembranous (arrow indicates prolapse of the aortic valve through the VSD). **C,** Inlet type. **D,** Midmuscular VSD. **E,** Multiple muscular VSD, "Swiss-cheese" type.

Medical Management

Medical management is directed at the pathophysiologic consequences of the left-to-right shunt, the management of increased pulmonary vascular resistance, and prophylactic antibiotic administration for endocarditis.

Infants with congestive heart failure often respond to digitalis, diuretic therapy, and afterload reduction. Supplemental nutritional support may be necessary because of poor feeding and failure to thrive. Optimal antibiotic therapy will be required for recurrent pulmonary infections. These supportive measures often allow delay of surgical treatment and may promote spontaneous restriction or closure of the VSD. When these measures are not effective, surgical closure should be undertaken. Occasionally, a patient may require assisted ventilation and inotropic support to treat decompensated congestive heart failure as a bridge to surgical therapy. Under these conditions, a thorough evaluation should be undertaken to determine causes for the decompensation, such as subaortic stenosis, coarctation, persistent PDA, or infection.

Older patients with pulmonary hypertension and elevated pulmonary vascular resistance require cardiac catheterization to determine the pulmonary arterial pressure, along with the response to inspired oxygen and other vasodilators such as amrinone, isoproterenol, nitroglycerin, nitroprusside, inhaled nitric oxide, and prostaglandin E1. An increase in left-to-right shunting and/or a decrease in the mean pulmonary arterial pressure are considered responses favoring VSD closure. These same agents can be administered postoperatively to promote resolution of reversible pulmonary hypertension.

Patient Selection

The selection of patients for VSD closure centers around the size and type of the defect as determined by echocardiography and/or cardiac catheterization, the natural history, the intervening symptoms caused by the VSD, and complicating factors.

Patients with Large Ventricular Septal Defects

Infants with large VSDs and severe, intractable congestive heart failure should undergo surgical closure at any time during the first 3 months of life. If, however, these patients respond to medical therapy, then conservative follow-up is warranted up to about 6 months of age. Spontaneous closure of large VSDs becomes less probable after this time (Figure 17.13) [16,30,48,51,62], while the incidence of progressive pulmonary vascular obstructive disease increases. Closure should be undertaken at this time, especially if the pulmonary vascular resistance is high, greater

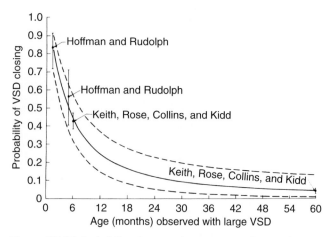

Figure 17.13 Probability of eventual spontaneous closure of a large VSD according to the age at which the patient is observed. The broken lines enclose the 70% CLs around the solid probability line. The specific ratios, with the 70% CLs reported by Hoffman and Rudolph [62] (1966) and Keith and associates [51] (1971), are shown centered on the mean or assumed ages of patients in their reports ($p < 0.001$). (Reproduced with permission from Blackstone *et al.* [48].)

than 4 units/m² [2,62] or if the ratio of pulmonary to systemic flows exceeds 2:1.

Older patients with large VSDs occasionally present with varying degrees of established pulmonary vascular obstructive disease. Predictably, these patients have a history of some antecedent clinical improvement due to the decreased left-to-right shunt in response to the increased pulmonary vascular resistance. Patients with a dominant right-to-left shunt and calculated pulmonary vascular resistance higher than 8 units/m² and who show no response to pulmonary arterial vasodilatation are not considered candidates for surgical closure. Some centers have depended on lung biopsy to evaluate the degree of pulmonary vascular changes, but this has now fallen from favor [63–65]. There has been limited experience with VSD closure and single- or double-lung transplantation for those patients with progressive pulmonary vascular disease. The results of this therapy are discussed in Chapter 43, *Heart, Lung and Heart-lung Transplantation in Children*.

Patients with Small Defects

Infants shown by echocardiography and physical examination to have small VSDs require little or no medical therapy. They are followed with the expectation that the VSDs may get smaller and/or undergo spontaneous closure. After the first year of life, asymptomatic patients with small perimembranous or muscular defects can be re-evaluated on a timely basis for physiologic and anatomic signs that would suggest indications for surgical closure. Recent data have led to questions regarding the validity of historical indications for surgical closure [66]. The proposed, more liberal indications are any evidence of aortic valvar prolapse (even without regurgitation), a history of prior endocarditis, and any evidence of ventricular dilation, even if the left-to-right shunt is less than 2:1. A review from our institution from 1980 to 1991 revealed 141 patients with a Qp/Qs ratio of less than 2:1 who had undergone surgical closure for one or more of the above indications [66]. There were no operative or late deaths, no instances of heart block, and no reoperations for residual shunting. Transatrial or transpulmonary repair was feasible in all. These data, although presently mildly controversial, suggest that the surgical risk of closing a restrictive VSD permitting a high-velocity turbulent jet is less than the combined lifetime risk of bacterial endocarditis, aortic valvar prolapse that may lead to aortic insufficiency, and tricuspid regurgitation [67,68].

Patients with Defects Opening Directly Beneath the Pulmonary Valve (Conal Ventricular Septal Defects)

These patients have a high probability of developing aortic valvar prolapse and aortic insufficiency, especially after 5 years of age (Figure 17.14) [30,69]. Early surgical intervention may control or prevent the progression of aortic insufficiency [69–75]. Because of the known natural history and the impact of surgery, all doubly committed and juxta-arterial defects (conal VSDs) should be closed regardless of the magnitude of the left-to-right shunt.

Surgical Considerations

Preoperative demonstration of the location of the VSD determines the options available with regard to the cardiac incisions needed for exposure, avoidance of injury to the conduction pathways, and the operative technique needed to secure closure when part of the perimeter of the defect is formed by the leaflets of the atrioventricular or arterial valves.

In general, there are five operative approaches for VSD closure: right atrial, transpulmonary, transaortic, right ventricular, and left ventricular. Mixed and multiple VSDs, or those that have extensive involvement of more than one region of the septum, may require a combined approach.

Right Atrial Approach

This surgical approach (Figure 17.15) [30] is the most frequently used and is usually applicable to perimembranous defects, all those opening to the inlet of the right ventricle, most muscular defects, and the Gerbode types. Closure of muscular defects is usually first attempted through the right atrium. With some types, nonetheless, such as those opening at the right ventricular apex or the Swiss-cheese variant, a limited left apical ventricular incision may be required.

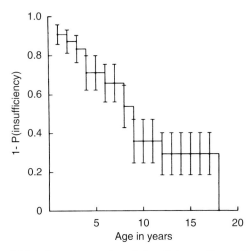

Figure 17.14 Onset curve of aortic insufficiency. Comparison of age versus probability of being free of aortic insufficiency in patients before operation for conal VSD (Kaplan-Meier technique). (Reproduced with permission from Backer *et al.* [69].)

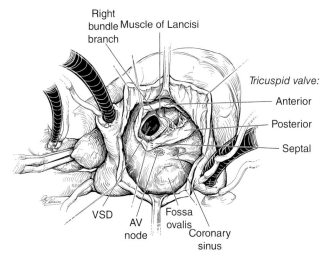

Figure 17.15 Right atrial approach for VSD closure after aortobicaval cannulation and aortic cross-clamp with cardioplegia. The tricuspid valvar leaflets are retracted to expose the VSD and the important surrounding structures. Interrupted pledget-supported sutures can be placed on the right ventricular side of the septum while avoiding injury to the aortic valve, the tricuspid valve leaflets, and the conduction system. (Ao, aorta; AV, atrioventricular; VSD, ventricular septal defect.)

In addition to the general tenets regarding the cavitary incision and the conduct of extracorporeal circulation, many established techniques may be helpful in facilitating exposure with these different approaches during surgical VSD closure. The use of aortic cross-clamping, cardioplegia, hypothermia, and a left ventricular vent are important not only to protect the myocardium and provide a relatively bloodless intracardiac surgical field but also to relax the myocardium in order to optimize exposure. The view through the tricuspid valvar orifice may not be sufficient to effect complete and simultaneous exposure of all areas and the extent of the defect. When the heart is relaxed, changing the direction and tension of retractors will permit viewing the lesion one sector at a time.

It is usual to close the defect with 5-0 double-armed sutures, with buttressing pledgets, placed 2–3 mm away from its edge on the right ventricular side, permitting a wider contact area between the patch and the myocardium, helping to avoid injury to the conduction bundle that often runs near the crest of the defect, usually on the left ventricular side. Frequently the defects in the perimembranous area may be covered by the septal leaflet of the TV and may not be visualized immediately. This occurs particularly in those cases when the cordal attachments of the TV to the edges of the defect are short and tight, or when there is formation of a pouch by redundant or accessory valvar tissue. In these instances, a clue to the location may be a depression in the TV tissue being sucked into the defect by the action of the left ventricular vent. At times, the surgeon may be misled to believe that a small opening in the valvar tissue represents the total extent of the VSD (Figures 17.16, 17.17) [30,76]. In this circumstance, there may be a temptation to use simple direct closure with a suture, thus leaving the defect open behind the leaflet. This may result in residual shunting through another unrecognized open part of the defect. In order to avoid this pitfall, the hinge of the tricuspid valvar leaflets should be opened in a radial fashion (Figure 17.18) [30], thus exposing the true perimeter of the defect, which should always be closed with a patch.

When incising the TV, it is essential to proceed carefully from the free edge toward an area 3–4 m from the annulus, gradually increasing the size of the opening in the leaflet depending on the needed exposure. The incision should be made meticulously, keeping the leaflets of the aortic valve constantly in view, in part because of their proximity on the upper rim but also because the aortic valvar leaflets may have prolapsed to varying degrees in this area. Radial incision of the TV has been shown to have minimal long-term influence on valvar function, validating the use of this technique [76]. Some authors prefer a circumferential inci-

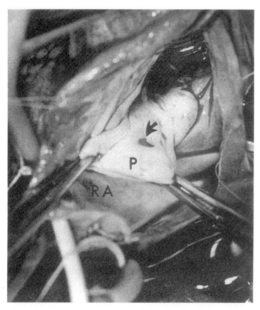

Figure 17.16 Operative photograph showing the right atrium opened to expose a tricuspid pouch, which is pulled with forceps to show a single orifice defect (black arrow). (P, tricuspid pouch; RA, right atrium.) (Reproduced with permission from Idriss *et al.* [76].)

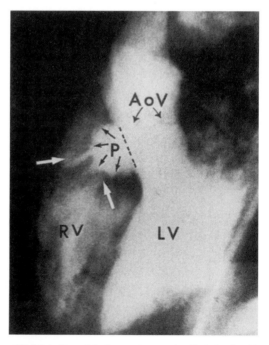

Figure 17.17 Left ventricular angiogram in diastole of a tricuspid pouch with multiple small jets (white arrows). The dotted line delineates the true ventricular defect. Note the proximity of the defect to the aortic valve. (AoV, aortic valve; LV, left ventricle; P, tricuspid pouch; RV, right ventricle.) (Reproduced with permission from Idriss *et al.* [76].)

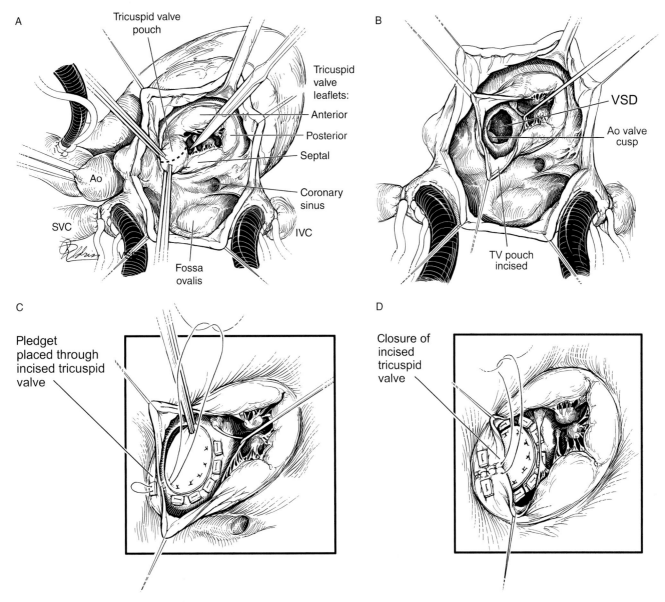

A

Tricuspid valve
pouch

Tricuspid
valve
leaflets:

Anterior

Posterior

Septal

Coronary
sinus

Ao

SVC

IVC

Fossa
ovalis

B

VSD

Ao valve
cusp

TV pouch
incised

C

Pledget
placed through
incised tricuspid
valve

D

Closure of
incised
tricuspid
valve

Figure 17.18 A, Tricuspid valve pouch exposed through a right atrial incision and retracted with sutures. The dotted line outlines the proposed incision site. **B,** The tricuspid valve pouch has been incised toward the annulus and retracted exposing the actual extent of the VSD; **C,** Pledget placed through incised tricuspid valve; **D,** Completed VSD closure showing repair of the incised tricuspid valve. (Ao, aorta; SVC, superior vena cava; IVC, inferior vena cava.)

sion for VSD exposure [77–80]. We have used such a circumferential incision to expose large perimembranous VSDs opening primarily to the inlet of the right ventricle (Figures 17.19–17.24) [81].

To avoid injury to the conduction system, the sutures should be placed superficially and carefully along the inferior and posterior margins of the defect beginning from the area of insertion of the muscle of Lancisi and continuing to the annulus of the TV near the region of the apex of the triangle of Koch (Figure 17.25) [30]. At this junction, buttressed sutures should be placed from the right atrium inward through the septal leaflet of the TV, keeping the

needle about 1–2 mm away from the annulus. This suturing technique is continued superiorly until the transitional area, where the superior edge of the VSD begins to be formed by muscle of the outlet septum. Here, the risk of injury to the conduction system is minimal, while the hazard of damage to the aortic valve is increased. It may be tempting to place the sutures through the membranous flap, which represents the remnant of the interventricular part of the membranous septum, often found in the posteroinferior angle of the defect. We do not recommend this technique because of the possibility of injury to the conduction system. We also avoid the temptation to place sutures

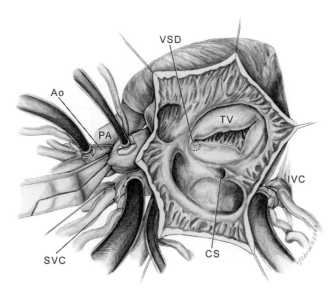

Figure 17.19 A perimembranous ventricular septal defect (circular dotted line) is represented behind the septal leaflet of the tricuspid valve that oftentimes extends toward the anterior leaflet. When complex chordal attachments are present, retraction and optimal exposure may result in chordal disruption and tricuspid insufficiency. It is for these reasons that a circumferential incision is performed to visualize the ventricular septal defect. (Ao, aorta; CS, coronary sinus; IVC, inferior vena cava; PA, pulmonary artery; SVC, superior vena cava; TV, tricuspid valve; VSD, ventricular septal defect.) (Reproduced with permission from Mavroudis *et al.* [81].)

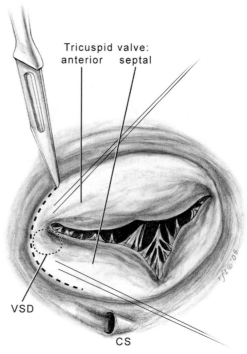

Figure 17.20 The circumferential incision (dashed line) is performed to detach that portion of the tricuspid valve in order to optimally expose the ventricular septal defect, thereby avoiding the possibility of chordal rupture. Great care is taken to avoid injury to the subtended aortic valve leaflets, which are in close proximity to the projected tricuspid incision. Oftentimes, a dose of antegrade cardioplegia can help in identifying the aortic leaflets through this approach. (CS, coronary sinus; VSD, ventricular septal defect.) (Reproduced with permission from Mavroudis *et al.* [81].)

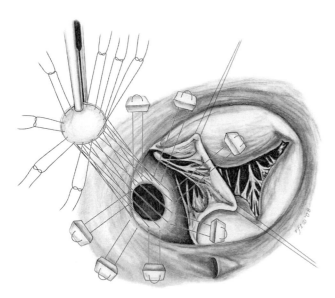

Figure 17.21 The tricuspid valve is retracted, which results in excellent exposure. Pledgeted sutures are place around the edges of the defect with special care to avoid injury to the tricuspid valve, the aortic valve, and the conduction system. At least two pledgeted sutures are placed through the tricuspid annulus from the right atrial cavity to anchor the polytetrafluoroethylene patch. These sutures are then placed through the patch, which can be tied in place, thereby closing the ventricular septal defect. (Reproduced with permission from Mavroudis *et al.* [81].)

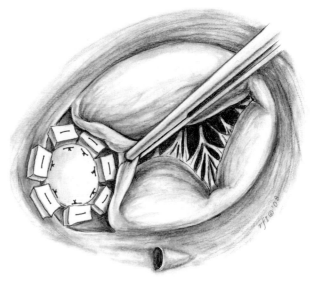

Figure 17.22 The closure of the ventricular septal defect is completed showing the tied pledgeted sutures anchoring the polytetrafluoroethylene patch in place. (Reproduced with permission from Mavroudis *et al.* [81].)

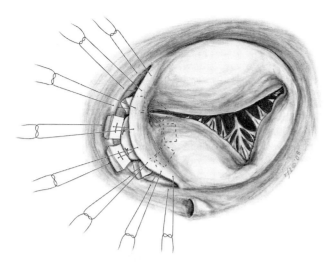

Figure 17.23 The tricuspid valve is reattached using the interrupted suture technique, which theoretically has the advantage of allowing annular growth. (Reproduced with permission from Mavroudis *et al.* [81].)

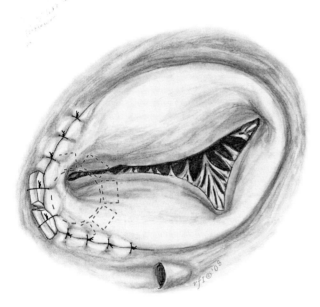

Figure 17.24 The completed ventricular septal defect closure using the circumferential tricuspid incision technique is shown. (Reproduced with permission from Mavroudis *et al.* [81].)

through any fibrous accretions on the crest of the muscular septum, because in our experience such tissue lacks holding qualities.

Transpulmonary Arterial Approach

This technique is usually used for repair of the doubly committed and juxta-arterial defects (conal VSDs) or for muscular defects opening in the subpulmonary area (Figure 17.26) [30]. The techniques for bypass and myocardial

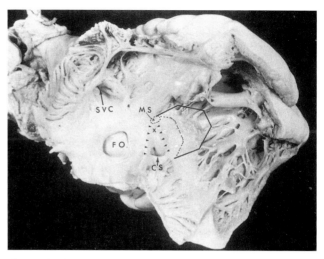

Figure 17.25 Preserved gross specimen showing the right atrium and right ventricle after an atrioventricular transannular incision for exposure. The solid and dotted lines show the inlet portion of the interventricular septum. The black triangles along with the coronary sinus (CS) mark the borders of the triangle of Koch in which lie the atrioventricular node and the bundle of His (X). (FO, foramen ovale; MS, membranous septum; SVC, superior vena cava.)

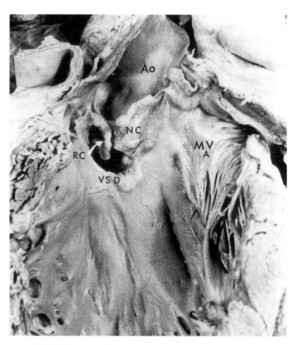

Figure 17.26 Preserved gross specimen showing a doubly committed juxta-arterial VSD with aortic valve prolapse. The left ventricle and aorta have been opened. The VSD is intimately related to the aortic valve and the right coronary cusp (RC) of the aortic valve is prolapsing into the defect. (Ao, aorta; MV$_A$, mitral valve anterior leaflet; NC, noncoronary cusp.)

preservation are the same as for the right atrial approach. Exposure is accomplished through a vertical incision in the pulmonary trunk (Figure 17.27) [30]. These defects are closed using a patch, which helps support the prolapsing leaflets of the aortic valve, preventing continued downward pressure on the leaflets. Complete closure of the defect eliminates the Venturi effect that initially pulls the aortic leaflet into the VSD. A particularly treacherous situation may exist should the prolapsing leaflet partially occlude the defect. In this circumstance, the defect itself may appear small and seem amenable to direct suture. It is important to recognize this pitfall, avoiding injury to the aortic valvar leaflet by using an appropriately sized patch and placing the sutures around the true perimeter of the defect rather than the small false opening (Figure 17.27) [30].

The superior aspect of these defects is formed by fibrous continuity between the leaflets of the aortic and pulmonary

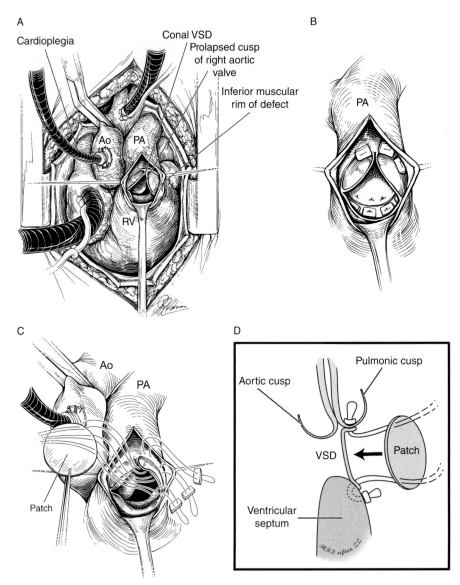

Figure 17.27 A, Operative view of the doubly committed and juxta-arterial (conal) VSD after cardiopulmonary bypass, aortic cross-clamping, and cardioplegic arrest have been established. The exposure is through the longitudinally opened pulmonary artery showing the right cusp of the aortic valve prolapsing into the defect and partially occluding it. **B,** Interrupted pledget-supported sutures are placed circumferentially around the defect and then through a PTFE. **C,** Anterior projection shows that at the superior portion of the defect, the sutures are placed through the base of the pulmonary valve leaflets because there is no muscular septum between the leaflets of the aortic and pulmonic valves. **D,** Lateral projection showing the relationship of the sutures to the pulmonary valve. (Ao, aorta; RV, right ventricle; PA, pulmonary artery; PTFE, polytetrafluoroethylene.)

valves, but the fibrous margin is frequently unsuitable for anchorage of sutures. In this circumstance, a few sutures must be anchored through the base of the leaflets of the pulmonic valve at their junction with the valvar sinuses where the small pledgets will rest against the arterial wall, decreasing the chances of the sutures tearing the thin valvar tissue (Figure 17.27C) [30]. Some have advocated a combined transaortic and transpulmonary approach for concomitant surgical repair of aortic insufficiency [82].

The patch should not interfere with the function of the pulmonary valve and should provide support to the previously prolapsed leaflets of the aortic valve (Figure 17.27D) [30]. The pulmonary trunk is closed primarily.

Transaortic Approach

Closure of VSDs via an aortic incision (Figure 17.28) [30] is usually performed when there is need for concomitant correction of associated lesions, such as aortic valvoplasty for prolapsed leaflets or for relief of valvar or subvalvar stenosis. An obliquely curved incision is made, starting on the anterior aspect of the ascending aorta at a level above the center of the right coronary aortic sinus. The surgeon

should keep in mind that orifices of the coronary arteries may occasionally arise high in the aortic sinuses or above the sinotubular junction and could be injured by the aortic incision. The incision is carried inferiorly and to the right under direct vision toward the center of the noncoronary aortic sinus. The incision may be extended as needed transversely toward the left. Alternatively, the aorta can be transected 1–2 mm above the sinotubular junction. This maneuver permits anterior mobilization of the proximal aorta, thus maximizing the transaortic view. The aortic valvar leaflets are retracted carefully to expose the defect. Often there is absence of a superior muscular or fibrous rim to the defect, making placement of sutures difficult. In this situation, mattress sutures buttressed with pledgets may be taken through the aortic wall from the inside of the aortic valvar sinuses. This exposure has also been used for the subaortic VSDs encountered in the setting of double-outlet right ventricle [83].

Right Ventricular Approach

This incision (Figure 17.29) [30] is now infrequently used for closure of isolated VSDs, as the majority can safely be

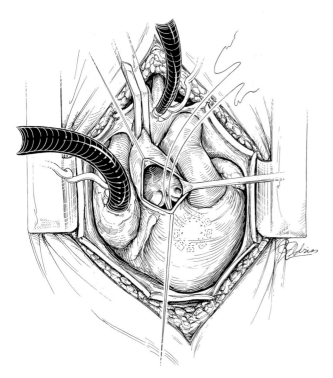

Figure 17.28 Transaortic approach to VSD closure can be applied if the VSD is subarterial and if other indications warrant intra-aortic exposure. Because of the increased risk of heart block, most surgeons prefer the other approaches for VSD closure.

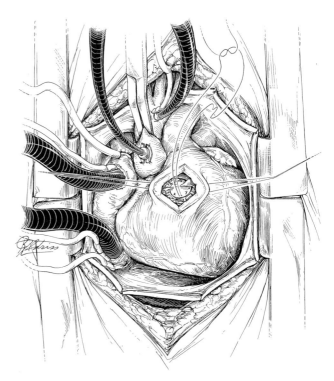

Figure 17.29 Diagram of VSD closure through a right ventriculotomy using aortobicaval cannulation, aortic cross-clamp with cardioplegia, and interrupted pledget-supported sutures.

approached through the right atrial, transpulmonary, or transaortic routes. Should the incision be required, it can be transverse or vertical. The transverse incision may have the advantage of limiting injury to the myocytes aggregated in circular fashion in the subpulmonary infundibulum, albeit that the exposure may be restricted. It is also inadequate when it proves necessary to enlarge the infundibulum with a patch.

The vertical incision should be limited to the infundibular area. Under direct vision, it is usually started in the middle of the anterior infundibular wall between traction sutures and extended upward in the direction of the pulmonary trunk or downward toward the apical component of the right ventricle.

The epicardial distribution of the coronary arteries should be established before beginning the ventriculotomy, in particular the origin of the left anterior descending artery from the main left coronary artery. On occasion, this artery arises as a branch of the right coronary artery and crosses the infundibular wall. At other times, there can be dual supply, with one branch originating from the left coronary artery and the other as an extension of a large conal artery arising from the right coronary artery. In either of these situations, a ventriculotomy is dangerous and should be avoided because of the possibility of injury to the myocardium supplied by the left anterior descending coronary artery. Infrequently, these arteries crossing the infundibulum are intramyocardial and may not clearly be seen. The coronary arterial distribution may also be obscured by adhesions resulting from previous surgery.

The indications for right ventricular incisions include inaccessibility from the right atrium or pulmonary trunk, the presence of a defect opening directly into the infundibular area, optimization of exposure in the presence of obstructive infundibular muscle bundles, and difficulty exposing the inferior margin of an outlet defect. A ventricular incision may optimize exposure in the presence of abnormal and obstructive infundibular muscle bundles that may require resection. Oftentimes these muscle bundles cannot be excised adequately from a right atrial incision, especially when enlargement of the infundibulum with a patch is deemed necessary. A ventricular incision may also be necessary should difficulty be encountered in exposing the inferior margin of an outlet defect due to absence of the subpulmonary infundibulum. A small infundibular incision will help in securing the patch to the inferior border of the VSD. At times this may be accomplished through the right atrium without ventriculotomy.

Left Ventricular Approach

This approach (Figure 17.30) [30] is rarely used. It is limited to closure of certain types of apical muscular defects, par-

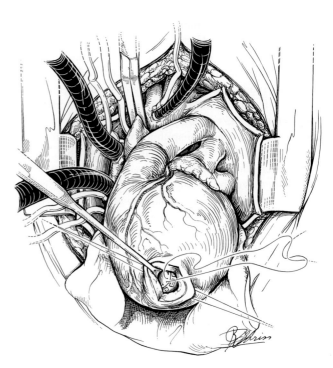

Figure 17.30 Diagram of left ventricular exposure for an apical muscular VSD using aortobicaval cannulation, aortic cross-clamp with cardioplegia, and interrupted pledget-supported sutures. Care is taken to limit the left ventriculotomy to the apex away from the converging coronary arteries. Midmuscular VSDs, on the other hand, are best approached through a right atriotomy to avoid left ventricular dysfunction, which is associated with larger and higher left ventriculotomies.

ticularly those with multiple sieve-like perforations. These defects may be easier to patch from the left ventricular side because of the relatively smooth septum, unlike the right ventricle with its coarse trabeculations and attachments of papillary muscles. The muscular defects, when viewed from the right side, may be hidden or divided by the ventricular trabeculations, thus appearing as multiple openings on the right side, but having a single opening when seen from the left side of the septum.

There are two types of left ventricular incisions. The more frequently employed vertical incision [84] starts in the relatively avascular left ventricular apical area and requires limited extension superiorly. The alternative is to make a transverse incision [85]. In either case, attention to the distribution of the coronary arteries is essential to minimize injury. Left ventricular incisions, except for the small apical incisions that are well tolerated, should be avoided whenever possible to minimize the possibility of associated significant long-term ventricular dysfunction [86].

Relationship of the Conduction Pathways to Different Types of Ventricular Septal Defects

The relationship of the atrioventricular bundle to isolated VSDs was determined by the early work of Lev [87], Truex and Bishof [88], and more recently by Kurosawa and Becker [89], and Milo and colleagues [90]. These contributions enhanced surgical knowledge and awareness of the location of the pathways for atrioventricular conduction, and decreased the incidence of intraoperative injury. Damage to the atrioventricular node, the penetrating bundle, or its right or left branches may result from a suturing needle, from snaring by the suture material, by fibrosis, from hemorrhage, or by anoxic insult. Direct pressure and trauma from rough handling of surgical instruments may also contribute to the occurrence of atrioventricular and intraventricular conduction disturbances [91,92].

When the intracardiac anatomy is viewed through the most commonly used right atrial approach, the location of the atrioventricular node is indicated by the apex of the triangle of Koch (Figure 17.25) [30]. This location does not vary appreciably with the different types of isolated VSDs, aside from the VSD associated with straddling and overriding of the TV. The surgeon can identify the area by the depression or concavity felt by palpation above the coronary sinus and between it and the attachment of the septal leaflet of the TV. From the apex of the triangle, the atrioventricular bundle penetrates the central fibrous body to reach the crest of the muscular ventricular septum. There are variations, however, in the course of the conduction bundle, its depth within the ventricular myocardium, and its relationship to the septal crest.

Avoiding Conduction Injury During Closure of Different Types of Ventricular Septal Defects

Defects Having a Muscular Posteroinferior Rim
Such muscular rims are found in muscular outlet VSDs and in the majority of doubly committed and juxta-arterial VSDs. In the presence of such a muscular rim, the conduction bundle is usually at a safe distance from the margin of the defect. Although the sutures for closure of the defect can be placed with minimal fear of injury to conduction axis, conduction disturbances can occur due to careless introduction of instruments, such as a suction tip, into the right ventricle. In some large VSDs, however, with minimal formation of the caudad limb of the septal band, the inferior rim of the defect may be very close to the bundle of His.

Perimembranous Ventricular Septal Defects
The major danger area for all perimembranous VSDs, apart from those associated with straddling and overriding of the TV, is the inferior and posterior region of the defect as seen

from the right atrium through the tricuspid valvar orifice. The region is generally between the area of the medial papillary muscle of the conus (Lancisi) and the corner where the defect meets the tricuspid annulus, near the remnant of the membranous septum. In the type of defects that have some extension toward the inlet of the right ventricle, the medial papillary muscle may be more anterior and superior in location than usual.

Inlet Ventricular Septal Defects
In the VSDs opening to the inlet of the right ventricle, the medial papillary muscle is usually located more superiorly in relation to the edge of the defect. A consistent guide to the location of the penetrating bundle remains the apical area of the triangle of Koch. From this point the common bundle courses around the inferior aspect of the defect. This type of defect can be distinguished from the muscular inlet type by absence of a muscular ridge in the inlet (Figure 17.3).

Muscular Ventricular Septal Defects
Muscular VSDs opening to the apical part of the right ventricle are unrelated directly to the conduction bundles, and those opening to the outlet are protected from the conduction axis by the caudad limb of the septal band. For muscular defects opening to the inlet of the right ventricle, the conduction axis is found anterosuperiorly relative to the defect (Figure 17.3).

Gerbode Ventricular Septal Defects
The rare left-ventricular-to-right atrial defects located in the atrioventricular portion of the atrial septum are at less risk to the conduction system during closure [40]. Some perimembranous defects, however, may simulate the LV-to-RA defects by shunting through an opening in the TV septal leaflets and have the same risk of injury to the conduction system as other perimembranous VSDs.

The Conduction System and the Transaortic approach

In the normal heart, the nonbranching part of the atrioventricular bundle passes under the fibrous triangle interposed between the noncoronary and right coronary leaflets of the aortic valve. In the presence of a VSD, however, the bundle can be located near the left corner and left inferior border of the defect, close to the junction of the central fibrous body, the remnant of the membranous septum and the mitral valve, and directly beneath the noncoronary leaflet of the aortic valve. Hence, the area extending from under the noncoronary leaflet toward the zone of apposition with the right coronary leaflet and extending toward the middle of the right coronary leaflet should be considered a danger zone with regard to the possibility of surgical injury to the conduction system.

Surgical Management of Ventricular Septal Defects with Associated Lesions

Patent Ductus Arteriosus

Closure of persistent PDA should not present a significant technical difficulty at the time of repair of an associated VSD. Early in the history of surgical management of this combination, correction was performed in two stages. First, ligation of the patent duct coupled with banding of the pulmonary trunk was performed early in infancy, followed at an older age by a second-stage definitive closure of the VSD, debanding of the pulmonary trunk, and arterioplasty.

This early approach has been generally abandoned in favor of a single-stage repair. Infrequently, the two-stage approach is indicated in small sick infants with severe ventricular failure due to multiple muscular or Swiss-cheese VSDs, which may present significant technical difficulties with incomplete closure and unsatisfactory results when primary repair is attempted.

The PDA is easily isolated through the median sternotomy. After opening the pericardium, dissection along the pulmonary trunk carried distally leads to the duct, which is situated in the space near the pulmonary arterial bifurcation between the left pulmonary artery and the aorta.

Several precautionary steps should be taken. During dissection to expose the patent duct, the surgeon should be cognizant at all times of the intimate relationship with the recurrent laryngeal nerve. Hugging too close to the aortic wall during dissection at the aortoductal junction or too close to the sometimes very friable ductal wall should be avoided. The surgeon should carefully clarify the margins of the duct and its aortic and pulmonary relationship before passing an instrument or a ligature around it in order to prevent the possibility of accidental ligation of the left pulmonary artery.

The duct itself should be ligated before initiation of bypass whenever feasible, or exposed enough to be readily closed as soon as bypass is started. Presence of a large open duct during extracorporeal circulation will produce a steal from the aorta into the lower-resistance pulmonary circulation, causing difficulties in maintaining perfusion pressure and possibly causing pulmonary congestion and hemorrhage.

Ventricular Septal Defect with Aortic Insufficiency

Aortic insufficiency (AI) is known to be associated with either the doubly committed subarterial VSDs or perimembranous VSDs opening to the outlet of the right ventricle [69,93–96].

In general, it is the right coronary leaflet of the aortic valve that prolapses into the VSD when the defect is doubly committed (conal VSDs), while the noncoronary leaflet is prolapsed with perimembranous VSDs. At times, the right coronary leaflet near its zone of apposition with the noncoronary leaflet, as well as the noncoronary leaflet itself, protrudes into the defect. The left coronary leaflet is rarely involved [97].

Concomitant repair of the prolapsing leaflet during closure of the VSD depends on the extent of prolapse and the severity of aortic regurgitation. In patients with aortic prolapse and/or mild aortic insufficiency, closing the defect with a patch at a relatively early age has the effect of treating the prolapse by supporting the leaflet and eliminating the windsock or Venturi effect through the open VSD.

In patients with moderate-to-severe aortic regurgitation, consideration should be given to performing an aortic valvoplasty, especially in the older child with long-standing prolapse and a markedly distorted and stretched aortic valvar leaflet. Transaortic exposure is usually employed for aortic valvoplasty, while the VSD itself can be closed through either the transaortic or right atrial approach. Yacoub [98] has advocated a transaortic approach to repair the prolapsing leaflet and suggests closing the VSD using sutures but without inserting a patch. The principles of repair center on reefing of the redundant aortic leaflet and approximation of the inferior rim of the VSD with the hinge of the leaflet from the valvar sinus.

In the presence of moderate-to-severe aortic valve regurgitation, there is a large steal of blood flow from the aortic cannula to the left ventricle during bypass. This will tend to diminish the effectiveness of extracorporeal circulation, distend the left ventricle, and interfere with myocardial perfusion. Left ventricular distention becomes especially severe when the heart fibrillates. Important and rapid sequential steps need to be taken on initiation of bypass to prevent this situation.

On initiation of bypass and positioning of a left ventricular vent, the aorta is cross-clamped and opened. General body cooling is simultaneously begun with cold cardioplegia directly injected into the orifices of the coronary arteries. Alternatively or in combination, retrograde cardioplegia may also be employed. The left ventricular outflow tract is explored to evaluate the location of the VSD, and to determine if closure can be performed through the aorta, or in combination with another type of intracardiac exposure.

Aortic valvar competence is achieved by making the length of the stretched free margin of the prolapsed leaflet equal to that of the adjacent normal leaflets. The center of all three leaflets is approximated through the corresponding body of Arantius with a temporary suture that allows accurate comparison of the opposing three leaflets and helps determine the extent of the needed plication.

Shortening and anchoring of the prolonged leaflet can be accomplished by reefing, plication, or by closing part of the zone of apposition with the adjacent leaflets [97–103]. Although coaptation of the repaired valve may appear quite satisfactory at termination of the procedure, there is a tendency for disruption, continued stretching, and recurrence of regurgitation, particularly in those with long-standing prolapse. The technique of shortening the leaflet and fixing the folded portion of the redundant leaflet to the aortic wall between buttressed sutures [97] provides a relatively secure repair (Figure 17.31) [30]. Often more than one technical maneuver will be needed to accomplish successful and stable correction.

In extreme cases, where the aortic valve has been badly distorted and damaged with fibrosis, calcifications, and hemodynamic changes, replacement may be the only satisfactory solution. Under these circumstances, the surgeon may elect to implant a prosthetic or biologic valve. We believe that early repair [69] of the doubly committed (conal, subarterial) or perimembranous VSDs should be undertaken whenever a prolapsing aortic leaflet is identified, even before the onset of aortic regurgitation, and even though the left-to-right shunt may be hemodynamically small. This treatment policy will prevent progression to the more extreme stages of valvar distortion that necessitate eventual replacement of the aortic valve.

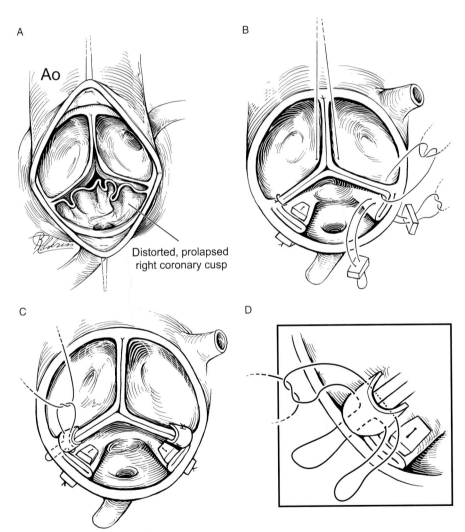

Figure 17.31 Diagram of aortic valve repair. **A**, Elongated free margin of prolapsed right leaflet. **B**, Suture in corpora arantii allowing accurate comparison with apposing leaflets to determine extent of plication. Suture at commisure to maintain correct leaflet length. **C**, Fold of excess valve securely sandwiched against aortic wall by pledget-supported mattress sutures. **D**, Commisure reinforced with hood of pericardium.

Ventricular Septal Defects with Coarctation of the Aorta

Coarctation of the aorta is often associated with VSDs, albeit with varying incidence in reported series. In one study at the Hospital for Sick Children [104] in London, a VSD was found in one-sixth of a cohort of infants and children operated for repair of coarctation, with similar findings reported from the Royal Brompton Hospital, also in London [105]. A study of 100 autopsied specimens from subjects with coarctation of the aorta revealed that patients under 6 months of age with coarctation and VSD frequently had associated tubular hypoplasia of the aortic arch [106].

The morphology of the VSDs associated with coarctation of the aorta has been the focus of several autopsy studies [107,108] and echocardiographic investigations [109]. These showed that the outlet septum could be deviated rightward with aortic overriding or leftward alignment to narrow the subaortic area. In the majority of cases studied, narrowing of the left ventricular outflow tract was present due to hypertrophic muscle bundles, anomalous attachments of the mitral or TVs, septal bulges, or fibrous ridges. These findings give credence to the hypothesis that coarctation of the aorta is induced by a compromise of flow to the ascending aorta during fetal life. When coarctation is associated with a VSD, the surgeon may be faced with more complex problems, and there are several options for surgical management.

One option is to repair the coarctation only. This is applicable when the VSD is small and likely to close spontaneously, or if it is moderate in size and can be managed medically [110,111]. This option has limited applicability to patients with hemodynamically insignificant defects. Although some success can be attained in medical management of infants with more significant VSDs after repair of coarctation of the aorta, it is difficult to select the patient in advance.

Another option, repair of the coarctation and banding the pulmonary trunk [112,113], has been used extensively in infants with large left-to-right shunts and severe heart failure. The surgical approach is through a left thoracotomy incision. The coarctation is repaired and the pulmonary trunk is then banded. There is a trend toward avoiding banding because of several disadvantages. Scarring of the pulmonary trunk may necessitate extensive arterioplasty at the time of debanding, leaving the child subject to restenosis. Obstruction to the right ventricle, in cases where the VSD is spontaneously becoming smaller while waiting for the second-stage repair, is especially dangerous if there is recurrence of the coarctation, or if it is associated with narrowing of the left ventricular outflow tract. This situation results in obstruction to the outflow from both the left and right ventricles, which often leads to significant heart failure.

Still another option is to perform concomitant repair of both lesions using two incisions [114]. The coarctation is repaired first through a left thoracotomy, followed by repair of the VSD through the standard median sternotomy. The clinical results with this approach have been excellent. The proponents of this approach cite better exposure for repair of the coarctation with the left thoracotomy, avoidance of circulatory arrest that is necessary to adequately repair the coarctation from the front, and the excellent tolerance infants have for the double incision.

Simultaneous repair of the VSD and coarctation can also be achieved through a median sternotomy. Historically, this method produced suboptimal results [15,16,19,110]. Recent experience, however, has been more favorable, now making the combined approach the procedure of choice [115–120]. The procedure can be performed with deep hypothermia and circulatory arrest. While cooling the infant, extensive dissection of the great vessels and descending aorta is performed that permits coarctectomy and extended end-to-end anastomosis. This maneuver also corrects the frequent problem of hypoplasia of the transverse aortic arch. Most surgeons prefer to perform the coarctectomy and extended end-to-end anastomosis during a brief period lasting from 15 to 20 minutes of deep hypothermia circulatory arrest, followed by closure of the VSD once cardiopulmonary bypass is re-established [121]. Others [122,123] have used low-flow perfusion via the brachiocephalic artery to achieve the same results. There are similar differences in the technique used to close the VSD. While some surgeons prefer to repair the coarctation and close the VSD during one period of deep hypothermia and circulatory arrest, most, having repaired the coarctation, have used perfusion to close the VSD. This method is in keeping with recent trends to limit, as much as possible, the period of circulatory arrest when there are reasonable alternatives [124–127].

Complications

Complications of closure of VSDs are generally related to injury to the anatomic structures, inadequate exposure, and the conduct of cardiopulmonary bypass.

The anatomic structures that are at risk during VSD closure are the conduction system and the leaflets of the tricuspid and aortic valves. Transient arrhythmias are not uncommon after closure and can be associated with close contact with the atrioventricular node and His bundle during administration of cardioplegia. Right bundle branch block, not usually found in patients undergoing transatrial closure, is a frequent finding in those undergoing transventricular closure. This is not related to subsequent serious conduction disturbances [128,129]. Complete heart block requiring a pacemaker should now be avoidable, albeit often reported in 1–2% of cases [130]. Injury to the aortic valve can occur during closure due to inappropriate incision of the TV, placement of sutures, or both. These problems can result in aortic insufficiency. Hemolysis has also been reported in these circumstances with the insufficient aortic jet striking the VSD patch [131]. Tricuspid insufficiency can occur if the cords are foreshortened by the VSD patch. If severe, the aortic and/or tricuspid valvar defects should be repaired.

Incomplete closure can be due to inadequate exposure, disruption of sutures placed in immature or diseased myocardium, and bacterial endocarditis. This complication occurs in less than 5% of cases, and reoperation is indicated if the residual left-to-right shunt is greater than 1.5 to 1. The introduction [132] and routine use of intraoperative epicardial and, later, transesophageal echocardiography has given the surgeon the capability visually to evaluate the closure and to intervene, if necessary, to close residual or undiagnosed defects. Intraoperative echocardiography has been instrumental in decreasing the incidence of residual shunts and has been shown to be cost effective despite the increased resources that are necessary for its routine use [133–135].

Complications related to the conduct of cardiopulmonary bypass are usually the result of deep hypothermia and circulatory arrest. The incidence of neurologic complications is directly related to the period required for circulatory arrest. While some have noted few deleterious neurologic and developmental effects with deep hypothermia and circulatory arrest [136,137], others [124–127, 138–140] have noted significant motor and intellectual abnormalities not generally seen in those who had continuous cardiopulmonary bypass. We prefer continuous cardiopulmonary bypass whenever possible, even in babies weighing 2 kg or less, with short periods of very low flow, using hypothermic circulatory arrest only when absolutely necessary.

Results

Operative mortality for VSD closure has decreased considerably over the past two decades because of improved techniques of cardiopulmonary bypass, myocardial preservation, and postoperative care. In older patients with uncomplicated VSDs the mortality should now approach zero [66]. Mortality in infants, which had been higher [141,142] due to the severity of the left-to-right shunt and their size, has steadily improved allowing surgeons to perform cardiopulmonary bypass safely and close VSDs successfully in premature infants weighing as little as 700 g [143].

Over a span of 14 years, from 1990 to 2004, we closed isolated defects in 358 infants and children at Children's Memorial Hospital, Chicago. These numbers include patients with an atrial septal defect and/or a persistent

PDA. The classification of the VSD at the time of surgery and corresponding percentages are shown in Table 17.1. None of our patients died. Heart block occurred in seven patients (1.9%). In six of these, the patients had Down syndrome with inlet VSDs. There were no residual VSDs. Postoperative complications are shown in Table 17.2. These results are consistent with other published series [144,145] and underline the current effectiveness of surgical closure in infants and children.

Transcatheter/Transventricular Device Closure

The introduction of transcatheter closure of atrial and ventricular septal defects has been associated with therapeutic controversies comparing catheter and surgical techniques [146–154]. The development of VSD occluders has undergone many iterations that have resulted in improved delivery systems and higher rates of complete closure [146–154]. Device closure of VSDs has been applied to muscular [155–158] and perimembranous [146–154] subtypes, with the

Table 17.1 Surgical classification of VSD (1990–2004), Children's Memorial Hospital.

Type	Patients	%
Perimembranous (type II, paramembranous, Conoventricular)	284	79
Doubly committed juxta-arterial (type I, subarterial, supracristal, conal septal defect, infundibular)	34	9
Muscular	16	4
Atrioventricular septal defect with exclusively ventricular shunting (type III, inlet, atrioventricular canal type)	12	3
Multiple defects	12	3
Direct Gerbode defect	6	1.7
TOTAL	358	

Table 17.2 Complications of VSD closure during the period from 1990 to 2004 at Children's Memorial Hospital.

Type	Patients	%
Death	0	0
Heart block requiring pacemaker	7*	1.9
Reoperation for bleeding	4	1.0
Significant residual shunting	0	0

*6 of 7 had Down syndrome.

devices delivered either by transcutaneous or perventricular techniques [158].

Perhaps the least controversial therapeutic application of transcutaneous or perventricular closure is in patients with muscular VSDs. Apical and anterior muscular defects can be difficult to visualize by surgical techniques owing to obstructing trabeculations and uncertainty regarding the detection of the margins. Self-centering devices have been used effectively in these situations, because identification is enhanced by flow velocity and absence of confounding trabeculations on the left ventricular side. In addition to effective identification, transcatheter or perventricular techniques allow closure without cardiopulmonary bypass or aortic cross-clamping. Disadvantages of this technique are unwanted disruption of atrioventricular tendinous cords, device embolization, hemolytic anemia, and the yet to be determined long-term effects of a large metallic mass in the heart. In particular, heart block for closure of muscular VSDs is rare. Open surgical closure, on the other hand, has the distinct advantage of avoidance of cannulation of the femoral vessels and allows the surgeon to address other hemodynamic problems such as additional VSDs, a significant atrial septal defect, or coarctation of the aorta.

Significant controversy exists with transcatheter closure of perimembranous defects compared with open surgical techniques. During the development and clinical application of transcatheter closure, significant problems were encountered such as aortic insufficiency, hemolytic anemia, tricuspid regurgitation, device embolization, endocarditis [159], and complete heart block. In particular, the incidence of complete heart block requiring a pacemaker has been reported to be 5.7% [146] and as high as 22% [160], which compares unfavorably to surgical closure and ideally should now be zero. The impact of life-long pacer therapy for children undergoing transcatheter closure cannot be overemphasized, as this enduring complication can be associated with pacer-induced cardiomyopathy and an abbreviated life span.

The difficulty with transcatheter closure of perimembranous VSDs is the basic anatomy relative to the conduction system. Most self-centering devices are firm and by necessity hug the left ventricular lip of the VSD, exactly the location of the bundle of His. This fact will always challenge transcatheter techniques, as complete heart block can occur acutely or remotely and potentially result in sudden death. At the present time, most clinicians consider the rate of complete heart block following transcatheter closure of perimembranous VSDs to be unacceptable [160].

Conclusions

In summary, the results of operative closure of VSD are very good. The risk of mortality for all patients including those with pulmonary arterial hypertension is less than 1%. The risk of major morbidity, atrioventricular block requiring a pacemaker, emergent reoperation, and significant residual shunting are all approximately 1%. Thus over 96% of patients have excellent outcomes when surgeons have used the surgical techniques outlined in this chapter.

References

1. Mitchell SC, Korones SB, Berendes HW. (1971) Congenital heart disease in 56,109 births. Incidence and natural history. Circulation 43, 323–332.
2. Fyler DC. (1992) Ventricular septal defect. In: Fyler DC, ed. *Nadas' Pediatric Cardiology*. Philadelphia, PA: Hanley & Belfus.
3. Wells WJ, Lindesmith GG. (1985) Ventricular septal defect. In: Arciniegas E, ed. *Pediatric Cardiac Surgery*. Chicago, Ill: Year Book Medical Publishers.
4. Roger H. (1879) Recherches cliniques sur la communication congenitale de deux coeurs: pars inocclusion de septum interventriculaire. Bull Acad Natl Med 8, 1074.
5. Eisenmenger V. (1897) Die angeborenen Defecte der Kammerscheidewand des Herzens. Z Kim Med (suppl 32):1.
6. Abbott ME. (1936) *Atlas of Congenital Cardiac Disease*. New York, NY: American Heart Association.
7. Selzer A. (1949) Defect of the ventricular septum; summary of 12 cases and review of the literature. Arch Intern Med (Chic) 84, 798–823.
8. Muller WH Jr, Dammann JF Jr. (1952) The treatment of certain congenital malformations of the heart by the creation of pulmonic stenosis to reduce pulmonary hypertension and excessive pulmonary blood flow; a preliminary report. Surg Gynecol Obstet 95, 213–219.
9. Lillehei CW, Cohen M, Warden HE, *et al.* (1955) The results of direct vision closure of ventricular septal defects in eight patients by means of controlled cross circulation. Surg Gynecol Obstet 101, 446–466.
10. DuShane JW, Kirklin JW, Patrick RT, *et al.* (1956) Ventricular septal defects with pulmonary hypertension; surgical treatment by means of a mechanical pump-oxygenator. J Am Med Assoc 160, 950–953.
11. Stirling GR, Stanley PH, Lillehei CW. (1957) The effects of cardiac bypass and ventriculotomy upon right ventricular function; with report of successful closure of ventricular septal defect by use of atriotomy. Surg Forum 8, 433–438.
12. Kirklin JW, Dushane JW. (1961) Repair of ventricular septal defect in infancy. Pediatrics 27, 961–966.
13. Sigmann JM, Stern AM, Sloan HE. (1967) Early surgical correction of large ventricular septal defects. Pediatrics 39, 4–13.
14. Okamoto Y. (1969) [Clinical studies on open heart surgery in infants with profound hypothermia]. Nippon Geka Hokan 38, 188–207.
15. Barratt-Boyes BG, Neutze JM, Clarkson PM, *et al.* (1976) Repair of ventricular septal defect in the first two years of life using profound hypothermia-circulatory arrest techniques. Ann Surg 184, 376–390.

16. Kirklin JW, Barratt-Boyes BG. (1993) Ventricular septal defect. In: *Cardiac Surgery*, 2nd ed. New York, NY: Churchill Livingstone.

17. Pinkley K, Stoesz PA. (1981) Ventricular septal defect. Morb Mortal Wkly Rep 30, 609–610.

18. Rothman KJ, Fyler DC. (1976) Association of congenital heart defects with season and population density. Teratology 13, 29–34.

19. Ando M, Takao A. (1979) Racial differences in the morphology of common cardiac anomaloes. Jpn Bull Heart Inst, 47.

20. Momma K, Toyama K, Takao A, *et al.* (1984) Natural history of subarterial infundibular ventricular septal defect. Am Heart J 108, 1312–1317.

21. Whittemore R, Hobbins JC, Engle MA. (1982) Pregnancy and its outcome in women with and without surgical treatment of congenital heart disease. Am J Cardiol 50, 641–651.

22. Newman TB. (1985) Etiology of ventricular septal defects: an epidemiologic approach. Pediatrics 76, 741–749.

23. Moe DG, Guntheroth WG. (1987) Spontaneous closure of uncomplicated ventricular septal defect. Am J Cardiol 60, 674–678.

24. Capelli H, Andrade JL, Somerville J. (1983) Classification of the site of ventricular septal defect by 2-dimensional echocardiography. Am J Cardiol 51, 1474–1480.

25. Edwards JE. (1960) Congenital malformations of the heart and great vessels. In: Gould SE, ed. *Pathology of the Heart*. Springfield, Ill: Charles C Thomas.

26. Goor DA, Lillehei CW, Rees R, *et al.* (1970) Isolated ventricular septal defect. Development basis for various types and presentation of classification. Chest 58, 468–482.

27. Hagler DJ, Edwards WD, Seward JB, *et al.* (1985) Standardized nomenclature of the ventricular septum and ventricular septal defects, with applications for two-dimensional echocardiography. Mayo Clin Proc 60, 741–752.

28. Lincoln C, Jamieson S, Joseph M, *et al.* (1977) Transatrial repair of ventricular septal defects with reference to their anatomic classification. J Thorac Cardiovasc Surg 74, 183–190.

29. Soto B, Becker AE, Moulaert AJ, *et al.* (1980) Classification of ventricular septal defects. Br Heart J 43, 332–343.

30. Mavroudis C, Backer CL, Jacobs JP. (2003) Ventricular septal defect. In: Mavroudis C, Backer CL, eds. *Pediatric Cardiac Surgery*, 3rd ed. Philadelphia, PA: Mosby Inc.

31. Cooley DA, Garrett HE, Howard HS. (1962) The surgical treatment of ventricular septal defect: an analysis of 300 consecutive surgical cases. Prog Cardiovasc Dis 4, 312–323.

32. Lue HC. (1985) Is subpulmonic ventricular septal defect an Oriental disease? In: Lue HC, Takao A, eds. *Subpulmonic Ventricular Septal Defect*. Tokyo, Japan: Springer.

33. Tatsuno K, Ando M, Takao A, *et al.* (1975) Diagnostic importance of aortography in conal ventricular-septal defect. Am Heart J 89, 171–177.

34. Van Praagh R, Geva T, Kreutzer J. (1989) Ventricular septal defects: how shall we describe, name and classify them? J Am Coll Cardiol 14, 1298–1299.

35. Agmon Y, Connolly HM, Olson LJ, *et al.* (1999) Noncompaction of the ventricular myocardium. J Am Soc Echocardiogr 12, 859–863.

36. Seddio F, Reddy VM, McElhinney DB, *et al.* (1999) Multiple ventricular septal defects: how and when should they be repaired? J Thorac Cardiovasc Surg 117, 134–139; discussion 139–140.

37. Kelle AM, Young L, Kaushal S, *et al.* (2009) The Gerbode defect: a ventriculo-atrial defect. CTSNet: www.ctsnet.org/sections/clinicalresources/congenital/article-24.html

38. Buhl (1857), cited by Meyer H. Uber angeborene Enge oder Verschluss der Lungenarterienbahn. Virchow's Arch Path Anat 12, 532.

39. Kirby CK, Johnson J, Zinsser HF. (1957) Successful closure of a left ventricular-right atrial shunt. Ann Surg 145, 392–394.

40. Gerbode F, Hultgren H, Melrose D, *et al.* (1958) Syndrome of left ventricular-right atrial shunt; successful surgical repair of defect in five cases, with observation of bradycardia on closure. Ann Surg 148, 433–446.

41. McKay R, Battistessa SA, Wilkinson JL, *et al.* (1989) A communication from the left ventricle to the right atrium: a defect in the central fibrous body. Int J Cardiol 23, 117–123.

42. Riemenschneider TA, Moss AJ. (1967) Left ventricular-right atrial communication. Am J Cardiol 19, 710–718.

43. Wilcox BR, Anderson RH. (1992) *Surgical Anatomy of the Heart*, 2nd ed. London, England: Gower Medical Publishing.

44. Castaneda AR, Jonas RA, Mayer JE, *et al.* (1994) *Cardiac Surgery of the Neonate and Infant*. Philadelphia, PA: WB Saunders Co.

45. Jacobs JP, Quintessenza JA, Burke RP, *et al.* (2000) Congenital Heart Surgery Nomenclature and Database Project: atrial septal defect. Ann Thorac Surg 69, S18–S24.

46. Jacobs JP, Burke RP, Quintessenza JA, *et al.* (2000) Congenital Heart Surgery Nomenclature and Database Project: ventricular septal defect. Ann Thorac Surg 69, S25–S35.

47. Wagenvoort CA, Neufeld HN, Dushane JW, *et al.* (1961) The pulmonary arterial tree in ventricular septal defect. A quantitative study of anatomic features in fetuses, infants. and children. Circulation 23, 740–748.

48. Blackstone EH, Kirklin JW, Bradley EL, *et al.* (1976) Optimal age and results in repair of large ventricular septal defects. J Thorac Cardiovasc Surg 72, 661–679.

49. Collins G, Calder L, Rose V, *et al.* (1972) Ventricular septal defect: clinical and hemodynamic changes in the first five years of life. Am Heart J 84, 695–705.

50. Hoffman JI, Rudolph AM. (1965) The natural history of ventricular septal defects in infancy. Am J Cardiol 16, 634–653.

51. Keith JD, Rose V, Collins G, *et al.* (1971) Ventricular septal defect. Incidence, morbidity, and mortality in various age groups. Br Heart J 33, 81–87.

52. Alpert BS, Mellits ED, Rowe RD. (1973) Spontaneous closure of small ventricular septal defects. probability rates in the first five years of life. Am J Dis Child 125, 194–196.

53. Auld PA, Johnson AL, Gibbons JE, *et al.* (1963) Changes in pulmonary vascular resistance in infants and children with left-to-right intracardiac shunts. Circulation 27, 257–260.

54. Clarkson PM, Frye RL, DuShane JW, *et al.* (1968) Prognosis for patients with ventricular septal defect and severe pulmonary vascular obstructive disease. Circulation 38, 129–135.

55. Heath D, Edwards JE. (1958) The pathology of hypertensive pulmonary vascular disease; a description of six grades of structural changes in the pulmonary arteries with special reference to congenital cardiac septal defects. Circulation 18, 533–547.

56. Lucas RV Jr, Adams P Jr, Anderson RC, *et al.* (1961) The natural history of isolated ventricular septal defect. A serial physiologic study. Circulation 24, 1372–1387.

57. Campbell M. (1971) Natural history of ventricular septal defect. Br Heart J 33, 246–257.

58. Citak M, Rees A, Mavroudis C. (1992) Surgical management of infective endocarditis in children. Ann Thorac Surg 54, 755–760.

59. Corone P, Doyon F, Gaudeau S, *et al.* (1977) Natural history of ventricular septal defect. A study involving 790 cases. Circulation 55, 908–915.

60. Pacifico AD, Kirklin JW, Kirklin JK. (1990) Surgical treatment of ventricular septal defect. In: Sabiston DC, Spencer FC, eds. *Surgery of the Chest*, 5th ed. Philadelphia, PA: WB Saunders Co.

61. Shah P, Singh WS, Rose V, *et al.* (1966) Incidence of bacterial endocarditis in ventricular septal defects. Circulation 34, 127–131.

62. Hoffman JI, Rudolph AM. (1966) Increasing pulmonary vascular resistance during infancy in association with ventricular septal defect. Pediatrics 38, 220–230.

63. Braunlin EA, Moller JH, Patton C, *et al.* (1986) Predictive value of lung biopsy in ventricular septal defect: long-term follow-up. J Am Coll Cardiol 8, 1113–1118.

64. Rabinovitch M, Haworth SG, Castaneda AR, *et al.* (1978) Lung biopsy in congenital heart disease: a morphometric approach to pulmonary vascular disease. Circulation 58, 1107–1122.

65. Rabinovitch M, Keane JF, Norwood WI, *et al.* (1984) Vascular structure in lung tissue obtained at biopsy correlated with pulmonary hemodynamic findings after repair of congenital heart defects. Circulation 69, 655–667.

66. Backer CL, Winters RC, Zales VR, *et al.* (1993) Restrictive ventricular septal defect: how small is too small to close? Ann Thorac Surg 56, 1014–1018.

67. Malm JR. (1993) A reason to close ventricular septal defect? Ann Thorac Surg 56, 1013.

68. Waldman JD. (1993) Why not close a small ventricular septal defect? Ann Thorac Surg 56, 1011–1012.

69. Backer CL, Idriss FS, Zales VR, *et al.* (1991) Surgical management of the conal (supracristal) ventricular septal defect. J Thorac Cardiovasc Surg 102, 288–295; discussion 295–296.

70. Chang CH, Lee MC, Shieh MJ. (1988) Surgical treatment of supracristal type of ventricular septal defect. Scand J Thorac Cardiovasc Surg 22, 221–225.

71. de Leval M, Pozzi M, Starnes V, *et al.* (1988) Surgical management of doubly committed subarterial ventricular septal defects. Circulation 78, III40–III46.

72. Komai H, Naito Y, Fujiwara K, *et al.* (1997) Surgical strategy for doubly committed subarterial ventricular septal defect with aortic cusp prolapse. Ann Thorac Surg 64, 1146–1149.

73. Moreno-Cabral RJ, Mamiya RT, Nakamura FF, *et al.* (1977) Ventricular septal defect and aortic insufficiency. Surgical treatment. J Thorac Cardiovasc Surg 73, 358–365.

74. Pugliese G, Luisi VS, Santi C, *et al.* (1982) Ventricular septal defect associated with aortic regurgitation. Surgical considerations. G Ital Cardiol 12, 46–51.

75. Schmidt KG, Cassidy SC, Silverman NH, *et al.* (1988) Doubly committed subarterial ventricular septal defects: echocardiographic features and surgical implications. J Am Coll Cardiol 12, 1538–1546.

76. Idriss FS, Muster AJ, Paul MH, *et al.* (1992) Ventricular septal defect with tricuspid pouch with and without transposition. Anatomic and surgical considerations. J Thorac Cardiovasc Surg 103, 52–59.

77. Gaynor JW, O'Brien JE Jr, Rychik J, *et al.* (2001) Outcome following tricuspid valve detachment for ventricular septal defects closure. Eur J Cardiothorac Surg 19, 279–282.

78. Hudspeth AS, Cordell AR, Meredith JH, *et al.* (1962) An improved transatrial approach to the closure of ventricular septal defects. J Thorac Cardiovasc Surg 43, 157–165.

79. Pridjian AK, Pearce FB, Culpepper WS, *et al.* (1993) Atrioventricular valve competence after takedown to improve exposure during ventricular septal defect repair. J Thorac Cardiovasc Surg 106, 1122–1125.

80. Tatebe S, Miyamura H, Watanabe H, *et al.* (1995) Closure of isolated ventricular septal defect with detachment of the tricuspid valve. J Card Surg 10, 564–568.

81. Mavroudis C, Backer CL. (2010) Technical tips for three congenital heart operations: modified Ross-Konno procedure, optimal ventricular septal defect exposure by tricuspid valve incision, coronary unroofing and endarterectomy for anomalous aortic origin of the coronary artery. Oper Tech Thorac Cardiovasc Surg 15, 18–40.

82. Dietl CA, Torres AR. (1993) Combined transaortic-transpulmonary approach for surgical repair of aortic insufficiency associated with ventricular septal defect. Cardiovasc Surg 1, 638–642.

83. Sakamoto K, Charpentier A, Popescu S, *et al.* (1997) Transaortic approach in double-outlet right ventricle with subaortic ventricular septal defect. Ann Thorac Surg 64, 856–858.

84. Binet JP, Conso JF, Langlois J, *et al.* (1970) [Closure of certain low congenital interventricular communications by left ventricular approach]. Arch Mal Coeur Vaiss 63, 1345–1351.

85. Aaron BL, Lower BR. (1975) Muscular ventricular septal defect repair made easy. Ann Thorac Surg 19, 568–570.

86. DiBernardo LR, Kirshbom PM, Skaryak LA, *et al.* (1998) Acute functional consequences of left ventriculotomy. Ann Thorac Surg 66, 159–165.

87. Lev M. (1960) The architecture of the conduction system in congenital heart disease. III. Ventricular septal defect. Arch Pathol 70, 529–549.

88. Truex RC, Bishof JK. (1958) Conduction system in human hearts with interventricular septal defects. J Thorac Surg 35, 421–439.

89. Kurosawa H, Becker AE. (1984) Modification of the precise relationship of the atrioventricular conduction bundle to the margins of the ventricular septal defects by the trabec-

ula septomarginalis. J Thorac Cardiovasc Surg 87, 605–615.

90. Milo S, Ho SY, Wilkinson JL, *et al.* (1980) Surgical anatomy and atrioventricular conduction tissues of hearts with isolated ventricular septal defects. J Thorac Cardiovasc Surg 79, 244–255.

91. Lev M, Fell EH, Arcilla R, *et al.* (1964) Surgical injury to the conduction system in ventricular septal defect. Am J Cardiol 14, 464–476.

92. Titus JL, Daugherty GW, Kirklin JW, *et al.* (1963) Lesions of the atrioventricular conduction system after repair of ventricular septal defect. Relation to heart block. Circulation 28, 82–88.

93. Kawashima Y, Danno M, Shimizu Y, *et al.* (1973) Ventricular septal defect associated with aortic insufficiency: anatomic classification and method of operation. Circulation 47, 1057–1064.

94. Nadas AS, Thilenius OG, Lafarge CG, *et al.* (1964) Ventricular septal defect with aortic regurgitation: medical and pathologic aspects. Circulation 29, 862–873.

95. Tatsuno K, Konno S, Sakakibara S. (1973) Ventricular septal defect with aortic insufficiency. Angiocardiographic aspects and a new classification. Am Heart J 85, 13–21.

96. Van Praagh R, McNamara JJ. (1968) Anatomic types of ventricular septal defect with aortic insufficiency. Diagnostic and surgical considerations. Am Heart J 75, 604–619.

97. Trusler GA, Moes CA, Kidd BS. (1973) Repair of ventricular septal defect with aortic insufficiency. J Thorac Cardiovasc Surg 66, 394–403.

98. Yacoub MH, Khan H, Stavri G, *et al.* (1997) Anatomic correction of the syndrome of prolapsing right coronary aortic cusp, dilatation of the sinus of Valsalva, and ventricular septal defect. J Thorac Cardiovasc Surg 113, 253–260; discussion 261.

99. Garamella JJ, Cruz AB Jr, Heupel WH, *et al.* (1960) Ventricular septal defect with aortic insufficiencyl Successful surgical correction of both defects by the transaortic approach. Am J Cardiol 5, 266–272.

100. Hitchcock JF, Suijker WJ, Ksiezycka E, *et al.* (1991) Management of ventricular septal defect with associated aortic incompetence. Ann Thorac Surg 52, 70–73.

101. Plauth WH Jr, Braunwald E, Rockoff SD, *et al.* (1965) Ventricular septal defect and aortic regurgitation: clinical, hemodynamic and surgical considerations. Am J Med 39, 552–567.

102. Spencer FC, Doyle EF, Danilowicz DA, *et al.* (1973) Long-term evaluation of aortic valvuloplasty for aortic insufficiency and ventricular septal defect. J Thorac Cardiovasc Surg 65, 15–31.

103. Starr A, Menashe V, Dotter C. (1960) Surgical correction of aortic insufficiency associated with ventricular septal defect. Surg Gynecol Obstet 111, 71–76.

104. Tawes RL Jr, Aberdeen E, Waterston DJ, *et al.* (1969) Coarctation of the aorta in infants and children. A review of 333 operative cases, including 179 infants. Circulation 39, I173–184.

105. Shinebourne EA, Tam AS, Elseed AM, *et al.* (1976) Coarctation of the aorta in infancy and childhood. Br Heart J 38, 375–380.

106. Becker AE, Becker MJ, Edwards JE. (1970) Anomalies associated with coarctation of aorta: particular reference to infancy. Circulation 41, 1067–1075.

107. Anderson RH, Lenox CC, Zuberbuhler JR. (1983) Morphology of ventricular septal defect associated with coarctation of aorta. Br Heart J 50, 176–181.

108. Moene RJ, Gittenberger-de Groot AC, Oppenheimer-Dekker A, *et al.* (1987) Anatomic characteristics of ventricular septal defect associated with coarctation of the aorta. Am J Cardiol 59, 952–955.

109. Smallhorn JF, Anderson RH, Macartney FJ. (1983) Morphological characterisation of ventricular septal defects associated with coarctation of aorta by cross-sectional echocardiography. Br Heart J 49, 485–494.

110. Neches WH, Park SC, Lenox CC, *et al.* (1977) Coarctation of the aorta with ventricular septal defect. Circulation 55, 189–194.

111. Park JK, Dell RB, Ellis K, *et al.* (1992) Surgical management of the infant with coarctation of the aorta and ventricular septal defect. J Am Coll Cardiol 20, 176–180.

112. Fishman NH, Bronstein MH, Berman W Jr, *et al.* (1976) Surgical management of severe aortic coarctation and interrupted aortic arch in neonates. J Thorac Cardiovasc Surg 71, 35–48.

113. Hammon JW Jr, Graham TP Jr, Boucek RJ Jr, *et al.* (1985) Operative repair of coarctation of the aorta in infancy: results with and without ventricular septal defect. Am J Cardiol 55, 1555–1559.

114. Tiraboschi R, Alfieri O, Carpentier A, *et al.* (1978) One stage correction of coarctation of the aorta associated with intracardiac defects in infancy. J Cardiovasc Surg (Torino) 19, 11–16.

115. Bove EL, Minich LL, Pridjian AK, *et al.* (1993) The management of severe subaortic stenosis, ventricular septal defect, and aortic arch obstruction in the neonate. J Thorac Cardiovasc Surg 105, 289–295; discussion 295–296.

116. DeLeon SY, Idriss FS, Ilbawi MN, *et al.* (1981) Transmediastinal repair of complex coarctation and interrupted aortic arch. J Thorac Cardiovasc Surg 82, 98–102.

117. Hazekamp MG, Quaegebeur JM, Singh S, *et al.* (1991) One stage repair of aortic arch anomalies and intracardiac defects. Eur J Cardiothorac Surg 5, 283–286; discussion 287.

118. Hirooka K, Fraser CD Jr. (1997) One-stage neonatal repair of complex aortic arch obstruction or interruption. Recent experience at Texas Children's Hospital. Tex Heart Inst J 24, 317-321.

119. Sandhu SK, Beekman RH, Mosca RS, *et al.* (1995) Single-stage repair of aortic arch obstruction and associated intracardiac defects in the neonate. Am J Cardiol 75, 370–373.

120. Tchervenkov CI, Tahta SA, Jutras L, *et al.* (1998) Single-stage repair of aortic arch obstruction and associated intracardiac defects with pulmonary homograft patch aortoplasty. J Thorac Cardiovasc Surg 116, 897–904.

121. Backer CL, Mavroudis C, Zias EA, *et al.* (1998) Repair of coarctation with resection and extended end-to-end anastomosis. Ann Thorac Surg 66, 1365–1370; discussion 1370–1371.

122. Asou T, Kado H, Imoto Y, *et al.* (1996) Selective cerebral perfusion technique during aortic arch repair in neonates. Ann Thorac Surg 61, 1546–2548.

123. Pigula FA, Siewers RD, Nemoto EM. (1999) Regional perfusion of the brain during neonatal aortic arch reconstruction. J Thorac Cardiovasc Surg 117, 1023–1024.

124. Bellinger DC, Jonas RA, Rappaport LA, *et al.* (1995) Developmental and neurologic status of children after heart surgery with hypothermic circulatory arrest or low-flow cardiopulmonary bypass. N Engl J Med 332, 549–555.

125. Hickey PR. (1998) Neurologic sequelae associated with deep hypothermic circulatory arrest. Ann Thorac Surg 65, S65–S69.

126. Jonas R, Wernovsky G, Ware J. (1992) The Boston Circulatory Arrest Study: perioperative neurological and developmental outcome after the arterial switch operation. Circulation 86, I360.

127. Newburger JW, Jonas RA, Wernovsky G, *et al.* (1993) A comparison of the perioperative neurologic effects of hypothermic circulatory arrest versus low-flow cardiopulmonary bypass in infant heart surgery. N Engl J Med 329, 1057–1064.

128. Boccanelli A, Wallgren CG, Zetterqvist P. (1980) Ventricular dynamics after surgical closure of VSD. Scand J Thorac Cardiovasc Surg 14, 153–157.

129. Hobbins SM, Izukawa T, Radford DJ, *et al.* (1979) Conduction disturbances after surgical correction of ventricular septal defect by the atrial approach. Br Heart J 41, 289–293.

130. Tamiya T, Yamashiro T, Matsumoto T, *et al.* (1985) A histological study of surgical landmarks for the specialized atrioventricular conduction system, with particular reference to the papillary muscle. Ann Thorac Surg 40, 599–613.

131. Wada J, Yokoyama M, Imai Y, *et al.* (1979) Hemolysis due to aortic insufficiency following closure of ventricular septal defect. Int Surg 64, 53–56.

132. Ungerleider RM, Greeley WJ, Kanter RJ, *et al.* (1992) The learning curve for intraoperative echocardiography during congenital heart surgery. Ann Thorac Surg 54, 691–696; discussion 696–698.

133. Leung MP, Chau KT, Chiu C, *et al.* (1996) Intraoperative TEE assessment of ventricular septal defect with aortic regurgitation. Ann Thorac Surg 61, 854–860.

134. Randolph GR, Hagler DJ, Connolly HM, *et al.* (2002) Intraoperative transesophageal echocardiography during surgery for congenital heart defects. J Thorac Cardiovasc Surg 124, 1176–1182.

135. Ungerleider RM, Kisslo JA, Greeley WJ, *et al.* (1995) Intraoperative echocardiography during congenital heart operations: experience from 1,000 cases. Ann Thorac Surg 60, S539–S542.

136. Clarkson PM, MacArthur BA, Barratt-Boyes BG, *et al.* (1980) Developmental progress after cardiac surgery in infancy using hypothermia and circulatory arrest. Circulation 62, 855–861.

137. Tharion J, Johnson DC, Celermajer JM, *et al.* (1982) Profound hypothermia with circulatory arrest: nine years' clinical experience. J Thorac Cardiovasc Surg 84, 66–72.

138. Mavroudis C, Greene MA. (1992) Cardiopulmonary bypass and hypothermic circulatory arrest in infants. In: Jacobs ML, Norwood WI, eds. *Pediatric Cardiac Surgery: Current Issues.* Stoneham, MA: Butterworth-Heinemann.

139. Wells FC, Coghill S, Caplan HL, *et al.* (1983) Duration of circulatory arrest does influence the psychological development of children after cardiac operation in early life. J Thorac Cardiovasc Surg 86, 823–831.

140. Wright JS, Hicks RG, Newman DC. (1979) Deep hypothermic arrest: observations on later development in children. J Thorac Cardiovasc Surg 77, 466–468.

141. McNicholas KW, Bowman FO, Hayes CJ, *et al.* (1978) Surgical management of ventricular septal defects in infants. J Thorac Cardiovasc Surg 75, 346–353.

142. Richardson JV, Schieken RM, Lauer RM, *et al.* (1982) Repair of large ventricular septal defects in infants and small children. Ann Surg 195, 318–322.

143. Reddy VM, McElhinney DB, Sagrado T, *et al.* (1999) Results of 102 cases of complete repair of congenital heart defects in patients weighing 700 to 2500 grams. J Thorac Cardiovasc Surg 117, 324–331.

144. Hardin JT, Muskett AD, Canter CE, *et al.* (1992) Primary surgical closure of large ventricular septal defects in small infants. Ann Thorac Surg 53, 397–401.

145. Meijboom F, Szatmari A, Utens E, *et al.* (1994) Long-term follow-up after surgical closure of ventricular septal defect in infancy and childhood. J Am Coll Cardiol 24, 1358–1364.

146. Butera G, Carminati M, Chessa M, *et al.* (2007) Transcatheter closure of perimembranous ventricular septal defects: early and long-term results. J Am Coll Cardiol 50, 1189–1195.

147. Butera G, Chessa M, Carminati M. (2007) Percutaneous closure of ventricular septal defects. State of the art. J Cardiovasc Med (Hagerstown) 8, 39–45.

148. Carminati M, Butera G, Chessa M, *et al.* (2005) Transcatheter closure of congenital ventricular septal defect with Amplatzer septal occluders. Am J Cardiol 96, 52L–58L.

149. Fu YC, Bass J, Amin Z, *et al.* (2006) Transcatheter closure of perimembranous ventricular septal defects using the new Amplatzer membranous VSD occluder: results of the U.S. phase I trial. J Am Coll Cardiol 47, 319–325.

150. Knauth AL, Lock JE, Perry SB, *et al.* (2004) Transcatheter device closure of congenital and postoperative residual ventricular septal defects. Circulation 110, 501–507.

151. Kramoh EK, Dahdah N, Fournier A, *et al.* (2008) Invasive measurements of atrioventricular conduction parameters prior to and following ventricular septal defect closure with the amplatzer device. J Invasive Cardiol 20, 212–216.

152. Masura J, Gao W, Gavora P, *et al.* (2005) Percutaneous closure of perimembranous ventricular septal defects with the eccentric Amplatzer device: multicenter follow-up study. Pediatr Cardiol 26, 216–219.

153. Michel-Behnke I, Le TP, Waldecker B, *et al.* (2005) Percutaneous closure of congenital and acquired ventricular septal defects–considerations on selection of the occlusion device. J Interv Cardiol 18, 89–99.

154. Szkutnik M, Qureshi SA, Kusa J, *et al.* (2007) Use of the Amplatzer muscular ventricular septal defect occluder for

closure of perimembranous ventricular septal defects. Heart 93, 355–358.

155. Holzer R, Balzer D, Cao QL, *et al.* (2004) Device closure of muscular ventricular septal defects using the Amplatzer muscular ventricular septal defect occluder: immediate and mid-term results of a U.S. registry. J Am Coll Cardiol 43, 1257–1263.

156. Jameel AA, Arfi AM, Arif H, *et al.* (2006) Retrograde approach for device closure of muscular ventricular septal defects in children and adolescents, using the Amplatzer muscular ventricular septal defect occluder. Pediatr Cardiol 27, 720–728.

157. Lim DS, Forbes TJ, Rothman A, *et al.* (2007) Transcatheter closure of high-risk muscular ventricular septal defects with the CardioSEAL occluder: initial report from the CardioSEAL VSD registry. Catheter Cardiovasc Interv 70, 740–744.

158. Vasilyev NV, Melnychenko I, Kitahori K, *et al.* (2008) Beating-heart patch closure of muscular ventricular septal defects under real-time three-dimensional echocardiographic guidance: a preclinical study. J Thorac Cardiovasc Surg 135, 603–609.

159. Scheuerman O, Bruckheimer E, Marcus N, *et al.* (2006) Endocarditis after closure of ventricular septal defect by transcatheter device. Pediatrics 117, e1256–e1258.

160. Predescu D, Chaturvedi RR, Friedberg MK, *et al.* (2008) Complete heart block associated with device closure of perimembranous ventricular septal defects. J Thorac Cardiovasc Surg 136, 1223–1228.

CHAPTER 18

Atrioventricular Canal Defects

Carl L. Backer[1] and Constantine Mavroudis[2]

[1]Ann & Robert H. Lurie Children's Hospital of Chicago, formerly Children's Memorial Hospital, Chicago, IL, USA
[2]Florida Hospital for Children, Orlando, FL, USA

The atrioventricular canal defects, also referred to as atrioventricular septal defects or endocardial cushion defects encompass a wide spectrum of anatomic findings. The pathognomonic feature of this group of hearts is a *common atrioventricular junction* [1]. The complete atrioventricular canal defect consists of a large ventricular septal defect beneath the plane of the atrioventricular (AV) valves, an atrial septal defect immediately superior to the plane of the AV valves, and instead of two AV valve orifices, a single or common AV valve orifice. Atrioventricular canal defects account for 4% of all congenital cardiac malformations and over half of the cardiac defects seen in children with trisomy 21 [2,3]. There can be varying degrees of incomplete development of the septal tissue surrounding the AV valve, along with varying degrees of abnormalities of the AV valves themselves, leading to the broad classification of partial, intermediate, and complete AV canal defects [4].

The first successful repair of a complete atrioventricular canal defect was reported by Lillehei and colleagues in 1955, using cross-circulation and direct suture of the atrial rim of the septal defect to the crest of the ventricular septum [5]. The early experience with surgical correction of complete atrioventricular canal had a high mortality and a high incidence of complications such as complete AV block, residual AV valve insufficiency, and subaortic stenosis. Developments in the understanding of the precise anatomic details of this lesion and refinements in operative technique have led to substantial improvement in patient outcome [6]. A significant advance occurred in 1958 when Maurice Lev described the location of the bundle of His in patients with complete AV canal [7]. This understanding resulted in a significant reduction in the incidence of postoperative heart block. In 1962, James Maloney and Frank Gerbode independently described a single-patch technique

suspending the AV valve tissue to a single patch that closed both the atrial and ventricular septal defects [8,9]. Giancarlo Rastelli and colleagues at the Mayo Clinic described a classification system of complete atrioventricular canal in 1966 that emphasized the heterogeneity of this lesion and the different approaches required by different anatomic findings [10]. The two-patch technique was first reported by George Trusler in 1975 [11]. This technique employed a Dacron patch to close the ventricular septal defect component, suturing the valve leaflets to the crest of the ventricular septal defect patch, closing the left AV valve zone of apposition, and using a pericardial patch to close the atrial septal defect component. Most recently, Ben Wilcox from the University of North Carolina at Chapel Hill [12] and Graham Nunn from Sydney Children's Hospital [13] have reported a technique of repair that does not use a patch for the ventricular septal defect closure. Congenital heart surgeons should be familiar with all techniques and in point of fact, different anatomic morphology in different patients often lends itself to one of these three techniques.

Historically, pulmonary artery banding played a role in the management of infants with atrioventricular canal who presented early with severe congestive heart failure. However, this strategy of an initial pulmonary artery band followed later by complete repair has been abandoned by most centers. Pulmonary artery banding often results in an increase in AV valve insufficiency and hence does not ameliorate the congestive heart failure [14]. Improvements in neonatal and infant techniques of cardiopulmonary bypass, anesthesia, and postoperative intensive care unit medical management have allowed earlier repair of atrioventricular canal defects with, in nearly all instances, improvement in outcome by earlier date of operation. Most centers currently recommend complete repair of atrioventricular canal defects at the age of 3–5 months.

Pathology and Anatomy

Atrioventricular canal defect represents a spectrum of cardiac anomalies subdivided into partial, intermediate, and complete atrioventricular canal [4,15–17]. Partial atrioventricular canal (also referred to as partial atrioventricular septal defect) has an atrial septal defect adjacent to the AV valves along with a trifoliate left AV valve leading to varying degrees of left AV valve insufficiency (Figure 18.1) [17]. The atrial septal defect is a crescent-shaped defect in the inferior portion of the atrial septum immediately adjacent to the AV valves. Complete atrioventricular canal defect (also known as complete atrioventricular septal defect) has both an atrial septal defect and a defect in the ventricular septum below the common AV valve (Figure 18.2) [17]. In complete atrioventricular canal defect there is a common AV valve that bridges both the right and left sides of the heart, creating superior (anterior) and inferior (posterior) bridging leaflets. These patients always have a "bare area" at the crest of the ventricular septum. Intermediate atrioventricular canal (also known as transitional atrioventricular canal) is "intermediate" between the partial and complete lesions: there are two distinct left and right AV valve orifices, an atrial septal defect adjacent to the AV valves, and a ventricular septal defect below the AV valves [18]. The ventricular septal defect in these patients is usually in the inlet septum, and there is *no* "bare area"

at the crest of the ventricular septal defect. These anatomic variations are merely different phenotypic expressions of the same underlying genotype.

The Rastelli classification (Figure 18.3) [4] describes three types of complete atrioventricular canal based on the morphology of the anterior (superior) bridging leaflet, its degree of bridging, and its chordal attachments [10]. The Rastelli classification does *not* relate to the anatomy of the posterior common leaflet or inferior bridging leaflet. In a Rastelli type A defect, the common superior (anterior) bridging leaflet is effectively split in two "halves" at the septum. The left superior leaflet is entirely over the left ventricle and the right superior leaflet is similarly entirely over the right ventricle. This division of the common anterior leaflet into left and right components is caused by extensive attachment of the superior bridging leaflet to the crest of the ventricular septum by chordae tendineae. This morphologic finding effectively divides the anterior common AV valve into right and left components for the surgeon at the time of reconstruction. The anterior common leaflet is "divided and attached." Rastelli type B is quite rare and describes an anomalous papillary muscle attachment from the right side of the ventricular septum to the left side of the common anterior bridging leaflet. In Rastelli type C defects, there is marked bridging of the ventricular

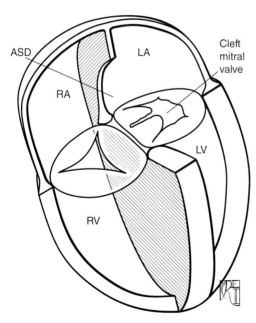

Figure 18.1 Partial AV canal defect. There is an atrial septal defect (ASD) immediately adjacent to the right AV valve and the left AV valve is trifoliate. (LA, RA, left, right atrium; LV, RV, left, right ventricle.)

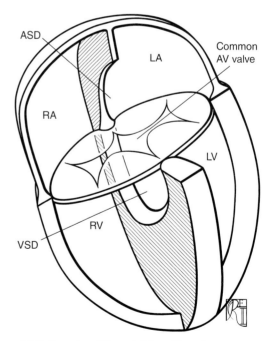

Figure 18.2 Complete AV canal defect. There is a common (single) AV valve with an atrial septal defect (ASD) "above" and a large ventricular septal defect (VSD) "below." There is a common atrioventricular junction. (LA, RA, left, right atrium; LV, RV, left, right ventricle.)

A B C

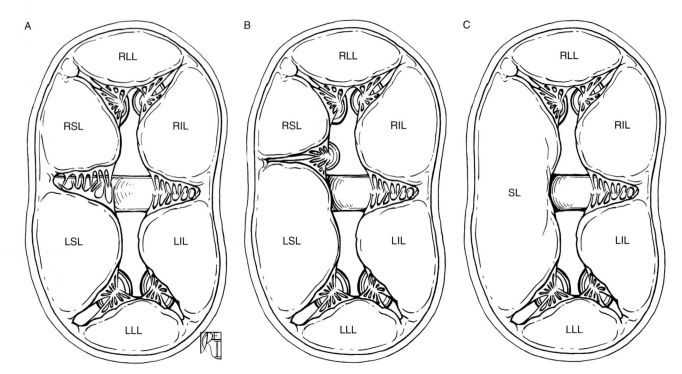

Figure 18.3 Rastelli classification. **A,** In a Rastelli type A defect, the common superior (anterior) bridging leaflet is effectively split in two at the septum; the left superior (anterior) leaflet (LSL) is entirely over the left ventricle, and the right superior (anterior) leaflet (RSL) is similarly entirely over the right ventricle. **B,** Rastelli type B is rare and involves anomalous papillary muscle attachment from the right side of the ventricular septum to the left side of the common superior (anterior) bridging leaflet. **C,** In Rastelli type C defects there is marked bridging of the ventricular septum by the superior (anterior) bridging leaflet (SL). The superior (anterior) bridging leaflet is generally not divided and floats without chordal attachment to the crest of the ventricular septum. The posterior common leaflet may be divided (as shown), or undivided, but nearly always is well attached (as shown). (LIL, RIL, left, right inferior (posterior) leaflets; LLL, RLL, left, right lateral leaflets). (Reproduced with permission from Jacobs *et al.* [4].)

septum by the anterior (superior) bridging leaflet. The anterior (superior) bridging leaflet is *not* divided and floats freely over the ventricular septum without chordal attachment to the crest of the ventricular septum. The anterior common leaflet is "not divided and not attached." In our series of AV canal patients, the Rastelli classification breakdown in 110 patients was Rastelli A, 76 patients (69%), Rastelli B, 10 patients (9%), and Rastelli C, 24 patients (22%) [19].

There is a definite association of complete atrioventricular canal and other conotruncal anomalies, particularly tetralogy of Fallot, double-outlet right ventricle, and transposition of the great arteries. The most common conotruncal anomaly associated with atrioventricular canal defect is tetralogy of Fallot. It is encountered in 6% of cases of atrioventricular canal [20]. The pathophysiology in these patients is dictated by the degree of right ventricular outflow tract obstruction, which causes varying degrees of cyanosis. Congestive heart failure is infrequent in these patients because of the restricted pulmonary blood flow. Double-outlet right ventricle in association with complete atrioventricular canal is also rare (34 of 507 pathology spec-

imens – 6%), and transposition of the great arteries is even rarer (17 of 507 specimens – 3%) [20]. Other anomalies associated with complete atrioventricular canal defect are patent ductus arteriosus (10%), persistent left superior vena cava (3%), and left ventricular outflow tract obstruction (3%) from discrete subaortic stenosis or redundant AV valve tissue.

Deficiencies in the atrioventricular septum in patients with AV canal defects result in displacement of the atrioventricular conduction tissue (Figure 18.4) [7,21,22]. The AV node is more posterior and inferior (near the coronary sinus ostium) than normal. The bundle of His usually courses along the inferior rim of the ventricular septal defect and therefore the bundle branches arise more inferiorly. It is this displacement of the AV node that causes the northwest axis on electrocardiogram.

Hemodynamics/Natural History

Patients with an atrioventricular canal defect initially have excessive pulmonary blood flow resulting from left-to-right shunting at the atrial and ventricular levels. If there

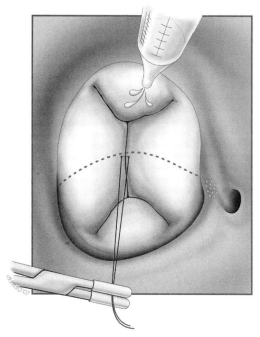

Figure 18.4 This is an illustration of a common atrioventricular valve in a patient with complete AV canal defect. The coronary sinus and the AV node are identified. The dotted line indicates where the AV valve will be divided into right and left components. (Reproduced with permission from Backer *et al.* [22].)

is no interventricular communication, the hemodynamics are similar to those of a large atrial septal defect, with increased right ventricular stroke volume. As the AV valve insufficiency through the left AV valve increases over time these patients may develop a larger left-to-right shunt. In some cases, the regurgitation from the left AV valve proceeds directly into the right atrium. These patients develop progressive cardiomegaly and congestive heart failure that is definitely more significant than in a patient with an atrial septal defect without left AV valve insufficiency.

In patients with a complete atrioventricular canal defect, the large left-to-right shunt causes right ventricular and pulmonary artery pressures to be the same as the systemic pressure. These patients have significant pulmonary hypertension from birth which is unrelenting until they have complete intracardiac repair. These patients can have a relatively rapid progression of their pulmonary vascular disease [23]. Trisomy 21 appears to be associated with accelerated development of pulmonary hypertension [24]. Within a few months of birth the pulmonary vascular resistance is frequently significantly elevated. In our series of AV canal patients, the mean PVR (u/m^2) at 0–3 months was 2.1 ± 0.9, at 4–6 months was 4.0 ± 2.6, and at 7–17 months was 5.7 ± 3.0 [19]. The pulmonary hypertension and congestive heart failure is compounded by the presence of AV valve insufficiency, which increases the ven-

tricular volume overload. It is the rapid elevation of pulmonary vascular resistance and progression of pulmonary vascular obstructive disease that makes early repair of complete atrioventricular canal defects so important.

Diagnosis

Patients with a complete atrioventricular canal defect typically have all the classic symptoms of congestive heart failure in infants. This includes frequent upper respiratory tract infections, poor feeding and inadequate weight gain, and sweating with feeds. On physical examination, these patients will have tachycardia, tachypnea, dyspnea, and hepatomegaly. On cardiac examination the precordium is hyperactive and if there is significant AV valve insufficiency a loud systolic murmur will be present. Chest X-ray will demonstrate cardiomegaly with biventricular enlargement and increased pulmonary vascular markings. Electrocardiographic findings include biventricular hypertrophy, a prolonged P-R interval, and a characteristic northwest or leftward and superior axis.

Two-dimensional echocardiography with Doppler color interrogation has become the standard for diagnosis of atrioventricular canal defects [25,26]. Two-dimensional echocardiography can identify and characterize valvular abnormalities, atrial and ventricular septal defect morphology, and associated anomalies (e.g., left superior vena cava, patent ductus arteriosus, left ventricular outflow tract obstruction). Color flow Doppler imaging provides accurate information regarding the degree of interatrial and interventricular shunting and assessment of AV valve insufficiency. It is more and more frequent now for the diagnosis of complete atrioventricular valve defect to be made on a prenatal ultrasound. Cardiac catheterization was previously frequently used to evaluate patients with complete atrioventricular canal defects. However, because most of these patients are known to have systemic pulmonary artery pressures, the use of cardiac catheterization is now more frequently limited to those patients presenting late in life where there can be a question as to whether or not the pulmonary vascular resistance has elevated to a point where repair is no longer indicated. In our practice, the most common indication for cardiac catheterization is as noted above or to evaluate other associated defects such as tetralogy of Fallot and double-outlet right ventricle. The characteristic "goose neck" deformity is seen in both the partial and complete forms of atrioventricular canal (Figure 18.5) [27]. This is caused by the "unwedging" of the aorta [1].

Indications and Timing of Operation

In patients with a partial atrioventricular canal defect, surgical repair is usually performed electively between 1 and

4 years of age [28,29]. Exceptions to this may occur if there is significant mitral valve regurgitation or hypoplastic left-sided cardiac structures (coarctation of the aorta, abnormal mitral valve, subaortic stenosis) [30]. Patients with complete atrioventricular canal defect usually present with congestive heart failure within the first 1–3 months of infancy. These children should be operated on between the ages of 3 and 5 months [19,31]. Failure to perform the operation until after 6–9 months of age can be associated with the risk of developing elevated pulmonary vascular resistance that is not reversible. Although in most surgical series patients with associated tetralogy of Fallot and sig-

nificant right ventricular outflow tract stenosis were initially palliated with a preliminary modified Blalock–Taussig shunt, several authors [32–34] have advocated early primary repair.

Operative Management and Results

As mentioned in the introduction, pulmonary artery banding was previously used for many patients with a complete atrioventricular canal defect [14,35]. The problem with pulmonary artery banding is that it often makes the left AV valve insufficiency worse and does not result in effective palliation. Most centers have now adopted early primary repair as the procedure of choice. Pulmonary artery banding is only used in exceptional cases where the use of cardiopulmonary bypass must be avoided (cerebrovascular accident, sepsis, etc.). Closure of the partial atrioventricular canal defect is reviewed in Chapter 16, *Atrial Septal Defect, Partial Anomalous Pulmonary Venous Connection, and Scimitar Syndrome.*

The principles of operative management of complete atrioventricular canal defect include closure of the atrial septal defect, closure of the ventricular septal defect, creation of two nonstenotic, competent AV valves, and avoidance of damage to the AV node and bundle of His. Repair of complete atrioventricular canal defects has been described using single-patch, two-patch, and modified single-patch techniques (Figure 18.6) [17]. The method of cardiopulmonary bypass is similar for the different techniques. We have routinely used continuous cardiopulmonary bypass with moderate hypothermia (28–32 °C) and intermittent antegrade cold blood cardioplegia for myocardial protection. In many cases we cannulate the superior

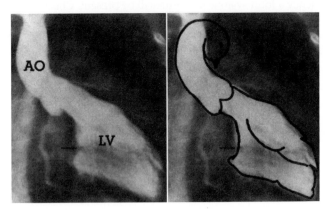

Figure 18.5 Frontal view of a left ventriculogram of a patient with a partial AV canal defect showing a goose-neck deformity. The left ventricular outflow tract is elongated and narrowed. The arrows point to the left AV valve zone of apposition. (Reproduced from Park [27].)

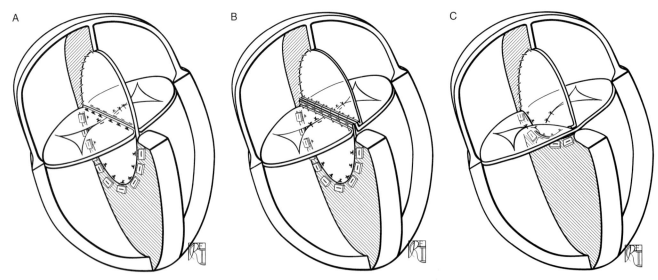

Figure 18.6 Schematic three-dimensional reconstruction of the three different surgical techniques: single-patch (**A**), two-patch (**B**), and modified single-patch (**C**).

vena cava directly with a right angle cannula to improve exposure within the right atrium. We have used a vent placed in the right superior pulmonary vein after beginning cardiopulmonary bypass. This vent can be pulled back into the atrium during the time of the left-sided AV valve repair. It is then reinserted into the left ventricle as the atrial septal defect is closed and the right-sided AV valve repair is performed. We have emphasized a long, medial atriotomy (parallel to the right coronary artery) that extends to a point medial to the inferior vena cava. This offers excellent exposure of the defect to facilitate the repair (Figure 18.7) [17]. Some surgeons are using both antegrade and retrograde cardioplegia [36]. Other centers use deep hypothermia and circulatory arrest, particularly for the younger and smaller infants. We and others use transesophageal echocardiographic assessment for all cases of AV canal [37].

One of the keys to successful repair of atrioventricular canal defects using any technique is a careful inspection of the intracardiac anatomy. This includes an assessment of the right and left ventricular size, the size and shape of the atrial and ventricular septal defect components, the number and location of papillary muscles, and the arrangement of the chordal structures including their attachment to the ventricular septum. The ventricular chambers should be gently filled with cold saline prior to the procedure to float the AV valve leaflets to their closed position. Floating the

valvar leaflets with saline helps to identify the line of apposition between the anterior and posterior common leaflets (Figure 18.4) [22]. Careful inspection of the leaflet tissue identifies the line that divides the valves into the right and left components. Some techniques employ division of the common AV valves, some do not.

Single-Patch Technique

The single-patch technique has been described using a pericardial, polytetrafluoroethylene (PTFE), or Dacron patch. The pericardial patch is most commonly used, especially for smaller infants, but carries some risk of aneurysm development at the ventricular level [38]. This can be corrected by fixing the patch in glutaraldehyde. The Dacron patch, although somewhat more malleable than PTFE, runs the risk of postoperative hemolysis should the jet of mitral or tricuspid valve insufficiency strike the Dacron. The patch dimensions are determined by the size and shape of the ventricular septal defect, the distance between the anterior and posterior margins of the AV valve annulus, and the dimensions of the atrial septal defect. This repair is started by floating the AV valve leaflets into the closed position. The line of apposition of the anterior and posterior common leaflets is noted and an imaginary line demarcating the tricuspid and mitral valve components is created by marking the coaptation of the anterior and posterior common leaflets with a horizontal mattress suture (Figure 18.8) [17]. The crest of the ventricular septum is then

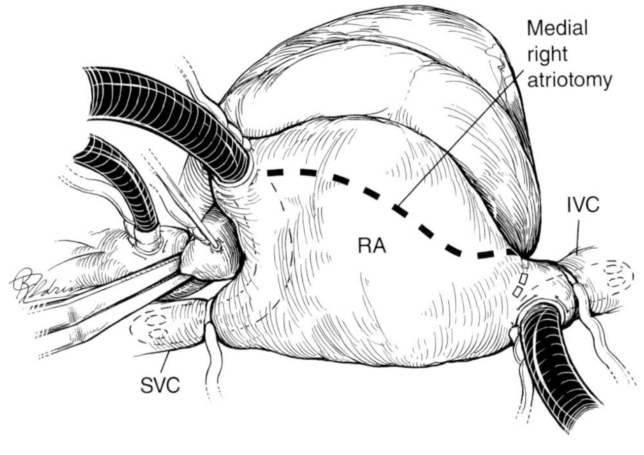

Figure 18.7 Atrial incision. Aortic and bicaval venous cannulation has been accomplished. The aorta has been cross-clamped and cold blood cardioplegia is being administered. The caval tapes have been snared. The dotted line indicates the medial right atrial incision. This incision extends from the right atrial appendage parallel to the right AV groove and the right coronary artery. Note the most inferior extent of the incision which is between the inferior vena cava (IVC) and the right coronary artery and coronary sinus. This incision allows excellent mobilization of the ventricle and resultant exposure of the AV valves. (RA, right atrium; SVC, superior vena cava.)

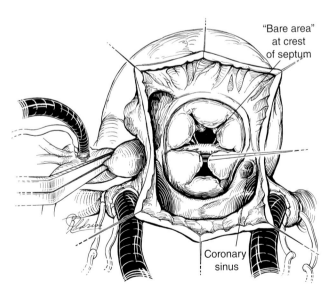

Figure 18.8 Single-patch technique in a Rastelli type A patient. Long medial atriotomy facilitates exposure. The zone of apposition of the superior and inferior bridging components of the left AV valve is approximated with a horizontal mattress suture. This defines the portion of the valve that will become the left AV valve.

A   B

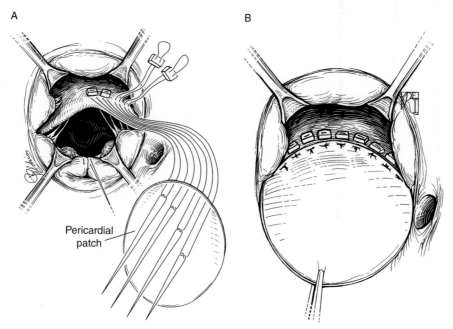

Pericardial
patch

Figure 18.9 A, Pledget-supported horizontal mattress sutures are inserted on the right side of the ventricular septum and passed through the base of the pericardial patch. **B,** The patch is lowered down to the septum and these sutures are then tied.

sutured to the inferior aspect of the patch with multiple interrupted horizontal mattress sutures (Figure 18.9) [17]. It may be necessary to weave the patch carefully around chordal structures. The leftward components of the common AV valve tissue are then secured to the patch in the appropriate plane with multiple interrupted mattress sutures. This may require division of the common AV valve. The left AV valve zone of apposition closure is illustrated in Figure 18.10 [17]. Whenever possible, these same sutures can be used to anchor the right AV valve components to the patch (Figure 18.11) [17]. The atrial portion of the defect is then closed by suturing the superior rim of the patch to the lower rim of the atrial septal defect (Figure 18.12) [17]. Care is taken to avoid injuring the conduction system and the bundle of His by carrying this suture line into the left atrium adjacent to the mitral valve in the region of the coronary sinus. Superficial bites are taken in this region. Some authors recommend displacing the coronary sinus into the left atrium by carrying the suture line of the atrial septal defect up and around the coronary sinus. Both techniques have a similar (low) incidence of complete atrioventricular heart block [19].

Two-Patch Technique

The two-patch repair, as first described by George Trusler [11], uses a patch of Dacron or PTFE to close the ventricular septal defect. The valve leaflets are sutured to the top of the ventricular septal defect patch. The left AV valve zone

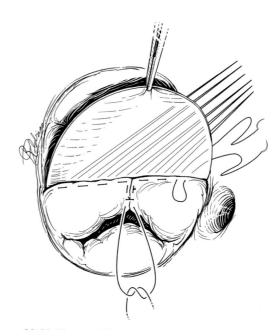

Figure 18.10 The patch has now been reflected anteriorly and a row of horizontal mattress sutures attaches the left AV valve tissue to the patch at the appropriate level. The zone of apposition of the left AV valve becomes apparent as shown and can be closed as indicated.

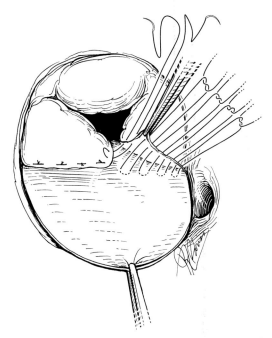

Figure 18.11 The sutures that pass through the left AV valve and through the patch are now passed through the edge of the right-sided AV valve. These sutures, once tied, anchor the valves to the patch at an appropriate height above the ventricular crest.

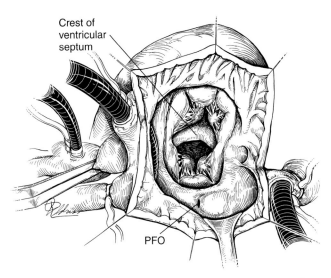

Figure 18.13 Two-patch technique. Exposure of atrioventricular canal defect, Rastelli type A. The right atrium has been opened with the medial atriotomy and stay sutures have been placed. The pertinent anatomic findings are a single common AV valve and the "bare" area at the crest of the ventricular septum that divides the right and left ventricles. In this particular patient there is a patent foramen ovale (PFO). Spatial relationships are demonstrated in Figure 18.14.

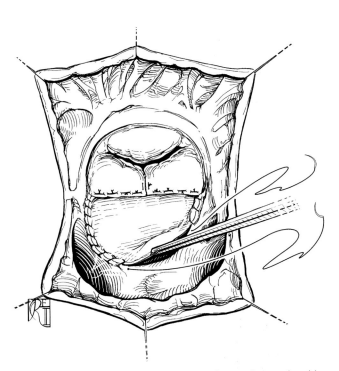

Figure 18.12 The single-patch closure technique is completed by using the pericardial patch to close the atrial septal component of the AV canal with a running suture technique.

of apposition is sutured closed, and a separate pericardial patch is used to close the atrial septal defect. Again, exposure is obtained through a long medial atriotomy (Figure 18.13) [17]. The distance between the superior aspect of what will become the left AV valve and the crest of the ventricular septum (extent of the ventricular septal defect) is assessed to accurately fashion a PTFE patch for the ventricular septal defect component (Figure 18.14) [17]. This will place the AV valves at the proper height above the septum and theoretically prevent subaortic stenosis. The ventricular component of the atrioventricular canal defect is closed with a PTFE patch anchored with interrupted pledget-supported sutures (Figure 18.15) [17]. These sutures are placed on the right ventricular side of the septum to avoid the left bundle and the AV node. In some cases the posterior common leaflet must be divided to fully expose the ventricular septal defect. The left AV valve is then suspended from the PTFE patch after approximating the left superior and inferior leaflets centrally (Figure 18.16) [17]. The left AV valve is sandwiched between the ventricular (PTFE) and atrial (pericardial) patches, as a buttressing measure to prevent sutures from cutting through the valve leaflets, thereby minimizing the chance of valve dehiscence (Figure 18.17) [17,39]. The zone of apposition of the left AV valve created between the left superior and left inferior leaflets is closed with simple interrupted polypropylene sutures (Figure 18.18) [17]. This closure is carried to the insertion site of the first order chordae tendineae at the free

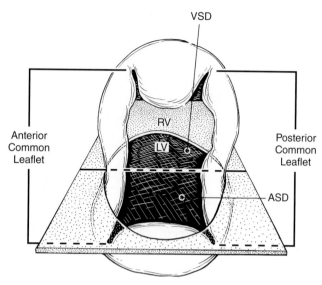

Figure 18.14 A schematic representation of the three-dimensional relationship of the ventricular and atrial septal defects and their location in regard to the AV valve tissue is an important concept to grasp. The imaginary line spatially divides the ventricular septal defect from the atrial septal defect. Standard surgical nomenclature refers to the anterior and posterior common AV valve leaflets as illustrated.

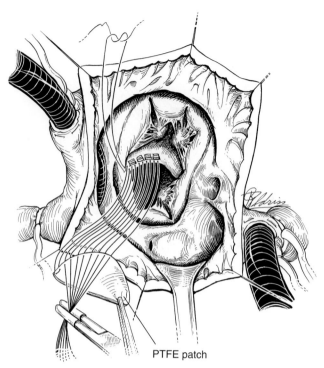

Figure 18.15 Ventricular septal defect closure; two-patch technique. A series of pledget-supported sutures are being placed on the crest of the ventricular septum and then passed through a polytetrafluoroethylene (PTFE) patch. Sutures are placed on the right ventricular side of the septum. A separate horizontal mattress suture at the very corner of the patch passes underneath the anterior common leaflet into the atrium to anchor the corner of the ventricular septal defect patch. The ventricular septal defect patch is cut in a crescent shape with a flat top where the AV valve tissue will be suspended to the patch.

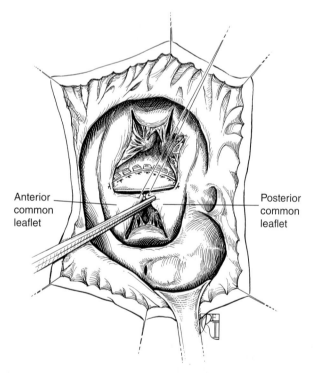

Figure 18.16 The anterior and posterior common leaflets have been brought together in the midline above the crest of the ventricular septal defect patch that has now been tied in place. This sets up the attachment of the left AV valve to the crest of the ventricular septal defect patch and also the location for the zone of apposition closure.

edge of the left AV valve leaflet. Competency of the left-sided AV valve is assessed by irrigating the left ventricle with sterile saline solution through a bulb syringe (Figure 18.19) [17]. An autologous pericardial patch is used to close the atrial septal defect (Figure 18.20) [17]. We have used a running polypropylene suture to anchor the atrial septal defect patch (Figure 18.21) [17]. Care is taken in the area of the AV node to place superficial sutures that extend close to the left-sided AV valve and thus away from the conduction system. The coronary sinus is kept on the right atrial side of the patch. The right AV valve is repaired in a similar fashion to the left-sided AV valve by closing the zone of apposition between the right superior and inferior leaflets (Figure 18.22) [17] and approximating the valve edge to the atrial septal defect patch (Figure 18.23) [17]. This valve is also irrigated with saline to assess competency.

We currently employ intraoperative transesophageal echocardiography in all patients with a partial, intermediate, or complete atrioventricular canal defect. Transesophageal

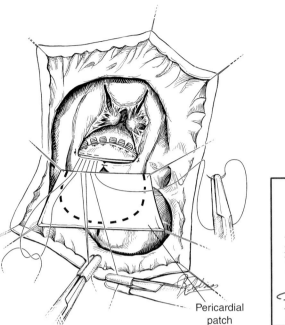

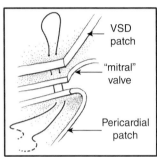

Figure 18.17 Atrial septal defect closure. Separate horizontal mattress sutures of polypropylene are passed through the crest of the ventricular septal defect patch, through the left AV valve leaflet tissue, and then through the pericardial patch that had previously been harvested. The small inset shows how the left AV valve is sandwiched between the ventricular septal defect patch of PTFE and the pericardial atrial septal defect patch. This reduces the incidence of valve dehiscence following the procedure.

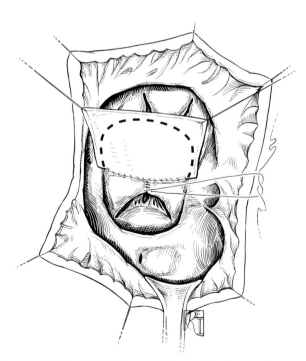

Figure 18.18 Left AV valve zone of apposition closure. The pericardial patch has been reflected anteriorly and separate interrupted polypropylene sutures have been placed to close the "zone of apposition" between the anterior and posterior common leaflets. The extent of this closure is to the insertion of the primary chordae at the edge of the left AV valve leaflet.

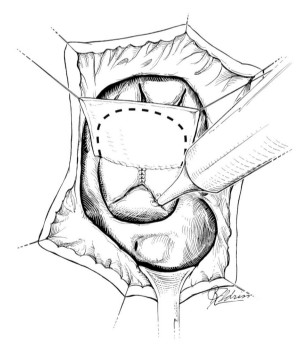

Figure 18.19 Valve assessment. The reconstructed left AV valve is tested intraoperatively with a bulb syringe. The bulb syringe is passed into the ventricle and cold saline is injected. As the ventricle fills and the valve becomes competent, the bulb syringe is removed. As the ventricle recoils against the cold saline, left AV valve insufficiency can be assessed. Often, a small residual jet can be eliminated by an additional suture in the zone of apposition.

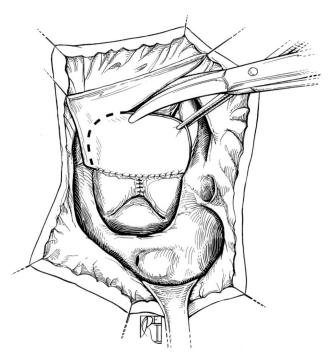

Figure 18.20 Atrial septal defect closure. The pericardial patch is being trimmed to an appropriate shape to approximate the extent of the atrial component of the defect.

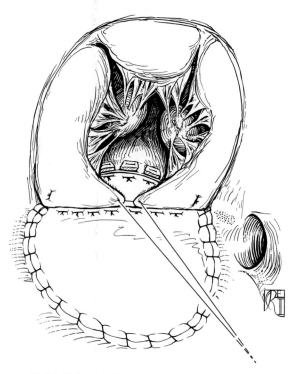

Figure 18.22 Right AV valve repair. The right AV valve is reconstructed by first approximating the anterior and posterior leaflets in the midline.

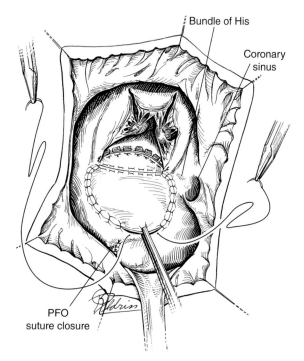

Figure 18.21 Two separate suture lines are used to complete the atrial septal defect closure. Each begins at the corner of the ventricular septal defect patch (running polypropylene). In the region of the bundle of His, the suturing is carried down into the left atrium immediately adjacent to the left AV valve in an effort to avoid creating heart block. Prior to completing the suture lines and tying the knot, the left side of the heart is de-aired.

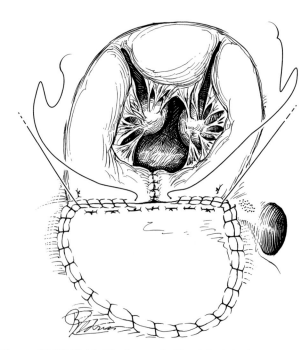

Figure 18.23 Right AV valve repair. The right AV valve is sutured to the confluence of the ventricular septal defect patch and the atrial septal defect pericardial patch. The right AV valve is irrigated with cold saline to see if there is any evidence of insufficiency that may be amenable to further suturing of the zone of apposition.

echocardiography is used to evaluate the preoperative anatomy, particularly the right and left ventricular sizes, the anatomy of the common AV valve, straddling or other unusual chordal issues, and the extent of preoperative AV valve insufficiency. Postoperatively, the transesophageal echocardiography can be used to evaluate for residual ventricular septal defect, residual atrial septal defect, subaortic stenosis, and right and left AV valve insufficiency or stenosis. All of these can be potential indications for an immediate re-repair of the noted abnormality.

Modified Single-Patch Technique

We perform this operation with continuous cardiopulmonary bypass, moderate hypothermia, and multi-dose cold blood antegrade cardioplegia. The ventricular septal defect is closed by placing a series of pledget-supported 5-0 sutures on the right side of the crest of the interventricular septum (Figure 18.24) [17]. These sutures are then

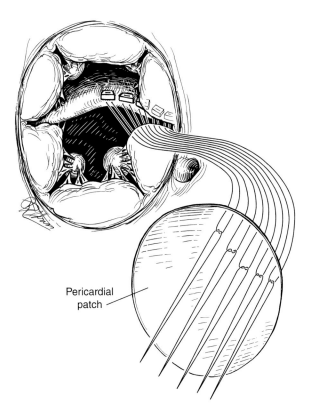

Pericardial patch

Figure 18.24 Modified single-patch technique in a Rastelli type A patient. A series of pledget-supported sutures are placed on the right ventricular side of the crest of the ventricular septum. The sutures are passed through the left AV valve component of the common AV valve, and then through the pericardial patch.

passed sequentially through the anterior and posterior common leaflets at a site predetermined to separate the right and left AV valves. The visualization of the division of the valve leaflets into right and left components is facilitated by insufflating the ventricles with cold saline and marking the midportion of the valves with a prolene suture (Figure 18.4) [22]. In most cases, we begin with the central suture and then progress first toward the AV node and then toward the aortic valve. When in doubt, we "give" valve tissue to the left AV valve. After all the sutures are placed through the leaflets, Nunn advocates passing them through a thin strip of Dacron, aiming to reduce the length of the septal crest sufficiently to create an increased central coaptation of the anterior and posterior leaflet components [13]. We have *not* incorporated the use of a Dacron strip in our patients having the modified single-patch technique. The sutures are then placed through the edge of a patch of autologous pericardium (Figure 18.25) [17]. These sutures are then tied, effectively eliminating the VSD and converting the remaining pathology to that of a partial AV canal. Now the zone of apposition of the left AV valve component created by apposition of the anterior and posterior common leaflets is closed (Figure 18.26) [17]. Closure of the zone of apposition is to the point where chordal attachments from the papillary muscles reach the free edges of the leaflet. The reconstructed valve is tested for competence with saline irrigation. The atrial component of the AV canal defect is then closed with the pericardial patch (Figure 18.27) [17]. This is performed with a running monofilament suture that follows the edge of the defect except in the region of the AV node. Here the suture line skirts down into the left atrium adjacent to the mitral annulus and close to the mitral leaflet tissue until a point lateral to the triangle of Koch is reached. The suture line then crosses up to the edge of the remaining atrial septum allowing the coronary sinus to normally drain into the right atrium. Separate secundum atrial septal defects are either covered by the same patch or sutured closed directly or closed with a separate pericardial patch if they are large and remote from the AV canal defect.

AV Canal with Tetralogy of Fallot

The presence of tetralogy of Fallot imposes some modifications in the technique used for atrioventricular canal repair. Most surgeons prefer to use a double-patch technique for these patients, and the patch needs to be wider near the subaortic area to allow enough redundancy at the anterosuperior end of the ventricular septal defect and thus avoid left ventricular outflow tract obstruction. With the two-patch technique, the ventricular septal defect patch is

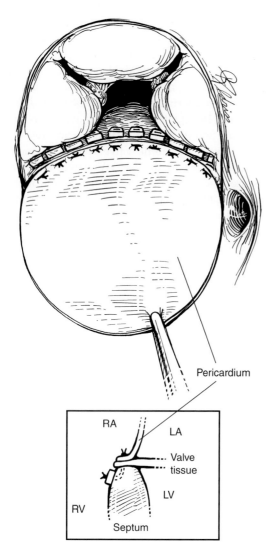

Figure 18.25 The sutures have now been tied, eliminating the ventricular septal defect by approximating the left AV valve to the crest of the ventricular septal defect between the pledgets and the pericardial patch. Inset shows the relationship between the pledget-supported suture, the left AV valve, and the pericardial patch. (LA, RA, left, right atrium; LV, RV, left, right ventricle.)

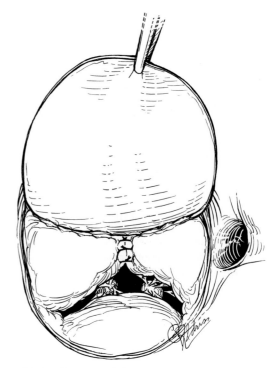

Figure 18.26 The pericardial patch is reflected anteriorly and the zone of apposition of the left AV valve is being closed.

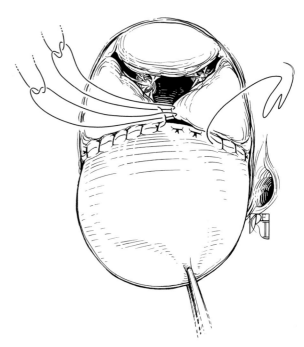

Figure 18.27 Right AV valve reconstruction and pericardial patch closure of ASD. The anterior and posterior common leaflet portion that is to become the right AV valve is sutured to the confluence of the pericardial patch, left AV valve tissue, and crest of the VSD. The interrupted sutures in the center are closing the right AV valve zone of apposition.

"comma"-shaped. The VSD component in these patients is frequently very large. The current trend in these patients is to avoid palliation and repair the patients primarily with a transatrial/transpulmonary approach [40]. Palliation with a shunt is reserved for severely cyanotic neonates and patients with small pulmonary arteries [41]. Palliation with a shunt will result in volume loading of the ventricles and the potential (desirable in this case) for annular dilation making partitioning of the common AV valve easier [42]. The review by Najm and associates would suggest that primary repair does have the best results [33].

Results

The results of the three main techniques described above can be best evaluated by examining the operative mortality and the reoperation rates for mitral insufficiency, pacemaker, left ventricular outflow tract obstruction, and residual atrial or ventricular septal defect. A comparison summary of selected recent series of AV canal repairs is shown in Table 18.1 [12,19,43–54]. In comparing the results of these series one must keep in mind the fact that some of the results have an era effect. The modified single-patch technique has been more frequently applied in the recent era as compared to the two-patch technique and classic single-patch technique where the results go back, in some cases, nearly 20 years. Despite that era effect we believe that the modified single-patch technique offers distinct advantages over the other techniques. In comparing operative mortality the modified single-patch technique at 2% was less than the two-patch technique at 3.5%, and the single-patch technique at 4.8%. This may be partially reflected by the era effect as I mentioned previously, but I believe it is also a tribute to the ease with which the modified single-patch technique can be performed. The modified single-patch technique has been shown to have shorter cross-clamp and cardioplegia times than the other techniques. In our comparison the mean cross-clamp time was shorter by 26 minutes and the mean cardiopulmonary bypass time was shorter by 29 minutes [45]. Another reason the mortality rate may be lower in the patients with the modified single-patch technique is that this operation lends itself well to the smaller infant. In our series the mean age at the time of repair has dropped from 6 months to under 4 months. Operating on these babies earlier in life, prior to the progression of pulmonary vascular disease and atrioventricular valve insufficiency is advantageous.

It is the reoperation rate for left AV valve insufficiency that has the most dramatically different outcome when comparing the three techniques. The modified single-patch technique reoperation rate was 2%, the two-patch technique was 7.2%, and the classic single-patch technique was 9.7%. This has always been the "Achilles' heel" of complete AV canal repair. In his landmark review of a single surgeon's experience of over 25 years using the single-patch technique, Fred Crawford stated, "Unfortunately what has not improved and what continues to be the limiting factor of this procedure, especially insofar as long-term results are concerned, is left atrioventricular valve competence" [52]. Crawford collected 13 operative series reported from 1997 to 2006 and examined the incidence of reoperation for left AV valve regurgitation. He found that the incidence of reoperation ranged from 3.5–19.7% and was in fact remarkably constant at approximately 7–8%. Kanani and associates recently stated the following in a review of mechanisms for late incompetence of the left AV valve after repair of

Table 18.1 A comparison summary of selected recent series of AV canal repairs. (NS, not stated.)

Author	Number of patients	Operative mortality	Late mortality	Left AV valve reoperation	Heart block
Modified single-patch technique					
Wilcox [12]	12	1	0	0	0
Nunn [43]	128	2	0	3	0
Jonas [44]	34	0	NS	0	1
Backer [45]	26	1	0	1	0
	200	4 (2%)	0	4 (2%)	1 (0.5%)
Two-patch technique					
Litwin [46]	222	6	6	13	3
Backer [45,19,47]	173	10	2	14	7
Lacour-Gayet [48]	110	4	2	7	3
Masuda [49]	64	2	3	5	NS
Ten Harkel [50]	111	3	3	10	2
Fortuna [51]	209	6	3	15	2
	889	31 (3.5%)	19 (2.1%)	64 (7.2%)	17 (2%)
Classic single-patch technique					
Crawford [52]	88	0	0	9	3
Reddy [53]	72	1	1	2	0
Prifti [54]	190	16	13	23	5
	350	17 (4.8%)	14 (4%)	34 (9.7%)	8 (2.3%)

atrioventricular valve defect, "Mortality following repair of atrioventricular septal defects has fallen dramatically in the last four decades, but reoperation for late regurgitation across the left atrioventricular valve has remained disconcertingly stagnant" [55].

This problem of reoperation of the left AV valve after AV canal repair is we believe addressed and altered significantly by the modified single-patch technique. This may be the single most important reason why the modified single-patch technique is now our operation of choice for patients with complete AV canal defect. There are several reasons for this improvement in outcome. The modified single-patch technique, because of its simplicity, is well suited for repair in the young infant. In Nunn's series the median age of patients at operation was 63 days, just over 2 months [45]. In our series the mean age is 4 months [46]. Dr Lacour-Gayet and colleagues have reported the importance of operating on these patients at 2–4 months of age [47]. This avoids the complications of pulmonary vascular obstructive disease and progressive dilatation of the common AV junction leading to regurgitation across the left AV valve.

Another explanation for the success of the modified single-patch technique is that the complexity of the repair is considerably reduced by avoiding the VSD patch. When this patch is placed it has the potential to be too short, too wide, too tall, or too long. Any one of these combinations can affect the coaptation of the left AV valve. This exact sizing of the ventricular patch is avoided with the modified single-patch technique. A third explanation for the success of the modified single-patch technique is that it is performed without dividing the AV valve leaflets. When the leaflets are divided, they must be reapproximated to the top of the VSD patch or to the midportion of the classic single patch. The very act of splitting the common leaflet and reattaching the left and right components by necessity sacrifices valve tissue. Although this may not be significant in older children, it becomes important in infants in whom the sacrificed valve tissue comprises a greater portion of the whole. Moreover, the potential for patch disruption of the reattached mitral and tricuspid components is avoided if the common leaflets are not split [56].

Fortuna and colleagues at the Hospital for Sick Children in Toronto reviewed their results with the two-patch technique in 209 children [51]. They demonstrated that division of the bridging leaflets obligates a portion of the leaflet tissue to the repair whether using one or two patches. This loss of leaflet tissue may lead to distortion of the remaining valve tissue and an increase in tension on the zone of apposition closure, leading to the potential for valve regurgitation and increased risk of valve dehiscence. They concluded that the division of the bridging leaflets is a risk factor for AV valve regurgitation during the first year after repair. In contrast, preservation of the bridging leaflet integrity improves valve competency, decreases the need for future

reoperation, and eliminates some causes of operative mortality.

One possible complication of the modified single-patch technique is the potential for left ventricular outflow tract obstruction in the patient with a very large ventricular component or "scoop." Adachi and colleagues have shown that in addition to the VSD size, the degree of anterosuperior extension of the VSD is also important in assessing the risk of late left ventricular outflow tract obstruction [57]. This "potential" complication does not seem to be a major clinical problem. In Nunn's recent review he applied the modified single-patch technique sequentially to all patients regardless of VSD size (n = 128) [43]. The long-term follow-up of the modified single-patch technique in Nunn's series would appear to refute and to answer the question regarding the possible risk of late left ventricular outflow tract obstruction. Nunn now has 26 patients with more than 10–15 years of follow-up, and no patient has required reoperation for left ventricular outflow tract obstruction. Similarly in our own series, no patient has developed significant left ventricular outflow tract obstruction, a finding replicated in the series from Jonas [44]. In fact, the synthetic material placed in the two-patch technique in the left ventricular outflow tract may encourage fibrotic obstruction in the naturally narrow left ventricular outflow tract. It may also contribute to increased rigidity in the posterior wall of the left ventricle outlet by its very presence, and in doing so may promote turbulence on the left ventricular outflow tract during systolic contraction in a manner similar to that seen in asymmetric septal hypertrophy. We have elected not to apply the modified single-patch technique only in the unusual case when the ventricular septal defect is >12 mm in diameter as measured from the crest of the VSD to the level of the common AV valve during end diastole by transesophageal echocardiogram [58].

It would appear that all three techniques have a very low risk of third-degree atrioventricular heart block. In the modified single-patch technique we have not seen a patient with heart block at our institution. In over 200 total reported patients there was only one incidence noted of complete heart block. In the two-patch technique and the classic single-patch technique the incidence as reported in the literature is 2–2.5%. Again, the removal of the rigid PTFE or Dacron patch from the VSD closure portion of the repair may lend itself to a lower incidence of AV block, although this would be difficult to demonstrate statistically with its low overall incidence.

In summary, the modified single-patch technique, which was first performed in a significant amount of patients beginning in the mid-1990s is now in our opinion the procedure of choice for atrioventricular canal repair. The operative mortality rate is very low (<2%), the late mortality rate is very low (<1%), and the incidence of left AV valve reoperation is very low at 2%; significantly lower than any reported repairs with the classic single-patch or two-patch techniques. The modified single-patch technique has results that are superior to the classic two-patch technique and can be applied in very young infants (2–3 months of age). This facilitates AV canal repair before progression of pulmonary hypertension, AV valve dilatation, and AV valve insufficiency.

Risk Factors

Age at Operation

It was previously thought that delaying operation until a later age would increase operative survival. This in fact is incorrect, and earlier age at operation, particularly operating on these patients at less than 6 months of age, is associated with increased survival based primarily on decreased incidence of significant postoperative pulmonary hypertension. [19,48,59]. In the recent series from Michigan [59], the median age at operation for complete atrioventricular canal was 4.8 months.

Preoperative AV Valve Incompetence

The presence of severe preoperative left AV valve regurgitation, and its contribution to the development of pulmonary hypertension and changes in pulmonary vascular resistance is a significant factor in increased risk of hospital death after repair.

Double Orifice Left AV Valve

Approximately 5% of patients with complete atrioventricular canal or partial atrioventricular canal will have a double orifice left AV valve [60]. The left AV valve component will have two separate orifices. These orifices are typically abnormal holes in essentially normal leaflets, not abnormal fibrous bridges or adhesions across commissures. The key to repair is not dividing the tissue bridging between these two orifices as this will cause severe valvar insufficiency. This can be an area of preoperative assessment confusion as the orifice can be assessed as "too small," not considering the fact that there are actually two orifices for the left AV valve.

Zone of Apposition

The nomenclature of the left AV valve has changed dramatically as our understanding of this valve has increased. We formerly referred to the area between the superior and inferior bridging leaflets as the "mitral valve cleft." Professor Robert Anderson in particular has demonstrated for us that the left AV valve in these patients is not anatomically a mitral valve. The surgical approximation of the superior and inferior bridging leaflets is really bringing together what should more accurately be called, "the zone of apposition" [61]. In the late 1970s and early 1980s some

surgeons believed that this valve should be treated as a trifoliate valve and that the superior and inferior bridging leaflets should not be joined. However, not closing the zone of apposition is associated with an increased incidence of late left AV valve insufficiency [54,62]. Now, almost all surgeons approximate the zone of apposition at the time of partial or complete atrioventricular septal defect repair. We have been routinely closing the zone of apposition since 1985.

Trisomy 21

In many series the presence of trisomy 21 has been associated with redundant AV valve tissue available for reconstruction. This helps to decrease the incidence of significant postoperative AV valve insufficiency and has been associated with a better outcome as far as reducing the incidence of left AV valve reoperation [31]. The great majority of patients with atrioventricular canal (86% in our series) will have trisomy 21. In a recent article from Masuda and colleagues, the incidence of reoperation on the left AV valve was 4% in the trisomy 21 group and 15% in the non-trisomy 21 group [63]. In another recent review, the presence of trisomy 21 was protective of the need for reoperation [64].

Postoperative Management

We routinely manage our postoperative complete atrioventricular canal patients with paralysis, sedation, and hyperventilation. This helps to avoid pulmonary hypertensive crises and optimizes cardiac output in the critical first 24–48 hours postoperatively. Factors that are known to trigger pulmonary hypertensive crisis such as hypoxia, hypercapnia, acidosis, pain, and hypothermia, are minimized by this strategy. The sedation and paralysis is continued usually for a minimum of 24 hours, often 48 hours, and sometimes 72 hours, depending on the age of the patient and the expected degree of pulmonary hypertension. Studying the pulmonary artery pressures of these patients postoperatively in the operating room, many of them after a good repair have essentially normal pulmonary artery pressures with the use of the above strategies. However, we would treat patients who have any evidence of residual pulmonary hypertension with inhaled nitric oxide [65]. Cardiac output in these patients is optimized by routine administration of low-dose dopamine (2.5–5 μg/kg/min) and low-dose dobutamine (2.5–5 μg/kg/min). In addition, we have used milrinone (0.5–0.7 μg/kg/min), a phosphodiesterase inhibitor, in all patients.

Conclusion

Atrioventricular canal defects represent a spectrum of intracardiac anomalies. The pathognomonic feature is a common atrioventricular junction. This ranges from a partial atrioventricular canal (atrial septal defect, trifoliate left AV valve) to intermediate atrioventricular canal (atrial septal defect, trifoliate left AV valve, ventricular septal defect beneath two separate AV valve orifices), to complete atrioventricular canal (atrial and ventricular septal defects and a common AV valve). The complete atrioventricular canal defects are divided into three categories, Rastelli A, B, and C. Patients with partial atrioventricular canal defects are treated much like patients with a large atrial septal defect and can be operated on electively between the ages of 1 and 4 years. Patients with a complete atrioventricular canal defect should undergo operative repair before 6 months of age. Surgical techniques currently employed for complete atrioventricular canal include the single-patch technique, the two-patch technique, and the modified single-patch technique. In the current era, repair is facilitated by the use of intraoperative transesophageal echocardiography in all patients. Postoperative management centers on proactive management of pulmonary hypertension. The most common late complication is residual or recurrent left AV valve insufficiency. Long-term survival and functional outcome are excellent for most of those patients. Our current operation of choice for the great majority of patients with complete atrioventricular canal defect is the modified single-patch technique.

References

1. Anderson RH, Ho SY, Falcao S, *et al.* (1998) The diagnostic features of atrioventricular septal defect with common atrioventricular junction. Cardiol Young 8, 33–49.

2. Mitchell SC, Korones SB, Berendes HW. (1984) Congenital heart disease in 56,109 live births. Incidence and natural history. Circulation 43, 323–332.

3. Spicer RL. (1984) Cardiovascular disease in Down syndrome. Pediatr Clin North Am 31, 1331–1343.

4. Jacobs JP, Burke RP, Quintessenza JA, *et al.* (2000) Congenital Heart Surgery Nomenclature and Database Project: atrioventricular canal defect. Ann Thorac Surg 69(suppl), S36–S43.

5. Lillehei CW, Cohen M, Warden HE, *et al.* (1955) The direct-vision intracardiac correction of congenital anomalies by controlled cross-circulation: results in thirty-two patients with ventricular septal defects, tetralogy of Fallot, and atrioventricularis communis defects. Surgery 38, 11–29.

6. Backer CL, Stewart RD, Mavroudis C. (2007) Overview: history, anatomy, timing, and results of complete atrioventricular canal. Semin Thorac Cardiovasc Surg Pediatr Card Surg Annu 10, 3–10.

7. Lev M. (1958) The architecture of the conduction system in congenital heart disease. I. Common atrioventricular orifice. AMA Arch Pathol 65, 174–191.

8. Maloney JV Jr, Marable SA, Mulder DG. (1962) The surgical treatment of common atrioventricular canal. J Thorac Cardiovasc Surg 43, 84–96.

9. Gerbode F. (1962) Surgical repair of endocardial cushion defect. Ann Chir Thorac Cardiovasc 1, 753–755.

10. Rastelli G, Kirklin JW, Titus JL. (1966) Anatomic observations on complete form of persistent common atrioventricular canal with special reference to atrioventricular valves. Mayo Clin Proc 41, 296–308.

11. Trusler GA (1976) Discussion of Mills NL, Ochsner JL, King TD. Correction of type C complete atrioventricular canal. Surgical considerations. J Thorac Cardiovasc Surg 71, 2028.

12. Wilcox BR, Jones DR, Frantz EG, *et al.* (1997). Anatomically sound, simplified approach to repair of "complete" atrioventricular septal defect. Ann Thorac Surg. 64, 487–493.

13. Nicholson IA, Nunn GR, Sholler GF, *et al.* (1999) Simplified single patch technique for the repair of atrioventricular septal defect. J Thorac Cardiovasc Surg 118, 642–646.

14. Epstein ML, Moller JH, Amplatz K, *et al.* (1979) Pulmonary artery banding in infants with complete atrioventricular canal. J Thorac Cardiovasc Surg 78, 28–31.

15. Wakai CS, Edwards JE. (1958) Pathologic study of persistent common atrioventricular canal. Am Heart J 56, 779–794.

16. Titus JL, Rastelli GC. (1976) Anatomic features of persistent common atrioventricular canal. In: Feldt RH, McGoon DC, eds. *Atrioventricular Canal Defects.* Philadelphia, PA: Saunders.

17. Backer CL, Mavroudis C. (2003) Atrioventricular canal defect. In: Mavroudis C, Backer CL, eds. *Pediatric Cardiac Surgery*, 3rd ed. Philadelphia, PA: Mosby.

18. Bharati S, Lev M, McAllister HA Jr. (1980) Surgical anatomy of the atrioventricular valve in the intermediate type of common atrioventricular orifice. J Thorac Cardiovasc Surg 79, 884–889.

19. Backer CL, Mavroudis C, Alboliras ET, *et al.* (1995) Repair of complete atrioventricular canal defects: results with the two-patch technique. Ann Thorac Surg 60, 530–537.

20. Bharati S, Kirklin JW, McAllister HA Jr, *et al.* (1980) The surgical anatomy of common atrioventricular orifice associated with tetralogy of Fallot, double outlet right ventricle and complete regular transposition. Circulation 61, 1142–1149.

21. Feldt RH, Titus JL. (1976) The conduction system in persistent common atrioventricular canal. In: Feldt RH, McGoon DC, eds. *Atrioventricular Canal Defects.* Philadelphia, PA: Saunders.

22. Backer CL, Stewart RD, Mavroudis C. (2007) What is the best technique for repair of complete atrioventricular canal? Semin Thorac Cardiovasc Surg 19, 249–257.

23. Newfeld EA, Sher M, Paul MH, *et al.* (1977) Pulmonary vascular disease in complete atrioventricular canal defect. Am J Cardiol 39, 721–726.

24. Clapp S, Perry BL, Farooki ZQ, *et al.* (1990) Down's syndrome, complete atrioventricular canal, and pulmonary vascular obstructive disease. J Thorac Cardiovasc Surg 100, 115–121.

25. Minich LA, Snider AR, Bove EL, *et al.* (1992) Echocardiographic evaluation of atrioventricular orifice anatomy in children with atrioventricular septal defect. J Am Coll Cardiol 19, 149–153.

26. Zellers TM, Zehr R, Weinstein E, *et al.* (1994) Two-dimensional and Doppler echocardiography alone can adequately define preoperative anatomy and hemodynamic status before repair of complete atrioventricular septal defect in infants <1 year old. J Am Coll Cardiol 24, 1565–1570.

27. Park MK. (2002) *Pediatric Cardiology for Practitioners*, 4th ed. St. Louis, MO: Mosby.

28. Sadeghi AM, Laks H, Pearl JM. (1997) Primum atrial septal defect. Semin Thorac Cardiovasc Surg 9, 2–7.
29. Najm HK, Williams WG, Chuarantanaphong S, et al. (1998) Primum atrial septal defect in children: early results, risk factors, and freedom from reoperation. Ann Thorac Surg 66, 829–835.
30. Manning PB, Mayer JE Jr, Sanders SP, et al. (1994) Unique features and prognosis of primum ASD presenting in the first year of life. Circulation 90, II30–II35.
31. Weintraub RG, Brawn WJ, Venables AW, et al. (1990) Two-patch repair of complete atrioventricular septal defect in the first year of life. Results and sequential assessment of atrioventricular valve function. J Thorac Cardiovasc Surg 99, 320–326.
32. McElhinney DB, Reddy VM, Silverman NH, et al. (1998) Atrioventricular septal defect with common valvar orifice and tetralogy of Fallot revisited: making a case for primary repair in infancy. Cardiol Young 8, 455–461.
33. Najm HK, Van Arsdell GS, Watzka S, et al. (1998) Primary repair is superior to initial palliation in children with atrioventricular septal defect and tetralogy of Fallot. J Thorac Cardiovasc Surg 116, 905–913.
34. Karl TR. (1997) Atrioventricular septal defect with tetralogy of Fallot or double-outlet right ventricle: surgical considerations. Semin Thorac Cardiovasc Surg 9, 26–34.
35. Silverman N, Levitsky S, Fisher E, et al. (1983) Efficacy of pulmonary artery banding in infants with complete atrioventricular canal. Circulation 68, II148–II153.
36. Crawford FA Jr, Stroud MR. (2001) Surgical repair of complete atrioventricular septal defect. Ann Thorac Surg 72, 1621–1629.
37. Cohen GA, Stevenson JG. (2007) Intraoperative echocardiography for atrioventricular canal: decision-making for surgeons. Semin Thorac Cardiovasc Surg Pediatr Card Surg Annu 10, 47–50.
38. Burkhart HM, Moody SA, Ensing GJ, et al. (1996) Ventricular septal aneurysm after atrioventricular septal repair with pericardium. Ann Thorac Surg 61, 1838–1839.
39. Katz NM, Blackstone EH, Kirklin JW, et al. (1981) Suture techniques for atrioventricular valves: experimental study. J Thorac Cardiovasc Surg 81, 528–536.
40. Hoohenkerk GJ, Schoof PH, Bruggemans EF, et al. (2008) 28 years' experience with transatrial–transpulmonary repair of atrioventricular septal defect with tetralogy of Fallot. Ann Thorac Surg 85, 1686–1689.
41. Prifti E, Bonacchi M, Bernabei M, et al. (2004) Repair of complete atrioventricular septal defect with tetralogy of Fallot: our experience and literature review. J Card Surg 19, 175–183.
42. Mitchell ME, Litwin SB, Tweddell JS. (2007) Complex atrioventricular canal. Semin Thorac Cardiovasc Surg Pediatr Card Surg Annu 10, 32–41.
43. Nunn GR. (2007) Atrioventricular canal: single patch technique. Semin Thorac Cardiovasc Surg Pediatr Card Surg Annu 10, 28–31.
44. Jonas RA. (2004) Complete atrioventricular canal. In: Jonas RA, DiNardo J, Lausen PC, et al. eds. *Comprehensive Surgical Management of Congenital Heart Disease*. London: Arnold Publishers, pp. 397–398.

45. Backer CL, Stewart RD, Bailliard F, et al. (2007) Complete atrioventricular canal: comparison of modified single-patch technique with two-patch technique. Ann Thorac Surg 84, 2038–2046.
46. Litwin SB, Tweddell JS, Mitchell ME, et al. (2007) The double patch repair for complete atrioventricularis communis. Semin Thorac Cardiovasc Surg Ped Card Surg Annu 10, 21–27.
47. Mavroudis C, Backer CL. (1997) The two-patch technique for complete atrioventricular canal. Semin Thorac Cardiovasc Surg 9, 35–43.
48. Lacour-Gayet F, Campbell DN, Mitchell M, et al. (2006) Surgical repair of atrioventricular septal defect with common atrioventricular valve in early infancy. Cardiol Young 16 (suppl 3), 52–58.
49. Masuda M, Kado H, Tamoue Y, et al. (2005) Does Down syndrome affect the long-term results of complete atrioventricular septal defect when the defect is repaired during the first year of life? Eur J Cardiothorac Surg 27, 405–409.
50. Ten Harkel AD, Cromme-Dijkhuis AH, Heinerman BC, et al. (2005) Development of left atrioventricular valve regurgitation after correction of atrioventricular septal defect. Ann Thorac Surg 79, 607–612.
51. Fortuna RS, Ashburn DA, DeOliveira NC, et al. (2004) Atrioventricular septal defects: effect of bridging leaflet division on early valve function. Ann Thorac Surg 77, 895–902.
52. Crawford FA. (2007) Atrioventricular canal: single-patch technique. Semin Thorac Cardiovasc Surg Pediatr Card Surg Annu 10, 11–20.
53. Reddy VM, McElhinney DB, Brook MM, et al. (1998) Atrioventricular valve function after single patch repair of complete atrioventricular septal defect in infancy: how early should repair be attempted? J Thorac Cardiovasc Surg 115, 1032–1040.
54. Prifti E, Bonachi M, Bernabei M, et al. (2004) Repair of complete atrioventricular septal defects in patients weighing less than 5 kg. Ann Thorac Surg 77, 1717–1726.
55. Kanani M, Elliott M, Cook A, et al. (2006) Late incompetence of the left atrioventricular valve after repair of atrioventricular septal defects: the morphologic perspective. J Thorac Cardiovasc Surg 132, 640–646.
56. Mavroudis C, Weinstein G, Turley K, et al. (1982) Surgical management of complete atrioventricular canal. J Thorac Cardiovasc Surg 83, 670–679.
57. Adachi I, Ho SY, McCarthy KP, et al. (2009) Ventricular scoop in atrioventricular septal defect: relevance to simplified single-patch method. Ann Thorac Surg 87, 198–203.
58. Backer CL. (2009) Invited Commentary: Ventricular scoop in atrioventricular septal defect: relevance to simplified single-patch method. Ann Thorac Surg 87, 203.
59. Suzuki T, Bove EL, Devaney EJ, et al. (2008) Results of definitive repair of complete atrioventricular septal defect in neonates and infants. Ann Thorac Surg 86, 596–603.
60. Bano-Rodrigo A, Van Praagh S, Trowitzseh E, et al. (1988) Double-orifice mitral valve: a study of 27 postmortem cases with developmental, diagnostic and surgical considerations. Am J Cardiol 61, 152–160.
61. Wetter J, Sinzobahamvya N, Blaschczok C, et al. (2000) Closure of the zone of apposition at correction of complete

atrioventricular septal defect improves outcome. Eur J Cardiothorac Surg 17, 146–153.

62. Najm HK, Coles JG, Endo M, *et al.* (1997) Complete atrioventricular septal defects: results of repair, risk factors, and freedom from re-operation. Circulation 96, 829–835.

63. Masuda M, Kado H, Tanoue Y, *et al.* (2005) Does Down syndrome affect the long-term results of complete atrioventricular septal defect when the defect is repaired during the first year of life? Eur J Cardiothorac Surg 27, 405–409.

64. Al-Hay AA, MacNeill SJ, Yacoub M, *et al.* (2003) Complete atrioventricular septal defect, Down syndrome, and surgical outcome: risk factors. Ann Thorac Surg 75, 412–421.

65. Curran RD, Mavroudis C, Backer CL, *et al.* (1995) Inhaled nitric oxide for children with congenital heart disease and pulmonary hypertension. Ann Thorac Surg 60, 1765–1771.

CHAPTER 19

Truncus Arteriosus

Constantine Mavroudis[1] and Carl L. Backer[2]

[1]Florida Hospital for Children, Orlando, FL, USA
[2]Ann & Robert H. Lurie Children's Hospital of Chicago, formerly Children's Memorial Hospital, Chicago, IL, USA

Truncus arteriosus is a congenital malformation in which a single arterial trunk arises from the heart, overrides the interventricular septum, and supplies the systemic, pulmonary, and coronary circulations. With truncus arteriosus there are no remnants of a separate pulmonary valve or ventricular-to-pulmonary artery continuity and thus this lesion can be distinguished from the severe forms of tetralogy of Fallot with pulmonary atresia. Truncus arteriosus is relatively uncommon, representing 0.21–0.34% of patients with congenital heart disease [1–4].

Embryologic and Anatomic Features

During embryonic life, the truncus arteriosus normally begins to separate and spiral into a distinguishable anterior pulmonary artery and posterior aorta. Persistent truncus arteriosus, therefore, represents an arrest in embryonic development at this stage [5,6]. Other implicated embryologic events include absence of truncal spiraling and division, twisting of the dividing truncus due to ventricular looping, subinfundibular atresia, and abnormal location of the semilunar valve anlages [1,7–9]. Experimental studies in chick embryos have shown that ablation of the neural crest results in persistent truncus arteriosus [10,11]. The neural crest also develops into the pharyngeal pouches and thence the thymus and parathyroids. This association explains the prevalence of truncus arteriosus with DiGeorge syndrome [12]. Recent studies [13–15] have demonstrated the association of DiGeorge syndrome (chromosome 22q11.2 microdeletion) with conotruncal malformations, including truncus arteriosus. They found a higher incidence of complex cardiovascular anatomy in association with depressed immunologic status, pulmonary vascular reactivity, neonatal hypocalcemia, bronchomalacia and bronchospasm, laryngeal web, and a tendency to airway bleeding.

The most striking characteristic of truncus arteriosus is the single arterial trunk arising from the heart, more or less overriding the ventricular septum, being dominantly positioned over the right ventricle in 42%, the left ventricle in 16%, and equally shared in 42% [16]. Anatomic classifications, however, have been based on the pulmonary artery origin from the truncus. Collett and Edwards [17] subdivided truncus arteriosus into type I – a short main pulmonary artery arising from and to the left of the truncus; type II – separate but closely positioned pulmonary arteries arising from the posterior truncus; type III – widely separated pulmonary arteries arising laterally from the truncus; and type IV – pulmonary arteries arising from the descending aorta (Figure 19.1) [18]. This classification, although helpful, has not explained entirely the more frequently found anatomic variations and is rarely used today.

Van Praagh [9] has offered a modified classification (Figure 19.1) [18]. Type A1 is similar to type I; type A2 more accurately combines types II and III since type III is exceedingly rare. In clinical practice one is more apt to see a continuum between types A1 and A2 (types I, II, III) depending on the site of origin of the right pulmonary artery. Van Praagh's A3 describes a single pulmonary artery origin from the truncus (usually the right pulmonary artery) with either a ductus or collateral vessels supplying the contralateral side. The A4 classification is truncus arteriosus with an interrupted aortic arch. Type IV truncus (Collett and Edwards) or pseudotruncus classifications ought to be abandoned as they are not true forms of truncus arteriosus and are, more accurately, ventricular septal defect with pulmonary atresia and major aortopulmonary collateral arteries. In addition to these aforementioned truncus arteriosus types are a number of variants including absence of a pulmonary artery [1], crossed pulmonary arteries [19], and various abnormalities of the brachiocephalic arteries [20,21]. Recently Russell, Jacobs, Mavroudis, Anderson,

Pediatric Cardiac Surgery, Fourth Edition. Edited by Constantine Mavroudis and Carl L. Backer.
© 2013 Blackwell Publishing Ltd. Published 2013 by Blackwell Publishing Ltd.

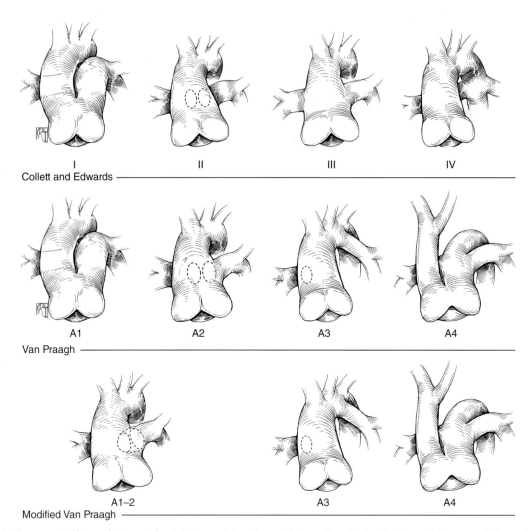

Figure 19.1 There are similarities between the Collett and Edwards and the Van Praagh classifications of truncus arteriosus. Type I is the same as A1. Types II and III are grouped as a single type A2 because they are not significantly distinct embryologically or therapeutically. Type A3 denotes unilateral pulmonary artery with collateral supply to the contralateral lung. Type A4 is truncus associated with interrupted aortic arch (13% of all cases of truncus arteriosus).

and associates have redefined truncus arteriosus as common arterial trunk with either predominantly aortic or pulmonary artery characteristics [22]. This definition allows for description of all the anatomic possibilities associated with this entity (Figure 19.2) [22]. Jacobs [23] developed an extensive and inclusive nomenclature database system by expanding Van Praagh's classification into a stepwise, computerized hierarchical system that allows for all variants and associated anomalies of truncus arteriosus. Such a system can be used world-wide in order to monitor incidence, document surgical results, and develop risk stratification models.

The truncal valve is often insufficient owing to abnormally thickened and deformed leaflets [16]. Very rarely the valve is stenotic. The truncal valve is usually tricuspid (60%), quadricuspid (25%), or bicuspid (5%). The aortic arch is right-sided in 18–36% of patients with truncus arteriosus and is usually associated with mirror-image branching of the brachiocephalic arteries [1,9,16,24]. A patent ductus arteriosus is sometimes encountered and may be associated with interrupted aortic arch, which is present in 11–14% of patients with truncus arteriosus [1,9,16,25]. The ventricular septal defect is usually located in an anterosuperior position, lying between the two superior limbs of the trabecula septomarginalis [21] remote from the conduction tissue (Figure 19.3) [18]. Occasionally the ventricular septal defect extends to the membranous septum closer to the conduction tissue, and will require more careful consideration during patch closure to avoid surgical heart block [26].

Anomalous coronary artery origin and distribution are not uncommon in truncus arteriosus and may impact unfa-

A
B

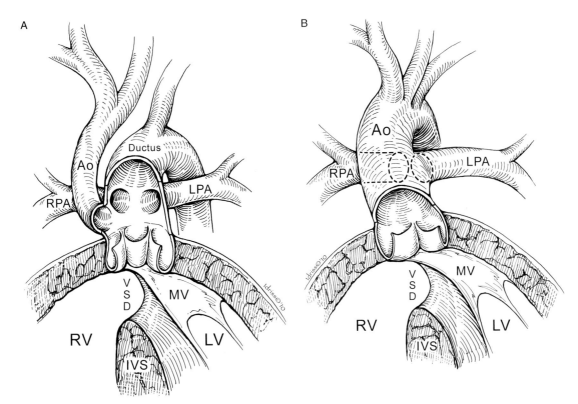

Figure 19.2 The essential features of pulmonary versus aortic dominance as observed in our autopsied specimens with common arterial trunk. **A**, Interruption of the aortic arch. Only in this setting, and in hearts with severe aortic coarctation, did we find origin of the pulmonary arteries from either side of the intrapericardial pulmonary trunk. **B**, The salient features of aortic dominance with the pulmonary arteries arising separately but next to each other from the leftward and dorsal aspect of the common trunk. We also find pulmonary arteries arising more anteriorly and then crossing as they extended toward the pulmonary hilums. (Ao, aorta; IVS, interventricular septum; LPA, RPA, left, right pulmonary arteries; LV, RV, left, right ventricle; MV, mitral valve; VSD, ventricular septal defect.) (Reproduced with permission from Russell *et al.* [22].)

vorably on surgical corrections. Single origins of the left and right coronary arteries have been reported [27,28] as well as abnormally high osteal takeoff above the sinuses of Valsalva [1,24] among others [29]. Clearly, the anomalous coronary arteries must be identified and preserved during neoaortic construction after removal of the pulmonary artery trunk [30,31].

Physiology and Clinical Findings

The overwhelming abnormal pathophysiologic feature of truncus arteriosus is a large left-to-right shunt that increases after the neonatal period as the pulmonary vascular resistance falls. Truncal valve regurgitation is present in about 50% of patients and may cause pressure overload to the already volume-overloaded ventricles. Pulmonary vascular obstructive disease may develop as early as 6 months of age, leading to poor results after late surgical correction.

The clinical manifestations of truncus arteriosus usually become apparent within the first weeks of life because of a murmur, tachypnea, and costosternal retractions. The patients are sometimes cyanotic, but the progressive signs of congestive heart failure are most prominent, including tachypnea, hepatomegaly, sweating with feeding, failure to thrive, bounding pulses, a pansystolic murmur at the left sternal border, and sometimes a diastolic murmur if significant truncal regurgitation is present. The second heart sound is predictably single.

The electrocardiogram shows sinus rhythm and biventricular hypertrophy. Left ventricular forces may predominate in the case of large pulmonary flow, while right ventricular forces may predominate if pulmonary vascular obstructive disease develops. The chest roentgenogram shows cardiomegaly, increased pulmonary vascular markings, and an absent pulmonary artery segment. A right aortic arch can be appreciated in about one-third of cases. Unequal vascularity may denote unilateral pulmonary artery atresia, while bilaterally decreased pulmonary markings often reflect long-standing pulmonary vascular obstructive disease.

The various views of two-dimensional echocardiography combined with pulsed-Doppler or Doppler color-flow

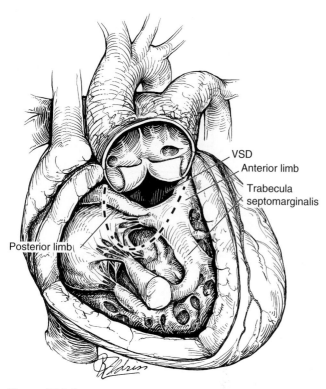

VSD
Anterior limb
Trabecula
septomarginalis

Posterior limb

Figure 19.3 In truncus arteriosus the location of the ventricular septal defect (VSD) can be variable. Shown here is the high and anterior type, which is surrounded by the two limbs of the trabecula septomarginalis. Other VSD types resemble those seen in patients with tetralogy of Fallot. These VSDs extend toward the paramembranous area (dotted line).

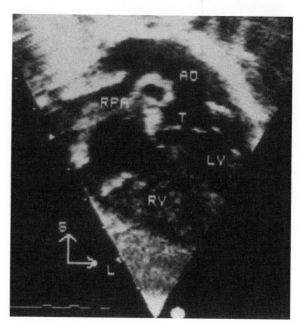

Figure 19.4 Subcostal two-dimensional echocardiographic view of left ventricular outflow in a different patient with truncus arteriosus. This patient has a right aortic arch and right pulmonary artery arising from the truncal vessel. The left pulmonary artery was hypoplastic and originated from isolated ductus arteriosus. (AO, aorta; LV, left ventricle; RPA, right pulmonary artery; RV, right ventricle; T, truncal vessel; arrows: S, superior; L, left.)

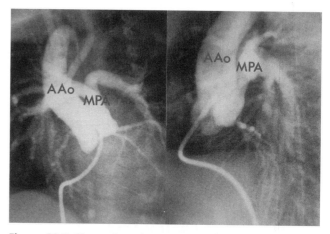

Figure 19.5 Cinecardioangiogram (anteroposterior and lateral views) of a patient with type A1 (type I) truncus arteriosus. (AAo, ascending aorta; MPA, main pulmonary artery.)

mapping can usually provide sufficient information to determine the type of truncus arteriosus, the origin of the coronary arteries and their proximity to the pulmonary trunk, the character of the truncal valve, and to some extent, the degree of truncal insufficiency, if present (Figure 19.4) [18]. The newer and less invasive diagnostic methods of magnetic resonance imaging and computed tomography (Plate 19.1, see plate section opposite p. 594) have helped to provide more accurate anatomic details such as coronary artery location and pulmonary artery origins, which can help in planning the operation and avoiding complications. Despite these advances in imaging techniques, cardiac catheterization is sometimes indicated to further evaluate truncal insufficiency, confirm anatomic details (Figures 19.5 and 19.6) [18], and measure pulmonary vascular resistance, especially in the case of late presentation.

Natural History

Untreated patients with truncus arteriosus have a dismal prognosis with a 65% 6-month and 75% 1-year mortality rate [17]. Occasionally some children will develop a mild degree of increased pulmonary vascular resistance to balance their systemic and pulmonary circulations and live to 10 years and more [32,33]. The greater number, however, fall victim to congestive heart failure due to the large left-to-right shunt or develop accelerated pulmonary vascular obstructive disease with progressive cyanosis. Surgeons now perform complete repair in the first 1–2 weeks of life, which has resulted in improved early and late survival.

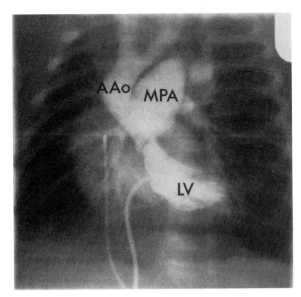

Figure 19.6 Cinecardioangiogram of a patient with truncus arteriosus, interrupted aortic arch (type A4) and truncal valve stenosis. (AAo, ascending aorta; LV, left ventricle; MPA, main pulmonary artery.)

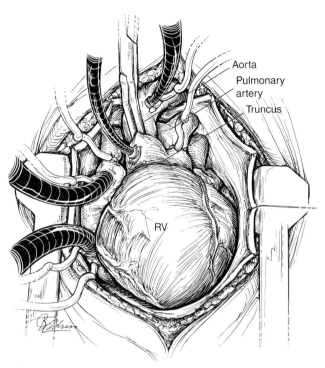

Figure 19.7 Diagrammatic representation of a patient with truncus arteriosus after aorto-bicaval cardiopulmonary bypass, pulmonary artery constriction, and aortic cross-clamping with cardioplegic arrest.

Management

Most infants with truncus arteriosus develop early congestive heart failure and failure to thrive despite medical treatment with digoxin, diuretics, and vasodilator therapy. Early experience with pulmonary artery banding resulted in ineffective palliation and high mortality [34–37]. Complete repair was first accomplished by McGoon and his associates [38] based on the experimental work of Rastelli [39], who introduced the idea that ventricular-to-pulmonary artery continuity could be established by a valved conduit. Early successes occurred in older children, leading surgeons to delay repair. However, many patients decompensated and died while waiting to achieve greater size and weight. Ebert and colleagues [40] demonstrated that operative intervention for complete repair could be undertaken in infants less than 6 months of age with excellent short- and long-term results. Other authors [41–44] have achieved similar results even with concomitant truncal valve repair or replacement in young infants and newborns [45–51]. This has led to early surgical intervention, well before the patient exhibits decompensated congestive cardiac failure, increased pulmonary vascular resistance, or cardiac cachexia.

Operative Technique

The operative techniques for truncus arteriosus repair have undergone evolutionary advances relating to: cannulation and perfusion techniques, myocardial preservation, and types of extracardiac conduits. Early strategies stressed the

importance of simplified perfusion techniques and management of postoperative hemorrhage. Ebert [40] achieved his outstanding results with aorto-uniatrial cannulation, no ventricular vent, no cardioplegia, and a 12-mm stiff porcine Dacron conduit despite a high perioperative reoperation rate for bleeding. Wider availability of cryopreserved homografts, improvements with blood cardioplegia, and newer cannulas have allowed the surgeon to perform this operation under more favorable conditions [41–53]. In particular, improved results with transmediastinal interrupted aortic arch reconstruction [54–62] and truncal valve repair [63–68] have positively influenced perioperative survival and long-term outcome. These techniques are discussed in this section.

We prefer high aortic cannulation to allow enough room for the aortic clamp, pulmonary trunk detachment, and aortic reconstruction. Bicaval cannulation and left ventricular venting are employed to minimize venous line air, maximize intraventricular exposure, and enhance the myocardial preservation effects of cold blood cardioplegia (Figures 19.7–19.9) [18]. Cardiopulmonary bypass is commenced as the pulmonary trunk is constricted by a tourniquet. This technique can also be used for patients with interrupted aortic arch since the descending aorta is in continuity with the arterial cannula through the patent ductus arteriosus and pulmonary trunk. A notable difference in techniques is that at the onset of cardiopulmonary bypass, patients

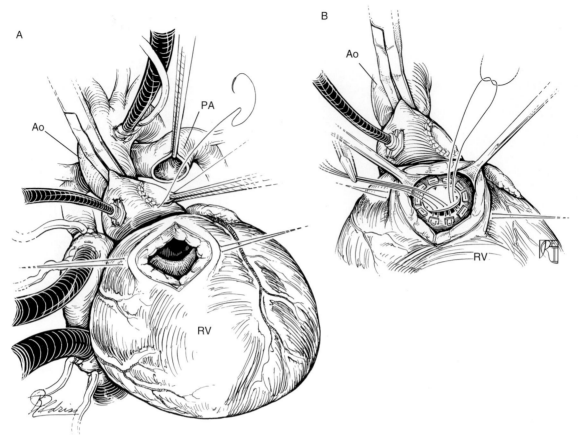

Figure 19.8 A, Pulmonary artery has been disconnected from the arterial trunk, and the aorta has been reconstructed with a PTFE patch to avoid coronary flow complications. **B,** Transventricular closure of the ventricular septal defect is shown with interrupted pledgeted sutures and a Dacron patch. (Ao, aorta; PA, pulmonary artery; RV, right ventricle.)

with intact aortic arch can undergo pulmonary trunk constriction while patients with interrupted aortic arch will require separate pulmonary artery constriction to maintain flow through the patent ductus arteriosus. The conduct of the operation for patients with interrupted aortic arch diverges at this point from patients with intact aortic arch due to the requirement for arch reconstruction which is performed first during a period of deep hypothermia and circulatory arrest or regional perfusion techniques [69]. This part of the procedure will be discussed separately.

For patients without interrupted aortic arch the progression of the operation is straightforward. After left ventricular vent placement, the cross-clamp is applied and followed by antegrade administration of cold blood cardioplegia. In those patients with severe truncal insufficiency, antegrade cardioplegia may not be applicable thereby necessitating direct coronary perfusion or retrograde coronary sinus perfusion (in these circumstances, we prefer retrograde cold blood cardioplegia). The pulmonary artery trunk is then removed with special attention to the coronary artery anatomy and the truncal valve, which are inspected. If the truncal valve is incompetent, valve repair

techniques or truncal valve replacement can be undertaken at this point [52,63–68,70]. These techniques will be discussed separately. Aortic closure can be performed directly or with polytetrafluoroethylene (PTFE) patch (we prefer a patch to minimize coronary flow complications). A separate pericardial patch can be placed over the PTFE patch to minimize bleeding if indicated. The distal valved conduit-to-pulmonary artery anastomosis is then performed. Depending on the relative sizes of the conduit and pulmonary artery, incisions can be made in the pulmonary arteries to accommodate the graft. In the event that a Dacron valved conduit is used, care is taken to perform the anastomosis to the Dacron graft close to the valve commissures. This will position the valve distally, thereby minimizing coronary artery and heart compression by the bioprosthetic valve stent [71]. Similar techniques should be used with homografts and heterografts. This is followed by right ventriculotomy, ventricular septal defect closure, and cross-clamp removal. The patent foramen is generally left alone unless the interatrial communication is large. Leaving the patent foramen ovale will help with the postoperative hemodynamics as the right ventriculotomy often

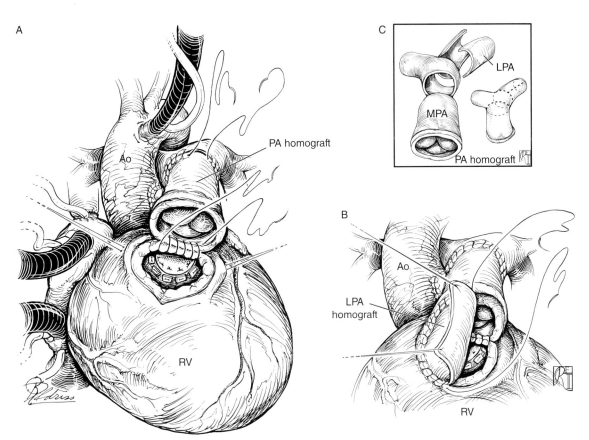

Figure 19.9 A, Distal pulmonary homograft is sutured to the pulmonary artery, and the posterior one-third portion of the homograft annulus is sutured directly to the superior rim of the right ventriculotomy. **B,** Homograft hood technique. The previously harvested left pulmonary artery homograft segment (C) is sutured to the annulus of the proximal homograft and to the remaining portion of the right ventriculotomy. **C,** Pulmonary homograft. The pulmonary bifurcation is separated from the main pulmonary artery and fashioned for the hood technique. (Ao, aorta; LPA, MPA, left, main pulmonary artery; PA, pulmonary artery; RV, right ventricle.)

leads to temporary right ventricular dysfunction. The patent foramen ovale can serve as a "pop-off" to maintain cardiac output when decreased right ventricular compliance limits diastolic filling. The resultant right-to-left atrial shunt during these episodes maintains cardiac output but causes an obligatory mild cyanosis that is usually well tolerated [72]. The patient is then rewarmed while the proximal conduit-to-right ventricular anastomosis is completed. Air and vent removal are followed by separation from cardiopulmonary bypass.

Right ventricular-to-pulmonary artery reconstruction has undergone many changes in the evolution of this repair. Excellent results have been achieved with the relatively stiff 12-mm commercially available porcine-valved Dacron grafts. Accelerated neointimal hyperplasia (Figure 19.10) [18], calcification, and porcine valve degeneration have led surgeons to use cryopreserved homografts and more recently glutaraldehyde-preserved bovine valved internal jugular veins. Because the biological grafts are more pliable, the distal pulmonary anastomosis is less likely to bleed, and can be downsized in the event that the repair need be per-

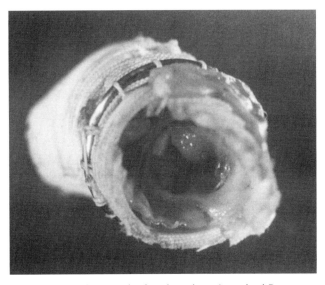

Figure 19.10 Photograph of explanted porcine valved Dacron right ventricular-to-pulmonary artery conduit shows the neointimal peel of fibrous tissue.

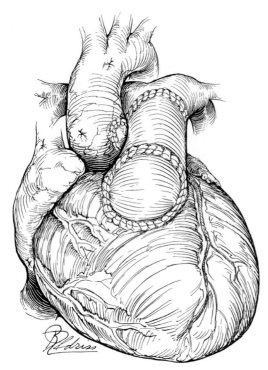

Figure 19.11 Completed homograft hood technique. The homograft hood is used to ensure a generous opening from the right ventricle to the pulmonary artery.

formed in a newborn infant less than 1 month old. Second, homograft or prosthetic material extensions can be employed to minimize the size of the ventriculotomy when desirable. The homograft extension technique has the added benefit of choice between aortic and pulmonary homografts. We and others [52,73,74] have used the Microvel Hemashield (Meadox Medicals, Inc., Oakland, NJ) graft as an extension because of favorable hemostatic properties. However, owing to accelerated neointimal hyperplasia, we have abandoned this technique in favor of homograft hood augmentation techniques using pericardium, homograft material, or PTFE (Figures 19.7–19.9, 19.11) [18]. At the present time, we prefer to use pulmonary homografts and the hood extension technique for right ventricular-to-pulmonary artery continuity. Pulmonary homografts are preferred because they have been shown to resist calcification more than aortic homografts [75,76]. The hood extension technique using PTFE or homograft material allows for a portion of the proximal anastomosis to be performed directly between the right ventricle and the pulmonary homograft, which should limit proximal tubular stenosis. The PTFE hood that completes the reconstruction with rigid material will also limit unwanted cavitary entry in the case of resternotomy for conduit replacement.

Recent technological advances have made available the use of the glutaraldehyde-preserved valved bovine internal jugular graft (Contegra; Medtronic Inc, Minneapolis,

MN). While some authors have experienced distal anastomotic stenoses [77–81] with this graft, others have found great utility owing to its accessibility and midterm preservation of valve function [82]. Clearly the comparative long-term benefits and disadvantages of both conduit options will have to be assessed before any informed recommendation can be made.

Repair of Truncus with Interrupted Aortic Arch

After aorto-bicaval cardiopulmonary bypass with separate pulmonary artery constriction is established, the patient is cooled to 18 °C using pH-stat strategy [83,84]. A left ventricular vent is placed; the brachiocephalic vessels are dissected, mobilized, and controlled with snuggers; so too is the descending aorta dissected and mobilized taking care to preserve the recurrent laryngeal nerve. After cardioplegic arrest, a short period (15–30 minutes) of circulatory arrest is used to resect the ductal tissue and perform a direct anastomosis between the proximal and distal aorta thereby performing the arch reconstruction (Figure 19.12) [18]. Cardiopulmonary bypass can then be reinstituted during which time the rest of the operation can proceed. Many variations on this theme have been reported [54–62], both with cardiopulmonary bypass strategies and resultant anatomic configurations. Regional perfusion techniques have been gaining favor since circulatory arrest can be eliminated [85], although there have been no controlled studies to substantiate the utility of this method. Specifically, a Gore-Tex graft is connected, end-to-side, into the innominate or carotid artery (in the case of anomalous descending aorta take-off of the subclavian artery). Cardiopulmonary bypass is commenced with separate pulmonary artery constriction. At 18–20 °C, the proximal brachiocephalic arteries are controlled with snuggers, the descending aorta is clamped, and antegrade cardioplegia is administered. The systemic arterial flow is lowered, allowing direct perfusion to the brain and indirect perfusion to the lower extremity through collateral arteries. The ascending, transverse, and proximal descending aorta is now isolated and can be repaired, segmented, or transposed as necessary. Once the aortic arch reconstruction is completed, whole-body perfusion can be reinstituted through the Gore-Tex graft. After separation from cardiopulmonary bypass, the graft can be clipped, leaving the stump in place. Most anatomic variations use the Lecompte maneuver to transpose the pulmonary artery from the retroaortic area and thus prevent right pulmonary artery compression (Figure 19.12) [18]. Others have used aortic extension techniques to create a larger retroaortic space for the pulmonary artery [62]. Pulmonary artery autologous flaps have also been used for interrupted aortic arch repair [59]. More recent series have documented the high mortality associated with truncus arteriosus and interrupted aortic arch.

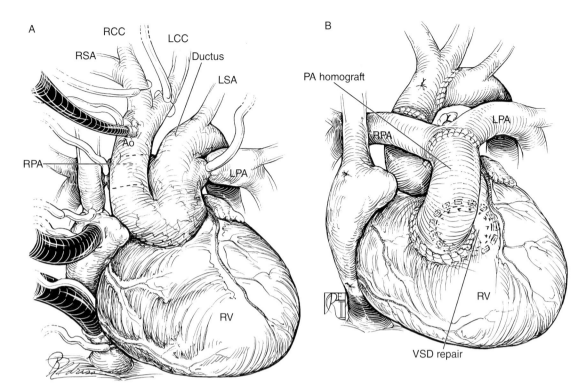

Figure 19.12 Diagrammatic representation shows a patient with truncus arteriosus and interrupted aortic arch. **A,** Aortobicaval cardiopulmonary bypass is established with bilateral pulmonary artery constriction (enforced snuggers). Lower extremity flow is accomplished through the patent ductus arteriosus. **B,** Completed repair of truncus arteriosus with interrupted aortic arch. Direct aortic reconstruction is performed without foreign material. The maneuver of Lecompte facilitates right ventricular-to-pulmonary artery continuity. (Ao, aorta; LCC, RCC, left, right common carotid artery; LPA, RPA, left, right pulmonary artery; LSA, RSA, left, right subclavian artery; PA, pulmonary artery; RV, right ventricle; VSD, ventricular septal defect.)

Konstantinov and the members of the Congenital Heart Surgeons Society reported on 472 neonates between 1987 and 1997 and found the overall mortality to be 44%, 39%, and 31% at 6 months, 1 year, and 10 years respectively [86,87]. Miyamoto and associates [88] reported an operative mortality of 50% owing to the high incidence of truncal valve regurgitation, coronary artery anomalies, and DiGeorge syndrome. They concluded that to improve outcome in these high-risk patients, preoperative management should be optimized, repair should not be delayed, and regurgitant truncal valves should be repaired or replaced. It is clear that surgical repair of truncus arteriosus with interrupted aortic arch is controversial and will require further clinical study if outcomes are to be optimized [55,56]. The surgeon should be cognizant of all repairs and use the best reconstruction for the appropriate circumstance.

Truncal Valve Repair/Replacement

The early surgical solutions to severe truncal insufficiency were prosthetic valve replacement or homograft valve replacement as an aortic root replacement with coronary reimplantation [52,68,70,89,90]. The acute and chronic results were less than satisfactory owing to the increased complexity of the initial and subsequent operations that are necessary because of somatic growth. Truncal valve repair, using a number of techniques, has gained favor over the last few years with excellent results [63–66,68]. Early successful techniques included suturing of partially developed commissures, suspension of cusps, resection of redundant portions of the cusps, annuloplasty of the commissures, and resection of excrescences on the surface of valve leaflets (Figures 19.13 and 19.14) [64,67]. Reports by Jonas [66], Mavroudis and Backer [67], and Mee [65] have emphasized these techniques with excellent short- and mid-term results. Recently, Henaine and associates [91] have analyzed their long-term results with truncus arteriosus repair with special reference to the fate of the truncal valve. They performed truncal valve repair (n = 6) or replacement (n = 3) and achieved a freedom from truncal valve reoperation rate of 96%, 82.3%, and 62.7% at 1, 10, and 18 years postoperatively, respectively, with a low risk for mortality.

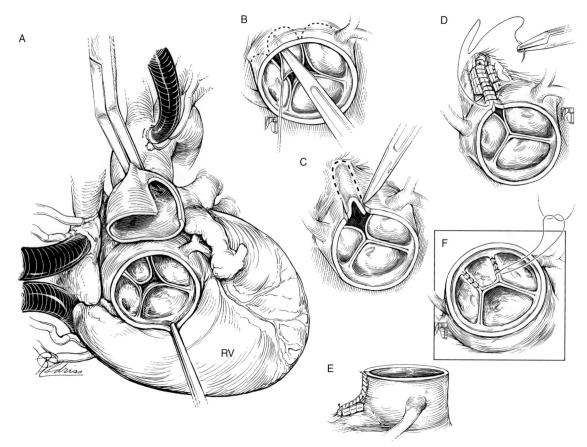

Figure 19.13 Series of diagrams shows two examples of truncal valve repair by (1) leaflet excision and annular remodeling (A to E) and (2) valve suture technique (F). **A,** Translocation of the common arterial trunk shows incompetent quadricuspid truncal valve. Usually one leaflet is grossly prolapsed. In this case, the small prolapsed leaflet does not involve the coronary sinus of Valsalva. **B,** Prolapsed leaflet is removed, care being taken to leave the neighboring leaflets attached. **C,** Sinus of Valsalva truncal wall is resected in preparation for the remodeling procedure. **D,** Pledget-supported sutures are used to tighten the annulus and bring the remaining leaflets together. The rest of the truncal wall is approximated, and the truncal valve is remodeled into a smaller, competent, and nonstenotic neoaortic valve. **E,** Lateral view of the remodeled neoaortic valve. **F,** The suture valvuloplasty technique performed by attaching the edges of the prolapsed leaflet to either one or both adjacent leaflets using fine sutures, thereby creating a functional tricuspid or bicuspid semilunar valve. (Reproduced with permission from Mavroudis *et al.* [67].)

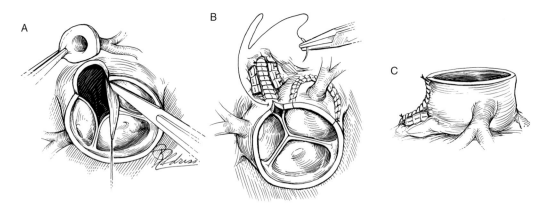

Figure 19.14 The prolapsed leaflet occasionally involves the coronary sinus of Valsalva. Under these circumstances the coronary artery can be reimplanted into the neighboring sinus of Valsalva, and prolapsed leaflet resection and annular remodeling become possible. **A,** Coronary button has been removed from the affected sinus of Valsalva. The prolapsing leaflet is excised. **B,** Annulus is tightened (see Figure 19.13D) and the coronary artery button is reimplanted, using much the same technique as is used for the arterial switch operation. **C,** Lateral projection of the annular remodeling technique. (Reproduced with permission from Mavroudis *et al.* [67].)

Results of Total Correction

The idea that a valved conduit could establish right ventricular-to-pulmonary artery continuity [39] was followed by refinements in infant cardiopulmonary bypass, myocardial protection, and cryopreserved homograft/heterograft availability, which have been instrumental in the evolution of the excellent results that have been achieved. Early perioperative survival, therefore, depends mostly on the amount of increased pulmonary vascular resistance, degree of truncal valve insufficiency, and associated cardiac anomalies rather than perioperative bleeding, coronary compression, or other technical mishaps. The most significant factor responsible for these gains is the steady trend toward earlier correction, which provides a patient with reversible pulmonary vascular obstructive disease and preserved myocardial function.

The early results of complete repair were reported by Marcelletti and colleagues [92], who reviewed the course of 92 patients between 1967 and 1972. They achieved a 75% survival rate, which improved significantly in subsequent reports. Less favorable results were reported by other authors during this time period [93–95]. Ebert's [96] report of 91% survival in 77 infants less than 6 months old showed that improved results were possible. Later reports by Bove [45,52], Pearl [43,44], Hanley [42,49], McKay [53], and others [47,48,51,97–99] confirmed these findings and showed that excellent results are possible even at younger ages and when truncal insufficiency or interrupted aortic arch are also present.

The mid- and long-term survival after complete repair is determined by the degree of truncal insufficiency and the incidence of pulmonary artery conduit replacement. The incidence of truncal valve repair or replacement at the initial repair is low [52]. Subsequent truncal valve repair or replacement may become necessary for progressive truncal valve insufficiency. The intermediate-term surgical results of truncal insufficiency favor repair [66]. This therapy, while not always fully reparative, allows for improved valvar function, avoidance of anticoagulation in the case of prosthetic valve replacement, and somatic growth. The amount of subsequent truncal insufficiency can be re-evaluated either before or at the time of conduit replacement. The truncal valve can be re-repaired or replaced at that time, as noted earlier [91].

Right ventricular-to-pulmonary artery conduit longevity has been the focus of numerous reports that center around the problems of conduit size, valve degeneration, and neointimal hyperplasia [100-120]. Xenograft woven Dacron conduits developed stenosis because of valve calcification and often severe pseudointimal proliferation [100,103,121]. Intimal peel fenestration caused localized dissection, neointimal detachment, and thrombus formation between the intimal peel and the Dacron conduit, which accelerated pseudointimal thickening [100,101]. This process was thought to be the result of low porosity of the woven Dacron graft, which does not allow tight anchoring of the peel to the graft by fibroblastic tissue growth [101,107]. When Dacron low-porosity grafts were used as an extension for homografts, a similar obstructive process was observed [106,114,115]. Kay and Ross [114] reported that the major cause of late homograft obstruction was attributed to peel formation in the composite woven Dacron graft. Bull and associates [106] also showed that conduit obstruction was more often related to the Dacron component than to the homograft portion of the composite graft. Because of these findings, knitted Dacron grafts were employed with the idea that the initial intimal peel would be firmly attached to the graft, thus avoiding constant neointimal detachments, hyperplasia, and obstruction. In animal models, various biologic sealants were used for knitted Dacron grafts to avoid excessive bleeding at the time of implant [104,110,113]. The biologic sealant, in theory, would prevent bleeding in the immediate perioperative period and then be replaced by transitional interstitial ingrowth of fibroblastic tissue into the graft. This would result in a firm neointimal attachment not subject to the forces of disruption that are prevalent in woven grafts. Animal studies confirmed this hypothesis and showed a less than 1-mm neointimal peel when knitted Dacron grafts were used [110]. However, in human studies with Dacron knitted grafts and biologic sealant, the neointimal peel became much thicker, even though the peel was densely and firmly attached to the Dacron graft [73,74]. For these reasons, biologic extension techniques with homografts, PTFE, and pericardial hoods appear to offer the best chance for increased conduit longevity, which should be limited by actual size and not neointimal hyperplasia.

Over the last 10 years, a considerable amount of experience has been gained with use of homograft conduits. The homograft conduits have been shown to have a positive impact on neonatal repair, postoperative bleeding, and perioperative survival when compared with Dacron-housed porcine valves [122]. The durability and replacement statistics of the homograft valves have also been studied. Weipert and associates [123] have noted that reoperation for conduit replacement is dependent on the initial conduit size and somatic growth. They found that all homografts with valve sizes less than 15.0 mm required replacement within 7 years. When the homograft was larger than 15.0 mm, replacement was necessary in 20% at 10 years. Chan and colleagues [124] have closely followed their postoperative truncus arteriosus patients with serial echocardiograms and found that 50% of conduits implanted before 18 months of age could be predicted to stenose by 21.8 months postoperatively compared with only 5% of those implanted after 18 months of age. These data indicate that somatic growth is the discriminating factor that determines the need for conduit replacement.

More recent reports have emphasized that longer intervals between conduit operations can be achieved by valveless right ventricular to pulmonary artery conduits [125–127]. In general, these authors found no difference in operative mortality between the valved conduits and the nonvalved conduits and speculated that early repair will result in less pulmonary hypertension, thereby allowing improved right ventricular tolerance of the valveless strategy. Mayer and coworkers [128,129] have used tissue engineering techniques in experimental animals to "grow" a valved conduit from the animal's own endothelial cells. These conduits have been shown to grow appropriately with the animal and resist degeneration and calcification since the cells are genetically identical to the host. The possibility exists therefore that this strategy could result in only one reparative operation for patients with truncus arteriosus. Further studies and yet undiscovered innovative techniques will surely impact favorably on the long-term therapeutic outcome of these patients.

It appears that patients with successful repair of truncus arteriosus will have to be followed closely for aortic (truncal) insufficiency and right ventricular-to-pulmonary artery conduit failure and can be expected to undergo at least two subsequent open-heart procedures. Fortunately, the results of conduit replacement have been excellent thus far. New areas of clinical research should ameliorate and resolve the problems of neointimal hyperplasia and valve degeneration. These patients can then look forward to longer intervals between operations and fewer complications.

References

1. Calder L, Van Praagh R, Van Praagh S, *et al.* (1976) Truncus arteriosus communis. Clinical, angiocardiographic, and pathologic findings in 100 patients. Am Heart J 92, 23–38.
2. Fyler DC. (1992) *Truncus arteriosus*. In: Fyler DC, ed. *Nadas' Pediatric Cardiology*. Philadelphia, PA: Hanley & Belfus.
3. Rowe RD, Freedom RM, Mehrizi A, *et al.* (1981) *The Neonate with Congenital Heart Disease*. Philadelphia, PA: WB Saunders.
4. Schaff HV, Danielson GK, Puga FJ. (1985) Truncus arteriosus. In: Arciniegas E, ed. *Pediatric Cardiac Surgery*. Chicago, IL: Year Book Medical.
5. De La Cruz MV, Da Rocha JP. (1956) An ontogenetic theory for the explanation of congenital malformations involving the truncus and conus. Am Heart J 51, 782–805.
6. Hernanz-Schulman M, Fellows KE. (1985) Persistent truncus arteriosus: pathologic, diagnostic and therapeutic considerations. Semin Roentgenol 20, 121–129.
7. Bartelings MM, Gittenberger-de Groot AC. (1988) The arterial orifice level in the early human embryo. Anat Embryol (Berl) 177, 537–542.
8. Van Mierop LH, Patterson DF, Schnarr WR. (1978) Pathogenesis of persistent truncus arteriosus in light of observations made in a dog embryo with the anomaly. Am J Cardiol 41, 755–762.
9. Van Praagh R, Van Praagh S. (1965) The anatomy of common aorticopulmonary trunk (truncus arteriosus communis) and its embryologic implications. A study of 57 necropsy cases. Am J Cardiol 16, 406–425.
10. Kirby ML. (1988) Nodose placode provides ectomesenchyme to the developing chick heart in the absence of cardiac neural crest. Cell Tissue Res 252, 17–22.
11. Kirby ML, Gale TF, Stewart DE. (1983) Neural crest cells contribute to normal aorticopulmonary septation. Science 220, 1059–1061.
12. Radford DJ, Perkins L, Lachman R, *et al.* (1988) Spectrum of Di George syndrome in patients with truncus arteriosus: expanded Di George syndrome. Pediatr Cardiol 9, 95–101.
13. Carotti A, Digilio MC, Piacentini G, *et al.* (2008) Cardiac defects and results of cardiac surgery in 22q11.2 deletion syndrome. Dev Disabil Res Rev 14, 35–42.
14. Kyburz A, Bauersfeld U, Schinzel A, *et al.* (2008) The fate of children with microdeletion 22q11.2 syndrome and congenital heart defect: clinical course and cardiac outcome. Pediatr Cardiol 29, 76–83.
15. Ziolkowska L, Kawalec W, Turska-Kmiec A, *et al.* (2008) Chromosome 22q11.2 microdeletion in children with conotruncal heart defects: frequency, associated cardiovascular anomalies, and outcome following cardiac surgery. Eur J Pediatr 167, 1135–1140.
16. Butto F, Lucas RV Jr, Edwards JE. (1986) Persistent truncus arteriosus: pathologic anatomy in 54 cases. Pediatr Cardiol 7, 95–101.
17. Collett RW, Edwards JE. (1949) Persistent truncus arteriosus; a classification according to anatomic types. Surg Clin North Am 29, 1245–1270.
18. Mavroudis C, Backer CL. (2003) Truncus arteriosus. In: Mavroudis C, Backer CL, eds. *Pediatric Cardiac Surgery*, 3rd ed. Philadelphia, PA: Mosby, Inc.
19. Becker AE, Becker MJ, Edwards JE. (1970) Malposition of pulmonary arteries (crossed pulmonary arteries) in persistent truncus arteriosus. Am J Roentgenol Radium Ther Nucl Med 110, 509–514.
20. Bhan A, Gupta M, Kumar MJ, *et al.* (2006) Persistent truncus arteriosus with double aortic arch. Pediatr Cardiol 27, 378–380.
21. Crupi G, Macartney FJ, Anderson RH. (1977) Persistent truncus arteriosus. A study of 66 autopsy cases with special reference to definition and morphogenesis. Am J Cardiol 40, 569–578.
22. Russell HM, Jacobs ML, Anderson RH, *et al.* (2011) A simplified categorization for common arterial trunk. J Thorac Cardiovasc Surg 141, 645–653.
23. Jacobs ML. (2000) Congenital Heart Surgery Nomenclature and Database Project: truncus arteriosus. Ann Thorac Surg 69(4 Suppl):S50–S55.
24. Bharati S, McAllister HA Jr, Rosenquist GC, *et al.* (1974) The surgical anatomy of truncus arteriosus communis. J Thorac Cardiovasc Surg 67, 501–510.
25. Thiene G, Bortolotti U, Gallucci V, *et al.* (1976) Anatomical study of truncus arteriousus communis with embryological and surgical considerations. Br Heart J 38, 1109–1123.
26. Bharati S, Karp R, Lev M. (1992) The conduction system in truncus arteriosus and its surgical significance. A study of five cases. J Thorac Cardiovasc Surg 104, 954–960.

27. Anderson KR, McGoon DC, Lie JT. (1978) Surgical significance of the coronary arterial anatomy in truncus arteriosus communis. Am J Cardiol 41, 76–81.

28. Shrivastava S, Edwards JE. (1977) Coronary arterial origin in persistent truncus arteriosus. Circulation 55, 551–554.

29. Daskalopoulos DA, Edwards WD, Driscoll DJ, et al. (1983) Fatal pulmonary artery banding in truncus arteriosus with anomalous origin of circumflex coronary artery from right pulmonary artery. Am J Cardiol 52, 1363–1364.

30. Lenox CC, Debich DE, Zuberbuhler JR. (1992) The role of coronary artery abnormalities in the prognosis of truncus arteriosus. J Thorac Cardiovasc Surg 104, 1728–1742.

31. Oddens JR, Boger AJ, Witsenburg M, et al. (1994) Anatomy of the proximal coronary arteries as a risk factor in primary repair of common arterial trunk. J Cardiovasc Surg (Torino) 35, 295–299.

32. Espinola-Zavaleta N, Munoz-Castellanos L, Gonzalez-Flores R, et al. (2008) [Common truncus arteriosus in adults]. Arch Cardiol Mex 78, 210–216.

33. Marcelletti C, McGoon DC, Mair DD. (1976) The natural history of truncus arteriosus. Circulation 54, 108–111.

34. Oldham HN Jr, Kakos GS, Jarmakani MM, et al. (1972) Pulmonary artery banding in infants with complex congenital heart defects. Ann Thorac Surg 13, 342–350.

35. Poirier RA, Berman MA, Stansel HC Jr. (1975) Current status of the surgical treatment of truncus arteriosus. J Thorac Cardiovasc Surg 69, 169–182.

36. Singh AK, De Leval MR, Pincott JR, et al. (1976) Pulmonary artery banding for truncus arteriosus in the first year of life. Circulation 54(6 Suppl):III17–III19.

37. Smith GW, Thompson WM Jr, Dammann JF Jr, et al. (1964) Use of the pulmonary artery banding procedure in treating type Ii truncus arteriosus. Circulation 29, 108–113.

38. McGoon DC, Rastelli GC, Ongley PA. (1968) An operation for the correction of truncus arteriosus. JAMA 205, 69–73.

39. Rastelli GC, Titus JL, McGoon DC. (1967) Homograft of ascending aorta and aortic valve as a right ventricular outflow. An experimental approach to the repair of truncus arteriosus. Arch Surg 95, 698–708.

40. Ebert PA, Turley K, Stanger P, et al. (1984) Surgical treatment of truncus arteriosus in the first 6 months of life. Ann Surg 200, 451–456.

41. Castaneda AR. (1989) Truncus arteriosus. Ann Thorac Surg 47, 491–492.

42. Hanley FL, Heinemann MK, Jonas RA, et al. (1993) Repair of truncus arteriosus in the neonate. J Thorac Cardiovasc Surg 105, 1047–1056.

43. Pearl JM, Laks H, Drinkwater DC Jr, et al. (1992) Repair of conotruncal abnormalities with the use of the valved conduit: improved early and midterm results with the cryopreserved homograft. J Am Coll Cardiol 20, 191–196.

44. Pearl JM, Laks H, Drinkwater DC Jr, et al. (1991) Repair of truncus arteriosus in infancy. Ann Thorac Surg 52, 780–786.

45. Bove EL, Lupinetti FM, Pridjian AK, et al. (1993) Results of a policy of primary repair of truncus arteriosus in the neonate. J Thorac Cardiovasc Surg 105, 1057–1065; discussion 1065-1066.

46. Heinemann MK, Hanley FL, Fenton KN, et al. (1993) Fate of small homograft conduits after early repair of truncus arteriosus. Ann Thorac Surg 55, 1409–1411; discussion 1411–1412.

47. Lacour-Gayet F, Serraf A, Komiya T, et al. (1996) Truncus arteriosus repair: influence of techniques of right ventricular outflow tract reconstruction. J Thorac Cardiovasc Surg 111, 849–856.

48. Losay J, Planche C, Lacour-Gayet F, et al. (1991) [Immediate and mid-term results of complete repair of truncus arteriosus during the first year of life]. Arch Mal Coeur Vaiss 84, 691–695.

49. Rajasinghe HA, McElhinney DB, Reddy VM, et al. (1997) Long-term follow-up of truncus arteriosus repaired in infancy: a twenty-year experience. J Thorac Cardiovasc Surg 113, 869–878; discussion 878–879.

50. Slavik Z, Keeton BR, Salmon AP, et al. (1994) Persistent truncus arteriosus operated during infancy: long-term follow-up. Pediatr Cardiol 15, 112–115.

51. Urban AE, Sinzobahamvya N, Brecher AM, et al. (1998) Truncus arteriosus: ten-year experience with homograft repair in neonates and infants. Ann Thorac Surg 66(6 Suppl):S183–S188.

52. Bove EL, Beekman RH, Snider AR, et al. (1989) Repair of truncus arteriosus in the neonate and young infant. Ann Thorac Surg 47, 499–505; discussion 506.

53. McKay R, Miyamoto S, Peart I, et al. (1989) Truncus arteriosus with interrupted aortic arch: successful correction in a neonate. Ann Thorac Surg 48, 587–589.

54. Berdjis F, Wells WJ, Starnes VA. (1996) Truncus arteriosus with total anomalous pulmonary venous return and interrupted arch. Ann Thorac Surg 61, 220–222.

55. Cohen DM. (1995) Lecompte maneuver for truncus arteriosus with type B arch interruption: is this a panacea? Ann Thorac Surg 60, 229.

56. Haydar S. (1996) Lecompte maneuver in truncus arteriosus repair: potential risks! Ann Thorac Surg 62, 1241.

57. Lacour-Gayet F, Serraf A, Galletti L, et al. (1997) Biventricular repair of conotruncal anomalies associated with aortic arch obstruction: 103 patients. Circulation 96(9 Suppl): II328–II334.

58. Mohamed G, Ott DA. (1993) Anterior translocation of the pulmonary confluence in the surgical treatment of truncus arteriosus. Tex Heart Inst J 20, 285–287.

59. Nakae S, Kawada M, Kasahara S, et al. (1995) Truncus arteriosus with interrupted aortic arch: successful correction using autologous flap. Ann Thorac Surg 60, 697–698.

60. Pretre R, Friedli B, Rouge JC, et al. (1996) Anterior translocation of the right pulmonary artery to prevent bronchovascular compression in a case of truncus arteriosus and type A interrupted aortic arch. J Thorac Cardiovasc Surg 111, 672–674.

61. Rao IM, Swanson JS, Hovaguimian H, et al. (1995) Anterior pulmonary translocation for repair of truncus arteriosus with interrupted arch. Ann Thorac Surg 59, 216–218.

62. Tlaskal T, Hucin B, Kostelka M, et al. (1998) Successful reoperation for severe left bronchus compression after repair of persistent truncus arteriosus with interrupted aortic arch. Eur J Cardiothorac Surg 13, 306–309.

63. Black MD, Adatia I, Freedom RM. (1998) Truncal valve repair: initial experience in neonates. Ann Thorac Surg 65, 1737–1740.

64. Elami A, Laks H, Pearl JM. (1994) Truncal valve repair: initial experience with infants and children. Ann Thorac Surg 57, 397–401; discussion 402.

65. Imamura M, Drummond-Webb JJ, Sarris GE, et al. (1999) Improving early and intermediate results of truncus arteriosus repair: a new technique of truncal valve repair. Ann Thorac Surg 67, 1142–1146.

66. Jahangiri M, Zurakowski D, Mayer JE, et al. (2000) Repair of the truncal valve and associated interrupted arch in neonates with truncus arteriosus. J Thorac Cardiovasc Surg 119, 508–514.

67. Mavroudis C, Backer CL. (2001) Surgical management of severe truncal insufficiency: experience with truncal valve remodeling techniques. Ann Thorac Surg 72, 396–400.

68. McElhinney DB, Reddy VM, Rajasinghe HA, et al. (1998) Trends in the management of truncal valve insufficiency. Ann Thorac Surg 65, 517–524.

69. Hoffman GM, Stuth EA, Jaquiss RD, et al. (2004) Changes in cerebral and somatic oxygenation during stage 1 palliation of hypoplastic left heart syndrome using continuous regional cerebral perfusion. J Thorac Cardiovasc Surg 127, 223–233.

70. De Leval MR, McGoon DC, Wallace RB, et al. (1974) Management of truncal valvular regurgitation. Ann Surg 180, 427–432.

71. Daskalopoulos DA, Edwards WD, Driscoll DJ, et al. (1983) Coronary artery compression with fatal myocardial ischemia. A rare complication of valved extracardiac conduits in children with congenital heart disease. J Thorac Cardiovasc Surg 85, 546–551.

72. Laudito A, Graham EM, Stroud MR, et al. (2006) Complete repair of conotruncal defects with an interatrial communication: oxygenation, hemodynamic status, and early outcome. Ann Thorac Surg 82, 1286–1291; discussion 1291.

73. Angelini GD, Witsenburg M, Ten Kate FJ, et al. (1989) Severe stenotic scar contracture of the Microvel Hemashield right-sided extracardiac conduit. Ann Thorac Surg 48, 714–716.

74. Kobayashi J, Backer CL, Zales VR, et al. (1993) Failure of the Hemashield extension in right ventricle-to-pulmonary artery conduits. Ann Thorac Surg 56, 277–281.

75. Niwaya K, Knott-Craig CJ, Lane MM, et al. (1999) Cryopreserved homograft valves in the pulmonary position: risk analysis for intermediate-term failure. J Thorac Cardiovasc Surg 117, 141–146; discussion 146–147.

76. Yankah AC, Alexi-Meskhishvili V, Weng Y, et al. (1995) Performance of aortic and pulmonary homografts in the right ventricular outflow tract in children. J Heart Valve Dis 4, 392–395.

77. Calvaruso D, Rubino A, Ocello S, et al. (2008) Images in cardiovascular medicine: right ventricular outflow tract reconstruction with contegra bovine valved conduit. Circulation 118, e519–e520.

78. Gober V, Berdat P, Pavlovic M, et al. (2005) Adverse mid-term outcome following RVOT reconstruction using the Contegra valved bovine jugular vein. Ann Thorac Surg 79, 625–631.

79. Kocher TZ, Pestaner JP, Koutlas TC. (2006) Early complication after repair of truncus arteriosus with Contegra conduit. Ann Thorac Surg 82, 1949.

80. Meyns B, Van Garsse L, Boshoff D, et al. (2004) The Contegra conduit in the right ventricular outflow tract induces supravalvular stenosis. J Thorac Cardiovasc Surg 128, 834–840.

81. Tiete AR, Sachweh JS, Roemer U, et al. (2004) Right ventricular outflow tract reconstruction with the Contegra bovine jugular vein conduit: a word of caution. Ann Thorac Surg 77, 2151–2156.

82. Hickey EJ, McCrindle BW, Blackstone EH, et al. (2008) Jugular venous valved conduit (Contegra) matches allograft performance in infant truncus arteriosus repair. Eur J Cardiothorac Surg 33, 890–898.

83. du Plessis AJ, Jonas RA, Wypij D, et al. (1997) Perioperative effects of alpha-stat versus pH-stat strategies for deep hypothermic cardiopulmonary bypass in infants. J Thorac Cardiovasc Surg 114, 991–1000; discussion 1001.

84. Skaryak LA, Chai PJ, Kern FH, et al. (1995) Blood gas management and degree of cooling: effects on cerebral metabolism before and after circulatory arrest. J Thorac Cardiovasc Surg 110, 1649–1657.

85. Tlaskal T, Hucin B, Kucera V, et al. (2005) Repair of persistent truncus arteriosus with interrupted aortic arch. Eur J Cardiothorac Surg 28, 736–741.

86. Konstantinov IE. (2006) Repair of persistent truncus arteriosus with interrupted aortic arch: what did we learn? Eur J Cardiothorac Surg 29, 635–636; author reply 636–637.

87. Konstantinov IE, Karamlou T, Blackstone EH, et al. (2006) Truncus arteriosus associated with interrupted aortic arch in 50 neonates: a Congenital Heart Surgeons Society study. Ann Thorac Surg 81, 214–222.

88. Miyamoto T, Sinzobahamvya N, Kumpikaite D, et al. (2005) Repair of truncus arteriosus and aortic arch interruption: outcome analysis. Ann Thorac Surg 79, 2077–2082.

89. Conte S, Jensen T, Jacobsen JR, et al. (1997) Double-homograft repair of truncus arteriosus with severe truncal valve dysfunction. Scand Cardiovasc J 31, 245–247.

90. Elkins RC, Steinberg JB, Razook JD, et al. (1990) Correction of truncus arteriosus with truncal valvar stenosis or insufficiency using two homografts. Ann Thorac Surg 50, 728–733.

91. Henaine R, Azarnoush K, Belli E, et al. (2008) Fate of the truncal valve in truncus arteriosus. Ann Thorac Surg 85, 172–178.

92. Marcelletti C, McGoon DC, Danielson GK, et al. (1977) Early and late results of surgical repair of truncus arteriosus. Circulation 55, 636–641.

93. Appelbaum A, Bargeron LM Jr, Pacifico AD, et al. (1976) Surgical treatment of truncus arteriosus, with emphasis on infants and small children. J Thorac Cardiovasc Surg 71, 436–440.

94. Parenzan L, Crupi G, Alfieri O, et al. (1980) Surgical repair of persistent truncus arteriosus in infancy. Thorac Cardiovasc Surg 28, 18–20.

95. Stark J, Gandhi D, de Leval M, et al. (1978) Surgical treatment of persistent truncus arteriosus in the first year of life. Br Heart J 40, 1280–1287.

96. Ebert PA. (1983) Truncus arteriosus. In: Glenn WWL, Baue AE, Geha AS, eds. *Thoracic and Cardiovascular Surgery*, 4th ed. Norwalk, CT: Appleton-Century-Crofts.

97. Kalavrouziotis G, Purohit M, Ciotti G, *et al.* (2006) Truncus arteriosus communis: early and midterm results of early primary repair. Ann Thorac Surg 82, 2200–2206.

98. Thompson LD, McElhinney DB, Reddy M, *et al.* (2001) Neonatal repair of truncus arteriosus: continuing improvement in outcomes. Ann Thorac Surg 72, 391–395.

99. Ullmann MV, Gorenflo M, Sebening C, *et al.* (2003) Long-term results after repair of truncus arteriosus communis in neonates and infants. Thorac Cardiovasc Surg 51, 175–179.

100. Agarwal KC, Edwards WD, Feldt RH, *et al.* (1981) Clinicopathological correlates of obstructed right-sided porcine-valved extracardiac conduits. J Thorac Cardiovasc Surg 81, 591–601.

101. Agarwal KC, Edwards WD, Feldt RH, *et al.* (1982) Pathogenesis of nonobstructive fibrous peels in right-sided porcine-valved extracardiac conduits. J Thorac Cardiovasc Surg 83, 584–589.

102. Berger K, Sauvage LR, Rao AM, *et al.* (1972) Healing of arterial prostheses in man: its incompleteness. Ann Surg 175, 118–127.

103. Bisset GS 3rd, Schwartz DC, Benzing G 3rd, *et al.* (1981) Late results of reconstruction of the right ventricular outflow tract with porcine xenografts in children. Ann Thorac Surg 31, 437–443.

104. Borst HG, Haverich A, Walterbusch G, *et al.* (1982) Fibrin adhesive: an important hemostatic adjunct in cardiovascular operations. J Thorac Cardiovasc Surg 84, 548–553.

105. Bowman FO Jr, Hancock WD, Malm JR. (1973) A valve-containing dacron prosthesis. Its use in restoring pulmonary artery-right ventricular continuity. Arch Surg 107, 724–728.

106. Bull C, Macartney FJ, Horvath P, *et al.* (1987) Evaluation of long-term results of homograft and heterograft valves in extracardiac conduits. J Thorac Cardiovasc Surg 94, 12–19.

107. Edwards WD, Agarwal KC, Feldt RH, *et al.* (1983) Surgical pathology of obstructed, right-sided, porcine-valved extracardiac conduits. Arch Pathol Lab Med 107, 400–405.

108. Fontan F, Choussat A, Deville C, *et al.* (1984) Aortic valve homografts in the surgical treatment of complex cardiac malformations. J Thorac Cardiovasc Surg 87, 649–657.

109. Fry WJ, Deweese MS, Kraft RO, *et al.* (1964) Importance of porosity in arterial prostheses. Arch Surg 88, 836–842.

110. Haverich A, Oelert H, Maatz W, *et al.* (1984) Histopathological evaluation of woven and knitted Dacron grafts for right ventricular conduits: a comparative experimental study. Ann Thorac Surg 37, 404–411.

111. Hoots AV, Watson DC Jr. (1989) Construction of an aortic homograft conduit for right ventricle to pulmonary artery continuity. Ann Thorac Surg 48, 731–732.

112. Jonas RA, Freed MD, Mayer JE Jr, *et al.* (1985) Long-term follow-up of patients with synthetic right heart conduits. Circulation 72, II77–II83.

113. Jonas RA, Schoen FJ, Ziemer G, *et al.* (1987) Biological sealants and knitted Dacron conduits: comparison of collagen and fibrin glue pretreatments in circulatory models. Ann Thorac Surg 44, 283–290.

114. Kay PH, Ross DN. (1985) Fifteen years' experience with the aortic homograft: the conduit of choice for right ventricular outflow tract reconstruction. Ann Thorac Surg 40, 360–364.

115. Kirklin JW, Blackstone EH, Maehara T, *et al.* (1987) Intermediate-term fate of cryopreserved allograft and xenograft valved conduits. Ann Thorac Surg 44, 598–606.

116. McGoon DC, Danielson GK, Puga FJ, *et al.* (1982) Late results after extracardiac conduit repair for congenital cardiac defects. Am J Cardiol 49, 1741–1749.

117. Naito Y, Fujita T, Manabe H, *et al.* (1980) The criteria for reconstruction of right ventricular outflow tract in total correction of tetralogy of Fallot. J Thorac Cardiovasc Surg 80, 574–581.

118. Ross DN, Somerville J. (1966) Correction of pulmonary atresia with a homograft aortic valve. Lancet 2, 1446–1447.

119. Schaff HV, DiDonato RM, Danielson GK, *et al.* (1984) Reoperation for obstructed pulmonary ventricle-pulmonary artery conduits. Early and late results. J Thorac Cardiovasc Surg 88, 334–343.

120. Wesolowski SA. (1965) The healing of vascular prostheses. Surgery 57, 319–324.

121. Boyce SW, Turley K, Yee ES, *et al.* (1988) The fate of the 12 mm porcine valved conduit from the right ventricle to the pulmonary artery. A ten-year experience. J Thorac Cardiovasc Surg 95, 201–207.

122. Reddy VM, Rajasinghe HA, McElhinney DB, *et al.* (1995) Performance of right ventricle to pulmonary artery conduits after repair of truncus arteriosus: a comparison of Dacron-housed porcine valves and cryopreserved allografts. Semin Thorac Cardiovasc Surg 7, 133–138.

123. Weipert J, Meisner H, Mendler N, *et al.* (1995) Allograft implantation in pediatric cardiac surgery: surgical experience from 1982 to 1994. Ann Thorac Surg 60(2 Suppl), S101–S104.

124. Chan KC, Fyfe DA, McKay CA, *et al.* (1994) Right ventricular outflow reconstruction with cryopreserved homografts in pediatric patients: intermediate-term follow-up with serial echocardiographic assessment. J Am Coll Cardiol 24, 483–489.

125. Chen JM, Glickstein JS, Davies RR, *et al.* (2005) The effect of repair technique on postoperative right-sided obstruction in patients with truncus arteriosus. J Thorac Cardiovasc Surg 129, 559–568.

126. Danton MH, Barron DJ, Stumper O, *et al.* (2001) Repair of truncus arteriosus: a considered approach to right ventricular outflow tract reconstruction. Eur J Cardiothorac Surg 20, 95–103 discussion 104.

127. Derby CD, Kolcz J, Gidding S, *et al.* (2008) Outcomes following non-valved autologous reconstruction of the right ventricular outflow tract in neonates and infants. Eur J Cardiothorac Surg 34, 726–731.

128. Sodian R, Hoerstrup SP, Sperling JS, *et al.* (2000) Evaluation of biodegradable, three-dimensional matrices for tissue engineering of heart valves. Asaio J 46, 107–110.

129. Stock UA, Nagashima M, Khalil PN, *et al.* (2000) Tissue-engineered valved conduits in the pulmonary circulation. J Thorac Cardiovasc Surg 119, 732–740.

Aortopulmonary Window and Aortic Origin of a Pulmonary Artery

Stephanie Fuller[1,2] and J. William Gaynor[1]
[1]The Children's Hospital of Philadelphia, Philadelphia, PA, USA
[2]University of Pennsylvania School of Medicine, Philadelphia, PA, USA

Introduction

Aortopulmonary (AP) window is a rare congenital heart defect resulting from abnormal separation of the truncus arteriosus into the aorta and pulmonary artery [1–3]. An AP window is found in 0.2% of patients with congenital heart disease [2]. A variety of terms have been applied to this defect, including AP fistula, aortic septal defect, AP septal defect, and AP fenestration. A closely related defect is origin of a pulmonary artery (either the right or the left) from the ascending aorta. The term *hemitruncus* has been used for aortic origin of a pulmonary artery, but this term is inaccurate and should be avoided.

Historical Aspects

Aortopulmonary window was first described by Elliotson in 1830 [4]. Cotton reported the first case in the United States in 1899 [5]. Abbott's classic review of 1000 cases of congenital heart disease included only 10 cases of AP window [6]. In 1948, Gross successfully ligated an AP window in a patient undergoing thoracotomy for closure of a patent ductus arteriosus but noted that this method would be dangerous in many patients [7]. Scott and Sabiston described a closed method for division of AP window [8]. In 1957, Cooley and associates reported the first successful division of AP window during cardiopulmonary bypass [9]. A variety of techniques [2,7,10,13–15,17,18,20,21] have since been described for repair of AP window (Table 20.1).

Aortic origin of a pulmonary artery was first reported by Fraentzel in 1868 [22]. Armer and associates in 1961 reported the first successful repair of aortic origin of the right pulmonary artery by means of an interposition graft

[23]. Kirkpatrick and colleagues in 1967 reported the first successful repair [24].

Embryology and Anatomy

In the truncus arteriosus, two opposing truncal cushions form on the right superior and left inferior walls and fuse to form the proximal portion of the septum between the aortic and pulmonary channels [25]. Distally, the fourth aortic arches align with the aortic channel. The distal AP septum, which fuses with the proximal truncal cushion, is formed by the wall between the origins of the fourth and sixth aortic arches. Failure of fusion or malalignment of the truncal cushions can result in a proximal defect in the AP septum. Abnormal migration of the sixth aortic arches can result in distal AP window or aortic origin of a pulmonary artery [26,27].

Most commonly, AP window is a single defect beginning a few millimeters above the semilunar valves on the left wall of the aorta [3,25,28]. Both AP window and aortic origin of a pulmonary artery usually are associated with two normal semilunar valves, differentiating these defects from truncus arteriosus. The defect can be very small or as large as several centimeters in diameter. Aneurysmal dilatation may be seen in large defects. There is usually minimal length to the defect, as the term *window* implies. However, a ductus-like structure occasionally is present.

Either the right or left pulmonary artery may arise from the ascending aorta. Aortic origin of a pulmonary artery should be differentiated from absence of the proximal portion of a pulmonary artery with the distal artery supplied by either a patent ductus arteriosus or AP collateral vessels [27]. The anomalously arising pulmonary artery

---

Pediatric Cardiac Surgery, Fourth Edition. Edited by Constantine Mavroudis and Carl L. Backer.

Table 20.1 Surgical repair of aortopulmonary window.

Year	Surgeon	Method
1948	Gross [7]	Ligation
1953	Scott and Sabiston [8]	Division without cardiopulmonary bypass
1957	Cooley et al. [9]	Division with cardiopulmonary bypass
1966	Putnam and Gross [2]	Transpulmonary patch closure
1967–1968	Negre et al. [17]	Anterior sandwich patch closure
	Aberg [10]	
	Johansson et al. [14]	
1968	Wright et al. [20]	Transaortic suture closure
1969	Deverall et al. [13]	Transaortic patch closure
1987	Shatapathy et al. [18]	Pulmonary artery flap closure
1992	Matsuki et al. [15]	Anterior pulmonary artery flap closure

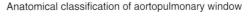

Anatomical classification of aortopulmonary window

Type I proximal defect   Type II distal defect   Type III total defect

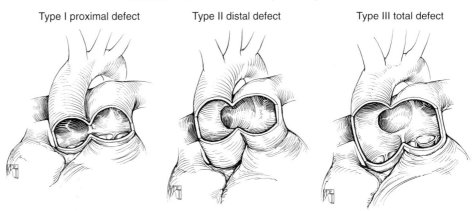

Figure 20.1 Classification of aortopulmonary window.

(commonly the right) usually originates from the posterior aspect of the ascending aorta a short distance above the sinotubular junction. The anomalous pulmonary artery usually is opposite the laterality of the aortic arch, and there is no defect between the ascending aorta and the main pulmonary artery.

In the classification of AP window proposed by Richardson and associates, type I AP window is a proximal defect on the medial wall of the ascending aorta immediately above the sinus of Valsalva [3]. Type II AP window is a more distal defect on the posterior wall of the ascending aorta, usually near the origin of the pulmonary artery. Type III AP window is actually anomalous origin of either pulmonary artery from the ascending aorta. Mori et al. proposed an alternative classification (Figure 20.1) [21,29]. Types I and II defects are the same as in Richardson's classification; however, type III AP window is defined as complete absence of the AP septum. Aortic origin of a pulmonary artery is not considered a type of AP window. The Congenital Heart Surgery Nomenclature and Database Project [30] uses a classification system for AP window

similar to that proposed by Mori et al. [29]. Aortic origin of either pulmonary artery is classified as a separate defect.

Aortopulmonary window is frequently found as an isolated defect. Associated cardiac lesions, including patent ductus arteriosus [31], interruption of the aortic arch [32–34], ventricular septal defect [35], and tetralogy of Fallot [36], are present in one-third to one-half of patients with AP window.

Unlike the common form of interrupted aortic arch, the ventricular septum usually is intact in patients with AP window and aortic arch interruption. Subaortic obstruction is rare in these patients. Diversion of aortic blood into the pulmonary circulation *in utero* with decreased flow to the arch has been proposed as the cause of this combination of defects. When AP window is found in association with interruption of the aortic arch, the arch anatomy usually is that of type A interrupted aortic arch. In a review of the cases of 46 patients with AP window and interruption of the aortic arch, 30 patients were found to have type A interrupted aortic arch, seven patients had type B, and the arch anatomy was not described in nine cases [32]. Associated ventricular septal defect is more common with AP window and type B interrupted aortic arch. Other associated anomalies include atrial septal defect and systemic venous anomalies.

The association of the tetralogy of Fallot and AP window is unusual, and the diagnosis can be difficult [36]. The left-to-right shunt through the AP window may provide adequate palliation for tetralogy of Fallot until significant pulmonary vascular disease develops. The presence of a right aortic arch with AP window may indicate the presence of tetralogy of Fallot. Ventriculoarterial concordance usually is present, although in rare instances transposition of the great arteries has been reported in association with AP window [37]. In some patients with AP window (5.1% in one series) [35], anomalous origin of either coronary artery from the pulmonary artery is found [38–41]. The orifice usually is found within a few millimeters of the AP window. Unlike the situation for isolated origin of a coronary artery from the pulmonary artery, the coronary artery is exposed to aortic pressure and oxygenated blood. Thus myocardial ischemia is not present, and shunting through the coronary artery does not occur. Chen *et al.* described in 2005 the first reported case of left pulmonary artery sling and AP window [42]. Although narrowed by external compression, the airway was left untreated as no segmental stricture was found [42].

In rare instances, AP window is found in association with extracardiac anomalies, including the VATER complex (vertebral defects, imperforate anus, tracheoesophageal fistula with esophageal atresia, and radial and renal dysplasia). Despite the frequency of associated AP window and interrupted aortic arch, no consistent association of AP window and DiGeorge syndrome has been found. Aortic origin of a pulmonary artery can occur as an isolated defect; however, as with AP window, associated anomalies, including patent ductus arteriosus, interrupted aortic arch, ventricular septal defect, atrial septal defect, and tetralogy of Fallot, may be present.

Clinical Features and Natural History

The physiology of AP window is similar to that of patent ductus arteriosus, ventricular septal defect, and truncus arteriosus. The magnitude of the shunt is related mainly to the size of the defect and to pulmonary vascular resistance. Small defects are associated with small left-to-right shunts and minimal or no symptoms. The defect often is large, and a marked left-to-right shunt is present, resulting in congestive heart failure, pulmonary hypertension, and early development of pulmonary vascular obstructive disease. Cyanosis usually is absent unless severe pulmonary vascular disease has developed, but poor feeding, delayed growth, and repeated respiratory infections are frequently present. At cardiac examination, the heart is enlarged, and a systolic murmur frequently is heard in the third or fourth left intercostal space. Unlike patients with patent ductus

arteriosus, a continuous murmur is unusual. The peripheral pulses are bounding. The clinical course is thought to be similar to that of untreated patients with large ventricular septal defect; however, the shunt during diastole (at the expense of systemic and coronary perfusion) may produce earlier symptoms in patients with AP window. Patients with a large AP window usually do not survive infancy. Children and young adults with AP window are occasionally encountered and frequently have congestive heart failure, gradual development of irreversible pulmonary hypertension, and death by Eisenmenger's syndrome. Le Bret *et al.* report a case of a patient diagnosed late at 17 years old with an AP window considered irreparable because of severe pulmonary hypertension, who then presented at 31 years of age with acute dissection and rupture of the pulmonary artery [43].

Aortic origin of a pulmonary artery also results in a large left-to-right shunt and exposes the lung to systemic pressure. The contralateral lung receives the entire right ventricular output. Pulmonary vascular disease may develop at an early age, particularly in the lung exposed to systemic flow. Of interest is that pulmonary hypertension usually is present in the contralateral lung.

Diagnosis

The differential diagnosis of AP window and aortic origin of a pulmonary artery includes patent ductus arteriosus, ventricular septal defect, persistent truncus arteriosus, and ruptured aneurysm of the sinus of Valsalva. The chest radiograph usually reveals cardiomegaly and increased pulmonary vascularity. Echocardiography can show the location and size of the defect (Figure 20.2) and is useful for evaluation of associated anomalies [44,45]. Echocardiography is excellent at depicting the AP window, but the diagnosis can be difficult if the patient has associated anomalies. It may be difficult to differentiate AP window from persistent truncus arteriosus. To confirm the diagnosis, the presence of two separate semilunar valves must be demonstrated. In rare cases, aortic or pulmonary atresia has been reported in association with AP window. Patients with this combination of defects have only one semilunar valve. Although the diagnosis can be difficult, the two conditions are differentiated from those with persistent truncus arteriosus by the presence of two arterial trunks (one with an atretic valve) arising from the base of the heart. The electrocardiogram commonly reveals left ventricular or biventricular hypertrophy. Cardiac catheterization is rarely necessary but may be useful for assessment of pulmonary vascular resistance in older patients and in the evaluation of associated cardiac anomalies.

Surgical Treatment

Surgical repair is indicated in the treatment of all patients with AP window or aortic origin of a pulmonary artery. In

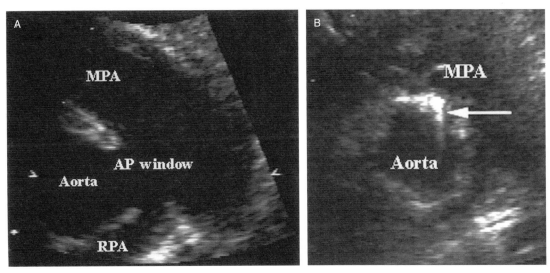

Figure 20.2 A, Preoperative parasternal short-axis echocardiogram shows relations between the aorta, main pulmonary artery (MPA), right pulmonary artery (RPA), and aortopulmonary window. **B,** Postoperative parasternal short-axis echocardiogram shows patch (arrow) between aorta and MPA after anterior sandwich patch repair. (Echocardiograms courtesy of William Mahle, MD.)

rare instances, if the patient has a small asymptomatic defect, an elective operation may be performed after infancy. For most patients, however, repair should be undertaken at the time of diagnosis because of the risk of pulmonary vascular occlusive disease. In patients with associated anomalies, single-stage repair of all defects should be performed.

A variety of techniques have been suggested for repair of AP window. Simple ligation has been used, but there is risk of fatal intraoperative bleeding, incomplete closure, and recanalization. Thus, this method cannot be recommended. Backer and Mavroudis described their single institution experience over a 40-year period in which the mortality for the first 16 patients who underwent simple AP window division was 37% [46]. Attempts at division or suture without the use of cardiopulmonary bypass can result in fatal hemorrhage because the fistula walls are friable and thin.

Other techniques have been described for obliteration of the defect without the use of cardiopulmonary bypass. These procedures, however, are less than satisfactory and cannot be recommended. In general, patch closure of the defect should be performed. Some small defects can be closed primarily. With large defects, direct suture closure may narrow either the pulmonary artery or the aorta and should be avoided. Division of an AP window with simple closure of the aorta and pulmonary artery also can result in stenosis of the vessels. If division is used, patch repair of the resulting defects in the aorta and pulmonary artery should be performed. Backer and Mavroudis describe no deaths in their more recent experience with patients undergoing transaortic patch closure of AP window.

At a maximum of 8 years of follow-up, all of these patients demonstrate normal pulmonary artery and aortic growth.

There have been reports of transcatheter closure of AP window [19,47]. Tulloh and Rigby reported successful closure in an 8-kg infant [19]. The surgeons used a double umbrella device. Other reports have documented successful closure in older children and adults. Transcatheter closure may be appropriate in patients with small defects located distal to the semilunar valves and in whom the coronary arteries can be adequately visualized. However, the long-term outcome of transcatheter closure, especially the degree of residual shunting and risk of pulmonary artery stenosis, is not known.

Closure should be performed through a median sternotomy and with cardiopulmonary bypass (Figure 20.3) [21]. The aortic cannula should be inserted as distally as possible on the ascending aorta, well away from the defect, so that placement of the cross-clamp does not interfere with the repair. Single venous or bicaval cannulation may be used, depending on the need for repair of associated anomalies. The pulmonary arteries should be controlled with tourniquets and occluded when cardiopulmonary bypass is instituted. The repair may be performed with either continuous cardiopulmonary bypass or, in small infants, deep hypothermic circulatory arrest. The presence or absence of associated anomalies can alter the operative plan. The anterior wall of the AP window is opened vertically. The coronary ostia must be carefully visualized and included on the aortic side of the patch. If a coronary artery originates from the pulmonary artery, the patch should be positioned to ensure that the coronary ostia remain on the aortic side.

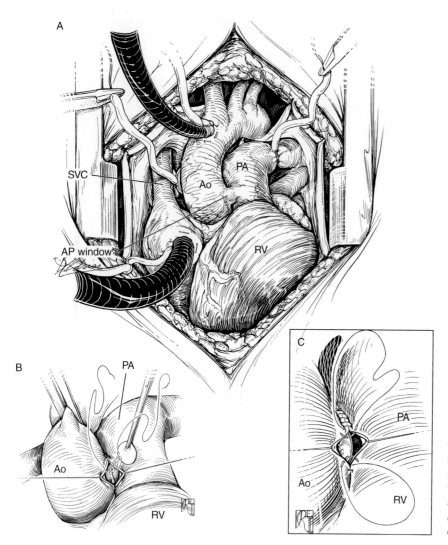

Figure 20.3 Anterior sandwich patch closure of aortopulmonary window. **A,** The aorta is cross-clamped after institution of cardiopulmonary bypass. **B,** The defect is opened anteriorly, and a prosthetic patch is sutured to the superior, posterior, and inferior rims. **C,** The patch is incorporated in the closure of the anterior incision. (Ao, aorta; AP, aortopulmonary; PA, pulmonary artery; RV, right ventricle; SVC, superior vena cava.)

Coronary transfer as in the arterial switch operation may occasionally be required. Repair usually is performed with the anterior sandwich patch technique. A prosthetic patch is sewn to the superior, posterior, and inferior rims of the defect (Figure 20.3) [21]. The incision is closed, incorporating the patch in the anterior suture line. Transpulmonary closure is not recommended because of difficulty in visualizing the fistula and coronary ostia. Transaortic patch closure is an acceptable alternative.

Cannulation for repair of AP window with interrupted aortic arch is the same as that for repair of isolated AP window (Figure 20.4) [21]. A single aortic cannula is positioned in the ascending aorta, and the pulmonary arteries are occluded with snares after institution of cardiopulmonary bypass. Perfusion of the lower body is maintained through the AP window and the ductus arteriosus. The cerebral vessels are controlled with tourniquets and occluded after adequate cooling and institution of deep hypothermic circulatory arrest. There often is little distance

between the AP window and the origin of the cerebral vessels. The AP window is divided and the incision carried superiorly onto the left subclavian artery (type A interrupted aortic arch) or the left carotid artery (type B). The ductus is ligated and all ductal tissue is excised. The superior portion of the descending aorta is anastomosed to the superior aspect of the incision in the aorta and subclavian artery. A homograft patch is used to augment the underside of the aorta and extended proximally for closure of the defect caused by the AP window in the ascending aorta. The pulmonary artery is reconstructed with a separate patch to avoid stenosis.

Patients with aortic origin of a pulmonary artery should undergo repair by direct anastomosis of the anomalous pulmonary artery to the main pulmonary artery (Figure 20.5) [21] The use of prosthetic grafts should be avoided. Cannulation and the conduct of cardiopulmonary bypass are similar to those for repair of AP window. The anomalous pulmonary artery is divided at its origin from the

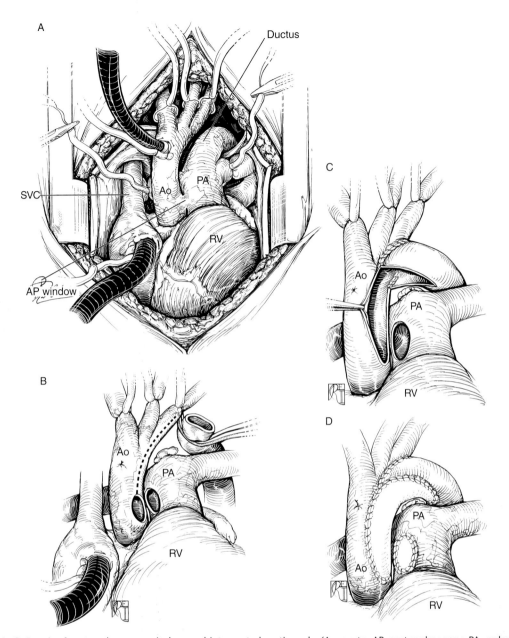

Figure 20.4 A–C, Repair of aortopulmonary window and interrupted aortic arch. (Ao, aorta; AP, aortopulmonary; PA, pulmonary artery; RV, right ventricle; SVC, superior vena cava.)

aorta, and the defect is closed with a patch. An incision is made in the main pulmonary artery. The right pulmonary artery is positioned posterior to the ascending aorta, and the anastomosis is completed. It may be helpful to use a flap of main pulmonary artery to reduce tension on the anastomosis.

Postoperative Course

The postoperative course usually is routine after closure of AP window. Intraoperative transesophageal echocardiog-

raphy is useful for confirming complete closure of the defect and ensuring that the pulmonary arteries have not been narrowed. In some cases, however, severe pulmonary hypertension occurs. These episodes can occur suddenly in the postoperative period and are characterized by increased pulmonary artery pressure, hypoxia, hypotension, and worsening peripheral perfusion. Therapy consists of sedation, paralysis, and hyperventilation with 100% oxygen. In refractory cases, treatment with inhaled nitric oxide or support with extracorporeal membrane oxygenation may be useful.

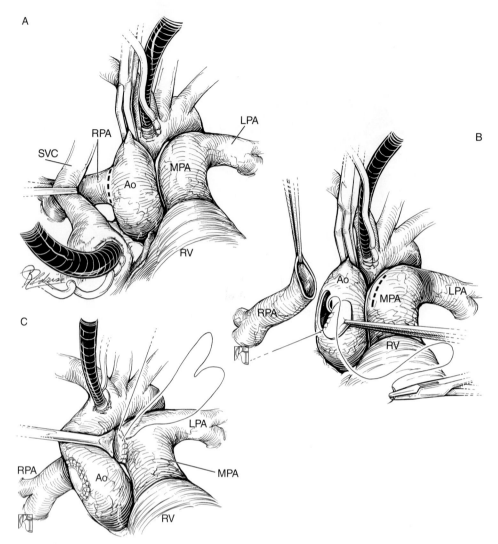

Figure 20.5 Repair of aortic origin of right pulmonary artery. (Ao, aorta; LPA, left pulmonary artery; MPA, main pulmonary artery; RPA, right pulmonary artery; RV, right ventricle; SVC, superior vena cava.)

Outcome After Surgery

Tkebuchava and colleagues reported on the outcome of repair of AP window in 11 children who, between 1971 and 1993 underwent repair by a variety of techniques at a mean age of 31 months [48]. There was one operative death of a neonate with AP window and interrupted aortic arch, and there were no late deaths. One patient needed reoperation for recurrent AP window and one for pulmonary artery stenosis. Di Bella and Gladstone reported on repair of AP window in six infants between 1993 and 1995 [49]. Four patients with isolated AP window underwent repair with an anterior pulmonary artery flap technique. In two infants with AP window and interrupted aortic arch, the distal aorta was anastomosed directly to the aortic defect after division of the AP window. There were no hospital or late deaths, and no child had needed reintervention after a mean follow-up period of 30 months.

McElhinney and associates reported on outcome after reports of AP window in 24 patients younger than 6 months [28]. Isolated AP window was present in 12 patients, associated interrupted aortic arch in nine, and other anomalies in three. There were no early or late deaths of patients with isolated AP window. There were five early deaths of patients with associated lesions. All patients who survived repair of AP window and interrupted aortic arch had recurrent arch obstruction, but only two needed reintervention.

The operative mortality for repair of isolated AP window or aortic origin of a pulmonary artery approaches zero, even among infants. For patients without associated anomalies, the late results of surgical correction of AP window are excellent. The risk of recurrent fistula formation is unknown but should be low with patch closure or division of the AP window. Limited data are available on long-term outcome after repair of aortic origin of a pulmonary artery. The patients must be observed closely for development of pulmonary artery stenosis. For patients with complex associated anomalies, the prognosis is determined largely by the presence of associated anomalies. For older patients, outcome depends largely on pulmonary vascular resistance at the time of repair.

References

1. Neufeld HN, Lester RG, Adams P Jr, *et al.* (1962) Aorticopulmonary septal defect. Am J Cardiol 9, 12–25.
2. Putnam TC, Gross RE. (1966) Surgical management of aortopulmonary fenestration. Surgery 59, 727–735.
3. Richardson JV, Doty DB, Rossi NP, *et al.* (1979) The spectrum of anomalies of aortopulmonary septation. J Thorac Cardiovasc Surg 78, 21–27.
4. Elliotson J. (1830) Case of malformation of the pulmonary artery and aorta. Lancet 1, 247–251.
5. Cotton A. (1899) Report of a case of anuria. Trans Am Pediatr Soc 11, 137.
6. Abbott M. (1936) *Atlas of Congenital Heart Disease.* New York: American Heart Association.
7. Gross RE. (1952) Surgical closure of an aortic septal defect. Circulation 5, 858–863.
8. Scott HW Jr, Sabiston DC Jr. (1953) Surgical treatment for congenital aorticopulmonary fistula; experimental and clinical aspects. J Thorac Surg 25, 26–39.
9. Cooley DA, McNamara DG, Latson JR. (1957) Aorticopulmonary septal defect: diagnosis and surgical treatment. Surgery 42, 101–120; discussion 120.
10. Aberg T. (1979) Reply: aortopulmonary window. Ann Thorac Surg 28, 493.
11. Clarke CP, Richardson JP. (1976) The management of aortopulmonary window: advantages of transaortic closure with a dacron patch. J Thorac Cardiovasc Surg 72, 48–51.
12. Daily PO, Sissman NJ, Lipton MJ, *et al.* (1975) Correction of absence of the aortopulmonary septum by creation of concentric great vessels. Ann Thorac Surg 19, 180–190.
13. Deverall PB, Lincoln JC, Aberdeen E, *et al.* (1969) Aortopulmonary window. J Thorac Cardiovasc Surg 57, 479–486.
14. Johansson L, Michaelsson M, Westerholm CJ, *et al.* (1978) Aortopulmonary window: a new operative approach. Ann Thorac Surg 25, 564–567.
15. Matsuki O, Yagihara T, Yamamoto F, *et al.* (1992) New surgical technique for total-defect aortopulmonary window. Ann Thorac Surg 54, 991–992.
16. Negre E. (1979) Aortopulmonary window. Ann Thorac Surg 28, 493.
17. Negre E, Chaptal PA, Mary H. (1968) [Aortopulmonary fistulae: technical details of their closure]. Ann Chir Thorac Cardiovasc 7, 65–68.
18. Shatapathy P, Madhusudhana Rao K, Krishnan KV. (1987) Closure of aortopulmonary septal defect. J Thorac Cardiovasc Surg 93, 789–791.
19. Tulloh RM, Rigby ML. (1997) Transcatheter umbrella closure of aorto-pulmonary window. Heart 77, 479–480.
20. Wright JS, Freeman R, Johnston JB. (1968) Aorto-pulmonary fenestration. A technique of surgical management. J Thorac Cardiovasc Surg 55, 280–283.
21. Gaynor JW. (2003) Aortopulmonary window and aortic origin of a pulmonary artery. In: Mavroudis C, Backer CL, eds. *Pediatric Cardiac Surgery*, 3rd ed. Philadelphia, PA: Mosby.
22. Fraentzel O. (1868) Ein fall von abnormer communication der aorta mit der arteria pulmonalis. Virchows Arch Pathol Anat 43, 420–426.
23. Armer RM, Shumacker HB, Klatte EC. (1961) Origin of the right pulmonary artery from the ascending aorta. Report of a surgically corrected case. Circulation 24, 662–668.
24. Kirkpatrick SE, Girod DA, King H. (1967) Aortic origin of the right pulmonary artery. Surgical repair without a graft. Circulation 36, 777–782.
25. Kutsche LM, Van Mierop LH. (1987) Anatomy and pathogenesis of aorticopulmonary septal defect. Am J Cardiol 59, 443–447.
26. Kutsche LM, Van Mierop LH. (1988) Anomalous origin of a pulmonary artery from the ascending aorta: associated anomalies and pathogenesis. Am J Cardiol 61, 850–856.
27. Penkoske PA, Castaneda AR, Fyler DC, *et al.* (1983) Origin of pulmonary artery branch from ascending aorta. Primary surgical repair in infancy. J Thorac Cardiovasc Surg 85, 537–545.
28. McElhinney DB, Reddy VM, Tworetzky W, *et al.* (1998) Early and late results after repair of aortopulmonary septal defect and associated anomalies in infants <6 months of age. Am J Cardiol 81, 195–201.
29. Mori K, Ando M, Takao A, *et al.* (1978) Distal type of aortopulmonary window. Report of 4 cases. Br Heart J 40, 681–689.
30. Jacobs JP, Quintessenza JA, Gaynor JW, *et al.* (2000) Congenital Heart Surgery Nomenclature and Database Project: aortopulmonary window. Ann Thorac Surg 69(4 Suppl), S44–S49.
31. Berry TE, Bharati S, Muster AJ, *et al.* (1982) Distal aortopulmonary septal defect, aortic origin of the right pulmonary artery, intact ventricular septum, patent ductus arteriosus and hypoplasia of the aortic isthmus: a newly recognized syndrome. Am J Cardiol 49, 108–116.
32. Braunlin E, Peoples WM, Freedom RM, *et al.* (1982) Interruption of the aortic arch with aorticopulmonary septal defect. An anatomic review. Pediatr Cardiol 3, 329–335.
33. Chiemmongkoltip P, Moulder PV, Cassels DE. (1971) Interruption of the aortic arch with aortico-pulmonary septal defect and intact ventricular septum in a teenage girl. Chest 60, 324–327.
34. Konstantinov IE, Karamlou T, Williams WG, *et al.* (2006) Surgical management of aortopulmonary window associated with interrupted aortic arch: a Congenital Heart Surgeons Society study. J Thorac Cardiovasc Surg 131, 1136–1141 e2.
35. Faulkner SL, Oldham RR, Atwood GF, *et al.* (1974) Aortopulmonary window, ventricular septal defect, and membranous pulmonary atresia with a diagnosis of truncus arteriosus. Chest 65, 351–353.

36. Castaneda AR, Kirklin JW. (1977) Tetralogy of Fallot with aorticopulmonary window. Report of two surgical cases. J Thorac Cardiovasc Surg 74, 467–468.

37. Krishnan P, Airan B, Sambamurthy, *et al.* (1991) Complete transposition of the great arteries with aortopulmonary window: surgical treatment and embryologic significance. J Thorac Cardiovasc Surg 101, 749–751.

38. Agius PV, Rushworth A, Connolly N. (1970) Anomalous origin of left coronary artery from pulmonary artery associated with an aorto-pulmonary septal defect. Br Heart J 32, 708–710.

39. Burroughs JT, Schmutzer KJ, Linder F, *et al.* (1962) Anomalous origin of the right coronary artery with a orticopulmonary window and ventricular septal defect. Report of a case with complete operative correction. J Cardiovasc Surg (Torino) 3, 142–147.

40. Corno A, Pierli C, Lisi G, *et al.* (1988) Anomalous origin of the left coronary artery from an aortopulmonary window. J Thorac Cardiovasc Surg 96, 669–671.

41. Luisi SV, Ashraf MH, Gula G, *et al.* (1980) Anomalous origin of the right coronary artery with aortopulmonary window: functional and surgical considerations. Thorax 35, 446–448.

42. Chen HM, Tseng HI, Huang JW, *et al.* (2005) Coexistence of left pulmonary artery sling and aortopulmonary window complicated with difficult airway-a rare congenital cardiopulmonary defect. Eur J Cardiothorac Surg 28, 900–902.

43. Le Bret E, Lupoglazoff JM, Bachet J, *et al.* (2004) Pulmonary artery dissection and rupture associated with aortopulmonary window. Ann Thorac Surg 78, e67–e68.

44. Balaji S, Burch M, Sullivan ID. (1991) Accuracy of cross-sectional echocardiography in diagnosis of aortopulmonary window. Am J Cardiol 67, 650–653.

45. Rice MJ, Seward JB, Hagler DJ, *et al.* (1982) Visualization of aortopulmonary window by two-dimensional echocardiography. Mayo Clin Proc 57, 482–487.

46. Backer CL, Mavroudis C. (2002) Surgical management of aortopulmonary window: a 40-year experience. Eur J Cardiothorac Surg 21, 773–779.

47. Jureidini SB, Spadaro JJ, Rao PS. (1998) Successful transcatheter closure with the buttoned device of aortopulmonary window in an adult. Am J Cardiol 81, 371–372.

48. Tkebuchava T, von Segesser LK, Vogt PR, *et al.* (1997) Congenital aortopulmonary window: diagnosis, surgical technique and long-term results. Eur J Cardiothorac Surg 11, 293–297.

49. Di Bella I, Gladstone DJ. (1998) Surgical management of aortopulmonary window. Ann Thorac Surg 65, 768–770.

CHAPTER 21

Isolated Right Ventricular Outflow Tract Obstruction

John M. Karamichalis,[1] Jeffrey R. Darst,[2] Max B. Mitchell,[3] and David R. Clarke[4]

[1]University of California, San Francisco, San Francisco, CA, USA
[2]Children's Hospital Colorado, Aurora, CO, USA
[3]Children's Hospital Colorado Heart Institute, Aurora, CO, USA
[4]University of Colorado Denver, Aurora, CO, USA

Isolated right ventricular outflow tract obstruction involves a broad spectrum of lesions ranging from mild valvar pulmonary stenosis to pulmonary atresia with associated secondary right-sided cardiac defects. As indicated by the title, this chapter considers only lesions in which right ventricular outflow tract obstruction occurs in the presence of an intact ventricular septum with normal ventriculoarterial connections. The variety of congenital lesions accompanied by right ventricular outflow tract obstruction is addressed in other chapters. Specifically, this chapter focuses on the surgical management of pulmonary atresia with intact ventricular septum (PA-IVS), neonatal critical pulmonary stenosis, and valvar pulmonary stenosis beyond the neonatal period. Isolated supravalvar pulmonary artery stenosis and subvalvar right ventricular outflow tract obstruction are also discussed. Reference is also made to catheter intervention treatment modalities.

Pulmonary Atresia with Intact Ventricular Septum

Incidence, Definition, and Etiology

Pulmonary atresia with intact ventricular septum is an uncommon lesion with an incidence of approximately 4.5 cases per 100 000 live births [1,2]. As such this lesion represents fewer than 1% of all congenital heart defects [3,4]. The name of this lesion is derived from the fact that there is no physiologic communication between the right ventricle and the pulmonary arteries. Although conceptually simple, PA-IVS is frequently complicated by substantial associated morphologic abnormalities of the right side of

the heart and coronary arteries [5]. The degree of right heart development varies widely from minor hypoplasia of the right ventricle to severe underdevelopment with right ventricular-dependent coronary circulation. This spectrum of morphologic variation mandates individualized management that can involve biventricular or univentricular strategies.

The cause of PA-IVS is unknown. Kutsche and Van Mierop [6] postulated that this lesion occurs relatively late in embryologic development after cardiac septation. Variations in the timing of the insult that causes the pulmonary valve to become atretic may account for the spectrum of associated morphologic lesions of the pulmonary valve annulus, right ventricular myocardium, tricuspid valve, and coronary arteries. Conceptually, pulmonary atresia occurring very soon after cardiac septation would result in a completely undeveloped pulmonary valve, a diminutive right ventricle, and extensive right ventricular-to-coronary artery communications. Conversely, pulmonary atresia occurring later in gestation would result in a larger right ventricle, absence of coronary artery anomalies, a pulmonary valve with three developed sinuses of Valsalva, and three distinct, completely fused leaflets. Kutsche and Van Mierop [6] also hypothesized that the etiologic insult is a prenatal inflammatory process. However, histopathologic studies of fetuses and neonates with pulmonary atresia have not demonstrated evidence of inflammation [7].

In most cases the main pulmonary artery is well developed, and the ductus arteriosus is present, a finding suggesting that at some time in utero antegrade right ventricular blood flow was present [4]. Studies with fetal echocardiography have shown antegrade flow across the pulmonary valve in fetuses that have subsequently developed pulmonary atresia [8]. This finding suggests that altered hemodynamics may be a primary cause of pulmonary atresia. Increased left-heart loading owing to changes in the tricuspid valve, foramen ovale, and patent ductus arteriosus during early development could lead to left-to-right ductal flow with lack of right heart ejection. The result is fusion of the pulmonary valve leaflets as development proceeds [9].

Other authors have proposed a genetic cause of PA-IVS [10–14]. A recent report of PA-IVS occurring in monozygotic twins [11], points to a genetic etiology of this disorder. The significance of the array comparative genomic hybridization (aCGH) results, which show a 55-kb deletion in 20q13.12 involving the WFDC8 and WFDC9 genes in both of these patients is unclear, however they suggest that a combination of genetic and environmental factors may be responsible for some cases of PA-IVS.

A different study [10], showed for the first time an association of 22q11.2 deletion with PA-IVS and absent pulmonary arteries, discussing a possible role of the deletion in pulmonary artery arborization, and also increasing the spectrum of deletion 22q11.2 associated cardiac malformations. Autosomal dominant inheritance with incomplete penetrance of PA-IVS was suggested by a report of two first cousins with PA-IVS [13]. The authors suggest a genetic cause that is mitochondrial, autosomal dominant with incomplete penetrance or multifactorial. Laterality defects (heterotaxy) have been associated with connexin43 mutations, and mice lacking connexin43 developed PA-IVS [12].

Morphology

Pulmonary atresia with intact ventricular septum almost always occurs in hearts with a situs solitus position that have concordant atrioventricular and ventriculoarterial connections [15]. The branch pulmonary arteries are confluent and arborize normally in the lungs. In most cases a single ductus arteriosus connects the pulmonary arteries to the systemic circulation. The confluence of the main pulmonary artery with the branches usually is normal, and a well developed main pulmonary artery tapers proximally to an atretic valve. The pulmonary valve may vary from a minuscule fibrous dimple with long segment muscular atresia to a fused trileaflet valve with well developed commissures and sinuses (Figure 21.1) [16].

Although the right-sided structures distal to the atretic valve are relatively normal, structures proximal to the valve often are markedly abnormal. The heart usually is enlarged owing to right atrial dilatation. In the presence of severe tricuspid regurgitation, the heart may be massively enlarged and resemble a severe form of Ebstein anomaly. Secundum atrial septal defect or patent foramen ovale must be present to allow *in utero* development and subsequent live birth. The tricuspid valve is nearly always

abnormal [17]. Tricuspid regurgitation is present in essentially all cases; severe regurgitation is present in approximately 25% of cases [18]. The tricuspid annulus is typically hypoplastic. The tricuspid valve leaflets are dysplastic, having shortened chordae and restricted leaflet motion. In other cases concomitant Ebstein anomaly occurs and is characterized by a dilated tricuspid annulus, redundant sail-like anterior leaflet, and downward displacement of the septal and posterior leaflets. In rare instances, severe deficiency of tricuspid leaflet tissue leaves the tricuspid orifice essentially unguarded [19].

The right ventricle is abnormal. In 90% of cases it is hypertrophied and hypoplastic (Figure 21.2) [16,18].

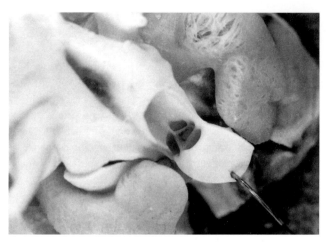

Figure 21.1 Pathologic specimen from a neonate with pulmonary atresia with intact ventricular septum viewed from main pulmonary artery. Developed sinuses and valve commissures are evident.

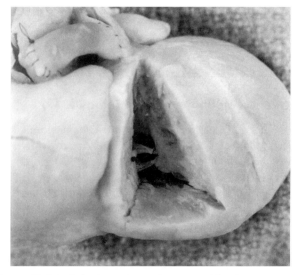

Figure 21.2 Pathologic specimen of neonate with pulmonary atresia with intact ventricular septum. Hypertrophy of right ventricular wall and marked reduction of ventricular cavity are evident.

Ventricular cavity size is severely reduced in more than 50% of cases [16,18]. Less commonly the right ventricle is thinned and markedly dilated. This situation occurs only with more severe degrees of tricuspid regurgitation, particularly when Ebstein anomaly or unguarded tricuspid valve orifice is present [19]. In the usual case of a small right ventricle, the degree of hypoplasia varies. The size of the right ventricle correlates very closely with the size of the tricuspid valve annulus [16,18]. In an effort to direct appropriate treatment choices, Bull and colleagues [20] categorized right ventricular morphology in PA-IVS as unipartite (inlet part only), bipartite (inlet and outlet parts), and tripartite (inlet, outlet, and trabecular parts). This classification has been questioned on a developmental basis because even very small right ventricles are thought to have all three components with massive hypertrophy obliterating the trabecular and/or outlet portions. The importance of this distinction is that even very hypoplastic ventricles composed of all three parts can grow and eventually function normally after decompression [21,22].

A spectrum of intramural and extramural coronary artery abnormalities can occur with PA-IVS. These abnormalities can be congenital or acquired, and many of them are specific to hearts with PA-IVS [7]. More than one half of all cases are accompanied by some form of coronary artery abnormality [18]. Fistulas between the right ventricle and the coronary arteries are the most common abnormality. When a fistula is present, the coronary artery tree usually communicates with the right ventricular cavity through endothelium-lined channels, known as sinusoids, within the right ventricular muscle mass. When a coronary fistula enters a sinusoid, this is also known as coronary-cameral fistula. Sinusoids most likely represent remnants of sinusoidal channels that provide myocardial blood before formation of the coronary arteries during development. In many cases localized areas of myointimal hyperplasia result in development of coronary artery stenosis and, more rarely, complete interruption. These lesions have been identified in fetuses as well as newborns with PA-IVS. Interestingly, the coronary stenosis does not occur in the absence of ventriculocoronary connections. When present the stenotic lesions are near the fistulas. Furthermore, these lesions occur in association with PA-IVS only when the right ventricle is a thick-walled high-pressure chamber [7]. These findings suggest that the cause of the stenotic coronary lesions in PA-IVS may be acquired intimal injury secondary to turbulent competitive blood flow from the high-pressure right ventricle through the fistulas into the coronary arteries [5,7,23].

In rare cases there is no proximal aortocoronary connection, and all coronary perfusion is supplied from the right ventricular cavity. This type of coronary lesion usually is remote from the ventriculocoronary connection, and the cause of such a lesion is thought to be congenital. The importance of concomitant coronary stenosis or obstruction and ventriculocoronary connections is that perfusion of the myocardium distal to stenotic lesions may depend on desaturated venous blood from the high-pressure right ventricular cavity. Importantly the presence and physiologic implications of ventriculocoronary connections correlate closely with small tricuspid valve diameter, small right ventricular cavity, and increased right ventricular pressure [18,24].

Myocardial abnormalities are the rule with PA-IVS [5]. In most cases there is severe right ventricular hypertrophy with reduced cavity volume. Myocardial fiber disarray is a distinctive histopathologic finding associated with the hypertrophy present in this lesion [25]. Ischemic changes with infarction and diffuse fibrosis may occur in the myocardium [26]. In severe cases endocardial fibroelastosis may occur. Sinusoids with or without concomitant coronary artery fistulas occur in as many as 50% of cases [18] but only when there is a thick-walled high pressure right ventricle. In the approximately 5–10% of cases with severe tricuspid valve incompetence, dilatation and marked thinning of the right ventricle are common. In such cases sinusoids and coronary fistulas do not occur [7].

Natural History

In the absence of medical therapy and surgical intervention during the newborn period, survival of patients with PA-IVS is rare [27]. Within 2 weeks of life mortality is approximately 50% and by 6 months mortality is approximately 85% [27]. Survival beyond the neonatal period requires an alternative source of pulmonary blood flow. In rare cases patients have survived to the third decade because of the presence of a patent ductus arteriosus or aortopulmonary collateral vessels [28,29].

Pathophysiology

Infants born with PA-IVS depend on the ductus arteriosus for pulmonary blood flow, and systemic venous return enters the left atrium through a nonrestrictive atrial level communication. Consequently, all of these children are cyanotic to some degree. Closure of the ductus arteriosus produces profound hypoxemia, acidosis, and hemodynamic collapse. Prostaglandin E (PGE$_1$) infusion is required to maintain ductal patency. In unusual cases restriction at the atrial septal defect causes elevated central venous pressure, diminished left heart loading, and hypotension. In most cases, however, shunting at the atrial level is unrestricted, and cardiac output is preserved as long as the ductus arteriosus remains patent.

Cardiac output is markedly elevated because the left ventricle must also provide pulmonary blood flow. The ratio of pulmonary to systemic blood flow ranges between 2:1 and 4:1 depending on the relative resistance of the two circulations. Systemic oxygen saturation depends on pulmonary blood flow and usually ranges from 70–90%.

Saturation greater than 90% suggests pulmonary overcirculation. The low-resistance runoff into the pulmonary circulation results in a widened pulse pressure. In the absence of severe tricuspid regurgitation, the hypoplastic right ventricular cavity has systemic or suprasystemic systolic pressure and elevated diastolic pressure. Less commonly a dilated right ventricle, present when there is gross tricuspid incompetence, has lower intracavitary pressure.

Myocardial perfusion is perturbed relative to that in a normal heart, in which most perfusion occurs during diastole and myocardial oxygen consumption is near maximal. Oxygen transport is limited by cyanosis. Tachycardia, common in these infants, shortens the diastolic time interval and increases myocardial oxygen demand. Elevated wall tension in the right ventricle also increases myocardial oxygen demand and limits perfusion because of the decreased gradient between aortic diastolic pressure and the right ventricular coronary bed. This situation is further compounded by decreased aortic diastolic pressure, which occurs in the presence of a patent ductus arteriosus. Consequently, such patients have markedly decreased coronary reserve.

Coronary reserve is even more limited in the presence of ventriculocoronary connections with right ventricle-dependent coronary circulation. In some cases coronary blood flow may even be retrograde into the ascending aorta (Figure 21.3) [16]. Regions of myocardium supplied by coronary arteries distal to interruptions or areas of marked stenosis depend on desaturated blood supplied by the high-pressure right ventricle, which always is present in this circumstance. Despite elevated right ventricular systolic and diastolic pressure, intracavitary diastolic pressure usually is lower than normal aortic diastolic pressure. Therefore in contrast to the normal situation, perfusion of right ventricle-dependent myocardium may not occur primarily during diastole. Any reduction in right ventricular pressure, owing to hypovolemia, right ventricular outflow tract decompression, or balloon disruption of the tricuspid valve, can compromise the extremely marginal coronary reserve in these patients and have disastrous consequences. Varying configurations of coronary fistulas and proximal coronary stenosis may result in lesser degrees of myocardial dependence on right ventricular coronary blood flow with important but less severe consequences from right ventricular decompression.

Moderate to severe tricuspid valve regurgitation occurs in most cases because of elevated right ventricular pressure

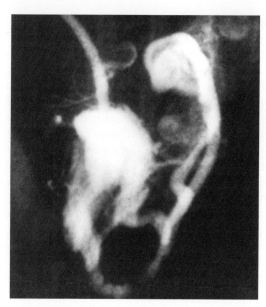

Figure 21.3 Right ventricular angiogram of a neonate with pulmonary atresia with intact ventricular septum shows severe right ventricular hypoplasia and multiple ventriculocoronary connections. Retrograde flow of contrast material from the coronary bed into the ascending aorta is evident. (Courtesy Dr K Chan Chen, University of Colorado, Denver, CO, USA.)

and anatomic abnormalities of the leaflets, chordae, and papillary muscles [17]. In cases of deficiency of leaflet tissue or concomitant Ebstein anomaly, regurgitation is massive.

Clinical Presentation and Diagnosis

Most infants with PA-IVS are born at term. Soon after birth, progressive cyanosis develops. With closure of the ductus arteriosus, profound hypoxemia unresponsive to supplemental oxygen occurs. Even with appropriate resuscitation and PGE_1 infusion, such infants usually have tachycardia and tachypnea. Auscultation reveals a systolic murmur of ductal flow and single first and second heart sounds. Depending on the degree of severity, a pansystolic murmur of tricuspid regurgitation may be heard at the left sternal border. The electrocardiogram demonstrates dominant left ventricular forces in contrast to the usual dominant right ventricular forces found in the neonate. On a chest radiograph the cardiac silhouette appears normal unless severe tricuspid regurgitation and associated right atrial and ventricular enlargement are present. Pulmonary vascular markings are diminished but may become more normal with resuscitation. Echocardiography demonstrates absence of the right ventricular outflow tract and is the primary diagnostic modality. Right ventricular cavity size and function (Figure 21.4) [16], tricuspid valve dimensions

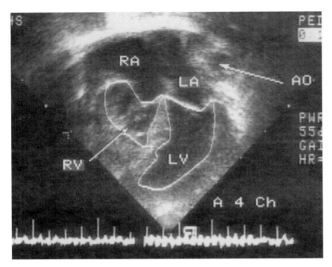

Figure 21.4 Two-dimensional echocardiogram in apical four-chamber view shows pulmonary atresia with intact ventricular septum at end diastole. Hypoplasia of right ventricular cavity is evident. (AO, aorta; LA, RA, left, right atrium; LV, RV, left, right ventricle.)

and function, and right-to-left atrial level shunting as well as patency of the ductus arteriosus all can be reliably assessed. In some cases echocardiography documents coronary artery fistulas (Plate 21.1, see plate section opposite p. 594) [16]. Echocardiography and cardiac catheterization are complementary, and both studies should be performed in all cases. Cardiac catheterization is the only means of conclusively defining coronary anatomy and demonstrating the presence or absence of ventriculocoronary fistulas. In some cases interventional catheterization may play a stabilizing or even therapeutic role. For example, balloon atrial septostomy may be necessary in a patient with a restrictive atrial level shunt.

The differential diagnosis of PA-IVS includes neonatal conditions marked by cyanosis, soft systolic murmur, and decreased pulmonary vascular markings. The diagnostic possibilities include critical pulmonary stenosis, tetralogy of Fallot, pulmonary atresia with ventricular septal defect, neonatal Ebstein anomaly, tricuspid atresia with pulmonary atresia, and complex univentricular heart with pulmonary atresia.

Management

Preintervention Medical Management

The initial medical treatment of a patient with PA-IVS usually must begin before a specific diagnosis can be established. Therefore treatment is similar to that of any neonate with suspected cyanotic congenital heart disease. Vascular

access should be established, and PGE_1 infusion should be initiated to maintain ductal patency. Metabolic acidosis should be corrected, and inotropic support should be initiated if perfusion is inadequate. Mechanical ventilation and pharmacologic paralysis may be necessary for very ill neonates.

Choice of Initial Therapy

The diagnosis of PA-IVS is in itself an indication for surgical or in some cases catheter-based intervention. Because this lesion manifests with such a wide degree of morphologic variability, the choice of therapy is complex. The primary options for initial therapy include decompression of the right ventricle alone by surgical or transcatheter valvotomy or transannular patch, construction of a systemic-pulmonary artery shunt alone, or a combination of a pulmonary outflow tract procedure and shunt. Possible outcomes encompass a gamut that includes biventricular repair, the perceived middle ground of the so-called one-and-a-half ventricular repair, and univentricular management. Cardiac transplantation has been advocated in severe cases.

A study of 210 consecutive patients with PA-IVS concluded that outcomes have improved over time [30]. This study also indicated that careful initial management, and better selection, are still needed for those patients destined to undergo biventricular repair.

Appropriate management must balance the operative risk of the initial therapeutic choice with long-term functional outcome. The primary goals of initial therapy should be to minimize mortality and simultaneously optimize the likelihood of eventual biventricular repair. One difficulty is that the strategy that achieves the lowest initial mortality (systemic-pulmonary artery shunt alone [18]) may prevent achieving biventricular repair. Several reports have indicated that patients with severely hypoplastic right ventricle can be treated with medium-term mortality equivalent to that of patients with less severe morphology; however, precise management algorithms are difficult to derive from these reports [31,32]. The long-term goal of achieving biventricular repair in the maximum number of patients may be offset by the reasonable clinical outcome of management schema in which a larger number of patients undergo univentricular management [31,32].

Most single-center reports of surgical outcome of PA-IVS either describe too few patients or are too vague to provide useful morphologic criteria for the initial treatment of these patients. Several centers have proposed various morphologic criteria for guiding the choice of initial management [24,33–37]. Most of these reports describe some measure of right ventricular size or morphology. More recently, fetal tricuspid valve Z score and rate of growth have been suggested to predict postnatal outcome [38]. One simple approach has been to attempt right ventricular decompression with pulmonary valvotomy and construct a systemic-pulmonary artery shunt in all patients found to have a right ventricular infundibulum. Patients without an infundibulum or those having right ventricle-dependent coronary circulation undergo shunt alone. Results with this strategy have been mixed. The need for eventual biventricular, intermediate, or univentricular repair is determined on the basis of subsequent right ventricular development [22,24,37,39]. Unfortunately, there is considerable morphologic variability in patients who have a right ventricular infundibulum, and this strategy may subject some patients to an unnecessary shunting procedure with the obligatory need to occlude the shunt at a later date.

There is no consensus on the therapeutic intervention most appropriate in all cases [24,31–33,37,40–51]. This lesion is rare, and individual institutional experiences are relatively limited. Ideal therapeutic management depends on the morphologic and physiologic substrate of the individual patient. The recognition that right heart growth may occur in markedly hypoplastic right ventricles after establishment of right ventricular-to-pulmonary artery continuity has added further complexity to initial decision making, largely because accurate guidelines for predicting eventual right heart functional capacity are limited [21,22,52–56]. There are cases at the worst end of the morphologic spec-

trum in which univentricular physiology is the only possible course. There are also cases at the most favorable end in which biventricular repair is likely. The most difficult decisions must be made for patients with intermediate cases, that is, most patients. For the intermediate group it is simpler to understand that without decompression of the right ventricle and establishment of antegrade flow into the pulmonary arteries early in the neonatal period, right heart growth is unlikely to occur, and biventricular circulation is not attainable [21,22,46]. Therefore it is logical to approach intermediate cases in a manner that does not preclude the possibility of eventual biventricular physiology as long as the mortality risk of the initial procedure does not exceed the mortality of a procedure that would likely preclude biventricular repair in the future.

The only study of sufficient size to provide a reliable morphologic basis on which to base appropriate initial management is the prospective multicenter study conducted by the Congenital Heart Surgeons Society (CHSS) consisting of 171 neonates treated between 1987 and 1991 [18]. Although there was considerable management variability among participating institutions, initial management was categorized into three basic procedures: relief of right ventricular outflow tract obstruction alone, relief of right ventricular outflow tract obstruction plus systemic-pulmonary artery shunt, and systemic-pulmonary artery shunt alone. The overall survival rate in this study was 81%

A

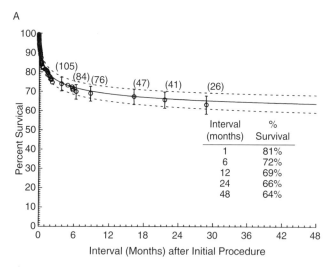

B

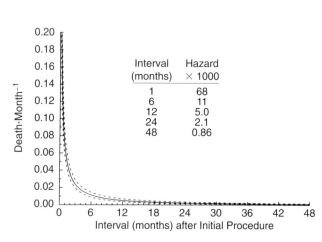

Figure 21.5 Survival (determined by life table methods and parametrically) after the initial procedure (performed, on average, at 3 days of age) of neonates with pulmonary atresia and intact ventricular septum (n = 171). Patients with abnormally large right ventricles with or without Ebstein anomaly and those who did not undergo a procedure are not included. The depiction is of 153 patients. Numbers in parentheses represent the number of patients available for follow-up study after the actuarial estimate. Patients

were not censored at any subsequent procedure. Circles represent each death and are positioned along the horizontal axis at the time of death and actuarially along the vertical axis. Vertical bars represent 70% confidence interval. Solid line represents the parametrically determined continuous point estimate. Dashed lines enclose 70% confidence interval. **A,** Survivorship. **B,** Hazard function. (Reproduced with permission from Hanley *et al.* [18].)

at 1 month and 64% at 4 years (Figure 21.5) [18]. An important finding in this study was that the size of the tricuspid valve (expressed as Z value) correlated very closely to right ventricular cavity volume. Second, smaller tricuspid Z value, marked right ventricular coronary artery dependency, and choice of initial procedure were important risk factors for death (Table 21.1) [18]. However, a smaller tricuspid Z value was a risk factor for death only when the initial procedure included right ventricular decompression either by valvotomy or transannular patch. If a systemic-pulmonary artery shunt alone was performed, the size of the tricuspid valve (right ventricle) did not influence survival. The outcome of the three initial procedures as a function of the severity of right ventricular hypoplasia expressed as the tricuspid valve Z value was determined in this study (Figure 21.6) [18]. The need for secondary nondefinitive procedures was considerable. Of the patients who underwent valvotomy as the initial right ventricular outflow tract procedure, 55% required a subsequent transannular patch within 3 years. Similarly, 51% of patients not receiving a systemic-pulmonary artery shunt at the initial procedure needed a shunt within 1 month.

The initial report of the CHSS study suggested that eventual biventricular repair may be achieved in some patients with tricuspid annulus Z values as small as –4. In addition, the early risk of a combined pulmonary outflow procedure and systemic-pulmonary shunt in this group

Table 21.1 Multivariable risk factor equation for death after the initial procedure for pulmonary atresia with intact ventricular septum. (Reproduced with permission from Hanley *et al.* [18].)

Incremental risk factor for death after initial procedure	Single hazard phase *p* value
Patient	
(Lower) birth weight	<.0001
Diameter (Z value) of tricuspid valve*	.03†
Right ventricular dependency of coronary circulation Procedural	.03
Procedural	
(Earlier) date of procedure‡	.002

Summary excludes 13 patients with Ebstein anomaly or large right ventricle. Variables with footnotes are interaction terms, not true risk factors.
*Interaction term that applies only when the initial procedure involved valvotomy or transannular patch but not when it was shunt alone.
†*p* value was .001 if valvotomy or transannular patch was performed without a shunt.
‡Interaction term that applies only to isolated systemic-pulmonary artery shunt without atrial septectomy but not to any other initial procedure.

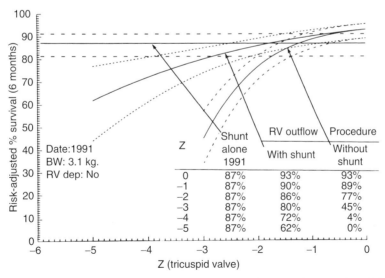

Figure 21.6 Nomogram shows a specific solution of a multivariable equation illustrating the effect on survival of the diameter (Z value) of the tricuspid valve and the type of initial procedure on neonates with pulmonary atresia and intact ventricular septum. Right ventricular outflow procedure includes both valvotomy and transannular patching. A Z value of zero represents the normal mean value of the diameter of the tricuspid valve. A Z value of –1 represents a diameter one standard deviation below the normal mean value; + 1 represents one standard deviation above normal, and so on. (Reproduced with permission from Hanley *et al.* [18].)

versus shunt alone was similar at or above a tricuspid Z value of −4 [18]. Consequently, the recommendation for patients with moderate right ventricular hypoplasia (tricuspid Z value −1 to −4) was a combined pulmonary outflow tract procedure with shunt. More recent analysis of the CHSS data, including a total of 247 patients with more follow-up time, suggested that patients with tricuspid Z values less than −3 have a higher initial mortality for combined pulmonary outflow procedure and shunt than for shunt alone [9]. No patient in this group underwent biventricular repair. These findings suggest that the recommendations for initial therapeutic intervention made in the original report should be modified. The following recommendations have been made by Reddy and colleagues [9] and are based on the more recent analysis of the patients accrued by the CHSS.

Mild right ventricular hypoplasia. Patients with mild hypoplasia of the right ventricle have a tricuspid Z value ranging from 0 to −2. The goal of treatment of these patients is to promote right ventricular growth and to minimize intervention. Initial treatment of this group should consist of decompressing the right ventricle by means of establishing right ventricular to pulmonary artery continuity. In rare cases with very mild right ventricular hypoplasia, radio frequency valve perforation and balloon valvuloplasty may obviate initial surgical intervention for some patients [44,45,48,50]. Reports of long-term outcome for such patients are scant, and there is insufficient information to allow comparison with the outcome among surgically treated patients with similar anatomy. Most patients with mild right ventricular hypoplasia should undergo either valvotomy or transannular patch. Valvotomy alone does not require cardiopulmonary bypass, but a number of patients need infundibular muscle resection and transannular patch to relieve residual outflow tract obstruction. Initial transannular patching achieves more long-standing right ventricular outflow tract decompression, but this advantage is offset by more serious pulmonary insufficiency, which may have deleterious early and long-term effects on right ventricular function. There are no data indicating that one approach is superior to the other. Regardless of the initial outflow tract procedure, the atrial septal defect should be left open to allow early right-to-left decompression, because almost all cases require time before right ventricular function becomes capable of carrying the entire cardiac output. In addition, severe postoperative hypoxemia may necessitate the addition of a systemic-pulmonary artery shunt in as many as 50% of cases [18].

Moderate right ventricular hypoplasia. Moderate right ventricular hypoplasia is a tricuspid Z value ranging from −2 to −3. These patients have the potential to achieve future biventricular repair, and the probability of this outcome is directly related to the size of the right ventricle. Because a

pulmonary outflow tract procedure and a systemic-pulmonary artery shunt carry a mortality risk similar to that of a shunt alone, a combined procedure is favored [9,18]. This approach preserves the chance that the right ventricle will grow and allows subsequent biventricular repair. This approach also minimizes the need for subsequent procedures. Options for the right ventricular outflow tract procedure are the same as for management of mild right ventricular hypoplasia and carry the same risks and benefits.

Severe right ventricular hypoplasia. Severe right ventricular hypoplasia is a tricuspid annulus Z value less than or equal to −3. No patient in the CHSS study in this group successfully underwent biventricular repair [9]. Second, the early mortality risk of a combined pulmonary outflow tract procedure and shunt was significantly higher than that for a shunt alone in this category (see Figure 21.6) [18]. Third, many of these patients have extensive coronary fistulas or marked right ventricle-dependent coronary circulation. Patients in this category should undergo systemic-pulmonary artery shunt alone.

In a more recent report from Japan [57], patients were treated according to a management protocol based on a quantitative assessment of right ventricular morphology with good results. For initial palliation the right ventricular development index (RVDI) was determined. Right ventricular end-diastolic volume (RVEDV) expressed a percentage of expected normal volumes (%N), and tricuspid valve diameter (TVD) measured in end diastole expressed as a percentage of the predicted diameter (%N) were derived. The diameter of the right ventricular outflow (RVOD) tract was measured at the narrowest portion in the lateral projection at end-diastole. RVDI was then calculated according to the equation:

$$RVDI = RVEDV(\%N) * TVD(\%N) * RVOD(mm) * 10^{-5}/BSA(m^2)$$

For patients with RVDI>0.7, open transpulmonary valvotomy was recommended as an initial palliation. When RVDI is between 0.35 and 0.7, beta blocker therapy was added to valvotomy. When RVDI is lower than 0.35, concomitant valvotomy and systemic to pulmonary shunt was done. For patients with muscular atresia of the right ventricular outflow tract or right ventricle dependent coronary circulation only a shunt was performed [57].

For later definitive operation the right ventricle-tricuspid valve (RV-TV) index based on measurements in end diastole is calculated:

$$RV\text{-}TV \text{ index} = RVEDV(\%N) * TVD(\%N) * 10^{-4}$$

Complete biventricular repair is accomplished in patients with the RV-TV index >0.4. For patients with RV-TV index ranging between 0.2 and 0.4, a biventricular repair with partial closure of atrial septal defect was recommended.

When RV-TV index is between 0.1 and 0.2, one and half ventricular repair was chosen. For patients with RV-TV index of lower than 0.1, univentricular definitive palliation was used [57].

Right Ventricle-Dependent Coronary Circulation

There is uniform agreement that patients with complete right ventricle-dependent coronary circulation (RVDCC) should not undergo decompression of the right ventricle [18,58,59]. These patients should undergo systemic-pulmonary artery shunt alone. Some centers recommend consideration for cardiac transplantation. However, for lesser degrees of right ventricular dependency, opinions vary widely. One difficulty is that the description of what constitutes "significant" right ventricular dependency is subjective. Consequently, careful analysis of various management protocols is difficult because of uncertainty regarding the comparability of patient populations. An important distinction is the existence of fistulas with or without concomitant stenosis or obstruction. Most patients who have coronary artery fistulas alone may undergo decompression safely [58]. The risk of death upon right ventricular decompression increases significantly if one of three major coronary arteries (left anterior descending, left circumflex, right coronary artery) contains fistulous connections and is obstructed. The likelihood of mortality is very high if two major arteries are affected [58].

One method of decision making allows for decompression of the right ventricle unless two major vessels are obstructed, complete atresia of the coronary ostia is demonstrated, or a significant portion of the left ventricular myocardium is supplied by coronary fistulas from the right ventricle, regardless of proximal stenosis [60]. This approach assumes reasonable right ventricular size and no additional anatomic confounders. As most patients with significant right ventricular coronary dependency have severe right ventricular hypoplasia, the recommendation for initial treatment (systemic-pulmonary artery shunt alone) can be based on tricuspid Z value only.

Precise definition of coronary arterial anatomy remains imperative to the management of neonates with PA-IVS. Early mortality among such patients appears to be related to coronary ischemia at or around the time of initial palliation. In an early study, 12 patients with PA-IVS-RVDCC who underwent single ventricle palliation between 1986 and 1997 were found to have an 83% 5-year actuarial survival. The two deaths (17%) in that series occurred within 4 months after the systemic to pulmonary shunt from presumed coronary ischemia [59]. The results of single ventricle palliation from a more recent retrospective review [61], were practically identical, with 18.8% overall mortality and 81.3% 5, 10, and 15 year actuarial survival. All deaths in this series occurred within 3 months of the shunt from

presumed coronary ischemia. In both series there were no perioperative or late deaths after bidirectional Glenn or Fontan. It is clear that in patients surviving the initial shunt, single ventricle palliation yields excellent mid- to long-term survivals with well preserved LV systolic function and should be the preferred management strategy for the majority of these patients. Longer follow-up will be necessary to assess whether these patients will be at risk either from sudden death owing to ventricular dysrhythmias or for ventricular dysfunction as a result of coronary perfusion with subnormal saturated blood.

Neonates with aortocoronary atresia, the most extreme form of RVDCC, or those with significant left ventricular dysfunction should undergo cardiac transplantation [61]. Patients listed for transplant may wait weeks to months and face significant risk during this time. Prolonged PGE_1 administration, ductal stenting, or systemic to pulmonary shunt can be used to manage patients on the waiting list.

Severe Tricuspid Regurgitation

Patients with Ebstein anomaly or unguarded tricuspid orifice usually have an enlarged tricuspid annulus and a dilated, poorly contractile right ventricle. From a clinical standpoint these patients are similar to neonates with severe cyanosis and Ebstein anomaly (see Chapter 29, *Ebstein Anomaly*). The mortality in this group is high, and right ventricular outflow tract procedures combined with tricuspid valve repair have poor results. In fact, patients with pulmonary atresia and Ebstein anomaly have been demonstrated to have a higher risk of in-hospital mortality [62]. Nearly all surviving patients with severe tricuspid regurgitation need univentricular management, which is only avoided by primary cardiac transplantation. Currently, most centers attempt initial therapy with a systemic-pulmonary artery shunt alone. Another alternative is conversion of the anatomy to tricuspid atresia with construction of a systemic-pulmonary artery shunt [63].

Other Procedures

Other procedures, including tricuspid valve disruption, tricuspid valve closure, right ventricular thromboexclusion, ligation of coronary fistula, and attempts at tricuspid valve repair for regurgitation, have been advocated in the initial treatment of neonates with PA-IVS. The use of these procedures is not supported by evidence of a favorable effect on outcome.

Subsequent Surgical Management

All patients with PA-IVS need close follow-up care after initial treatment. Nearly all surviving patients need at least one secondary intervention, and the timing and selection of subsequent interventions are complicated. Patients initially undergoing systemic-pulmonary artery shunt alone who are anticipated to need subsequent univentricular management should undergo cardiac catheterization between 3 and 6 months of age in preparation for a bidirectional superior cavopulmonary shunt and systemic-pulmonary artery shunt takedown. Ideally, this procedure should be completed before the age of 12 months. Between the ages of 2 and 4 years, depending on patient growth, a total cavopulmonary connection (Fontan procedure) should be completed. In patients with significant right ventricle-dependent coronary circulation, the Fontan procedure should involve a modification that allows maintenance of right ventricular pressure, directs oxygenated blood into the right ventricle, and allows drainage of coronary sinus blood into the low-pressure atrial chamber. Options include the lateral tunnel and extra cardiac modifications of the Fontan procedure. Although not widely practiced, another solution is concomitant Fontan procedure and construction of an aortic-to-right ventricular conduit to maintain coronary perfusion [64,65]. There is no evidence to support the superiority of this approach over conventional total cavopulmonary connection. In patients with known right ventricle-dependent coronary circulation, even temporary decompression of the right ventricle that occurs with standard cardiopulmonary bypass techniques can cause lethal myocardial ischemia; therefore altered perfusion strategies may be needed during a Fontan procedure on these patients [66].

Patients with mild right ventricular hypoplasia who have successfully undergone right ventricular outflow tract decompression (balloon valvuloplasty, surgical valvotomy, or transannular patch) without a systemic-pulmonary artery shunt should undergo echocardiography and cardiac catheterization between 3 and 6 months of age. Right ventricular function and the degree of residual right ventricular outflow tract obstruction should be assessed during temporary occlusion of the atrial septal defect. Right atrial pressure, systemic arterial pressure, and mixed venous oxygen saturation should be measured to determine whether the right ventricle is capable of carrying the entire systemic output. In addition, simultaneous recording of right atrial and right ventricular pressure, when technically feasible, can evaluate tricuspid valve stenosis. In cases of only valvar pulmonary outflow tract obstruction and good right ventricular function, balloon valvuloplasty may be used, and closure of the atrial septum can be accomplished with a catheter-delivered device. In the most favorable situation, catheter-based closure of the atrial septal defect may be all that is needed to achieve biventricular physiology.

Though not always the case, criteria for determination of a suitable right heart that can sustain full cardiac output over the long-term is frequently unclear. More commonly, residual right ventricular outflow tract obstruction is not amenable to balloon valvuloplasty, and surgical treatment is needed. Appropriate surgical intervention consists of infundibular muscle resection with repeated valvotomy or

a transannular patch. In either case the atrial septal defect should be closed concomitantly. If right ventricular function is borderline and there is residual outflow tract obstruction, the atrial septal defect may be left open at the time of right ventricular outflow tract enlargement and reassessed for delayed closure either surgically or with a catheter-based device. Some authorities advocate the use of an adjustable atrial septal defect closure method to allow simple closure of the atrial septal communication either in the early postoperative period or at a later date [65].

In patients with borderline right heart development, a newer approach has been to construct a bidirectional superior cavopulmonary connection with or without right ventricular outflow tract enlargement. This option is known as the one-and-a-half ventricular approach. Total separation of the two circulations can be achieved if the patient tolerates concomitant closure of the atrial septal defect. If the atrial septal defect cannot be closed because of inadequate left-sided filling, the defect can be restricted in anticipation of delayed closure. The one-and-a-half ventricular approach has been used more commonly because it seems intuitively superior to total cavopulmonary connection [67,68]. However, there is no long-term evidence that demonstrates superiority of the one-and-a-half ventricular repair over univentricular circulation [69].

Patients with moderate right ventricular hypoplasia necessitating an initial combined systemic-pulmonary artery shunt and outflow tract procedure should undergo echocardiography at approximately 3 months of age for assessment of growth of the right ventricle and the tricuspid valve. Patients with growth of the right heart structures should undergo cardiac catheterization at 6 months of age. At catheterization the systemic-pulmonary artery shunt should be temporarily occluded. If adequate arterial oxygen saturation is maintained, permanent coil occlusion can be accomplished at this time. In addition, temporary closure of the atrial septal defect can be performed to determine whether the right ventricle is capable of carrying the entire cardiac output. Management options then become identical to those in the treatment of patients with mild right ventricular hypoplasia necessitating only an initial outflow tract procedure, as discussed in the preceding paragraph.

There are several options for patients with moderate hypoplasia who do not have adequate right ventricular growth to allow biventricular repair. The patient can be committed to univentricular circulation consisting of a bidirectional superior cavopulmonary shunt and takedown of the systemic-pulmonary artery shunt. Thereafter, suitability for completion Fontan versus one-and-a-half ventricular repair consisting of atrial septal defect closure with or without right ventricular outflow tract enlargement can be determined. A second option is to proceed with planned one-and-a-half ventricular repair at this stage. This approach consists of bidirectional superior caval anastomosis (with or without right ventricular outflow tract enlargement) and atrial septal defect closure. If atrial septal defect closure is not tolerated, the defect may be left restrictive with the intent of achieving closure at a subsequent procedure. A third option is the right ventricular overhaul approach advocated by Mee and colleagues [24]. This strategy consists of a second-stage procedure with cardiopulmonary bypass to perform tricuspid valvotomy with or without repair, infundibular muscle resection with repeated pulmonary valvotomy or transannular patch, and enlargement of the trabecular portion of the right ventricle by division of hypertrophied muscle bundles. The systemic-pulmonary artery shunt is left open at this time, and the atrial septal defect is restricted to enhance flow across the tricuspid valve to promote right ventricular growth. If right ventricular development is later judged adequate, the systemic-pulmonary artery shunt is occluded, and the atrial septal defect is closed to achieve biventricular repair. If inadequate right heart development occurs, then a one-and-a-half repair or univentricular approach is pursued. Although this approach has not been widely reported, impressive results with this strategy have been obtained in a few centers [24,37].

Surgical Technique

Relief of Right Ventricular Outflow Tract Obstruction

The main pulmonary artery and ductus arteriosus are dissected through a standard median sternotomy. If valvotomy is the intended procedure, it can be accomplished with or without cardiopulmonary bypass. If cardiopulmonary bypass or a concomitant systemic-pulmonary artery shunt is not planned, the distal pulmonary artery is clamped just proximal to the pulmonary artery bifurcation to allow pulmonary blood flow through the ductus arteriosus. Longitudinal pulmonary arteriotomy is performed, and the atretic pulmonary valve is examined. Stay sutures of 7-0 monofilament are placed at both ends of the arteriotomy to assist in clamp placement after valvotomy. A no. 11 blade scalpel is used to perforate the valve plate, and a hemostat is inserted to dilate the annulus. A side-biting vascular clamp is applied to control the arteriotomy, and the distal pulmonary artery clamp is released. The arteriotomy is then closed with the previously placed stay sutures.

When transannular patch is the intended procedure, venous drainage through a single right atrial cannula is sufficient if the atrial septal defect is adequate. Cardiopulmonary bypass is initiated, and the ductus arteriosus is temporarily occluded. Normothermic normocalcemic perfusion is maintained because aortic clamping is not necessary. The distal main pulmonary artery is clamped to enhance exposure, and the pulmonary artery is opened longitudinally. The pulmonary valve plate is incised in an anteroposterior direction, and the pulmonary artery incision is extended proximally across the annulus and carried into the right ventricular free wall until the communication into the right ventricular cavity is slightly smaller than normal. An opening of 7–8 mm is typical for the usual neonate. A dilator of the desired luminal diameter of the outflow tract is placed in the transannular incision, and an oval patch of 0.4-mm polytetrafluoroethylene is cut to the appropriate length and width to close the defect. The patch is sutured to the edges of the incision to complete the procedure. The patient is weaned from cardiopulmonary bypass. If systemic saturations are adequate, the ductus arteriosus is ligated.

Systemic-Pulmonary Artery Shunt

If a systemic-pulmonary artery shunt is to be performed alone, the modified Blalock-Taussig shunt can be approached through a right thoracotomy or median sternotomy. The thoracotomy allows spontaneous closure of the ductus arteriosus while the sternotomy enables ductal ligation if indicated. The distal innominate artery is dissected, and the proximal right subclavian artery is exposed. The pericardium is opened parallel to the phrenic nerve and anterior to the right pulmonary artery. The upper lobe branch and continuation of the right pulmonary artery are encircled with silk ligatures. An appropriately sized polytetrafluoroethylene conduit (usually 4 or 5 mm) is selected and beveled on one end. The patient is then given systemic heparin (100 units/kg). The beveled end of the conduit is sutured end to side to an arteriotomy in the proximal right subclavian artery. Thereafter the conduit is cut to the appropriate length without a bevel. The proximal right pulmonary artery is clamped, and tension is placed on the silk ligatures to control the distal branches of the pulmonary artery. The distal end of the shunt is sutured end to side into an arteriotomy placed proximal to the upper lobe branch of the right pulmonary artery. Shunt flow is established, and prostaglandin infusion is discontinued.

When a systemic-pulmonary artery shunt is performed concomitantly with a right ventricular outflow tract procedure, the technique is similar (modified Blalock-Taussig shunt) except that a median sternotomy approach is used. If cardiopulmonary bypass is intended, it is technically easier to perform the shunt during bypass, either before or after the right ventricular outflow tract procedure. After completion of the procedure, shunt flow is established, and the patient is weaned from cardiopulmonary bypass. The ductus arteriosus is ligated after adequate systemic oxygen saturation is confirmed. When cardiopulmonary bypass is not used, it is prudent to construct the shunt as the initial procedure. The rationale for this is that exposure during pulmonary valvotomy is improved by temporary occlusion of the ductus arteriosus and individual control of the branch pulmonary arteries; a clamp on the distal pulmonary artery is unnecessary. Single right lung perfusion is maintained through the shunt during the brief time required to perform the valvotomy, which is performed as described previously. When antegrade flow is established and adequate systemic saturation is confirmed, the ductus arteriosus is ligated.

Transcatheter Valvotomy

If the right ventricle is of adequate size, and the atretic valve has the usual membrane-like configuration, perforation of the pulmonary valve can be performed in the catheterization lab. Hand injections from both the infundibulum and the main pulmonary artery (retrograde via the ductus arteriosus) are usually adequate to characterize the anatomy of the right ventricular outflow tract. A catheter can be manipulated into position just below the valve. In some cases, a pinhole of antegrade flow can be demonstrated and a wire can be passed across the "atretic" valve. If no flow is appreciated, radiofrequency perforation can be performed [70]. Alternatively, the stiff end of a wire can be used if radiofrequency is not available or not successful. Obviously, the risk of unintended perforation outside the heart or pulmonary artery is not trivial and must be recognized immediately. Pericardiocentesis or surgical intervention may be required.

Recently, other innovative methods of decompressing the right heart have been described. Hybrid approaches, with valvuloplasty performed via a subxiphoid incision to access the right heart, have been used with success [71]. This approach was first employed during emergent treatment of perforation of the outflow tract during transcatheter radiofrequency perforation. Patients selected for this hybrid approach are first evaluated in standard fashion with a cardiac catheterization. The angle of catheter course to the right ventricular outflow tract via the tricuspid valve is evaluated. If deemed unsuitable for safe radiofrequency valve perforation, the hybrid method is employed from the subxiphoid approach. A sheath and dilator are introduced, rather than a ventriculotomy incision, and perforation and balloon dilation can be performed over a more direct course. The angle of approach from the base of the heart allows excellent alignment of the radiofrequency catheter with the infundibulum and valve plate. Similar to traditional transcatheter perforation, this does not necessarily obviate the need for additional intervention such as additional valvuloplasty or shunt placement, depending on the clinical course of the patient. Of the three patients in which this has been described, one required PV dilation and another returned for a shunt.

A report in 2006 concluded that balloon valvotomy alone for PA-IVS rarely obviates the need for an additional source of pulmonary blood flow provided by either a shunt or ductal stenting [72,73]. If shunt placement is needed after valvuloplasty, mid-term results from at least one center suggest eventual two, or one-and-one-half ventricle repair are often achievable in this population [74]. Anatomy that mandates a shunt at the outset, however, may be associated with early mortality. Similarly a study published in 2007 found that catheter interventions rarely avoid surgical repair and that right ventricle-dependent coronary circulation and Ebstein anomaly were associated with high mortality. These authors concluded that the single-ventricular pathway is likely a better strategy for these patient populations [62].

Intervention in the yet unborn child has been employed to potentially alter the course of congenital disease [75]. Attempted relief of right-sided obstruction by pulmonary valve dilation in utero is a newer technique that is under investigation at a limited number of centers. Evaluation of procedural success and longer-term outcomes is ongoing, and time will tell if fetal intervention has a role in management of right ventricular outflow obstruction.

Valvar Pulmonary Stenosis

Unlike PA-IVS, isolated pulmonary valvar stenosis is not commonly accompanied by major associated architectural anomalies of the other right heart components. Although pulmonary stenosis can be viewed as occupying the more favorable end of the spectrum of right heart obstructive lesions, the lack of major associated tricuspid valve and right ventricular structural abnormalities greatly simplifies diagnostic and therapeutic decision making relative to pulmonary atresia and intact septum. In reality, pulmonary stenosis represents an entity clinically distinct from PA-IVS. Pulmonary stenosis does, however, manifest with widely varying degrees of severity, and secondary infundibular hypertrophy can contribute to right ventricular obstruction. Unlike PA-IVS, which almost always manifests during the neonatal period, valvar pulmonary stenosis can manifest at any age. In subsequent discussion, the diagnosis and treatment of patients with pulmonary stenosis are considered separately for patients with disease manifesting in the neonatal period and for those who come to medical attention after the neonatal period.

Incidence and Etiology

Isolated pulmonary valvar stenosis is one of the most common cardiac defects, accounting for between 8% and 10% of all cases of congenital heart disease [76]. Patients with isolated severe pulmonary stenosis who need emergency intervention as neonates or young infants are only a small fraction of these patients [77]. The cause of pulmonary valvar stenosis is not known. Most theories are similar to those previously discussed for the cause of PA-IVS

[78,79]. Genetic factors play an important role in the patho-genesis of some cases. There is an increased prevalence of congenital heart disease among siblings of patients with isolated pulmonary valvar stenosis [80]. Familial cases of pulmonary stenosis have been described [81]. A number of clearly defined chromosomal abnormalities and genetic syndromes are accompanied by pulmonary valvar steno-sis, including Noonan's syndrome, trisomy 18, multiple lentigines (leopard syndrome), Watson syndrome, neurofi-bromatosis, and others [82–85].

Morphology

The morphology of the pulmonary valve in isolated valvar pulmonary stenosis has been categorized into six distinct anatomic subgroups [86]. These subgroups include domed, tricuspid, bicuspid, unicommissural, dysplastic, and hypo-plastic annulus. Regardless of subgroup the leaflets are almost always thickened, and in most types there is com-missural fusion. An important exception is the dysplastic type, which comprises approximately 10–20% of all cases of isolated valvar pulmonary stenosis. Most syndrome-associated cases of valvar pulmonary stenosis are of the dysplastic type. The dysplastic valve usually has three redundant and thickened leaflets, but the commissures are not fused. The annulus is hypoplastic, and both the infundibulum below the valve and the pulmonary artery above the valve are narrowed. Microscopic examination shows dysplastic valves are myxomatous with a paucity of elastic fibers [86]. Obstruction is because of the narrowing of the lumen at all levels of the pulmonary outflow tract and the excess bulk of the leaflet tissue. This finding has important therapeutic implications, which are addressed later.

Other associated right heart findings with pulmonary stenosis most likely represent secondary changes owing to valvar obstruction [78]. Poststenotic dilatation of the main pulmonary artery is common with most types, the notable exception being dysplastic valve. The degree of post-stenotic pulmonary artery dilatation does not correspond to the severity of valvar obstruction. Poststenotic dilatation is frequently more marked in older patients with relatively moderate degrees of obstruction. Right ventricular hyper-trophy is caused by the increased pressure load imposed on the right ventricle. This pressure overload is the funda-mental factor underlying the pathophysiologic mechanism of this lesion. Significant infundibular muscular obstruc-tion having both fixed and dynamic components frequently develops. Increased stress on the tricuspid valve may lead to chordal lengthening, annular dilatation, and tricuspid regurgitation. In neonates with critical pulmonary valvar stenosis, the tricuspid valve and right ventricle often are hypoplastic, and severe tricuspid regurgitation is common [87]. The right atrium often is dilated, the degree of dilata-tion corresponding to the degree of tricuspid regurgitation, and often is thickened [78]. A patent foramen ovale or atrial septal defect almost always is present in younger babies. In older infants and children, a patent foramen ovale or atrial septal defect is present more than two thirds of the time [88]. With very severe pulmonary valvar obstruction, subendocardial ischemia in the right ventricle can produce areas of myocardial infarction and fibrosis [89].

Critical Pulmonary Stenosis of the Neonate

Severe pulmonary valvar stenosis manifesting as cyanosis in the neonatal period is commonly called critical pulmo-nary stenosis. This term denotes both the severity of valvar obstruction and the critically ill nature of babies born with this condition. In a strict sense this clinical entity is defined by fetal pulmonary stenosis severe enough to limit right heart output and lead to a larger than normal right-to-left atrial level shunt in utero [76,77]. In most cases the pulmo-nary valve is tricuspid, and commissural fusion results in a small orifice. The dysplastic type valve rarely presents with critical pulmonary stenosis. There usually is only mild hypoplasia of the pulmonary annulus [87]. During fetal development, right heart growth may be limited by low flow through the right ventricle. Consequently, hypoplasia of the tricuspid valve and right ventricle is present in approximately 50% of neonates with critical pulmonary stenosis, and there usually is severe right ventricular hypertrophy [87]. Severe hypoplasia of the right ventricle is uncommon. Coronary fistulas are uncommon with criti-cal pulmonary stenosis, and right ventricular coronary dependency is encountered in only a small fraction of cases.

Pathophysiology and Natural History

Severe obstruction of right ventricular output and right ventricular hypertrophy are accompanied by decreased diastolic compliance and elevated right ventricular diasto-lic pressure. Tricuspid regurgitation usually is present. These factors combine to produce elevated right atrial pres-sure and a right-to-left shunt at the atrial level through the patent foramen ovale or atrial septal defect. Severely reduced right ventricular output renders the left side of the heart dependent on loading through the atrial level shunt. Marked restriction at the atrial level results in left heart preload inadequate to sustain adequate cardiac output. As with PA-IVS, pulmonary blood flow depends on the ductus arteriosus. Left heart output must be several times normal to supply adequate systemic and pulmonary perfusion. Consequently, left ventricular myocardial oxygen demand is increased. Similarly, right ventricular oxygen demand is increased owing to elevated wall tension resulting from severe pressure overload. Simultaneously, myocardial oxygen supply is compromised by the cyanosis resulting from the obligatory right-to-left atrial level shunt. Lower diastolic coronary perfusion pressure resulting from low-resistance runoff into the pulmonary circulation through the patent ductus arteriosus further compromises myocardial oxygen supply. Consequently, neonates with critical pulmonary stenosis are born in a precarious hemodynamic state. If the lesion is not detected soon after birth, closure of ductus arteriosus leads to decreased pulmonary blood flow, progressive hypoxemia, acidosis, cardiovascular collapse, and death. Not surprisingly, patients with this entity die within the first days to weeks of life. Longer survival is possible only when the ductus arteriosus remains patent and there is minimal restriction of atrial level shunting.

Presentation and Diagnosis

In the absence of associated syndromes, the body habitus is normal. Infants with critical pulmonary stenosis are cyanotic at birth and have systemic or suprasystemic right ventricular pressure. Most infants with this defect have an adequate atrial level shunt that allows maintenance of cardiac output. Patients come to medical attention in much the same way as infants with PA-IVS. If ductal closure ensues, the degree of cyanosis increases with progressive hemodynamic deterioration. Depending on the degree of pulmonary valve narrowing, antegrade flow of blood into the pulmonary arteries may be sufficient to allow relative stability in some patients. Tachypnea and tachycardia are typically present, and respiratory distress develops as cyanosis and metabolic deterioration progress before resuscitation. Auscultation may reveal a loud systolic ejection murmur at the upper left sternal border; however, in critically ill infants the murmur is often much softer because of diminished cardiac output and shunting of blood at the atrial level. Tricuspid insufficiency is commonly present and produces a holosystolic murmur at the lower left sternal border. A murmur associated with the ductus arteriosus may be heard in the upper sternal region. Cardiomegaly owing to right atrial enlargement may be evident on precordial palpation. Chest radiography confirms cardiomegaly and may show diminished vascular markings depending on the state of the ductus arteriosus. In most cases the electrocardiogram shows right axis deviation and right ventricular strain indicative of right ventricular hypertrophy.

Two-dimensional echocardiography with color Doppler examination is the diagnostic modality of choice. The anatomy and function of the pulmonary valve, tricuspid valve, and right ventricle, and patency of the foramen ovale and ductus arteriosus can be determined. Cardiac catheterization is complementary (Figure 21.7) [16] and is indicated when echocardiographic findings suggest the

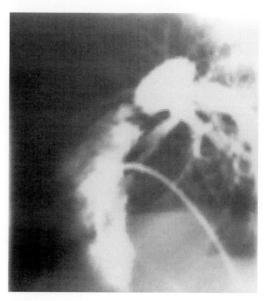

Figure 21.7 Angiographic representation of critical pulmonary stenosis. Well developed pulmonary arteries are evident.

diagnosis of critical pulmonary stenosis. Catheterization best shows pulmonary and coronary arterial morphology. Percutaneous balloon valvuloplasty is the management of choice of critical pulmonary stenosis [76,78,90,91]. Angiocardiography defines the severity and location of the obstructing components of pulmonary stenosis. The pulmonary valve annulus may be nearly normal or may be hypoplastic, and the right ventricle may be hypoplastic with filling defects, findings that indicate marked hypertrophy.

In most cases the diagnosis of critical pulmonary stenosis is readily made with the combination of physical examination and echocardiography. The differential diagnosis of critical pulmonary stenosis includes PA-IVS, tetralogy of Fallot, and severe Ebstein anomaly.

Management of Critical Pulmonary Stenosis

Most children born with critical pulmonary stenosis should eventually be able to undergo biventricular repair. As discussed later, this may necessitate interventional catheter techniques, surgery, or a combination of these modalities. Preinterventional management of critical pulmonary stenosis mirrors that of pulmonary atresia and intact septum. Intravenous access should be established and PGE_1 infusion initiated even before establishment of a definite diagnosis. Mechanical ventilation, inotropic support, and management of metabolic acidosis should be provided as needed. In unusual cases a restrictive atrial septal communication may mandate urgent or even emergency balloon atrial septostomy.

A surgical procedure for pulmonary stenosis in older children was first performed in the late 1940s [92–94]. The history of surgical pulmonary valvotomy is fascinating for the ingenuity involved and the number of notable cardiac surgeons who made contributions in this area [95–97]. A variety of techniques were developed, including closed techniques and open techniques with surface cooling, inflow occlusion, and cardiopulmonary bypass [98–101]. As surgical management of pulmonary stenosis evolved, it was used to treat younger and younger children, including neonates with critical pulmonary stenosis [87,98,102,103]. In the timeframe before percutaneous balloon valvuloplasty, the mortality associated with surgery for critical pulmonary stenosis was considerable and would no doubt be much lower today with state-of-the-art perioperative techniques. In 1982 the first successful outcome of percutaneous balloon valvuloplasty of congenital pulmonary stenosis was reported for an older child [90]. This treatment was quickly adapted to younger patients, including neonates [104–108]. Interventional catheter techniques with outcome equivalent to that of surgery have supplanted initial surgical management of this disease, and balloon valvuloplasty is now the treatment of choice [43,87,105,109–114]. There are no surgical series with which to compare outcome of balloon valvuloplasty during the same time period. Given that outcomes were nearly equivalent for the two techniques (6% mortality and similar gradient reduction) in the multicenter CHSS study [87] reported in 1993 and that balloon valvuloplasty has low morbidity, there has been no stimulus for further comparison.

The diagnosis of critical pulmonary stenosis is the indication for prompt treatment. After resuscitation, the urgency of the intervention is dependent on the patient's clinical status. If right ventricular function is preserved with an adequate atrial septal communication and patent ductus arteriosus, and the patient demonstrates hemodynamic stability, catheterization may be performed semi-electively on the first day or two of life. If the above is not true, and the baby is unstable, he or she should be taken immediately to the catheterization suite for diagnostic angiography followed by balloon valvuloplasty. Concurrent balloon atrial septostomy may be performed at this time when indicated. After successful decompression of the right ventricle, many patients continue to be cyanotic and need continued PGE_1 infusion to maintain adequate pulmonary blood flow. Diastolic compliance and right ventricular dysfunction may take considerable time to improve before adequate antegrade blood flow is achieved. Thereafter, the child should be weaned from PGE_1 infusion. Mild to moderate cyanosis may persist for weeks or even months after initial therapy because of continued right-to-left shunting at the atrial level. In most cases, dynamic right ventricular outflow tract obstruction owing to infundibular

muscle hypertrophy gradually regresses, diastolic compliance improves, and antegrade blood flow increases [115,116]. In some cases early recatheterization may be indicated on the basis of serial echocardiographic findings, and repeated balloon valvuloplasty may be used. Less commonly, cyanosis persists, and a surgical systemic-pulmonary artery shunt is needed to alleviate the need for PGE_1 infusion [87].

By 1 year of age, catheterization should be repeated for assessment of hemodynamics in children who remain cyanotic. Balloon occlusion of the atrial septum may determine whether complete separation of the two circulations is feasible, as described previously for PA-IVS. Thereafter the atrial septal defect can be closed either surgically or with a percutaneous atrial septal defect occlusion device. Management is similar for patients who need an early surgical systemic-pulmonary artery shunt, except that at repeated catheterization, test occlusion of the shunt should be performed to determine whether the shunt can be safely closed. If oxygenation remains adequate, coil occlusion can be accomplished percutaneously. Simultaneous test occlusion of the atrial septal defect should then be performed. If right atrial pressure does not increase, superior vena caval oxygen content remains stable, and systemic blood pressure is maintained, the atrial septal defect can usually be closed. In the situation in which surgical closure of the atrial septal defect is required, division of the shunt can be performed concomitantly. The atrial septal defect occasionally cannot be closed at this time, and assessment should be repeated within 6 months. If the shunt cannot be closed, a univentricular or one-and-a-half ventricular treatment strategy may be required. Decision making regarding these options is similar to that previously discussed for PA-IVS.

The primary indication for surgical treatment is unsuccessful balloon valvuloplasty. Because expertise with balloon valvuloplasty is widespread, the inability to transfer a child to an experienced center is now an uncommon indication for surgical intervention. In rare cases the pulmonary annulus or right ventricle may be markedly hypoplastic. Although the need for initial surgical management can be argued, the perception that balloon valvuloplasty does not prevent subsequent surgical intervention is prevalent, and almost all neonates undergo percutaneous treatment as the initial therapy. In the unusual circumstance in which initial surgical management is selected, there is no consensus about the appropriate surgical method or procedure. Options include open valvotomy, either under inflow occlusion or with cardiopulmonary bypass, and closed valvotomy. Reports comparing these options are now relatively outdated [98]. Given the safety and ability to perform a precise valvotomy, most surgeons favor the use of cardiopulmonary bypass. It is clear, however, that in the absence of severe right heart hypoplasia, initial treatment should include only direct relief of pulmonary stenosis [87]. The ductus arteriosus should be not be ligated so that PGE$_1$ infusion may be reinitiated in the event that antegrade blood flow is inadequate. A surgical shunt should be necessary in fewer than 10% of cases [87]. However, patients now referred for surgical treatment are likely to have marked pulmonary annulus and right ventricular hypoplasia. As with PA-IVS, establishment of antegrade right ventricular blood flow is required for right heart growth [55,87,117]. A transannular patch with surgical shunt may be required as initial treatment for patients with marked hypoplasia of the pulmonary annulus (Z value less than −3). This approach requires cardiopulmonary bypass. In any case the atrial septal defect should be left open initially. Subsequent evaluation and intervention are similar to those described for initial balloon valvuloplasty. Should right ventricular growth prove inadequate for biventricular repair, univentricular or one-and-a-half ventricular repair options must be assessed.

In the rare circumstance in which critical pulmonary stenosis is accompanied by coronary fistulas, management is not altered unless coronary artery stenosis or evidence of substantial right ventricle-dependent coronary circulation is present. In the latter case right ventricular decompression is contraindicated, and a surgical systemic-pulmonary artery shunt should be performed in anticipation of univentricular management. A similar approach should be considered for patients with concomitant Ebstein anomaly.

Outcome in Critical Pulmonary Stenosis

The only prospective, multicenter trial assessing outcome among infants with critical pulmonary stenosis was conducted by the CHSS, and the results were reported in 1993 [87]. The investigators evaluated 101 neonates from 27 institutions. The patients were initially treated by balloon valvuloplasty or one of a variety of surgical techniques. The overall survival rate was 89% at 1 month and 81% at 4 years (Figure 21.8) [87]. After initial treatment the right ventricular-to-pulmonary artery gradient was less than 30 mmHg in 81% of patients, and there were no differences between surgical and balloon valvuloplasty. There were no identifiable morphologic or other patient-specific risk factors for death. The lack of identified risk factors was probably because of the morphologic homogeneity of patients with critical pulmonary stenosis evaluated in this trial. Open pulmonary valvotomy without cardiopulmonary bypass or inflow occlusion was the only procedure that proved to be a risk factor for early death (Table 21.2) [87]. The survival rate after balloon valvuloplasty, open valvotomy (with cardiopulmonary bypass or inflow occlusion), and closed valvotomy was 94%. Reintervention of any type was necessary in 26% of cases and was similar for surgical and balloon valvuloplasty. Risk factors for requiring a systemic-pulmonary artery shunt were small right ventricular cavity and use of closed surgical valvotomy. Only two patients underwent subsequent Fontan proce-

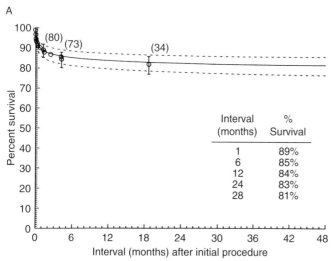

A

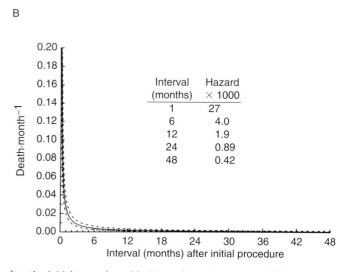

B

Figure 21.8 Survival and hazard function for death after the first procedure. Each circle represents an individual death, positioned along the horizontal axis at the time of death and actuarially (Kaplan-Meier) along the vertical axis. Vertical bars indicate 70% confidence interval of the actuarial estimates. Numbers in parentheses are the number of patients available for follow-up evaluation after the actuarial estimate. (By 24, 36, and 48 months

after the initial procedure, 29, 14, and 1 patient were still being observed.) Solid line indicates the continuous point estimate of survival (or hazard function in B obtained by a separate hazard function regression analysis). Dashed line encloses 70% confidence interval. **A,** Survival. **B,** Hazard function. (Reproduced with permission from Hanley *et al.* [87].)

dures, and 85% of patients had undergone correction to two-ventricle circulation within 48 months of study entry. All other patients in this study were predicted to be able to undergo biventricular repair within 6 years of study entry.

Because of the excellent results of balloon valvuloplasty, this intervention has become the dominant initial treatment strategy for patients with pulmonary stenosis, including critical pulmonary stenosis. Smaller and technically improved balloon catheters and increased experience with this technique have contributed to this trend. Unfortunately, few reports have detailed the long-term outcome among patients treated as neonates. The initial success, procedural survival, and likelihood of sustained relief of right ventricular outflow tract obstruction are higher for older children treated by balloon valvuloplasty than for neonates [112,118–120]. Successful balloon valvuloplasty can be achieved by experienced interventionalists in 90–95% of neonatal patients [111,120,121]. Approximately 5–10% of patients need a subsequent systemic-pulmonary artery shunt. The procedural mortality of balloon valvuloplasty in neonates is approximately 3–5%, and major complications occur in approximately 10% of cases [118,120,122,123]. In patients with pulmonary annulus hypoplasia necessitating a transannular patch, the risk of mortality is increased if a concomitant systemic-pulmonary artery shunt is not performed (Table 21.2) [87]. In this scenario, use of a combined transannular patch and systemic-pulmonary artery shunt is advised.

The rate of long-term freedom from reintervention, excluding patients who need an early systemic-pulmonary artery shunt, has been approximately 85% at 3–8 years [118,120]. Severe pulmonary valve insufficiency is uncommon in older children, but one report indicated that the use of oversized balloons in neonates carries substantial risk of late severe pulmonary valve insufficiency [124].

Surgical Technique for Critical Pulmonary Stenosis

The most common indication for surgical relief of critical pulmonary stenosis is unsuccessful balloon valvuloplasty. Lack of success usually is associated with the presence of extremely tight valvar obstruction, in which crossing the pinhole-like pulmonary valve can be very difficult.

Surgical valvotomy is achieved with a standard median sternotomy. Inflow caval occlusion or preferably cardiopulmonary bypass should be used. The aorta is cannulated in the standard manner. A single right atrial cannula is satisfactory for venous drainage because the atrial septal communication should be left alone. Before bypass is initiated, the ductus arteriosus is encircled with a tourniquet. Aortic occlusion is not necessary and should be avoided; therefore normothermic normocalcemic perfusion is used. After bypass is initiated, the ductus arteriosus is snared. Occlusion of each branch pulmonary artery facilitates exposure. The main pulmonary artery is opened longitudinally and the pulmonary valve is exposed. Careful commissurotomies are performed with a sharply pointed scalpel so that each commissure is incised into the wall of the pulmonary artery (Figure 21.9) [16]. The commissures frequently are tethered to the wall of the pulmonary artery so that valve motion is limited. Valve function is improved by careful release of each commissure from the sinus wall by precise sharp dissection. The main pulmonary artery is then closed. The branch pulmonary arteries are released, and cardiopulmonary bypass is discontinued. The ductus arteriosus should not be ligated permanently because temporary ductal patency may be necessary to allow adequate pulmonary blood flow until right ventricular function recovers. The results of balloon valvuloplasty indicate that aggressive transannular patching, subvalvar resection, and concomitant systemic-pulmonary artery shunts are only rarely necessary.

Table 21.2 Incremental risk factors for death any time after the initial accomplished procedure. (Reproduced with permission from Hanley *et al.* [87].)

Procedure	Single hazard phase *p* value
Open pulmonary valvotomy without inflow stasis or cardiopulmonary bypass	<.0001
Transannular patching without a shunt*	
(Smaller) Dimension of the right ventricular–pulmonary trunk junction	.01
(Greater) Degree of tricuspid incompetence	.0002
(Earlier) Date of procedure	.04

*Variables are interaction terms.

Valvar Pulmonary Stenosis in Older Infants and Children

Pathophysiology and Natural History

The pathophysiology of valvar pulmonary stenosis is directly related to the severity of obstruction of right ventricular output. The delayed presentation of this lesion in older children results from the progression of obstruction and secondary morphologic changes that occur if sustained elevation of right ventricular pressure is not corrected. Progression from moderate to severe valvar obstruction is

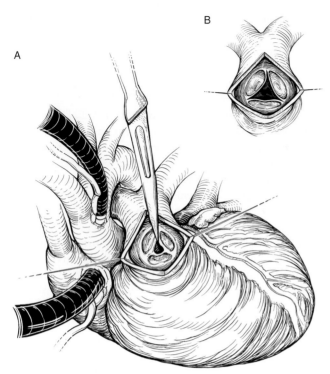

Figure 21.9 Technique of pulmonary valvulotomy. **A,** Fused leaflet commissures are incised to the pulmonary artery wall. **B,** Completed valvulotomy.

not usually because of relative underdevelopment of the pulmonary annulus, because the annular dimensions in older children and adults with this lesion are only mildly decreased in most cases. Progression of stenosis does not occur in all patients, and the underlying mechanism of progression is not known. Possible mechanisms of progression include increased demand for cardiac output owing to somatic growth with maintenance of a constant and reduced pulmonary valve orifice area [125]. The development of infundibular hypertrophy may contribute to the progression of obstruction. Increased pressure overload of the right ventricle causes muscle hypertrophy and increases myocardial oxygen demand while oxygen delivery is limited by decreased cardiac output. This condition can lead to subendocardial ischemia and myocardial infarction. As right heart failure ensues, right ventricular compliance decreases, and right atrial pressure increases. In the presence of atrial level communication, right-to-left flow can occur at the atrial level and produce cyanosis.

Early studies of the natural history of pulmonary stenosis were biased by selection criteria limited to patients undergoing cardiac catheterization [126,127]. These studies indicated that younger children were more likely than older children to have progression of stenosis and that rapid progression was more common among younger patients. Mody [126] found that more than one half of

children with moderate pulmonary stenosis diagnosed before 1 year of age had severe stenosis by the age of 5 years. Results of more recent studies with two-dimensional echocardiography with Doppler and color-flow mapping techniques confirmed that younger children are more likely to have lesions that progress to severe obstruction, although the likelihood of progression is lower than reported in older studies [128,129]. Most studies have shown that the degree of stenosis at initial diagnosis correlates with the progression of obstruction [130]. It has not been possible, however, to identify which children at a given age or with a given level of obstruction will have disease progression. One study conducted with serial echocardiographic examinations showed that 58% of children with mild or moderate stenosis actually had a decreasing degree of stenosis [131].

Presentation and Diagnosis

Most patients with isolated valvar pulmonary stenosis have no symptoms and exhibit normal growth. Asymptomatic lesions typically manifest when a pathologic heart murmur is detected at a physical examination performed for other reasons. Syndromic valvar pulmonary stenosis, such as Noonan's syndrome, commonly is identified early because of the recognized association of these syndromes with pulmonary stenosis. This lesion should be specifically sought in such patients. The onset of symptoms usually occurs after infancy and even into adulthood when the severity of stenosis and secondary right ventricular hypertrophy begins to limit cardiac output. Symptoms are absent in patients with mild and even moderate stenosis but become evident with exertion in some patients with moderate stenosis. Early symptoms include fatigue and exertional dyspnea. Only one fourth of patients with severe pulmonary stenosis are free of symptoms [78]. Patients with longstanding severe obstruction may have right-sided congestive heart failure. Patients with advanced right ventricular obstruction and a large atrial septal defect may have cyanosis. Other less common presenting symptoms associated with severe pulmonary stenosis include chest pain, syncope, and ventricular arrhythmias.

The differential diagnosis of isolated mild or moderate pulmonary stenosis in symptom-free children includes mild aortic stenosis, atrial septal defect, idiopathic dilatation of the main pulmonary artery, peripheral pulmonary artery stenosis, mitral valve prolapse, and innocent heart murmur. The differential diagnosis of severe pulmonary stenosis includes ventricular septal defect, ventricular septal defect with pulmonary stenosis, and moderate aortic stenosis [76,78].

Auscultatory findings include a normal first heart sound followed by a characteristic ejection click in patients with mild or moderate stenosis. As the severity of stenosis increases, the ejection click occurs earlier in systole until it merges with the first heart sound and may become inaudible in patients with severe stenosis. A prominent systolic ejection murmur is heard maximally at the upper left sternal border with radiation to the entire precordium, neck, and back. In general the intensity of the ejection murmur is proportional to the severity of stenosis, except in patients with advanced right-heart failure, in whom the murmur may be relatively soft owing to diminished cardiac output. The second heart sound usually is split, and the degree of splitting corresponds to the severity of stenosis. A wide, fixed, split second heart sound is indicative of associated atrial septal defect. Jugular venous distention occurs with a prominent A-wave pulse in cases of severe obstruction. In such patients hepatic enlargement and pulsation usually are present. At precordial examination a prominent right ventricular heave is present, and a systolic thrill usually is palpable in the left second intercostal space or at the suprasternal notch.

Abnormal electrocardiographic findings are present in most patients with moderate pulmonary stenosis and in almost all patients with severe stenosis. Right axis deviation occurs, and there is evidence of right ventricular hypertrophy. The height of the R wave in lead V_1 correlates with the degree of right ventricular hypertension. Heart size on chest radiographs usually is normal, although impressive cardiomegaly may be present in advanced cases. The most distinctive radiographic finding is prominence of a main pulmonary artery segment caused by the poststenotic dilatation present in most patients after infancy. The pulmonary vasculature usually is normal, but the lungs may appear oligemic in severe cases.

Two-dimensional echocardiography with color Doppler examination is the primary definitive diagnostic technique and should be used for all patients. This modality allows accurate assessment of both the valvar and subvalvar components of obstruction and is a noninvasive means of quantifying the severity of stenosis. Other cardiac lesions can be excluded. The morphology of the valve can be assessed, and in most cases the dysplastic pulmonary valve type can be identified. Right ventricular function and the degree of right ventricular hypertrophy can be evaluated. Tricuspid valve anatomy and function can be defined, and when tricuspid regurgitation is present, right ventricular pressure can be estimated. Acceleration of blood flow across the pulmonary valve allows estimation of the peak instantaneous pressure gradient between the right ventricle and the pulmonary artery. Last, the presence of atrial septal defect can be confirmed, and Doppler evaluation can be used to determine the direction of shunting at the atrial level. Findings at echocardiographic assessment of the severity of obstruction have been shown to correlate well with direct hemodynamic measurements obtained at cardiac catheterization [132].

The ability to accurately diagnose and grade the severity of pulmonary stenosis has made cardiac catheterization a technique primarily reserved for therapeutic intervention rather than a diagnostic tool. However, the grading criteria for severity of valvar pulmonary stenosis were established with hemodynamic measurements, and angiography still contributes useful anatomic details in the evaluation of patients for whom either operative or percutaneous intervention is warranted. Angiography illustrates the anatomy of the right ventricular outflow tract, and doming of the pulmonary valve is a characteristic finding. Angiography is useful in assessing the anatomy of the main and branch pulmonary arteries. The grading scale of pulmonary stenosis is based on the measurements of right and left ventricular pressure and the peak-to-peak gradient measured across the right ventricular outflow tract. These definitions are based on the assumption that the patient is in the resting state and has normal cardiac output. In a healthy patient, resting right ventricular systolic pressure is 30 mmHg or less, and the gradient across the pulmonary valve is less than 10 mmHg. Mild pulmonary stenosis is defined as a right ventricular outflow tract pressure gradient less than 40 mmHg and a right ventricular-to-left ventricular pressure ratio of 0.5 or less. Moderate stenosis is defined as a pressure gradient greater than 40 mmHg but less than 80 mmHg and a right ventricular-to-left ventricular pressure ratio greater than 0.5 but less than 1.0. Severe stenosis is defined as a pressure gradient of 80 mmHg or greater and a right ventricular-to-left ventricular pressure ratio of 1.0 or greater [78].

Management of Pulmonary Stenosis

Percutaneous Balloon Valvuloplasty

Percutaneous balloon valvuloplasty is the treatment of choice for nearly all patients who need intervention for isolated valvar pulmonary stenosis. All patients with symptoms should undergo intervention. Specific treatment is not indicated if the patient has asymptomatic mild pulmonary stenosis. These patients need only careful surveillance with serial physical examinations and echocardiography for detection of progression of obstruction. Cardiac catheterization is indicated if symptoms develop or echocardiography shows progression of obstruction. Older studies with long-term follow-up evaluation of patients with pulmonary valvar gradients ranging from 50–79 mmHg who were treated medically showed that most of these patients eventually needed intervention [130]. Balloon valvuloplasty after the neonatal period carries very low risk of morbidity and mortality and is highly efficacious. Consequently, most authorities recommend that any patient with a pulmonary valve gradient greater than 50 mmHg undergo balloon valvuloplasty. It seems logical to intervene at this stage to avoid the long-term deleterious effects of right ventricular hypertrophy that may lead to the development of myocardial fibrosis [76]. Patients in whom recurrent pulmonary stenosis develops after previous percutaneous or surgical intervention also need repeated balloon valvuloplasty as the first-line treatment.

Management of dysplastic pulmonary valvar stenosis is controversial. In this type there usually is no commissural fusion. The mechanism of balloon valvuloplasty is the splitting of fused leaflet tissue present in the other types of pulmonary stenosis. In the dysplastic type, subannular narrowing, annular hypoplasia, lack of commissural fusion, unusual leaflet tethering, and the mass of dysplastic valvar tissue all contribute to obstruction and complicate balloon valvuloplasty. Early results of balloon valvuloplasty for this type of valve revealed a high failure rate; however, adequate relief has been reported in 35–65% of cases [112,133,134]. Consequently, balloon pulmonary valvuloplasty usually is still recommended for first-line management of dysplastic pulmonary valvar stenosis [76,78]. Surgical therapy is reserved for patients who do not respond to balloon valvuloplasty.

The intermediate results of balloon valvuloplasty in children and adults with pulmonary valvar stenosis have been excellent [111,112,133,135,136]. Predictors of poor intermediate outcome of balloon valvuloplasty include smaller pulmonary annulus size and a higher immediate residual gradient. Long-term results of balloon pulmonary valvuloplasty remain limited. Compared with patients treated surgically, patients undergoing balloon valvuloplasty have had a lower incidence of late moderate or severe pulmonary insufficiency requiring pulmonary valve replacement [136]. However, there have been no direct comparisons of patients treated percutaneously with surgical patients over a contemporaneous period. The long-term survival rate after surgical intervention for this disease is 97% at 25 years. It is reasonable to assume that survival after balloon valvuloplasty will be equally excellent [130].

Surgical Management

Surgery for pulmonary valvar stenosis has been supplanted by balloon valvuloplasty. There have been no recent reports of early results of surgery for this lesion, because surgery now is used only rarely. The early mortality of surgical valvotomy in the most recently published surgical series has ranged from 0–4% [27,102,137]. Consequently, it is reasonable to state that surgery in the current era carries very low risk. The primary indications for surgical pulmonary valvotomy are failure of balloon valvotomy and anatomy unsuitable for successful valvotomy. The most common type managed surgically is dysplastic pulmonary valve. Because annular hypoplasia is a substantial component of obstruction, pulmonary valvotomy or valvectomy alone is rarely sufficient operative management, and a transannular patch

with subvalvar resection is more commonly needed. Nearly all such patients have at least moderate pulmonary insufficiency. In general this condition is well tolerated in the medium term. However, the long-term deleterious effects of unmanaged clinically significant pulmonary insufficiency have been recognized, and replacement of the pulmonary valve may be necessary for many of these patients.

Surgical Technique

Standard median sternotomy with bicaval and aortic cannulation is used for surgical pulmonary valvotomy. This approach allows the surgeon to close any associated atrial septal communication and facilitates transatrial resection of obstructing infundibular muscle bundles and precise valvotomy. Cardioplegia is not necessary for cases in which simple valvotomy or transannular patching is performed. However, if transatrial resection of obstructing muscle bundles is to be performed, cardioplegic arrest is required. In the unusual circumstance of operation for simple valvar pulmonary stenosis with typical poststenotic dilatation, a transverse pulmonary arteriotomy is made, and commissural fusion is sharply divided back into the wall of the pulmonary artery. Valvar tethering is released with sharp dissection, and thickened valve edges are trimmed. Primary closure of the pulmonary artery is then performed with monofilament suture. More commonly, marked annular hypoplasia is present (diameter two standard deviations below normal or smaller), and a transannular incision is needed. In this case longitudinal arteriotomy is preferred. Commissural fusion when present is addressed as described previously. The arteriotomy is extended through the anteriorly located commissure and crosses the annulus into the right ventricular muscle just until a dilator of appropriate size can be passed retrograde through the valve. Obstructive infundibular muscle bundles are divided to further relieve right ventricular outflow tract obstruction. In the case of a dysplastic pulmonary valve with no commissural fusion, the valve is resected, and a transannular incision is made as necessary. After muscle resection, the transannular incision is closed with a patch of autologous pericardium or 0.4 mm polytetrafluoroethylene with an appropriately sized dilator for judging the width of patch necessary to provide adequate relief of obstruction. Before the right ventricular outflow tract is closed, the heart is either arrested with cardioplegia or electrically fibrillated, and the atrial septal defect or patent foramen ovale is closed. Closure of the right ventricular outflow tract can be accomplished during reperfusion. If there is marked right ventricular dysfunction or hypoplasia, the atrial septal defect should not be completely closed. In the case of patent foramen ovale the atrial communication should be left open at this time. The patient is then weaned from cardiopulmonary bypass. Intraoperative transesophageal echocardiography is recommended to aid in assessing residual gradients, valvar insufficiency, shunt direction at the atrial septum when left open, and ventricular function.

Other Forms of Isolated Right Ventricular Outflow Tract Obstruction

Supravalvar Pulmonary Artery Stenosis

Supravalvar main pulmonary artery stenosis is a very rare lesion. It occurs most commonly in association with Noonan's syndrome and occasionally with Williams' syndrome. In rare instances this form of arterial stenosis occurs in the absence of an associated syndrome. The indications for management of such stenosis mirror those for isolated pulmonary stenosis. However, the primary mode of management is surgical, as supravalvar narrowing is frequently resistant to balloon angioplasty. In most cases simple patch enlargement is all that is needed.

Peripheral pulmonary artery stenosis is much more common and can affect the branch or intraparenchymal pulmonary arteries. In most cases balloon angioplasty with or without intravascular stenting, often on a recurrent basis, is preferred when treatment is needed.

Primary Infundibular Stenosis

Primary infundibular stenosis accounts for approximately 5% of all cases of isolated right ventricular outflow tract obstruction [76]. This entity manifests similarly to isolated pulmonary valvar stenosis after the neonatal period. The diagnosis is made with echocardiography. The indications for treatment are identical to those for valvar pulmonary stenosis. Unlike pulmonary valvar stenosis, management of primary infundibular stenosis is surgical. There are two distinct types of primary infundibular stenosis. In one type there is fibromuscular thickening in the wall of the right ventricular infundibulum. This process exists immediately below the pulmonary valve and can extend into the proximal portion of the infundibulum. Treatment consists of longitudinal infundibulotomy with patch enlargement. In most cases the pulmonary valve is normal, therefore, the incision must be kept below the annulus of the pulmonary valve to avoid damage to the valve. Recently, stent placement in the right ventricular outflow tract has been used as a palliative modality to enable patient growth before definitive surgical repair [138].

The other type of primary infundibular stenosis is characterized by an obstructive fibrous muscle band at the junction of the main right ventricular cavity and the proximal infundibulum. This lesion is often referred to as double-chambered right ventricle. Surgical treatment can usually be accomplished by transatrial resection of the obstructing band, but in some cases a right ventriculotomy is needed [139].

Conclusion

The category *isolated right ventricular outflow tract obstruction* encompasses a wide range of complexity from lesions that are among the easiest to treat to anomalies that are the most difficult to manage successfully. It is clear that catheter intervention alone or combined with surgery is currently and increasingly important among the therapeutic alternatives for these abnormalities. Frequently associated pathologies of the right ventricle, tricuspid valve, and coronary arteries continue to negatively impact outcomes in these patients. In a small group of the most complex cases, cardiac transplantation is the most reasonable option.

References

1. Daubeney PE, Sharland GK, Cook AC, *et al.* (1998) Pulmonary atresia with intact ventricular septum: impact of fetal echocardiography on incidence at birth and postnatal outcome. UK and Eire Collaborative Study of Pulmonary Atresia with Intact Ventricular Septum. Circulation 98, 562–566.
2. Leonard H, Derrick G, O'Sullivan J, *et al.* (2000) Natural and unnatural history of pulmonary atresia. Heart 84, 499–503.
3. Ferencz C, Rubin JD, McCarter RJ, *et al.* (1985) Congenital heart disease: prevalence at livebirth. The Baltimore-Washington Infant Study. Am J Epidemiol 121, 31–36.
4. Zuberbuhler JR, Anderson RH. (1979) Morphological variations in pulmonary atresia with intact ventricular septum. Br Heart J 41, 281–288.
5. Freedom RM. (1989) *Pulmonary Atresia with Intact Ventricular Septum*. Mt Kisco, NY: Futura.
6. Kutsche LM, Van Mierop LH. (1983) Pulmonary atresia with and without ventricular septal defect: a different etiology and pathogenesis for the atresia in the 2 types? Am J Cardiol 51, 932–935.
7. Freedom RM, Nykanen DG. (2001) Pulmonary atresia and intact ventricular septum. In: Allen HD, Clarke DR, Gutgesell HP, *et al.*, eds. *Moss and Adams' Heart Disease in Infants, Children, and Adolescents*, 6th ed. Philadelphia, PA: Lippincott Williams & Wilkins.
8. Allan LD, Crawford DC, Tynan MJ. (1986) Pulmonary atresia in prenatal life. J Am Coll Cardiol 8, 1131–1136.
9. Reddy VM, Ungerleider RM, Hanley FL. (1998) Pulmonary valve atresia with intact ventricular septum. In: Garson AG Jr, Bricker JT, Fischer DJ, eds. *The Science and Practice of Pediatric Cardiology*, 2nd ed. Baltimore, MD: Williams & Wilkins.
10. Li C, Chudley AE, Soni R, *et al.* (2003) Pulmonary atresia with intact ventricular septum and major aortopulmonary collaterals: association with deletion 22q11.2. Pediatr Cardiol 24, 585–587.
11. De Stefano D, Li P, Xiang B, *et al.* (2008) Pulmonary atresia with intact ventricular septum (PA-IVS) in monozygotic twins. Am J Med Genet A 146A, 525–528.

12. Gelb BD. (1997) Molecular genetics of congenital heart disease. Curr Opin Cardiol 12, 321–328.

13. Grossfeld PD, Lucas VW, Sklansky MS, *et al.* (1997) Familial occurrence of pulmonary atresia with intact ventricular septum. Am J Med Genet 72, 294–296.

14. Chitayat D, McIntosh N, Fouron JC. (1992) Pulmonary atresia with intact ventricular septum and hypoplastic right heart in sibs: a single gene disorder? Am J Med Genet 42, 304–306.

15. Fricker FL, Zuberbuhler JR. (1987) Pulmonary atresia with intact ventricular septum. In: Anderson RH, Macartney FJ, Shinebourne EA, eds. *Pediatric Cardiology.* White Plains, NY: Churchill Livingstone.

16. Mitchell MB, Clarke DR. (2003) Isolated right ventricular outflow tract obstruction. In: Mavroudis C, Backer CL, eds. *Pediatric Cardiac Surgery*, 3rd ed. Philadelphia, PA: Mosby, Inc.

17. Choi YH, Seo JW, Choi JY, *et al.* (1998) Morphology of tricuspid valve in pulmonary atresia with intact ventricular septum. Pediatr Cardiol 19, 381–389.

18. Hanley FL, Sade RM, Blackstone EH, *et al.* (1993) Outcomes in neonatal pulmonary atresia with intact ventricular septum. A multiinstitutional study. J Thorac Cardiovasc Surg 105, 406–423, 424–427; discussion 423–424.

19. Anderson RH, Silverman NH, Zuberbuhler JR. (1990) Congenitally unguarded tricuspid orifice: its differentiation from Ebstein's malformation in association with pulmonary atresia and intact ventricular septum. Pediatr Cardiol 11, 86–90.

20. Bull C, de Leval MR, Mercanti C, *et al.* (1982) Pulmonary atresia and intact ventricular septum: a revised classification. Circulation 66, 266–272.

21. Lewis AB, Wells W, Lindesmith GG. (1986) Right ventricular growth potential in neonates with pulmonary atresia and intact ventricular septum. J Thorac Cardiovasc Surg 91, 835–840.

22. Shaddy RE, Sturtevant JE, Judd VE, *et al.* (1990) Right ventricular growth after transventricular pulmonary valvotomy and central aortopulmonary shunt for pulmonary atresia and intact ventricular septum. Circulation 82(5 Suppl), IV157–IV163.

23. Gittenberger-de Groot AC, Sauer U, Bindl L, *et al.* (1988) Competition of coronary arteries and ventriculo-coronary arterial communications in pulmonary atresia with intact ventricular septum. Int J Cardiol 18, 243–258.

24. Pawade A, Capuani A, Penny DJ, *et al.* (1993) Pulmonary atresia with intact ventricular septum: surgical management based on right ventricular infundibulum. J Card Surg 8, 371–383.

25. Bulkley BH, D'Amico B, Taylor AL. (1983) Extensive myocardial fiber disarray in aortic and pulmonary atresia. Relevance to hypertrophic cardiomyopathy. Circulation 67, 191–198.

26. Fyfe DA, Edwards WD, Driscoll DJ. (1986) Myocardial ischemia in patients with pulmonary atresia and intact ventricular septum. J Am Coll Cardiol 8, 402–406.

27. Kirklin JW, Barratt-Boyes BG. (1993) Pulmonary atresia and intact ventricular septum. In: Kirklin JW, Barratt-Boyes BG, eds. *Cardiac Surgery*, 2nd ed. New York, NY: Churchill Livingstone.

28. McArthur JD, Munsi SC, Sukumar IP, *et al.* (1971) Pulmonary valve atresia with intact ventricular septum. Report of a case with long survival and pulmonary blood supply from an anomalous coronary artery. Circulation 44, 740–745.

29. Robicsek F, Bostoen H, Sanger PW. (1966) Atresia of the pulmonary valve with normal pulmonary artery and intact ventricular septum in a 21 year-old woman. Angiology 17, 896–901.

30. Dyamenahalli U, McCrindle BW, McDonald C, *et al.* (2004) Pulmonary atresia with intact ventricular septum: management of, and outcomes for, a cohort of 210 consecutive patients. Cardiol Young 14, 299–308.

31. Jahangiri M, Zurakowski D, Bichell D, *et al.* (1999) Improved results with selective management in pulmonary atresia with intact ventricular septum. J Thorac Cardiovasc Surg 118, 1046–1055.

32. Rychik J, Levy H, Gaynor JW, *et al.* (1998) Outcome after operations for pulmonary atresia with intact ventricular septum. J Thorac Cardiovasc Surg 116, 924–931.

33. de Leval M, Bull C, Hopkins R, *et al.* (1985) Decision making in the definitive repair of the heart with a small right ventricle. Circulation 72, II52–II60.

34. Giglia TM, Jenkins KJ, Matitiau A, *et al.* (1993) Influence of right heart size on outcome in pulmonary atresia with intact ventricular septum. Circulation 88, 2248–2256.

35. McCaffrey FM, Leatherbury L, Moore HV. (1991) Pulmonary atresia and intact ventricular septum. Definitive repair in the neonatal period. J Thorac Cardiovasc Surg 102, 617–623.

36. Minich LL, Tani LY, Ritter S, *et al.* (2000) Usefulness of the preoperative tricuspid/mitral valve ratio for predicting outcome in pulmonary atresia with intact ventricular septum. Am J Cardiol 85, 1325–1328.

37. Sano S, Ishino K, Kawada M, *et al.* (2000) Staged biventricular repair of pulmonary atresia or stenosis with intact ventricular septum. Ann Thorac Surg 70, 1501–1506.

38. Salvin JW, McElhinney DB, Colan SD, *et al.* (2006) Fetal tricuspid valve size and growth as predictors of outcome in pulmonary atresia with intact ventricular septum. Pediatrics 118, e415–e420.

39. Hawkins JA, Thorne JK, Boucek MM, *et al.* (1990) Early and late results in pulmonary atresia and intact ventricular septum. J Thorac Cardiovasc Surg 100, 492–497.

40. Amodeo A, Keeton BR, Sutherland GR, *et al.* (1991) Pulmonary atresia with intact ventricular septum: is neonatal repair advisable? Eur J Cardiothorac Surg 5, 17–21.

41. Bowman FO Jr, Malm JR, Hayes CJ, *et al.* (1971) Pulmonary atresia with intact ventricular septum. J Thorac Cardiovasc Surg 61, 85–95.

42. de Leval M, Bull C, Stark J, *et al.* (1982) Pulmonary atresia and intact ventricular septum: surgical management based on a revised classification. Circulation 66, 272–280.

43. Jureidini SB, Rao PS. (1996) Critical pulmonary stenosis in the neonate: role of transcatheter management. J Invasive Cardiol 8, 326–331.

44. Justo RN, Nykanen DG, Williams WG, *et al.* (1997) Transcatheter perforation of the right ventricular outflow tract as initial therapy for pulmonary valve atresia and intact ventricular septum in the newborn. Cathet Cardiovasc Diagn 40, 408–413.

45. Latson LA. (1991) Nonsurgical treatment of a neonate with pulmonary atresia and intact ventricular septum by transcatheter puncture and balloon dilation of the atretic valve membrane. Am J Cardiol 68, 277–279.

46. Lewis AB, Wells W, Lindesmith GG. (1983) Evaluation and surgical treatment of pulmonary atresia and intact ventricular septum in infancy. Circulation 67, 1318–1323.

47. Milliken JC, Laks H, Hellenbrand W, *et al.* (1985) Early and late results in the treatment of patients with pulmonary atresia and intact ventricular septum. Circulation 72, II61–II69.

48. Ovaert C, Qureshi SA, Rosenthal E, *et al.* (1998) Growth of the right ventricle after successful transcatheter pulmonary valvotomy in neonates and infants with pulmonary atresia and intact ventricular septum. J Thorac Cardiovasc Surg 115, 1055–1062.

49. Trusler GA, Yamamoto N, Williams WG, *et al.* (1976) Surgical treatment of pulmonary atresia with intact ventricular septum. Br Heart J 38, 957–960.

50. Wang JK, Wu MH, Chang CI, *et al.* (1999) Outcomes of transcatheter valvotomy in patients with pulmonary atresia and intact ventricular septum. Am J Cardiol 84, 1055–1060.

51. Williams WG, Burrows P, Freedom RM, *et al.* (1991) Thromboexclusion of the right ventricle in children with pulmonary atresia and intact ventricular septum. J Thorac Cardiovasc Surg 101, 222–229.

52. Metzdorff MT, Pinson CW, Grunkemeier GL, *et al.* (1986) Late right ventricular reconstruction following valvotomy in pulmonary atresia with intact ventricular septum. Ann Thorac Surg 42, 45–51.

53. Patel RG, Freedom RM, Moes CA, *et al.* (1980) Right ventricular volume determinations in 18 patients with pulmonary atresia and intact ventricular septum. Analysis of factors influencing right ventricular growth. Circulation 61, 428–440.

54. Rao PS, Liebman J, Borkat G. (1976) Right ventricular growth in a case of pulmonic stenosis with intact ventricular septum and hypoplastic right ventricle. Circulation 53, 389–394.

55. Weldon CS, Hartmann AF Jr, McKnight RC. (1984) Surgical management of hypoplastic right ventricle with pulmonary atresia or critical pulmonary stenosis and intact ventricular septum. Ann Thorac Surg 37, 12–24.

56. Graham TP Jr, Bender HW, Atwood GF, *et al.* (1974) Increase in right ventricular volume following valvulotomy for pulmonary atresia or stenosis with intact ventricular septum. Circulation 50(2 Suppl), II69–II79.

57. Yoshimura N, Yamaguchi M, Ohashi H, *et al.* (2003) Pulmonary atresia with intact ventricular septum: strategy based on right ventricular morphology. J Thorac Cardiovasc Surg 126, 1417–1426.

58. Giglia TM, Mandell VS, Connor AR, *et al.* (1992) Diagnosis and management of right ventricle-dependent coronary circulation in pulmonary atresia with intact ventricular septum. Circulation 86, 1516–1528.

59. Powell AJ, Mayer JE, Lang P, *et al.* (2000) Outcome in infants with pulmonary atresia, intact ventricular septum, and right ventricle-dependent coronary circulation. Am J Cardiol 86, 1272–1274, A9.

60. Bergersen L, Foerster S, Marshall AC, *et al.* (2009) Pulmonary atresia with intact ventricular septum (PA-IVS). *Congenital Heart Disease: The Catheterization Manual.* Boston, MA: Springer Science and Business Media, LLC.

61. Guleserian KJ, Armsby LB, Thiagarajan RR, *et al.* (2006) Natural history of pulmonary atresia with intact ventricular septum and right-ventricle-dependent coronary circulation managed by the single-ventricle approach. Ann Thorac Surg 81, 2250–2257; discussion 2258.

62. Hirata Y, Chen JM, Quaegebeur JM, *et al.* (2007) Pulmonary atresia with intact ventricular septum: limitations of catheter-based intervention. Ann Thorac Surg 84, 574–579; discussion 579–580.

63. Starnes VA, Pitlick PT, Bernstein D, *et al.* (1991) Ebstein's anomaly appearing in the neonate. A new surgical approach. J Thorac Cardiovasc Surg 101, 1082–1087.

64. Freeman JE, DeLeon SY, Lai S, *et al.* (1993) Right ventricle-to-aorta conduit in pulmonary atresia with intact ventricular septum and coronary sinusoids. Ann Thorac Surg 56, 1393–1395.

65. Laks H, Gates RN, Grant PW, *et al.* (1995) Aortic to right ventricular shunt for pulmonary atresia and intact ventricular septum. Ann Thorac Surg 59, 342–347.

66. Asou T, Matsuzaki K, Matsui K, *et al.* (2000) Veno-venous bypass to prevent myocardial ischemia during right heart bypass operation in PA, IVS, and RV dependent coronary circulation. Ann Thorac Surg 69, 955–956.

67. Kreutzer C, Mayorquim RC, Kreutzer GO, *et al.* (1999) Experience with one and a half ventricle repair. J Thorac Cardiovasc Surg 117, 662–668.

68. Miyaji K, Shimada M, Sekiguchi A, *et al.* (1995) Pulmonary atresia with intact ventricular septum: long-term results of "one and a half ventricular repair". Ann Thorac Surg 60, 1762–1764.

69. Hanley FL. (1999) The one and a half ventricle repair-we can do it, but should we do it? J Thorac Cardiovasc Surg 117, 659–661.

70. Lee ML, Tsao LY, Chiu HY, *et al.* (2009) Outcomes in neonates with pulmonary atresia and intact ventricular septum underwent pulmonary valvulotomy and valvuloplasty using a flexible 2-French radiofrequency catheter. Yonsei Med J 50, 245–251.

71. Burke RP, Hannan RL, Zabinsky JA, *et al.* (2009) Hybrid ventricular decompression in pulmonary atresia with intact septum. Ann Thorac Surg 88, 688–689.

72. McLean KM, Pearl JM. (2006) Pulmonary atresia with intact ventricular septum: initial management. Ann Thorac Surg 82, 2214–2219; discussion 2219–2220.

73. Michel-Behnke I, Akintuerk H, Thul J, *et al.* (2004) Stent implantation in the ductus arteriosus for pulmonary blood supply in congenital heart disease. Catheter Cardiovasc Interv 61, 242–252.

74. Hannan RL, Zabinsky JA, Stanfill RM, *et al.* (2009) Midterm results for collaborative treatment of pulmonary atresia with intact ventricular septum. Ann Thorac Surg 87, 1227–1233.

75. Tworetzky W, Marshall AC. (2004) Fetal interventions for cardiac defects. Pediatr Clin North Am 51, 1503–1513, vii.

76. Latson LA, Prieto LR. (2001) Pulmonary stenosis. In: Allen HD, Clark EB, Gutgesell HP, *et al.*, eds. *Moss and Adams' Heart Disease in Infants, Children, and Adolescents*, 6th ed. Philadelphia, PA: Lippincott Williams & Wilkins.

77. Freed MD, Rosenthal A, Bernhard WF, *et al.* (1973) Critical pulmonary stenosis with a diminutive right ventricle in neonates. Circulation 48, 875–881.

78. Cheatham JP. (1998) Pulmonary stenosis. In: Garson AGJ, Bricker JT, Fischer DJ, eds. *The Science and Practice of Pediatric Cardiology*, 2nd ed. Baltimore, MD: Williams & Wilkins.

79. Oka M, Angrist A. (1967) Mechanism of cardiac valvular fusion and stenosis. Am Heart J 74, 37–47.

80. Campbell M. (1962) Factors in the aetiology of pulmonary stenosis. Br Heart J 24, 625–632.

81. Klinge T, Laursen HB. (1975) Familial pulmonary stenosis with underdeveloped or normal right ventricle. Br Heart J 37, 60–64.

82. Gorlin RJ, Anderson RC, Blaw M. (1969) Multiple lentigenes syndrome. Am J Dis Child 117, 652–662.

83. Noonan J, O'Connor W. (1996) Noonan syndrome: a clinical description emphasizing the cardiac findings. Acta Paediatr Jpn 38, 76–83.

84. Rosenquist GC, Krovetz LJ, Haller JA Jr, *et al.* (1970) Acquired right ventricular outflow obstruction in a child with neurofibromatosis. Am Heart J 79, 103–108.

85. Watson GH. (1967) Pulmonary stenosis, cafe-au-lait spots, and dull intelligence. Arch Dis Child 42, 303–307.

86. Gikonyo BM, Lucas RV, Edwards JE. (1987) Anatomic features of congenital pulmonary valvar stenosis. Pediatr Cardiol 8, 109–116.

87. Hanley FL, Sade RM, Freedom RM, *et al.* (1993) Outcomes in critically ill neonates with pulmonary stenosis and intact ventricular septum: a multiinstitutional study. Congenital Heart Surgeons Society. J Am Coll Cardiol 22, 183–192.

88. Roberts WC, Shemin RJ, Kent KM. (1980) Frequency and direction of interatrial shunting in valvular pulmonic stenosis with intact ventricular septum and without left ventricular inflow or outflow obstruction. An analysis of 127 patients treated by valvulotomy. Am Heart J 99, 142–148.

89. Franciosi RA, Blanc WA. (1968) Myocardial infarcts in infants and children. I. A necropsy study in congenital heart disease. J Pediatr 73, 309–319.

90. Kan JS, White RI Jr, Mitchell SE, *et al.* (1982) Percutaneous balloon valvuloplasty: a new method for treating congenital pulmonary-valve stenosis. N Engl J Med 307, 540–542.

91. Tynan M, Jones O, Joseph MC, *et al.* (1984) Relief of pulmonary valve stenosis in first week of life by percutaneous balloon valvuloplasty. Lancet 1, 273.

92. Blalock A, Kieffer RF Jr. (1950) Valvulotomy for the relief of congenital valvular pulmonic stenosis with intact ventricular septum; report of 19 operations by the Brock method. Ann Surg 132, 496–516.

93. Brock RC. (1948) Pulmonary valvulotomy for the relief of congenital pulmonary stenosis; report of three cases. Br Med J 1, 1121–1126.

94. Sellers TH. (1948) The surgery of pulmonary stenosis. Lancet 1, 988.

95. Swan H, Cleveland HC, Mueller H, *et al.* (1954) Pulmonic valvular stenosis; results and technique of open valvuloplasty. J Thorac Surg 28, 504–515.

96. Hessel EA 2nd, Dillard DH, Winterscheid LC, *et al.* (1965) Surgical treatment of pulmonic stenosis with intact ventricular septum with the use of cardiopulmonary bypass. Report of 26 cases and a review of the literature. J Thorac Cardiovasc Surg 49, 796–812.

97. Tandon R, Nadas AS, Gross RE. (1965) Results of open-heart surgery in patients with pulmonic stenosis and intact ventricular septum. A report of 108 cases. Circulation 31, 190–201.

98. Awariefe SO, Clarke DR, Pappas G. (1983) Surgical approach to critical pulmonary valve stenosis in infants less than six months of age. J Thorac Cardiovasc Surg 85, 375–387.

99. Daskalopoulos DA, Pieroni DR, Gingell RL, *et al.* (1982) Closed transventricular pulmonary valvotomy in infants. J Thorac Cardiovasc Surg 84, 187–191.

100. Mistrot J, Neal W, Lyons G, *et al.* (1976) Pulmonary valvulotomy under inflow stasis for isolated pulmonary stenosis. Ann Thorac Surg 21, 30–37.

101. Sade RM, Crawford FA, Hohn AR. (1982) Inflow occlusion for semilunar valve stenosis. Ann Thorac Surg 33, 570–575.

102. Jonas RA, Castaneda AR, Norwood WI, *et al.* (1985) Pulmonary valvotomy under normothermic caval inflow occlusion. Aust N Z J Surg 55, 39–44.

103. Srinivasan V, Konyer A, Broda JJ, *et al.* (1982) Critical pulmonary stenosis in infants less than three months of age: a reappraisal of closed transventricular pulmonary valvotomy. Ann Thorac Surg 34, 46–50.

104. Ali Khan MA, al-Yousef S, Huhta JC, *et al.* (1989) Critical pulmonary valve stenosis in patients less than 1 year of age: treatment with percutaneous gradational balloon pulmonary valvuloplasty. Am Heart J 117, 1008–1014.

105. Hofbeck M, Singer H, Buheitel G, *et al.* (1999) Balloon valvuloplasty of critical pulmonary valve stenosis in a premature neonate. Pediatr Cardiol 20, 147–149.

106. Ladusans EJ, Qureshi SA, Parsons JM, *et al.* (1990) Balloon dilatation of critical stenosis of the pulmonary valve in neonates. Br Heart J 63, 362–367.

107. Rey C, Marache P, Francart C, *et al.* (1988) Percutaneous transluminal balloon valvuloplasty of congenital pulmonary valve stenosis, with a special report on infants and neonates. J Am Coll Cardiol 11, 815–820.

108. Zeevi B, Keane JF, Fellows KE, *et al.* (1988) Balloon dilation of critical pulmonary stenosis in the first week of life. J Am Coll Cardiol 11, 821–824.

109. Cheung YF, Leung MP, Lee JW, *et al.* (2000) Evolving management for critical pulmonary stenosis in neonates and young infants. Cardiol Young 10, 186–192.

110. Fedderly RT, Beekman RH 3rd. (1995) Balloon valvuloplasty for pulmonary valve stenosis. J Interv Cardiol 8, 451–461.

111. Fedderly RT, Lloyd TR, Mendelsohn AM, *et al.* (1995) Determinants of successful balloon valvotomy in infants with critical pulmonary stenosis or membranous pulmonary atresia with intact ventricular septum. J Am Coll Cardiol 25, 460–465.

112. McCrindle BW. (1994) Independent predictors of long-term results after balloon pulmonary valvuloplasty. Valvuloplasty and Angioplasty of Congenital Anomalies (VACA) Registry Investigators. Circulation 89, 1751–1759.

113. Rao PS. (1996) Balloon valvuloplasty in the neonate with critical pulmonary stenosis. J Am Coll Cardiol 27, 479–480.

114. Thanopoulos B, Triposkiadis F, Tsaousis GS. (1997) Single-stage balloon valvuloplasty for critical pulmonary valve stenosis in the neonate. Cathet Cardiovasc Diagn 40, 322–325.

115. Fontes VF, Esteves CA, Sousa JE, *et al.* (1988) Regression of infundibular hypertrophy after pulmonary valvuloplasty for pulmonic stenosis. Am J Cardiol 62, 977–979.

116. Thapar MK, Rao PS. (1989) Significance of infundibular obstruction following balloon valvuloplasty for valvar pulmonic stenosis. Am Heart J 118, 99–103.

117. Merrill WH, Shuman TA, Graham TP Jr, *et al.* (1987) Surgical intervention in neonates with critical pulmonary stenosis. Ann Surg 205, 712–718.

118. Colli AM, Perry SB, Lock JE, *et al.* (1995) Balloon dilation of critical valvar pulmonary stenosis in the first month of life. Cathet Cardiovasc Diagn 34, 23–28.

119. Stanger P, Cassidy SC, Girod DA, *et al.* (1990) Balloon pulmonary valvuloplasty: results of the Valvuloplasty and Angioplasty of Congenital Anomalies Registry. Am J Cardiol 65, 775–783.

120. Tabatabaei H, Boutin C, Nykanen DG, *et al.* (1996) Morphologic and hemodynamic consequences after percutaneous balloon valvotomy for neonatal pulmonary stenosis: medium-term follow-up. J Am Coll Cardiol 27, 473–478.

121. Velvis H, Raines KH, Bensky AS, *et al.* (1997) Growth of the right heart after balloon valvuloplasty for critical pulmonary stenosis in the newborn. Am J Cardiol 79, 982–984.

122. Gildein HP, Kleinert S, Goh TH, *et al.* (1996) Treatment of critical pulmonary valve stenosis by balloon dilatation in the neonate. Am Heart J 131, 1007–1011.

123. Gournay V, Piechaud JF, Delogu A, *et al.* (1995) Balloon valvotomy for critical stenosis or atresia of pulmonary valve in newborns. J Am Coll Cardiol 26, 1725–1731.

124. Berman W Jr, Fripp RR, Raisher BD, *et al.* (1999) Significant pulmonary valve incompetence following oversize balloon pulmonary valveplasty in small infants: a long-term follow-up study. Catheter Cardiovasc Interv 48, 61–65; discussion 66.

125. Danilowicz D, Hoffman JI, Rudolph AM. (1975) Serial studies of pulmonary stenosis in infancy and childhood. Br Heart J 37, 808–818.

126. Mody MR. (1975) The natural history of uncomplicated valvular pulmonic stenosis. Am Heart J 90, 317–321.

127. Nugent EW, Freedom RM, Nora JJ, *et al.* (1977) Clinical course in pulmonary stenosis. Circulation 56(1 Suppl), I38–I47.

128. Anand R, Mehta AV. (1997) Natural history of asymptomatic valvar pulmonary stenosis diagnosed in infancy. Clin Cardiol 20, 377–380.

129. Rowland DG, Hammill WW, Allen HD, *et al.* (1997) Natural course of isolated pulmonary valve stenosis in infants and children utilizing Doppler echocardiography. Am J Cardiol 79, 344–349.

130. Hayes CJ, Gersony WM, Driscoll DJ, *et al.* (1993) Second natural history study of congenital heart defects. Results of treatment of patients with pulmonary valvar stenosis. Circulation 87(2 Suppl), I28–I37.

131. Gielen H, Daniels O, van Lier H. (1999) Natural history of congenital pulmonary valvar stenosis: an echo and Doppler cardiographic study. Cardiol Young 9, 129–135.

132. Currie PJ, Hagler DJ, Seward JB, *et al.* (1986) Instantaneous pressure gradient: a simultaneous Doppler and dual catheter correlative study. J Am Coll Cardiol 7, 800–806.

133. Masura J, Burch M, Deanfield JE, *et al.* (1993) Five-year follow-up after balloon pulmonary valvuloplasty. J Am Coll Cardiol 21, 132–136.

134. Rao PS. (1988) Balloon dilatation in infants and children with dysplastic pulmonary valves: short-term and intermediate-term results. Am Heart J 116, 1168–1173.

135. McCrindle BW, Kan JS. (1991) Long-term results after balloon pulmonary valvuloplasty. Circulation 83, 1915–1922.

136. O'Connor BK, Beekman RH, Lindauer A, *et al.* (1992) Intermediate-term outcome after pulmonary balloon valvuloplasty: comparison with a matched surgical control group. J Am Coll Cardiol 20, 169–173.

137. Kopecky SL, Gersh BJ, McGoon MD, *et al.* (1988) Long-term outcome of patients undergoing surgical repair of isolated pulmonary valve stenosis. Follow-up at 20–30 years. Circulation 78, 1150–1156.

138. Dohlen G, Chaturvedi RR, Benson LN, *et al.* (2009) Stenting of the right ventricular outflow tract in the symptomatic infant with tetralogy of Fallot. Heart 95, 142–147.

139. Alva C, Ho SY, Lincoln CR, *et al.* (1999) The nature of the obstructive muscular bundles in double-chambered right ventricle. J Thorac Cardiovasc Surg 117, 1180–1189.

CHAPTER 22

Tetralogy of Fallot

Robert D. Stewart,[1] Constantine Mavroudis,[2] and Carl L. Backer[3]

[1]Cleveland Clinic Children's Hospital, Cleveland, OH, USA
[2]Florida Hospital for Children, Orlando, FL, USA
[3]Ann & Robert H. Lurie Children's Hospital of Chicago, formerly Children's Memorial Hospital, Chicago, IL, USA

Definition, Morphology, and Nomenclature

Arthur Louis Etienne Fallot was born in 1850 in southern France, and after studying medicine in Marseilles, went on to become Professor of Hygiene and Legal Medicine. In 1888, he published a 104-page treatise entitled "Contribution a 'l'anatomie pathologique de la maladie bleue [1]." He used "tetralogie" to refer to the aggregate of four features of the anatomy seen in the majority of specimens coming into his autopsy service from patients with "la maladie bleue": pulmonary artery stenosis, ventricular septal communication, rightward deviation of the aorta's origin, and hypertrophy of the right ventricle (Figure 22.1) [2]. This characteristic morphology had in fact been recognized and illustrated long before Fallot's description. The first published report is from 1671 by the Danish monk, Niels Stenson, famous for his description of the parotid duct, who described the association of lesions after observing the findings in an ectopic heart from a fetus [3]. The first attribution to Fallot came from Ambrose Birmingham, a Professor of Anatomy at the Catholic University in Dublin, Ireland. He called the constellation of lesions "Pentalogy of Fallot" in 1892, adding the common presence of an atrial septal defect (ASD) [4]. However, widespread use of the term tetralogy of Fallot (TOF) did not follow until its use by Maude Abbott in an article on the classification of congenital heart defects published by Dawson and Abbott in 1924 [5].

More recently, attempts have been made to identify one of the four anatomic features as being paramount. This, of course, acknowledges that it is most likely that the four features of pathologic anatomy are collectively secondary consequences of a common pathway of altered cardiac development, as opposed to the possibility that they rep-resent four "coincident" errors of morphogenesis. Van Praagh and his colleagues asserted that it was underdevelopment of the subpulmonary infundibulum that was the primary feature, stating that this part of the heart was "too narrow, too shallow, and too short" [6,7]. Anderson and associates observed that the infundibulum is unequivocally narrow and hypoplastic, but that its length is variable, and that in many hearts with TOF the infundibulum is longer than normal [8,9]. They suggested that anterocephalad deviation of the insertion of the infundibular septum relative to the septomarginal trabeculation was the key feature. Further investigation suggested that this was not a completely satisfactory unifying hypothesis. First, the outlet septum could be deviated in anterocephalad fashion without producing subpulmonary obstruction, as in the Eisenmenger defect [10]. Second, in some hearts, there could be subpulmonary obstruction when the outlet septum was fibrous, rather than muscular. A more satisfactory explanation does involve anterocephalad deviation of the outlet septum, be it muscular or fibrous, but requires an abnormal relation of the outlet septum to the septoparietal trabeculations, producing subpulmonary obstruction [11].

The ventricular septal defect (VSD) occurs as a result of the anterocephalad malalignment and deviation of the insertion of the infundibular septum relative to the limbs of the septomarginal trabeculation. The resulting hole between the ventricles is directly beneath the overriding aortic valvar orifice. Thus, Anderson considers it an outlet defect [11], while others refer to it as a malaligned cono-ventricular defect. The VSD in TOF is large and, in nearly all instances, physiologically nonrestrictive. In most cases, the ventriculoinfundibular fold stops short of the posteroinferior limb of the septomarginal trabeculation, resulting in fibrous continuity between the aortic and tricuspid

Pediatric Cardiac Surgery, Fourth Edition. Edited by Constantine Mavroudis and Carl L. Backer.
© 2013 Blackwell Publishing Ltd. Published 2013 by Blackwell Publishing Ltd.

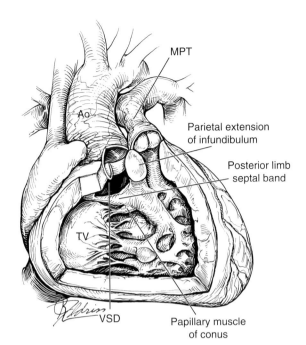

Figure 22.1 Pathologic anatomy of tetralogy of Fallot demonstrating a nonrestrictive malalignment VSD with aortic override. Right ventricular outflow tract obstruction caused by hypertrophied parietal and septal bands and the hypoplastic main pulmonary trunk and valve. (Ao, aorta; MPT, main pulmonary trunk; VSD, ventricular septal defect; TV, tricuspid valve.)

valves. Such defects are accurately described as perimembranous. Less often, there is muscular continuity throughout the right ventricular margins of the defect. In such cases, the muscular fold located inferoposteriorly, together with the membranous septum, separates the conduction tissues from the crest of the ventricular septum. There is then yet a third variety of defect, characterized by presence of a fibrous rather than a muscular outlet septum. This is the doubly committed and juxta-arterial defect, by far the least common in the western world, but commoner in the Far East and South America.

In addition to the variability described above with respect to the limits of the VSD, the spectrum of TOF with pulmonary stenosis (as opposed to atresia) is characterized by several other important anatomic variants, as well as associated malformations. Anterior and cephalad deviation of the outlet septum results in varying degrees of right ventricular outflow tract (RVOT) obstruction, related to hypoplasia of the right ventricular infundibulum and the presence of prominent septoparietal muscle bands or trabeculations, which tend to undergo progressive hypertrophy postnatally. A localized narrowing, or os infundibulum, frequently occurs at the inferior border of the right ventricular infundibulum. In most cases, the pulmonary

valve morphology is abnormal, frequently with thickened immobile leaflets, often with commissural fusion and/or tethering of leaflets to the pulmonary artery wall. The pulmonary valve ring or annulus is hypoplastic in comparison to normal hearts, and the pulmonary valve is bicuspid in more than half of cases [12]. More distal levels of RVOT obstruction include hypoplasia or discrete stenoses within the main pulmonary trunk and/or the branch pulmonary arteries. Not uncommonly there is a discrete narrowing with a fibrous shelf within the left branch pulmonary artery at a level corresponding to the site of insertion of the ductus arteriosus.

Other anatomical variants include the presence of one or more additional VSDs, which occur in approximately 5% of cases [13]. Most commonly, the secondary defects are located anteriorly, within the muscular septum. Variants of coronary artery anatomy are seen in TOF, with the most common being origin of the anterior descending coronary artery from the right coronary artery [14,15]. In such cases the anterior descending artery traverses the anterior surface of the RVOT a short distance below the pulmonary annulus. It is susceptible to injury if a ventriculotomy incision is required to affect repair. Less commonly, there is dual supply to the anterior interventricular septum, with branches originating from both the right coronary artery and the left main coronary artery. Rarer still is origin of all coronary branches from a single ostium within the right sinus of Valsalva. Other TOF-associated congenital heart defects include complete atrioventricular septal defect (AVSD; described in more detail later in this chapter), patent foramen ovale (PFO) or ostium secundum type ASD, patent ductus arteriosus (PDA), persistent left superior vena cava, ductal origin of one branch pulmonary artery (most often the left pulmonary artery), and right-sided aortic arch, which is seen in 15–25% of patients [16].

Pulmonary atresia is present in approximately 7% of patients with TOF [17]. An important distinction is made between those with a PDA and those without. When there is a PDA in the setting of TOF with pulmonary atresia, it is most often the only source of pulmonary blood flow. In such cases, there may be varying degrees of hypoplasia of the pulmonary arteries, but it is most often the case that all or nearly all lung segments are supplied by branches arborizing from the right and left pulmonary arteries. In the absence of a PDA, pulmonary artery arborization is much less predictable, and varying amounts of pulmonary parenchyma are supplied partially or entirely by multiple major aortopulmonary collateral arteries (MAPCAs). The clinical presentation and natural history of this variant is considerably different from that of the more typical TOF, and a variety of distinctive treatment strategies have evolved. Pulmonary atresia with VSD and MAPCAs is described in detail in Chapter 23, *Surgical Treatment of Pulmonary Atresia with Ventricular Septal Defect.*

In view of the contemporary understanding of the path-ologic anatomy, the issue of a unifying definition of TOF was debated by the International Working Group for Mapping and Coding of Nomenclatures for Pediatric and Congenital Cardiac Disease in 2008. The following consensus definition was adopted: *Tetralogy of Fallot is defined as a group of malformations with biventricular atrioventricular alignments or connections characterized by anterosuperior deviation of the conal or outlet septum or its fibrous remnant, narrowing or atresia of the pulmonary outflow, a ventricular septal defect of the malalignment type, and biventricular origin of the aorta. Hearts with tetralogy of Fallot will always have a ventricular septal defect, narrowing or atresia of the pulmonary outflow, and aortic override; hearts with tetralogy of Fallot will most often have right ventricular hypertrophy* [18]. The diagnostic choices used for coding in the contemporary version of the Society of Thoracic Surgeons Congenital Heart Surgery Database are listed in Table 22.1 [19]. In the database, however, pulmonary atresia with VSD is not linked in a hierarchical fashion to TOF, acknowledging that not all cases of pulmonary atresia with VSD can be conclusively said to fall within the category of TOF.

Tetralogy of Fallot and associated variants are thought to constitute as much as 10% of all forms of congenital heart disease, and TOF is the most common form of cyanotic congenital heart disease with an incidence of 421 cases per million live births [20]. In a recent report of the Society of Thoracic Surgeons Congenital Heart Surgery Database outcomes of 67 596 operations on 59 163 patients between July 2004 and June 2008, 3518 (5.2%) of all operations were performed on patients with a primary diagnosis of TOF (exclusive of pulmonary atresia with VSD) [21].

Genetic syndromes are identified in at least 20% of TOF patients. The most common associated syndrome is DiGeorge syndrome, which results from one of several known deletions on chromosome 22 (del 22q11). In one

study looking specifically at associated genetic syndromes in 306 patients with TOF, 28% had genetic defects or syndromes, of which 32% were del 22q11, 15% were trisomy 21, and 14% were VACTERL [22].

History of Surgical Management

One of the most significant and exciting accomplishments by any of the pioneers of congenital heart surgery is the historical "blue baby operation" by Dr. Alfred Blalock in 1944 [23]. Helen Taussig, the physician in charge of the pediatric cardiology clinic at Johns Hopkins Hospital hypothesized that creation of an arterial duct would confer significant relief of the hypoxemia of patients with TOF. Taussig took her idea to Blalock, who had previously proposed an operation to bypass coarctation of the aorta based on turning down the divided distal end of the left subclavian artery. Coincidentally, Vivien Thomas, the research assistant in Blalock's surgical laboratory had created a canine model to study pulmonary arterial hypertension in which the divided distal end of a branch of the subclavian artery was connected to a pulmonary artery. Ironically, while this model failed to reliably create pulmonary arterial hypertension, it was precisely the equivalent of the artificial duct sought by Taussig. On November 29, 1944, Alfred Blalock performed the first operation on a cyanotic 1-year-old child with TOF. The Blalock-Taussig shunt had a high rate of success, and by 1950, 1000 such operations had been performed by Blalock and his team [24].

In the same timeframe, other surgical pioneers of the time devised a variety of related closed-heart procedures, either to address obstruction within the RVOT or to augment pulmonary blood flow by creation of a systemic-to-pulmonary arterial shunt. In London in 1948, Thomas Holmes Sellors and Russell Claude Brock separately described the use of genitourinary sounds to probe and dilate the RVOT [25,26]. Charles Bailey later reported treating eight patients with TOF in Philadelphia with the Brock procedure [27]. In Chicago, Willis Potts created an anastomosis between the descending thoracic aorta and the left pulmonary artery [28]. Alternatively, David Waterston developed posterior anastomosis of the ascending aorta to the right pulmonary artery [29]. These side-to-side connections were touted as being more easily created than the Blalock-Taussig shunt in very small infants. Thousands of patients benefited from the Potts shunts and Waterston shunts, which at the time were intended as definitive palliation. Unfortunately, they also posed a significant challenge to take down.

The first intracardiac repair of TOF was by C. Walton Lillehei and his team at the University of Minnesota during their remarkable series of 45 cross-circulation cases that started on March 26, 1954 [30]. On August 31 of that same year, Lillehei, Varco, and Warden performed the first suc-

Table 22.1 The diagnostic short list of the version of The International Pediatric and Congenital Cardiac Code. Derived from the International Congenital Heart Surgery Nomenclature and Database Project of The European Association for Cardio-Thoracic Surgery and The Society of Thoracic Surgeons. (AVC, atrioventricular canal; AVSD, atrioventricular septal defect; DORV, double-outlet right ventricle; PA, pulmonary atresia; VSD, ventricular septal defect; VSD-MAPCA, ventricular septal defect–multiple aortopulmonary collateral artery.)

TOF (tetralogy of Fallot)
TOF, Pulmonary stenosis
TOF, Absent pulmonary valve
TOF, AVC (AVSD)
DORV, TOF type
Pulmonary atresia, VSD (including TOF, PA)
Pulmonary atresia, VSD-MAPCA (pseudotruncus)

cessful repair of TOF on a 10-year-old boy [31]. Unique among the cross-circulation cases, this operation was the first where cross-circulation did not involve the parent or a relative as the circulatory donor, but rather a random volunteer with compatible blood type who was recruited by the Red Cross. The patient was the first of 10 patients with TOF who underwent repair using cross-circulation, and he was one of six survivors, a remarkable feat given the ground-breaking nature of the endeavor [32]. An additional technical milestone developed by Lillehei and his team was the development of a patch to close the VSD. This patch was used in the last three patients after the experience of primary VSD closure in the initial seven. One year after the Lillehei team's success, John Kirklin performed the first successful repair of TOF using extracorporeal support with a mechanical pump oxygenator at the Mayo Clinic in 1955 [33].

Presentation and Diagnosis

Tetralogy of Fallot is a common cyanotic congenital heart defect [20], however, only a small percentage of patients present with deep cyanosis in the neonatal period following closure of the PDA. These are colloquially referred to as "blue TETs" in contradistinction to the acyanotic "pink TETs." Among the group of acyanotic TOF patients, a few may have normal arterial oxygen saturation measurements and even present with signs of pulmonary overcirculation if the pulmonary stenosis is mild. More typically there is initial mild desaturation in the range of 80–90% depending on the presence of a PDA and the degree of pulmonary stenosis. The infants with profound cyanosis typically have severe valvar level stenosis, or near atresia. Occasionally, these patients remain undiagnosed in the presence of a moderate to large PDA and can present days or weeks after birth with profound cyanosis after ductal closure. When this presentation is at a time where ductal patency cannot be re-established with prostaglandin infusion, it represents an emergent surgical situation to establish adequate pulmonary blood flow. The most common natural progression of acyanotic TOF patients is slowly decreasing baseline saturations as they develop progressive right ventricular hypertrophy and subvalvar stenosis. Close follow-up of acyanotic TOF patients is required to provide appropriate timing of intervention before the development of moderate to severe cyanosis. Acyanotic and mildly cyanotic TOF patients can also develop episodic profound hypercyanosis. These "TET spells" result from dynamic changes in the relative pulmonary and systemic resistances leading to severe right to left shunting through the VSD with systemic oxygen saturations often dropping well below 50%. The most commonly touted, though unproven, etiology for hypercyanotic spells is infundibular muscle spasms leading to a large dynamic

increase in the subvalvar obstruction with resulting right-to-left shunting through the VSD.

Clinical exam is notable for varying degrees of cyanosis, from slight pallor to marked generalized cyanosis. Clubbing can occasionally be seen in advanced cases. Auscultation reveals a systolic murmur from the right ventricular outflow obstruction. During a "TET spell" this murmur will soften or disappear as a result of the limited flow through the RVOT. Because of the large size of the VSD and systemic level pressure in the right ventricle, little or no VSD murmur is typically appreciated. The second heart sound is usually not split as the small, abnormal pulmonary valve and low poststenotic pulmonary pressures often do not create a sound. Electrocardiography shows marked right ventricular hypertrophy and a right axis deviation, however, these findings are neither specific nor diagnostic. Chest X-rays may show the classic "boot-shaped" heart resulting from right ventricular hypertrophy and small pulmonary arterial knob (Figure 22.2). The right aortic arch present in 15–25% of patients with TOF may be appreciated on chest X-ray. The lung fields are generally dark as a result of relative hypoperfusion. Echocardiography is the primary diagnostic modality in the vast majority of cases (Figure 22.3). The combination of M-mode and Doppler echocardiography provides a complete evaluation of the TOF anatomy [34,35] including estimations of the pressure gradient at the subvalvar, valvar, and supravalvar levels of the RVOT. Echocardiography has been shown to reliably determine the coronary pattern in the majority of cases, including left anterior descending artery from the right coronary artery [36]. Prenatal echocardiography increasingly makes the in utero diagnosis of TOF and has a high degree of accuracy, though it cannot fully determine the degree of pulmonary stenosis [37]. There is no clear evidence that prenatal diagnosis benefits long-term survival [38].

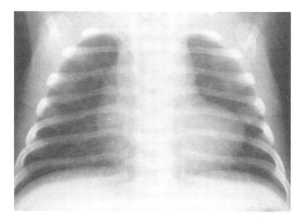

Figure 22.2 Typical chest radiograph of the boot-shaped heart in a patient with tetralogy of Fallot. This appearance results from right ventricular hypertrophy and hypoplasia of the main pulmonary artery.

Three-dimensional echocardiography has yet to prove any substantial benefit over two-dimensional studies for diagnosis and preoperative assessment. However, three-dimensional echocardiography may prove an important modality for long-term follow-up of morphological and functional changes to the right ventricle in repaired TOF [39]. Cardiac catheterization was the gold standard for diagnosis of TOF before the advancements in echocardiography and Doppler technology. Most patients with TOF currently do not require cardiac catheterization before reparative surgery (Figure 22.4). The most common current indications for cardiac catheterization are unclear anatomy of the branch pulmonary arteries and confirmation of the presence of a left anterior descending artery from the right coronary crossing anterior to the RVOT. This is particularly important in any patient who had a palliative operation where the branch pulmonary artery architecture may be distorted and where the postoperative adhesions on the right ventricle may obscure an unsuspected anomalous coronary artery. Axial imaging with three-dimensional reconstruction, including computed tomography (CT) scan and magnetic resonance imaging (MRI), have an important role in the evaluation of TOF. Before complete repair, these modalities can be used as an alternative to cardiac catheterization as they may reveal branch pulmonary artery and aortic arch anatomy and also delineate coronary anomalies. Cardiac magnetic resonance imaging (CMR) is emerging as one of the most useful studies for long-term evaluation of the repaired TOF patient (Figure 22.5) [2].The volumetric measurements of the right ventricle and quantification of pulmonary regurgitant fraction and right ventricular function are superior to those obtained by means of two-dimensional echocardiography [40–42]. Such CMR measurements are becoming the benchmarks for timing of reinterventions, most importantly regarding the timing of pulmonary valve insertion or replacement [43,44]. Finally, postnatal screening with pulse oximetry has been used to detect unsuspected congenital heart defects including TOF, but has failed to demonstrate cost effectiveness [45,46].

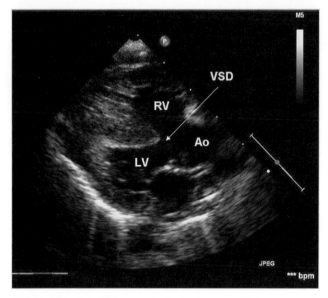

Figure 22.3 Two-dimensional echocardiogram with a parasternal long access view of a patient with tetralogy of Fallot. The large unrestrictive malalignment ventricular septal defect is clearly evident with significant aortic override. (Ao, aorta; LV, left ventricle; RV, right ventricle; VSD, ventricular septal defect.)

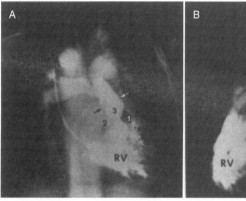
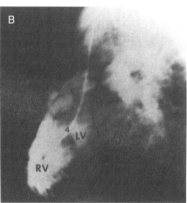
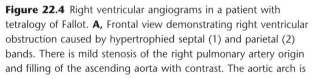

Figure 22.4 Right ventricular angiograms in a patient with tetralogy of Fallot. **A,** Frontal view demonstrating right ventricular obstruction caused by hypertrophied septal (1) and parietal (2) bands. There is mild stenosis of the right pulmonary artery origin and filling of the ascending aorta with contrast. The aortic arch is on the right and the left Blalock-Taussig shunt is visible. **B,** The lateral view demonstrates the right ventricular obstruction with anterior displacement of the infundibular (conal) septum. The stenotic pulmonary valve is seen. Contrast material outlines the VSD (4) and the left ventricle (LV). (RV, right ventricle.)

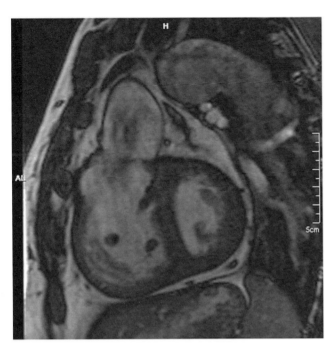

Figure 22.5 Cardiac magnetic resonance image with a sagittal view of a patient with long-standing repaired tetralogy of Fallot. The right ventricle is significantly dilated, and there is severe pulmonary insufficiency.

Medical Management

There is no long-term medical solution for TOF, and the definitive treatment is surgical repair. However, there are a few significant medical adjuncts; most important of these being the use of prostaglandin E1 (PGE₁) to maintain ductal patency in profoundly cyanotic neonates with TOF [47]. Administered as a continuous intravenous infusion at a dose of 0.01–0.1 μg/kg/min, PGE₁ will open and maintain the ductus arteriosus thus providing blood flow until surgical correction or establishment of a systemic to pulmonary shunt. The use of PGE₁ is primarily limited to the first week of life. Administration of PGE₁ to infants presenting after that point is less likely to result in opening of the duct, with success after 2 weeks being rare. The most significant unwanted side effect of PGE₁ infusion is apnea, which often necessitates endotracheal intubation and mechanical ventilation. The majority of other medical treatments are aimed at preventing or treating "TET spells." Beta-blockade is used by some cardiologists, with the theoretical objective of reducing the incidence of spasm of the infundibular muscle of the RVOT. There is conflicting evidence concerning the effectiveness of this therapy [48,49]. The downside of continued use of beta-blockade in TOF patients is that it has been shown to increase the need for inotrope use and temporary pacing following surgical repair [50]. These findings favor earlier surgical intervention for patients who

require beta-blockade for paroxysmal spells. Acute medical management for a hypercyanotic patient includes supplemental oxygen, sedation, volume resuscitation, and the alpha-receptor antagonist phenylephrine. Phenylephrine increases systemic resistance through direct vasoconstriction and has been shown to decrease right-to-left shunting, resulting in increased pulmonary blood flow [51,52]. However, any TOF patient who requires such therapy should be referred for urgent surgical palliation or repair.

Surgical Repair

Surgical timing remains a debated topic centered on two issues regarding neonates and TOF. First, should symptomatic neonates and infants below a certain age or size be palliated before complete repair or should all TOF patients have a primary repair regardless of size or age? The second controversy relates to acyanotic neonates and young infants and whether they should be repaired at diagnosis. Proponents of early primary repair offer the following rationales: early repair avoids a longer period of cyanosis that might distress neurologic development; early repair decreases right ventricular hypertrophy; pulmonary artery and pulmonary alveolar development may be adversely affected; any palliative procedure by definition means the patient and family are subjected to multiple procedures [53]. There is evidence demonstrating that early operations, including those in very small neonates can be performed with low mortality [54–61]. However, others have reported increased morbidity with increased requirement for inotropes and prolonged mechanical ventilation after very early repair [62,63]. The reported rate of early reinterventions and reoperations in infants who undergo primary repair under 1 month of age is high [64]. More concerning to advocates of selective staged management of neonates and infants with TOF is the elevated use of a transventricular approach to closure of the VSD and increased use of transannular patch or pulmonary homografts. Reports of repair for patients less than 3 months of age have transannular patch rates at least 50% [63,65], but the use of either a transannular patch or homograft in true neonates (less than 1 month old), range from 84–100% [56,57,61,64]. Also in neonates, the vast majority of VSD repairs are via a transventricular approach. Advocates of selective staged management feel that preserving pulmonary valve function and avoiding transventricular approach to VSD closure outweighs the concerns of delaying primary repair or a staged operation. Within the era of neonatal surgery, the transatrial-transpulmonary approach with selective shunting of symptomatic neonates continues to be advocated with excellent results [66–68]. Evidence shows decreased ventricular arrhythmias and improved right ventricular function with the transatrial-transpulmonary approach when compared with the transventricular approach [69]. Authors have reported the use of pulmonary valve-sparing techniques in 80% of patients [68]. There are reports of long-term tolerance of significant pulmonary valve regurgitation related to use of the transannular patch based on clinical symptoms [70] and overall mortality [71]. However, the deleterious long-term effects of pulmonary insufficiency (PI) including increased incidence of arrhythmia, decreased right ventricular function, and risk of sudden death have been well documented and are discussed in detail later in this chapter [72–75].

The necessity of a palliative procedure is questioned by advocates of early neonatal repair. There is evidence that the use of selective shunting may positively affect ability to preserve the pulmonary valve. In the authors' series [68], only 40% of previously shunted patients required transannular patch, which compares favorably with the reported rates near 100% if they were repaired primarily. Although we did not demonstrate that the pulmonary annulus grew after placement of the shunt, there is evidence for such growth. In a report from Paris involving 56 TOF patients younger than 6 months of age, eight patients had palliative shunts and went on to complete repair. The Z-score of the pulmonary annulus in these eight patients had increased by a mean of 2.2 and only one of eight infants repaired after shunt required a transannular patch [76]. There was no shunt-related mortality in this series, which reflects the experience of recent series [66,68].

Palliative Procedures

The most common palliative procedure is the modified Blalock-Taussig shunt (MBTS), which has supplanted the classic Blalock-Taussig shunt [77]. While some surgeons still prefer to perform the MBTS via thoracotomy, we use median sternotomy for the following reasons. Median sternotomy allows for the use of cardiopulmonary bypass in cases of hemodynamic collapse or severe hypoxia, allows for examination of the coronary anatomy, and leaves the patient with a single incision after eventual complete repair. The relative comfort of performing a resternotomy that has developed from numerous staged procedures for single-ventricle repair has minimized the rationale of avoiding the sternotomy for MBTS. The majority of procedures are performed without cardiopulmonary bypass. A 3.5- or 4-mm Gore-Tex shunt is anastomosed end to side to the innominate artery and to the ipsilateral branch pulmonary artery. Typically the shunt is placed on the side opposite that of the aortic arch; thus a patient with a left aortic arch receives a right-sided MBTS. Ligation of ductus arteriosus confirms the adequacy of the shunt and may decrease the chances of occurrence of branch pulmonary artery coarctation that can accompany natural constriction of the duct.

A transannular patch without repair of the VSD in small infants with very small pulmonary arteries has been reported with success, but is generally reserved for extreme situations [78,79]. Right ventricular outflow tract and pulmonary valve percutaneous balloon plasty and stenting have also been reported. This has been shown to be helpful in very small infants, and proponents have demonstrated growth of the branch pulmonary arteries [80,81]. However, these reports of pulmonary valve stenting show that effective relief of stenosis is achieved at the cost of irreversible damage to the pulmonary valve [82].

Complete Repair

Anesthetic induction of the patient with TOF is of particular concern as many anesthetic agents cause systemic vasodilation, which can greatly exacerbate any right-to-left shunting, possibly leading to profound hypoxia and potential hemodynamic collapse. The important basic principles include maintaining adequate volume status with a hemoglobin level of at least 10 mg/dL, use of a high inspired oxygen level, and avoidance of inhalational agents as they have a significant vasodilatory affect. Induction of anesthesia with intravenous agents including narcotics [83] and ketamine [84] can minimize unwanted vasodilation. It is also imperative to use extreme care to avoid introducing any air bubbles through the venous lines as the right-to-left shunt may allow these bubbles to reach the systemic circulation, where they can cause myocardial ischemia or stroke [85]. Transesophageal echocardiography should be performed in every patient (if the size of the patient permits) and should be interpreted preoperatively and postoperatively by a pediatric cardiologist.

A median sternotomy is performed and the size of the thymus should be noted before subtotal excision because of the association between TOF and DiGeorge syndrome. If a prior shunt was performed it is carefully isolated following systemic heparinization and aortic and bicaval cannulation. Cardiopulmonary bypass is initiated with moderate hypothermia (28 °C). If a shunt is present, it is ligated proximally and distally and divided to avoid any future tenting of the branch pulmonary artery. If the pulmonary artery is narrowed at the site of the shunt, the shunt is excised from the pulmonary artery and a patch augmentation using fresh autologous pericardium is performed. A left ventricular vent is inserted via the right superior pulmonary vein. The aorta is cross-clamped and cold-blood cardioplegia is delivered in an antegrade fashion through a cardioplegia cannula inserted into the aortic root. The cardioplegia should be readministered every 15–20 minutes or at any sign of cardiac activity. Topical slush saline is placed on the heart in conjunction with the cardioplegia. The cavae are snared, and a generous medial right atriotomy is made (Figure 22.6) [2]. The

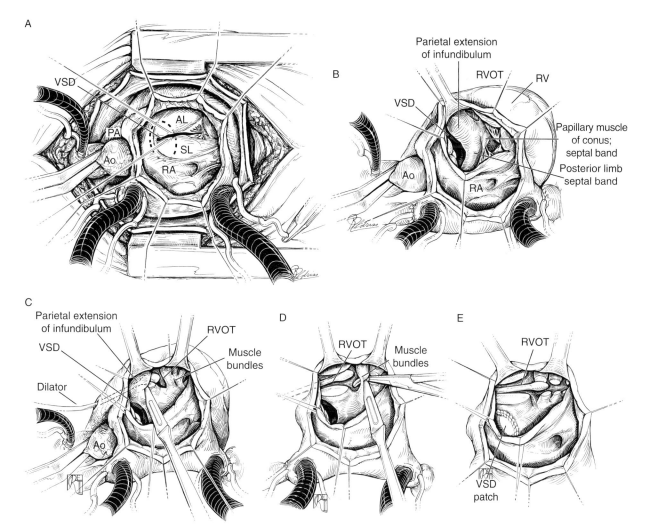

Figure 22.6 The surgical anatomy as viewed through a right atriotomy. The free edge of the atrial wall is retracted with stay sutures. The location of the VSD is denoted by the dashed line. **A,** Stay sutures are placed in the septal and anterior leaflets of the tricuspid valve for retraction. **B,** The tricuspid valve leaflets have been retracted and a single valve retractor is in place to aid exposure. The inferior margin of the VSD can be seen superior to posterior limb of the septal band. **C,** A dilator placed through the pulmonary annulus delineates the course of the right ventricular outflow tract. The parietal extension of the infundibulum is visible at the tip of the dilator. The parietal extension can be resected at its origin from the infundibular septum, dissected up toward the free wall, and amputated at the free wall. **D,** Division of the obstructing muscle bundles along the anterior limb of the septal band. **E,** View through the right atriotomy and tricuspid valve following patch closure of the VSD. (AL, atrial leaflet; Ao, aorta; PA, pulmonary artery; RV, right ventricle; RVOT, right ventricular outflow tract; SL, septal leaflet; VSD, ventricular septal defect.)

RVOT is examined. Resection involves careful excision of any endocardial fibroelastic tissue, which represents areas of turbulent flow. The hypertrophic muscle bundles projecting from the septomarginal and septoparietal bands can be divided or partially excised. Smaller trabecular muscles that are causing obstruction can be completely excised. Care must be taken to avoid excessive resection in the septal portion of the RVOT, which can damage the septal perforating coronary arteries, as well as in the area of the free wall of the right ventricle, which can result in a coronary fistula from the conal branches. The subvalvar apparatus of the tricuspid valve must be carefully noted and preserved during resection. While most of the RVOT resection can be performed through the right atrium and tricuspid valve, additional resection can be performed through the pulmonary valve, if necessary. In the presence of severe tunnel stenosis of the RVOT, a small infundibular incision, approximately 10–12 mm in length, placed immediately below the pulmonary valve annulus, may be required to establish adequate relief of obstruction. This infundibular incision is closed with a thin-walled (0.4 mm) Gore-Tex patch.

A longitudinal pulmonary arteriotomy is made and carried into the two anterior sinuses in the case of a tri-leaflet valve or into the lateral sinuses of a vertically oriented bicuspid valve. For a horizontally oriented bicuspid valve, the incision is not bifurcated but rather carried straight up to the annulus, or more accurately, to the right ventricle-pulmonary artery junction. A pulmonary valvotomy is performed using a number 11 blade, dividing the typically partially fused commissures back to the level of the arterial wall, allowing for maximal opening through the preserved annulus. A probe is inserted and if the size is larger than −3 Z score, the annulus is left intact. The pulmonary arteriotomy is then closed with a pantaloon pericardial patch, which maximizes the size of the pulmonary root completely relieving supravalvar obstruction (Figure 22.7) [68]. Inspection of the orifice of the branch pulmonary arteries, especially the left pulmonary artery, should be done as this is frequently stenotic in TOF patients and can be corrected with an extension of the pericardial patch onto the branch PA or a separate patch if necessary.

The VSD is closed by placing a series of interrupted horizontal mattress sutures using 5-0 Ethibond with Teflon pledgets around the circumference of the defect. Superiorly these sutures should be placed close to the aortic annulus to avoid residual defects through the trabeculations. Between the muscle of Lancisi and the tricuspid valve annulus inferiorly, avoiding deep suture bites is critical to avoid damage to the AV node and bundle of His. Several of the sutures are usually placed from the right atrial side of the tricuspid annulus bridging the superiorly and inferiorly placed sutures. A Gore-Tex patch is cut generously

to slightly oversize the defect as this avoids potential subaortic narrowing resulting from the anterior malalignment of the VSD. The tricuspid valve is tested and a PFO, which is almost always present, is closed primarily with 5-0 Prolene suture. The PFO is often left open when the repair is performed in the neonatal period. The right atrial incision is closed using two layers of running Prolene suture. The heart is carefully de-aired and the cross-clamp is removed.

After separation from cardiopulmonary bypass, direct measurements of the right ventricle and left ventricle pressures are made using a 21-gauge spinal needle attached to a pressure transducing line. If the right ventricle/left ventricle (RV/LV) pressure ratio is greater than 0.7 [64,68], the transesophageal echocardiography is carefully assessed for level of residual obstruction. If it is predominately at the annulus, then bypass is recommended and a transannular patch is created. If the stenosis is subvalvar, then only an infundibular patch is inserted starting immediately below the annulus and extending approximately 10–12 mm. Owing to the relatively high incidence of junctional ectopic tachycardia (JET) following TOF repair, regardless of the rhythm after separation from bypass, temporary atrial and ventricular pacing wires are placed.

Results

Mortality

The mortality rate for complete repair of TOF has decreased sharply since the 40% mortality rate initially reported by Dr Lillehei [32]. Between 1955 and 1960, the early mortality rate among 251 patients operated on for TOF at the Mayo

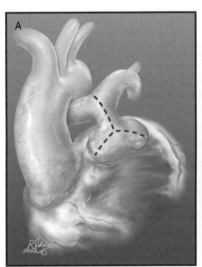
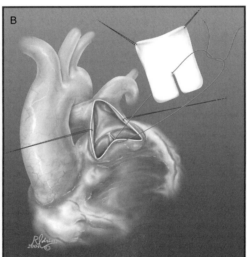
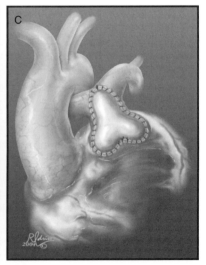

Figure 22.7 A, Pulmonary arteriotomy. **B,** Autologous pantaloon pericardial patch. **C,** Completed pulmonary artery pantaloon patch. (Reproduced with permission from Stewart *et al.* [68].)

clinic was 20% [86]. The mortality rate further decreased to 4.9% among 309 patients operated on at Stanford from 1960 to 1982 [87]. However, the average age at repair of TOF in that era was older. The mean age among 658 patients who underwent repair of TOF between 1958 and 1977 in one large series was 12.2 years [88]. There was a higher mortality initially with the advent of infant and neonatal surgery first championed by Paul Ebert [89,90], Brian Barrett-Boyes [91], and Aldo Castenada [92]. One of the first series of TOF repairs in infants and young children at Boston Children's Hospital between 1972 and 1977 was noteworthy for the excellent long-term results, but also for the 14% early mortality [70]. However, advances made over the last three decades in surgical technique, anesthetic management, and perioperative care have drastically reduced the mortality of infant and neonatal repair of TOF. Roger Mee and colleagues reported a 0.5% hospital mortality among 366 patients with TOF between 1980 and 1991 using a transatrial, transpulmonary approach [67]. There were no mortalities in our series of 102 cases (average age: 5.9 months) at Children's Memorial Hospital in Chicago between 1997 and 2004 [68]. Most recent reports of infant and neonatal TOF have equally low rates of mortality ranging from 0 to 3% [54,57,58,60–63].

The long-term survival rate of patients with TOF is excellent, even for patients who were operated on in the earliest era. The 32-year actuarial survival among 163 patients who had survived 30 days after complete repair of TOF at the Mayo Clinic before 1960 was 86%, with an expected rate of 96% in a control population matched for age and sex [86]. Similarly, a 1997 report on a group of 658 patients with repaired TOF found an 89% 30-year actuarial survival [93].

Morbidity

The most significant complications following repair of TOF are arrhythmias, early reoperation or catheter reintervention, residual VSD, and heart block. Heart block requiring a pacemaker is reported between 0 and 2% and occurs occasionally late after the operation [94]. It is noted that early postoperative transient heart block is a risk factor for the development of late heart block [95]. Other complications include phrenic nerve injury, chylothorax, and delayed sternal closure.

Early Reoperation and Reinterventions

The right ventricle can tolerate the volume load of PI for a number of years, thus reoperation for PI, while being very significant late after repair, is a rare early event. The most common indication for early reoperation after repair of TOF is residual RVOT obstruction. Residual stenosis can be

at the infundibular level, valvar level, or in the branch pulmonary arteries. When present in the branch PAs, these are often amenable to catheter-based balloon plasty and/or stent placement. The incidence of reoperation varies greatly with the patient population. The collective experience with electively repaired patients shows that the reoperation rate is relatively low. Mee and colleagues in Australia reported in 1991 a 5- and 10-year freedom from reoperation of 95% [67]. The group from Texas Children's Hospital reported a 3% early reoperative rate [66]. In a series of 90 patients who underwent primary repair of TOF at less than 4 months of age, the reoperation rate was 8%, and 14% required catheter reintervention at a mean follow-up of 4.7 years [61]. Conversely, in a series of primary repair on symptomatic neonates, the reoperative rate has been reported as high as 30% [64]. However, a comparison study of reoperative rates on the RVOT at 20 years for primary repairs versus staged repairs found that the freedom from reoperation is not statistically different [96].

The amount of residual obstruction at the conclusion of initial repair, as assessed by the RV/LV pressure ratio, is directly related to the incidence of reoperation. A study from the University of Alabama, Birmingham in 1982 demonstrated that an RV/LV pressure ratio greater than 0.85 was associated with a 2.5 times increased risk of death and a 7.3 times increased risk of reoperation [97]. But they also showed a decrease in the RV/LV pressure ratio with time, with the greatest reduction seen in those patients with the highest immediate postoperative ratios. In our series, four of seven reoperations were in patients who had an RV/LV pressure ratio between 0.7 and 0.8 [68]. In contrast, a group from Spain reported accepting a RV/LV pressure ratio up to 0.9 in order to preserve more pulmonary valves. Only one of 24 patients required reoperation at one year for annular stenosis, and the group with RV/LV ratios between 0.7 and 0.9 showed a greater reduction in pressure ratio compared with those with RV/LV <0.7 at 32 months follow-up [98].

Other indications for early reoperation include residual VSD, residual ASD, RVOT aneurysm, severe tricuspid regurgitation, heart block, phrenic nerve injury, and chylothorax. Interestingly, while most series report few reoperations for residual VSD, a large series from Germany found that among the 102 reoperations at 12.8 years after repair in 914 patients, half of the reoperations were for residual VSD [99].

Arrhythmias and Sudden Death

Arrhythmias and conduction disturbances are significant both for their prevalence and serious consequences. In fact, the most common cause of mortality late after TOF repair is sudden death, presumably attributable to ventricular arrhythmias [72]. In the early postoperative period, the most common disturbance is right bundle branch block, which results from RVOT and/or sutures from the VSD repair. In cases where a ventriculotomy is performed, right bundle branch block is seen in up to 90% of patients [100]. In contradistinction, complete heart block is a relatively uncommon complication of TOF repair, with reported incidence being 1–3% [57,59,61,62]. The most common early arrhythmia following repair is JET. The incidence of JET varies greatly based on age at surgery and surgical approach. In a series of patients under 3 months of age undergoing a transventricular repair, 29% had postoperative arrhythmias of which 48% were JET and 17% had some form of supraventricular tachycardia (SVT) [59]. Conversely, in our series of 102 patients repaired at a mean age of 6 months by a transatrial/transpulmonary approach, the incidence of JET was 12% [68]. In another group of patients repaired at a mean age of 1 year by the same approach, the incidence of JET was only 6% [66]. Junctional ectopic tachycardia can result in major hemodynamic instability in the immediate postoperative period. Treatment includes correction of electrolytes, mild hypothermia (33–35 °C), reduction or elimination of catecholaminergic infusions, sedation, and treatment with amiodarone. While 5 mg/kg as a single bolus is recommended by some, we favor multiple boluses of only 1 mg/kg over 20–30 minutes to avoid the negative inotropic effect of amiodarone.

Late arrhythmias after TOF repair include both atrial and ventricular tachycardias (VT). The Alliance for Adult Research in Congenital Cardiology conducted a multi-institutional retrospective study of 556 previously repaired TOF patients and found 43% had a history of arrhythmias [101]. Atrial tachyarrhythmias were present in 20% and ventricular tachyarrhythmias in 15%. This may be an overestimation of the incidence of arrhythmias in a selected population. Sustained SVT was documented in 12% of a cohort of 242 adult patients late after repair [102]. In a multi-institutional study of 793 patients studied at a mean of 21 years after repair, Gatzoulis and colleagues found an incidence of atrial and ventricular tachyarrhythmias of approximately 4% [72]. However, they also found an alarming incidence of sudden death: 2%. Conversely, the incidence of paroxysmal atrial tachyarrhythmias has been found to be as high as one-third of patients [103]. By far the most common type of SVT seen in TOF patients is atrial re-entry tachycardia. The most common site of slow conduction is in the area of the isthmus between the tricuspid valve and the inferior vena cava [104]. Re-entrant circuits also develop in scar areas around atrial incisions. See Chapter 41, *Surgical Therapy of Cardiac Arrhythmias* for a detailed explanation of the mechanisms of re-entry tachycardia. The prevalence of SVT has been shown to be related to older age at surgery, the presence of moderate or severe tricuspid regurgitation, right atrial enlargement, PI, poor right ventricular function, and hypertension [101–105].

While not as life threatening as VTs, supraventricular arrhythmias are perhaps responsible for more morbidity including decreased exercise capacity, heart failure, and stroke. Treatment for atrial arrhythmias includes pharmacologic agents, transcatheter ablation, and surgical ablation. Because of the success with the maze operation in controlling atrial re-entry arrhythmias in patients with congenital heart disease [106,107], we feel that all patients who require reoperation, particularly for pulmonic valve insertion or replacement, should be evaluated for presence of arrhythmias with a 24-hour Holter monitor. If there is any index of suspicion including any history of palpitations, patients should be evaluated by a formal electrophysiologic study to elicit and characterize re-entry pathways in the right or left atrium that can be obliterated with incision, cryotherapy, or radiofrequency ablation at the time of surgery.

The risk factors that have been associated with ventricular arrhythmias include older age at repair, ventriculotomy, transannular patch, severe pulmonary regurgitation, poor right ventricle function, poor left ventricle function, right ventricle enlargement, and elongated QRS duration [72,102,108,109]. The risk of sudden death includes QRS duration greater than 180 msec, older age at repair, severe pulmonary regurgitation, history of sustained VT, and left ventricle systolic dysfunction [72,110].

Long-term Complications Following Repair of Tetralogy of Fallot

The major late complications of repaired TOF result from the deranged physiology of the right ventricle. The long-term effect of volume overload from PI, and tricuspid regurgitation as well as any residual shunts is additive to any pressure load resulting from residual pulmonary stenosis. The sequelae include right ventricular dysfunction, atrial and ventricular arrhythmias, sudden death, late left ventricular dysfunction, and aneurysmal dilation of the aorta. The majority who suffer these complications have been shown to have long-standing PI as the primary etiology. This is directly related to the use of the transannular patch. There have been several studies demonstrating good long-term functional outcomes after repair of TOF with a transannular patch [70,71]. Bacha and colleagues reported long-term outcomes of 45 patients operated on for TOF as infants at Boston Children's Hospital and showed that the functional status as measured by New York Heart Association class was similar for transannular patch and valve-sparing procedures [70]. Kirklin's group at the University of Alabama, Birmingham examined 814 patients and found that the risk of reoperation for PI at 20 years was 7%; they ascribed this low rate of reoperation, despite a significant incidence of PR, to the adaptive properties of the right ventricle [71]. They also found no difference in New York Heart Association class between transannular patch and valve-sparing approaches. These findings are contradicted by other studies showing the deleterious effects of PI on the right ventricle when more sensitive measurements are made [41,73]. Exercise testing has shown that functional status is impaired in TOF patients with long-term PI [73,111]. Cardiac magnetic resonance cine examination of TOF patients late after repair have demonstrated that PI is closely associated with the transannular patch and that PI results in significant right ventricular dysfunction, even in asymptomatic patients [41,112]. The group at Great Ormond Street has used tissue Doppler assessments of isovolumetric myocardial acceleration to more accurately assess right ventricular function in the face of highly variable loading conditions that exist with PI [113]. They found in a group of 124 patients in which the use of transannular patch highly correlated with PI and PI was associated with both right ventricular and left ventricular dysfunction [113]. The late effect of transannular patch and PI on both right ventricle and patient functional status are further documented by the growing number of reports on the ventricular improvement and symptomatic relief achieved with pulmonary valve insertion late after TOF repair [114–116].

Pulmonary Valve Replacement

Despite reports of functional improvement after pulmonary valve replacement (PVR) in patients with severe PI late after TOF repair, the timing and effect of PVR remains controversial. While no data show overall improvement in survival, in a study of matched cohorts of 82 patients with and without PVR, there were no sudden deaths in the PVR group [117]. The effect of PVR on VT, the substrate for sudden death, is also unclear. One study showed a decrease in the incidence of VT from 23% to 9% after PVR [118] while a matching cohort study of 98 patients showed that PVR did not decrease the incidence of VT or death [119]. The effect of PVR on the duration of the QRS is variable. Therrien reported that PVR stabilized the duration of the QRS while not decreasing it [118]. Others have shown that the QRS decreases early after PVR, and the decrease correlates with the decrease in right ventricular end-diastolic volume (RVEDV) as measured by CMR [120]. Still another report showed only a transient decrease in QRS with an eventual increase in duration to >180 msec. This late increase in QRS duration was more likely for those with a QRS >180 msec before PVR [121]. Pulmonary valve replacement has been shown to improve right ventricular function and to decrease the size of the right ventricle [120,122], but this improvement appears to be limited when the right ventricle has reached a critical size. In an analysis of patients after PVR, there was an improvement in RVEDV and right ventricle end-systolic volume (RVESV); however, no patient with RVEDV >170 mL/m^2 or a RVESD >85 mL/m^2 achieved a normal RVEDV or RVESV while 90% of those with RVEDV <170 mL/m^2 before PVR had normal post-PVR in right ventricular volumes [43].

Because of the myriad of findings after PVR, there are no universally accepted indications. However, most consider that PVR is an important intervention late after TOF repair but that if executed too late, may fail to achieve optimal benefit. Geva and colleagues have recommended general criteria for PVR in patients with moderate to severe PI [123]. The presence of any two of the following represents an indication for PVR: RVEDD index >160 mL/m^2; RVESD index >70 mL/m^2; LVEDV index >65 mL/m^2; RVEF <45%; RVOT aneurysm; clinical symptoms or signs including syncope and VT [123]. These indications will certainly evolve as more data are analyzed.

The technical aspects of PVR include homograft replacement, valved conduit replacement, and bioprosthetic valve insertion in the orthotopic location with the creation of RVOT hood using Gore-Tex or heterograft pericardium [124–126]. All of these techniques have been successful without clear advantage of any particular technique. Others have used stentless porcine valves for RVOT reconstruction with success [127], and there are reports of mechanical valves being used for PVR, though most avoid these valves because of the risk of thrombosis and indication for anticoagulation [128]. An alternative method for PVR involves the percutaneous insertion of a bovine jugular valve sewn to an expandable stent [129]. This technique, introduced by Bonhoeffer, has the clear advantage of avoiding a redo sternotomy. At the present time the approved indications limit its use to circumstances of failure (obstruction or regurgitation) of a previously implanted conduit (with some constraints related to minimum and maximum size of the RVOT conduit). The risk of coronary artery compression is also present with percutaneous PVR. The use of percutaneous PVR will certainly become more prevalent as the engineering of the devices improves. The indications for percutaneous PVR should be the same as for surgical PVR.

Neurological Outcomes

Evaluations of children with repaired TOF have demonstrated inferior full-scale IQ than the general age-matched population [130]. However, when repaired TOF children were stratified by presence of a genetic lesion or syndrome, those without any identified defects had scores within the normal limits for age [131]. It has also been recognized that the incidence of stroke is higher in adults with repaired TOF than the general population, though no clear etiology for this finding has been demonstrated [132].

Aortic Complications

Aortic valve and aortic root complications have become well recognized late after TOF repair. In a study of 59 patients, Zahka and colleagues evaluated PI at a mean of 18 years after repair and noted that 21% of patients had important aortic regurgitation [133]. This finding has been reported by others late after repair [134], but has been shown to begin in childhood and to be associated with a high level of elastic fiber fragmentation seen in the aorta of children with TOF [135]. Another study of the autopsy specimens from patients with TOF found that the aorta had elastic fragmentation in 59%, medionecrosis in 29%, cystic medial necrosis in 35%, and fibrosis in 82% [136]. These aorta histologic derangements can lead to the development of aortic aneurysms [137] and aortic dissection [138] late after TOF repair. These aneurysms require surgical intervention with the same criteria as aneurysms in nontetralogy patients [139].

Special Circumstances

Tetralogy of Fallot with Absent Pulmonary Valve

Approximately 2.5% of cases of TOF have a unique variant of the morphologic features, characterized by near absence of the pulmonary valve leaflets [140]. Rather than the semilunar cusps of a more typical pulmonary valve, these valves have very rudimentary leaflets, completely lacking three-dimensional cusp-like anatomy. In addition to having limited mobility, these cusps are centrally deficient so that there is a large coaptation gap. The combination of annular hypoplasia, leaflet immobility, and the central deficiency of valvar tissue create the anatomic substrate for combined pulmonary stenosis and insufficiency. The infundibulum tends to be somewhat elongated and tubular, and muscular right ventricular outflow obstruction is not commonly a major element. In some cases the main pulmonary trunk and central right and left branch pulmonary arteries are markedly dilated (Figure 22.8) [2]. The aneurysmal features of the central pulmonary arteries may extend into the pulmonary hilum, in which case only segmental branches can be identified emanating from the bulbous central aneurysm. An important feature of these cases is compression of the tracheal-bronchial tree by the enlarged central pulmonary arteries. In the most extreme instances, severe respiratory distress is present from birth. The name "tetralogy of Fallot with absent pulmonary valve syndrome" has been applied, in recognition of the unique presentation and pathophysiology. Anatomically, there is complete absence of a patent ductus or ductal ligament in the vast majority of cases, and this has been invoked as a consequential stimulus accounting for the in utero development of the aneurysmal pathology of the central pulmonary arteries. These infants are frequently ventilator-dependent at birth and require early intervention. Those with less severe symptoms might allow for elective repair in the first 6 months of life. The classic repair involves a homograft valve replacement, closure of the VSD, and pulmonary arterioplasty to reduce their size and relieve bronchial compression. Alternatives to this repair now include a transannular patch without a homograft valve. The rationale for such an approach relates to a significantly longer interval before a required reoperation as any infant will outgrow a homograft within the first few years of life [141]. In cases where the bronchial compression cannot be ameliorated by a pulmonary reduction arterioplasty, the addition of the Lecompte maneuver to the repair has been reported. By transferring the dilated branch pulmonary arteries anterior

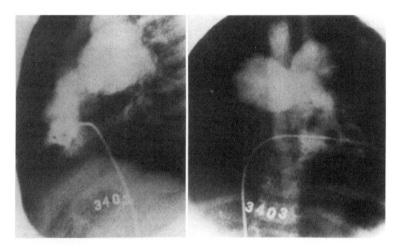

Figure 22.8 Angiogram in a patient with tetralogy of Fallot and absent pulmonary valve. There is marked aneurysmal dilatation of the main, right, and left pulmonary arteries and absent pulmonary valve.

to the aorta and thus away from the bronchi, the Lecompte maneuver has been shown to provide substantial relief from bronchial compression [142]. Others have replaced the entire proximal pulmonary artery, including the dilated branches, with a pulmonary homograft that includes the branch pulmonary arteries [143].

Mortality from repair of TOF with absent pulmonary valve is approximately 5% [144,145] and more often than not occurs in the most critically ill infants with substantial pulmonary disease related to bronchial compression and persistent bronchial malacia.

Tetralogy of Fallot and Atrioventricular Septal Defect

After ASD and PDA, the condition most commonly associated with TOF is complete AVSD. The combination of TOF and AVSD (TOF-AVSD) occurs in approximately 3% of all TOF cases. While less than 10% of patients with TOF have trisomy 21, the majority of TOF-AVSD patients have trisomy 21, similar to isolated AVSD [146]. Unlike isolated AVSD, the incidence of early pulmonary hypertension is limited by the protective effects of RVOT obstruction. The associated AVSD is usually Rastelli type C, with an absence of cordal attachments from the anterior bridging leaflet to the crest of the ventricular septum. Repair is usually undertaken between 4 and 6 months of age. Using a transatrial approach, a two-patch technique is most commonly used with a modified VSD patch in the shape of a comma [147]. This patch combines the geometry of the crescentic VSD patch of an isolated AVSD, which extends under the posterior bridging leaflet, with that of the large round patch of a typical TOF anterior malalignment VSD extending under the anterior bridging leaflet. The RVOT obstruction is treated as in isolated TOF. Historically, TOF-AVSD has a higher morbidity and a mortality of up to 10%, but more recent series have shown a substantial reduction in both, including a recent report with no mortality in 20 patients [148].

Conclusion

Tetralogy of Fallot is the most common cyanotic congenital heart lesion. Surgical repair has a high rate of success, and long-term survival with excellent functional outcome has been well demonstrated. While there is general consensus that repair in infancy is superior, controversy persists regarding neonatal repair versus staged repair. Late complications include right ventricular dysfunction, atrial and ventricular arrhythmias, and sudden death. The effectiveness of late pulmonary valve repair in ameliorating these complications is being actively studied, and intervention criteria are evolving.

References

1. Fallot E. (1888) Contribution a l'anatomie pathologique de la maladie bleue. Marseille Med 25, 77–93, 138–158, 207–223, 270–286, 341–354, 403–420.
2. Hirsch JC, Bove EL. (2003) Tetralogy of Fallot. In: Mavroudis C, Backer CL, eds. *Pediatric Cardiac Surgery*, 3rd ed. Philadelphia, PA: Mosby, Inc.
3. Steno N. (1671) Anatomicus regij Hafniensis, Embryo monstro affinis Parisiis dissectus. In: Bartholin T, ed. *Acta Medica et Philosophia Hafniencia*, pp. 200–203.
4. Birmingham A. (1892) Extreme anomaly of the heart and great vessels. Trans Roy Acad Ire 27, 139–150.
5. Abbott ME, Dawson WT. (1924) The clinical classification of congenital cardiac disease. Int Clin 4, 156–188.
6. Van Praagh R. (1989) Etienne-Louis Arthur Fallot and his tetralogy: a new translation of Fallot's summary and a modern reassessment of this anomaly. Eur J Cardiothorac Surg 3, 381–386.
7. Van Praagh R, Van Praagh S, Nebesar RA, *et al*. (1970) Tetralogy of Fallot: underdevelopment of the pulmonary infundibulum and its sequelae. Am J Cardiol 26, 25–33.
8. Becker AE, Connor M, Anderson RH. (1975) Tetralogy of Fallot: a morphometric and geometric study. Am J Cardiol 35, 402–412.
9. Howell CE, Ho SY, Anderson RH, *et al*. (1990) Variations within the fibrous skeleton and ventricular outflow tracts in tetralogy of Fallot. Ann Thorac Surg 50, 450–457.
10. Eisenmenger V. (1897) Die angeborenen Defekte der Kammerscheidewande des Herzens. Zeitsch Klin Med 32(suppl), 1–28.
11. Anderson RH, Weinberg PM. (2005) The clinical anatomy of tetralogy of fallot. Cardiol Young 15, 38–47.
12. Altrichter PM, Olson LJ, Edwards WD, *et al*. (1989) Surgical pathology of the pulmonary valve: a study of 116 cases spanning 15 years. Mayo Clin Proc 64, 1352–1360.
13. Dickinson DF, Wilkinson JL, Smith A, *et al*. (1982) Variations in the morphology of the ventricular septal defect and disposition of the atrioventricular conduction tissues in tetralogy of Fallot. Thorac Cardiovasc Surg 30, 243–249.
14. Dabizzi RP, Caprioli G, Aiazzi L, *et al*. (1980) Distribution and anomalies of coronary arteries in tetralogy of fallot. Circulation 61, 95–102.
15. van Son JA. (1995) Repair of tetralogy of Fallot with anomalous origin of left anterior descending coronary artery. J Thorac Cardiovasc Surg 110, 561–562.
16. Suzuki A, Ho SY, Anderson RH, *et al*. (1990) Further morphologic studies on tetralogy of Fallot, with particular emphasis on the prevalence and structure of the membranous flap. J Thorac Cardiovasc Surg 99, 528–535.
17. Chiariello L, Meyer J, Wukasch DC, *et al*. (1975) Intracardiac repair of tetralogy of Fallot. Five-year review of 403 patients. J Thorac Cardiovasc Surg 70, 529–535.
18. Beland MJ, Franklin RC, Jacobs JP, *et al*. (2004) Update from the International Working Group for Mapping and Coding of Nomenclatures for Paediatric and Congenital Heart Disease. Cardiol Young 14, 225–229.

19. Jacobs ML. (2000) Congenital Heart Surgery Nomenclature and Database Project: tetralogy of Fallot. Ann Thorac Surg 69(4 Suppl), S77–S82.

20. Hoffman JI, Kaplan S. (2002) The incidence of congenital heart disease. J Am Coll Cardiol 39, 1890–1900.

21. Jacobs JP, Jacobs ML, Mavroudis C, *et al.* (2008) Executive Summary: The Society of Thoracic Surgeons Congenital Heart Surgery Database Ninth Harvest (July 1, 2004 to June 30, 2008). Durham, NC: The Society of Thoracic Surgeons and Duke Clinical Research Institute.

22. Michielon G, Marino B, Formigari R, *et al.* (2006) Genetic syndromes and outcome after surgical correction of tetralogy of Fallot. Ann Thorac Surg 81, 968–975.

23. Blalock A, Taussig HB. (1945) The surgical treatment of malformations of the heart in which there is pulmonary stenosis or pulmonary atresia. JAMA 128, 189–202.

24. Taussig HB. (1979) Neuhauser Lecture: Tetralogy of Fallot: early history and late results. Am J Roentgenol 133, 422–431.

25. Brock RC. (1948) Pulmonary valvulotomy for the relief of congenital pulmonary stenosis; report of three cases. Br Med J 1, 1121–1126.

26. Sellors TH. (1948) Surgery of pulmonary stenosis; a case in which the pulmonary valve was successfully divided. Lancet 1, 988.

27. Downing DF, Bailey CP, Glover RP. (1951) Brock procedure for the relief of pulmonary stenosis in the tetralogy of Fallot. Pediatrics 7, 230–239.

28. Potts WJ, Smith S, Gibson S. (1946) Anastomosis of the aorta to a pulmonary artery in certain types of congenital heart disease. Case Rep Child Meml Hosp Chic 5, 704–718.

29. Waterston DJ. (1962) [Treatment of Fallot's tetralogy in children under 1 year of age]. Rozhl Chir, 41, 181–183.

30. Warden HE, Cohen M, Read RC, *et al.* (1954) Controlled cross circulation for open intracardiac surgery: physiologic studies and results of creation and closure of ventricular septal defects. J Thorac Surg 28, 331–341; discussion 341–343.

31. Gott VL. (1990) C. Walton Lillehei and total correction of tetralogy of Fallot. Ann Thorac Surg 49, 328–332.

32. Lillehei CW, Cohen M, Warden HE, *et al.* (1955) Direct vision intracardiac surgical correction of the tetralogy of Fallot, pentalogy of Fallot, and pulmonary atresia defects; report of first ten cases. Ann Surg 142, 418–442.

33. Kirklin JW, Dushane JW, Patrick RT, *et al.* (1955) Intracardiac surgery with the aid of a mechanical pump-oxygenator system (gibbon type): report of eight cases. Proc Staff Meet Mayo Clin 30, 201–206.

34. Dadlani GH, John JB, Cohen MS. (2008) Echocardiography in tetralogy of Fallot. Cardiol Young 18(Suppl 3), 22–28.

35. Gatzoulis MA, Soukias N, Ho SY, *et al.* (1999) Echocardiographic and morphological correlations in tetralogy of Fallot. Eur Heart J 20, 221–231.

36. Need LR, Powell AJ, del Nido P, *et al.* (2000) Coronary echocardiography in tetralogy of Fallot: diagnostic accuracy, resource utilization and surgical implications over 13 years. J Am Coll Cardiol 36, 1371–1377.

37. Tongsong T, Sittiwangkul R, Chanprapaph P, *et al.* (2005) Prenatal sonographic diagnosis of tetralogy of Fallot. J Clin Ultrasound 33, 427–431.

38. Lee W, Smith RS, Comstock CH, *et al.* (1995) Tetralogy of Fallot: prenatal diagnosis and postnatal survival. Obstet Gynecol 86, 583–588.

39. Kjaergaard J, Petersen CL, Kjaer A, *et al.* (2006) Evaluation of right ventricular volume and function by 2D and 3D echocardiography compared to MRI. Eur J Echocardiogr 7, 430–438.

40. Geva T, Powell AJ, Crawford EC, *et al.* (1998) Evaluation of regional differences in right ventricular systolic function by acoustic quantification echocardiography and cine magnetic resonance imaging. Circulation 98, 339–345.

41. Roest AA, Helbing WA, Kunz P, *et al.* (2002) Exercise MR imaging in the assessment of pulmonary regurgitation and biventricular function in patients after tetralogy of Fallot repair. Radiology 223, 204–211.

42. van den Berg J, Wielopolski PA, Meijboom FJ, *et al.* (2007) Diastolic function in repaired tetralogy of Fallot at rest and during stress: assessment with MR imaging. Radiology 243, 212–219.

43. Therrien J, Provost Y, Merchant N, *et al.* (2005) Optimal timing for pulmonary valve replacement in adults after tetralogy of Fallot repair. Am J Cardiol 95, 779–782.

44. Knauth A, Gauvreau K, Landzberg M. (2005) Right ventricular size and function and age at repair predict major adverse outcomes late after tetralogy of Fallot repair (abstr). Circulation 112, II681.

45. Koppel RI, Druschel CM, Carter T, *et al.* (2003) Effectiveness of pulse oximetry screening for congenital heart disease in asymptomatic newborns. Pediatrics 111, 451–455.

46. Sendelbach DM, Jackson GL, Lai SS, *et al.* (2008) Pulse oximetry screening at 4 hours of age to detect critical congenital heart defects. Pediatrics 122, e815–e820.

47. Elliott RB, Starling MB, Neutze JM. (1975) Medical manipulation of the ductus arteriosus. Lancet 1, 140–142.

48. Cumming GR, Carr W. (1966) Relief of dyspnoeic attacks in Fallot's tetralogy with propanolol. Lancet 1, 519–522.

49. Garson A Jr, Gillette PC, McNamara DG. (1981) Propranolol: the preferred palliation for tetralogy of Fallot. Am J Cardiol 47, 1098–1104.

50. Graham EM, Bandisode VM, Bradley SM, *et al.* (2008) Effect of preoperative use of propranolol on postoperative outcome in patients with tetralogy of Fallot. Am J Cardiol 101, 693–695.

51. Nudel DB, Berman MA, Talner NS. (1976) Effects of acutely increasing systemic vascular resistance on oxygen tension in tetralogy of Fallot. Pediatrics 58, 248–251.

52. Tanaka K, Kitahata H, Kawahito S, *et al.* (2003) Phenylephrine increases pulmonary blood flow in children with tetralogy of Fallot. Can J Anaesth 50, 926–929.

53. Jonas RA. (2009) Early primary repair of tetralogy of Fallot. Semin Thorac Cardiovasc Surg Pediatr Card Surg Annu 12, 39–47.

54. Derby CD, Pizarro C. (2005) Routine primary repair of tetralogy of Fallot in the neonate. Expert Rev Cardiovasc Ther 3, 857–863.

55. Di Donato RM, Jonas RA, Lang P, *et al.* (1991) Neonatal repair of tetralogy of Fallot with and without pulmonary atresia. J Thorac Cardiovasc Surg 101, 126–137.

56. Hennein HA, Mosca RS, Urcelay G, *et al.* (1995) Intermediate results after complete repair of tetralogy of Fallot in neonates. J Thorac Cardiovasc Surg 109, 332–344; discussion 342–343.

57. Kolcz J, Pizarro C. (2005) Neonatal repair of tetralogy of Fallot results in improved pulmonary artery development without increased need for reintervention. Eur J Cardiothorac Surg 28, 394–399.

58. Parry AJ, McElhinney DB, Kung GC, *et al.* (2000) Elective primary repair of acyanotic tetralogy of Fallot in early infancy: overall outcome and impact on the pulmonary valve. J Am Coll Cardiol 36, 2279–2283.

59. Pigula FA, Khalil PN, Mayer JE, *et al.* (1999) Repair of tetralogy of Fallot in neonates and young infants. Circulation 100(19 Suppl), II157–II161.

60. Reddy VM, Liddicoat JR, McElhinney DB, *et al.* (1995) Routine primary repair of tetralogy of Fallot in neonates and infants less than three months of age. Ann Thorac Surg 60(6 Suppl), S592–S596.

61. Tamesberger MI, Lechner E, Mair R, *et al.* (2008) Early primary repair of tetralogy of Fallot in neonates and infants less than four months of age. Ann Thorac Surg 86, 1928–1935.

62. Kanter KR, Kogon BE, Kirshbom PM, *et al.* (2010) Symptomatic neonatal tetralogy of Fallot: repair or shunt? Ann Thorac Surg 89, 858–863.

63. van Dongen EI, Glansdorp AG, Mildner RJ, *et al.* (2003) The influence of perioperative factors on outcomes in children aged less than 18 months after repair of tetralogy of Fallot. J Thorac Cardiovasc Surg 126, 703–710.

64. Hirsch JC, Mosca RS, Bove EL. (2000) Complete repair of tetralogy of Fallot in the neonate: results in the modern era. Ann Surg 232, 508–514.

65. Gustafson RA, Murray GF, Warden HE, *et al.* (1988) Early primary repair of tetralogy of Fallot. Ann Thorac Surg 45, 235–241.

66. Fraser CD Jr, McKenzie ED, Cooley DA. (2001) Tetralogy of Fallot: surgical management individualized to the patient. Ann Thorac Surg 71, 1556–1561; discussion 1561–1563.

67. Karl TR, Sano S, Pornviliwan S, *et al.* (1992) Tetralogy of Fallot: favorable outcome of nonneonatal transatrial, transpulmonary repair. Ann Thorac Surg 54, 903–907.

68. Stewart RD, Backer CL, Young L, *et al.* (2005) Tetralogy of Fallot: results of a pulmonary valve-sparing strategy. Ann Thorac Surg 80, 1431–1438; discussion 1438–1439.

69. Stellin G, Milanesi O, Rubino M, *et al.* (1995) Repair of tetralogy of Fallot in the first six months of life: transatrial versus transventricular approach. Ann Thorac Surg 60(6 Suppl), S588–S591.

70. Bacha EA, Scheule AM, Zurakowski D, *et al.* (2001) Long-term results after early primary repair of tetralogy of Fallot. J Thorac Cardiovasc Surg 122, 154–161.

71. Kirklin JK, Kirklin JW, Blackstone EH, *et al.* (1989) Effect of transannular patching on outcome after repair of tetralogy of Fallot. Ann Thorac Surg 48, 783–791.

72. Gatzoulis MA, Balaji S, Webber SA, *et al.* (2000) Risk factors for arrhythmia and sudden cardiac death late after repair of tetralogy of Fallot: a multicentre study. Lancet 356, 975–981.

73. Horneffer PJ, Zahka KG, Rowe SA, *et al.* (1990) Long-term results of total repair of tetralogy of Fallot in childhood. Ann Thorac Surg 50, 179–183; discussion 183–185.

74. Ilbawi MN, Idriss FS, DeLeon SY, *et al.* (1987) Factors that exaggerate the deleterious effects of pulmonary insufficiency on the right ventricle after tetralogy repair. Surgical implications. J Thorac Cardiovasc Surg 93, 36–44.

75. Marie PY, Marcon F, Brunotte F, *et al.* (1992) Right ventricular overload and induced sustained ventricular tachycardia in operatively "repaired" tetralogy of Fallot. Am J Cardiol 69, 785–789.

76. Sousa Uva M, Lacour-Gayet F, Komiya T, *et al.* (1994) Surgery for tetralogy of Fallot at less than six months of age. J Thorac Cardiovasc Surg 107, 1291–1300.

77. de Leval MR, McKay R, Jones M, *et al.* (1981) Modified Blalock–Taussig shunt. Use of subclavian artery orifice as flow regulator in prosthetic systemic-pulmonary artery shunts. J Thorac Cardiovasc Surg 81, 112–119.

78. Korbmacher B, Heusch A, Sunderdiek U, *et al.* (2005) Evidence for palliative enlargement of the right ventricular outflow tract in severe tetralogy of Fallot. Eur J Cardiothorac Surg 27, 945–948.

79. Seipelt RG, Vazquez-Jimenez JF, Sachweh JS, *et al.* (2002) Antegrade palliation for diminutive pulmonary arteries in tetralogy of Fallot. Eur J Cardiothorac Surg 21, 721–724; discussion 724.

80. Laudito A, Bandisode VM, Lucas JF, *et al.* (2006) Right ventricular outflow tract stent as a bridge to surgery in a premature infant with tetralogy of Fallot. Ann Thorac Surg 81, 744–746.

81. Wu ET, Wang JK, Lee WL, *et al.* (2006) Balloon valvuloplasty as an initial palliation in the treatment of newborns and young infants with severely symptomatic tetralogy of Fallot. Cardiology 105, 52–56.

82. Dohlen G, Chaturvedi RR, Benson LN, *et al.* (2009) Stenting of the right ventricular outflow tract in the symptomatic infant with tetralogy of Fallot. Heart 95, 142–147.

83. Barankay A, Richter JA, Henze R, *et al.* (1992) Total intravenous anesthesia for infants and children undergoing correction of tetralogy of Fallot: sufentanil versus sufentanil-flunitrazepam technique. J Cardiothorac Vasc Anesth 6, 185–189.

84. Tugrul M, Camci E, Pembeci K, *et al.* (2000) Ketamine infusion versus isoflurane for the maintenance of anesthesia in the prebypass period in children with tetralogy of Fallot. J Cardiothorac Vasc Anesth 14, 557–561.

85. Horrow JC, Laucks SO. (1982) Coronary air embolism during venous cannulation. Anesthesiology 56, 212–214.

86. Murphy JG, Gersh BJ, Mair DD, *et al.* (1993) Long-term outcome in patients undergoing surgical repair of tetralogy of Fallot. N Engl J Med 329, 593–599.

87. Zhao HX, Miller DC, Reitz BA, *et al.* (1985) Surgical repair of tetralogy of Fallot. Long-term follow-up with particular

emphasis on late death and reoperation. J Thorac Cardiovasc Surg 89, 204–220.

88. Nollert GD, Dabritz SH, Schmoeckel M, *et al.* (2003) Risk factors for sudden death after repair of tetralogy of Fallot. Ann Thorac Surg 76, 1901–1905.

89. Ebert PA, Turley K. (1983) Surgery for cyanotic heart disease in the first year of life. J Am Coll Cardiol 1, 274–279.

90. Turley K, Mavroudis C, Ebert PA. (1982) Repair of congenital cardiac lesions during the first week of life. Circulation 66, I214–I219.

91. Barratt-Boyes BG, Neutze JM. (1973) Primary repair of tetralogy of Fallot in infancy using profound hypothermia with circulatory arrest and limited cardiopulmonary bypass: a comparison with conventional two stage management. Ann Surg 178, 406–411.

92. Castaneda AR, Freed MD, Williams RG, *et al.* (1977) Repair of tetralogy of Fallot in infancy. Early and late results. J Thorac Cardiovasc Surg 74, 372–381.

93. Nollert G, Fischlein T, Bouterwek S, *et al.* (1997) Long-term survival in patients with repair of tetralogy of Fallot: 36-year follow-up of 490 survivors of the first year after surgical repair. J Am Coll Cardiol 30, 1374–1383.

94. Friedli B. (1999) Electrophysiological follow-up of tetralogy of Fallot. Pediatr Cardiol 20, 326–330.

95. Hokanson JS, Moller JH. (2001) Significance of early transient complete heart block as a predictor of sudden death late after operative correction of tetralogy of Fallot. Am J Cardiol 87, 1271–1277.

96. Knott-Craig CJ, Elkins RC, Lane MM, *et al.* (1998) A 26-year experience with surgical management of tetralogy of Fallot: risk analysis for mortality or late reintervention. Ann Thorac Surg 66, 506–511.

97. Katz NM, Blackstone EH, Kirklin JW, *et al.* (1982) Late survival and symptoms after repair of tetralogy of Fallot. Circulation 65, 403–410.

98. Boni L, Garcia E, Galletti L, *et al.* (2009) Current strategies in tetralogy of Fallot repair: pulmonary valve sparing and evolution of right ventricle/left ventricle pressures ratio. Eur J Cardiothorac Surg 35, 885–889; discussion 889–890.

99. Tirilomis T, Friedrich M, Zenker D, *et al.* (2010) Indications for reoperation late after correction of tetralogy of Fallot. Cardiol Young 20, 396–401.

100. Friedli B. (1996) [Arrhythmia after surgery for congenital cardiopathies. What studies? What treatment?] Arch Mal Coeur Vaiss 89, 351–357.

101. Khairy P, Aboulhosn J, Gurvitz MZ, *et al.* (2010) Arrhythmia burden in adults with surgically repaired tetralogy of Fallot. A multi-institutional study. Circulation 122, 868–875.

102. Harrison DA, Siu SC, Hussain F, *et al.* (2001) Sustained atrial arrhythmias in adults late after repair of tetralogy of Fallot. Am J Cardiol 87, 584–588.

103. Roos-Hesselink J, Perlroth MG, McGhie J, *et al.* (1995) Atrial arrhythmias in adults after repair of tetralogy of Fallot. Correlations with clinical, exercise, and echocardiographic findings. Circulation 91, 2214–2219.

104. Le Gloan L, Guerin P, Mercier LA, *et al.* (2010) Clinical assessment of arrhythmias in tetralogy of Fallot. Expert Rev Cardiovasc Ther 8, 189–197.

105. Wessel HU, Bastanier CK, Paul MH, *et al.* (1980) Prognostic significance of arrhythmia in tetralogy of Fallot after intracardiac repair. Am J Cardiol 46, 843–848.

106. Deal BJ, Mavroudis C, Backer CL. (2003) Beyond Fontan conversion: surgical therapy of arrhythmias including patients with associated complex congenital heart disease. Ann Thorac Surg 76, 542–553; discussion 553–554.

107. Stulak JM, Dearani JA, Puga FJ, *et al.* (2006) Right-sided Maze procedure for atrial tachyarrhythmias in congenital heart disease. Ann Thorac Surg 81, 1780–1784; discussion 1784–1785.

108. Dietl CA, Cazzaniga ME, Dubner SJ, *et al.* (1994) Life-threatening arrhythmias and RV dysfunction after surgical repair of tetralogy of Fallot. Comparison between transventricular and transatrial approaches. Circulation 90, II7–II12.

109. Khairy P, Landzberg MJ, Gatzoulis MA, *et al.* (2004) Value of programmed ventricular stimulation after tetralogy of Fallot repair: a multicenter study. Circulation 109, 1994–2000.

110. Ghai A, Silversides C, Harris L, *et al.* (2002) Left ventricular dysfunction is a risk factor for sudden cardiac death in adults late after repair of tetralogy of Fallot. J Am Coll Cardiol 40, 1675–1680.

111. Carvalho JS, Shinebourne EA, Busst C, *et al.* (1992) Exercise capacity after complete repair of tetralogy of Fallot: deleterious effects of residual pulmonary regurgitation. Br Heart J 67, 470–473.

112. Singh GK, Greenberg SB, Yap YS, *et al.* (1998) Right ventricular function and exercise performance late after primary repair of tetralogy of Fallot with the transannular patch in infancy. Am J Cardiol 81, 1378–1382.

113. Frigiola A, Redington AN, Cullen S, *et al.* (2004) Pulmonary regurgitation is an important determinant of right ventricular contractile dysfunction in patients with surgically repaired tetralogy of Fallot. Circulation 110(Suppl 1), II153–II157.

114. Discigil B, Dearani JA, Puga FJ, *et al.* (2001) Late pulmonary valve replacement after repair of tetralogy of Fallot. J Thorac Cardiovasc Surg 121, 344–351.

115. Eyskens B, Reybrouck T, Bogaert J, *et al.* (2000) Homograft insertion for pulmonary regurgitation after repair of tetralogy of Fallot improves cardiorespiratory exercise performance. Am J Cardiol 85, 221–225.

116. Warner KG, O'Brien PK, Rhodes J, *et al.* (2003) Expanding the indications for pulmonary valve replacement after repair of tetralogy of Fallot. Ann Thorac Surg 76, 1066–1071; discussion 1071–1072.

117. Gengsakul A, Harris L, Bradley TJ, *et al.* (2007) The impact of pulmonary valve replacement after tetralogy of Fallot repair: a matched comparison. Eur J Cardiothorac Surg 32, 462–468.

118. Therrien J, Siu SC, Harris L, *et al.* (2001) Impact of pulmonary valve replacement on arrhythmia propensity late after repair of tetralogy of Fallot. Circulation 103, 2489–2494.

119. Harrild DM, Berul CI, Cecchin F, *et al.* (2009) Pulmonary valve replacement in tetralogy of Fallot: impact on survival and ventricular tachycardia. Circulation 119, 445–451.

120. van Huysduynen BH, van Straten A, Swenne CA, *et al.* (2005) Reduction of QRS duration after pulmonary valve replacement in adult Fallot patients is related to reduction of right ventricular volume. Eur Heart J 26, 928–932.

121. Oosterhof T, Vliegen HW, Meijboom FJ, *et al.* (2007) Long-term effect of pulmonary valve replacement on QRS duration in patients with corrected tetralogy of Fallot. Heart 93, 506–509.

122. van Straten A, Vliegen HW, Lamb HJ, *et al.* (2005) Time course of diastolic and systolic function improvement after pulmonary valve replacement in adult patients with tetralogy of Fallot. J Am Coll Cardiol 46, 1559–1564.

123. Geva T. (2006) Indications and timing of pulmonary valve replacement after tetralogy of Fallot repairs. Semin Thorac Cardiovasc Surg Pediatr Card Surg Annu 9, 11–22.

124. Champsaur G, Robin J, Curtil A, *et al.* (1998) Long-term clinical and hemodynamic evaluation of porcine valved conduits implanted from the right ventricle to the pulmonary artery. J Thorac Cardiovasc Surg 116, 793–804.

125. Chan KC, Fyfe DA, McKay CA, *et al.* (1994) Right ventricular outflow reconstruction with cryopreserved homografts in pediatric patients: intermediate-term follow-up with serial echocardiographic assessment. J Am Coll Cardiol 24, 483–489.

126. Homann M, Haehnel JC, Mendler N, *et al.* (2000) Reconstruction of the RVOT with valved biological conduits: 25 years experience with allografts and xenografts. Eur J Cardiothorac Surg 17, 624–630.

127. Hawkins JA, Sower CT, Lambert LM, *et al.* (2009) Stentless porcine valves in the right ventricular outflow tract: improved durability? Eur J Cardiothorac Surg 35, 600–604; discussion 604–605.

128. Deorsola L, Abbruzzese PA, Aidala E, *et al.* (2010) Pulmonary valve replacement with mechanical prosthesis: long-term results in 4 patients. Ann Thorac Surg 89, 2036–2038.

129. Khambadkone S, Coats L, Taylor A, *et al.* (2005) Percutaneous pulmonary valve implantation in humans: results in 59 consecutive patients. Circulation 112, 1189–1197.

130. Miatton M, De Wolf D, Francois K, *et al.* (2007) Intellectual, neuropsychological, and behavioral functioning in children with tetralogy of Fallot. J Thorac Cardiovasc Surg 133, 449–455.

131. Zeltser I, Jarvik GP, Bernbaum J, *et al.* (2008) Genetic factors are important determinants of neurodevelopmental outcome after repair of tetralogy of Fallot. J Thorac Cardiovasc Surg 135, 91–97.

132. Chow CK, Amos D, Celermajer DS. (2005) Cerebrovascular events in young adults after surgical repair of tetralogy of Fallot. Cardiol Young 15, 130–132.

133. Zahka KG, Horneffer PJ, Rowe SA, *et al.* (1988) Long-term valvular function after total repair of tetralogy of Fallot. Relation to ventricular arrhythmias. Circulation 78, III14–III19.

134. Niwa K, Siu SC, Webb GD, *et al.* (2002) Progressive aortic root dilatation in adults late after repair of tetralogy of Fallot. Circulation 106, 1374–1378.

135. Chong WY, Wong WH, Chiu CS, *et al.* (2006) Aortic root dilation and aortic elastic properties in children after repair of tetralogy of Fallot. Am J Cardiol 97, 905–909.

136. Tan JL, Davlouros PA, McCarthy KP, *et al.* (2005) Intrinsic histological abnormalities of aortic root and ascending aorta in tetralogy of Fallot: evidence of causative mechanism for aortic dilatation and aortopathy. Circulation 112, 961–968.

137. Dimitrakakis G, Von Oppell U, Bosanquet D, *et al.* (2009) Aortic aneurysm formation five decades after tetralogy of Fallot repair. Ann Thorac Surg 88, 1000–1001.

138. Kim WH, Seo JW, Kim SJ, *et al.* (2005) Aortic dissection late after repair of tetralogy of Fallot. Int J Cardiol 101, 515–516.

139. Crestanello JA, Cook S, Daniels C, *et al.* (2010) Medial necrosis in aortic root aneurysm after repair of tetralogy of Fallot. J Card Surg 25, 230–232.

140. Zucker N, Rozin I, Levitas A, *et al.* (2004) Clinical presentation, natural history, and outcome of patients with the absent pulmonary valve syndrome. Cardiol Young 14, 402–408.

141. Chen JM, Glickstein JS, Margossian R, *et al.* (2006) Superior outcomes for repair in infants and neonates with tetralogy of Fallot with absent pulmonary valve syndrome. J Thorac Cardiovasc Surg 132, 1099–1104.

142. Hraska V, Photiadis J, Schindler E, *et al.* (2009) A novel approach to the repair of tetralogy of Fallot with absent pulmonary valve and the reduction of airway compression by the pulmonary artery. Semin Thorac Cardiovasc Surg Pediatr Card Surg Annu 59–62.

143. Hew CC, Daebritz SH, Zurakowski D, *et al.* (2002) Valved homograft replacement of aneurysmal pulmonary arteries for severely symptomatic absent pulmonary valve syndrome. Ann Thorac Surg 73, 1778–1785.

144. Alsoufi B, Williams WG, Hua Z, *et al.* (2007) Surgical outcomes in the treatment of patients with tetralogy of Fallot and absent pulmonary valve. Eur J Cardiothorac Surg 31, 354–359; discussion 359.

145. Brown JW, Ruzmetov M, Vijay P, *et al.* (2006) Surgical treatment of absent pulmonary valve syndrome associated with bronchial obstruction. Ann Thorac Surg 82, 2221–2226.

146. Gatzoulis MA, Shore D, Yacoub M, *et al.* (1994) Complete atrioventricular septal defect with tetralogy of Fallot: diagnosis and management. Br Heart J 71, 579–583.

147. Delius RE, Kumar RV, Elliott MJ, *et al.* (1997) Atrioventricular septal defect and tetralogy of Fallot: a 15-year experience. Eur J Cardiothorac Surg 12, 171–176.

148. Hoohenkerk GJ, Schoof PH, Bruggemans EF, *et al.* (2008) 28 years' experience with transatrial-transpulmonary repair of atrioventricular septal defect with tetralogy of Fallot. Ann Thorac Surg 85, 1686–1689.

CHAPTER 23

Surgical Treatment of Pulmonary Atresia with Ventricular Septal Defect

Vadiyala Mohan Reddy and Frank L. Hanley
Lucile Packard Children's Hospital, Stanford University, Stanford, CA, USA

Introduction

Pulmonary atresia with ventricular septal defect (PA-VSD) is perhaps best characterized as being at the extreme end of tetralogy of Fallot and differs from regular tetralogy of Fallot in having obligatory extracardiac sources of pulmonary blood flow. Within PA-VSD is a spectrum of lesions distinguished by a dramatic heterogeneity of pulmonary blood supply [1–3], which makes it difficult to characterize the exact incidence of each of these subsets.

Somewhere between 35% and 70% of patients with PA-VSD have a "duct-dependent" pulmonary circulation in which blood supply to the lungs is entirely through true pulmonary arteries supplied via the ductus arteriosus. The remaining 30–65% of patients, who constitute perhaps the most challenging subset of patients with this anomaly, derive pulmonary blood flow entirely or in large part from major aortopulmonary collateral arteries (MAPCAs) [4,5]. These collaterals, which are thought to arise from the embryonic splanchnic plexus, can originate from the aorta, the subclavian or carotid arteries, the coronaries, or the bronchial arteries. Each collateral may supply as little as one lung segment or as much as an entire lung and may be characterized by extrapulmonary and intraparenchymal stenoses. In such patients, true pulmonary arteries are typically either hypoplastic or absent altogether [1–3,6,7].

Although variations in pulmonary blood supply constitute a spectrum, it is practical to consider pulmonary blood flow in patients with pulmonary atresia as either "duct-dependent" or "MAPCA-dependent" because the timing and technique of surgical management differ across this division. Several reports have looked at patients with tetralogy of Fallot, pulmonary atresia, and hypoplastic confluent pulmonary arteries as a separate category of patients [8]. However, these patients almost always have collaterals contributing to pulmonary blood flow by feeding the true pulmonary arteries.

Another important morphologic feature that differs among patients with pulmonary atresia is the form of atresia: the pulmonary arteries may be separated from the right ventricle by a long-segment atresia or, occasionally, by an imperforate membrane. The primary surgical relevance of this difference relates to the method of right ventricular outflow tract reconstruction. Whereas membranous atresia may be repaired with an outflow tract patch and valvotomy or resection of the atretic valve, long-segment atresia generally requires creation or implantation of a conduit.

The cardiac morphology in these patients is almost always similar to tetralogy of Fallot with a single conoventricular type of ventricular septal defect and anterior maligned conal septum with aortic override. The presence of an atrial-septal communication, coronary anomalies, and left superior vena cava is similar to tetralogy of Fallot. The incidence of right aortic arch and retroaortic innominate vein seems to be higher in our experience. In a small percentage of patients there may be communication between the pulmonary arteries and the coronary arteries, which provide a source of pulmonary blood flow.

Clinical Features

Pulmonary atresia with ventricular septal defect accounts for approximately 1–2% of children born with congenital heart defects. A prevalence of 0.07 per 1000 live births was reported in one study [9] where 1.4% of all children born with congenital heart disease and 20.3% of all children born

Pediatric Cardiac Surgery, Fourth Edition. Edited by Constantine Mavroudis and Carl L. Backer.
© 2013 Blackwell Publishing Ltd. Published 2013 by Blackwell Publishing Ltd.

with tetralogy of Fallot had PA-VSD. The risk of PA-VSD is higher in siblings (2.5–3%) and in children of adults with tetralogy of Fallot (1.2–8.3%).

The incidence of extracardiac anomalies is significant, and the common associations are 22q deletion syndromes, DiGeorge syndrome, VATER (vertebrae, anus, trachea, esophagus, and renal) syndrome, and Alagille syndrome. There is also a relatively high incidence of bronchus suis (right upper-lobe bronchus originating from the trachea). Often the tracheobronchial compression may result from a large aorta, especially with a right aortic arch and right descending aorta. Commonly associated cardiac anomalies include atrial septal defects (ASDs), multiple ventricular septal defects, coronary artery abnormalities, left superior vena cava, and retroaortic innominate vein. Clinical presentation is variable because of the unpredictable nature of the pulmonary blood supply.

A predictable patient population is the one in which there are duct-dependent, confluent, and normal pulmonary arteries. Patients become cyanotic as the duct starts to close and require resuscitation with prostaglandin (PGE) if they have not been diagnosed prenatally. In patients with MAPCAs, cyanosis is the most common clinical presentation, and many of these infants are asymptomatic until they become progressively more cyanotic. However, some infants may present with signs of pulmonary overcirculation and congestive heart failure (CHF). Cyanotic spells are uncommon but may occur probably owing to a drop in systemic vascular resistance resulting in decreased pulmonary blood flow. In late-presenting patients previously undiagnosed, clubbing and polycythemia may be present, and sometimes stroke or cerebral abscess may be presenting features.

Increasingly with widespread use of fetal echocardiography as a prenatal screening modality, more and more children born with congenital heart disease are diagnosed prenatally. Pulmonary atresia with ventricular septal defect is relatively easy to diagnose in the fetus, although it is difficult to identify the sources of pulmonary blood flow. Nevertheless, if the ductus arteriosus is not seen in a fetus with PA-VSD, then the likelihood of MAPCAs is high. All prenatally diagnosed neonates with this condition should undergo a thorough diagnostic evaluation postnatally.

Diagnostic Evaluation

In the current era, a chest X-ray and electrocardiogram are probably less useful as diagnostic tools and more useful in patient management. Echocardiography is useful for complete delineation of the intracardiac anatomy and identifying any associated anomalies, such as confluent pulmonary arteries, duct-dependent circulation, ASDs, multiple ventricular septal defects, left superior vena cava, retroaortic innominate, and coronary anomalies. Especially in neonates and infants, a thorough echocardiographic evaluation can

identify patients who will need further investigation to identify the sources of pulmonary blood flow. However, older infants or children with PA-VSD will need additional studies to evaluate the pulmonary circulation.

It is essential to determine all sources of pulmonary blood flow in all patients before surgery. The pressure in each collateral needs to be measured, and the blood flow to all segments of the lung should be defined. Cardiac catheterization and angiography is currently our standard to evaluate these sources and the health of the pulmonary microvasculature. Often direct injection and catheter entry into each collateral is necessary. The true pulmonary arteries can be defined if the patient has a patent ductus arteriosus or if a collateral is communicating with them. Occasionally pulmonary venous wedge angiography may be necessary to define the true pulmonary arteries and/or the blood supply to some segments of the lung. If dual supply to a lobe or some segments is suspected it is important to determine the exact anatomy and the reliability of the connection between the true pulmonary arteries and the collaterals. In 10–30% of patients, true pulmonary arteries are completely absent.

Computed tomographic (CT) angiography and magnetic resonance imaging (MRI) are increasingly being used to define the collateral anatomy. Indeed, in our institution all neonates with PA-VSD undergo CT angiography to identify the sources of pulmonary blood flow and serve as a road map for cardiac catheterization before surgical intervention. With the current level of sophistication, these modalities have the advantage of being less invasive and providing a three-dimensional reconstruction of the pulmonary blood supply. This detail can be useful in planning the dissection and rerouting of the collaterals for unifocalization. However, they do not provide the hemodynamic data.

In patients who have undergone previous palliation or unifocalization but not intracardiac repair, cardiac catheterization is essential. In these patients, the pressures in the collaterals and the calculation of pulmonary-to-systemic blood flow ratio (Qp:Qs) together with the morphology is needed to determine if complete repair can be performed. If the Qp:Qs is greater than 2:1 then a complete repair can be safely performed. However, a lower Qp:Qs does not rule out complete repair if the collaterals are well developed or have grown well from previous palliation but have surgically treatable stenosis accounting for the low Qp:Qs ratio. During cardiac catheterization reactivity of the pulmonary vascular bed can also be tested with oxygen and inhaled nitric oxide.

Surgical Management

Pulmonary atresia with ventricular septal defect with duct-dependent circulation was initially managed by palliation with a systemic-pulmonary arterial shunt [10]. In 1954

Lillehei reported the use of a technique for repairing PA by anastomosing the pulmonary artery directly to an infundibulotomy [11]. Subsequently, repair using a nonvalved conduit was first reported in 1965, and repair using a valved allograft conduit was first reported in 1966 [12].

Because an enormous variety of lesions exists within the spectrum of PA-VSD, particularly with regard to pulmonary artery size, origin, course, and site of obstruction, a convenient scheme to divide PA-VSD patients into anatomic subtypes may be used for operative planning:

• **Group 1:** in this group, the patients all have large-sized duct-dependent pulmonary arteries that connect to all bronchopulmonary segments and arborize normally. It is rare to discover diminutive PAs in this group of patients.
• **Group 2:** this group of PA-VSD patients consists of infants with diminutive pulmonary arteries that supply some or all lung segments, while a variable number of MAPCAs feed the hypoplastic pulmonary arteries or are the sole supply to some segments.
• **Group 3:** in this group, all bronchopulmonary segments are supplied by MAPCAs. These patients have no true pulmonary arteries that course through the mediastinum. This group represents the most severe form of PA-VSD and has traditionally required multiple staged operations to unifocalize the MAPCAs into the pulmonary arterial system.

As with simple tetralogy of Fallot, for patients in group 1 (duct-dependent normal pulmonary arteries) the issue of palliation versus primary complete repair in the neonatal period remains purely an institution- and surgeon-dependent choice. Our bias is to repair and not perform systemic-to-pulmonary artery shunt with rare exceptions. Older age at repair was found by Kirklin et al. [13] to be the most important incremental risk factor for death after repair of tetralogy with PA in the constant hazard phase.

In contrast, the management of group 2 and 3 patients with PA-VSD and MAPCA-dependent pulmonary blood flow is much more controversial. MAPCAs are highly variable in terms of number, size, origin, course, arborization, and structure. They may constitute the sole source of pulmonary blood flow or may supply as little as a single lung segment. Until the mid-1970s medical management was considered the only option, with surgical treatment reserved for palliation, which generally consisted of one or more systemic-pulmonary arterial or systemic-collateral shunts, or with right ventricular outflow reconstruction and ligation of MAPCAs [14–17]. Based on the morphologic and physiologic studies of the variable pulmonary blood supply, Haworth and Macartney postulated that pulmonary blood supply in these patients might be normalized by unifocalizing the individual pulmonary arteries and MAPCAs to a single source [2,18].

Since then, a number of surgeons and institutions have developed strategies for the management of this lesion. Most of these have been based on the concept of staged unifocalization, with the initial phase(s) of management typically designed to increase flow to the true pulmonary arteries in an effort to stimulate growth [19–25]. These strategies have served to advance the field and have provided good results for a select group of patients. However, very few if any have cohorts of infants, and most leave a substantial proportion of patients without complete repair. As Bull and colleagues [26] observed in their article, *"Infancy is the period of greatest attrition for complex pulmonary atresia, without and with attempts at palliation ... any surgical focus aiming to make an impact on the overall mortality of this condition must alter the pattern of attrition in infancy."* Most reports do not address this most difficult group of patients. Taking into account natural attrition, which is highest in infancy [26], it is logical to conclude that only 20–30% of a cohort of newborns with tetralogy of Fallot and MAPCAs will achieve complete repair with acceptable right ventricular hemodynamics if a delayed, staged approach is taken.

The definitive goal of surgical therapy in PA-VSD with MAPCAs is to normalize circulatory physiology. Among patients surviving complete repair, the most important physiologic indicator of outcome is peak right ventricular pressure, with lower pressures being more favorable [13,27]. For a right ventricle pumping a single cardiac output, peak pressure is a direct function of pulmonary vascular input impedance, which is generally calculated as resistance. In addition to vascular resistance, which is inversely related to the total cross-sectional area of the distal pulmonary vascular bed, pulmonary arterial input impedance is also influenced by pulse-wave propagation characteristics and the presence or absence of arterial stenoses.

Given the importance of right ventricular pressure in predicting outcome, the most reliable means of ensuring that patients receive the optimal benefit from surgical therapy is to make every effort to minimize right ventricular afterload. This principle forms the basis for early complete unifocalization and repair in infancy. In patients with repaired tetralogy of Fallot and PA, the number of lung segments supplied by the pulmonary arterial system has been found to correlate strongly with pulmonary arterial pressure and calculated pulmonary vascular resistance [27]. Thus, in patients with multifocal pulmonary blood supply, it is critical to incorporate as many lung segments as possible into the unifocalized pulmonary vascular bed. In addition we have to ensure that resistance in a given pulmonary segment is as low as possible, which is largely a function of the health of the microvasculature. Presumably, the microvasculature of the lung in patients with MAPCAs is in its healthiest state at birth. The natural history of MAPCAs often follows a course of progressive stenosis and occlusion, sometimes precluding access to a given segment of lung at the time of unifocalization. Even if a severely stenosed collateral can be incorporated into the unifocalization, chronic hypoperfusion may lead to distal hypoplasia of the pulmonary vasculature and underdevelopment of alveoli [3]. Also, iatrogenic occlusion can occur when MAPCAs are unifocalized in stages using nonviable conduits, sometimes resulting in loss of segments. On the other hand, unrestricted flow through large collaterals without protective stenoses can lead to pulmonary vascular obstructive disease, which also effectively raises resistance. As experimental studies have shown, pulmonary vascular function and structure are altered after as little as 4 weeks of postnatal pulmonary hypertension with high pulmonary blood flow [28]. Similarly, staged unifocalization utilizing systemic-pulmonary arterial shunts may result in pulmonary vascular obstructive disease without necessarily stimulating compensatory flow-related growth [29]. Injuries to the distal pulmonary vasculature owing to both hypoperfusion and perfusion at systemic pressures are progressive, time-related processes. Thus, one of the keys to optimizing the health of the pulmonary vasculature, and hence the entire right heart complex, is to normalize the pulmonary circulation as early in life as possible, removing the pulmonary vascular bed from exposure to the inevitable hemodynamic vagaries associated with MAPCAs.

It is also important to preserve the growth potential of the pulmonary vascular bed. One means of accomplishing this goal is by maximizing the use of native pulmonary arterial tissue in the reconstruction and avoiding prosthetic material, especially circumferential conduits. Moreover, if the aim is to repair patients at as young an age as possible, preferably early infancy, growth potential is an important concern. Non-native tissue lacks such growth potential and is also susceptible to acquired stenosis and/or calcification. Moreover, although the mechanics of the pulmonary vasculature and its coupling with the right ventricle are not yet understood in their full complexity, especially in the context of the heterogeneous arborization and structural anomalies characteristic of tetralogy of Fallot with MAPCAs, this may also be an important issue in evaluating the health of the pulmonary circulation [30,31]. When circumferential conduits are employed in the central and hilar reconstruction of the pulmonary vasculature, the mechanical efficiency of right ventricle-pulmonary arterial coupling is likely to be impaired. Large pericardial manifolds or synthetic conduits, regularly incorporated into the reconstruction in many approaches to staged unifocalization [20–23,32,33], may produce extensive compliance and diameter mismatches in the pulmonary vascular bed, which can decrease the efficiency of right ventricle-pulmonary arterial coupling and predispose to shear stress-related vascular changes at anastomotic junctions [30,34].

There are other factors to consider in defining therapeutic goals of management for tetralogy of Fallot with MAPCAs. As discussed in Chapter 22, *Tetralogy of Fallot*, there are several benefits to early normalization of the circulation other than those affecting the pulmonary vasculature per se, including avoidance of right ventricular hypertrophy and fibrosis, avoidance of cyanotic spells and minimization of the consequences of cyanosis and polycythemia, and optimal preservation of left ventricular and aortic valvar function.

In light of the poor natural history of tetralogy of Fallot with MAPCAs and the inadequacy of staged approaches for achieving successful complete repair in the majority of patients, a strategy for managing this lesion that is founded on the principle of early total repair with one-stage unifocalization of all lung segments and maintenance of native tissue continuity seems appealing [35]. The aim of this strategy is to provide complete repair with optimum results for as many patients as possible. Keeping in mind the therapeutic goals outlined above, a complete repair in early infancy may be the ideal approach. This allows for early normalization of cardiovascular physiology, with preservation of the pulmonary vascular bed, recruitment of all lung segments, alleviation of cyanosis, and prevention of other cardiac sequelae. By performing the repair in a single stage, the number of operations required can be minimized and a greater proportion of patients is likely to be treated successfully.

The decision whether to close the ventricular septal defect at the time of unifocalization is critical to successful repair. An incorrect decision may lead to substantial morbidity, if not death. With respect to this issue, one-stage unifocalization differs significantly from staged approaches, as catheterization and angiographic data are not available following unifocalization but before closure of the ventricular septal defect. In several reports of staged unifocalization, criteria for ventricular septal defect closure based largely on angiographic measurement of the reconstructed pulmonary arteries and measurement of pulmonary vascular resistance have been suggested [21,23,27]. In patients undergoing one-stage unifocalization, such methods are not applicable, and the decision must be made intraoperatively. Angiographic measurements of the collaterals and pulmonary arteries preoperatively can be performed to estimate a neopulmonary artery index, which is the sum of the indexed cross-sectional areas of all vessels unifocalized [36]. Although we have found this method to be helpful in defining a neopulmonary artery index above which all patients can undergo closure of the ventricular septal defect ($200\,mm^2/m^2$), it is of little help in predicting suitability for closure in patients below this level. More useful is an intraoperative pulmonary flow study to estimate the resistance of the unifocalized pulmonary arterial bed [36].

Techniques of Repair

PA-VSD with Duct-Dependent Pulmonary Blood Flow

Exposure of the heart and great vessels and the initiation of cardiopulmonary bypass are performed in the same manner as described for tetralogy with pulmonary stenosis. Inevitably, right ventriculotomy is a necessary component of complete repair. Therefore, the ventricular septal defect may be closed and infundibular myectomy performed through an incision in the infundibulum rather than via a transatrial-transpulmonary approach. As such, a vertical incision is made in the right ventricular infundibulum, and the ventricular septal defect is exposed. Muscle bands bordering the incision may be resected both to ensure an unobstructed subpulmonary region and to aid in exposure. The ventricular septal defect is closed with an autologous pericardial patch using interrupted pledgeted sutures for tetralogy with pulmonary stenosis as described in Chapter 22, *Tetralogy of Fallot*. After closure of the defect,

the right ventricular outflow reconstruction is completed. In the majority of cases, a valved homograft conduit must be used to restore right ventricle–pulmonary arterial continuity. A nonvalved conduit, transannular patch with a monocusp valve, or valved conduits other than homografts can also be used. (Refer to Chapter 22, *Tetralogy of Fallot*, for more details.)

PA-VSD with MAPCA-Dependent Pulmonary Blood Flow

Surgical strategy can be categorized into four groups on the basis of morphologic variations in pulmonary blood supply:

• **Strategy A:** in patients where the size of the MAPCAs is adequate, the stenotic segments can be approached through sternotomy, and the distal bed is healthy, a complete unifocalization and intracardiac repair can be performed in one stage (Figure 23.1) [37].

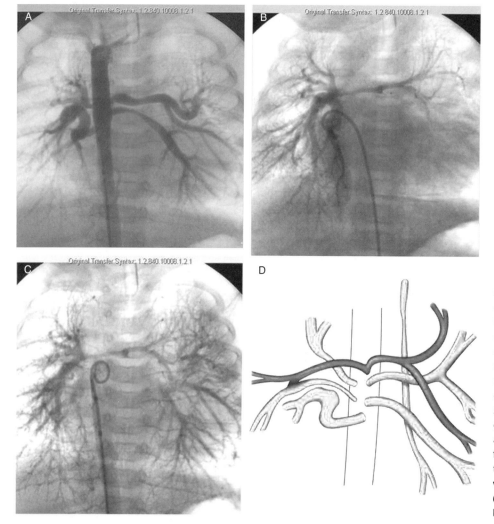

Figure 23.1 Surgical strategy A: one-stage unifocalization and intracardiac repair. **A–D** Representation of the anatomy conducive to a one-stage unifocalization and complete repair. These patients have well developed MAPCAs without significant distal stenoses. Light gray in **D** denotes MAPCAs, which are pulmonary arteries derived from the aorta. Dark gray denotes the main pulmonary arteries, which are undeveloped. (Reproduced with permission from Malhotra *et al.* [37].)

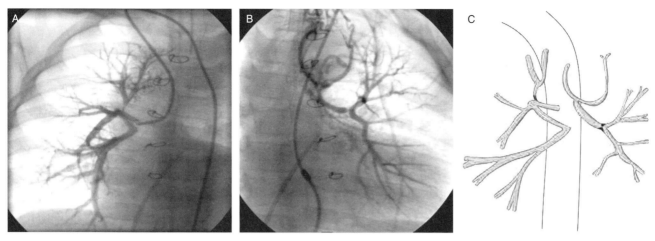

Figure 23.2 Surgical strategy B: one-stage unifocalization with shunt. The pulmonary angiograms (**A,B**) and diagram (**C**) depict small to moderate sized collaterals with proximal stenoses. This patient subgroup is amenable to one-stage complete unifocalization. However, intracardiac repair must be deferred because of elevated pulmonary arterial resistance. (Reproduced with permission from Malhotra *et al.* [37].)

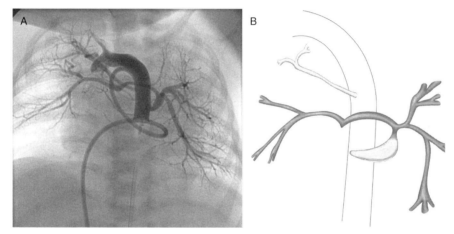

Figure 23.3 Surgical strategy C: aortopulmonary window. **A,B,** The morphology depicted is that of a well arborizing but hypoplastic true pulmonary arterial tree and poorly developed collaterals. This subgroup requires an initial aortopulmonary window to induce PA growth before completing repair. (Reproduced with permission from Malhotra *et al.* [37].)

- **Strategy B:** in patients where the MAPCAs are hypoplastic, the stenotic segments can be approached through sternotomy, and the distal bed is hypoplastic, a complete unifocalization can be performed in one stage but intracardiac repair is not feasible (Figure 23.2) [37].
- **Strategy C:** in patients where the true pulmonary arteries including the intraparenchymal vessels are hypoplastic but supply a majority of the lung segments (approximately 80%), an aortopulmonary window can be created and the collaterals feeding the true PAs can be ligated (Figure 23.3) [37].
- **Strategy D:** in patients where the MAPCAs have distal segmental stenotic areas that cannot be approached through sternotomy, a staged unifocalization through thoracotomy can be performed (Figure 23.4) [37].

Strategy A: Complete Unifocalization and Intracardiac Repair

The approach to one-stage unifocalization of pulmonary blood supply in tetralogy of Fallot with MAPCAs follows several basic principles: it is essential to control all collaterals before commencing cardiopulmonary bypass and to perform native tissue-tissue reconstruction whenever possible. A number of important techniques can aid in achieving these goals [35]. The mediastinum is entered through a median sternotomy, which is extended and retracted widely to improve exposure. Other investigators have described the use of a bilateral transsternal thoracotomy, which will also provide good exposure [38]. Collaterals are identified and dissected using a variety of approaches.

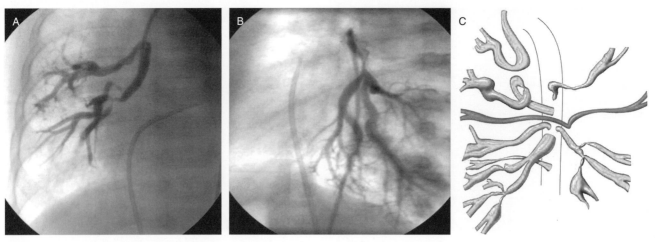

Figure 23.4 Surgical strategy D: staged thoracotomy. **A–C,** The dominant collateral system depicted has multiple stenoses at the segmental level. Sequential unilateral unifocalizations are required because of the distal extent of the obstructive lesions. Light gray denotes MAPCAs which are pulmonary arteries derived from the aorta. (Reproduced with permission from Malhotra *et al.* [37].)

Both pleural spaces are opened widely anterior to the phrenic nerves and the lungs are lifted out of their respective pleural cavities, allowing identification of collaterals at their aortic origins. Additional collaterals from the upper descending aorta are identified and dissected in the subcarinal space (between the tracheobronchial angle and the roof of the left atrium) by approaching between the right superior vena cava and the aorta (Figure 23.5) [35]. The floor of the pericardial reflection in the transverse sinus is opened and the posterior mediastinal soft tissues dissected to expose the aortic segment and the collaterals in this region. This is an important maneuver for gaining access to MAPCAs, which often arise from this location, and for providing a direct pathway for rerouting of MAPCAs to facilitate tissue-tissue anastomoses [35]. Collaterals arising from the aortic arch, brachiocephalic vessels, or coronary arteries are also exposed and dissected. To achieve controlled perfusion, collaterals are controlled before cardiopulmonary bypass and ligated at their origin before or immediately after commencing bypass.

As many collaterals as possible are ligated, mobilized, and unifocalized without cardiopulmonary bypass. Arterial oxygen saturation is followed with the ligation of each collateral, and it is possible to proceed with unifocalization off bypass until the cyanosis approaches a compromising level. At this point, partial cardiopulmonary bypass is instituted with the heart beating, and the remaining collaterals are unifocalized. The patient is cooled to 25 °C and a calcium-supplemented blood prime is used to maintain normal cardiac function. During the unifocalization process, emphasis is placed on avoiding nonviable conduits in the periphery and achieving unifocalization by native tissue-tissue anastomosis. Important concepts in

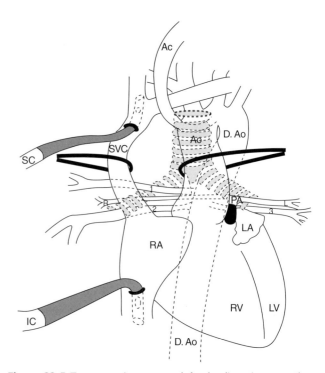

Figure 23.5 Transverse sinus approach for the dissection, rerouting, and unifocalization of the major AP collaterals. (Ac, aortic cannula; Ao, ascending aorta; DAo, descending aorta; IC, venous cannula in the inferior vena cava; L, true left pulmonary artery; LA, left atrium; LV, left ventricle; PA, long-segment pulmonary atresia; R, true right pulmonary artery; RA, right atrium; RV, right ventricle; SC, venous cannula in the superior vena cava; T, trachea; 1, 2, and 3, major AP collaterals.) (Reproduced with permission from Reddy *et al.* [35].)

achieving this type of unifocalization are flexibility regarding reconstruction, aggressive mobilization, maximizing length of the MAPCAs, and creative rerouting. Avenues for collateral rerouting are developed by opening the pleura on both sides posterior to the phrenic nerves in the hilar regions and by opening the subcarinal space through the transverse sinus. To meet the objective of complete unifocalization without peripheral conduits and with maximization of native tissue-tissue anastomosis, the following peripheral and central reconstructive techniques are employed (Figure 23.6):

- end-to-side or oblique end-to-side anastomosis of collaterals to other collaterals or to central pulmonary arteries (A);
- side-to-side or long onlay anastomosis of collaterals to the central pulmonary arteries (B);
- allograft patch augmentation of distal collateral stenoses (C);

- end-to-end or end-to-side anastomosis of collaterals to a central conduit (D);
- anastomosis of a descending aortic button giving off multiple unobstructed collaterals to true pulmonary arteries (E);
- allograft patch augmentation of the reconstructed central pulmonary arteries (F).

These techniques are used as necessary in a given patient and frequently combined, depending on the particular anatomy. Figure 23.7 [35] is an example of complex reconstruction using several of these methods. Direct tissue-tissue anastomoses are achieved by bringing collaterals through the transverse sinus, or below or above the lung hilum, utilizing as much of the collateral length as possible. Collateral length is given the highest priority so that tissue-tissue anastomosis can be achieved. For example, if a discrete stenosis is present in the mid-portion of a collateral, the entire collateral is still used, and the stenosis is relieved by side-to-side reconstruction with another collateral

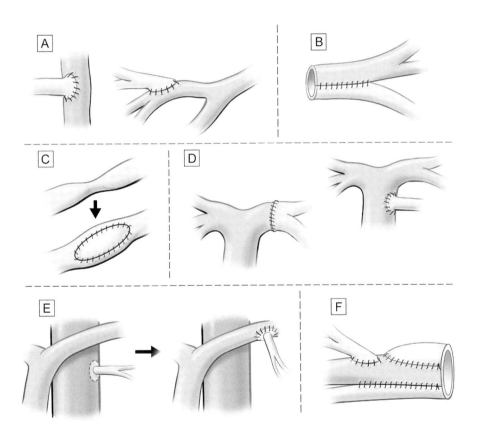

Figure 23.6 Techniques of unifocalization. To meet the objective of complete unifocalization without peripheral conduits and with maximization of native tissue-tissue anastomosis, the following peripheral and central reconstructive techniques are employed. **A,** End-to-side or oblique end-to-side anastomosis of collaterals to other collaterals or to central pulmonary arteries. **B,** Side-to-side or long onlay anastomosis of collaterals to the central pulmonary arteries. **C,** Allograft patch augmentation of distal collateral stenoses. **D,** End-to-end or end-to-side anastomosis of collaterals to a central conduit. **E,** Anastomosis of a descending aortic button giving off multiple unobstructed collaterals to true pulmonary arteries. **F,** Allograft patch augmentation of the reconstructed central pulmonary arteries. (Reprinted with permission, Cleveland Clinic Center for Medical Art & Photography © 2009–2012. All rights reserved).

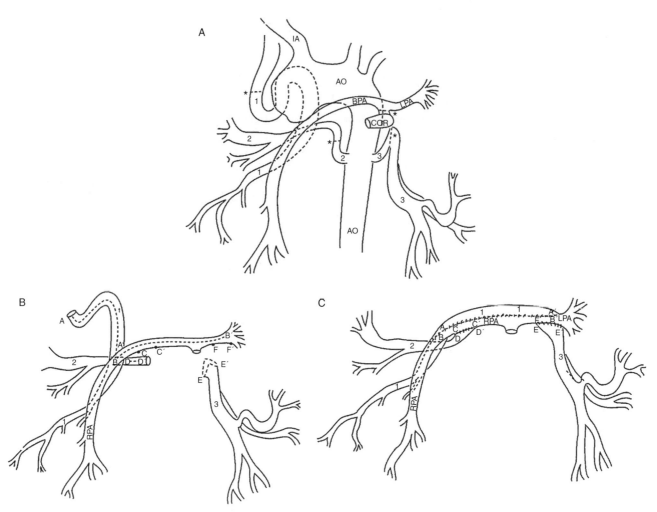

Figure 23.7 Diagrams of the anatomy of the major AP collaterals and true pulmonary arteries and the techniques of unifocalization in a 3.5-month-old infant weighing 3.5 kg. **A,** Schematic representation of the major AP collaterals and true pulmonary arteries. (AO, aorta; COR, coronary collateral; IA, innominate artery; LPA, left pulmonary artery; RPA, right pulmonary artery; 1, large and tortuous major AP collateral arising from the carotid artery; 2 and 3, major AP collaterals arising from the descending aorta. *Site of ligation and division of the major AP collaterals.) **B,** A-A', D-D', E-E', the major AP collaterals are filleted open along the broken lines; B-B', the true right and left pulmonary arteries are filleted open from hilum to hilum. **C,** A-A' to B-B', major AP collateral 1 is filleted open along its length all the way to the hilum and is anastomosed to the true pulmonary arteries, thereby augmenting the pulmonary arteries from hilum to hilum; C-C' to D-D' and F-F' to E-E', major AP collaterals 2 and 3 are anastomosed to the augmented true pulmonary arteries in an end-to-side fashion. Unifocalization and central pulmonary artery reconstruction are thus achieved without the need for non-native material. (Reproduced with permission from Reddy *et al.* [35].)

or true pulmonary artery, or by patch augmentation if necessary. All collaterals are incorporated into the reconstruction using these methods, including those that provide dual supply to a lung segment along with a true pulmonary artery, to build up the neopulmonary arteries with as much native tissue as possible.

In patients undergoing complete repair, blood flow to the unifocalized pulmonary arteries is provided via an aortic allograft valved conduit from the right ventricle to the central pulmonary arteries. Following unifocalization, the distal end of the allograft conduit is anastomosed to the central pulmonary arteries. If necessary, allograft tissue from the conduit can be extended distally to help augment the central branch pulmonary arteries. Before completing the proximal anastomosis, intracardiac repair is performed. The aorta is cross-clamped, and cardioplegia is administered. A longitudinal ventriculotomy is made in the right ventricular infundibulum and the hypertrophied muscle bundles are resected. In patients undergoing closure of the ventricular septal defect, this is performed with an autologous pericardial patch fixed in glutaraldehyde or a prosthetic patch using continuous or interrupted pledgeted sutures. The right atrium is opened to inspect the atrial septum. If an ASD or patent foramen ovale is present, it is closed partially to leave a small unidirectional interatrial communication for decompression of the right heart in the event of postoperative right ventricular dysfunction. In some cases with intact atrial septum, a small one-way interatrial communication is created. Following this the aortic cross-clamp is removed. During the rewarming period the right ventricular outflow tract reconstruction is completed by anastomosing the proximal conduit to the infundibulotomy.

In the vast majority of patients the ventricular septal defect can be closed based on the preoperative data. However, when in doubt, a pulmonary flow study can be performed [38] with the patient still on cardiopulmonary bypass. A pulmonary arterial catheter and perfusion cannula are placed into the reconstructed neopulmonary arterial system. While venting the left atrium vigorously, the lungs are perfused from the bypass pump with gradually increasing flow equivalent to at least one cardiac index ($2.5\,L/min/m^2$). In both laboratory and clinical studies, we have found this method to predict reliably mean pulmonary arterial pressure with the ventricular septal defect closed [38]. If the mean pulmonary arterial pressure is ≤25 mmHg in infants, the ventricular septal defect is usually closed. Otherwise, the defect is typically left open. In such situations in our early experience the authors performed a right ventricle-to-pulmonary artery conduit and left the ventricular septal defect open. However, the authors favor an aortopulmonary shunt instead. This avoids the need to cross-clamp and do a ventriculotomy, and the reconstructed pulmonary arterial suture lines are not exposed to systemic pressures, which can result in significant bleeding problems in some. Some groups have advocated the use of a fenestrated ventricular septal defect or its variations.

After separation from cardiopulmonary bypass, aortic, pulmonary arterial, and atrial pressures are measured continuously. Transesophageal echocardiography is performed to ensure that there are no significant residual defects. Bilateral pleural and mediastinal tube drains are placed and the sternum is closed. If bleeding or ventilation is an issue, the sternum is left open electively and the skin incision is closed with a Silastic patch. The sternum is then closed on the second or third postoperative day.

Strategy B: Complete Unifocalization to a Systemic-Pulmonary Artery Shunt

In this group of patients a complete unifocalization is performed using the same techniques as described earlier but the pulmonary blood flow is provided by constructing a central systemic-pulmonary artery shunt. The authors' preference is to place a Gore-Tex tube graft from the ascending aorta to the unifocalized neopulmonary arteries. The shunt is anastomosed using 7/0 or 6/0 polypropylene monofilament suture. The length of the shunt should be optimal without any kinks. The diameter of the shunt is determined by the quality of distal pulmonary bed and size of the patient. If the distal pulmonary bed is hypoplastic, a larger shunt may be necessary. To err on the larger side appears to be a safer option in this group of patients to allow for growth of the pulmonary bed with more flow. However, it is important to avoid excessive pulmonary flow resulting in low systemic output and pulmonary congestion. It may be necessary to reduce the size of the shunt by using hemoclips if the pulmonary blood is excessive resulting in hemodynamic compromise.

Strategy C: Creation of an Aortopulmonary Window

Creation of an aortopulmonary window involves direct anastomosis of the hypoplastic main pulmonary artery to the ascending aorta [39,40]. Through a median sternotomy approach the great arteries are carefully dissected. The main pulmonary artery is mobilized to its origin at the right ventricular infundibulum (Figure 23.8) [40]. The proximal left and right main pulmonary arteries are also adequately mobilized. Temporary neurovascular clips are placed on the branch pulmonary arteries, and the most proximal extent of the main pulmonary artery is divided as closely as possible to its infundibular origin. If needed, the proximal margin is oversewn or occluded with a surgical clip. The best location for the anastomosis of the hypoplastic main pulmonary artery to the aorta is generally to the left posterolateral aspect of the ascending aorta. Careful positioning is critical to avoid stretching and distorting the right pulmonary artery branch where it passes behind the ascending aorta. In occasional cases the pulmonary artery is better positioned by being anastomosed superiorly to the underside of the aortic arch. This decision may be heavily influenced by the anatomy of the ascending aorta and aortic arch, which can be quite variable in these patients.

The goal of a surgical aortopulmonary window is to create the largest anastomosis possible between the aorta and the diminutive main pulmonary artery trunk. The proximal end of the divided main pulmonary artery is spatulated at its open end with a longitudinal incision approximately twice the diameter of the main pulmonary artery. The incision is made on the aspect of the pulmonary artery directly adjacent to the aorta. Patients are given 150–200 units/kg of heparin before the pulmonary arteries are clamped. At completion of the anastomosis, the temporary neurovascular clips are removed from the pulmonary arteries and the partial-occluding aortic clamp is released. Diastolic blood pressure and systemic arterial saturations must be carefully monitored. Typically, the diastolic blood pressure drops by 5–10 mmHg, and the systemic arterial oxygen saturations rise by 5–10%. The heparin is not reversed. After hemodynamic stability has been ensured, the sternotomy incision is closed. Cardiopulmonary bypass

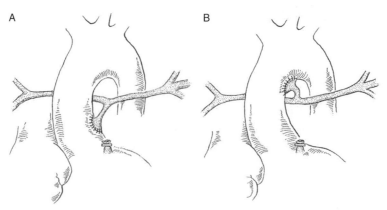

Figure 23.8 Surgical aortopulmonary window. Ideal location for anastomosis varies according to patient-specific anatomic variables and may be dictated not only by pulmonary artery anatomy but also by aortic size and position. **A,** Most common anastomotic position at left posterolateral aspect of ascending aorta, just above sinotubular junction. **B,** Less commonly, pulmonary artery confluence has better positional lie when located superiorly to undersurface of aortic arch. (Reproduced with permission from Rodefeld *et al.* [40].)

in general is not required unless the patient is severely cyanotic or hemodynamically unstable.

Strategy D: Staged Thoracotomy Unifocalization to a Systemic-Pulmonary Artery Shunt

In patients where MAPCAs are the predominant supply to the lungs but significant distal segmental stenoses are present that are not amenable for unifocalization through sternotomy, the strategy of traditional thoracotomy and unifocalization to a systemic-pulmonary artery shunt is most appropriate. Because the operation is typically performed without cardiopulmonary bypass, a posterolateral thoracotomy (through the fourth or fifth intercostal space) is performed on the side that has the worst morphology of MAPCAs so that patient's oxygenation is not affected significantly during the procedure. All the MAPCAs are dissected and controlled and then unifocalized applying the same principles as through the midline. Once the unifocalization is complete, the neopulmonary arteries are connected to the aorta or the subclavian artery using an expanded polytetrafluoroethylene (ePTFE) shunt. The unifocalized neopulmonary artery is brought close to the hilum and as close as possible centrally to facilitate later completion from the midline. The authors prefer an aortopulmonary shunt because of the ease of taking it down during the completion phase.

Postoperative Management

The postoperative management of these patients in general should follow the same principles involved in managing a complex cardiac patient following prolonged cardiopulmonary bypass. However, PA-VSD patients are prone to a certain set of special postoperative challenges. Pulmonary parenchymal reperfusion injury, parenchymal hemorrhage, and bronchospasm are commonly seen. Reperfusion injury is often seen in the regions that are underperfused preoperatively. This can result in opacification of an entire lobe or whole lung. All of these factors can sometimes make ventilating patients a challenge. A strategy of permissive hypercarbia and high positive end-expiratory pressure (PEEP) is often effective. Occasionally a ventilator may be employed and rarely venovenous extracorporeal membrane oxygenation (ECMO) may be needed until the lungs recover. It is important to restrain from escalating ventilatory peak pressures, for this can certainly result in further lung damage. Pulmonary parenchymal hemorrhage is self-resolving over time, but any coagulopathy should be promptly treated. Hemorrhage into the bronchial tree is not uncommon and usually should be managed with bronchoscopy and pulmonary toilet as indicated. Patients with bronchus suis also often need bronchoscopy for effective pulmonary toilet. Bronchospasm is often seen in the early postoperative period, especially in younger infants, possibly because of extensive dissection around the tracheobronchial tree. This usually resolves after the initial few days during which time broncholytic agents may be required. In patients who fail to extubate, phrenic nerve injury and any tracheobronchial compression should be entertained.

Postoperatively these patients require modest doses of dopamine, milrinone and calcium infusions, and sometimes epinephrine. In general in the first 48 hours after surgery the patients are well sedated and often paralyzed. Because all patients routinely have a right ventricular or pulmonary arterial catheter to monitor pressure, it is easy to observe the reactivity of pulmonary vasculature and use nitric oxide if indicated.

Bleeding can be another significant problem in the perioperative period. In the authors' experience, bleeding problems can be minimized with the use of small needles on 7/0 or 8/0 polypropylene suture and the routine use of epsilon-aminocaproic acid. If bleeding is still a concern at the end of the operation, the sternum can be left open and the mediastinum packed with thrombin-soaked Gelfoam and gauze. With this approach the risks of tamponade and re-exploration for bleeding are minimized.

Follow-Up Evaluation

At the time of discharge, in addition to the routine investigations, all patients undergo a lung perfusion scan to obtain a baseline distribution of blood to the right and left lungs and to various regions within each lung. Subsequently patients are followed closely by the cardiologist with echocardiograms and periodic lung perfusion scans. If there is clinical and echocardiographic suspicion of elevated right ventricular pressures, right ventricular dilatation, and/or depressed right ventricular function, a cardiac catheterization is performed. Nearly 30% of the patients will require additional pulmonary arterioplasty or balloon dilatation to keep the right ventricular pressure low and to encourage growth of the distal pulmonary bed by avoiding maldistribution of blood within the lungs. In this regard, the lung perfusion scan is also very important. Even in the presence of low right ventricular pressures, if there is gross maldistribution of blood between the right and left lungs or within each lung, a cardiac catheterization is performed to evaluate whether further intervention is needed to correct the stenotic areas in the reconstructed pulmonary arteries.

In patients with open ventricular septal defect, a cardiac catheterization is performed 3–4 months after unifocalization to assess the feasibility of repair. If the Qp:Qs ratio is more than 2:1 the ventricular septal defect can be closed safely. If not, the pulmonary arterial system is assessed with the goal of addressing any residual stenotic lesions that can be addressed by balloon dilation or surgery. The authors strongly discourage the use of stents in the pulmonary arterial system unless the goal is for future palliation only or if the stenoses cannot be approached by thoracotomy. Even after hemodynamically good repair, these patients should be closely followed to preserve right ventricular function with timely intervention for conduit changes or pulmonary arterioplasty.

Outcomes

In the current era, the outcomes for PA-VSD and confluent normally arborizing pulmonary arteries are almost as good as for regular tetralogy of Fallot except that these patients require multiple conduit changes over their life span; these are best considered along with tetralogy of Fallot. This section will focus on outcomes in patients with PA-VSD and MAPCAs.

Although there are numerous reports of early outcomes [19,20,22–25,32,33,35] there are very few reports of midterm [41] to long-term outcomes. This is because programmatic surgical unifocalization strategy was adopted in very few centers, and most of the cohorts include only older patients, often with preselected patients. Further, while the strategy of staged unifocalization has yielded good results in select patients [23,32,33], many of these programs did not initiate surgical treatment in early infancy when the attrition rate for infants born with PA-VSD is the highest.

In addition the variability of MAPCAs makes it difficult to compare results between institutions and between various approaches. The fact that many reports do not segregate the data of different patient groups further compounds the problem by making it difficult to discern the mortality, morbidity, and outcomes of different groups. For instance patients with hypoplastic central pulmonary arteries with a normally arborizing, good-sized intraparenchymal system would require patch augmentation of the central intrapericardial branch pulmonary arteries along with a conduit placement; in these patients the outcomes are almost as good as in tetralogy of Fallot with normal-sized central pulmonary arteries. Conversely, if the intraparenchymal pulmonary arteries are also hypoplastic, then the surgical management and results will change significantly. Patients with MAPCAs as the predominant source of pulmonary blood flow who require unifocalization of the collaterals also will have different outcomes.

Cho and Puga and associates [42] included all forms of PA-VSD in reviewing the Mayo clinic experience in 495 patients from 1977 to 1999. They reported that the presence of MAPCAs is a risk factor for mortality in unrepaired patients. In patients who were palliated with shunts and/or unifocalization but did not undergo complete repair, early mortality was 16.3% and late mortality was 23.1%. In patients who underwent complete repair (median age, 11.3 years), early mortality was 4.5% and late mortality was 16%. In 6.6% of patients the ventricular septal defects had to be reopened because of high right ventricle pressures. The risk factors for mortality at a mean follow-up of 11.4 years (standard deviation, 7.5 years) were male sex, nonconfluent central pulmonary arteries, reopening of the ventricular septal defect, and, surprisingly, postrepair conduit change. Actuarial survival at 20 years was 75%. At 22 years following initiation of PA-VSD management, 32.3% of the cohort and 27.6% of the survivors remained unrepaired.

In another report from Australia, the outcomes of staged unifocalization were evaluated in a cohort of 82 patients [43]. Approximately 65% were able to undergo complete repair, and overall survival at 12 years after complete repair was 51% (standard deviation, 14%).

A report from Toronto [44], examined a cohort of 185 surgical patients between 1975 and 2004 with only 53 patients having MAPCAs. Overall survival for the entire group at 10 years from the time of initial operation was 71%. Risk factors for death included younger age at surgery, earlier birth cohort, fewer bronchopulmonary segments supplied by native pulmonary arteries, and initial palliation with systemic-pulmonary artery shunt. Another report from Tokyo [45] is much more encouraging for staged unifocalization, with 7-year survival of 91.3% in the cohort of patients receiving late repair. Nevertheless, the patients' age in this group at first unifocalization was 3.9 years, again suggesting that many of the unifocalization programs do not initiate surgical management in early infancy where the attrition rate is high.

Between July 1992 and December 2007, the authors performed unifocalization procedures in 338 patients with PA-VSD and MAPCAs. The median age of the patients was 7.7 months (range, 10 days to 39 years; 65% of patients were infants). The median number of collateral arteries in these patients was 4 (range, 1 to 7). Collaterals supplied a median of 16.5 lung segments (range, 4 to 20), and 23.5% of patients had complete absence of true pulmonary arteries. Complete single-stage unifocalization and intracardiac repair was performed in 196 patients (58%), complete unifocalization to shunt or right ventricular conduit in 64 patients (19%), an aortopulmonary window in 37 patients (11%), and staged unifocalization via thoracotomy in 41 patients (12%). During this period complete repair was eventually achieved in 90% of the patients with perioperative right ventricle/left ventricle pressure ratio of 0.41 ± 0.12. In patients operated on since 1999, the ratio was 0.37 ± 0.11.

Overall early mortality was 5.6%. The mortality was lowest in patients with complete unifocalization and repair (3%; 6/96). Mortality with complete unifocalization to a shunt or conduit was 7.8% (5/64), with aortopulmonary window was 10.8% (4/37), and with staged thoracotomies was 10% (4/41).

Since 1999, overall mortality decreased to 2.3%. As the majority of patients were infants, conduit changes were required earlier and have been performed in 20% of the patients. In addition 22.6% of patients have undergone surgical reintervention for unifocalized pulmonary artery stenosis. Catheter intervention, predominantly balloon dilation, was performed in 19.7% of patients; in the majority of these patients, stenosis was addressed at the time of subsequent surgery. The authors have observed definitive growth in the unifocalized collaterals, also substantiated by the continued low right ventricle/pulmonary artery ratio of 0.37 ± 0.11.

Mid to late mortality was observed in 7.1% of patients (8.3% between 1992 and 1998; and 6.2% between 1999 and 2005). Late mortality was lowest in patients with complete unifocalization and repair (3%; 6/96). The mortality with complete unifocalization to a shunt or conduit was 10.4% (6/64), with aortopulmonary window was 13.5% (5/37), and with staged thoracotomies was 17% (7/41).

Total cumulative mortality was 12.7% (43/338) despite the fact that the majority of patients were infants and underwent complete unifocalization. At 10 years the actuarial survival for the whole group was 85.5%. Analysis of the data showed risk factors to be: year of surgery, and patients with both DiGeorge syndrome and gastroesophageal reflux.

More recently institutions that have adopted a programmatic approach to PA-VSD and MAPCAs have reported encouraging results.

References

1. Liao PK, Edwards WD, Julsrud PR, *et al.* (1985) Pulmonary blood supply in patients with pulmonary atresia and ventricular septal defect. J Am Coll Cardiol 6, 1343–1350.
2. Haworth SG, Macartney FJ. (1980) Growth and development of pulmonary circulation in pulmonary atresia with ventricular septal defect and major aortopulmonary collateral arteries. Br Heart J 44, 14–24.
3. Rabinovitch M, Herrera-deLeon V, Castaneda AR, *et al.* (1981) Growth and development of the pulmonary vascular bed in patients with tetralogy of Fallot with or without pulmonary atresia. Circulation 64, 1234–1249.
4. Hofbeck M, Sunnegardh JT, Burrows PE, *et al.* (1991) Analysis of survival in patients with pulmonic valve atresia and ventricular septal defect. Am J Cardiol 67, 737–743.
5. Shimazaki Y, Maehara T, Blackstone EH, *et al.* (1988) The structure of the pulmonary circulation in tetralogy of Fallot with pulmonary atresia. A quantitative cineangiographic study. J Thorac Cardiovasc Surg 95, 1048–1058.
6. DeRuiter MC, Gittenberger-de Groot AC, Poelmann RE, *et al.* (1993) Development of the pharyngeal arch system related to the pulmonary and bronchial vessels in the avian embryo. With a concept on systemic-pulmonary collateral artery formation. Circulation 87, 1306–1319.
7. Jefferson K, Rees S, Somerville J. (1972) Systemic arterial supply to the lungs in pulmonary atresia and its relation to pulmonary artery development. Br Heart J 34, 418–427.
8. Millikan JS, Puga FJ, Danielson GK, *et al.* (1986) Staged surgical repair of pulmonary atresia, ventricular septal defect, and hypoplastic, confluent pulmonary arteries. J Thorac Cardiovasc Surg 91, 818–825.
9. Perry LW, Neill CA, Ferencz C, *et al.* (1993) Infants with congenital heart disease: the cases. In: Ferencz C, Robbins JD, Loffredo CA, *et al.*, eds. *Perspectives in Pediatric Cardiology: Epidemiology of Congenital Heart Disease – The Baltimore-Washington Infant Study 1981–89.* Armonk, NY: Futura, pp. 33–62.
10. Blalock A, Taussig HB. (1945) The surgical treatment of malformations of the heart in which there is pulmonary stenosis or pulmonary atresia. JAMA 128, 189–202.
11. Lillehei CW, Cohen M, Warden HE, *et al.* (1955) Direct vision intracardiac surgical correction of the tetralogy of Fallot, pentalogy of Fallot, and pulmonary atresia defects; report of first ten cases. Ann Surg 142, 418–442.
12. Ross DN, Somerville J. (1966) Correction of pulmonary atresia with a homograft aortic valve. Lancet 2, 1446–1447.

13. Kirklin JW, Blackstone EH, Shimazaki Y, *et al.* (1988) Survival, functional status, and reoperations after repair of tetralogy of Fallot with pulmonary atresia. J Thorac Cardiovasc Surg 96, 102–116.

14. Doty DB, Kouchoukos NT, Kirklin JW, *et al.* (1972) Surgery for pseudotruncus arteriosus with pulmonary blood flow originating from upper descending thoracic aorta. Circulation 45(suppl 1), I121–I129.

15. McGoon DC, Baird DK, Davis GD. (1975) Surgical management of large bronchial collateral arteries with pulmonary stenosis or atresia. Circulation 52, 109–118.

16. Murphy DA, Sridhara KS, Nanton MA, *et al.* (1979) Surgical correction of pulmonary atresia with multiple large systemic-pulmonary collaterals. Ann Thorac Surg 27, 460–464.

17. Pacifico AD, Allen RH, Colvin EV. (1985) Direct reconstruction of pulmonary artery arborization anomaly and intracardiac repair of pulmonary atresia with ventricular septal defect. Am J Cardiol 55, 1647–1649.

18. Haworth SG, Rees PG, Taylor JF, *et al.* (1981) Pulmonary atresia with ventricular septal defect and major aortopulmonary collateral arteries. Effect of systemic pulmonary anastomosis. Br Heart J 45, 133–141.

19. Shimazaki Y, Kawashima Y, Hirose H, *et al.* (1983) Operative results in patients with pseudotruncus arteriosus. Ann Thorac Surg 35, 294–299.

20. Sullivan ID, Wren C, Stark J, *et al.* (1988) Surgical unifocalization in pulmonary atresia and ventricular septal defect. A realistic goal? Circulation 78, III5–III13.

21. Puga FJ, Leoni FE, Julsrud PR, *et al.* (1989) Complete repair of pulmonary atresia, ventricular septal defect, and severe peripheral arborization abnormalities of the central pulmonary arteries. Experience with preliminary unifocalization procedures in 38 patients. J Thorac Cardiovasc Surg 98, 1018–1028; discussion 1028–1029.

22. Sawatari K, Imai Y, Kurosawa H, *et al.* (1989) Staged operation for pulmonary atresia and ventricular septal defect with major aortopulmonary collateral arteries. New technique for complete unifocalization. J Thorac Cardiovasc Surg 98, 738–750.

23. Iyer KS, Mee RB. (1991) Staged repair of pulmonary atresia with ventricular septal defect and major systemic to pulmonary artery collaterals. Ann Thorac Surg 51, 65–72.

24. Rome JJ, Mayer JE, Castaneda AR, *et al.* (1993) Tetralogy of Fallot with pulmonary atresia. Rehabilitation of diminutive pulmonary arteries. Circulation 88, 1691–1698.

25. Marelli AJ, Perloff JK, Child JS, *et al.* (1994) Pulmonary atresia with ventricular septal defect in adults. Circulation 89, 243–251.

26. Bull K, Somerville J, Ty E, *et al.* (1995) Presentation and attrition in complex pulmonary atresia. J Am Coll Cardiol 25, 491–499.

27. Shimazaki Y, Tokuan Y, Lio M, *et al.* (1990) Pulmonary artery pressure and resistance late after repair of tetralogy of Fallot with pulmonary atresia. J Thorac Cardiovasc Surg 100, 425–440.

28. Reddy VM, Wong J, Liddicoat JR, *et al.* (1996) Altered endothelium-dependent responses in lambs with pulmonary hypertension and increased pulmonary blood flow. Am J Physiol 271, H562–H570.

29. Johnson RJ, Sauer U, Buhlmeyer K, *et al.* (1985) Hypoplasia of the intrapulmonary arteries in children with right ventricular outflow tract obstruction, ventricular septal defect, and major aortopulmonary collateral arteries. Pediatr Cardiol 6, 137–143.

30. Fourie PR, Coetzee AR, Bolliger CT. (1992) Pulmonary artery compliance: its role in right ventricular-arterial coupling. Cardiovasc Res 26, 839–844.

31. Kussmaul WG, Noordergraaf A, Laskey WK. (1992) Right ventricular-pulmonary arterial interactions. Ann Biomed Eng 20, 63–80.

32. Yagihara T, Yamamoto F, Nishigaki K, *et al.* (1996) Unifocalization for pulmonary atresia with ventricular septal defect and major aortopulmonary collateral arteries. J Thorac Cardiovasc Surg 112, 392–402.

33. Permut LC, Laks H. (1994) Surgical management of pulmonary atresia with ventricular septal defect and multiple aortopulmonary collaterals. Adv Card Surg 5, 75–95.

34. Weston MW, Rhee K, Tarbell JM. (1996) Compliance and diameter mismatch affect the wall shear rate distribution near an end-to-end anastomosis. J Biomech 29, 187–198.

35. Reddy VM, Liddicoat JR, Hanley FL. (1995) Midline one-stage complete unifocalization and repair of pulmonary atresia with ventricular septal defect and major aortopulmonary collaterals. J Thorac Cardiovasc Surg 109, 832–844; discussion 844–845.

36. Reddy VM, Petrossian E, McElhinney DB, *et al.* (1997) One-stage complete unifocalization in infants: when should the ventricular septal defect be closed? J Thorac Cardiovasc Surg 113, 858–866; discussion 866–868.

37. Malhotra SP, Hanley FL. (2009) Surgical management of pulmonary atresia with ventricular septal defect and major aortopulmonary collaterals: a protocol-based approach. Semin Thorac Cardiovasc Surg Pediatr Card Surg Annu 12, 145–151.

38. Moritz A, Marx M, Wollenek G, *et al.* (1996) Complete repair of PA-VSD with diminutive or discontinuous pulmonary arteries by transverse thoracosternotomy. Ann Thorac Surg 61, 646–650.

39. Watterson KG, Wilkinson JL, Karl TR, *et al.* (1991) Very small pulmonary arteries: central end-to-side shunt. Ann Thorac Surg 52, 1132–1137.

40. Rodefeld MD, Reddy VM, Thompson LD, *et al.* (2002) Surgical creation of aortopulmonary window in selected patients with pulmonary atresia with poorly developed aortopulmonary collaterals and hypoplastic pulmonary arteries. J Thorac Cardiovasc Surg 123, 1147–1154.

41. Reddy VM, McElhinney DB, Amin Z, *et al.* (2000) Early and intermediate outcomes after repair of pulmonary atresia with ventricular septal defect and major aortopulmonary collateral arteries: experience with 85 patients. Circulation 101, 1826–1832.

42. Cho JM, Puga FJ, Danielson GK, *et al.* (2002) Early and long-term results of the surgical treatment of tetralogy of Fallot with pulmonary atresia, with or without major aortopulmonary collateral arteries. J Thorac Cardiovasc Surg 124, 70–81.

43. d'Udekem Y, Alphonso N, Norgaard MA, *et al.* (2005) Pulmonary atresia with ventricular septal defects and major

aortopulmonary collateral arteries: unifocalization brings no long-term benefits. J Thorac Cardiovasc Surg 130, 1496–1502.

44. Amark KM, Karamlou T, O'Carroll A, *et al.* (2006) Independent factors associated with mortality, reintervention, and achievement of complete repair in children with pulmonary atresia with ventricular septal defect. J Am Coll Cardiol 47, 1448–1456.

45. Ishibashi N, Shin'oka T, Ishiyama M, *et al.* (2007) Clinical results of staged repair with complete unifocalization for pulmonary atresia with ventricular septal defect and major aortopulmonary collateral arteries. Eur J Cardiothorac Surg 32, 202–208.

CHAPTER 24

Ventricular to Pulmonary Artery Conduits

John W. Brown,[1] Osama M. Eltayeb,[2] Mark Ruzmetov,[1] Mark D. Rodefeld,[1] and Mark W. Turrentine[1]

[1]Indiana University School of Medicine, Indianapolis, IN, USA
[2]The Children's Hospital at Saint Francis, Tulsa, OK, USA

Valve pathology in infants and children poses numerous challenges to the pediatric cardiologist and cardiovascular surgeon. Valve reconstruction is the goal of all surgical intervention because restoration of anatomy and physiology employs native tissue that allows for growth and potentially better long-term outcome. When repair fails, or is not feasible, valve replacement becomes inevitable [1]. The valve pathology, patient size, and the requirement for growth all interrelate making valve replacement in neonates, infants, and children a challenging surgical procedure.

The pulmonary valve is the most common valve replaced in the congenital population. We have replaced more than 800 pulmonary valves in the past 25 years at our institution. Reconstruction of the right ventricular outflow tract (RVOT) is performed in patients with congenital heart disease when there is discontinuity between the right ventricle (RV) and the branch pulmonary arteries (PA) or in whom significant pulmonary valve stenosis or insufficiency is present. In 1964, Gian Rastelli and coworkers inserted a pericardial nonvalved tube as the first right ventricle-to-pulmonary artery (RV-PA) conduit in a child with pulmonary atresia [2]. Ross and Somerville [3] introduced the aortic valved allograft for RVOT reconstruction in 1966.

The extracardiac conduit has permitted routine repair of congenital anomalies that involve pulmonary atresia or hypoplasia of the RVOT. Such lesions include complex forms of tetralogy of Fallot (with or without pulmonary atresia), truncus arteriosus, pulmonary atresia without ventricular septal defect (VSD), transposition of the great arteries, VSD with pulmonary stenosis or atresia, certain subtypes of double outlet right ventricle, as well as pulmonary autograft replacement of the aortic root in the Ross operation. Many of these anomalies are routinely corrected in neonates—the most challenging environment for any prosthesis selected for RVOT reconstruction.

The porcine valve Dacron conduit was favored through the 1970s and early 1980s, but late obstructive complications, particularly the development of neointimal peel formation within the Dacron tube led to abandonment of this prosthesis [4]. The cryopreserved allograft (aortic and pulmonary) subsequently became the conduit of choice for RVOT reconstruction from the mid 1980s to the late 1990s. Development of cryopreservation techniques considerably improved availability and durability of allografts resulting in increased clinical use. Numerous valved conduits have since been introduced including aortic xenografts in Dacron tubes, stented bovine pericardial or porcine xenografts in pericardial tubes, glutaraldehyde fixed aortic and pulmonary roots, aortic and pulmonary allografts, and bovine jugular vein conduits [5–10].

In the following pages we will review monocusp reconstruction following transannular RVOT reconstruction, the various RV-PA conduits, isolated pulmonary valve replacement in older patients including transcatheter pulmonary valves, and finally the indications for intervention and reintervention on the RVOT in older patients who have had previous surgical and nonsurgical intervention.

Polytetrafluoroethylene Monocusp Right Ventricular Outflow Tract Reconstruction

Tetralogy of Fallot patients with significant pulmonary valve annulus and/or leaflet hypoplasia historically have been treated in one of two ways: 1) transannular patch or 2) valved conduit insertion. The transannular patch immediately relieves RV hypertension and enhances RV growth proportionally with patient growth, and reoperation for RVOT stenosis is generally uncommon. The disadvantage of transannular patching is acute pulmonary insufficiency (PI) resulting in sudden hemodynamic conversion of an

Pediatric Cardiac Surgery, Fourth Edition. Edited by Constantine Mavroudis and Carl L. Backer.
© 2013 Blackwell Publishing Ltd. Published 2013 by Blackwell Publishing Ltd.

obstructed pressure-loaded RV to a volume-loaded RV, which causes temporary and/or delayed RV dysfunction. Chronic RV volume overload can lead to late biventricular dysfunction and tricuspid insufficiency necessitating the need for pulmonary valve insertion [11,12].

The initial advantage of a valved conduit is immediate pulmonary valve competency. Conduit insertion is particularly useful in patients who have peripheral unrepaired pulmonary stenosis or elevated pulmonary vascular resistance (PVR >4 Wood units). The disadvantages of currently available valved conduits are their structural deterioration secondary to calcification, shrinkage, and lack of growth resulting in early and late valve dysfunction. These unsolved problems are manifested by the allograft conduit (AC) that became popular in the United States during the mid 1980s. Pulmonary allografts remain popular at present despite freedom from reoperation of 50% at 5 years in patients undergoing a non-Ross RVOT conduit insertion [10,12].

An attractive alternative strategy has been the concept of a monocusp RVOT patch reconstruction, which in certain patient populations has the potential advantages lacking in patients who require a transannular patch without pulmonary valve reconstruction or placement of a valved conduit that may interrupt RV-PA continuity. A monocusp valve can be placed in any sized patient when the monocusp leaflet is tailor-made to fit the RVOT that is being enlarged by a transannular outflow patch, is less expensive, and usually lasts longer than a valved conduit in an infant. The monocusp RVOT patch can be constructed with autologous or bovine pericardium [13,14], allograft pulmonary valve cusp [15], or a polytetrafluoroethylene (PTFE) membrane (0.1 mm PTFE cusp; W.L. Gore & Associates, Inc, Flagstaff, AR; off-label use) traditionally employed as a pericardial substitute [16–20]. Each of these materials have demonstrated good immediate postoperative valve competency and reduced early PI [17,19–21].

In 1993, Yamagishi and Kurosawa [18] and Oku and colleagues [19] independently introduced 0.1 mm PTFE pericardial membrane as readily available material with good handling characteristics for monocusp valve construction and found it superior when compared to biologic leaflet materials. Our animal studies suggest that 0.1 mm PTFE functioned as well as or better than fresh or glutaraldehyde-treated pericardium. Clinical application of this material in our patients with tetralogy of Fallot in whom transannular patching was necessary resulted in improved perioperative RV function as evidenced by a lower postoperative central venous pressure, less need for postoperative inotropic agents, less chest tube drainage, and a decreased intensive care unit (ICU) and hospital stay [22]. The PTFE membrane is now our material of choice for a monocusp construction and has been used in more than 250 patients with a wide range of RVOT obstructive and regurgitation defects. We particularly value its use in the small infant undergoing primary tetralogy of Fallot repair with and without pulmonary atresia in whom transannular patching is necessary.

Construction of a pericardial or PTFE monocusp is simple, relatively inexpensive, and reproducible. Allograft pulmonary valve cusps are considerably more expensive in the United States and may be difficult to custom fit into the RVOT. The potential disadvantage of a monocusp patch in comparison with insertion of a pulmonary valve or valved conduit is that PI may recur more quickly in some patients if the monocusp leaflet sticks in the open position as has been reported with some biologic monocusps [17,20,21]. Recurrent stenosis at the level of the monocusp valve is rarely seen with monocusp leaflet material of any type. The major advantage of the 0.1 mm PTFE is that it does not allow tissue ingrowth and remains mobile (functional) for a much longer period.

The technique of monocusp insertion at our institution has remained relatively constant over the last 16 years. The length and width of the monocusp leaflet are determined and the 0.1 mm PTFE membrane is sewn into the RVOT. To ensure monocusp leaflet coaptation to the conal septum and/or residual pulmonary leaflet tissue, the width and length of the patch is kept mildly redundant. A second patch of 0.4 mm PTFE is sewn across the entire RVOT onto the main PA with the second suture line. Patients with defects that include an intact pulmonary valve annulus are evaluated following pulmonary valvotomy. The annulus diameter is measured with a Hegar dilator and if the annular Z value was ≥–2, then transannular patching is not performed. In patients with moderate-to-severe annular hypoplasia (Z score <–2), or postvalvotomy RVOT gradient >30 mmHg and/or RV pressure >80% of systemic pressure, transannular patch repair with a monocusp valve insertion is used (Figures 24.1–24.3).

The PTFE monocusp with separate RVOT patch has been useful for our patients with tetralogy of Fallot or pulmonary atresia with VSD who require a transannular patch (35–40% of our tetralogy series) and in patients requiring a second RVOT procedure after failed initial conduit reconstruction. The monocusp valve has functioned well in most patients for the first 3–4 years and for up to 10–12 years in some patients. While the majority of patients developed some pulmonary regurgitation as the RV outflow tract grows, recurrent outflow obstruction at the leaflet level has not been observed. Another important indication for PTFE monocusp reconstruction is primary AC failure because inserting a second AC has been associated with accelerated structural failure [12].

The PTFE monocusp can be expected to retain adequate function in the early to mid postoperative period. The only anticoagulant used is aspirin (10 mg/kg day, up to a limit of 80 mg/day).

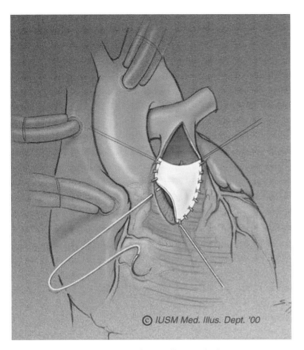

Figure 24.1 Technique for polytetrafluoroethylene monocusp insertion (monocusp inserted before outflow patch). (Reproduced with permission from Indiana University School of Medicine. Copyright © 2012 Indiana University Trustees.)

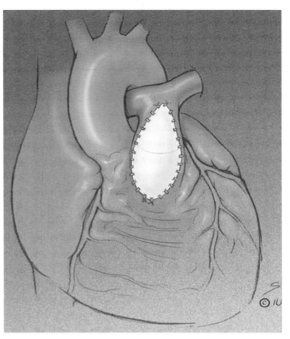

Figure 24.2 Technique for polytetrafluoroethylene monocusp insertion (complete right ventricular outflow tract patch). (Reproduced with permission from Indiana University School of Medicine. Copyright © 2012 Indiana University Trustees.)

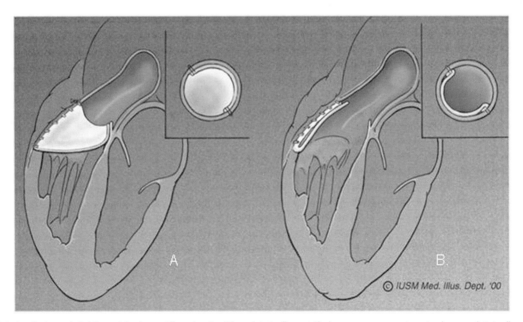

Figure 24.3 Lateral view of right ventricular outflow tract with polytetrafluoroethylene monocusp. Inserts show polytetrafluoroethylene monocusp in (**A**) closed and (**B**) open position. (Reproduced with permission from Indiana University School of Medicine. Copyright © 2012 Indiana University Trustees.)

From 1994 through 2006, 192 patients (mean age 3.3 ± 5.0 years) underwent RVOT reconstruction with a PTFE mono-cusp valve (192 patients; 202 implants), mean interval (4 to 9 ± 3.1 years) (range, 6 months to 12 years). The series was divided into three groups: patients undergoing initial repair of tetralogy or pulmonary atresia with VSD (group I); patients undergoing redo RVOT procedure (group II); and patients undergoing complex initial repair (group III).

There were four early and five late deaths (9 of 192 patients; 5%). The difference between the preoperative and postoperative peak RVOT gradients for the 192 patients was significant (71.2 versus 23.1; $p < .0001$). Twenty-five patients (13%) developed mild-to-moderate RVOT stenosis at one or more locations proximal and/or distal to the monocusp valve but not at the monocusp valve (mean gradient, 44.7 ± 20.3 mmHg). Freedom from increased PI greater than moderate was 86% at 1 year, 68% at 5 years, and 48% at 10 years (Figure 24.4) [23]. Twenty-five patients have undergone 35 PTFE monocusp reoperations 4.2 ± 3.1 years (range; 3 months to 10 years) after initial repair. Kaplan-Meier freedom from reoperation was 96% at 1 year, 89% at 5 years, and 82% at 10 years following surgery (Figure 24.5) [23]. Freedom from reoperation in group II (69%) was significantly higher when compared with group I (88%; $p = .01$) and group III (90%; $p = .02$) while there was no observed difference between groups I and III.

Several bicuspid PTFE reconstructions, conduits, and a folding monocusp PTFE leaflet have been recently introduced. Most incorporate a 0.1 mm pericardial PTFE membrane that is used "off label" for leaflet construction as described earlier [22,23]. Early results with these new modifications seem promising, but longer follow-up will be necessary to evaluate their durability.

Quintessenza and colleagues described a bicuspid RVOT outflow reconstruction [24]. Their early results (3 years) with the 0.1 mm PTFE are considerably better than those obtained with the 0.6 mm PTFE followed for up to 8 years. Nunn and colleagues described a folding monocusp using 0.1 mm PTFE and demonstrated less regurgitation across the RVOT at the expense of a higher gradient at mid-term follow-up than obtained with a simple horizontal monocusp [25]. Morell and colleagues have described a PTFE tube with a bicuspid PTFE valve constructed in the conduit [26]. Their initial results have been satisfactory in spite their short follow-up (<1 year).

Allograft Conduits

Cryopreserved pulmonary allografts were the "gold standard" in the United States from the mid-1980s through the late 1990s [5,6,10]. In most centers, pulmonary ACs were favored over aortic allografts as they are less prone to dysfunction and calcification [27]. The higher elastin content of aortic allografts may increase their propensity for early dense calcification and adherence to adjacent structures making conduit removal or revision challenging. In some patients, extracardiac pulmonary ACs are prone to significant valve regurgitation within months of insertion or can develop shrinkage leading to late conduit stenosis [12]. However, pulmonary allograft performance and longevity is significantly improved in the Ross operation because many of the patients are older and the oversized pulmonary allograft is inserted into the orthotopic position, which may alleviate the turbulent flow seen in extracardiac valved conduits.

The evaluation of AC durability is critical in determining the choice of prosthesis for pulmonary valve replacement. Forbess *et al.* [5] evaluated 185 consecutive pulmonary AC implanted at a single institution over 14 years in three separate age groups. Their univariate analysis demonstrated that smaller allograft size (<14 mm),

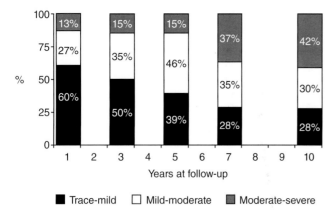

Figure 24.4 Degree of pulmonary insufficiency of polytetrafluoroethylene monocusps on echocardiography at different periods of follow-up. (Reproduced with permission from Brown *et al.* [23].)

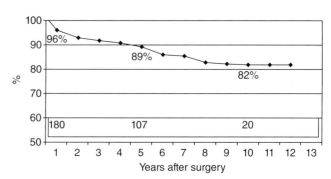

Figure 24.5 Kaplan-Meier estimated 12-year freedom from reoperation in patients with polytetrafluoroethylene monocusp. (Reproduced with permission from Brown *et al.* [23].)

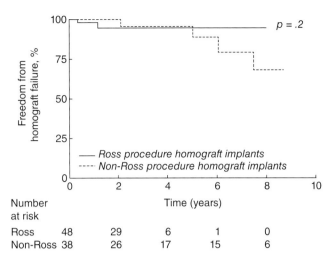

Figure 24.6 Kaplan-Meier freedom from pulmonary allograft failure for Ross and non-Ross right ventricular outflow tract reconstruction in patients more than 10 years of age. (Reproduced with permission from Forbess *et al.* [5].)

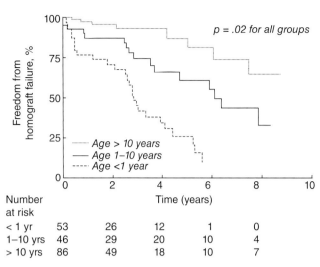

Figure 24.7 Kaplan-Meier freedom from allograft failure by age category. (Reproduced with permission from Forbess *et al.* [5].)

younger aged patients (<1 year), and diagnosis of truncus arteriosus were all risk factors for conduit failure while allograft size was the only predictor of failure in the multivariate analysis. Ross aortic valve replacement (AVR)-related implants had the best outcome with a 5-year AC survival of 94% (Figure 24.6) [5], while non-Ross AC implants in children >10 years of age had a 5-year graft survival of 76% (Figure 24.7) [5].

Dearani *et al.* published the largest series of pulmonary valve replacement and RV-PA conduits from the Mayo Clinic [6]. They described 1270 RVOT procedures in 1095 patients undergoing RV-PA conduit or pulmonary valve replacement over a 37-year period. The operative mortality was 3.7% in the most recent decade. Mean follow-up for the entire series was 10.9 years with a maximum of 29 years. Three types of conduits were implanted: 730 porcine valved Dacron conduits, 239 homografts, and 126 nonvalved conduits. Risk factors for conduit failure included pulmonary allografts, younger age (<4 years) at initial operation, and smaller conduit size (<19 mm) [6]. Survivorship free of reoperation for conduit failure was 84.1% ± 1.4% at 5 years, 55.5% ± 2.0% at 10 years, 39.6% ± 2.2% at 15 years, and 31.9% ± 2.7% at 20 years. In their series comparing the AC with the Dacron tube with a porcine xenograft they found the AC was less durable.

At our institution, 117 non-Ross patients received cryopreserved ACs (94 pulmonary and 23 aortic) between January 1985 and December 2003 for RVOT construction [30]. Ages ranged from 6 days to 43 years (mean, 8 months), and there were 57 children (49%) younger than 12 months of age. There were no device-related deaths. Overall patient survival was 80% at 15 years. Freedom from AC failure (valve explantation, balloon dilatation) was 60% at 5 years

and 43% at 15 years; freedom from AC failure was worse in infants (42% at 5 years and 34% at 15 years). Freedom from AC dysfunction (AC stenosis >40 mmHg and AC insufficiency more than moderate) was 40% at 5 years and 23% at 15 years; freedom from dysfunction was worse in infants (21% at 5 years and 16% at 15 years).

Univariate analysis identified younger age, smaller AC, diagnosis of truncus arteriosus, and presence of aortic AC as risk factors for AC dysfunction and failure. Multivariate analysis identified smaller AC size and the presence of truncus arteriosus as risk factors for AC dysfunction and failure (Figure 24.8 and Figure 24.9) [28]. A comparison of some published series of AC used for RVOT reconstruction is shown in Table 24.1 [7,8,10,28–34,72].

Pulmonary Allografts in Ross Aortic Valve Replacement Patients

In our experience the durability of RVOT reconstruction with a pulmonary AC in patients undergoing the Ross AVR is improved secondary to older age at implant, orthotopic positioning, and the ability to oversize the AC [35].

From 1993 at our institution, pulmonary allografts have been the RV-PA conduit of our choice for reconstruction in Ross AVR operation and remain so today with the exception of children younger than 5 years of age where the Contegra® conduit (Medtronic; Minneapolis, MN) is favored [35,36].

Aortic allografts calcify more quickly than pulmonary ACs when placed in the RVOT [8,10]. This is linked to the higher elastin content of the aortic AC wall [11]. The AC size was found to be a significant mechanical risk factor that influenced durability in many studies [5,8,36]. Our results

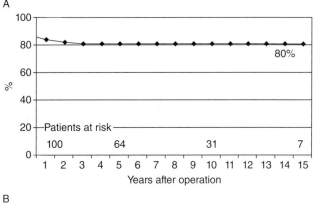

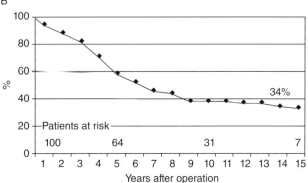

Figure 24.8 (**A**) Kaplan-Meier survival curve and (**B**) freedom from reoperation for 117 non-Ross patients undergoing allograft conduit reconstruction of the right ventricular outflow tract. (Reproduced with permission from Brown *et al.* [28].)

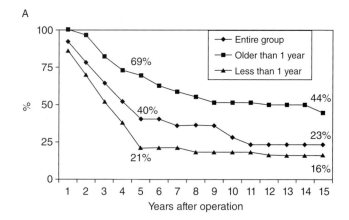

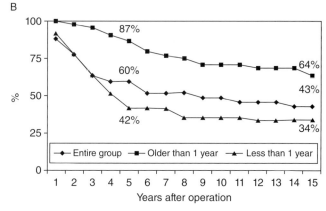

Figure 24.9 A, Kaplan-Meier freedom from pulmonary allograft dysfunction (gradient > 40 mmHg and/or > moderate allograft regurgitation). **B,** Kaplan-Meier freedom from pulmonary allograft failure (explantation of allograft or valve-related death). (Reproduced with permission from Brown *et al.* [28].)

Table 24.1 Results of surgical treatment in patients with RVOT allograft implantation: literature review. (AF, allograft conduit failure; AD, allograft conduit dysfunction.) (Reproduced with permission from Brown *et al.* [28].)

	No. of patients	Early death	Late death	Follow-up (mean)	Explant conduit	Freedom from AF Freedom from AD
Hawkins, Cincinnati, 1992 [29]	89 (non-Ross)	7 (8%)	9 (11%)	31 mo	8 (10%)	-
Bando *et al.*, Mayo, 1995 [10]	326 (non-Ross)	22 (6%)	24 (7%)	3.2 yr	32 (11%)	-
Yankah *et al.*, Berlin, 1995 [30]	53 (non-Ross)	15 (28%)	1 (3%)	26 mo	5 (13%)	-
Niwaya *et al.*, Oklahoma, 1999 [31]	369 (all)	38 (10%)	13 (4%)	3.8 yr	30 (9%)	62% at 8 yr 53% at 8 yr
Tweddell *et al.*, Milwaukee, 2000 [8]	178 (all)	22 (11%)	6 (4%)	3.6 yr	42 (27%)	54% at 10 yr 22% at 10 yr
Bielefeld *et al.*, Denver, 2001 [32]	223 (non-Ross)	31 (14%)	3 (9%)	6.0 yr	38 (20%)	-
Sinzobahamvya *et al.*, St. Augustin, 2001 [7]	76 (non-Ross)	7 (9%)	3 (4%)	54 mo	14 (20%)	65% at 10 yr 10% at 10 yr
Gerenstein *et al.*, Rotterdam, 2001 [72]	297 (all)	12 (4%)	15 (5%)	4 yr	24 (8%)	-
Brown *et al.*, Indianapolis, 2004 [28]	117	16 (14%)	7 (6%)	6.1 yr	43 (46%)	43% at 15 yr 23% at 15 yr
Askovich *et al.*, Salt Lake City, 2007 [33]	140 (all)	NA	NA	5.1 yr	77 (64%)	-
Boethig *et al.*, Hannover, 2007 [34]	79 (non-Ross)	NA	14 (18%)	6.6 yr	27 (34%)	-

are consistent with this observation as allograft diameter was found to be an independent predictor of late stenosis. This is especially true in the pediatric Ross AVR population. Children younger than 5 years of age have an accelerated growth and can quickly outgrow their valve conduit. For this reason, we aggressively oversize the implanted allograft in Ross AVR patients, regardless of the patients' pulmonary annulus size because size rather than patient age is the most important predictor for pulmonary allograft failure (defined as the need for graft replacement) [36].

Between June 1993 and May 2007, 183 consecutive patients at our institution underwent Ross AVR with RVOT reconstruction using a cryopreserved pulmonary allograft (n = 156), decellularized pulmonary homograft (n = 22), and bovine jugular vein conduit (n = 5). Ages ranged between 1 month and 61 years (mean age, 23.3 ± 15.2 years). Three patients (2%) died (two early and one late), 24 patients (13%) had a peak systolic RVOT gradient exceeding 20 mmHg, 5 (3%) had a gradient exceeding 40 mmHg, and 7 (4%) had more than 2+ PI. Eight patients (4%) underwent conduit replacement for RV dysfunction. Freedom from RVOT reoperation at 10 years is 96%. Freedom from RV conduit failure and dysfunction was 98% and 96% at 5 years and 96% and 93% at 10 years, respectively. Independent predictors of pulmonary allograft RV-PA conduit dysfunction are smaller (<14 mm) RVOT conduit size ($p = .03$) and follow-up exceeding 5 years ($p = .05$) (Figure 24.10) [35]. The most logical reasons for the superior performance of the allograft in Ross AVR patients are 1) orthotopic conduit position, 2) older implant age, and 3) the use an oversized homograft [35].

During the last decade demand has increased for a RV-PA conduit more durable than ACs for non-Ross RVOT reconstruction has increased [28,37]. In late 1999, we began implanting the bovine jugular vein conduit (Contegra® BJVC, Medtronic, Minneapolis, MN), porcine

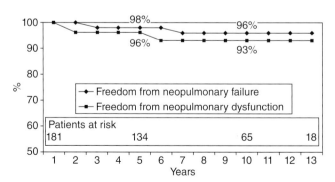

Figure 24.10 Kaplan-Meier freedom from neopulmonary conduit failure and dysfunction in patients following Ross aortic valve replacement. (Reproduced with permission from Brown *et al.* [35].)

stentless aortic root xenograft (Freestyle™, Medtronic), and the new decellularized pulmonary allograft (SynerGraft®, CyroLife, Kennesaw, GA) for non-Ross RVOT reconstruction [37–40].

Bovine Jugular Venous Valved Conduit

The limited availability and durability of ACs, especially in smaller sizes, supported the search for an alternative prosthesis to reconstruct the RVOT in patients with congenital heart disease (pulmonary allografts work well in Ross patients). In 1999, the Contegra BJVC was introduced as a potential alternative to allografts for RVOT reconstruction. The BJVC is a low-pressure, buffered glutaraldehyde fixed section of bovine jugular vein (12–15 cm in length and 12–22 mm in diameter). The three-cusp naturally occurring venous valves are in the center of the conduit, which possesses natural sinuses. The conduit wall is compliant with excellent suturability (Plate 24.1, see plate section opposite p. 594).

Early animal studies by Ichikawa and colleagues [41] and by our group [42] reported excellent results demonstrating good leaflet preservation and freedom from significant structural degeneration and valve regurgitation at 3 years. Herijgers and colleagues reported resistance of the Contegra BJVC to calcification when implanted in juvenile sheep, albeit for only 5 months [43].

These animal studies were confirmed in human clinical trials with up to 27 months (mean, 1.2 years) of follow-up reported by Breymann and colleagues [44] suggesting that the Contegra BJVC might represent a promising alternative to allograft. A report by Bove and colleagues [45] comparing a modified bicuspid pulmonary allografts and Contegra BJVC supported these findings in 41 patients (mean age 1.9 years) undergoing RVOT reconstruction. The BJVC demonstrated favorable hemodynamics as compared to allografts. Other advantages of the Contegra BJVC include greater shelf availability, natural continuity between valve and conduit, and no requirement for proximal extension.

The principles of Contegra BJVC insertion include: 1) the conduit is rinsed for 5 minutes with continuous manual agitation in four 500-cc baths of normal saline or Ringer's lactate before implantation; 2) the conduit is positioned into the main and left PA to avoid sternal compression; and 3) the outflow end of the conduit is cut so that the conduit valve is positioned as far distally as possible near the PA bifurcation to avoid valve distortion with sternal compression [7]. The inflow end of the conduit is spatulated and sewn with continuous monofilament suture to the edges of the right ventriculotomy without the use of additional prosthetic material.

Patients enrolled in this humanitarian device exemption (HDE) study had their surgical data and preoperative and postoperative catheterization and echocardiographic variables submitted to a core laboratory for analysis and review by the Contegra primary investigators, who make up the Contegra Scientific Advisory Board. The core laboratory analysis gave the data accuracy and consistency. Several European investigators have published their results, and their data are summarized along with ours in Table 24.2 [28,37,44–52]. Contegra was approved for HDE in the United States in November 2000, and more than 17 000 have been implanted to date.

The mid-term results of RVOT reconstruction using the Contegra BJVC in 153 patients at our institution were retrospectively analyzed [53]. Patient ages ranged from 2 weeks to 18 years (mean, 8.4 ± 7.4 years). The Contegra BJVC size varied in diameter between 12 and 22 mm (mean, 18.5 ± 3.7 mm). Actuarial survival, freedom from dysfunction, and freedom from failure were 95%, 85%, and 89%, respectively, at 3.7 ± 2.4 years' follow-up.

In our series, during 11 years of follow-up, we have not observed shrinkage of the Contegra BJVC using echocardiography. Conduit explantation, perhaps the most stringent measure of performance, was significantly better at 5 and 10 years with BJVC (when compared with allografts) [54]. Our experience is in agreement with the recent work of Boethig and coworkers who demonstrated a freedom from explantation at 5 years for Contegra BJVC at 90% and pulmonary allografts at 70% (p = .02) [55].

The Contegra BJVC is a promising alternative for RVOT reconstruction because early hemodynamic performance compares favorably with allografts, it is more readily available in smaller sizes (12–16 mm) than allografts, the location of the valve within the conduit permits proximal infundibular anastomosis without additional prosthetic material, and the cost of the bovine jugular venous valve is approximately one half that of many ACs. In addition, short-term freedom from dysfunction is at better than for most allografts. Since 1999, we have implanted 153 Contegra BJVC at Indiana University and have observed an 8-year freedom from conduit reintervention and explantation of 90% and 94% respectively, which is superior to our experience with allografts in non-Ross RVOT reconstruction (unpublished data). Although longer-term follow-up will determine durability of this conduit, in neonates, infants and young children, it is our prosthesis of choice for RVOT reconstruction (except in Ross AVR patients >5 years of age, where allografts are preferred) [46]. A listing of several reported series of Contegra BJVC conduits is shown in Table 24.2 [37,44–52].

Fiore, Brown, and colleagues compared the mid-term performance of BJVC with pulmonary homografts in children under 2 years of age [54]. At 5 and 10 years, freedom from dysfunction was significantly improved (BJVC, 90%

Table 24.2 RV-PA conduit with bovine jugular vein: literature review. (PR, pulmonary regurgitation.) (Reproduced with permission from Brown et al. [46].)

Authors	No. of patients	Age (mean)	Mortality (overall)	Postop reintervention	Follow-up Time	Gradient (>30 mmHg)	PR (>mild)
Breymann et al. (Bad Oeynhausen, Germany) [44]	71	3.4 yr	6 (8%)	7 (10%)	1.2 yr	valve - 10%	5 (7%)
						distal - 34 (47%)	
Corno et al. (Lausanne, Switzerland) [47]	26	13.5 yr	1 (4%)	1 (4%)	15 mo	NA	4 (16%)
Carrel et al. (Berne, Switzerland) [48]	21	NA	0	3 (14%)	NA	NA	NA
Bove et al. (Brussels, Belgium) [45]	41	1.9 yr	1 (2%)	0	NA	valve - 2 (13%)	4 (27%)
						distal - 6 (40%)	
Chatzis et al. (Athens, Greece) [49]	15	NA	0	1 (7%)	18.5 mo	NA	NA
Dave et al. (Zurich, Switzerland) [37]	13	NA	0	0	NA	NA	1 (8%)
Brown et al. (Indianapolis, USA) [46]	64	8.1 yr	6 (9%)	8 (13%)	25.7 mo	valve -1 (1.6%)	1 (1.6%)
						distal - 8 (13%)	
Rastan et al. (Leipzig, Germany) [50]	78	13 yr	2 (3%)	29 (38%)	31 mo	valve - 18 (24%)	12 (16%)
Morales et al. (Houston, USA) [51]	76	NA	2 (3%)	12 (16%)	20 mo	valve - 0	14 (19%)
Sekarski et al. (Lausanne, Switzerland) [52]	133	31 mo (median)	19 (14%)	26 (21%)	31 mo	valve - 2 (1.6%)	10 (8%)

and 85% versus pulmonary AC, 71% and 24%; $p < .05$); conduit failure trended lower (BJVC, 85% and 67% versus AC, 75% and 45%; $p = .06$), while freedom from explantation was significantly better for BJVC patients (BJVC, 85% and 67% versus AC, 75% and 45%; $p = .06$). Freedom from explantation, perhaps the most stringent measure of conduit durability was significantly better for BJVC patients (BJVC, 85% versus pulmonary AC, 47%; $p = .01$), while freedom from distal conduit and peripheral stenosis were similar in both cohorts.

Percutaneous Pulmonary Valves

In January 2010, the Melody® (Medtronic) stented bovine jugular venous valved RV-PA conduits were released in the United States under HDE to be placed percutaneously via venous access (Plate 24.2, see plate section opposite p. 594). More than 1400 have been used in other countries. Initial results are promising, but follow-up has been short.

Data of the first 99 patients enrolled in the Medtronic Melody study from January 2007 to December 2008 show that 90 of 99 patients enrolled were implanted [56]. Nine patients were excluded because of concern for coronary compression. Catheterization gradients decreased from 35 ± 16 mmHg to 14 ± 7 mmHg ($p < .001$) and all patients had less than trivial PI. Death occurred in 1 patient, and homograft rupture requiring surgery occurred in 1 patient. The RVOT gradient increased from 14 ± 7 mmHg at implant to 20 ± 8 mmHg at 6 months and 22 ± 10 mmHg at 1 year. Freedom from stent fracture was 89%, and freedom from surgical reintervention was 99% at 1 year.

Nonvalved Right Ventricular–Pulmonary Artery Conduits

Non-valved RV-PA conduits deserve mention and are still used in some centers. Early results are satisfactory but many patients develop late RV dilation within 10 years. Dearani and colleagues reported on 126 nonvalved RV-PA conduits and concluded that freedom from conduit failure was no different than for valved conduit [6]. They no longer use nonvalved conduit. We have not used non-valved conduits in more than 10 years.

Stented and Stentless Xenograft Valves in the Right Ventricular–Pulmonary Artery Position

The Contegra BVJC is under HDE category and cannot be inserted in patients over 18 years of age due to patent restrictions. The optimal prosthesis to implant in older children (>18 years) and adults is still an area of controversy. Fiore, Brown, and colleagues [54] retrospectively reviewed the performance of the Mosaic® (Medtronic) porcine,

bovine pericardial, and homograft prostheses for pulmonary valve replacement to correct chronic PI. The mean age of patients receiving the prostheses was 22.7 years. All three prostheses significantly reduced chronic PI, but late insufficiency was higher with allografts [57]. Late valve dysfunction (defined as a gradient >40 mmHg or >2+ regurgitation) was highest with homografts (54%), followed by porcine (19%) and pericardial (5.5) valves ($p < .05$). Fiore *et al.* concluded that all three prostheses performed similarly for 3 years. Pulmonary regurgitation developed more rapidly and frequently in homografts, albeit there was longer follow-up in the homograft group (Figure 24.11) [54].

We reviewed 85 patients who underwent pulmonary valve replacement using a stentless (n = 61) or a stented (n = 24) porcine aortic bioprosthesis [58]. All patients except two had prior RVOT reconstruction, and patients' median age was 21 years (range, 2 to 66 years; mean, 24.7 ± 13.0 years). We found that freedom from RVOT reintervention and porcine bioprosthetic explantation was 94% and 99% at 10 years, respectively. Univariate and multivariate analyses identified none of the tested variables as a risk factor for reoperation. Freedom from RV failure and dysfunction were 97% and 96% at 5 years and 96% and 93% at 10 years, respectively. In comparing stented and stentless porcine aortic valves in the RV-PA position, we found no significant difference between the groups in postoperative data, including survival rate, follow-up resting pulmonary gradient, freedom from reintervention and explantation, dysfunction and failure (Table 24.3) [58]. These data were surprising to us because the stentless valve has a one-third larger effective orifice area.

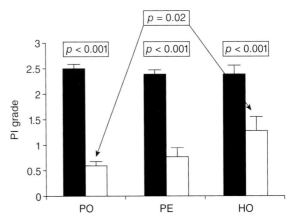

Figure 24.11 The change in pulmonary insufficiency (PI) before pulmonary valve replacement (solid bars) and at latest follow-up (open bars). PI grade: 1, mild; 2, moderate; 3, severe. HO, homograft; PE, pericardial; PO, porcine. (Reproduced with permission from Fiore *et al.* [54].)

Table 24.3 Follow-up data of patients with stented and stentless porcine aortic valves in the RV-PA position. (NYHA, New York Heart Association; PR, pulmonary regurgitation.) (Reproduced with permission from Brown *et al.* [58].)

Variable	Stentless (n = 61)	Stented (n = 24)	P value
Mortality (number of patients)	2 (3%)	3 (13%	0.13
Valve explantation (number of patients)	0	1 (4%)	0.28
Reintervention (number of patients)	4 (7%)	1 (4%)	1.00
Moderate PR (number of patients)	4 (7%)	1 (4%)	1.00
Follow-up pulmonary gradient (mmHg)	23.1+11.5	21.1+6.1	0.49
Pulmonary gradients >40 mmHg	5 (8%)	0	0.31
NYHA class III (number of patients)	1 (2%)	1 (4%)	0.49

Hawkins and colleagues reported on 150 patients with a stentless porcine xenograft (Medtronic Freestyle) of >19 mm in diameter between 1998 and 2008 [59]. The patients' mean weight was 50 kg and mean age was 16 years. The RVOT gradient was 13 ± 12 mmHg at 1 year and 25 ± 11 mmHg at 5 years. One hundred forty-five patients had mild or no PI, and five had moderate PI. Freedom from reoperation was 100% at 1 year and 95% at 5 years.

We concluded that the porcine aortic bioprosthesis remains an ideal valve choice for older teenagers (>18 years) and young adults with congenital abnormalities of the RVOT, especially for situations requiring reintervention [58]. We recommend using a stentless valve if a size ≥25 mm stented valve cannot be implanted.

Our current technique for stented valves is to implant them in situ in the RVOT as distally as possible and to roof them over with a small gusset of bovine pericardium if necessary. Our technique for stentless porcine valve (Freestyle) is to resect a short section of the old conduit or native PA and insert the Freestyle valve in situ with end-to-end proximal and distal suture lines to eliminate as much RVOT turbulence as possible.

Mechanical Valves in the Pulmonary Position

Mechanical valves have been used for PVR in a few centers [60,61]. Most centers recommend relatively large doses of Warfarin (International Normalised Ratio 3.5–4.5) and several reports of thromboses have been documented. We have used three mechanical valves in our population of nearly 800 pulmonary valve replacements. The only time we would consider a mechanical valve for PVR would be in an adult patient who has another mechanical heart valve that also requires Warfarin. Table 24.4 shows the reported series of mechanical valves used in the RVOT position [6, 60–67].

Bioengineered Valved Conduits for Right Ventricular Outflow Tract Reconstruction

Bioengineered valved conduits hold promise for RV-PA reconstruction. Biodegradable and biologic scaffolds have been constructed and host cells are said to populate the scaffolds; in some cases the scaffolds later disappear. To date we are not aware of valve-bearing bioengineered conduits in patients with other than short-term durability.

Gottlieb and colleagues demonstrated autologous, engineered tissue, valved conduits that function well at implantation, with subsequent monitoring of dimensions and function in real time by magnetic resonance imaging [68]. In vivo valves underwent structural and functional remodeling without stenosis, but with worsening PI after 6 weeks. Insights into mechanisms of in vivo remodeling are valuable for future iterations of engineered heart valves [68].

Critical to the current approaches to tissue-engineered heart valves is scaffold design, which must simultaneously provide immediate function (valves must function from the time of implant) as well as stress transfer to the new extracellular matrix. From a bioengineering point of view, a hierarchy of approaches will be necessary to connect the organ-tissue relationships with underpinning cellular and subcellular events [69].

When to Operate for Right Ventricular Outflow Tract Dysfunction

Right ventricular outflow tract dysfunction in children and adults is defined as moderate RVOT obstruction (≥40 mmHg) and/or greater than moderate (2+) PI. Patients with less than moderate dysfunction may remain asymptomatic or minimally symptomatic for many years. Detection of RV dysfunction before symptoms occur has become increasingly important because RV recovery may be incomplete if reconstruction is performed late. Preintervention RV volumes were independently associated with RV remodeling. Despite the substantial decrease in patients with very high preoperative RV volumes, normalization could be achieved when preoperative RV end-

Table 24.4 Literature review of mechanical PVR.

Authors/Institutions	No. of patients	Age (mean)	Valve type	Mortality	Thromboembolism	Comments
For						
Rosti et al., Italy (1998) [62]	8	10.1 yr	6 one-leaflet 2 bileaflet	0	No	6.4 yr of follow-up
Haas et al., Netherlands (2005) [61]	14	24.8 yr	All bileaflet	0	No	2.9 yr of follow-up
Dearani et al., Mayo (2005) [6]	17	Adults	NA	NA	No	8.3 yr of follow-up
Waterbolk et al., Netherlands (2006) [63]	27	33 yr	All bileaflet	2 (8%)	1	5.5 yr of follow-up, 1 pt has reoperated
Horer et al., Germany (2009) [60]	19	25.4 yr	All bileaflet	0	1	5.8 yr of follow-up, 2 pts have reoperated
Against						
Ilbawi et al., Chicago (1986) [64]	16	NA	All bileaflet	0	No	At 2 yr, 37% had valve dysfunction
Miyamura et al., Japan (1987) [65]	5	NA	All bileaflet	0	2	
Fleming et al., Omaha (1989) [66]	4	NA	All bileaflet	0	3	At 3.5 yr 3 pts have reoperated
Kiyota et al., Japan (1992) [67]	11	NA	All bileaflet	0	3	3 of 11 pts have reoperated

diastolic volume (EDV) was <160 mL/m^2 or RV end-systolic volume (ESV) <82 mL/m^2 [70].

The indications for intervention on a dysfunctional RVOT are controversial but patients with signs and symptoms of RV failure and objective evidence of significant RVOT dysfunction should undergo reintervention. Symptoms of RV failure include palpitations, decreased exercise tolerance, and fatigue. Signs include ascites, peripheral edema, atrial and ventricular arrhythmias, decreased RV ejection fraction, tricuspid valve insufficiency, progressive increase in RV EDV and, eventually, a decrease in left ventricular (LV) function.

Echocardiography can accurately quantitate pulmonary stenosis but is considerably less accurate in quantitating regurgitation and/or the degree of RV dilation. The introduction of cardiac magnetic resonance imaging (MRI) has permitted clinicians to quantify PI, which is expressed in cubic centimeters per meter squared and/or as a regurgitation fraction. This modality also permits accurate measurement of RV EDV, which can be compared to LV EDV.

The indications for intervention on a dysfunctional RVOT are evolving but currently include patients with moderate to severe PI and/or stenosis and any of the following problems [24,71,72]:

1. exertional symptoms of New York Heart Association class II or greater;
2. decreased performance capacity on exercise testing;
3. significant RV dilation (>150 mm/m^2 by MRI);
4. a RV/LV volume ratio >1.5 in the presence of symptoms and ≥2 in asymptomatic patients;
5. regurgitation fraction >35% on MRI;
6. significant RV dysfunction;
7. atrial and/or ventricular arrhythmias;
8. QRS duration >180 ms.

Conclusion

Pulmonary valve replacement and RVOT reconstruction with a valved conduit continues to be a "weak link" in our management of congenital heart disease. Nevertheless, progress continues to be made in this area. We recommend a variety of RVOT techniques that depend on the size of the patient and the anatomy of the RVOT. We preserve the pulmonary annulus and leaflets whenever possible. When a transannular RVOT patch is necessary in an infant with tetralogy, or one of the variants, we favor the PTFE monocusp RVOT reconstruction. When a RVOT conduit is required, we favor the Contegra BJVC in infants, children, and young adults, although patent restrictions currently limit its use in patients ≥18 years of age.

Currently in patients >18 years old who require a pulmonary valve replacement, we use the stentless porcine aortic root (Freestyle) or a stented biologic valve of at least 25 mm in diameter to achieve an adequate effective orifice area. The decellularized pulmonary homograft is our current conduit of choice for replacement of the pulmonary autograft in patients >5 years of age undergoing the Ross AVR. In the younger Ross group (<5 years old), we favor the Contegra conduit.

Regardless of the valve type, we recommend closure of the pericardium with a PTFE pericardial membrane so the RVOT or conduit does not adhere to the underside of the sternum. Our current preference is a low-porosity, 0.1 mm PTFE pericardial membrane. We have considered some other biologic materials but to date have not used them.

Our patients with complex congenital heart disease have benefited greatly by worldwide efforts to improve reconstructive options for the RVOT. Progress has been and will continue to be made in this field because the pulmonary valve is important and is the most common valve requiring replacement in children.

References

1. Husain SA, Brown JW. (2007) When reconstruction fails or is not feasible: valve replacement options in the pediatric population. Semin Thorac Cardiovasc Surg Pediatr Card Surg Annu 117–124.

2. Rastelli GC, Ongley PA, Davis GD, Kirklin JW. (1965) Surgical repair for pulmonary valve atresia with coronary-pulmonary artery fistula: report of case. Mayo Clin Proc 40, 521–527.

3. Ross DN, Somerville J. (1966) Correction of pulmonary atresia with a homograft aortic valve. Lancet 2, 1446–1447.

4. Jonas RA, Freed MD, Mayer JEJ, et al. (1985) Long-term follow-up of patients with synthetic right heart conduits. Circulation 72, II77–II83.

5. Forbess JM, Shah AS, St Louis JD, et al. (2001) Cryopreserved homografts in the pulmonary position: determinants of durability. Ann Thorac Surg 71, 54–59; discussion 59–60.

6. Dearani JA, Danielson GK, Puga FJ, et al. (2003) Late follow-up of 1095 patients undergoing operation for complex congenital heart disease utilizing pulmonary ventricle to pulmonary artery conduits. Ann Thorac Surg 75, 399–410; discussion 411.

7. Sinzobahamvya N, Wetter J, Blaschczok HC, et al. (2001) The fate of small-diameter homografts in the pulmonary position. Ann Thorac Surg 72, 2070–2076.

8. Tweddell JS, Pelech AN, Frommelt PC, et al. (2000) Factors affecting longevity of homograft valves used in right ventricular outflow tract reconstruction for congenital heart disease. Circulation 102(Suppl 3), III130–III135.

9. Chan KC, Fyfe DA, McKay CA, et al. (1994) Right ventricular outflow reconstruction with cryopreserved homografts in pediatric patients: intermediate-term follow-up with serial echocardiographic assessment. J Am Coll Cardiol 24, 483–489.

10. Bando K, Danielson GK, Schaff HV, et al. (1995) Outcome of pulmonary and aortic homografts for right ventricular outflow tract reconstruction. J Thorac Cardiovasc Surg 109, 509–517; discussion 517–518.

11. Feier H, Collart F, Ghez O, et al. (2005) Risk factors, dynamics, and cutoff values for homograft stenosis after the Ross procedure. Ann Thorac Surg 79, 1669–1675; discussion 1675.

12. Wells WJ, Arroyo H Jr, Bremner RM, et al. (2002) Homograft conduit failure in infants is not due to somatic outgrowth. J Thorac Cardiovasc Surg 124, 88–96.

13. Raanani E, Yau TM, David TE, et al. (2000) Risk factors for late pulmonary homograft stenosis after the Ross procedure. Ann Thorac Surg 70, 1953–1957.

14. Discigil B, Dearani JA, Puga FJ, et al. (2001) Late pulmonary valve replacement after repair of tetralogy of Fallot. J Thorac Cardiovasc Surg 121, 344–351.

15. Gundry SR. (1999) Pericardial and synthetic monocusp valves: Indication and results. Semin Thorac Cardiovasc Surg Pediatr Card Surg Annu 2, 77–82.

16. Ando M, Imai Y, Takanashi Y, et al (1997) Fate of trileaflet equine pericardial extracardiac conduit used for the correction of anomalies having pulmonic ventricle-pulmonary arterial discontinuity. Ann Thorac Surg 64, 154–158.

17. Bogers AJ, Roofthooft M, Pisters H, et al. (1994) Long-term results of the gamma-irradiation-preserved homograft monocusp for transannular reconstruction of the right-ventricular outflow tract in tetralogy of Fallot. Thorac Cardiovasc Surg 42, 337–339.

18. Yamagishi M, Kurosawa H. (1993) Outflow reconstruction of tetralogy of Fallot using a Gore-Tex valve. Ann Thorac Surg 56, 1414–1416; discussion 1416–1417.

19. Oku H, Matsumoto T, Kitayama H, et al. (1993) Semilunar valve replacement with a cylindrical valve. J Card Surg 8, 666–670.

20. Turrentine MW, McCarthy RP, Vijay P, et al. (2002) PTFE monocusp valve reconstruction of the right ventricular outflow tract. Ann Thorac Surg 73, 871–879; discussion 879–880.

21. Gundry SR, Razzouk AJ, Boskind JF, et al. (1994) Fate of the pericardial monocusp pulmonary valve for right ventricular outflow tract reconstruction. Early function, late failure without obstruction. J Thorac Cardiovasc Surg 107, 908–912; discussion 912–913.

22. Turrentine MW, McCarthy RP, Vijay P, et al. (2002) Polytetrafluoroethylene monocusp valve technique for right ventricular outflow tract reconstruction. Ann Thorac Surg 74, 2202–2205.

23. Brown JW, Ruzmetov M, Vijay P, et al. (2007) Right ventricular outflow tract reconstruction with a polytetrafluoroethylene monocusp valve: a twelve-year experience. J Thorac Cardiovasc Surg 133, 1336–1343.

24. Quintessenza JA, Jacobs JP, Chai PJ, et al. (2010) Polytetrafluoroethylene bicuspid pulmonary valve implantation: experience with 126 patients. World J Ped Congenital Heart Surg 1, 20–27.

25. Nunn GR, Bennetts J, Onikul E. (2008) Durability of hand-sewn valves in the right ventricular outlet. J Thorac Cardiovasc Surg 136, 290–296.

26. Dur O, Yoshida M, Manor P, *et al.* (2010) In vitro evaluation of right ventricular outflow tract reconstruction with bicuspid valved polytetrafluoroethylene conduit. Artif Organs 34, 1010–1016.

27. Perron J, Moran AM, Gauvreau K, *et al.* (1999) Valved homograft conduit repair of the right heart in early infancy. Ann Thorac Surg 68, 542–548.

28. Brown JW, Ruzmetov M, Rodefeld MD, *et al.* (2005) Right ventricular outflow tract reconstruction with an allograft conduit in non-Ross patients: risk factors for allograft dysfunction and failure. Ann Thorac Surg 80, 655–663; discussion 663–664.

29. Hawkins JA, Bailey WW, Dillon T, *et al.* (1992) Midterm results with cryopreserved allograft valved conduits from the right ventricle to the pulmonary arteries. J Thorac Cardiovasc Surg 104, 910–916.

30. Yankah AC, Alexi-Meskhishvili V, Weng Y, *et al.* (1995) Accelerated degeneration of allografts in the first two years of life. Ann Thorac Surg 60(2 Suppl), S71–S76; discussion S76–S77.

31. Niwaya K, Knott-Craig CJ, Lane MM, *et al.* (1999) Cryopreserved homograft valves in the pulmonary position: risk analysis for intermediate-term failure. J Thorac Cardiovasc Surg 117, 141–146; discussion 146–147.

32. Bielefeld MR, Bishop DA, Campbell DN, *et al.* (2001) Reoperative homograft right ventricular outflow tract reconstruction. Ann Thorac Surg 71, 482–487; discussion 487–488.

33. Askovich B, Hawkins JA, Sower CT, *et al.* (2007) Right ventricle-to-pulmonary artery conduit longevity: is it related to allograft size? Ann Thorac Surg 84, 907–911; discussion 911–912.

34. Boethig D, Goerler H, Westhoff-Bleck M, *et al.* (2007) Evaluation of 188 consecutive homografts implanted in pulmonary position after 20 years. Eur J Cardiothorac Surg 32, 133–142.

35. Brown JW, Ruzmetov M, Rodefeld MD, *et al.* (2008) Right ventricular outflow tract reconstruction in Ross patients: does the homograft fare better? Ann Thorac Surg 86, 1607–1612.

36. Brown JW, Ruzmetov M, Shahriari A, *et al.* (2009) Midterm results of Ross aortic valve replacement: a single-institution experience. Ann Thorac Surg 88, 601–607; discussion 607–608.

37. Dave H, Kadner A, Bauersfeld U, *et al.* (2003) Early results of using the bovine jugular vein for right ventricular outflow reconstruction during the Ross procedure. Heart Surg Forum 6, 390–392.

38. Schmid FX, Keyser A, Wiesenack C, *et al.* (2002) Stentless xenografts and homografts for right ventricular outflow tract reconstruction during the Ross operation. Ann Thorac Surg 74, 684–688.

39. Marino BS, Wernovsky G, Rychik J, *et al.* (1999) Early results of the Ross procedure in simple and complex left heart disease. Circulation 100(19 Suppl), II162–II166.

40. Elkins RC, Dawson PE, Goldstein S, *et al.* (2001) Decellularized human valve allografts. Ann Thorac Surg 71(5 Suppl), S428–S432.

41. Ichikawa Y, Noishiki Y, Kosuge T, *et al.* (1997) Use of a bovine jugular vein graft with natural valve for right ventricular

42. Scavo VA Jr, Turrentine MW, Aufiero TX, *et al.* (1999) Valved bovine jugular venous conduits for right ventricular to pulmonary artery reconstruction. ASAIO J 45, 482–487.

43. Herijgers P, Ozaki S, Verbeken E, *et al.* (2002) Valved jugular vein segments for right ventricular outflow tract reconstruction in young sheep. J Thorac Cardiovasc Surg 124, 798–805.

44. Breymann T, Thies WR, Boethig D, *et al.* (2002) Bovine valved venous xenografts for RVOT reconstruction: results after 71 implantations. Eur J Cardiothorac Surg 21, 703–710; discussion 710.

45. Bove T, Demanet H, Wauthy P, *et al.* (2002) Early results of valved bovine jugular vein conduit versus bicuspid homograft for right ventricular outflow tract reconstruction. Ann Thorac Surg 74, 536–541; discussion 541.

46. Brown JW, Ruzmetov M, Rodefeld MD, *et al.* (2006) Valved bovine jugular vein conduits for right ventricular outflow tract reconstruction in children: an attractive alternative to pulmonary homograft. Ann Thorac Surg 82, 909–916.

47. Corno AF, Hurni M, Griffin H, *et al.* (2002) Bovine jugular vein as right ventricle-to-pulmonary artery valved conduit. J Heart Valve Dis 11, 242–247; discussion 248.

48. Carrel T, Berdat P, Pavlovic M, *et al.* (2002) The bovine jugular vein: a totally integrated valved conduit to repair the right ventricular outflow. J Heart Valve Dis 11, 552–556.

49. Chatzis AC, Giannopoulos NM, Bobos D, *et al.* (2003) New xenograft valved conduit (Contegra) for right ventricular outflow tract reconstruction. Heart Surg Forum 6, 396–398.

50. Rastan AJ, Walther T, Daehnert I, *et al.* (2006) Bovine jugular vein conduit for right ventricular outflow tract reconstruction: evaluation of risk factors for mid-term outcome. Ann Thorac Surg 82, 1308–1315.

51. Morales DL, Braud BE, Gunter KS, *et al.* (2006) Encouraging results for the Contegra conduit in the problematic right ventricle-to-pulmonary artery connection. J Thorac Cardiovasc Surg 132, 665–671.

52. Sekarski N, van Meir H, Rijlaarsdam ME, *et al.* (2007) Right ventricular outflow tract reconstruction with the bovine jugular vein graft: 5 years' experience with 133 patients. Ann Thorac Surg 84, 599–605.

53. Brown JW, Ruzmetov M, Eltayeb O, *et al.* (2011) Contegra versus pulmonary homografts for right ventricular outflow tract reconstruction: a 10-year single institution comparison [abstract]. Presented at: *47th Annual Meeting of the Society of Thoracic Surgeons.* San Diego, CA.

54. Fiore AC, Rodefeld M, Turrentine M, *et al.* (2010) Pulmonary Valve Replacement: A Comparison of Three Biological Valves. Ann Thorac Surg 85, 1712–1718.

55. Boethig D, Thies WR, Hecker H, *et al.* (2005) Mid term course after pediatric right ventricular outflow tract reconstruction: a comparison of homografts, porcine xenografts and Contegras. Eur J Cardiothorac Surg 27, 58–66.

56. Vincent JA, Hellenbrand WE, Zahn EM, *et al.* (2009) Implantation of the Medtronic Melody Transcatheter pulmonary valve for dysfunctional right ventricular outflow conduits: clinical results of initial 99 patients in the US Investigational Device Exemption Trial. Circulation 120, S930–S931.

57. Fiore AC, Rodefeld M, Turrentine M, *et al.* (2008) Pulmonary valve replacement: a comparison of three biological valves. Ann Thorac Surg 85, 1712–1718; discussion 1718.

58. Brown JW, Ruzmetov M, Yurdakok O, *et al.* (In press) Intermediate follow-up of porcine xenografts for right ventricular outflow tract reconstruction in children and adults. Ann Thorac Surg.

59. Hawkins JA, Sower CT, Lambert LM, *et al.* (2009) Stentless porcine valves in the right ventricular outflow tract: improved durability? Eur J Cardiothorac Surg. 35, 600–604; discussion 604–605.

60. Horer J, Vogt M, Stierle U, *et al.* (2009) A comparative study of mechanical and homograft prostheses in the pulmonary position. Ann Thorac Surg 88, 1534–1539.

61. Haas F, Schreiber C, Horer J, *et al.* (2005) Is there a role for mechanical valved conduits in the pulmonary position? Ann Thorac Surg 79, 1662–1667; discussion 1667–1668.

62. Rosti L, Murzi B, Colli AM, *et al.* (1998) Pulmonary valve replacement: a role for mechanical prostheses? Ann Thorac Surg 65, 889–890.

63. Waterbolk TW, Hoendermis ES, den Hamer IJ, *et al.* (2006) Pulmonary valve replacement with a mechanical prosthesis. Promising results of 28 procedures in patients with congenital heart disease. Eur J Cardiothorac Surg 30, 28–32.

64. Ilbawi MN, Lockhart CG, Idriss FS, *et al.* (1987) Experience with St. Jude Medical valve prosthesis in children. A word of caution regarding right-sided placement. J Thorac Cardiovasc Surg 93, 73–79.

65. Miyamura H, Kanazawa H, Hayashi J, *et al.* (1987) Thrombosed St. Jude Medical valve prosthesis in the right side of the heart in patients with tetralogy of Fallot. J Thorac Cardiovasc Surg 94, 148–150.

66. Fleming WH, Sarafian LB, Moulton AL, *et al.* (1989) Valve replacement in the right side of the heart in children: long-term follow-up. Ann Thorac Surg 48, 404–408.

67. Kiyota Y, Shiroyama T, Akamatsu T, *et al.* (1992) In vitro closing behavior of the St. Jude Medical heart valve in the pulmonary position. Valve incompetence originating in the prosthesis itself. J Thorac Cardiovasc Surg 104, 779–785.

68. Gottlieb D, Kunal T, Emani S, *et al.* (2010) In vivo monitoring of function of autologous engineered pulmonary valve. J Thorac Cardiovasc Surg 139, 723–731.

69. Sacks MS, Schoen FJ, Mayer JE. (2009) Bioengineering challenges for heart valve tissue engineering. Annu Rev Biomed Eng 11, 289–313.

70. Oosterhof T, van Straten A, Vliegen HW, *et al.* (2007) Preoperative thresholds for pulmonary valve replacement in patients with corrected tetralogy of Fallot using cardiovascular magnetic resonance. Circulation 116, 545–551.

71. Frigiola A, Tsang V, Nordmeyer J, *et al.* (2008) Current approaches to pulmonary regurgitation. Eur J Cardiothorac Surg 34, 576–580; discussion 581–582.

72. Gerestein CG, Takkenberg JJ, Oei FB, *et al.* (2001) Right ventricular outflow tract reconstruction with an allograft conduit. Ann Thorac Surg 71, 911–917; discussion 917–918.

CHAPTER 25

Double-Outlet Ventricles

Henry L. Walters III[1] and Constantine Mavroudis[2]

[1]Children's Hospital of Michigan, Detroit, MI, USA
[2]Florida Hospital for Children, Orlando, FL, USA

DOUBLE-OUTLET RIGHT VENTRICLE

Introduction

Definition

Double-outlet right ventricle (DORV) represents a complex spectrum of congenital cardiac malformations that morphologically lie between ventricular septal defect (VSD) with overriding aorta and transposition of the great arteries (TGA) with VSD. DORV remains controversial both in terms of its anatomical definition and surgical management and it presents with multiple phenotypes, including a rich spectrum of different anatomical and physiological forms. The frequently associated cardiac malformations that are seen with DORV contribute to its overall complexity. We define DORV as a type of ventriculoarterial connection in which both great vessels arise entirely or predominantly from the right ventricle [1,2]. Hearts with DORV and subpulmonary VSD (Taussig-Bing malformation) are considered a subset of DORV until the pulmonary artery arises more than 90% from the left ventricle; they are then considered a subset of TGA with VSD [3,4]. DORV is usually associated with concordant atrioventricular connections. Rarely, it is associated with discordant [5] or univentricular [6] atrioventricular connections, atrioventricular valve atresia, or atrial isomerism. This chapter focuses on the forms of DORV with two functional ventricles.

Controversies

Whether the definition of DORV should include the presence of *aortic-mitral discontinuity* is controversial. Lev and associates [1] define DORV as that condition in which both arterial trunks emerge almost completely or completely from the right ventricle, and there may or may not be aortic-mitral or pulmonic-mitral continuity. Although exclusion of cases with aortic-mitral and pulmonic-mitral continuity is semantically pure and provides a sharp dividing point between cases of tetralogy of Fallot and DORV with subaortic VSD, this concept does not satisfy the pathologic data. In the transition from tetralogy of Fallot to DORV with subaortic VSD, there is, in the pathological data, a gradual diminution in the extent of normal aortic-mitral continuity until it is completely lost. Also, the pathologist sees a gradual transition from the Taussig-Bing heart without the pulmonary trunk overriding the interventricular septum, to those with an overriding pulmonary trunk, to those with the pulmonary trunk emerging equally from both ventricles, to those with the pulmonary trunk arising more from the left ventricle, and, finally, to those with complete TGA and VSD. During this process there is a gradual development of pulmonic-mitral continuity.

Another related controversy is whether bilateral coni must be present in order to categorize a lesion as DORV. This issue may have arisen from the original description of the Taussig-Bing heart [7,8], which did, indeed, have bilateral and well developed subpulmonary and subaortic muscular coni. That may have encouraged the application of these criteria to the definition of all hearts with DORV. This concept was supported by the radiographic studies of Baron [9] and Hallerman *et al.* [10]; they used the criteria of separation of the aortic and mitral valve leaflets to distinguish radiologically between DORV and tetralogy of Fallot. Howell and his colleagues [11], in an analysis of a selected group of hearts with an unequivocally complete origin of both great arteries from the morphologic right ventricle, stated that only 37.5% exhibited complete muscular and bilateral coni. They concluded that this criterion was a useful morphologic descriptor but was not mandatory for classification as DORV.

History

Peacock [12] and Rokitansky [13] documented cases of DORV in the mid-nineteenth century. In 1952 Braun and colleagues [14] coined the term, *double outlet ventricle*, in their postmortem description of the heart of a 19-year-old male with complete dextroposition of the aorta, subaortic VSD, and pulmonary stenosis. The first correct intraoperative recognition and surgical repair of DORV was at the Mayo Clinic in May of 1957. This 18-month-old male died 2 hours postoperatively of low cardiac output, perhaps owing to inadequate myocardial protection and subaortic stenosis [15]. Witham [16] published a postmortem, morphologic description of four cases of what he termed double-outlet right ventricle 1 month later. Engle *et al.* [17,18] emphasized the surgical importance of preoperative angiocardiography to distinguish DORV (with subaortic VSD and no pulmonary stenosis) from simple VSD and suggested angiographic criteria to differentiate between the two diagnoses. Neufeld and colleagues [19,20,21] published detailed clinicopathological descriptions of two distinct subsets of patients with "origin of both great vessels from the right ventricle," those with [19], and those without [20,21] pulmonary stenosis. He described the similarities of the pathophysiology of DORV with pulmonary stenosis to that of tetralogy of Fallot and underscored the importance of distinguishing between the two diagnoses in planning for surgical repair [19]. In a paper on DORV without pulmonary stenosis, Neufeld *et al.* [20] described the location and pathophysiology of VSDs committed to the aorta, the pulmonary artery and doubly committed VSDs. This insight laid the foundation for a classification of the VSDs associated with DORV. Lev, Bharati, and colleagues [1] built on these observations when they emphasized the importance of the relationship of the VSD to the great arteries: subaortic, subpulmonary, noncommitted and doubly committed. Angelini and Leachman [22], Wilcox *et al.* [23], Piccoli *et al.* [3], and Anderson and colleagues [24] demonstrated the importance of the positional relationships of the great arteries to each other.

While Pernkopf [25] mentioned DORV with subpulmonary VSD in 1926, Helen Taussig and Richard Bing [7] were the first to provide a complete clinical, angiographic, and pathophysiologic discussion of this disorder in 1949. In the postmortem examination of their 5½-year-old patient they described complete transposition of the aorta, slight levoposition of the pulmonary artery over a subpulmonary VSD, and a muscular ridge separating the pulmonary artery from the aorta. They correctly suggested that streaming accounted for the higher oxygen saturation in the pulmonary artery compared with that in both the right ventricle and the aorta. Later reports [26,27] of similar cases classified the Taussig-Bing malformation as a subset of complete TGA with VSD because the physiology of the two disorders was identical. Neufeld *et al.* [20] recognized that the Taussig-Bing heart was an anatomic subset of DORV even though it was more similar to TGA with VSD physiologically. This was confirmed when Van Praagh [8] analyzed the original Taussig-Bing heart and defined the Taussig-Bing malformation as DORV with semilunar valves side-by-side and approximately at the same height, a bilateral conus, and a subpulmonary VSD. Lev *et al.* [1] deemphasized the importance of the presence of bilateral coni and more simply defined the Taussig-Bing heart as DORV with a subpulmonary VSD. Daicoff and Kirklin [28] and Hightower and colleagues [29] performed the first successful surgical repairs of the Taussig-Bing malformation by tunneling the VSD to the pulmonary artery and performing an atrial switch (Mustard procedure). Patrick and McGoon [30] and Kawashima *et al.* [31] performed the first intraventricular tunnel repair of this disorder.

Embryology

The embryogenesis of DORV is controversial [22,32–39]. Anderson and his colleagues [33] studied the morphogenesis of a group of hearts with bulboventricular malformations. This collection included specimens with tetralogy of Fallot, DORV, and TGA with VSD. They contend that the development of this spectrum of hearts with abnormal ventriculoarterial connections is explained by departures from the normal development of portions of the bulboventricular loop. Conal malrotation, changes in the position of the anterior portion of the muscular interventricular septum, and differential conal absorption form the basis of their hypothesis.

Morphology

Sakata *et al.* [40] and Lecompte *et al.* [41] state that the classification and terminology of this complex group of patients with disorders of ventriculoarterial connection is less important than a precise definition of the preoperative anatomic criteria that are useful in determining the best type of surgical repair. Nonetheless, efforts to accurately categorize patients with DORV are necessary to make valid inferences regarding the results of different surgical treatments [3,24] for comparable anatomic subsets.

Atrioventricular and Ventriculoarterial Relationships

Atrial and Ventricular Situs
Approximately 86% of surgical patients with DORV have concordant atrioventricular connections [42]. Atrioven-

tricular discordance is present in 11% [5,42–44]. There may be atrial situs solitus, situs inversus or left/right atrial isomerism [43,45]. Hearts with DORV may have a muscular conus located beneath each of the semilunar valves (bilateral conus), a single conus beneath one of the semilunar valves or, more rarely, no conus at all.

Great Artery Relationships

There are three basic patterns of the relationship of the great arteries to each other in DORV [23]. In most cases the great arteries are normally related to one another – the aortic trunk is situated posteriorly and to the right of the pulmonary trunk, and the two great arteries spiral around each other as they leave the base of the heart. In the second group the aorta is to the right of the pulmonary artery, but these two vessels lie parallel to each other (do not spiral). They are usually side by side, although there can be any degree of anteroposterior variation. The third major group is the least common and consists of parallel trunks with the aorta anterior and to the left of the pulmonary artery (L-malposition). While it was once thought that the relationship of the VSD to the great arteries could be predicted with a reasonable degree of certainty from the relationship

of the great arteries to each other [24], this has been disputed by Kirklin and associates [6].

Characteristics of the Ventricular Septal Defect

The VSD, which represents the only outflow tract for the left ventricle, is usually unrestrictive (diameter equal to or larger than the diameter of the aortic annulus). In 10% of the cases [6] the VSD is restrictive [28,46–53]. Very rarely there is no interventricular communication (Figure 25.1F) [46,54–60]. When there is no VSD, mitral valvar and left ventricular hypoplasia usually coexist. A small atrial septal defect (ASD) serves as the only source of a left-to-right shunt. In one isolated case of DORV without an interventricular communication, the anterior leaflet of the mitral valve closed the VSD. Blood shunted left-to-right through a small ASD, and a small opening in the anterior leaflet of the mitral valve allowed blood to flow from the left atrium directly into the right ventricle. In 13% of cases of DORV the VSDs are multiple [6].

Location of the VSD

The actual anatomic location of the VSD in DORV is fairly constant. Most of these defects are conoventricular; they lie

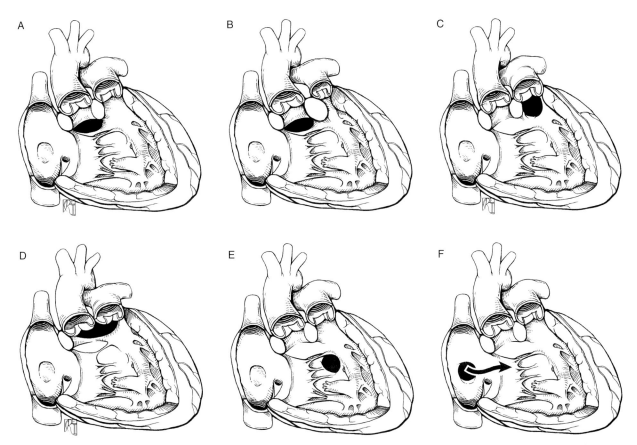

Figure 25.1 The relationship of the ventricular septal defect (VSD) to the great arteries in double-outlet right ventricle. **A,** Subaortic VSD without pulmonary stenosis. **B,** Subaortic VSD with pulmonary stenosis. **C,** Subpulmonary VSD (Taussig-Bing malformation). **D,** Doubly committed VSD. **E,** Noncommitted (remote) VSD. **F,** Intact interventricular septum.

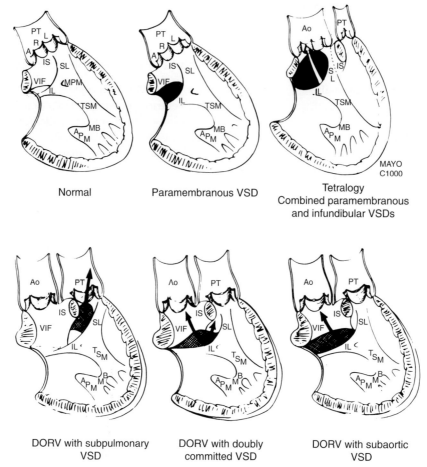

Normal Paramembranous VSD Tetralogy
Combined paramembranous
and infundibular VSDs

DORV with subpulmonary DORV with doubly DORV with subaortic
VSD committed VSD VSD

Figure 25.2 Diagrammatic representation of the location of the ventricular septal defect in hearts with an isolated perimembranous ventricular septal defect (VSD), tetralogy of Fallot, double-outlet right ventricle (DORV) with subpulmonary VSD, DORV with doubly committed VSD, and DORV with subaortic VSD. Note the location of the VSD nestled within the limbs of the trabeculoseptomarginalis (TSM). (APM, anterior tricuspid papillary muscle; IL, inferior (posterior) limb of TSM; IS, infundibular (conal) septum; MB, moderator band; PT, pulmonary trunk; SL, superior (anterior) limb of TSM; VIF, ventriculoinfundibular fold.) (Adapted with permission from Edwards [61].)

nestled within the anterior and posterior limbs of the trabeculoseptomarginalis (TSM or septal band) (Figure 25.2) [24,61]. These VSDs are not conoventricular when they are located in the inlet septum, the trabecular portion of the muscular interventricular septum, or when a perimembranous VSD extends inferiorly to occupy the inlet septum [24]. In these rare cases the VSD is typically non-committed, challenging to repair with an intraventricular tunnel, and can be associated with any relationship of the great arteries [24].

Relationship of the VSD to the Great Arteries

The VSD in DORV is usually described in relational terms as subaortic, subpulmonary, doubly committed or non-committed [1,19,24,57]. This relationship of the VSD to the great vessels has special surgical, rather than anatomic or embryologic, significance. These terms do not imply that

the VSD moves around within the interventricular septum. To the contrary, this important relationship of the VSD to the great arteries depends more on the highly variable relationships of the great arteries to each other and on the orientation and size of the infundibular (conal) septum [24]. In DORV the terms *subaortic* or *subpulmonary* can, but do not necessarily, demand that one of the borders of the VSD is formed by a semilunar valve (juxtaarterial). This distinction between the location of the VSD within the interventricular septum and its relationship to the great arteries is important to complete understanding of this disorder.

Subaortic VSD

Subaortic VSDs (Figure 25.1A,B) [60] are the most common type and occur in approximately 50% of surgical patients with DORV [4,62]. They are located beneath the aortic

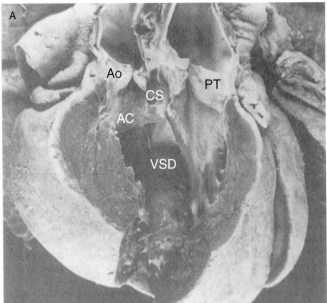 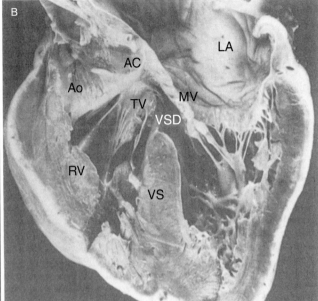

Figure 25.3 Double-outlet right ventricle with subaortic ventricular septal defect (VSD). **A,** A coronal section of the right ventricle through the aortic and pulmonary valves shows the side-by-side relationship of the great vessels. The VSD is related to the aortic valve but is separated from it by the subaortic conus. **B,** A sagittal section across the VSD demonstrates its subaortic commitment. The VSD serves as the only outlet for the left ventricle. The subaortic conus is interposed between the aortic valve and the anterior leaflet of the mitral valve. (AC, subaortic conus; Ao, aorta; CS, conal (infundibular) septum; LA, left atrium; LV, left ventricle; MV, mitral valve; PT, pulmonary trunk; RV, right ventricular free wall; TV, tricuspid valve; VS, interventricular septum.) (Adapted with permission from Neufeld *et al.* [19].)

valve and are separated from the valve by a variable distance depending on the presence and length of the subaortic conus. When a subaortic conus is absent (by definition aortic-mitral continuity is present), the left cusp of the aortic valve or the base of the anterior leaflet of the mitral valve forms the actual posterosuperior margin of the VSD (juxtaaortic) [6]. Typical subaortic VSDs in hearts with a right-sided aorta are located in the superior interventricular septum, posterior to the infundibular septum (Figure 25.3) [19,24]. The VSDs are usually perimembranous; they reach the annulus of the tricuspid valve at its anteroseptal commissure, and there is mitral-tricuspid continuity at the posteroinferior rim of the defect. Occasionally the posterior margin of the VSD is separated from the base of the tricuspid valve by a rim of muscular tissue. This represents fusion of the ventriculoinfundibular fold and the posterior limb of the TSM (Figure 25.4) [11,24,63]. The VSD can extend inferiorly from the perimembranous region to lie partly beneath the base of the septal leaflet of the tricuspid valve [63]. In an autopsy series 77% of patients with DORV and subaortic VSDs had bilateral coni, and 23% had only a subpulmonary conus [6]. Most hearts with aortic-mitral valvar continuity will have subaortic or doubly committed VSDs, and most with pulmonic-mitral valvar continuity will have subpulmonary VSDs [11].

DORV with L-Malposition of the Aorta

When DORV is associated with L-malposition of the aorta [64–68], the VSD is usually subaortic. Although still nestled within the limbs of the TSM, the VSD lies more anteriorly and superiorly within the muscular interventricular septum than it does when the aorta is on the right side (Figure 25.5) [57]. This is similar to the position of the VSD in the Taussig-Bing heart. Typically the superior border of the VSD is the aortic valve (juxtaaortic), and the anterior and posterior limbs of the TSM form its inferior and posterior borders, respectively. The VSD can extend to the annulus of the tricuspid valve posteriorly and be perimembranous. Rarely in DORV with L-malposition of the aorta, the VSD can be subpulmonary [69], noncommitted [70], or doubly committed [71].

Doubly Committed VSD

Doubly committed VSDs (Figure 25.1D) [60] occur in approximately 10% of surgical series of DORV [4,62]. The VSD lies within the divisions of the TSM superiorly in the interventricular septum and immediately beneath the leaflets of the aortic and pulmonary valves (juxtaarterial). The pulmonary and aortic valves generally are contiguous because the infundibular septum is deficient or absent. The semilunar valves form the superior border of this typically large VSD. The TSM, with its anterior and posterior

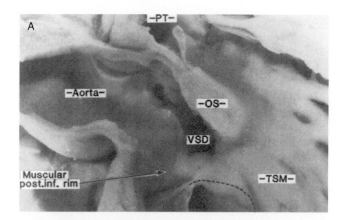

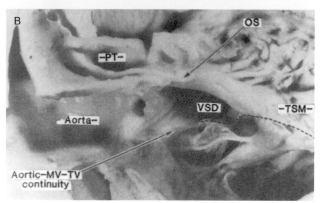

Figure 25.4 Comparison of two hearts with double-outlet right ventricle and subaortic ventricular septal defect (VSD). **A,** The posterior limb of the trabeculoseptomarginalis fuses with the ventriculoinfundibular fold to produce the muscular posterior margin of the VSD that protects the conduction tissue. **B,** In this specimen, there is no fusion of the posterior limb of the trabeculoseptomarginalis and ventriculoinfundibular fold. The VSD reaches the annulus of the tricuspid valve at its anteroseptal commissure where there is aortic–mitral–tricuspid valve continuity. The conduction tissue is vulnerable along the posteroinferior free margin of the VSD. (OS, outlet (infundibular, conal) septum; PT, pulmonary trunk; TSM, trabeculoseptomarginalis.) (Adapted with permission from Anderson *et al.* [24].)

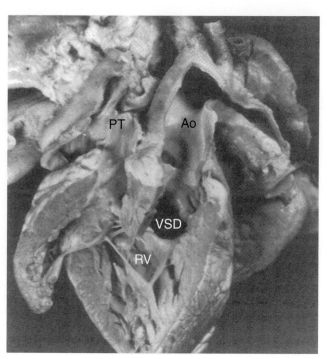

Figure 25.5 Double-outlet right ventricle with L-malposition of the great arteries and subaortic ventricular septal defect (VSD). Coronal section of the right ventricle through the aortic and pulmonary valves. The aorta is to the left and slightly anterior to the pulmonary valve (L-malposition). The VSD lies anteriorly and superiorly just beneath the aortic valve. This is similar to the position of the VSD in the Taussig-Bing malformation. (Ao, aorta; PT, pulmonary trunk; RV, right ventricle.) (Adapted with permission from Sridaromont *et al.* [57].)

divisions, makes up its anterior, inferior and posterior borders. There can be bilaterally deficient coni combined with an absent or deficient infundibular septum [6,72], or a single conus may exist beneath the two semilunar valves [6]. As both great arteries contribute to the superior border of the defect and override the interventricular septum to varying degrees, it is often difficult to determine from which ventricle the great arteries predominantly arise. For this reason Brandt and his colleagues [72] called this variant of DORV *double-outlet both ventricles.*

Subpulmonary VSD (Taussig-Bing)

Subpulmonary VSDs (Figure 25.1C) [60] are present in approximately 30% of patients in surgical series of DORV

(Taussig-Bing malformation) [4,62]. These VSDs are usually unrestrictive. They lie anteriorly and superiorly beneath the pulmonary valve in the interventricular septum and are cradled within the limbs of the TSM (Figure 25.6) [73]. This VSD position is similar to that described for DORV with L-malposition of the aorta (Figure 25.5) [57,63]. In the presence of a subpulmonary conus the VSD is separated from the pulmonary valve by a variable distance, and the conus forms the superior boundary of the VSD. If there is pulmonary-mitral continuity (no subpulmonary conus), the pulmonary valve will override the VSD to a variable extent and will form its superior border (juxtapulmonary). The infundibular (conal) septum is sagittally oriented and extends from the interventricular septum to the anterior wall of the right ventricle. So oriented, the infundibular septum does not actually constitute part of the interventricular septum but separates the VSD and subpulmonary region from the subaortic region. This commits the VSD to the pulmonary artery [74]. Hypertrophy of the infundibular septum and the parietal band can cause varying degrees of subaortic obstruction [74,75]. This may account for the relatively common occurrence of coarctation of the aorta

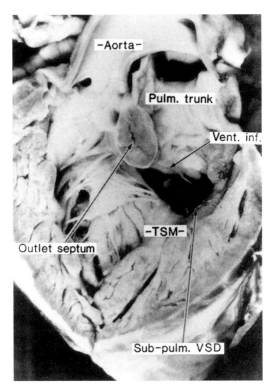

Figure 25.6 Coronal section of the right ventricle through the aortic and pulmonary valves in a heart with double-outlet right ventricle and subpulmonary ventricular septal defect (VSD) (Taussig-Bing malformation). The VSD is closely related to the pulmonary valve and is separated from the aortic valve by the outlet (infundibular, conal) septum. The ventricular septal defect extends to the tricuspid valve annulus posteriorly and, as such, is a perimembranous lesion. Note the sagittal orientation of the outlet (conal, infundibular) septum. (TSM, trabeculoseptomarginalis.) (Adapted with permission from Stellin *et al.* [73].)

(80%) in the Taussig-Bing malformation [74,76]. Bilateral coni or a single, subaortic conus each occur in approximately 50% of hearts with the Taussig-Bing malformation [6]. The pulmonary artery typically arises biventricularly. The aorta is usually to the right and is slightly anterior to or side-by-side with the pulmonary artery. These two great vessels are usually parallel; they do not spiral around each other as in the normal heart.

Noncommitted (Remote) VSD
Noncommitted [1] (remote [56]) VSDs (Figure 25.1E) [60] occur in 10–20% of patients in surgical series [4,62,77]. Lacour Gayet and associates have noted that the superior edge of these defects are located at least the distance of one aortic valve diameter from either arterial valve, both great vessels arise "200%" from the right ventricle and a double conus exists beneath both arterial valves [78,79,80]. These noncommitted VSDs are not nestled within the limbs of the TSM but rather are located within the inlet septum (without perimembranous extension) and/or the trabecular inter-

ventricular septum (Figure 25.7) [1,79,81–86]. A restrictive VSD and subaortic conus can frequently cause subaortic obstruction.

Right Ventricular Outflow Tract Obstruction
All of the variations of right ventricular outflow tract obstruction (RVOTO) that are present in hearts with tetralogy of Fallot can be present in hearts with DORV. Right ventricular outflow tract obstruction is most common in hearts with subaortic or doubly committed VSDs. It is extremely uncommon in patients with the Taussig-Bing malformation [74,87–93] and in those with noncommitted defects [1]. While RVOTO is most often infundibular, it can also be purely valvar with or without a small pulmonary valve annulus and hypoplasia of the central pulmonary arteries. Right ventricular outflow tract obstruction rarely can be caused by a diaphragm of muscle inserting between the inflow and outflow portions of the right ventricle. This produces a double-chambered right ventricle [50,94–97]. Other mechanisms of RVOTO: 1) straddling atrioventricular valve [98]; 2) accessory tissue tags; and 3) aneurysms of the membranous interventricular septum [99], occur uncommonly. Double-outlet right ventricle can rarely occur in association with pulmonary atresia.

Subaortic Stenosis
Subaortic stenosis is an uncommon, but clinically important, feature of DORV [56]. It occurs most often in those patients with subpulmonary VSD (35% of the Taussig-Bing hearts in Sondheimers series) [42]. It is especially common in Taussig-Bing hearts with aortic arch obstruction [100]. In this setting the subaortic stenosis is usually owing to a hypoplastic left ventricular outflow tract. Subaortic stenosis can also be caused by atrioventricular valve tissue, by accessory tissue tags, or by hypertrophied muscle bundles [75,101,102]. Aortic valvar stenosis [23,56] or atresia [103] can also be present.

Conduction System
In DORV with concordant atrioventricular connections, the atrioventricular node lies in the usual position in the muscular portion of the atrioventricular septum. The bundle of His penetrates the fibrous right trigone of the central fibrous body and lies along the posteroinferior margin of the VSD in lesions that are juxtatricuspid (perimembranous) whether the defect is subaortic, doubly committed, or subpulmonary. When muscle is interposed between the defect and the tricuspid valve, this muscle protects the bundle, which no longer runs along the posteroinferior free margin of the defect (Figure 25.4) [24].

Coronary Artery Anatomy
In the normal heart there are three aortic cusps. One is oriented posteriorly and is called the *noncoronary cusp*. The

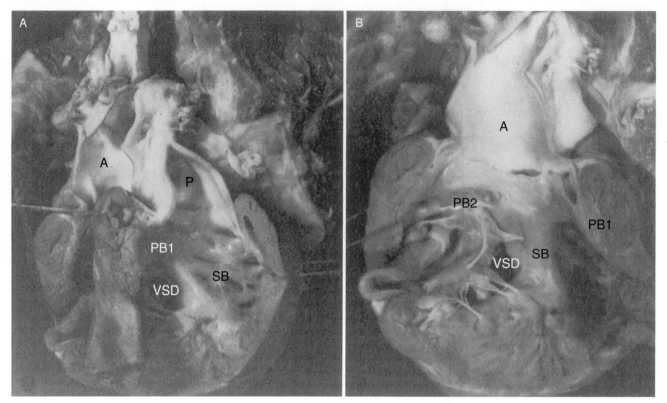

Figure 25.7 Double-outlet right ventricle with noncommitted atrioventricular canal type ventricular septal defect. **A,** Right ventricular view at the outflow tract of the pulmonary trunk. **B,** Right ventricular view at the outflow tract of the aorta. (A, aorta; P, pulmonary trunk; PB1, first parietal band; PB2, second parietal band; SB, septal band (trabeculoseptomarginalis); VSD, ventricular septal defect.) (Adapted with permission from Lev *et al.* [1].)

right anterior sinus gives rise to the right coronary artery (RCA), and the left anterior sinus gives rise to the left coronary artery. In most cases of DORV, the coronary orifices are rotated clockwise [104] as the observer looks from below. Hence, the left coronary artery arises more posteriorly and the RCA arises more anteriorly. With a right-sided and anterior aorta, the coronary artery pattern is similar to that seen in complete TGA. The RCA arises from the right posterior (facing) sinus (sinus 2), and the left coronary artery arises from the left posterior (facing) sinus (sinus 1) [104,105]. Nineteen (30%) of the patients with DORV in the series by Wilcox *et al.* [23] had coronary artery abnormalities. Two (3%) patients had a single coronary artery, one arising from sinus 1 and one from sinus 2. The branching pattern of the coronary arteries is usually normal [106]; however, in the series by Wilcox *et al.* [23] the left anterior descending coronary artery (LAD) arose from the RCA and ran anteriorly beneath the pulmonary valve across the RVOT in 16 (25%) patients. Gomes and colleagues [107,108] at the Mayo Clinic confirmed this finding. In the 3 (5%) hearts with L-malposition of the aorta in the series by Wilcox *et al.* [23], the RCA crossed anteriorly beneath the pulmonary valve on its way to the right atrioventricular groove.

Associated Cardiac Abnormalities

Almost any anomaly of the atrioventricular valves can complicate DORV and, when severe, create formidable obstacles to the performance of an anatomic repair. Examples of such anomalies include atrioventricular valve stenosis and atresia [23,55,56,109,110], straddling [23,111–117], and complete atrioventricular canal defect [118–121]. Coarctation of the aorta and other forms of left ventricular outflow tract obstruction are more common in hearts with the Taussig-Bing malformation [20,41,100,122,123]. Various other cardiac abnormalities including patent ductus arteriosus (PDA), ventricular hypoplasia (especially associated with atrioventricular valve abnormalities), unroofed coronary sinus syndrome, abnormalities of systemic venous return, juxtaposed atrial appendages, situs inversus totalis, dextrocardia, and ASD can occur.

Classification

As described earlier in the section on morphology, DORV has most often been classified anatomically in the literature according to the pure relational anatomy of the VSD to the semilunar valves: subaortic, doubly committed, subpulmonary, and noncommitted (remote). The Society of Thoracic Surgeons' (STS) Congenital Heart Surgery Nomenclature and Database Project Committee, the European Association of Cardiothoracic Surgery (EACTS) and the Association of European Pediatric Cardiologists (AEPC) have adopted a more practical and functional classification of DORV. While this nomenclature system groups these four classical anatomical subtypes into categories that convey a broad sense of the VSD relational anatomy, it also categorizes them according to their clinical presentation and the general approach to their surgical repair [124]. These categories include: 1) DORV, VSD type (subaortic and doubly committed VSDs without RVOTO); 2) DORV, tetralogy of Fallot type (subaortic and doubly committed VSDs with RVOTO); 3) DORV, TGA type (subpulmonary VSDs – Taussig-Bing); and 4) DORV, remote VSD type (uncommitted VSDs with or without RVOTO) [124,125]. A fifth group, DORV+ atrioventricular septal defect (AVSD) (AV canal), has also more recently been added to encompass DORV associated with complete AVSD. This especially complex subset of DORV patients is frequently associated with heterotaxy syndrome. These patients have frequent major associated cardiac lesions including some degree of RVOTO, total anomalous pulmonary venous connection (TAPVC), and partial anomalous systemic venous return (left SVC) along with right-sided atrial isomerism and asplenia. DORV, intact ventricular septum (IVS), though virtually nonexistent, has always been included in this classification for the sake of completeness.

Pathophysiology

Patients with DORV tend to present early in life at a mean age of 2 months (range, 1 day to 4 years) [42]. Without other major cardiac anomalies, the clinical presentation of patients with DORV depends on the relationship of the VSD to the great arteries and the presence or absence of pulmonary stenosis. These basic patterns of presentation for patients with DORV can be profoundly altered by the effect of major associated cardiac lesions [126].

Congestive Heart Failure

Patients with unrestricted subaortic doubly committed or noncommitted VSDs without pulmonary stenosis have unrestricted pulmonary blood flow and present with congestive heart failure. This presentation is indistinguishable from patients with an isolated and large VSD. Although these patients are usually mildly desaturated, they are not clinically cyanotic because the high pulmonary blood flow results in well saturated right ventricular blood owing to mixing with left ventricular blood through the VSD. There is also some preferential streaming of well saturated left ventricular blood into the aorta if the VSD is subaortic or doubly committed. Congestive heart failure can also be caused by left ventricular outflow tract obstruction and an obstructive left atrioventricular valve that produces pulmonary venous obstruction.

Cyanosis

Cyanosis can be produced in patients with DORV either by restriction to pulmonary blood flow, streaming, or a combination of both. In the Taussig-Bing malformation, highly saturated left ventricular blood is preferentially directed into the pulmonary artery by the sagittally oriented infundibular (conal) septum. Since relatively desaturated right ventricular blood tends to flow into the aorta, these Taussig-Bing patients mimic patients with TGA and VSD physiologically and present early in infancy with cyanosis and congestive heart failure. In the presence of significant pulmonary stenosis with any type of VSD, cyanosis can become severe owing to reduced pulmonary blood flow. These infants are similar to patients with tetralogy of Fallot in their presentation.

Diagnosis

Physical Examination, Electrocardiogram (ECG), Chest Radiograph

There are no physical findings or ECG criteria [127] that distinguish DORV from other congenital cardiac malformations with similar clinical presentations. The usual ECG findings are right axis deviation and right ventricular or biventricular hypertrophy. The chest radiograph findings are varied and nonspecific. They depend primarily on the amount of pulmonary blood flow and the presence of associated major cardiac anomalies. In any type of DORV with an unrestrictive VSD and without pulmonary stenosis, the chest radiograph will show evidence of pulmonary overcirculation. Conversely, patients with significant pulmonary stenosis will have relatively clear or oligopenic lung fields. Patients with L-malposition of the aorta can demonstrate a vertical left upper mediastinal aortic shadow on the posterolateral chest radiograph, although this is not a specific finding for DORV.

Echocardiogram

Echocardiography is the cornerstone of the diagnosis of DORV and, because of the subtleties and complexity of the diagnosis, it is often useful for the study to be performed in cooperation with the surgeon. Two-dimensional studies accurately define the diameter, location, number, and commitment of the VSD(s), the origin of both great arteries and their relationship to each other, semilunar-atrioventricular valve continuity or discontinuity, and absence of the normal left ventricular outflow tract. It also allows the accurate identification of: 1) right and left ventricular volumes; 2) pulmonary stenosis; 3) left ventricular outflow tract obstruction; 4) atrioventricular valve abnormalities such as straddling and/or overriding; 5) abnormal insertions of the tensor apparatus; 6) the distance between the tricuspid and the pulmonary valve annuli; 7) abnormalities of systemic and pulmonary venous return; 8) coronary artery abnormalities; and 9) the presence of complete atrioventricular canal defects [128–131].

Cardiac Catheterization and Cineangiography

Cineangiography with cardiac catheterization (Figure 25.8) [10,57] is not routinely performed unless there are anatomical features that are not adequately elucidated by the echocardiogram. If performed, these studies should be carefully examined for at least eight findings: 1) the size and relationship of the VSD to the great arteries; 2) the presence or absence of multiple VSDs; 3) the relationship of the great arteries to each other; 4) the presence or absence of pulmonary stenosis and the level(s) at which it occurs; 5) the coronary artery anatomy; 6) the presence and level(s) of left ventricular outflow tract obstruction; 7) the relationship of the atria to the ventricles (concordant or discordant); and 8) other associated cardiac anomalies. Because of the accuracy of two-dimensional echocardiography in defining most of the above features, cardiac catheterization is usually not essential for diagnosis and preopera-

tive planning. Rather, it is reserved to define associated cardiac anomalies that are not clearly identified by the echocardiogram (coronary artery anomalies, peripheral pulmonary artery stenoses, etc.), to provide an integrated image of the pulmonary arterial tree, and to identify irreversible pulmonary vascular disease. If cardiac catheterization is not performed in a given case, there should be no suspicion of pulmonary vascular disease or peripheral pulmonary artery stenoses, and the coronary anatomy should be clearly defined by the two-dimensional echocardiogram.

Cardiac catheterization of a patient with DORV, unrestrictive VSD, and no pulmonary or subaortic stenosis will demonstrate equal pressures in both ventricles and both great arteries. Pulmonary blood flow will be high in the presence of normal pulmonary vascular resistance, and both left atrial and left ventricular blood will be highly saturated. Saturations in the right ventricle will be lower owing to the admixture of left ventricular blood with the desaturated systemic venous return. Saturations in the great arteries will depend on the position of the VSD relative to each individual great artery and the streaming produced thereby. Patients with subaortic and doubly committed VSDs will tend to have higher aortic saturations than patients with subpulmonary VSDs. Patients with subpulmonary VSDs will tend to have pulmonary saturations equal to or higher than the systemic saturation [132].

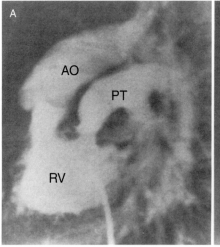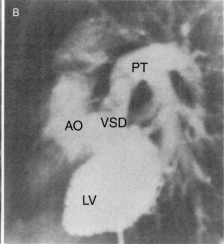

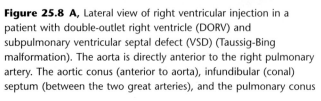

Figure 25.8 A, Lateral view of right ventricular injection in a patient with double-outlet right ventricle (DORV) and subpulmonary ventricular septal defect (VSD) (Taussig-Bing malformation). The aorta is directly anterior to the right pulmonary artery. The aortic conus (anterior to aorta), infundibular (conal) septum (between the two great arteries), and the pulmonary conus

(posterior to the pulmonary trunk) are well demonstrated.
B, Lateral view of a left ventricular injection in a patient with DORV and subpulmonary VSD (Taussig-Bing malformation). The VSD is located beneath the pulmonary artery. (Ao, aorta; LV, left ventricle; MV, mitral valve; PT, pulmonary trunk; RV, right ventricle.) (Adapted with permission from Sridaromont *et al.* [57].)

Magnetic Resonance Imaging

Magnetic resonance imaging can be useful in documenting the adequacy of the ventricular volumes for biventricular repair and in elucidating coexisting cardiac anatomy, such as abnormalities of systemic or pulmonary venous connections and other abnormalities, in some complex cases.

Natural History

The natural history of DORV with a subaortic, doubly committed or noncommitted VSD without pulmonary stenosis is similar to that of a large, isolated VSD except spontaneous closure of the VSD in DORV, a fatal event, is extremely rare [133]. The pulmonary vasculature of patients with DORV, pulmonary stenosis, and a subaortic, doubly committed or noncommitted VSD is relatively protected against the development of pulmonary vascular disease. The natural history of these patients is similar to that of patients with tetralogy of Fallot. The natural history of patients with DORV and subpulmonary VSD is similar to that of patients with TGA and VSD except for the tendency of the Taussig-Bing patients to develop pulmonary vascular disease earlier in life [6]. The natural history of any of these subsets of patients with DORV can be dramatically altered by major associated cardiac lesions such as left ventricular outflow tract obstruction and atrioventricular valve abnormalities with or without ventricular hypoplasia.

Treatment

The goal of the surgical treatment of DORV is complete anatomic repair. This is defined as connection of the left ventricle to the aorta, the right ventricle to the pulmonary artery, and closure of the VSD. In general, the timing of surgical intervention depends on the symptomatic state of the patient and the anatomy of and other cardiac anomalies associated with the DORV itself. The anatomy determines the ultimate, corrective surgical approach, which, in turn, influences the optimal age for definitive repair. The clinical state of the patient before the age at which definitive repair is planned will determine the need for initial palliative procedures. In general, a complete repair is undertaken at as early an age as possible.

Impediments to Complete Anatomic Repair

Anatomic repair of DORV can be contraindicated by the presence of ventricular hypoplasia, serious abnormalities of either atrioventricular valve, the presence of very remote and/or multiple VSDs, and the presence of irreversible pulmonary vascular disease. An atrioventricular valve with a diameter more than two standard deviations smaller than the mean normal value for the patient's body surface

area is usually attended by surgically important ventricular hypoplasia. In this situation successful anatomic repair is seldom possible. Severe straddling and/or overriding of either atrioventricular valve can render anatomic repair impossible. The presence of a single VSD far removed from either of the semilunar valves and the presence of multiple VSDs can render anatomical repair more difficult or ill-advised, depending on the anatomical situation. The presence of a borderline size right ventricular volume is a limiting factor for biventricular repair because the construction of the intracardiac right ventricular tunnel will reduce the right ventricular volume even more.

General Aspects of Surgical Repair

The anatomy is assessed through the tricuspid valve and a repair is planned. The repair is performed through the tricuspid valve and/or a vertical right ventriculotomy incision. Sometimes, when the repair is carried out entirely through the tricuspid valve, exposure of the most superior portion of the VSD is enhanced by performing a radial incision along the base of the septal and anterior leaflets of the tricuspid valve and/or by exerting gentle, external, inferior pressure at the aortoventricular junction.

DORV, VSD Type (Subaortic or Doubly Committed VSD Without Pulmonary Stenosis)

Timing of Surgical Repair

This variant represents approximately 25% of all DORV and in 20% the VSD can be restrictive [80,134]. These patients should undergo complete repair in early infancy [135] because the onset of pulmonary vascular disease is at least as rapid as it is in untreated patients with large, isolated VSDs. It has also been shown that young age, per se, is not a risk factor for hospital death [4,136,137].

Technique of Intraventricular Tunnel Repair

An intraventricular tunnel repair, connecting the left ventricle to the aorta, is preferred for patients with DORV, VSD type (Figure 25.9) [60]. Rarely, in patients with refractory congestive heart failure who are thought not to be immediate candidates for complete repair, pulmonary artery banding is required. This procedure is not recommended routinely; total correction should be performed in early infancy as soon as it is felt that the patient is a suitable candidate.

The size of the VSD, as well as its location relative to the aorta, is noted. If the VSD appears to be restrictive (diameter less than that of the aortic valve), it is enlarged by making an incision anterosuperiorly or by resecting a wedge of the interventricular septum in this area (Figure 25.9A) [53,60]. Care is taken not to injure the mitral valve

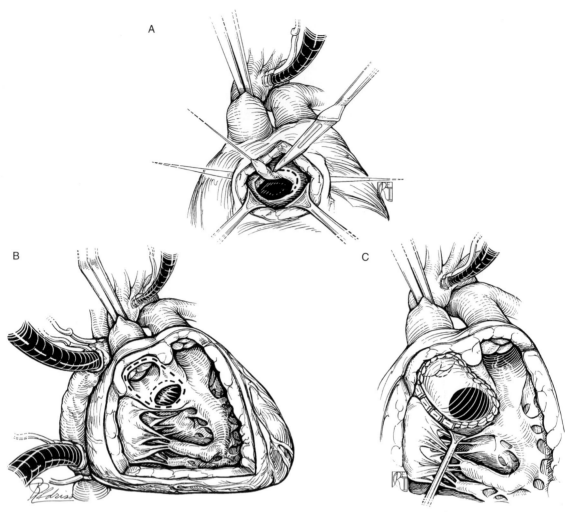

A

B

C

Figure 25.9 Intraventricular tunnel repair of double-outlet right ventricle with subaortic or doubly committed ventricular septal defect (VSD) without pulmonary stenosis. **A,** If the VSD is restrictive, it is enlarged by resection of the interventricular septum in the shaded area. Stippling indicates the portion of the infundibular septum that may require resection to prevent subaortic stenosis. (Inset shows the median sternotomy used for the repair.) **B,** Demonstrates the creation of a tunnel connecting the ventricular septal defect to the aorta (see text for details). **C,** The completed tunneling of the VSD to the aortic valve creating an unobstructed pathway for left ventricular blood to exit the heart.

or its tensor apparatus and to avoid injury to the anterior ventricular wall with its left anterior descending coronary artery and septal perforator [138].

Obstructive right ventricular muscle bundles are resected. Often a portion of the infundibular septum must be resected in order to construct a straight tunnel between the VSD and the aorta. It is usually possible to construct a tunnel from the left ventricle to the aorta without obstructing the pulmonary outflow tract if the minimal distance between the tricuspid valve annulus and the pulmonary valve annulus is equal to or greater than the diameter of the aortic valve annulus. Preoperatively, this distance can generally be estimated accurately with the subxyphoid view of the two-dimensional echocardiogram [40,41].

We create the intracardiac tunnel with an appropriately trimmed flat Gore-Tex patch (W.L. Gore and Associates, Inc, Flagstaff, AZ) secured with running or interrupted sutures. Alternatively, the tunnel can be constructed with a tailored dacron or Gore-Tex tube graft that takes advantage of the inherent graft curvature to create a naturally shaped and unobstructed intraventricular tunnel (Figure 25.9B,C) [60]. The long axis of the patch is oriented perpendicular to a line drawn through the center of the VSD and the center of the aortic orifice. The determination of the actual length of the patch long axis depends on the degree of dextroposition of the aorta. When the entire aorta is dextroposed into the right ventricular cavity, the patch length should be two thirds of the circumference of the aorta. One third of the circumference of the intraventricular tunnel so created will be composed of autogenous tissue and will, therefore, retain the capacity for growth. The width of the patch should extend from the inferior edge of the VSD to the superior margin of the aortic annulus. The suture line is carried well away from the edge of the VSD along its posteroinferior margin in order to avoid damage to the conduction tissue. Posteriorly, the patch is secured to the base of the septal leaflet of the tricuspid valve. If there is a ledge of muscle separating the posterior edge of the VSD from the tricuspid annulus, the VSD sutures can be placed on the right ventricular side of the free edge of this muscle bundle; the conduction tissue does not run in this muscle along the edge of the defect. That notwithstanding, we generally choose to suture the patch to the base of the septal leaflet of the tricuspid valve and to avoid the posteroinferior margin of the VSD entirely. Sometimes the dimensions of the right ventricular outflow tract must be augmented with an outflow patch because of the production of RVOTO by the intraventricular tunnel.

Complications After Intraventricular Tunnel Repair

Complications after the intraventricular tunnel repair of DORV, VSD type are infrequent. Complete heart block is uncommon, and the functional status of at least 87% of the survivors is New York Heart Association (NYHA) Class I [4]. Over 90% of patients who require only intraventricular tunnel repair for subaortic or doubly committed VSDs are free of reoperation at follow-up. Indications for reoperation should be rare but can include tunnel dehiscence, tunnel obstruction, residual VSD, and discrete, localized subaortic stenosis unrelated to the tunnel itself [4].

Results After Intraventricular Tunnel Repair

In the current era, the risk of death early after repair of DORV, VSD type is low [4,77]. The actuarial 15-year survival, including hospital death, is 96%. In an earlier era, younger age was a risk factor for death after repair. At the present time, the effect of younger age has been neutralized; however, older age has been shown to be a significant risk factor, possibly owing to the presence of increasing pulmonary vascular disease with age [4].

DORV, tetralogy of Fallot Type (Subaortic or Doubly Committed VSD with Pulmonary Stenosis)

Timing of Surgical Repair

This is the most frequent form of DORV and the pulmonary stenosis can range from a relatively mild valvar, subvalvar, and/or supravalvar pulmonary stenosis to frank pulmonary atresia. It may be difficult to differentiate between tetralogy of Fallot and DORV, tetralogy of Fallot type because of the significant anterior malposition of the aorta

in both. In the presence of DORV, tetralogy of Fallot type the techniques of repair are similar to those described for repair of tetralogy of Fallot except the VSD is closed with the tunnel technique rather than with a straight patch. Repair is generally advised by 6 months of age if the coronary artery anatomy is normal and if it is felt, with certainty, that an intraventricular repair can be performed. If the preoperative clinical condition of the patient is poor or if there are major associated noncardiac abnormalities, a palliative systemic-to-pulmonary artery shunt may be advisable before performing the definitive repair later in life. An initial systemic to pulmonary artery shunt may also be reasonably considered if the branch pulmonary arteries are severely hypoplastic and/or it is felt that an extracardiac conduit will be required for the final correction. Others advocate early primary repair for essentially all patients with DORV, thereby avoiding the need for palliative procedures with their attendant risks and complications [135].

Strategies of Surgical Repair

We prefer to avoid placement of a transannular patch. When a transannular patch is necessary (Figure 25.10A) [60] owing to pulmonary annular hypoplasia and/or pulmonary valve stenosis, the aggressive use of transatrial and transpulmonary endocardial resection of hypertrophied and obstructive muscle bundles is recommended. This allows the surgeon to limit the distance the transannular incision must be carried into the right ventricular outflow tract and to avoid possible right ventricular dysfunction associated therewith. When exposure of the VSD through the tricuspid valve is unsatisfactory, we do not hesitate to perform a right ventriculotomy. In patients with an anomalous coronary artery crossing the right ventricular outflow tract immediately beneath the pulmonary valve annulus and in patients with a suspected or measured elevation of pulmonary vascular resistance, it is necessary to place a valved, extracardiac conduit when endocardial resection alone will not relieve the RVOTO (Figure 25.10B) [60]. Patients with pure valvar pulmonary stenosis and a normal pulmonary annulus and arterial tree can undergo pulmonary valvotomy or valvectomy. Similar patients with mild-to-moderate pulmonary vascular disease may benefit from the orthotopic placement of a homograft pulmonary valve.

Results of Surgical Repair

The functional status of survivors of repair of DORV, tetralogy of Fallot type is excellent. The time-related actuarial freedom from reoperation after placement of a heterograft valved conduit from the right ventricle to the pulmonary artery is only 50% at 10 years [4]. Although antibiotic-sterilized, cryopreserved homografts are frequently used because of their excellent handling characteristics, it is not known with certainty whether they are more durable. The early and late survival of this group of patients is similar

A

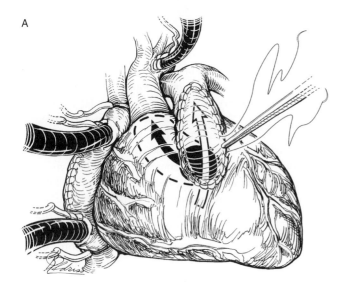

B

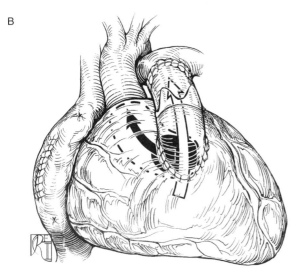

Figure 25.10 Reconstruction of the right ventricular outflow tract during repair of double-outlet right ventricle with subaortic or doubly committed ventricular septal defect. **A,** Patch enlargement of the right ventricular outflow tract with transannular extension into the main pulmonary artery. **B,** The use of a valved, extracardiac conduit to establish continuity between the right ventricle and pulmonary artery.

to that described for patients without pulmonary stenosis if the repair of the pulmonary stenosis did not require the placement of an extracardiac conduit or a transannular patch. In these latter two groups, the instantaneous risks of death in the early and late hazard phases are higher than when simpler forms of relief of RVOTO are used [4].

DORV, TGA Type (Subpulmonary VSD)

DORV, TGA type, as stated earlier, is frequently associated with aortic arch obstruction, subaortic obstruction, side-

by-side positioning of the great vessels, and a significant diameter mismatch of the great vessels, with the aortic valve diameter being significantly smaller than that of the pulmonary valve. Surgical repair of this complex subset of patients has evolved over the years: 1) patch tunneling of the VSD to the pulmonary artery combined with an atrial switch procedure (Mustard or Senning) [3,4,29,63,136,139,140]; 2) tunneling of the VSD to the pulmonary artery, aortopulmonary connection (Damus-Kaye-Stansel procedure) and placement of a valved extracardiac conduit from the right ventricle to the distal pulmonary artery [141–143]; 3) direct tunneling of the VSD to the aorta (Kawashima repair) [3,4,27,30,63,74,144–157]; 4) tunneling of the VSD to the pulmonary artery combined with an arterial switch procedure [62,158–160]; and, in select situations, 5) VSD closure to the aorta with placement of a right ventricular-to-pulmonary artery conduit (Rastelli procedure) [161,162], tunneling of the VSD to the aorta with translocation of the pulmonary artery (réparation à l'étage ventriculaire [REV] procedure of Lecompte) [40,41,163–169], or aortic translocation and biventricular outflow tract reconstruction (Nikaidoh procedure) [169–172]. Some of these surgical approaches are of historical importance only because they are no longer used clinically.

Intraventricular Tunnel Repair for the Taussig-Bing Malformation

One approach for the repair of DORV with subpulmonary VSD is a totally intraventricular repair without the need for the arterial switch operation or for the use of an extracardiac conduit. This type of repair has been accomplished using a number of techniques: 1) the posterior, tubular conduit repair of Abe and colleagues [151–153]; 2) the anterior, tubular conduit method of Doty [150]; 3) the anterior, spiral tunnel repair of Patrick and McGoon and colleagues [30,144,154]; and 4) the posterior, straight tunnel technique of Kawashima [31,144,147,156]. Of these four techniques, the Kawashima operation is the only totally intraventricular tunnel technique that is currently used by some surgeons to repair certain forms of the Taussig-Bing malformation.

The Kawashima Operation

When the great arteries are in a more or less side-by-side relationship with the aorta to the right of the pulmonary artery, the Kawashima [31,144,147,155–157] repair connects the left ventricle directly to the aorta with a tunnel that runs posterior to the pulmonary artery between the tricuspid and pulmonary valves (Figure 25.11) [60]. The infundibular (conal) septum must be resected in order to provide an unobstructed path for the tunnel (Figure 25.11B) [60]. The VSD is enlarged only if it is restrictive. Because this tunnel courses between the pulmonary and tricuspid valve annuli,

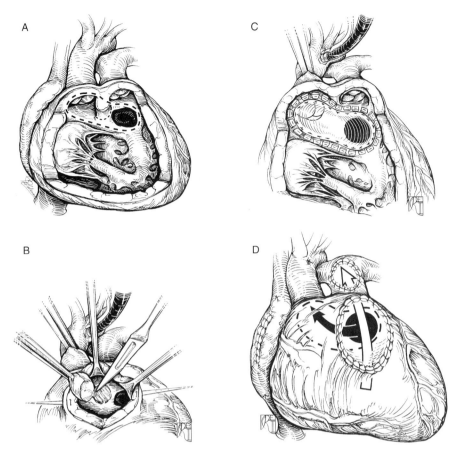

Figure 25.11 The Kawashima operation for double-outlet right ventricle with subpulmonary ventricular septal defect (VSD) (Taussig-Bing malformation). **A,** Inner, small dashed line indicates the portion of the infundibular (conal) septum that may require resection before construction of intraventricular tunnel (outer dashed line). **B,** A generous resection of the infundibular (conal) septum is performed in order to create an unobstructed path between the subpulmonary VSD and the aorta. **C,** The figure depicts the completed intraventricular tunnel repair. Note that there must be sufficient distance between the tricuspid valve and pulmonary valve annuli in order to create the tunnel successfully. **D,** It is sometimes necessary to augment the right ventricular outflow tract in order to relieve subpulmonary stenosis created by the tunnel or to relieve various preexisting pulmonary stenoses.

these two structures must be separated by a sufficient distance to make tunnel creation possible (Figure 25.11C) [60]. In patients with an oblique or anterior-posterior relationship of the great arteries, the tricuspid-pulmonary valve distance may not be great enough to allow the creation of this tunnel, and the arterial switch technique must be employed. The Kawashima repair can be performed either through the tricuspid valve or through a right ventriculotomy. Abnormal attachments of the tricuspid valve tensor apparatus onto the infundibular septum or straddling and/or overriding of the mitral valve may make this repair difficult or impossible.

Results of the Kawashima Operation

The series that report follow-up data on patients undergoing the Kawashima operation [31,74,144,155–157] is small;

however, all reported patients were alive and well. One report [155] documents a series of 10 patients out of 41 with the Taussig-Bing malformation who underwent a completely intraventricular repair. The relationship of the great arteries was side-by-side in nine patients and oblique in one patient. Average follow-up was 8 years and 4 months. There were no early or late deaths and reoperation was required in only one patient (residual pulmonary stenosis). Postoperative cardiac catheterization in eight patients showed no clinically significant subaortic stenosis. However, the right and left ventricular volumes were elevated, and the right ventricular ejection fraction was reduced. In summary, the Kawashima operation can be reasonably recommended in patients with a side-by-side relationship of the great arteries and, perhaps, in some with an oblique relationship. If elected, this operation should be performed as a primary procedure in early infancy. The trend, however, in most institutions has been toward the arterial switch operation even in those patients with side-by-side great vessel orientation.

The Arterial Switch Operation with Tunnel Closure of VSD

The most common approach to the repair of DORV with subpulmonary VSD is the arterial switch procedure combined with tunnel closure of the VSD to the pulmonary artery [157–160,173–177]. The advantage of this technique compared, for example, with the Kawashima operation is its flexibility in that it can be used successfully for the repair of Taussig-Bing hearts with any and all arrangements of the great arteries. The arterial switch operation is optimally performed in the first week of life before the patency of the ductus arteriosus is maintained by a prostaglandin infusion. A preoperative balloon atrial septostomy procedure is usually not required because of adequate mixing at the level of the PDA, the ASD, and the large subpulmonary VSD. In the absence of subaortic obstruction, palliation with aortic arch repair and pulmonary artery banding through a left thoracotomy incision may be considered. This is especially appropriate in cases of Swiss-cheese septum, concern over adequate size of the right ventricle, straddling of the atrioventricular valve or when serious, confounding medical conditions, like severe

prematurity, necrotizing enterocolitis or subarachnoid hemorrhage, are present. Otherwise, single-stage repair is preferred [177].

Initial phase (no aortic arch obstruction). Through a standard median sternotomy incision, the thymus is excised and the heart is suspended in a pericardial cradle. The ascending aorta, main pulmonary artery, and PDA are circumferentially dissected, and marking sutures are placed on the pulmonary artery (neoaorta) to mark the site at which coronary artery transfer is to occur. During the initial cooling phase of cardiopulmonary bypass the PDA is snared, the separation of the ascending aorta from the main pulmonary artery is completed, and the right and left pulmonary arteries are dissected circumferentially well beyond their branching points to achieve a tension-free mobilization. The ductus arteriosus is then suture ligated at its pulmonary and aortic ends and is divided. If the Lecompte maneuver is performed, it is facilitated by performing a relatively high aortic transection and a low transection of the main pulmonary artery. The technical details of the arterial switch operation in DORV, subpulmonary VSD (Taussig-Bing malformation) not associated with aortic arch obstruction are illustrated in Figures 25.12–25.14 [60].

Initial phase (aortic arch obstruction). When there is associated aortic arch obstruction with aortic arch hypoplasia and a small ascending aorta (80% of hearts with the Taussig-Bing anomaly) (Figure 25.15), a right radial arterial

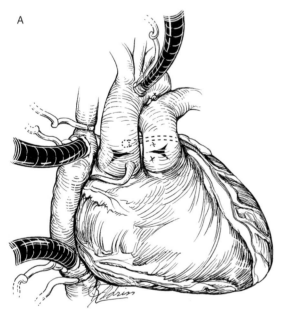
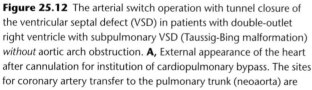
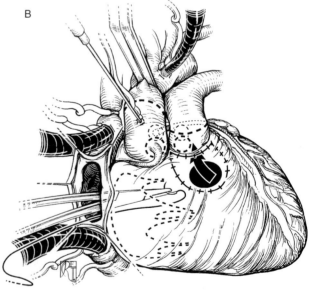

Figure 25.12 The arterial switch operation with tunnel closure of the ventricular septal defect (VSD) in patients with double-outlet right ventricle with subpulmonary VSD (Taussig-Bing malformation) *without* aortic arch obstruction. **A,** External appearance of the heart after cannulation for institution of cardiopulmonary bypass. The sites for coronary artery transfer to the pulmonary trunk (neoaorta) are marked with sutures. The ductus arteriosus has been ligated and divided. **B,** The VSD is closed transatrially or transventricularly. The levels for transection of the great arteries are marked with broken lines. It is assumed, in this illustration, that the Lecompte maneuver will not be used (see text for details of performing the Lecompte maneuver).

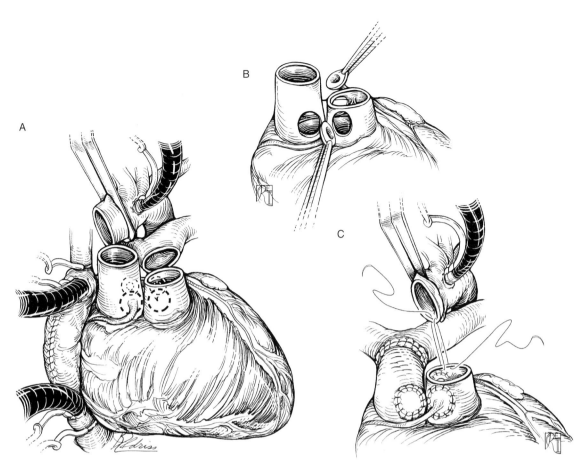

Figure 25.13 The arterial switch operation with tunnel closure of the ventricular septal defect in patients with double-outlet right ventricle with subpulmonary ventricular septal defect (Taussig-Bing malformation) *without* aortic arch obstruction. **A,** The great arteries are transected as if no Lecompte maneuver is to be performed (see text for details). **B,** The coronary artery orifices are excised with a button of native aortic wall. Ovals of the pulmonary artery (neoaortic root) are removed at the previously marked sites in preparation for coronary artery transfer. (Alternatively, these openings in the neoaortic root can be created as *U-shaped defects* or as medially hinged *trap-door* incisions. See Chapter 26, *Transposition of the Great Arteries.*) **C,** The defects in the aortic wall (neopulmonary root) are repaired with autologous pericardium. (Alternatively, this can be accomplished with a pantaloon patch. The mobilized coronary arteries are transferred to the neoaortic root and are sutured thereto without tension or kinking. The distal transected main pulmonary artery bifurcation is sutured to the neopulmonary root.

line and a femoral or umbilical arterial line are inserted preoperatively. The initial dissection is similar to that described above. A technique of dual arterial cannulation with antegrade cerebral perfusion is described in this chapter. An 8F arterial cannula is placed in the main pulmonary artery and is advanced through the PDA into the descending aorta. During the initial cooling phase of cardiopulmonary bypass the PDA is snared around the arterial cannula, the separation of the ascending aorta from the main pulmonary artery is completed, and the right and left pulmonary arteries are dissected circumferentially well beyond their branching points to achieve a tension-free mobilization. The entire transverse arch and brachiocephalic vessels are circumferentially dissected and fully mobilized during the initial cooling phase to 18 °C. During the cooling phase, a 3.5 mm Gore-Tex tube graft is sutured

to the innominate artery and is cannulated with a second 8F arterial cannula to mediate antegrade cerebral perfusion and to remove the second arterial cannula from the surgical field. This facilitates exposure and minimizes distortion of the aorta during the reconstruction.

After temporarily occluding the brachiocephalic vessels and during a brief period of deep hypothermic circulatory arrest (DHCA), the PDA is divided and then oversewn at its pulmonary end. The ascending aorta is divided (see details below in Coronary artery translocation). The aortic isthmus is divided at a point just beyond the origin of the left subclavian artery and all coarctation and ductal tissue are excised (Figure 25.16). A vascular clamp is placed across the transected, proximal descending thoracic aorta and antegrade cerebral perfusion is initiated. The proximal descending aorta is fully mobilized deep into the posterior

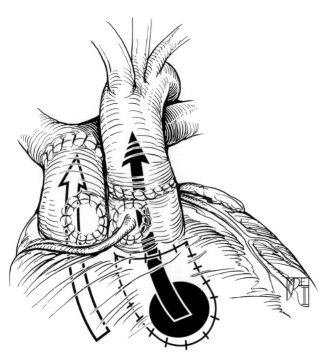

Figure 25.14 The arterial switch operation with tunnel closure of the ventricular septal defect in patients with double-outlet right ventricle with subpulmonary ventricular septal defect (Taussig-Bing malformation) *without* aortic arch obstruction. The neoaortic root is sutured to the distal transected ascending aorta to restore left ventriculoarterial concordance. The neopulmonary root was previously sutured to the distal transected main pulmonary artery bifurcation to restore right ventriculoarterial concordance.

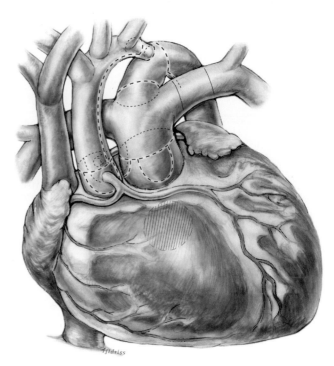

Figure 25.15 The arterial switch operation with tunnel closure of the ventricular septal defect (VSD) in patients with double-outlet right ventricle with subpulmonary VSD (Taussig-Bing malformation) *with* aortic arch obstruction. The great vessels are oriented in a side-by-side configuration. Note the mismatch in the diameter of the ascending aorta and main pulmonary artery. There is severe transverse aortic arch hypoplasia with a coarctation of the aorta. The hypoplastic distal transverse aortic arch inserts, at the point of the coarctation, into the patent ductus arteriosus. The right coronary artery (RCA), arising from the anterior facing sinus, gives rise to the left anterior descending (LAD) coronary artery. The LAD passes leftward and immediately inferior to the native pulmonary valve (neoaortic valve) annulus on its way to the anterior interventricular groove. The coronary artery arising from the posterior facing sinus is the circumflex coronary artery and it passes posterior to the pulmonary artery trunk. The dotted lines represent incisions for the proposed division and ligation of the patent ductus arteriosus, the aortic arch reconstruction and the arterial switch operation. The circular parallel lines represent the location of the subpulmonary VSD.

mediastinum, cauterizing and dividing intercostal vessels along the way, to facilitate mobilization of the descending aorta, and to ensure a tension-free aortic reconstruction. Once the mobilization of the descending thoracic aorta is complete, an incision is made in the inferior aspect of the transverse aortic arch and is extended proximally into the transected point of the ascending aorta. Part of the circumference of the transected proximal descending thoracic aorta is sutured to transected aortic isthmus. A 2 cm counter-incision is made into the inferior aspect of the proximal descending aorta (Figure 25.16). A pulmonary homograft patch is then used to augment the primary aortic anastomosis, the transverse aortic arch, and the distal ascending aorta (Figures 25.16, 25.17). The proximal width of this homograft patch augments the circumference of the transected ascending aorta to match the circumference of the native pulmonary (neoaortic) root. Care should be taken to avoid making the pulmonary homograft patch too wide proximally, thereby creating a bulbous aortic reconstruction that tends to kink or compress surrounding structures (Figure 25.17). The aorta is deaired while placing a cross-clamp above the cardioplegia needle. Antegrade cerebral perfusion through the Gore-Tex tube graft is then

transitioned to full-flow by removing the occluders on the brachiocephalic vessels and increasing the flows. The quality of the aortic arch reconstruction can be immediately assessed by comparing the umbilical/femoral pressures with the right radial arterial pressures.

An alternative approach to the technique described above consists of augmenting the entire length of aortic arch with a pulmonary homograft patch without dividing the aortic isthmus. After instituting DHCA, the PDA is divided, and its pulmonary end is oversewn. The proximal descending thoracic aorta is fully mobilized and a vascular

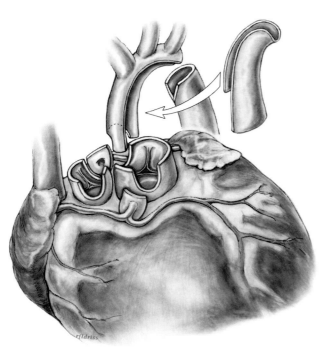

Figure 25.16 The arterial switch operation with tunnel closure of the ventricular septal defect (VSD) in patients with double-outlet right ventricle with subpulmonary VSD (Taussig-Bing malformation) *with* aortic arch obstruction. The patent ductus arteriosus is divided and the pulmonary end is oversewn. The ascending aorta and the aortic isthmus are divided. The descending thoracic aorta is mobilized and all coarctation/ductal tissues are excised. The aortic arch is repaired by partial direct anastomosis with patch (homograft) enlargement as depicted in the figure and as explained in detail in the text. Note the counter-incision in the posterior aspect of the distal, transected ascending aorta to accommodate the high insertion of the circumflex coronary artery.

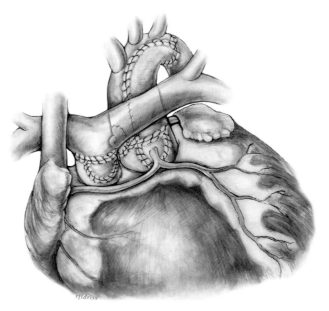

Figure 25.17 The arterial switch operation with tunnel closure of the ventricular septal defect (VSD) in patients with double-outlet right ventricle with subpulmonary VSD (Taussig-Bing malformation) *with* aortic arch obstruction. Note the partial direct anastomosis of the proximal descending thoracic aorta to the transected aortic isthmus and the augmentation of this anastomosis, the transverse aortic arch and the ascending aorta with the homograft patch. This completed aortic arch repair creates an excellent size match between the augmented ascending aorta and the neoaortic root. The circumflex coronary artery translocation is high relative to the right coronary artery translocation (see text for details). The defects in the neopulmonary root are filled with a pantaloon patch of fresh, autologous pericardium. When a Lecompte maneuver is used it is necessary to fashion a leftward shift in the anastomosis of the neopulmonary root to the pulmonary artery bifurcation (see text for details).

clamp is placed well distal to the aortic insertion of the PDA. Antegrade cerebral perfusion through the Gore-Tex tube graft is initiated. The ductal tissue is completely excised and the ascending aorta is transected at a previously marked point above the native aortic valve commissures. An incision is initiated at the medial aspect of the transected ascending aorta and is extended along the inferior aspect of the transverse aortic arch past the coarctation site and into the proximal, descending thoracic aorta to a point well beyond the aortic insertion of the excised PDA. The ascending aorta, transverse arch, and descending aorta are then augmented, in continuity, using a pulmonary homograft patch, as described above. The aorta is deaired, a cross-clamp is placed and standard cardiopulmonary bypass is resumed.

VSD closure. Owing to the malalignment of the conal septum, that is usually entirely located within the right ventricle, two orifices can be defined: the interventricular communication, which is the only outlet of the left ventricle, and the VSD, located between the conal septum and the muscular septum (Figure 25.18). It is the latter that is to be closed in tunneling the left ventricle to the pulmonary artery. The inferior and posterior margins of the VSD can frequently be closed using a transatrial approach through the tricuspid valve. A vertical right ventriculotomy incision is also frequently required to adequately visualize the anterior and, especially, the superior margins of the VSD. This also affords good visualization of the infundibular (conal) septum to facilitate relief of subaortic obstruction. Approaching the VSD through the native pulmonary valve (neoaortic orifice) is associated with the development of aortic valve regurgitation [188]. Closure of part of the VSD through the native aortic (neopulmonary) valve, after harvesting the coronary buttons is a safer approach. Once the VSD is closed, the patency of the newly reconstructed left ventricle outflow is ascertained through the pulmonary (neoaortic) valve.

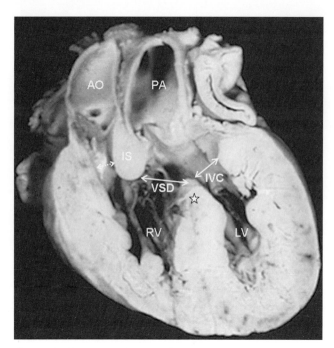

Figure 25.18 A sagittal section through a heart with double-outlet right ventricle with subpulmonary VSD (Taussig-Bing malformation) and subaortic obstruction. The aorta arises entirely from the RV. The PA overrides the crest of the ventricular septum. The anterior malalignment of the infundibular (conal) septum creates subaortic obstruction (dashed arrow). Two orifices are present. The interventricular communication is the only outlet of the left ventricle, and the VSD is the defect that must be closed (see text for details) in addition to performing an arterial switch operation. The RV is normal in size. There is a coexisting aortic arch obstruction that is not seen in this photograph. There are two coronary ostia, one located higher relative to the other. This higher location could indicate an intramural course. The location of the bundle of His is indicated with a star. (IVC, interventricular communication; VSD, ventricular septal defect; AO, aorta; PA, pulmonary artery; IS, infundibular (conal) septum; LV, left ventricle; RV, right ventricle.) (Courtesy of Norman Silverman MD, Stanford University, Stanford, CA, USA.)

Relief of RVOT obstruction. This phase of the operation is critical to avoid one of the most common early and late complications, subpulmonary obstruction. The RVOT is explored through the right ventriculotomy incision and through the native aortic (neopulmonary) valve through which obstructing muscle bundles are thoroughly excised. This phase of the operation is complicated by the presence of a coronary artery coursing across the RVOT and/or by marked hypoplasia of the neoaortic root. With the former, a lower ventriculotomy incision is created well below the level of the crossing coronary artery. Because RVOT hypoplasia is frequent the ventriculotomy incision should be

closed with a patch. A small, valved, homograft conduit or a nonvalved Gore-Tex conduit may be required in certain anatomical situations in which the neopulmonary annulus is severely hypoplastic and/or there is a crossing coronary artery.

Coronary artery translocation. The coronary artery translocation can be challenging because of frequent coronary abnormalities. A routine Lecompte maneuver is performed and is facilitated by performing a high aortic transection and a low transection of the main pulmonary artery. Others, however, argue against the routine use of this maneuver and report excellent results [178]. In the final analysis, it is probably safe to exclude the Lecompte maneuver if anterior coronary artery looping (right coronary artery from the left sinus or left anterior descending coronary artery from the right sinus) is not present. When the coronary artery anatomy is "usual" the technique of coronary artery translocation is identical to that of the usual arterial switch operation for TGA. However, in the Taussig-Bing malformation, deviation of the coronary artery anatomy from the "usual" situation is frequent. Therefore, when the RCA button gives rise to the left main coronary arterial trunk or to the circumflex coronary artery, it is placed in a superior position by creating a relatively high defect in the neoaortic root at the previously marked location and by interdigitating as much of the button into the aortic suture line and into a counter incision made in the distal, transected ascending aorta as is necessary to accommodate the remaining circumference of the button. The left coronary artery button is sutured into its corresponding defect created in the neoaortic root and is placed just high enough to avoid kinking of the translocated coronary artery (Figure 25.17).

Reconstructing the pulmonary artery. The defects in the neopulmonary artery root are filled with a generous pantaloon patch of fresh, autologous pericardium (Figure 25.17). While some prefer to do this part of the operation after removing the cross-clamp to reduce the myocardial ischemic time, deferring cross-clamp removal until after this phase of the operation improves precision and reduces the chance of coronary arterial injury. Also, when the RCA originates from the left sinus and loops anteriorly, this pantaloon patch should be placed before the left coronary artery translocation is performed because suturing the pantaloon patch to the left hemi-circumference of the neopulmonary root threatens injury to a left coronary artery button that has already been sutured to the neoaortic root. When a Lecompte maneuver is performed, an incision is made from the right side of the opening in the distal transected main pulmonary artery into the inferior aspect of the right pulmonary artery. The opening in the left side of the distal transected main pulmonary artery is closed with a patch promoting a rightward shift of the anastomosis of the neopulmonary root to the pulmonary bifurcation.

This improves the alignment of the pulmonary reconstruction and reduces the chance of compressing the RCA.

Results of the Arterial Switch Operation

The current hospital mortality of arterial switch for Taussig-Bing malformation ranges from 3–15%, with patients affected by aortic arch obstruction occupying the upper end of this range [157–160,173–178]. Planche and colleagues [174] studied 1200 patients who underwent the ASO, 79 of whom had Taussig-Bing malformation of whom 85% were 30-day survivors (n = 67). With a median follow-up of 4.5 years (range, 6 months to 17 years) the actuarial 10-year survival was 85% with no late deaths after 5 years. There was a 10% rate of reoperation, primarily for RVOTO. Patients with Taussig-Bing malformation and aortic arch obstruction are at particular risk (10–20%) for late subpulmonary stenosis because the hypoplastic native right ventricle outflow becomes the pulmonary outflow tract after the arterial switch operation [178–180]. Other causes of late reoperation are aortic valve regurgitation [181], aortic arch obstruction [177], and coronary obstruction [174].

DORV with Subpulmonary VSD and Pulmonary Stenosis

The arterial switch with VSD closure to the neoaorta, as described above, is contraindicated in patients with DORV, subpulmonary VSD, and pulmonary stenosis because this approach would create stenosis of the neoaortic valve. Three surgical techniques, therefore, have been developed over the last three decades to address this challenging and rare anatomical situation. One approach is the Rastelli procedure that consists of VSD closure to the aorta with placement of a right ventricular-to-pulmonary artery conduit (see Chapter 26, *Transposition of the Great Arteries*). The long-term results of the Rastelli procedure are not optimal, with a 20-year survival of only 52%. This probably relates to the intrinsic long-term liabilities of the anteriorly located right ventricular-to-pulmonary artery conduit, itself [161,162]. Lecompte introduced REV procedure in 1982 as an alternative to and an improvement of the Rastelli procedure by reconstructing the pulmonary outflow tract without having to use a right ventricular-to-pulmonary artery conduit [41,163–167]. His original operation has been modified by others to include harvesting the intact pulmonary root, rather than simply transecting the main pulmonary artery, to promote improved competency of the neopulmonary root [168,169]. Finally, Nikaidoh proposed a complex, aortic translocation and biventricular outflow tract reconstruction that creates more anatomically aligned left and right ventricular outflow tracts than either the Rastelli or the REV procedures [170]. His original procedure has been modified by other authors [169,171,172].

Techniques of the REV Procedure

(See Chapter 26, *Transposition of the Great Arteries*.) The initial stages of the REV procedure are the same as those used for the arterial switch procedure. The pulmonary arteries are dissected as far peripherally as possible. The aorta is completely freed from the pulmonary artery and from its pericardial attachments. After arresting the heart, the inferior portion of a vertical right ventriculotomy is performed, and this incision is carried superiorly, under direct vision, as close to the aortic valve as possible. The decision to perform the Lecompte maneuver should be made at the beginning of the operation. When the aortic and pulmonary arteries are side-by-side or when the aorta is slightly anterior to the pulmonary artery, it may not be necessary to perform this maneuver and, therefore, it is not necessary to transect the aorta. When the decision to perform the Lecompte maneuver has been made, the aorta is transected several millimeters above the aortic valve commissures. The intact pulmonary root is dissected and detached from its right ventricular attachments, using low-energy electrocautery, being careful to avoid injury to any adjacent coronary arteries. The infundibular (conal) septum, located between the two semilunar valves, is aggressively resected if its presence interferes with the construction of a tunnel from the VSD to the aorta. When the aorta is posterior and to the right of the pulmonary artery, the infundibular septum does not always interfere with the construction of the tunnel and may form its anterior wall. When the great arteries are in an anterior-posterior relationship, the infundibular septum typically is interposed between the VSD and the aorta and requires resection. Lecompte recommends inserting a dilator through the pulmonary artery into the left ventricle. This maneuver exposes the infundibular septum and protects the mitral valve apparatus during the infundibular resection. The infundibular septum is resected by making two vertical incisions parallel to the axis of the aorta. A third incision is made just beneath the aortic valve, joining each of the previous two incisions. Great care is taken to avoid injury to the aortic valve leaflets. When there are abnormal attachments of the tensor apparatus of the tricuspid valve to the infundibular septum, the latter can be reflected anteriorly, rather than resected, leaving these attachments intact. The VSD is then tunneled to the aorta, and the infundibular septal flap, with the attached tricuspid chordal attachments, is secured to the right ventricular surface of the patch. The main pulmonary artery and its confluence are translocated anterior to the previously transected aorta and the aorta is reconstructed (if the Lecompte maneuver was performed). If there is subpulmonary stenosis in the face of a nonobstructed pulmonary valve and main pulmonary artery, the posterior segment of the pulmonary annulus is anastomosed to the superior margin of the right ventriculotomy incision and the RVOT is reconstructed with a simple patch. If, on the other hand, the pulmonary valve and main pulmonary artery are obstructed, the posterior segment of the anteriorly opened pulmonary annulus is anastomosed to the superior margin of the right ventriculotomy incision. The RVOT can be reconstructed with a single-valved bovine jugular vein patch or an extemporaneous monocusp Gore-Tex or pericardial valve [41], placing the valve at the level of the native pulmonary valve leaflets, to help maintain a competent neopulmonary valve.

Technique of the Nikaidoh Procedure

The inspiration for the Nikaidoh procedure [170] was derived from the aortoventriculoplasty of the Konno [182] procedure and the aortic translocation procedure described by Bex and his colleagues [183] for the treatment of TGA with intact ventricular septum. As originally described, the Nikaidoh procedure consists of harvesting the aortic root from the right ventricle (with attached coronary arteries), relieving the LVOTO by dividing the outlet septum and excising the pulmonary valve, reconstructing the left ventricular outflow tract by closing the VSD and posteriorly translocating the aortic root, and reconstructing the right ventricular outflow tract with a pericardial patch [170]. More recently, however, important modifications have been reported by Hu *et al.* [169,171] and Morell and colleagues (Figure 25.19) [169,172]. The ascending aorta is divided just above its sinotubular junction. One or both coronary arteries are detached and mobilized in selected cases by Hu *et al.* [169,171] and both are routinely detached and mobilized by Morell and colleagues [172]. The aortic root is excised from the ventricle. The pulmonary root, itself, along with its semilunar valve, is also excised (when

it is no more than moderately stenotic) [169,171]. When the pulmonary root is more severely stenotic this modification can not be used and the pulmonary valve is simply excised in situ, the main pulmonary artery having been divided at its sinotubular junction [172]. The pulmonary annulus and underlying conal septum are divided to relieve the subvalvar pulmonary stenosis. A patch is used to close the VSD. The detached aortic root is translocated posteriorly to the position of the original pulmonary trunk and the coronary arteries are reimplanted. After performing the Lecompte maneuver, aortic continuity is reestablished. When the stenosis of the pulmonary root is no more than moderate, the detached pulmonary root, with its semilunar valve, is then translocated anteriorly and its posterior hemi-circumference is sutured to the RVOT. The anterior wall of the pulmonary root is incised and a single-valved bovine jugular vein patch or an extemporaneous monocusp Gore-Tex or pericardial valve is used to enlarge the RVOT, thereby still maintaining growth potential and pulmonary valve competence [169,171]. When the pulmonary root is more severely stenotic, pulmonary insufficiency can be minimized by reconstructing the RVOT with a pulmonary homograft [172]. The advantage of these modifications reported by Hu *et al.* [169,171] and Morrel and colleagues [172] is that they afford greater mobility of the aortic root for its posterior translocation because it is not tethered by one or both attached coronary arteries that may limit its mobility. This may reduce the possibility of producing coronary insufficiency during the posterior aortic translocation [172]. These modifications may also allow the Nikaidoh procedure to be used in the situation in which there is unusual and difficult coronary artery anatomy. Finally, as opposed to the original technique reported by Nikaidoh [170], these modifications reduce pulmonary insufficiency and, in the case of the Hu modification [169,171], allow for the possibility RVOT growth.

Results of the Rastelli, REV, and Nikaidoh Procedures

In general, larger series of the Rastelli, REV, and Nikaidoh procedures are not simply limited to patients with DORV, subpulmonary VSD, and pulmonary stenosis. Therefore, the results of the application of these three techniques to this particular anatomical substrate are not known with precision. In the Rastelli series from Boston Children's Hospital [161], the overall mortality was 7%, the freedom from reintervention for right-sided obstruction was 21% at 15 years, and there was a 10% incidence of LVOTO. The overall freedom from death or transplantation at 20 years was 52%. The Mayo clinic reported a similar experience [162] with a 59% survival at 20 years. For the REV procedure, the hospital mortality was 18% in an older series of 50 patients with anomalies of ventriculoarterial connection and VSD [166]. As usual, this series was not limited only to patients with DORV. The postoperative functional status

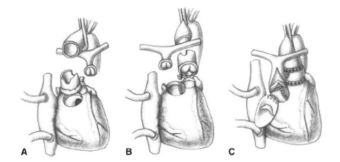

Figure 25.19 Double root translocation technique. **A,** Aortic and pulmonary root manipulation. Both the aortic and the pulmonary root are mobilized and excised. The ascending aorta is transected and the coronary arteries are detatched from the aortic sinus. **B,** Lecompte maneuver is performed in most cases. **C,** Restoration of left ventricle-aorta and right ventricle-pulmonary artery continuity. A single-valved bovine jugular vein patch was used to repair right ventricular outflow tract and enlarge the stenotic main pulmonary artery. (Reproduced with permission from Hu *et al.* [169].)

of this heterogeneous group of patients was excellent, and the left ventricular shortening fraction was normal at a mean follow-up time of 20 months. Assessment of right ventricular size and function was difficult to interpret owing to the lack of standard normal values for these variables in the presence of pulmonary insufficiency; however, the right ventricular size and contractility were considered normal in 83% of the 29 patients whose follow-up interval exceeded 1 year [166]. Despite its surgical complexity, reported results for the Nikaidoh procedure have been excellent with a 0% [169], 5% [184], and 8.3% [172] hospital mortality. In the largest reported series of Nikaidoh, himself, the median survival was 13.6 years (longest 23.0 years) in 19 patients [184]. Seven right ventricular outflow tract reoperations were required in five patients. No reoperations have been required on the LVOT or aortic valve.

When considering familiarity, applicability, and technical ease, the Rastelli procedure appears to be the "gold standard" for patients with DORV, subpulmonary VSD, and pulmonary stenosis. However, the Rastelli procedure stands alone when compared to the REV and Nikaidoh procedures, in producing an "ectopic" RVOT prone to sternal compression. Hu and his colleagues have also shown that both the Rastelli and the REV procedures share the same liability of producing a less anatomical and less laminar LVOT [169]. Though the Nikaidoh procedure is not guilty of producing either an "ectopic" and "vulnerable" RVOT or a long and tortuous LVOT, it is, by far, the most technically complex of the three procedures by virtue of its root translocation(s) and its potential for ischemic complications. Certainly, one could make a convincing argument for performing the Nikaidoh procedure in patients with inadequate anatomy for performing either a Rastelli or REV operation. Such relative contraindications might include coronary artery anomalies that interfere with a vertical right ventriculotomy incision, the presence of an inlet VSD, straddling atrioventricular valve or right ventricular hypoplasia. The argument for the Nikaidoh procedure is strengthened by the fact that it produces a more anatomical LVOT and RVOT than the Rastelli or REV procedures. Despite its theoretical advantages, caution should be exercised in strongly recommending the Nikaidoh procedure for DORV, subpulmonary VSD, and pulmonary stenosis since, of the cases reported in the literature, it has probably been used in fewer than seven patients worldwide [169, 184,185] with this anatomical substrate. Thus the ideal procedure for DORV/subpulmonary VSD/pulmonary stenosis, whether the Rastelli, REV or Nikaidoh procedures, remains elusive and requires further analysis.

DORV, Remote VSD Type

The goals of the two-ventricle repair of DORV with remote VSD with or without RVOTO is to construct an optimal intracardiac tunnel between the VSD and either one of the two arterial valves. The ideal tunnel should be as short as possible to avoid a long, noncontractile area on the surface of the interventricular septum. The tunnel should also be nonobstructive and avoid interfering with the tricuspid valve apparatus. Two-ventricle repair is best performed in early infancy rather than the neonatal period. Initial palliation with a systemic-to-pulmonary artery shunt or a pulmonary artery band may, therefore, be required.

Two-Ventricle Repair of DORV, Remote VSD Type (Without RVOTO)

There are two two-ventricle repair techniques to consider in patients with DORV, remote VSD without RVOTO: 1) intraventricular tunnel repair to the aorta; and 2) arterial switch with intraventricular tunnel to the pulmonary artery. The ability to perform the intraventricular tunnel repair to the aorta depends on the presence of an adequate distance between the tricuspid valve and the pulmonary valve as well as the ability to negotiate around the tricuspid subvalvar apparatus [78,79]. Tunnel repair to the aorta may require resection of the parietal band, reimplantation of the conal tricuspid papillary muscle on the tunnel patch, VSD enlargement superiorly/anteriorly, and resection of the subaortic conus [78,79,82]. If, for anatomical reasons, the VSD cannot be thus tunneled to the aorta, an arterial switch with tunneling of the VSD to the pulmonary artery may be preferable (Figures 25.20 and 25.21) [78,79]. This approach frequently results in the creation of a shorter tunnel and may result in less interference with the subvalvar apparatus of the tricuspid valve. The Lecompte maneuver is optional depending on the great vessel relationships. Surgical series of DORV with remote VSD are generally small [4,62,79,81–83] but the results have been improving over time with hospital mortality rates as low as 6.6% [77–79,82]. Longer-term results are needed to compare mortality, reintervention, exercise tolerance, and quality of life to other surgical approaches such as single-ventricle palliation.

Two-Ventricle Repair of DORV, Remote VSD Type (with RVOTO)

The RVOTO can be valvar, subvalvar or pulmonary atresia. If there is an isolated, muscular, subvalvar RVOT obstruction, then an intraventricular tunnel repair or an arterial switch with VSD closure (as described above) may be supplemented with a right ventricular infundibular patch augmentation to successfully repair the defect. When the RVOT obstruction is valvar and the VSD can be tunneled to the aorta, the pulmonary outflow tract is closed and a Rastelli-type or, preferably, an REV-type procedure is performed [166–169,186,187]. Hu and colleagues have recently reported no hospital deaths or reinterventions after a 22-month mean follow-up of six patients with DORV, remote VSD, and RVOTO treated with their modification

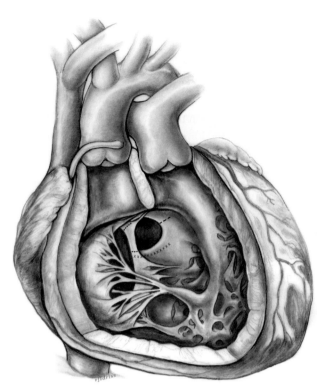

Figure 25.20 Intraventricular tunnel repair of double-outlet right ventricle, remote ventricular septal defect (VSD) type. The presence of tensor apparatus of the tricuspid valve makes the construction of a tunnel from the VSD to the aorta impossible. The VSD is enlarged superiorly when restrictive (anterosuperior dashed line). The VSD is tunneled to the pulmonary artery. Notice that the distance from the VSD to the infundibular ostium is relatively short. The intracardiac tunneling of the VSD to the pulmonary artery is followed by an arterial switch operation. The tricuspid valve and infundibular septum are spared.

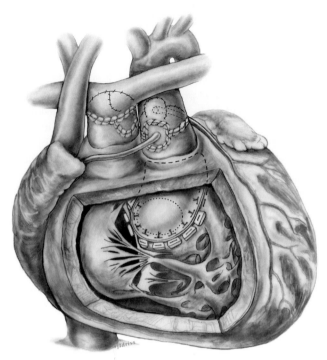

Figure 25.21 Intraventricular tunnel repair of double-outlet right ventricle, remote ventricular septal defect type. The left ventricle is tunneled to the pulmonary artery (neoaorta), which is depicted after completion of an arterial switch operation with a Lecompte maneuver.

of the Nikaidoh procedure adapted to address the anatomy of DORV, remote VSD [185]. This approach has yet to be substantiated by long-term results.

Single Ventricle Repair of DORV, Remote VSD Type (with or Without RVOTO)

Single ventricle palliation must be performed when neither of the two-ventricle repairs described above is feasible. This is especially true when there is significant ventricular hypoplasia, severe atrioventricular valve straddling or overriding and/or Swiss-cheese VSD. Significant cyanosis or pulmonary overcirculation is initially palliated with a systemic-to-pulmonary artery shunt or pulmonary artery band, respectively, until 6 months of age when a bidirectional cavopulmonary connection is performed. Palliation is completed with a total cavopulmonary connection procedure at 1.5–2 years of age. If tunnel closure of the VSD produces a critical reduction of the right ventricular

volume, a one and one-half ventricle repair can substitute for a Fontan procedure although some authors [188] have suggested that a total cavopulmonary connection is a superior surgical remedy. Late restriction of the VSD can occur after Fontan palliation in patients with DORV and remote VSD [189,190], leading to left ventricular exclusion and hypertension. Enlargement of a restrictive or borderline VSD at the time of Fontan palliation is, therefore, recommended [79,85,134,190,191].

DORV with AVSD

Two-Ventricle Repair of DORV with AVSD

This especially complex subset of DORV patients is frequently associated with the heterotaxy syndrome, most frequently a right isomerism with asplenia and abnormal systemic venous connections. These patients usually present with RVOTO (pulmonary stenosis to atresia), TAPVC, and frequent intestinal malrotation requiring a Ladd procedure. Compared with AVSD associated with tetralogy of Fallot, where Down syndrome is frequently associated, the patients with DORV-AVSD generally have a normal genotype [192]. The AVSD anatomy is typically Rastelli type C and the VSD is similar to the one found in tetralogy of Fallot-AVSD, with a large superior component extending close to the aortic valve annulus [23,84]. The distance from the superior edge of the subaortic component of the VSD to the aortic annulus varies but, in many instances, this distance is less than the diameter of the aortic annulus [131]; thus the term "noncommitted VSD" remains controversial to describe this subset of DORV.

Complete repair is performed after 6 months of age; therefore, in the presence of severe cyanosis a palliative systemic-to-pulmonary artery shunt is performed. Emergent repair of obstructed TAPVC is undertaken simultaneously with the performance of the systemic-to-pulmonary artery shunt. At the time of complete repair, incising the anterior bridging leaflet of the common atrioventricular valve enhances exposure of the aortic valve. Tunnel closure of the VSD is accomplished through a right atriotomy and ventriculotomy using a patch with a large anterior–superior extension. Postoperative pulmonary valve competence is desirable necessitating the placement of a right ventricular-to-pulmonary artery conduit when the intraventricular tunnel obstructs the RVOT. If the intraventricular tunnel causes a significant reduction in the right ventricular volume, a one and one-half ventricle repair can be performed.

Despite the technical complexity of performing a two-ventricle repair in DORV-AVSD, some groups advocate a two-ventricle repair based on superb early and intermediate-term results performing a complete repair in the majority of patients who present with DORV-AVSD [85,120,192].

Complex DORV with Straddling Atrioventricular Valves

Some authors [193] have documented better survival after Fontan palliation in patients with various complex forms of DORV including patients with straddling atrioventricular valves. Others [117] have successfully performed biventricular repairs in this high-risk group of patients.

Late Sudden Death in Survivors of Repair of DORV

It is interesting to note that Shen and his colleagues [194] found an 18% incidence of late sudden death when they analyzed 89 survivors of repair of DORV. Cox proportional hazards multivariate analysis demonstrated that older age at the time of operation, perioperative or postoperative ventricular tachyarrhythmias, and third-degree atrioventricular block were significant risk factors for late sudden death. This high incidence of late sudden death has not been reported in more recent surgical series of DORV.

DOUBLE-OUTLET LEFT VENTRICLE

Introduction

Double-outlet left ventricle (DOLV) is a rare congenital cardiac malformation of ventriculoarterial connection in which both great arteries arise wholly or in large part from the morphologic left ventricle [195–197].

History

In 1967, Sakakibara *et al.* [198] reported the first successful intraventricular repair of DOLV in a patient with two adequately sized ventricles. The wide morphologic variations of this disorder were established in subsequent case reports [72,194,199–201]. Kerr *et al.* [200] and Pacifico and colleagues [195] described the complete repair of DOLV with pulmonary stenosis using a valved extracardiac conduit to establish continuity between the right ventricle and the pulmonary artery. Sharratt *et al.* [202], in 1976, first reported the use of the Fontan procedure to correct DOLV with right ventricular hypoplasia.

Embryology

At one time it was thought that DOLV was an embryologic impossibility [37,203]. Goor and colleagues [203], however, demonstrated that a process of differential conal absorption draws the aorta over the cavity of the left ventricle. If this absorptive process continues, both coni are absorbed above the primitive ventricle. As a result, the pulmonary artery and aorta are drawn over the morphologic left ventricle to produce DOLV [203].

Morphology

General

Because of the great morphologic variability of DOLV, it is necessary to examine the segmental anatomy of each patient to understand the defect and to determine the optimal surgical approach [196]. Although DOLV occurs most commonly in the presence of atrial situs solitus with atrioventricular concordance, it has been described with situs inversus and/or atrioventricular discordance. The position of the aorta relative to the pulmonary artery can be to the right and posterior (normal), to the right and side-by-side, to the right and anterior (D-malposition) and to the left (L-malposition) [72,195,196,204].

Ventricular Septal Defect

Rarely, the interventricular septum is intact [196,199]. As with DORV, the VSDs of hearts with DOLV are conoventricular lesions that can be classified according to their relationship to the great arteries. In the series by Bharati *et al.* [196] of 45 cases 71% of the VSDs were subaortic, 18% were subpulmonic, 9% were doubly committed, and 2% were noncommitted. The subaortic VSD of DOLV can extend to the tricuspid annulus or be separated from it by a band of muscle, similar to hearts with DORV. When the VSD is juxtaaortic, the aorta can override the interventricular septum to a variable degree, and the lesion must be differentiated from TGA and VSD. When the VSD is doubly committed it is, by definition, juxtaarterial. In this case because both great arteries form the superior border of the defect and override the interventricular septum to a variable degree, it is often difficult to determine whether the heart lesion is DOLV or DORV. Brandt *et al.* [72] has called this *variant double-outlet both ventricles.*

Subaortic and Subpulmonary Coni

There is usually aortic-mitral continuity because of the absence of a subaortic conus. A subpulmonary conus is frequently present; however, when the subpulmonary conus is absent there is pulmonary-tricuspid continuity. Rarely, bilateral coni are present.

Associated Cardiac Lesions

Pulmonary stenosis affects the majority of patients with DOLV and can occur at the valvar and subvalvar levels. In the series by Bharati *et al.* [196], 38% of patients with DOLV had tricuspid valve and right ventricular hypoplasia. Tricuspid atresia [196,205], Ebstein anomaly [72], and mitral atresia [205] have also been associated with this disorder.

The Conduction System

The atrioventricular node and bundle of His are normally positioned in DOLV. When the VSD is juxtatricuspid, the bundle runs along its inferoposterior free edge and is at risk for injury during repair. When there is a band of muscle between the defect and the tricuspid valve annulus, the conduction tissue does not run along the free edge of the VSD. This relationship of the VSD to the conduction tissue is identical to that of DORV.

Pathophysiology

The clinical presentation of patients with DOLV is largely determined by the presence or absence of pulmonary stenosis. Since pulmonary stenosis is present in 85% of patients with DOLV, most patients present with varying degrees of cyanosis. Cyanosis can also be produced by the streaming of desaturated right ventricular blood into the aorta

through a subaortic VSD. When pulmonary stenosis is not present, the patient may present with congestive heart failure and, later in life, develop fixed pulmonary hypertension owing to pulmonary vascular disease.

Diagnosis

Biplane cineangiography with left and right ventricular injections profiling the septum will demonstrate the origin of both great vessels from the left ventricle, the position and number of VSDs, the presence and location of pulmonary stenosis, and the size and adequacy of the tricuspid valve and right ventricle (Figure 25.22) [72].

Natural History

When pulmonary stenosis coexists with DOLV, the natural history is similar to that of tetralogy of Fallot. In the absence of pulmonary stenosis, the natural history is similar to that of an isolated, large VSD except the VSD in DOLV does not have a tendency to close over time.

Treatment

General

The principles of cardiopulmonary bypass, myocardial protection, and avoidance of the conduction tissue are the same for hearts with DOLV as described for those with DORV. In general, a complete repair should be undertaken in early infancy if this can be accomplished. When an extracardiac conduit is to be employed, repair can be delayed until a later age when a larger conduit can be placed; however, there is no consensus regarding this point. As a general rule the use of palliative procedures, systemic to pulmonary artery shunts and pulmonary artery bands, should be minimized. Sparse follow-up data relating to the results of surgical repair in the current era are available for this rare entity.

DOLV with Pulmonary Stenosis

Complete Intraventricular Repair
When the pulmonary annulus is not obstructive and when the subpulmonary obstruction is localized, a completely intraventricular repair may be possible [198,206]. The subpulmonary obstruction is resected through the tricuspid valve, the pulmonary valve, and/or a right ventriculotomy. The VSD is tunneled to the pulmonary artery through a right ventriculotomy.

Pulmonary Artery Translocation
Usually, a completely intraventricular repair is not possible because the subpulmonary obstruction is long and

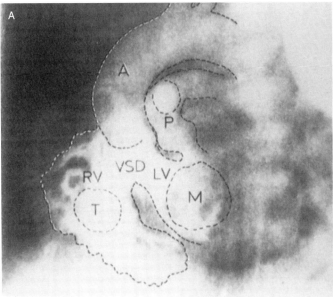 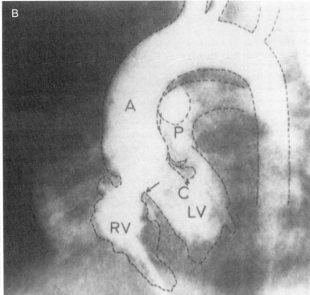

Figure 25.22 Cineangiogram of a patient with double-outlet left ventricle (DOLV). **A,** The right ventricular injection with left anterior oblique view demonstrates flow of contrast medium from the right ventricle, through the VSD into the left ventricle. The opacified aorta and pulmonary artery clearly arise from the left ventricle. **B,** The systolic frame of the same right ventricular injection demonstrates the subaortic VSD. The larger arrow demonstrates the inferior margin of the VSD and clearly shows that the entire aorta, except for the rightward anterior sinus, arises from the left ventricle. (A, aorta; LV, left ventricle; M, mitral valve; P, pulmonary artery; RV, right ventricle; T, tricuspid valve; VSD, ventricular septal defect.) (Adapted with permission from Brandt *et al.* [72].)

narrow. It is not possible to place a transannular patch because the left anterior descending coronary artery runs immediately inferior to the pulmonary valve ring. In this situation, when the pulmonary valve annulus and pulmonary valve are normal or near normal, a repair can be accomplished using pulmonary artery translocation (Figure 25.23) [60,206–208]. The right ventricle is opened with a vertical right ventriculotomy. The subpulmonary stenosis is closed through the VSD (Figure 25.23A) [60], and the VSD is closed with a simple patch (Figure 25.23B) [60]. The pulmonary artery trunk, with its intact valve, is removed from the base of the left ventricle, being careful to avoid injury to the adjacent left coronary artery branches (Figure 25.23B) [60]. The pulmonary outflow tract is then closed from the outside of the left ventricle. The intact pulmonary trunk is translocated anteriorly, and its posterior circumference is sutured to the superior aspect of the vertical right ventriculotomy (Figure 25.23C) [60]. The remainder of the right ventricle-to-pulmonary artery connection is completed with autologous pericardium (Figure 25.23D) [60]. This procedure has been reported in a 4-month-old patient [207]. There was a moderate right ventricular outflow tract gradient 14 days postoperatively, and there are no long-term follow-up data published to date.

REV Procedure

When, as is most common, a long and narrow subpulmonary obstruction is associated with a small and obstructive pulmonary annulus, the REV procedure may be used for repair (see Chapter 26, *Transposition of the Great Arteries*) [41,163–167]. While this does not involve translocation of the native pulmonary valve, it does provide an unobstructed repair without the need for an extracardiac conduit. The resultant pulmonary insufficiency should be well tolerated.

Rastelli Procedure

Alternatively, repair can be undertaken with a valved extracardiac conduit. Through a right ventriculotomy, the subpulmonary stenosis is viewed through the VSD and closed with pledgeted, horizontal mattress sutures. The VSD is patched and a valved, homograft extracardiac conduit is sutured to the pulmonary artery distally and then to the right ventriculotomy proximally.

DOLV Without Pulmonary Stenosis

In some cases an entirely intraventricular repair can be performed, as described above [182]. When this is not possible, repair with a valved extracardiac conduit is

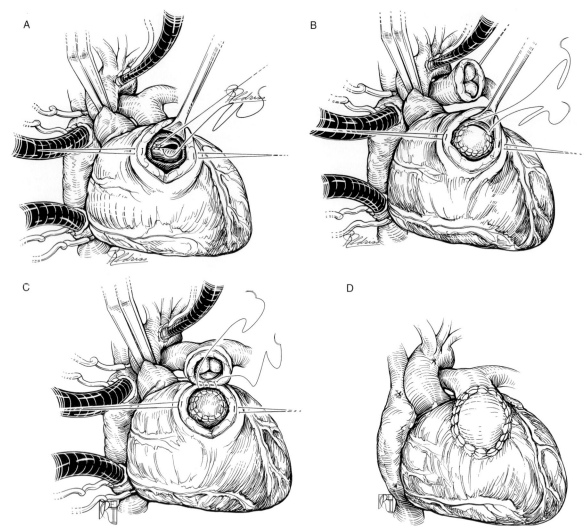

Figure 25.23 Pulmonary artery translocation for repair of double-outlet left ventricle (DOLV). **A,** The repair is performed through a vertical right ventriculotomy. The subpulmonary area is closed through the ventricular septal defect. **B,** The pulmonary artery trunk, with its intact valve, is removed from the base of the left ventricle. Care is taken to avoid injury to the adjacent coronary arteries. The ventricular septal defect is patched. **C,** The pulmonary trunk is translocated anteriorly, and its posterior circumference is sutured to the superior aspect of the right ventriculotomy. **D,** The connection of the right ventricle to the pulmonary artery is completed with an autologous pericardial patch.

recommended. It may be possible, under certain circumstances, to close the VSD so that the right ventricle ejects into the aorta. Ventriculoarterial concordance is restored with an arterial switch procedure. While the REV procedure theoretically could be employed in this situation, it is not recommended in patients without preoperative pulmonary stenosis. The postoperative pulmonary insufficiency is generally not well tolerated in such patients.

DOLV with Tricuspid and Right Ventricular Hypoplasia

When a two-ventricle repair cannot be performed, a bidirectional cavopulmonary anastomosis is performed at 6 months of age. This is followed by a total cavopulmonary connection at 1–2 years of age. Depending on the presence or absence of pulmonary stenosis, a systemic to pulmonary artery shunt or a pulmonary artery banding may have to be performed in early infancy as a brief prelude to the eventual two-staged Fontan procedures.

References

1. Lev M, Bharati S, Meng CC, *et al.* (1972) A concept of double-outlet right ventricle. J Thorac Cardiovasc Surg 64, 271–281.
2. Tynan MJ, Becker AE, Macartney FJ, *et al.* (1979) Nomenclature and classification of congenital heart disease. Br Heart J 41, 544–553.

3. Piccoli G, Pacifico AD, Kirklin JW, *et al.* (1983) Changing results and concepts in the surgical treatment of double-outlet right ventricle: analysis of 137 operations in 126 patients. Am J Cardiol 52, 549–554.

4. Kirklin JW, Pacifico AD, Blackstone EH, *et al.* (1986) Current risks and protocols for operations for double-outlet right ventricle. Derivation from an 18 year experience. J Thorac Cardiovasc Surg 92, 913–930.

5. Tabry IF, McGoon DC, Danielson GK, *et al.* (1978) Surgical management of double-outlet right ventricle associated with atrioventricular discordance. J Thorac Cardiovasc Surg 76, 336–344.

6. Kirklin JW, Barratt-Boyes BG. (1993) *Cardiac Surgery*, 2nd ed. Edinburgh: Churchill Livingstone, pp. 1469–1500.

7. Taussig HB, Bing RJ. (1949) Complete transposition of the aorta and a levoposition of the pulmonary artery; clinical, physiological, and pathological findings. Am Heart J 37, 551–559.

8. Van Praagh R. (1968) What is the Taussig-Bing malformation? Circulation 38, 445–449.

9. Baron MG. (1971) Radiologic notes in cardiology. Angiographic differentiation between tetralogy of Fallot and double-outlet right ventricle. Relationship of the mitral and aortic valves. Circulation 43, 451–455.

10. Hallermann FJ, Kincaid OW, Ritter DG, *et al.* (1970) Mitral-semilunar valve relationships in the angiography of cardiac malformations. Radiology 94, 63–68.

11. Howell CE, Ho SY, Anderson RH, *et al.* (1991) Fibrous skeleton and ventricular outflow tracts in double-outlet right ventricle. Ann Thorac Surg 51, 394–400.

12. Peacock TB. (1866) *Malformations of the Human Heart*, 2nd ed. London: J. Churchill and Sons.

13. Rokitansky K. (1875) *Die Defecte der Scheidewande des Herzens: Pathologisch-anatomische Abhandlung*. Wein: Wilhelm Braumuller.

14. Braun K, De Vries A, Feingold DS, *et al.* (1952) Complete dextroposition of the aorta, pulmonary stenosis, interventricular septal defect, and patent foramen ovale. Am Heart J 43, 773–780.

15. Kirklin JW, Harp RA, McGoon DC. (1964) Surgical treatment of origin of both vessels from right ventricle, including cases of pulmonary stenosis. J Thorac Cardiovasc Surg 48, 1026–1036.

16. Witham AC. (1957) Double outlet right ventricle; a partial transposition complex. Am Heart J 53, 928–939.

17. Engle MA, Holswade GR, Campbell WG, *et al.* (1960) Ventricular septal defect with transposition of aorta masquerading as a cyanotic ventricular septal defect. Circulation 22, 745 (abst).

18. Engle MA, Steinberg I. (1961) Angiocardiography in diagnosis of transposition of aorta with subaortic ventricular septal defect (origin of both great vessels from right ventricle). Circulation 24, 927 (abst).

19. Neufeld HN, Dushane JW, Edwards JE. (1961) Origin of both great vessels from the right ventricle. II. With pulmonary stenosis. Circulation 23, 603–612.

20. Neufeld HN, Lucas RV, Jr, Lester RG, *et al.* (1962) Origin of both great vessels from the right ventricle without pulmonary stenosis. Br Heart J 24, 393–408.

21. Neufeld HN, Dushane JW, Wood EH, *et al.* (1961) Origin of both great vessels from the right ventricle. I. Without pulmonary stenosis. Circulation 23, 399–412.

22. Angelini P, Leachman RD. (1976) The spectrum of double outlet right ventricle: an embryologic interpretation. Cardiovasc Dis 3, 127–149.

23. Wilcox BR, Ho SY, Macartney FJ, *et al.* (1981) Surgical anatomy of double-outlet right ventricle with situs solitus and atrioventricular concordance. J Thorac Cardiovasc Surg 82, 405–417.

24. Anderson RH, Becker AE, Wilcox BR, *et al.* (1983) Surgical anatomy of double-outlet right ventricle–a reappraisal. Am J Cardiol 52, 555–559.

25. Pernkopf E. (1926) Der partielle situs inversus der eingeweide beim menschen. Ztschr f Anat u Entwckingsgesch 79, 557 (Cited by Taussig HB, Bing RJ. (1949) Am Heart J 37, 551).

26. De Azevedo AC, Toledo AN, De Carvalho AA, *et al.* (1956) Transposition of the aorta and levoposition of the pulmonary artery (Taussig-Bing syndrome). Am Heart J 52, 249–256.

27. Beuren A. (1960) Differential diagnosis of the Taussig-Bing heart from complete transposition of the great vessels with a posteriorly overriding pulmonary artery. Circulation 21, 1071–1087.

28. Daicoff GR, Kirklin JW. (1967) Surgical correction of Taussig-Bing malformation. Report of three cases. Am J Cardiol 19, 125 (abst).

29. Hightower BM, Barcia A, Bargeron LM Jr, *et al.* (1969) Double-outlet right ventricle with transposed great arteries and subpulmonary ventricular septal defect: the Taussig-Bing malformation (abstr). Circulation 39 (suppl I), I207.

30. Patrick DL, McGoon DC. (1968) An operation for double-outlet right ventricle with transposition of the great arteries. J Cardiovasc Surg (Torino) 9, 537–542.

31. Kawashima Y, Fujita T, Miyamoto T, *et al.* (1971) Intraventricular rerouting of blood for the correction of Taussig-Bing malformation. J Thorac Cardiovasc Surg 62, 825–829.

32. Anderson RH. (1978) The morphogenesis of ventriculoarterial discordance. In: Van mierop LHS, Oppenheimer-Dekker A, Bruins CLD, eds. *Embryology and Tetralogy of the Heart and Great Arteries*. The Hague, The Netherlands: Leiden University Press.

33. Anderson RH, Wilkinson JL, Arnold R, *et al.* (1974) Morphogenesis of bulboventricular malformations. II. Observations on malformed hearts. Br Heart J 36, 948–970.

34. Goor DA, Lillehei CW. (1975) *Congenital Malformations of the Heart*. New York: Grune & Stratton.

35. Okamoto N. (1980) *Congenital Anomalies of the Heart. Embryologic, Morphologic and Experimental Teratology*. Tokyo: Igaku-Shoin.

36. van Praagh R. (1973) Conotruncal malformations. In: Barratt-Boyes BG, Neutze JM, Harris EA, eds. *Heart Disease in Infancy*. Edinburgh: Churchill Livingstone.

37. Vanmierop LH, Wiglesworth FW. (1963) Pathogenesis of transposition complexes. II. Anomalies due to faulty transfer of the posterior great artery. Am J Cardiol 12, 226–232.

38. Van Mierop LH, Gessner IH. (1972) Pathogenetic mechanisms in congenital cardiovascular malformations. Prog Cardiovasc Dis 15, 67–85.

39. Bartelings MM, Gittenberger-de Groot AC. (1989) The outflow tract of the heart–embryologic and morphologic correlations. Int J Cardiol 22, 289–300.

40. Sakata R, Lecompte Y, Batisse A, et al. (1988) Anatomic repair of anomalies of ventriculoarterial connection associated with ventricular septal defect. I. Criteria of surgical decision. J Thorac Cardiovasc Surg 95, 90–95.

41. Lecompte Y, Batisse A, DiCarlo D. (1993) Double-outlet right ventricle: A surgical synthesis. In *Advances in Cardiac Surgery*, Vol 4. St Louis: Mosby-Yearbook, Inc., pp. 109–136.

42. Sondheimer HM, Freedom RM, Olley PM. (1977) Double outlet right ventricle: clinical spectrum and prognosis. Am J Cardiol 39, 709–714.

43. Danielson GK, Tabry IF, Ritter DG, et al. (1978) Successful repair of double-outlet right ventricle, complete atrioventricular canal, and atrioventricular discordance associated with dextrocardia and pulmonary stenosis. J Thorac Cardiovasc Surg 76, 710–717.

44. Ruttenberg HD, Anderson RC, Elliott LP, et al. (1964) Origin of both great vessels from the arterial ventricle: A complex with ventricular inversion. Br Heart J 26, 631–641.

45. Alfieri O, Crupi G, Vanini V, et al. (1978) Successful surgical repair of double outlet right ventricle with situs inversus, l-loop, l-malposition and subaortic VSD in a 16-month-old patient. Eur J Cardiol 7, 41–47.

46. Edwards JE, James JW, Du SJ. (1952) Congenital malformation of the heart; origin of transposed great vessels from the right ventricle associated with atresia of the left ventricular outlet, double orifice of the mitral valve, and single coronary artery. Lab Invest 1, 197–207.

47. Lauer RM, Dushane JW, Edwards JE. (1960) Obstruction of left ventricular outlet in association with ventricular septal defect. Circulation 22, 110–125.

48. Cheng TO. (1962) Double outlet right ventricle: Diagnosis during life. Am J Med 32, 637–644.

49. Serratto M, Arevalo F, Goldman EJ, et al. (1967) Obstructive ventricular septal defect in double outlet right ventricle. Am J Cardiol 19, 457–463.

50. Mason DT, Morrow AG, Elkins RC, et al. (1969) Origin of both great vessels from the right ventricle associated with severe obstruction to left ventricular outflow. Am J Cardiol 24, 118–124.

51. Lavoie R, Sestier F, Gilbert G, et al. (1971) Double outlet right ventricle with left ventricular outflow tract obstruction due to small ventricular septal defect. Am Heart J 82, 290–299.

52. Marin-Garcia J, Neches WH, Park SC, et al. (1978) Double-outlet right ventricle with restrictive ventricular septal defect. J Thorac Cardiovasc Surg 76, 853–858.

53. Matsuoka Y, Akimoto K, Sennari E, et al. (1987) Double outlet right ventricle with severe left ventricular outflow tract obstruction due to small ventricular septal defect and anomalous adherence of the mitral valve to the ventricular septum. Jpn Circ J 51, 1335–1340.

54. McMahon JE, Lips M. (1964) Double outlet right ventricle with intact ventricular septum. Circulation 30, 745–748.

55. Ainger LE. (1965) Double-outlet right ventricle: intact ventricular septum, mitral stenosis, and blind left ventricle. Am Heart J 70, 521–525.

56. Zamora R, Moller JH, Edwards JE. (1975) Double-outlet right ventricle. Anatomic types and associated anomalies. Chest 68, 672–677.

57. Sridaromont S, Ritter DG, Feldt RH, et al. (1978) Double-outlet right ventricle. Anatomic and angiocardiographic correlations. Mayo Clin Proc 53, 555–577.

58. Pandit SP, Shah VK, Daruwala DF. (1987) Double outlet right ventricle with intact interventricular septum–a case report. Indian Heart J 39, 56–57.

59. Ikemoto Y, Nogi S, Teraguchi M, et al. (1997) Double-outlet right ventricle with intact ventricular septum. Acta Paediatr Jpn 39, 233–236.

60. Walters HL, 3rd, Pacifico AD. (2003) Double outlet ventricles. In: Mavroudis C, Backer CL, eds. *Pediatric Cardiac Surgery*, 3rd ed. Philadelphia, PA: Mosby Inc.

61. Edwards WD. (1981) Double-outlet right ventricle and tetralogy of Fallot. Two distinct but not mutually exclusive entities. J Thorac Cardiovasc Surg 82, 418–422.

62. Musumeci F, Shumway S, Lincoln C, et al. (1988) Surgical treatment for double-outlet right ventricle at the Brompton Hospital, 1973 to 1986. J Thorac Cardiovasc Surg 96, 278–287.

63. Stewart RW, Kirklin JW, Pacifico AD, et al. (1979) Repair of double-outlet right ventricle. An analysis of 62 cases. J Thorac Cardiovasc Surg 78, 502–514.

64. Danielson GK, Ritter DG, Coleman HN III, et al. (1972) Successful repair of double-outlet right ventricle with transposition of the great arteries (aorta anterior and to the left), pulmonary stenosis, and subaortic ventricular septal defect. J Thorac Cardiovasc Surg 63, 741–746.

65. Lincoln C, Anderson RH, Shinebourne EA, et al. (1975) Double outlet right ventricle with l-malposition of the aorta. Br Heart J 37, 453–463.

66. VanPraagh R, Perez-Trevino C, Reynolds JL, et al. (1975) Double outlet right ventricle (S,D,L) with subaortic ventricular septal defect and pulmonary stenosis. Report of six cases. Am J Cardiol 35, 42–53.

67. Paul MH, VanPraagh S, VanPraagh R. (1968) Transposition of the great arteries. In Watson H, ed. *Paediatric Cardiology*. London, Lloyd-Luke.

68. Blancquaert A, Defloor E, Bossaert L, et al. (1973) Double outlet right ventricle with L-malposition of the great arteries, ventricular D-loop and three fibrotic leaflets in a stenotic subpulmonary conus. Br Heart J 35, 770–773.

69. Shafer AB, Lopez JF, Kline IK, et al. (1967) Truncal inversion with biventricular pulmonary trunk and aorta from right ventricle (variant of Taussig-Bing complex). Circulation 36, 783–788.

70. Anderson RH, Pickering D, Brown R. (1975) Double outlet right ventricle with L-malposition and uncommitted ventricular septal defect. Eur J Cardiol 3, 133–142.

71. Mehrizi A. (1965) The origin of both great vessels from the right ventricle. I. With pulmonic stenosis. Clinico-

pathological correlation in 18 autopsied cases. Bull Johns Hopkins Hosp 117, 75.

72. Brandt PW, Calder AL, Barratt-Boyes BG, *et al.* (1976) Double outlet left ventricle. Morphology, cineangiocardiographic diagnosis and surgical treatment. Am J Cardiol 38, 897–909.

73. Stellin G, Zuberbuhler JR, Anderson RH, *et al.* (1987) The surgical anatomy of the Taussig-Bing malformation. J Thorac Cardiovasc Surg 93, 560–569.

74. Yacoub MH, Radley-Smith R. (1984) Anatomic correction of the Taussig-Bing anomaly. J Thorac Cardiovasc Surg 88, 380–388.

75. Thanopoulos BD, Dubrow IW, Fisher EA, *et al.* (1979) Double outlet right ventricle with subvalvular aortic stenosis. Br Heart J 41, 241–244.

76. Rudolph AM, Heymann MA, Spitznas U. (1972) Hemodynamic considerations in the development of narrowing of the aorta. Am J Cardiol 30, 514–525.

77. Belli E, Serraf A, Lacour-Gayet F, *et al.* (1998) Biventricular repair for double-outlet right ventricle. Results and long-term follow-up. Circulation 98(19 Suppl), II360–II365; discussion II365–II367.

78. Lacour-Gayet F, Haun C, Ntalakoura K, *et al.* (2002) Biventricular repair of double outlet right ventricle with non-committed ventricular septal defect (VSD) by VSD rerouting to the pulmonary artery and arterial switch. Eur J Cardiothorac Surg 21, 1042–1048.

79. Belli E, Serraf A, Lacour-Gayet F, *et al.* (1999) Double-outlet right ventricle with non-committed ventricular septal defect. Eur J Cardiothorac Surg 15, 747–752.

80. Lacour-Gayet F. (2008) Intracardiac repair of double outlet right ventricle. Semin Thorac Cardiovasc Surg Pediatr Card Surg Annu 39–43.

81. Luisi VS, Pasque A, Verunelli F, *et al.* (1980) Double outlet right ventricle, non-committed ventricular septal defect and pulmonic stenosis. Anatomical and surgical considerations. Thorac Cardiovasc Surg 28, 368–370.

82. Kirklin JK, Castaneda AR. (1977) Surgical correction of double-outlet right ventricule with noncommitted ventricular septal defect. J Thorac Cardiovasc Surg 73, 399–403.

83. Barbero-Marcial M, Tanamati C, Atik E, *et al.* (1999) Intraventricular repair of double-outlet right ventricle with noncommitted ventricular septal defect: advantages of multiple patches. J Thorac Cardiovasc Surg 118, 1056–1067.

84. Mahle WT, Martinez R, Silverman N, *et al.* (2008) Anatomy, echocardiography, and surgical approach to double outlet right ventricle. Cardiol Young 18(suppl 3), 39–51.

85. Artrip JH, Sauer H, Campbell DN, *et al.* (2006) Biventricular repair in double outlet right ventricle: surgical results based on the STS-EACTS International Nomenclature classification. Eur J Cardiothorac Surg 29, 545–550.

86. Freedom RM, Yoo SJ. (2000) Double-outlet right ventricle: Pathology and angiocardiography. Semin Thorac Cardiovasc Surg Pediatr Card Surg Annu 3, 3–19.

87. Lopez FN, Dobben GG, Rabinowitz M, *et al.* (1966) Taussig-Bing complex with pulmonary stenosis. Dis Chest 50, 1–12.

88. van Buchem FSP, van Wermeskerken Jl, Orie NG. (1950) Transposition of the aorta (Taussig's syndrome). Acta Med Scand 137, 66–77.

89. Campbell M, Suzman S. (1951) Transposition of the aorta and pulmonary artery. Circulation 4, 329–342.

90. Dubourg G, Castaing R, Bricaud H, *et al.* (1954) [Taussig–Bing syndrome; case history]. Arch Mal Coeur Vaiss 47, 75–81.

91. Bret J, Torner-Soler M. (1957) Complete transposition of the aorta; levoposition of the pulmonary artery with pulmonary stenosis; clinical and pathologic findings in three cases. Am Heart J 54, 385–395.

92. Edwards JE. (1960) Congenital malformations. In: Gould SE, ed. *Pathology of the Heart*, 2nd ed. Springfield, IL: Charles C Thomas Co.

93. Keith JD, Rowe RD, Vlad P. (1958) *Heart Disease in Infancy and Childhood*. New York: The Macmillan Co.

94. Judson JP, Danielson GK, Ritter DG, *et al.* (1982) Successful repair of coexisting double-outlet right ventricle and two-chambered right ventricle. J Thorac Cardiovasc Surg 84, 113–121.

95. Hindle WV Jr, Engle MA, Hagstrom JW. (1968) Anomalous right ventricular muscles: a clinicopathologic study. Am J Cardiol 21, 487–495.

96. Collan Y, Pesonen E. (1977) Double outlet right ventricle with extreme hypertrophy of muscle bundles associated with crista supraventricularis. A heart with three ventricles. Helv Paediatr Acta 31, 521–526.

97. Beitzke A, Anderson RH, Wilkinson JL, *et al.* (1979) Two-chambered right ventricle: simulating two-chambered left ventricle. Br Heart J 42, 22–26.

98. Van Praagh S, La Corte M, Fellows KE, *et al.* (1980) Supero-inferior ventricles: anatomic and angiographic findings in ten postmortem cases. In: van Praagh R, Takao A, eds. *Etiology and Morphogenesis of Congenital Heart Disease*. Mount Kisco, NY: Futura, pp. 317–378.

99. Freedom RM, Culham JAG, Moes CAF. (1984) *MacMillan Angiocardiography of Congenital Heart Disease*. New York: MacMillan.

100. Goor DA, Ebert PA. (1975) Left ventricular outflow obstruction in Taussig-Bing malformation. J Thorac Cardiovasc Surg 70, 69–75.

101. Pellegrino PA, Eckner FA, Meier MA, *et al.* (1973) Double outlet right ventricle with fibro-muscular obstruction to left ventricular outlet. J Cardiovasc Surg (Torino) 14, 253–260.

102. Golan M, Hegesh J, Massini C, *et al.* (1984) Double-outlet right ventricle associated with discrete subaortic stenosis. Pediatr Cardiol 5, 157–158.

103. Toews WH, Lortscher RH, Kelminson LL. (1975) Double outlet right ventricle with absent aortic valve. Chest 68, 381–382.

104. Lev M, Bharati S. (1975) Transposition of the arterial trunks in levocardia. In: Sommers SC, ed. *Cardiovascular Pathology Decennial 1966–1975*. Norwalk, CT: Appleton & Lange, p. 30.

105. Gittenberger-de Groot AC, Sauer U, Oppenheimer-Dekker A, *et al.* (1983) Coronary arterial anatomy in transposition of the great arteries: a morphologic study. Pediatr Cardiol 4(suppl I), 15–24.

106. Vlodaver Z, Neufeld HN, Edwards JE. (1975) *Coronary Arterial Variations in the Normal Heart and in Congenital Heart Disease.* New York: Academic Press, p. 121.

107. Gomes MM, Weidman WH, McGoon DC, *et al.* (1971) Double-outlet right ventricle without pulmonic stenosis. Surgical considerations and results of operation. Circulation 43(5 Suppl), I31–36.

108. Gomes MM, Weidman WH, McGoon DC, *et al.* (1971) Double-outlet right ventricle with pulmonic stenosis. Surgical considerations and results of operation. Circulation 43, 889–894.

109. Madhavan M, Narayanan PS. (1975) Tricuspid atresia with double outlet right ventricle (Beuren type). Report of a rare combination. Indian J Pediatr 42, 58–59.

110. Cameron AH, Acerete F, Quero M, *et al.* (1976) Double outlet right ventricle. Study of 27 cases. Br Heart J 38, 1124–1132.

111. Tandon R, Moller JH, Edwards JE. (1973) Communication of mitral valve with both ventricles associated with double outlet right ventricle. Circulation 48, 904–908.

112. Kitamura N, Takao A, Ando M, *et al.* (1974) Taussig-Bing heart with mitral valve straddling: case reports and postmortem study. Circulation 49, 761–767.

113. Muster AJ, Bharati S, Aziz KU, *et al.* (1979) Taussig-Bing anomaly with straddling mitral valve. J Thorac Cardiovasc Surg 77, 832–842.

114. Freedom RM, Culham G, Rowe RD. (1978) The criss-cross and superoinferior ventricular heart: an angiocardiographic study. Am J Cardiol 42, 620–628.

115. Aziz KU, Paul MH, Muster AJ, *et al.* (1979) Positional abnormalities of atrioventricular valves in transposition of the great arteries including double outlet right ventricle, atrioventricular valve straddling and malattachment. Am J Cardiol 44, 1135–1145.

116. Aeba R, Katogi T, Takeuchi S, *et al.* (2000) Surgical management of the straddling mitral valve in the biventricular heart. Ann Thorac Surg 69, 130–134.

117. Serraf A, Nakamura T, Lacour-Gayet F, *et al.* (1996) Surgical approaches for double-outlet right ventricle or transposition of the great arteries associated with straddling atrioventricular valves. J Thorac Cardiovasc Surg 111, 527–535.

118. Sridaromont S, Feldt RH, Ritter DG, *et al.* (1975) Double-outlet right ventricle associated with persistent common atrioventricular canal. Circulation 52, 933–942.

119. Bharati S, Kirklin JW, McAllister HA Jr, *et al.* (1980) The surgical anatomy of common atrioventricular orifice associated with tetralogy of Fallot, double outlet right ventricle and complete regular transposition. Circulation 61, 1142–1149.

120. Pacifico AD, Kirklin JW, Bargeron LM Jr. (1980) Repair of complete atrioventricular canal associated with tetralogy of Fallot or double-outlet right ventricle: report of 10 patients. Ann Thorac Surg 29, 351–356.

121. Imamura M, Drummond-Webb JJ, Sarris GE, *et al.* (1998) Double-outlet right ventricle with complete atrioventricular canal. Ann Thorac Surg 66, 942–944.

122. Tchervenkov CI, Tahta SA, Cecere R, *et al.* (1997) Single-stage arterial switch with aortic arch enlargement for trans-position complexes with aortic arch obstruction. Ann Thorac Surg 64, 1776–1781.

123. Lacour-Gayet F, Serraf A, Galletti L, *et al.* (1997) Biventricular repair of conotruncal anomalies associated with aortic arch obstruction: 103 patients. Circulation 96(9 Suppl), II328–334.

124. Walters HL III, Mavroudis C, Tchervenkov CI, *et al.* (2000) Congenital Heart Surgery Nomenclature and Database Project: double outlet right ventricle. Ann Thorac Surg 69(4 Suppl), S249–263.

125. Franklin RC, Anderson RH, Daniels O, *et al.* (2002) Report of the Coding Committee of the Association for European Paediatric Cardiology. Cardiol Young 12, 611–618.

126. Stark J. (1994) Double outlet ventricles. In Stark J, deLeval M, eds. *Surgery for Congenital Heart Defects*, 2nd ed. Philadelphia, WB Saunders Co.

127. Krongrad E, Ritter DG, Weidman WH, *et al.* (1972) Hemodynamic and anatomic correlation of electrocardiogram in double-outlet right ventricle. Circulation 46, 995–1004.

128. DiSessa TG, Hagan AD, Pope C, *et al.* (1979) Two-dimensional echocardiographic characteristics of double outlet right ventricle. Am J Cardiol 44, 1146–1154.

129. Sanders SP, Bierman FZ, Williams RG. (1982) Conotruncal malformations: diagnosis in infancy using subxiphoid two-dimensional echocardiography. Am J Cardiol 50, 1361–1367.

130. Hagler DJ, Tajik AJ, Seward JB, *et al.* (1981) Double-outlet right ventricle. Wide-angle two-dimensional echocardiographic observations. Circulation 63, 419–428.

131. Macartney FJ, Rigby ML, Anderson RH, *et al.* (1984) Double outlet right ventricle. Cross sectional echocardiographic findings, their anatomical explanation, and surgical relevance. Br Heart J 52, 164–177.

132. Sridaromont S, Feldt RH, Ritter DG, *et al.* (1976) Double outlet right ventricle: hemodynamic and anatomic correlations. Am J Cardiol 38, 85–94.

133. Marino B, Loperfido F, Sardi CS. (1983) Spontaneous closure of ventricular septal defect in a case of double outlet right ventricle. Br Heart J 49, 608–611.

134. Goldberg SP, McCanta AC, Campbell DN, *et al.* (2009) Implications of incising the ventricular septum in double outlet right ventricle and in the Ross-Konno operation. Eur J Cardiothorac Surg 35, 589–593; discussion 593.

135. Tchervenkov CI, Marelli D, Beland MJ, *et al.* (1995) Institutional experience with a protocol of early primary repair of double-outlet right ventricle. Ann Thorac Surg 60(6 Suppl), S610–613.

136. Luber JM, Castaneda AR, Lang P, *et al.* (1983) Repair of double-outlet right ventricle: early and late results. Circulation 68, II144–147.

137. Blackstone EH, Kirklin JW, Bradley EL, *et al.* (1976) Optimal age and results in repair of large ventricular septal defects. J Thorac Cardiovasc Surg 72, 661–679.

138. Edwards WD, Wilcox WD, Danielson GK, *et al.* (1980) Postoperative false aneurysm of left ventricle and obstruction of left circumflex coronary artery complicating enlargement of restrictive ventricular septal defect in double-outlet right ventricle. J Thorac Cardiovasc Surg 80, 141–147.

139. Ottino G, Kugler JD, McNamara DG, *et al.* (1980) Taussig-Bing anomaly: total repair with closure of ventricular septal defect through the pulmonary artery. Ann Thorac Surg 29, 170–176.
140. Wedemeyer AL, Lucas RV Jr, Castaneda AR. (1970) Taussig-Bing malformation, coarctation of the aorta, and reversed patent ductus arteriosus. Operative correction in an infant. Circulation 42, 1021–1027.
141. Smith EE, Pucci JJ, Walesby RK, *et al.* (1982) A new technique for correction of the Taussig-Bing anomaly. J Thorac Cardiovasc Surg 83, 901–904.
142. Binet JP, Lacour-Gayet F, Conso JF, *et al.* (1983) Complete repair of the Taussig-Bing type of double-outlet right ventricle using the arterial switch operation without coronary translocation. Report of one successful case. J Thorac Cardiovasc Surg 85, 272–275.
143. Ceithaml EL, Puga FJ, Danielson GK, *et al.* (1984) Results of the Damus-Stansel-Kaye procedure for transposition of the great arteries and for double-outlet right ventricle with subpulmonary ventricular septal defect. Ann Thorac Surg 38, 433–437.
144. Pacifico AD, Kirklin JK, Colvin EV, *et al.* (1986) Intraventricular tunnel repair for Taussig-Bing heart and related cardiac anomalies. Circulation 74, I53–60.
145. Kinsley RH, Ritter DG, McGoon DC. (1974) The surgical repair of positional anomalies of the conotruncus. J Thorac Cardiovasc Surg 67, 395–403.
146. Harvey JC, Sondheimer HM, Williams WG, *et al.* (1977) Repair of double-outlet right ventricle. J Thorac Cardiovasc Surg 73, 611–615.
147. Agarwala B, Doyle EF, Danilowicz D, *et al.* (1973) Double outlet right ventricle with pulmonic stenosis and anteriorly positioned aorta (Taussig-Bing variant). Report of a case and surgical correction. Am J Cardiol 32, 850–854.
148. Stewart S. (1977) Double-outlet right ventricle (S,D,D), VSD related to pulmonary artery, and pulmonic stenosis absent. Correction with an intraventricular conduit in infancy. J Thorac Cardiovasc Surg 74, 70–72.
149. Metras D, Coulibaly AO, Ouattara K. (1984) Successful intraventricular repair of Taussig-Bing anomaly in infancy: report of a case. J Thorac Cardiovasc Surg 88, 311–312.
150. Doty DB. (1986) Correction of Taussig-Bing malformation by intraventricular conduit. J Thorac Cardiovasc Surg 91, 133–138.
151. Abe T, Sugiki K, Izumiyama O, *et al.* (1984) A successful procedure for correction of the Taussig-Bing malformation. J Thorac Cardiovasc Surg 87, 403–409.
152. Danielson GK. (1984) A successful procedure for correction of the Taussig-Bing malformation. (Invited commentary). J Thorac Cardiovasc Surg 87, 403.
153. Pacifico AD. (1984) A successful procedure for correction of the Taussig-Bing malformation (Invited commentary). J Thorac Cardiovasc Surg 87, 403.
154. McGoon DC. (1972) Intraventricular repair of transposition of the great arteries. J Thorac Cardiovasc Surg 64, 430–434.
155. Kawashima Y, Matsuda H, Yagihara T, *et al.* (1993) Intraventricular repair for Taussig-Bing anomaly. J Thorac Cardiovasc Surg 105, 591–596; discussion 596–597.
156. Kawahira Y, Yagihara T, Uemura H, *et al.* (1999) Ventricular outflow tracts after Kawashima intraventricular rerouting for double outlet right ventricle with subpulmonary ventricular septal defect. Eur J Cardiothorac Surg 16, 26–31.
157. Mavroudis C, Backer CL, Muster AJ, *et al.* (1996) Taussig-Bing anomaly: arterial switch versus Kawashima intraventricular repair. Ann Thorac Surg 61, 1330–1338.
158. Kanter KR, Anderson RH, Lincoln C, *et al.* (1985) Anatomic correction for complete transposition and double-outlet right ventricle. J Thorac Cardiovasc Surg 90, 690–699.
159. Kanter K, Anderson R, Lincoln C, *et al.* (1986) Anatomic correction of double-outlet right ventricle with subpulmonary ventricular septal defect (the "Taussig-Bing" anomaly). Ann Thorac Surg 41, 287–292.
160. Masuda M, Kado H, Shiokawa Y, *et al.* (1999) Clinical results of arterial switch operation for double-outlet right ventricle with subpulmonary VSD. Eur J Cardiothorac Surg 15, 283–288.
161. Kreutzer C, De Vive J, Oppido G, *et al.* (2000) Twenty-five-year experience with Rastelli repair for transposition of the great arteries. J Thorac Cardiovasc Surg 120, 211–223.
162. Dearani JA, Danielson GK, Puga FJ, *et al.* (2001) Late results of the Rastelli operation for transposition of the great arteries. Semin Thorac Cardiovasc Surg Pediatr Card Surg Annu 4, 3.
163. Lecompte Y, Neveux JY, Leca F, *et al.* (1982) Reconstruction of the pulmonary outflow tract without prosthetic conduit. J Thorac Cardiovasc Surg 84, 727–733.
164. Lecompte Y, Zannini L, Hazan E, *et al.* (1981) Anatomic correction of transposition of the great arteries. J Thorac Cardiovasc Surg 82, 629–631.
165. Rubay J, Lecompte Y, Batisse A, *et al.* (1988) Anatomic repair of anomalies of ventriculo-arterial connection (REV). Results of a new technique in cases associated with pulmonary outflow tract obstruction. Eur J Cardiothorac Surg 2, 305–311.
166. Borromee L, Lecompte Y, Batisse A, *et al.* (1988) Anatomic repair of anomalies of ventriculoarterial connection associated with ventricular septal defect. II. Clinical results in 50 patients with pulmonary outflow tract obstruction. J Thorac Cardiovasc Surg 95, 96–102.
167. Vouhe PR, Tamisier D, Leca F, *et al.* (1992) Transposition of the great arteries, ventricular septal defect, and pulmonary outflow tract obstruction. Rastelli or Lecompte procedure? J Thorac Cardiovasc Surg 103, 428–436.
168. van Son JA, Sim EK. (1996) Lecompte operation with presevation of the pulmonary valve for anomalies of ventriculoarterial connection with ventricular septal defect and subpulmonary stenosis. Eur J Cardiothorac Surg 10, 585–589.
169. Hu S, Liu Z, Li S, *et al.* (2008) Strategy for biventricular outflow tract reconstruction: Rastelli, REV, or Nikaidoh procedure? J Thorac Cardiovasc Surg 135, 331–338.
170. Nikaidoh H. (1984) Aortic translocation and biventricular outflow tract reconstruction. A new surgical repair for transposition of the great arteries associated with ventricular septal defect and pulmonary stenosis. J Thorac Cardiovasc Surg 88, 365–372.

171. Hu SS, Li SJ, Wang X, *et al.* (2007) Pulmonary and aortic root translocation in the management of transposition of great arteries with ventricular septal defect and left ventricular outflow tract obstruction. J Thorac Cardiovasc Surg 133, 1090–1092.

172. Morell VO, Jacobs JP, Quintessenza JA. (2005) Aortic translocation in the management of transposition of the great arteries with ventricular septal defect and pulmonary stenosis: results and follow-up. Ann Thorac Surg 79, 2089–2092; discussion 2092–2093.

173. Soszyn N, Fricke TA, Wheaton GR, *et al.* (2011) Outcomes of the arterial switch operation in patients with Taussig-Bing anomaly. Ann Thorac Surg 92, 673–679.

174. Losay J, Touchot A, Serraf A, *et al.* (2001) Late outcome after arterial switch operation for transposition of the great arteries. Circulation 104(12 Suppl 1), I121–126.

175. Huber C, Mimic B, Oswal N, *et al.* (2011) Outcomes and re-interventions after one-stage repair of transpostition of great arteries and aortic arch obstruction. Eur J Cardiothorac Surg 39, 213–220.

176. Alsoufi B, Cai S, Williams WG, *et al.* (2008) Improved results with single-stage total correction of Taussig-Bing anomaly. Eur J Cardiothorac Surg 33, 244–250.

177. Griselli M, McGuirk SP, Ko C, *et al.* (2007) Arterial switch operation in patients with Taussig-Bing anomaly – influence of staged repair and coronary anatomy on outcome. Eur J Cardiothorac Surg 31, 229–235.

178. Wetter J, Sinzobahamvya N, Blaschczok HC, *et al.* (2004) Results of arterial switch operation for primary total correction of the Taussig-Bing anomaly. Ann Thorac Surg 77, 41–46; discussion 47.

179. Sinzobahamvya N, Blaschczok HC, Asfour B, *et al.* (2007) Right ventricular outflow tract obstruction after arterial switch operation for the Taussig-Bing heart. Eur J Cardiothorac Surg 31, 873–878.

180. Lacour-Gayet F. (2007) Arterial switch operation with ventricular septal defect repair and aortic arch reconstruction. Semin Thorac Cardiovasc Surg 19, 245–248.

181. Losay J, Touchot A, Capderou A, *et al.* (2006) Aortic valve regurgitation after arterial switch operation for transposition of the great arteries: incidence, risk factors, and outcome. J Am Coll Cardiol 47, 2057–2062.

182. Konno S, Imai Y, Iida Y, *et al.* (1975) A new method for prosthetic valve replacement in congenital aortic stenosis associated with hypoplasia of the aortic valve ring. J Thorac Cardiovasc Surg 70, 909.

183. Bex JP, Lecompte Y, Baillot F, *et al.* (1980) Anatomical correction of transposition of the great arteries. Ann Thorac Surg 29, 86–88.

184. Yeh T, Ramaciotti C, Leonard SR, *et al.* (2007) The aortic translocation (Nikaidoh) procedure: midterm results superior to the Rastelli procedure. J Thorac Cardiovasc Surg 133, 461–469.

185. Hu S, Xie Y, Li S, *et al.* (2010) Double-root translocation for double-outlet right ventricle with noncommitted ventricular septal defect or double-outlet right ventricle with subpulmonary ventricular septal defect associated with pulmonary stenosis: an optimized solution. Ann Thorac Surg 89, 1360–1365.

186. Rastelli GC. (1969) A new approach to "anatomic" repair of transposition of the great arteries. Mayo Clin Proc 44, 1–12.

187. Lecompte Y, Leca F, Neveux JY, *et al.* (1984) Anatomic correction of transposition of the great vessels with interventricular communication and pulmonary stenosis. Ann Pediatr 31, 621–624.

188. Lacour-Gayet F, Anderson RH. (2005) A uniform surgical technique for transfer of both simple and complex patterns of the coronary arteries during the arterial switch procedure. Cardiol Young 15(Suppl 1), 93–101.

189. Meadows J, Pigula F, Lock J, *et al.* (2007) Transcatheter creation and enlargement of ventricular septal defects for relief of ventricular hypertension. J Thorac Cardiovasc Surg 133, 912–918.

190. Lacour-Gayet F. (2009) Management of older single functioning ventricles with outlet obstruction due to a restricted "VSD" in double inlet left ventricle and in complex double outlet right ventricle. Semin Thorac Cardiovasc Surg Pediatr Card Surg Annu 130–132.

191. Serraf A, Lacour-Gayet F, Houyel L, *et al.* (1993) Subaortic obstruction in double outlet right ventricles. Surgical considerations for anatomic repair. Circulation 88, II177–182.

192. Lacour-Gayet F, Bonnet N, Piot D, *et al.* (1997) Surgical management of atrio ventricular septal defects with normal caryotype. Eur J Cardiothorac Surg 11, 466–472.

193. Kleinert S, Sano T, Weintraub RG, *et al.* (1997) Anatomic features and surgical strategies in double-outlet right ventricle. Circulation 96, 1233–1239.

194. Shen WK, Holmes DR Jr, Porter CJ, *et al.* (1990) Sudden death after repair of double-outlet right ventricle. Circulation 81, 128–136.

195. Pacifico AD, Kirklin JW, Bargeron LM Jr, *et al.* (1973) Surgical treatment of double-outlet left ventricle. Report of four cases. Circulation 48(1 Suppl), III19–23.

196. Bharati S, Lev M, Stewart R, *et al.* (1978) The morphologic spectrum of double outlet left ventricle and its surgical significance. Circulation 58, 558–565.

197. Tchervenkov CI, Walters HL, 3rd, Chu VF. (2000) Congenital Heart Surgery Nomenclature and Database Project: double outlet left ventricle. Ann Thorac Surg 69(4 Suppl), S264–269.

198. Sakakibara S, Takao A, Arai T, *et al.* (1967) Both great vessels arising from the left ventricle. Bull Heart Inst Japan 11, 66–86.

199. Paul MH, Muster AJ, Sinha SN, *et al.* (1970) Double-outlet left ventricle with an intact ventricular septum. Clinical and autopsy diagnosis and developmental implications. Circulation 41, 129–139.

200. Kerr AR, Barcia A, Bargeron LM Jr, *et al.* (1971) Double-outlet left ventricle with ventricular septal defect and pulmonary stenosis: report of surgical repair. Am Heart J 81, 688–693.

201. Anderson R, Galbraith R, Gibson R, *et al.* (1974) Double outlet left ventricle. Br Heart J 36, 554–558.

202. Sharratt GP, Sbokos CG, Johnson AM, *et al.* (1976) Surgical "correction" of solitus-concordant, double-outlet left ventricle with L-malposition and tricuspid stenosis with hypo-

plastic right ventricle. J Thorac Cardiovasc Surg 71, 853–858.

203. Goor DA, Dische R, Lillehei CW. (1972) The conotruncus. I. Its normal inversion and conus absorption. Circulation 46, 375–384.

204. van Praagh R, Calder AL, Delisle G. (1972) Transposition of the great arteries with overriding aorta and pulmonary stenosis. New entity and its surgical management (abstr). Circulation 46(suppl II), II96.

205. van Praagh R, Weinberg PM. (1983) Double outlet left ventricle. In: Adams FH, Emmanouilides GC, eds. *Heart Disease in Infants, Children, and Adolescents*, 3rd ed. Baltimore: Williams & Wilkins.

206. DeLeon SY, Ow EP, Chiemmongkoltip P, *et al*. (1995) Alternatives in biventricular repair of double-outlet left ventricle. Ann Thorac Surg 60, 213–216.

207. Chiavarelli M, Boucek MM, Bailey LL. (1992) Arterial correction of double-outlet left ventricule by pulmonary artery translocation. Ann Thorac Surg 53, 1098–1100.

208. McElhinney DB, Reddy VM, Hanley FL. (1997) Pulmonary root translocation for biventricular repair of double-outlet left ventricle with absent subpulmonic conus. J Thorac Cardiovasc Surg 114, 501–503.

26

Transposition of the Great Arteries

Constantine Mavroudis[1] and Carl L. Backer[2]

[1]Florida Hospital for Children, Orlando, FL, USA
[2]Ann & Robert H. Lurie Children's Hospital of Chicago, formerly Children's Memorial Hospital, Chicago, IL, USA

Transposition of the great arteries (TGA) is a congenital defect of the heart in which the anatomic relationship of the great arteries is reversed. Unlike in normal positioning, the aorta arises anterior to the pulmonary artery and from the right ventricle, while the pulmonary artery lies posterior to the aorta and arises from the left ventricle. In this chapter we will discuss patients with transposed great vessels who have undergone D-looping with two ventricles. Anatomic variations, which include tricuspid or mitral atresia, heterotaxy syndromes, and single ventricle, will be discussed in Chapter 28, *The Functionally Univentricular Heart and Fontan's Operation*. L-Loop transposition of the great arteries is discussed in Chapter 27, *Congenitally Corrected Transposition of the Great Arteries*.

Patients with TGA are subdivided into those with intact ventricular septum (50%), ventricular septal defect (VSD) (25%), and VSD with pulmonary stenosis (25%). Other frequently found cardiac anomalies include patent ductus arteriosus, coarctation of the aorta, and interrupted aortic arch. Transposition of the great vessels is the most common cyanotic heart defect in infancy and accounts for 9.9% of all cases of congenital heart disease [1].

Embryologic and Anatomic Considerations

After the description of TGA by Baillie in 1797 [2], numerous theories have been postulated concerning the morphogenesis of this abnormal relationship between the great arteries and the ventricles. These include 1) the straight truncoconal septum hypothesis, incriminating an abnormal septation of the aorta and pulmonary artery [3–9]; 2) the abnormal fibrous skeleton hypothesis in which pulmonary-mitral fibrous continuity instead of the normal aortic-mitral fibrous continuity occurs [10,11]; 3) the abnor-

mal embryonic hemodynamics hypothesis, caused by obstructive and alternative flow characteristics [12–18]; and 4) the inverted truncal swellings theory, citing the inverted development of the regions below the semilunar valves [19–21]. The latter interpretation resembles Van Praagh's analysis [22,23] in which he postulates that the subaortic conus persists and develops during the normal D-looping, while the subpulmonary conus undergoes absorption and eventual fibrous continuity with the mitral valve. As a result the aortic valve is anterior to the pulmonary valve, allowing both semilunar valves to align and connect respectively with the distal great vessels, without undergoing the usual twisting and untwisting that is hypothesized about normal hearts. The results of these events *in utero* lead to TGA.

Anatomic variations are encountered often. Although mesocardia and dextrocardia have been described [24], the heart is left-sided with atrial situs solitus in 95% of patients. The incidence of systemic venous anomalies is no greater than in other congenital heart defects. Left or right juxtaposition of the atrial appendages can be encountered and may signal other anomalies [25]. Most atrial communications are via a patent foramen ovale; a true ostium secundum defect is present in 10–20% of cases. A right-sided aortic arch is present in 4% of patients with TGA and intact ventricular septum and in 16% of those with VSD [26].

In patients with TGA and intact ventricular septum, functional obstruction of the left ventricular outflow tract may be present owing to septal bulging toward the mitral valve, which is caused by the differential in ventricular pressures. These defects, however, are resolved by anatomic correction. Rarely will a patient with TGA and intact ventricular septum have anatomic subvalvar stenosis [27–29].

Of patients with TGA, up to 50% will have a VSD, many of which close spontaneously. Theoretically VSDs can be

Pediatric Cardiac Surgery, Fourth Edition. Edited by Constantine Mavroudis and Carl L. Backer.
© 2013 Blackwell Publishing Ltd. Published 2013 by Blackwell Publishing Ltd.

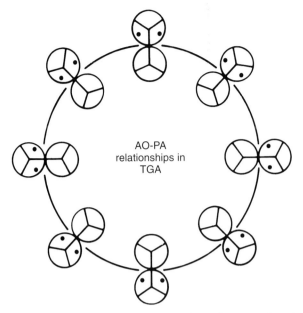

AO-PA
relationships in
TGA

Figure 26.1 Schematic diagram shows the wide range of spatial relationships between the great arteries in patients with "complete" transposition of the great arteries (TGA). (AO, aorta; PA, pulmonary artery.)

located anywhere in the ventricular septum, although most have been found in the infundibular and perimembranous locations [30,31]. Additional cardiac anomalies are more prevalent in patients with TGA and VSD. These include all levels of pulmonary stenosis, pulmonary atresia, overriding or straddling atrioventricular valves, coarctation of the aorta, and interruption of the aortic arch. Right ventricular outflow obstruction is exceedingly rare [32].

The spatial relationship between the great vessels is variable (Figure 26.1) [33,34], but most often the aorta is at the right and anterior to the pulmonary artery. Whatever the variation, in virtually every case the sinuses of Valsalva and coronary artery ostia face the corresponding pulmonary artery sinuses of Valsalva, favorable for a coronary transfer and arterial switch [33,35–39]; only a small number pose problems for an arterial switch (see section Special Coronary Problems).

Functional abnormalities of the mitral and tricuspid valves are infrequent [40–42] in patients who have an intact ventricular septum. In patients with VSD, tricuspid abnormalities resulting in straddling or overriding can occur. A straddling tricuspid valve has chordal attachments in the left ventricle, whereas an overriding tricuspid valve allows flow into the left ventricle without straddling chordae. Whether the tricuspid valve is straddling or overriding, the associated right ventricular hypoplasia carries with it major therapeutic implications regarding the choice of eventual repair [43,44].

Physiology

Transposition of the great arteries is characterized by two separate parallel circulations, in which the systemic venous blood passes through the right ventricle to the aorta while the pulmonary venous blood passes through the left ventricle, resulting in cyanosis [24,45,46]. Some mixing between the circulations is mandatory to sustain life and is dependent largely on the type of TGA.

Patients with TGA and intact ventricular septum survive because of aortopulmonary flow through a patent ductus arteriosus, often enhanced by prostaglandin E1 [47,48], and a left-to-right atrial shunt through a dilated patent foramen ovale caused by high left atrial pressure and an incompetent flap of the foramen ovale. This mixing, however, allows for only marginal tissue oxygenation, which is not improved with higher concentrations of inspired oxygen. Atrial balloon septostomy or surgical creation of an atrial septal defect improves systemic oxygen saturation and sets conditions for longer-term survival.

Patients with TGA and VSD have higher oxygen saturations by virtue of the anatomic defects, which allow more pulmonary flow and greater mixing at both the atrial and ventricular levels. There is, however, a spectrum of ventricular defects, from the small to the very large. Small defects allow minimal mixing and cyanosis indistinguishable from TGA and intact ventricular septum. Large defects also allow increased pulmonary flow and mixing, resulting in a pink patient who is subject to pulmonary overcirculation and the dangers of acquired pulmonary vascular hypertension.

Pulmonary outflow tract obstruction will alter the degree of cyanosis, more or less with the severity of the obstruction. In patients with intact ventricular septum, valvar stenosis is rare. The usual location of obstruction is subvalvar, owing to septal deviation caused by right ventricular distension. This problem is solved by an arterial switch, which eliminates the systemic right ventricular forces on the septum [49,50]. More often, subvalvar stenosis is associated with VSD. These patients usually have a more balanced physiology, resulting in mild cyanosis, and they tend to show symptoms of TGA later than other patients. When pulmonary stenosis becomes clinically significant, a systemic-to-pulmonary artery shunt is performed initially and followed by anatomic repair with a right ventricle-to-pulmonary artery conduit (Rastelli operation [51]), or the Lecompte or *réparation à l'étage ventriculaire* (REV) procedure [52,53], which allows anatomic repair without use of a conduit. Pulmonary vascular disease can occur in patients with TGA regardless of the presence of a VSD. Moreover, patients with TGA and VSD tend to develop pulmonary vascular disease earlier than patients who have VSD without TGA [54,55]. The reasons for these findings are speculative and may relate to differences in oxygen saturation, carbon dioxide content, and pulmonary arterial pH [46].

Clinical Presentation

Recent reports have demonstrated that antenatal diagnosis of TGA (fetal echocardiography) correlates with increased perioperative stability and improved surgical outcomes [56–59]. Unfortunately, prenatal detection rates depend on the institutional experience and can vary from 20% to 72% [56,59–63]. As a result, most infants with TGA will present with cyanosis, varying degrees of acidosis, and hemodynamic instability depending on the degree and type of associated anomalies [24,46]. Cyanosis is prevalent during the first days of life in patients with TGA and intact ventricular septum, whereas cyanosis may be less or not noticed in those with VSDs.

Infants with TGA may be at a higher risk for cerebral ischemic compromise resulting from chronically decreased oxygen delivery to the brain in fetal life [59]. Transposition of the great arteries causes oxygenated blood to preferentially flow into the lower body and not to the brain as occurs in the normal fetus. Park and associates [64] used proton magnetic resonance spectroscopy to show that cerebral metabolism was altered specifically in the parietal white matter, which suggested that a maturation delay rather than acute postnatal insult was responsible [59].

Cardiac examination reveals a mildly overactive precordium. Cardiac murmurs, when audible, are usually soft and occur during systole. The second heart sound is characteristically loud and single. The femoral pulses are normal or bounding when there is a large patent ductus arteriosus [24]. The liver may be enlarged, especially when there is a large systemic-to-pulmonary shunt, and the child may have tachypnea, intercostal and subcostal retractions, and inability to nurse successfully.

The electrocardiograph findings are usually within normal limits at birth, with progression to right ventricular hypertrophy with advancing age. The chest roentgenograph findings are also normal at birth except in those patients with large VSDs, who will have cardiomegaly, increased pulmonary vascularity, and evidence of congestive heart failure. In older infants, moderate cardiomegaly is often present with an "egg-on-its-side" appearance [24]. There may also be asymmetry of pulmonary blood flow, resulting in right-sided plethora owing to preferential right pulmonary artery flow.

The diagnosis of TGA generally can be made by echocardiography. A posterior great artery, dividing into right and left pulmonary arteries and arising from the left ventricle, along with an anterior aorta arising from the right ventricle, confirms the diagnosis (Figures 26.2 and 26.3) [34]. Doppler techniques can determine intercavitary shunting, which can occur from a ductus arteriosus, patent foramen

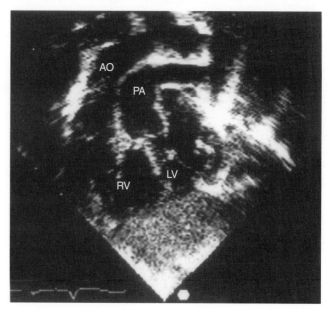

Figure 26.2 Subcostal sagittal view of an infant with transposition of the great arteries and intact ventricular septum. This view is obtained by positioning the transducer in the subcostal region, with the plane of sound tilted posteriorly to anteriorly to the level of the great vessels. (AO, aorta; PA, pulmonary artery; LV, left ventricle; RV, right ventricle.)

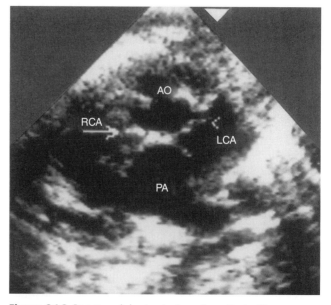

Figure 26.3 Parasternal short-axis view of a patient with transposition of the great arteries, intact ventricular septum, and normal coronary artery anatomy. The aorta is anterior, and the left main and right coronary arteries are visualized originating from the left and right coronary cusps, respectively. The pulmonary artery is posterior, and bifurcation of the left and right pulmonary arteries is demonstrated. This view is obtained with the transducer positioned in the left parasternal intercostal space, with the plane of sound directed from the left ventricular apex toward the head. (AO, aorta; RCA, right coronary artery; LCA, left coronary artery; PA, pulmonary artery.)

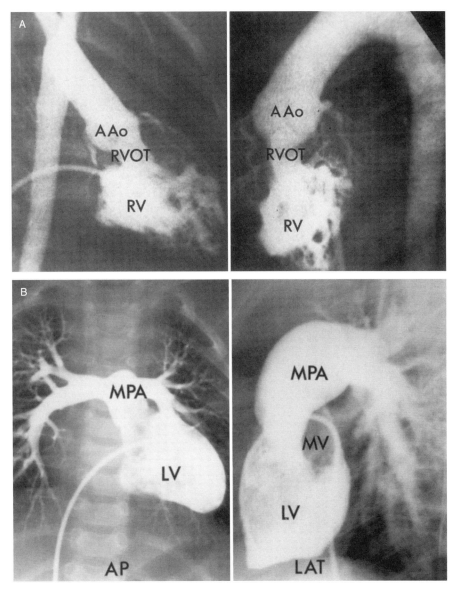

Figure 26.4 A, Right anterior oblique and left anterior oblique views of a trabeculated right ventriculogram in a patient with transposition of the great arteries and intact ventricular septum. **B,** Anterior (AP) and lateral (LAT) views of a smooth, nontrabeculated left ventriculogram in a patient with transposition of the great arteries and intact ventricular septum. (AAo, ascending aorta; LV, left ventricle; MPA, main pulmonary artery; MV, mitral valve; RV, right ventricle; RVOT, right ventricular outflow tract.)

ovale, or VSD [65]. Multiple views can determine the size and location of a VSD with reference to the infundibular septum, the nature of the atrial septal communication, the anatomy of the atrioventricular valves, the site and degree of pulmonary stenosis, and, in most cases, the course and anatomic variation of the coronary arteries [66].

Cardiac catheterization usually is reserved for those few patients in whom clinical instability demands Rashkind balloon atrial septostomy [67] or when more physiologic and anatomic data are required concerning the coronary arteries, the VSD, the degree of left ventricular outflow obstruction, or other anatomic variations such as interrupted aortic arch, coarctation, and the like (Figures 26.4 and 26.5) [34]. More often than not, however, these issues can be resolved with magnetic resonance imaging/magnetic resonance angiograpy (MRI/MRA) or computed tomography (CT) scans [68].

Medical Management of the Neonate

Medical management of neonates with TGA focuses on the stabilization and correction of physiologic aberrations

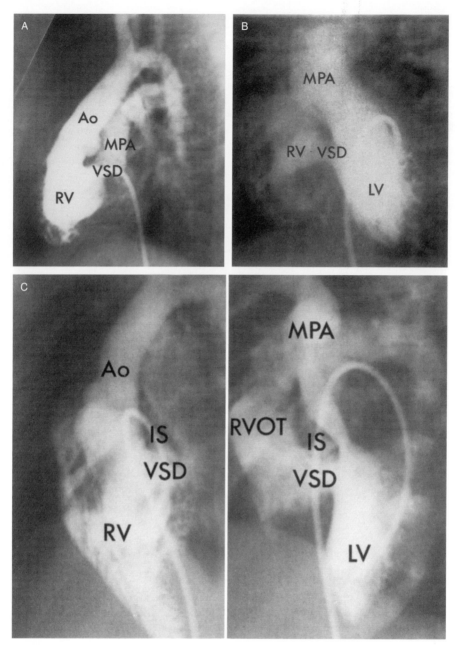

Figure 26.5 A, Cine cardioangiogram of a patient with transposition of the great arteries, nonmalalignment ventricular septal defect, and no pulmonary stenosis. **B,** Cine cardioangiogram of a patient with transposition of the great arteries, noncommitted, nonmalalignment ventricular septal defect, and no pulmonary stenosis. **C,** Cine cardioangiograms of a patient with transposition of the great arteries, ventricular septal defect, and subpulmonic stenosis caused by a posteriorly deviated infundibular septum. (Ao, aorta; IS, infundibular septum; LV, left ventricle; RV, right ventricle; MPA, main pulmonary artery; RVOT, right ventricular outflow tract.)

caused by cyanosis and poor perfusion. Correction of acid-base balance, maintenance of normothermia, prevention of hypoglycemia, and other routine supportive measures are undertaken. Prostaglandin E1 is administered to increase pulmonary blood flow and is usually followed by atrial balloon septostomy [67] to improve mixing. Whether balloon septostomy is used or not depends on the stability

of the patient and the operative decision concerning arterial switch. A recent multicenter study of the incidence and causes of preoperative death in isolated TGA revealed that 20 of 199 neonates (9.9%) with TGA died before surgery [69]. The authors concluded that the high preoperative mortality rate was mainly because of absent or small atrial shunt and furthermore that prenatal diagnosis of TGA with institution of prostaglandin E1 and balloon atrial septostomy immediately after birth could avoid a fatal outcome [69].

Surgical Management

The surgical management of TGA is determined by the associated lesions. Historically, numerous operations were introduced and employed until new therapeutic modalities limited their use.

The Blalock-Hanlon atrial septectomy was introduced in 1950 [70]. The operation, although associated with a high mortality rate, was successful in increasing atrial mixing at a time when balloon catheters and cardiopulmonary bypass were yet to be introduced. This procedure has been replaced largely by balloon septostomy, or open septectomy when necessary.

Pulmonary artery banding first was introduced for palliation in patients with VSD. The trend toward earlier corrective surgery and primary VSD closure has limited this operation to 1) patients with TGA and intact ventricular septum who, for one reason or another, did not undergo neonatal arterial switch and require left ventricular training; and 2) patients with TGA and right ventricular failure after an atrial baffle operation who might benefit from staged conversion to an arterial switch (see Arterial Switch). Internal pulmonary artery band placement has been used instead of classic banding to reduce the risk of pulmonary valve damage, pulmonary artery distortion, and pulmonary artery dilatation, with possible related coronary compression [71].

The Mustard [72] and Senning [73] atrial baffle procedures were created to reroute systemic venous return and pulmonary venous return to the ventricles that were associated with the appropriate great vessels. The pericardial baffle in the Mustard operation (Figure 26.6) [74] and the right atrial flap in the Senning operation (Figure 26.7) [34] direct systemic venous return to the left ventricle, pulmonary arteries, and the lungs for oxygenation. Oxygenated blood returns to the pulmonary atrium, right ventricle, aorta, and the systemic circulation. This obviously results in a physiologic correction but not an anatomic correction,

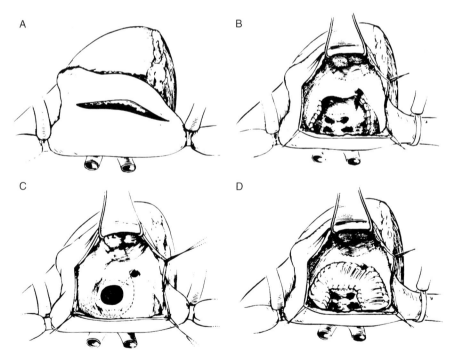

Figure 26.6 The Mustard operation. **A,** The right atrium is opened with a longitudinal incision well away from the sinoatrial node. **B,** The atrial septum is incised from the midpoint on a superior border of the atrial septal defect to the middle of the superior vena cava orifice. All the septum lateral to this incision is excised, avoiding the orifices of the right pulmonary veins. The ridge of the septum medially is preserved. **C,** The coronary sinus is cut back into the left atrium and all raw margins of atrial septum are oversewn. The *dotted line* indicates where the baffle will be sutured. **D,** Starting at the anterior lip of the left pulmonary vein orifices, the baffle is sutured in place, thus diverting the caval venous return to the mitral valve and the pulmonary venous return to the tricuspid valve. (Reproduced with permission from Trusler *et al.* [74].)

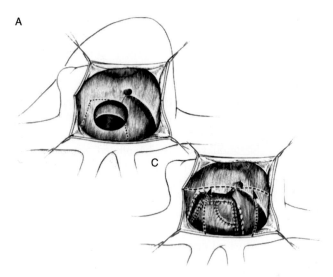

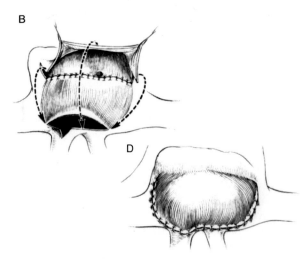

Figure 26.7 The Senning operation. **A,** The atrial septum is cut near the tricuspid valve, creating a flap attached posteriorly between the caval veins. **B,** The flap of atrial septum is sutured to the anterior lip of the orifices of the left pulmonary veins, effectively separating the pulmonary and systemic venous channels. **C,** The posterior edge of the right atrial incision is sutured to the remnant of atrial septum, diverting the systemic venous channel to the mitral valve. **D,** The anterior edge of the right atrial incision, lengthened by short incisions at each corner, is sutured around the cava above and below and to the lateral edge of the left atrial incision, completing the pulmonary channel and diversion of pulmonary venous blood to the tricuspid valve area.

because the systemic circulation is based on the right ventricle. The clinical results with these procedures were reproducible and associated with a low operative mortality rate (<5%). Long-term problems of superior vena caval obstruction, baffle leak, atrial and ventricular arrhythmias, tricuspid valve insufficiency, and right ventricular failure raised concerns with this approach [75,76]. The arterial switch operation has largely replaced the atrial baffle operations, with excellent mid- and long-term clinical results (see Arterial Switch).

Arterial Switch Operation for Transposition of the Great Arteries with Intact Ventricular Septum

The arterial switch operation has developed into the procedure of choice for TGA and associated great vessel malposition anomalies because of improved techniques of coronary transfer, myocardial protection, and neogreat vessel reconstruction [37,77–112]. These advances have resulted in improved survival statistics that compare favorably with the atrial baffle procedures [78,113–117]. The arterial switch operation results in left ventricle-to-aorta continuity and has not been associated with atrial arrhythmias, baffle stenoses, tricuspid insufficiency, right ventricular failure, and sudden death, all of which have been noted in patients who had atrial baffle repairs. Complications

after an arterial switch have thus far been infrequent. Coronary insufficiency is the most common cause of early death [118], and right ventricular outflow tract (RVOT) obstruction, supravalvar and subvalvar, is the most common long-term complication leading to reoperation [97,118–123]. A multicenter study [123] reported a risk-adjusted base incidence of 0.5% per year of reintervention for right-sided outflow obstruction. Akiba and associates [124] postulate that even subtle size mismatch between the proximal aorta and pulmonary trunk may initiate adaptive infundibular hypertrophy. Potential problems of semilunar valvar regurgitation and supravalvar neoaortic stenosis have been infrequent [123]. Recent studies [125] have identified patients with coronary artery obstruction that has been treated by proximal coronary arterioplasty and internal thoracic artery-to-coronary artery bypass. It seems, however, that these problems will prove to be infrequent in the long term (Figure 26.8) [34,126].

The principles of the arterial switch operation for TGA with intact ventricular septum (simple transposition) are similar for the more complex anatomic anomalies such as TGA with VSD, the Taussig-Bing type of double-outlet right ventricle with subpulmonic VSD, and staged conversion of the Mustard operation to arterial switch. For the latter more complex cases the arterial switch is combined with VSD closure, subvalvar muscular resection, or atrial baffle conversion.

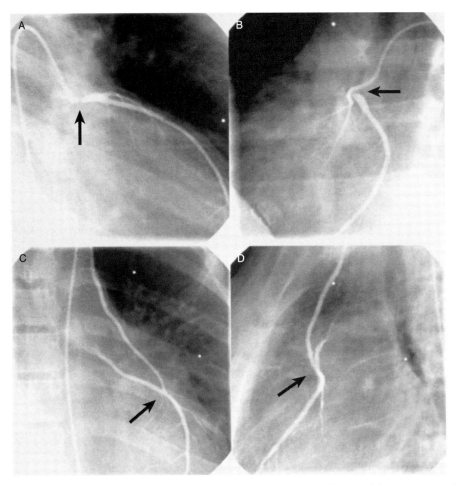

Figure 26.8 Cine cardioangiograms showing left main coronary artery stenosis 10 years after arterial switch. Arrows in **A** and **B** point to the areas of significant stenosis. **C, D,** Patent left internal thoracic artery to the middle left anterior descending coronary artery. Not shown is the proximal left main arterioplasty that was performed in concert with the coronary artery bypass graft.

An arterial switch for TGA can be divided into six stages, which include 1) pericardial harvest, evaluation, and dissection; 2) cannulation and cardiopulmonary bypass; 3) myocardial protection; 4) neoaortic reconstruction with coronary transfer; 5) neopulmonary artery reconstruction; and 6) separation from cardiopulmonary bypass and postoperative support.

Pericardial Harvest, Evaluation, and Dissection

After median sternotomy, pericardial harvest is performed for future neopulmonary artery reconstruction. Great care is taken to avoid injury to the phrenic nerves in the same manner as described for the Mustard operation [72,126]. The smooth visceral side should serve as the inner surface of the neopulmonary artery reconstruction. Some authors have recommended glutaraldehyde treatment [79,97] to stiffen and shrink the pericardium, thereby enhancing tech-

nical manipulation and preventing further pericardial shrinkage. We have avoided pericardial glutaraldehyde treatment because of anecdotal experience in a referred patient with significant and early supravalvar neopulmonary artery stenosis caused by pericardial shrinkage, which was confirmed at exploration. Presently we rely on a large redundant pantaloon pericardial patch with liberal tailoring, which has yielded a very low reoperation rate for neopulmonary artery stenosis.

The relationship of coronary artery distribution and origin to great vessel anatomy represents the most crucial planning stage of the arterial switch. Recognition of coronary anatomic patterns and ventricular flow distribution allows the surgeon to visualize the coronary transfer to the pulmonary artery-facing sinuses for the neoaortic reconstruction. During the developmental stages of neonatal arterial switch, some surgeons speculated that some coronary artery patterns could not be switched because of poor results having to do with coronary insufficiency. Others [84,85,104,110–112] have noted that the great majority of patients are candidates for arterial switch as long as favorable coronary transfer is performed, thereby avoiding the hazards of kinking and obstruction. This issue is still being debated because of wide variations in coronary anatomy [36,127–130], operative conditions relating to anatomic configurations, and the widely divergent experience of surgeons. Increasing experience with this operation, however, has resulted in improved results for patients with all types of coronary anatomy patterns [108,131–133]. This will obviously decrease the incidence of the bail-out atrial baffle procedure, which has a high complication rate under these circumstances [81,99].

Extensive and meticulous great vessel dissection aided by needle tip electrocautery is performed routinely before initiation of cardiopulmonary bypass, with great emphasis on freeing hilar attachments from the respective pulmonary arteries [37,80,84,86–88,90,91,93–95,99–101,110–112]. Failure to perform this part of the operation effectively may result in excessive tension, bleeding, and supravalvar neopulmonary artery stenosis after the maneuver of Lecompte [91].

Cannulation and Cardiopulmonary Bypass

Neonatal cannulation techniques for arterial switch are generally straightforward, varying slightly if deep hypothermia and circulatory arrest are employed. We place an 8-F arterial cannula (DLP, Inc., Grand Rapids, MI) near the innominate artery origin to maximize the available length of ascending aorta for neoaortic reconstruction and for the maneuver of Lecompte. Bicaval cannulation (Figure 26.9) [34] facilitates exposure to the atrial septal defect (patent foramen ovale or balloon septostomy tear) or VSD during continuous cardiopulmonary bypass without subjecting the patient to the hazards of circulatory arrest. In addition, the surgeon and perfusionist are spared the inconvenience of air in the venous line, which may occur with single venous atrial cannulation during the neopulmonary artery reconstruction. On the other hand, disadvantages of bicaval cannulation include small size and right atrial fragility, cannula-induced coronary artery tension, and atrial arrhythmias.

Single right atrial cannulation (Figure 26.10) [34] is simple and quick, and it provides effective venous drainage for cardiopulmonary bypass. The surgeon may elect to use deep hypothermia and circulatory arrest or various methods of continuous cardiopulmonary bypass during the stages of the arterial switch operation. Circulatory arrest during the atrial septal defect closure and neoaortic reconstruction frees the operative field of the left ventricular vent, two venous cannulas, and vena cava slings. Many authors [80,87,110–112] have reported excellent results with

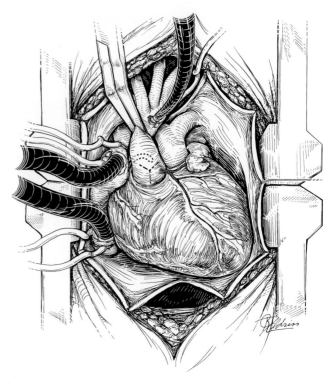

Figure 26.9 Aortobicaval cardiopulmonary bypass in a patient with transposition of the great arteries and intact ventricular septum. The aorta is cross-clamped in anticipation of antegrade cardioplegia and great vessel transection.

this technique. On the other hand, we feel that long periods of circulatory arrest (greater than 30 minutes) should be avoided if other reasonable means are available. Many studies [134–139] have emphasized that the safe period of deep hypothermia and circulatory arrest may be shorter than originally thought. Other recent experimental data have shown the superiority of hypothermia and low-flow states to deep hypothermia and circulatory arrest [140,141].

The Boston Circulatory Arrest Study Group [142–146], in a series of studies, has addressed the influence of hypothermic circulatory arrest versus low-flow cardiopulmonary bypass on the neurodevelopmental [142–145] and nonneurologic status [146] of neonates and infants who underwent surgical repair of TGA. Patients who had low-flow bypass had significantly greater weight gain and positive fluid balance while in the hospital after arterial switch; however this did not translate into a significant impact on duration of mechanical ventilation, intensive care unit stay, or hospital stay [146]. Duration of circulatory arrest was not associated with developmental outcome [143]. However, in a prospective study of infants undergoing arterial switch operation for TGA with or without VSD, circulatory arrest was associated with a higher risk of clinical seizures and overall greater central nervous system disturbance than a

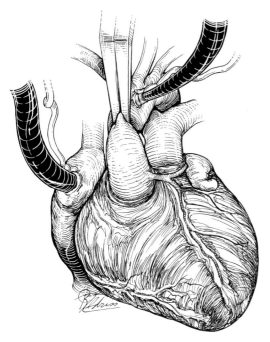

Figure 26.10 Aortouniatrial cardiopulmonary bypass in a patient with transposition of the great arteries with intact ventricular septum. The aorta is cross-clamped in anticipation of blood cardioplegia and great vessel transection. Special attention must be paid to the single atrial catheter position to avoid air introduction.

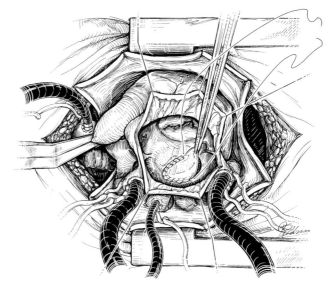

Figure 26.11 The atrial septal defect is repaired using bicaval cardiopulmonary bypass and cardioplegic arrest. Shown here is atrial septal reconstruction using a pericardial patch. Atriorrhaphy is then performed.

strategy of low-flow cardiopulmonary bypass [144]. Assessment at intermediate-term follow-up at 4 years of age and after arterial switch operation showed that the low-flow or circulatory arrest strategy choice and the duration of circulatory arrest did not significantly impact IQ scores or overall neurologic status, but use of circulatory arrest was associated with poorer motor coordination and planning [142]. Interestingly, the performance of the full cohort was below expected in IQ, expressive language, visual-motor integration, motor function, and oromotor control. Further longitudinal studies may help to identify critical factors for successful outcomes in neonates and infants who undergo repair of TGA.

Single venous cannulation does not necessarily require deep hypothermia and circulatory arrest for arterial switch. Low-flow states (0.2–$0.4\,L/min/m^2$) with systemic hypothermia ($22\,^\circ C$) and sucker bypass can be employed for atrial septal defect closure. After atriorrhaphy, single venous drainage can be reinstituted for the remainder of the operation. Three disadvantages of this technique include 1) unwanted air may enter the venous line during the neopulmonary artery reconstruction; 2) undrained atrial blood may enter the right ventricle and cause local myocardial warming during cardioplegic arrest; and 3)

undrained blood may enter the operative field and obscure landmarks and suture lines. We always have used continuous flow techniques with a bias toward bicaval venous cannulation for this operation. The initial extra time required to establish bicaval cannulation allows the surgeon uninterrupted time to perform the neogreat vessel reconstructions free from the inconveniences and potential hazardous episodes of venous line air, myocardial warming, and their attendant problems.

Conduct of Cardiopulmonary Bypass

Cardiopulmonary bypass is established with a standard blood prime, membrane oxygenator, and nonpulsatile perfusion. Flows are calculated at 2.0–$2.5\,L/min/m^2$ with systemic hypothermia ($22\,^\circ C$). Left ventricular drainage is by a 10-F catheter placed via the right superior pulmonary vein. Bicaval cannulation allows right atriotomy for atrial or VSD closure without sucker bypass and prevents venous line air during the reconstruction phase (Figure 26.11) [34]. Low-flow (0.2–$0.4\,L/min/m^2$) is used for short periods during neoaortic reconstruction to decrease venous return as necessary and increased gradually to $2.0\,L/min/m^2$ after myocardial reperfusion. Halfway through the neopulmonary artery reconstruction, the flow is increased further to $2.5\,L/min/m^2$ and the patient is rewarmed to $37\,^\circ C$ for separation from cardiopulmonary bypass.

Myocardial Protection

The evolution of neonatal myocardial protection techniques is based on sound experimental data [100,147–150].

We use antegrade single-dose blood cardioplegia, which in our practice is composed of cardiopulmonary bypass perfusate with 20 mEq/L of potassium chloride, 3 g/L of mannitol, 200 µg/L of nitroglycerin, and 12.5 g/L of albumin. In the event of unforeseen long cross-clamp time, retrograde coronary sinus cardioplegia infusion may be preferable to direct catheter coronary injection [151]. We also bathe the heart with iced saline slush during cardioplegic arrest to augment the benefits of blood cardioplegia [152].

Neoaortic Reconstruction and Coronary Artery Transfer

After aortic cross-clamping and cardioplegia are achieved, great vessel transection, the maneuver of Lecompte, and neoaortic reconstruction are performed. Adjustments for great vessel transection may be necessary based on the lengths of the vessels and their anatomic relationship.

Coronary artery excision from the respective sinuses of Valsalva is performed adjacent to the aortic commissures resulting in a large patch surrounding the coronary ostium, which will facilitate transfer and suture reconstruction (Figure 26.12) [34]. Fine-needle electrocautery and scissors

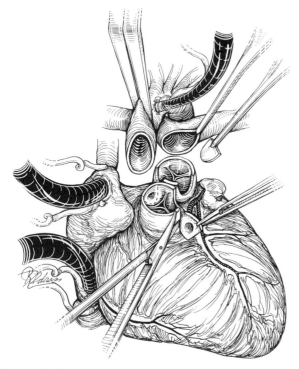

Figure 26.12 Fine scissor excision of the left coronary artery button from its sinus of Valsalva is shown. A liberal amount of aortic wall with the coronary artery is taken to facilitate the transfer to the neoaorta. Care is taken to avoid injury to coronary arteries.

are used to complete the dissection. The utmost care is exercised to avoid coronary injury during this part of the operation. Occasionally a small conal branch may require ligation to create more length for the coronary transfer. We have found, however, that careful and extensive dissection almost always obviates the need for ligation. The maneuver of Lecompte is then performed, translocating the pulmonary artery anterior to the aorta, along with repositioning of the aortic cross-clamp (Figure 26.13) [34]. Some surgeons have advocated side-by-side anatomic great vessel reconstruction [37], but most use the Lecompte maneuver, which minimizes neopulmonary artery tension.

The pulmonary artery–facing sinuses of Valsalva into which the coronary arteries are to be transferred have been prepared by punch excision [37,87,88,91,100,104], partial wall excision [93], and linear incision [79,84,85]. Some [79,153] advocate proximal pulmonary artery-to-distal aortic anastomosis before coronary transfer. This is followed by coronary patch alignment with the blood-filled neoaorta. The aortic clamp is then reapplied for the coronary patch transfer for a presumably more accurate reconstruction. We prefer to perform linear incisions, V-incisions, or U-shaped excisions into the facing sinuses, which allow for liberal excursion of the coronary patches thereby minimizing coronary kinking or obstruction. The coronary patches are placed in a "best lie" position for optimal flow after the reconstruction. The anastomotic lines are performed with running 8-0 monofilament suture (Figure 26.14) [34].

Special Coronary Problems

Anomalies of the coronary circulation in patients with TGA are common and varied [128,133,135,154–158]. In most cases there are two coronary ostia from the aortic sinuses of Valsalva, which favorably face the adjacent pulmonary artery sinuses of Valsalva (Figure 26.15) [159]. Special attention must be paid to coronary arteries arising from the nonfacing sinus (very rare), the single coronary artery, and the intramural coronary artery [39], which can traverse a commissure before emerging from the aortic wall. The rare circumstance of an artery arising from the nonfacing cusp is nontransferable unless prosthetic material or an internal mammary artery graft is used. Under these circumstances an atrial baffle operation may be preferable. The single coronary artery, however, is transferable by a number of techniques [102,130,155,160,161] depending on the anatomic relationships. Yacoub and Radley-Smith (Figure 26.16) [130] and Planche and associates (Figure 26.17) [102] have described methods to transfer the single coronary by the "trap door" technique employing aortic wall flaps for a favorable anastomosis. Sometimes the single coronary patch can be rotated in a "best lie" configuration, which can be managed by the aforementioned suture technique.

A   B

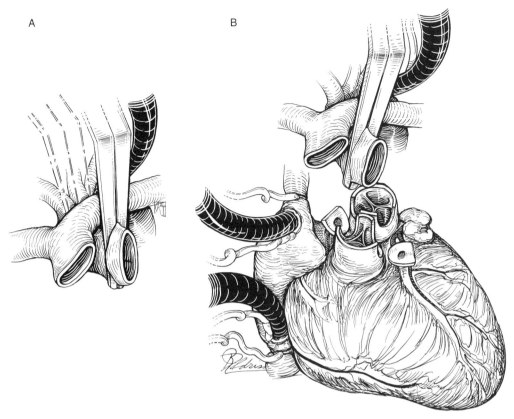

Figure 26.13 A, The maneuver of Lecompte (positioning the pulmonary artery anterior to the aorta) is shown, with aortic cross-clamp repositioning to retract the pulmonary artery during the neoaortic reconstruction. The phantom clamp represents the initial position on the aorta just before the administration of blood cardioplegia. The real clamp represents the new position on the aorta in order to retract the pulmonary artery after the maneuver of Lecompte. **B,** After the maneuver of Lecompte, the coronary artery buttons are mobilized in anticipation of anastomosis to the facing sinuses of the old pulmonary artery. After the reconstruction this will be called the *neoaorta*.

Whatever the circumstances the surgeon must be familiar with all these techniques in order to select the proper reconstruction for optimal coronary flow.

The intramural coronary artery [36,162,163] requires special attention and represents the greatest risk to the patient. The main principles for transfer are to recognize the anatomy before patch excision to avoid coronary transection, to accurately identify the intramural aortic wall entry and exit points, and to sacrifice valvar and commissural tissue in favor of the coronary artery anastomosis since the neopulmonary valve can be resuspended and reconstructed with pericardium to minimize the well tolerated possibility of neopulmonary valvar insufficiency. Oftentimes the orifice of the intramural branch coronary artery will require unroofing to prevent coronary hypoperfusion and resultant myocardial infarction [164,165]. New technical modifications have been introduced including the use of pericardial hoods [166], arterial switch with *in situ* coronary relocation [167], and arterial switch without coronary relocation [168] to meet the challenges of coronary artery anatomy in transposition.

Neopulmonary Artery Reconstruction

The goal of the neopulmonary artery reconstruction is to avoid the development of supravalvar stenosis. This is achieved by pericardial patch augmentation of the dissected sinuses of Valsalva of the old aorta, prevention of pulmonary artery distortion by extensive dissection to both pulmonary hili, and having direct continuity of native distal pulmonary artery and proximal neopulmonary artery for at least a portion of the anastomosis for eventual growth. Many methods have been described. Pacifico and colleagues [100] employed the posterior incision method, which depends on the distal pulmonary artery tissue to fill out the dissected sinuses of Valsalva without resorting to pericardium or graft material. Others [37,81,93,94] have advocated redundant double pericardial patches. We use the single pantaloon pericardial patch technique

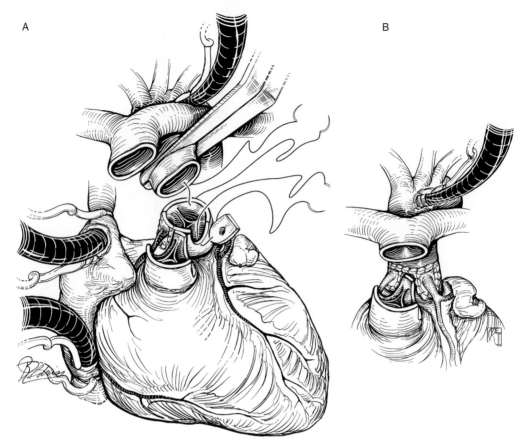

Figure 26.14 A, After the coronary patches are mobilized, they are sutured to the facing sinuses of Valsalva at the old pulmonary artery (neoaorta). **B,** Neoaortic reconstruction is completed with the end-to-end anastomosis between the proximal neoaorta and the ascending aorta. Coronary artery reperfusion is established after the cross-clamp is removed.

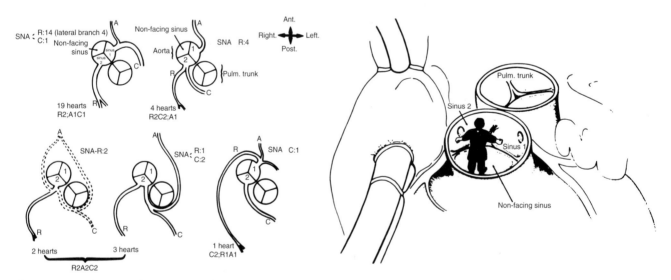

Figure 26.15 These two drawings show the convention for naming the aortic sinuses by Gittenberger-de Groot and colleagues. On the right, the two sinuses of the aorta face two sinuses of the pulmonary trunk and the third sinus is nonfacing. The figure in the diagram is standing in the nonfacing sinus and looking toward the pulmonary trunk. The coronary sinus to the right is sinus 1 and that to the left is sinus 2. On the left, the four patterns of coronary artery origin, including the origins of the sinus node artery (SNA) in each pattern, are noted. In all, the sinus node artery arose from the right coronary artery (R) in 25 hearts and from the circumflex artery (C) in three hearts. The coronary artery patterns are described using a simple system that takes into account the origins of the right coronary artery, the circumflex artery, and the anterior descending coronary artery (A) from either sinus 1 or sinus 2. The designation R2;A1C1, for example, describes the origin of the right coronary artery from sinus 2 and the latter two arteries from sinus 1. (Reproduced with permission from Rossi *et al.* [159].)

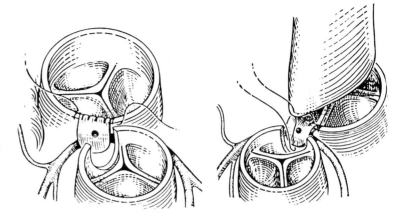

Figure 26.16 Yacoub's method of single coronary artery transfer. The coronary patch is turned 180 degrees and sutured upsidedown to the neoaorta. The distal aorta and the proximal aorta are then anastomosed to facilitate flow and avoid coronary obstruction. (Reproduced with permission from Yacoub *et al.* [130].)

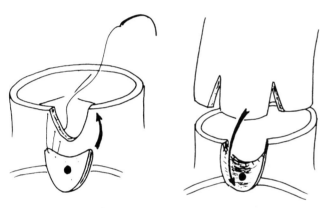

Figure 25.17 Planché's method of single coronary artery transfer. After the 180-degree coronary patch turn, a "trap door" is constructed at the distal aorta to form the neoaortic reconstruction without coronary kinking. (Reproduced with permission from Planché *et al.* [102].)

(Figure 26.18) [34,79,84,85]. A generous redundant pericardial patch is recommended without glutaraldehyde pretreatment. This method also allows the option of added posterior length, which may facilitate the repair and avoid coronary artery compression. The anterior portions of the distal pulmonary artery and the neopulmonary artery are always primarily anastomosed to allow for proportional growth.

Reconstruction of the neopulmonary artery for patients with Taussig-Bing anomaly or TGA with VSD and coarctation represents a significant challenge because of the associated small aorta, which is to become the neopulmonary artery. Hirata *et al.* [169] recently reviewed their experience with 51 patients and found that neonatal single-stage repair for TGA/coarctation achieves excellent survival without transannular patch at first operation. Although some of those patients had pressure gradients across the neo-RVOT, these lesions were amenable to reintervention in a small number of patients and with minimal morbidity. Sinzobahamvya and associates [170] advocate subaortic (subpulmonary artery) resection to treat this problem.

Separation from Cardiopulmonary Bypass and Postoperative Care

Separation from cardiopulmonary bypass is preceded by a careful evaluation of anastomotic suture lines and coronary perfusion. Coronary insufficiency can be suspected by qualitative regional wall dysfunction, high dose pressor requirements, and persistent ischemic electrocardiographic changes. In some cases filling of the heart during separation from cardiopulmonary bypass may result in coronary stretching, kinking, or occlusion. Other causes of coronary obstruction are neopulmonary artery compression, coronary malrotation, and intimal dissection. Corrective measures can be employed after reinstitution of cardiopulmonary bypass, including coronary pericardial patch augmentation [94], pulmonary artery suspension to treat coronary artery compression, and internal mammary artery grafting to the affected coronary artery [171]. Rarely extracorporeal membrane oxygenation (ECMO) may be necessary to support the stunned myocardium until recovery [172]. In general this form of circulatory support is most successful if the affected patient has had a period of circulatory stability before decompensation. It is important to correct the original problems that led to hemodynamic instability if a successful outcome is to be achieved.

The great majority of patients are separated from cardiopulmonary bypass with dobutamine (5µg/kg/min), dopamine (5µg/kg/min), and milrinone (.5µg/kg/min). Under these circumstances the patient's blood pressure can be expected to range between 65 and 85mmHg systolic with a wide pulse pressure and excellent peripheral perfusion. Drug doses may vary to achieve optimal levels of cardiac output, afterload reduction, and organ perfusion.

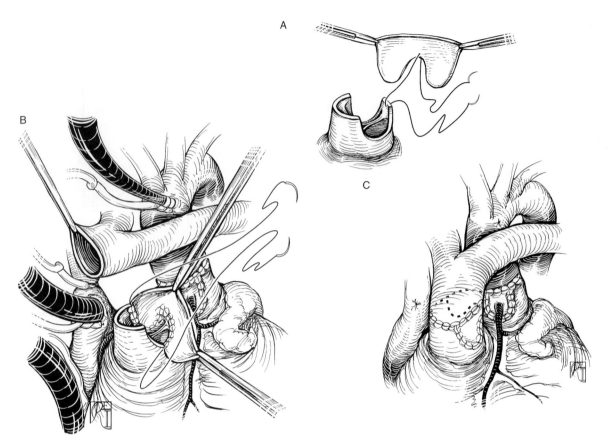

Figure 26.18 A, The "pantaloon" pericardial patch is shown being oriented to the old aorta (neopulmonary artery). **B,** During the rewarming stage the pantaloon pericardial patch can be sutured to the sinuses of Valsalva, thereby filling out the neopulmonary artery. **C,** The completed anastomosis is shown after separation from cardiopulmonary bypass.

Once hemodynamic stability has been ascertained, we employ a 10-minute period of modified ultrafiltration [173,174], which can be expected to yield 200–400 mL of transudate. This procedure was initially thought to remove myocardial depressant factors and harmful cytokines from the circulation, thereby enhancing myocardial performance. The more likely mechanism is that modified ultrafiltration has the effect of increasing the hematocrit and concentrating the pressor agents so that the effective doses in circulation tend to be higher. This allows for an elective decrease in pressor agents to achieve optimal hemodynamics. After sternal closure and transfer to the pediatric intensive care unit, repeated physical examination noting fontanelle fullness, liver edge level, strength of peripheral pulses, capillary filling time, and hourly urinary output will guide postoperative care. Ventilatory support is adjusted to maintain adequate oxygenation and mild respiratory alkalosis. The weaning process can then be started on the day following surgery or sooner if the program has instituted an early extubation policy.

Results and Analysis

The mid- and long-term survival rates of patients who had arterial switch for TGA are encouraging [103,106,108]. In the latest communication from the Congenital Heart Surgeons Society, 513 infants underwent an arterial switch repair [97]. The 1-month, 1-year, and 5-year survival rates were 84%, 82%, and 82%, respectively. Identified risk factors for death include origin of the left main coronary artery or only the left anterior descending or circumflex artery from the right posterior sinus (even stronger when an intramural course was present), multiple VSDs, longer global myocardial ischemic time, and total circulatory arrest time. Certain institutions were risk factors for death; with increasing experience, results improved in some centers while in others they worsened. These results were sustained in a follow-up study from the same cohort of patients [175].

Numerous other reports from large institutions have confirmed these results [79,102–104,106,108,176–185]. Supravalvar pulmonary stenosis was more likely in the early experience with arterial switch but became less prevalent after conversion to the autologous pantaloon-shaped pericardial patch to fill out the dissected sinuses of Valsalva of the neopulmonary artery [85]. Myocardial ischemia owing to coronary insufficiency is still the most common cause of perioperative death but has been decreasing with improved myocardial preservation and techniques for coronary transfer. Normal sinus rhythm is present in the vast majority of patients (>95%) and neoaortic regurgitation, when present (5–10%), is mild and nonprogressive.

The arterial switch operation for neonates with TGA and intact ventricular septum can be performed with a <5% operative mortality at most centers. The repair results in both anatomic and physiologic correction and appears to offer great expectations for excellent long-term results. Postoperative complications associated with the atrial baffle operations, which include atrial arrhythmias, ventricular dysfunction, and baffle obstructions, have been virtually eliminated. Moreover the incidence of anastomotic strictures, neoaortic insufficiency, and supravalvar pulmonary stenosis with the arterial switch operation has been quite low. Consequently the arterial switch operation for neonates with TGA and intact ventricular septum is the procedure of choice.

Arterial Switch and Ventricular Septal Defect Closure for Transposition of the Great Arteries and Ventricular Septal Defect

Arterial switch for TGA and intact ventricular septum required a learning curve for surgeons to achieve the survival statistics of the atrial baffle procedures [112]. Not so with arterial switch for TGA and VSD. The mortality rate for the atrial baffle procedures combined with VSD closure was so high (>21%) [109,186] that the initial reports by Jatene *et al.* (16% mortality) [37] and Pacifico and colleagues (0% mortality) [100] quickly established arterial switch and VSD closure as the procedure of choice and provided a more optimistic future for these patients who have become virtually free from the complications of arrhythmias, right ventricular failure, and late death.

With increasing experience, patient selection and timing of the operation have evolved. Initially arterial switch and VSD closure were delayed until 2–18 months of age while patients were treated medically or surgically (pulmonary artery band) for excessive pulmonary blood flow. Recently the trend has shifted toward earlier intervention. Bove [187] reported 12 infants (mean age, 19 days) with TGA and large VSD undergoing arterial switch and VSD closure with one early death and no late deaths. It appears that the limiting factor for early repair is patient size. The surgeon

may elect to perform pulmonary artery banding with subsequent anatomic repair at a later date in low-birthweight neonates.

Over the last 25 years the clinical results for arterial switch and VSD closure have been excellent [188]. Increasing experience and familiarity with the operation has resulted in earlier intervention without pulmonary artery banding. Likewise, there was a change from staged repair in those patients with coarctation or interrupted aortic arch to transmediastinal one-stage repair using extended end-to-end aortic anastomoses in addition to arterial switch and VSD closure.

Current Approach

The operative procedure for TGA and VSD is similar to that previously described with the obvious additional need for VSD closure. Aortobicaval cannulation is established to maximize exposure for right atrial, transpulmonary, or transaortic access to the VSD. We recommend that VSD closure be performed before the arterial switch. This is important as the neoaortic reconstruction cannot be disrupted by the retraction maneuvers required for intracardiac exposure of the VSD. Experimental studies [189,190] have supported the practice of cardioplegic arrest or reperfusion and subsequent cardioplegic arrest when used under these clinical conditions. Alternatively, multiple administrations of retrograde cardioplegia can be performed.

Our usual approach to VSD closure is transatrial (Figure 26.19) [34], but can also be through the pulmonary artery

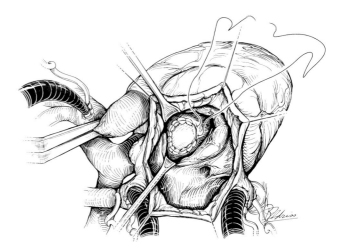

Figure 26.19 After arterial and bicaval venous cannulation, the ventricular septal defect is approached and closed through the right atrium under blood cardioplegic arrest. Running suture technique usually is performed. Alternatively, interrupted pledget-supported sutures can be used.

(Figure 26.20) [34] or the aorta when convenient. In our series of 28 patients, eight VSDs were closed through the pulmonary artery, 20 were closed through the right atrium, and none required ventriculotomy.

Many authors have reported excellent results with the arterial switch and VSD closure. Quaegebeur *et al.* [104] reported an 18% operative mortality rate in 1986, which was supported by the Congenital Heart Surgeons Society report [97] showing a 6–13% mortality rate at seven designated low-risk institutions. Reports by Yamaguchi and colleagues [191] and Planche *et al.* [192] showed that the arterial switch and VSD closure could be performed safely in neonatal and early infant time periods. The Society of Thoracic Surgeons National Congenital Heart Surgery Database Report revealed an overall mortality rate of 6.2% (22 deaths in 355 patients) in patients undergoing arterial switch for repair of TGA [193]. In the subgroup with TGA and VSD, the mortality rate was 6.3% (7 deaths in 111 patients) [193]. Follow-up studies [182,184] have confirmed the increased incidence of early mortality in patients with TGA and VSD when compared with mortality for arterial switch in patients with TGA and intact ventricular septum.

Staged Repair of Transposition of the Great Arteries with Intact Ventricular Septum

There are occasions when for one reason or another infants present late after the neonatal period when left ventricular pressure is low owing to decreased pulmonary vascular resistance. Under these circumstances a staged repair may be performed for ventricular training to induce left ventricular hypertrophy for adequate postoperative systemic circulatory support [194]. The staged repair, consisting of pulmonary artery banding, systemic-to-pulmonary artery shunt, and subsequent anatomic repair, was first described by Yacoub and colleagues in 1977 [112]. In our series of patients who have had an arterial switch, staged repair was more common among the earlier cases [195] owing to late referral or changing management (atrial switch to arterial switch) in older patients.

Surgical guidelines and techniques for left ventricular preparation at our institution have been previously published [86]. The exposure has changed from a left thoracotomy to a median sternotomy, which offers better exposure (Figure 26.21) [34]. The initial postoperative evaluation is determined by echocardiographic assessment of left ventricular wall thickness. Repeat cardiac catheterization is then performed before the arterial switch to measure

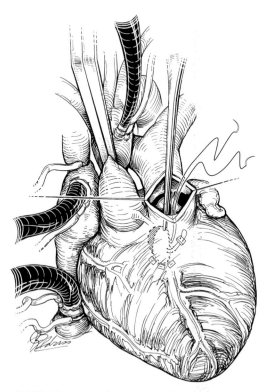

Figure 26.20 Diagrammatic representation of transposition of the great arteries and subpulmonic ventricular septal defect. The ventricular septal defect is closed with a Dacron patch and interrupted pledget-supported sutures through the pulmonary artery exposure.

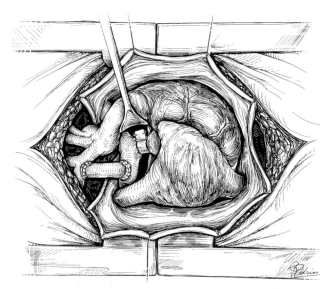

Figure 26.21 Diagrammatic representation of pulmonary artery band with a polytetrafluoroethylene systemic-to-pulmonary artery shunt for left ventricular training in preparation for arterial switch. With the band positioned but not tightened, a standard 5-mm modified Blalock-Taussig shunt (4 mm if infant's weight is <2.5 kg) is performed. The systemic blood pressure is monitored as the band is tightened sequentially until the proximal pulmonary artery approaches two thirds of the systemic pressure or until the oxygen saturation drops below 85%.

ventricular volumes, ejection fraction, and left ventricular muscle mass. Conditions favorable to successful arterial switch are 1) left ventricular wall thickness as indicated by echocardiography normal for the patient's age; 2) left ventricular to right ventricular pressure ratio greater than 70%; and 3) left ventricular volume and muscle mass normal for age.

Recent reports have advocated extending the boundaries of primary arterial switch operation in patients with TGA and intact ventricular septum outside the usual 2-week limit after birth [196,197] to as long as 2–3 months of age. This strategy has the advantage of eliminating preparatory pulmonary artery banding and systemic-pulmonary shunt, which is associated with pulmonary valve (neoaortic valve) dilatation and resultant neoaortic insufficiency after arterial switch. Adapting late arterial switch without left ventricular training, however, may lead to a period of mechanical support after arterial switch during which adaptation of the left ventricle takes place [198].

Arterial Switch Operation for Double-Outlet Right Ventricle and Subpulmonary Ventricular Septal Defect (Taussig-Bing Anomaly)

Taussig and Bing [15] first described an anatomic variation of TGA and VSD in a 5-year-old girl with a complex congenital cardiac malformation in which the aorta and pulmonary artery arose entirely from the right ventricle with the pulmonary artery overriding a VSD. This was redefined by Van Praagh [199] as a double-outlet right ventricle with semilunar valves side-by-side, a bilateral conus, and a subpulmonic VSD. Lev [200] expanded this definition to describe a spectrum of four types of hearts including the right-sided type without an overriding pulmonary trunk, the right-sided type with an overriding pulmonary trunk, an intermediate type, and the left-sided type.

A variety of operations have been used to repair the Taussig-Bing anomaly. Initial attempts at repair were aimed at anatomic correction to preserve left ventricular to aortic continuity, first described by Patrick and McGoon in 1968 [201]. This operation was refined by Kawashima *et al.* in 1971 [202], who described a similar intraventricular repair but emphasized the need for resection of the conal septum to avoid subaortic and subpulmonic stenosis. This technique may require enlargement of the VSD, tricuspid papillary muscle transfer, and/or an external valved conduit [203]. Experience with this repair is somewhat limited: Harvey and colleagues [204] reported four patients with one survivor; Kirklin *et al.* [205] reported nine patients, most of whom had external conduits, with no operative mortality and four late deaths; and Yacoub and Radley-Smith [206] reported two successful cases. We have used this intraventricular tunnel from the left ventricle to the

aorta successfully in four patients with side-by-side great vessel orientation [207]. In all cases the right ventricle-to-pulmonary artery continuity was restored without a conduit. Adequate conal septum resection was of paramount importance. Yacoub and Radley-Smith [206] and Van Praagh [208] have suggested that this repair should be limited to patients with side-by-side great vessels and should not be used for those with anteroposterior relationship of the great arteries who should have arterial switch and VSD closure instead.

Another therapeutic alternative was first described by Hightower and colleagues in 1968 [209] and later applied by others [204,205,210–213]. These authors performed VSD closure to establish right ventricular-to-aortic and left ventricular-to-pulmonary artery continuity that was accompanied by an atrial baffle procedure with variable results. However successful the initial results, these patients are still left with a physiologic but nonanatomic correction, which subjects them to the known complications of the atrial baffle procedures.

There are some patients with the Taussig-Bing anomaly in whom mitral straddling with abnormal valvar attachments to the crest of the VSD occurs. This group was identified as the left-sided or intermediate type [214]. Under these circumstances closure of the subpulmonic VSD and either arterial switch or atrial baffle may lead to death from subvalvar neoaortic obstruction and left ventricular failure. Preoperative evaluation and intraoperative confirmation can determine accurately the anatomy of the mitral valve attachments and their relationship to the VSD. If unfavorable anatomy is found, an atrial baffle operation, closure of the VSD, and a left ventricle-to-pulmonary artery conduit can be performed.

A third approach to the Taussig-Bing heart employs a modification of the technique described by Damus and coworkers [215], Stansel [216], and Kaye [217]. In this procedure the VSD is closed to connect the left ventricle to the pulmonary artery. The pulmonary trunk is divided, and the proximal pulmonary artery is connected end-to-side to the ascending aorta. A valved extracardiac conduit is then placed from the right ventricle to the distal pulmonary artery [218,219]. Ceithaml *et al.* reported four patients with three survivors [220]. Although this procedure has the advantage of left ventricle-to-aorta continuity, it has the disadvantage of requiring an extracardiac conduit, and the attendant problems of multiple conduit changes during a lifetime.

The fourth choice for repair of the Taussig-Bing anomaly is VSD closure and arterial switch, which was first reported by Freedom *et al.* in 1981 [82] and by Yacoub and Radley-Smith in 1984 [206]. Our early experience with the Taussig-Bing anomaly relied on preparatory palliative operations before arterial switch and VSD closure. The initial survival was excellent but several patients required late neoaortic valve replacements, recoarctation repair, and pulmonary outflow procedures [165,188]. Our more recent experience favors transmediastinal one-stage repair to perform arterial switch and VSD closure with or without coarctation repair and arch augmentation (see Chapter 25, *Double-Outlet Ventricles*).

Other authors [104,192,221] have had similar favorable results. An association between coarctation and Taussig-Bing anatomy has been noted previously by Parr and colleagues [222]. In their review of 105 Taussig-Bing heart patients, coarctation and/or aortic outflow tract obstruction was noted in 56 (53%); six of nine surgically treated for Taussig-Bing heart also had coarctation of the aorta.

This combined surgical experience shows that an arterial switch can be performed successfully for patients with both side-by-side and anteroposterior orientation of the great vessels, although Quaegebeur [223] cautioned that the Lecompte maneuver may not be helpful when the great arteries are side by side. In some cases it may be easier to slide the redundant pulmonary artery behind the new aorta for a direct anastomosis. He also noted that the coronary artery anatomy in the Taussig-Bing anomaly is similar to that in classic TGA. The same principles for coronary artery transfer therefore can be applied.

The arterial switch and VSD closure for the Taussig-Bing anomaly have distinct advantages of low mortality, anatomic and physiologic connections, no need for extracardiac conduits, and applicability to most patients despite the variability in coronary anatomy and great vessel orientation [224].

Staged Arterial Switch Operation for Right Ventricular Failure After the Atrial Baffle Procedures

Right ventricular failure after an atrial baffle procedure can occur in up to 10% of patients in the long-term [225] and more if patients had an associated VSD [76]. Nearly all of these have associated severe tricuspid insufficiency with varying amounts of pulmonary hypertension [226]. Surgical options for these patients include tricuspid valve replacement, staged conversion to arterial switch, and cardiac transplantation. Our experience with tricuspid valve replacement has been dismal. Of six patients who had tricuspid valve replacement for right ventricular dysfunction and tricuspid insufficiency, four died, one had subsequent cardiac transplantation, and only one had a good hemodynamic result. These results indicate that tricuspid insufficiency in these patients is a manifestation of right ventricular failure for which valve replacement has few beneficial effects. The preferable alternatives appear to be staged conversion to arterial switch or orthotopic cardiac transplantation.

Staged conversion of an atrial baffle procedure to arterial switch was first performed and reported by Mee [227] in

12 patients with the idea that pulmonary artery banding could induce left ventricular mass development in preparation for subsequent takedown of the atrial baffle, takedown of the pulmonary artery band, and an arterial switch. Twelve patients underwent pulmonary artery banding with two deaths from this procedure alone. Six patients subsequently had conversion to arterial switch with two deaths, and three patients underwent orthotopic cardiac transplantation with one late death. In a later series from the same center [228], 12 patients with failed atrial switch were reported, of whom nine proceeded to arterial switch operation with Senning or Mustard takedown and atrial resepation. There were two postoperative deaths and one patient underwent cardiac transplantation 3 months after surgery. Others [229–231] have performed arterial switch without preparatory pulmonary artery banding in selected patients with pulmonary venous obstruction complicating a Mustard procedure. Left ventricular retraining was serendipitous as a consequence of pulmonary venous obstruction; systemic level pressure was present in the pulmonary ventricle and provided the opportunity to perform a one-stage arterial switch successfully.

Our experience [232] with staged conversion is limited to 11 patients who underwent 15 preparatory pulmonary artery banding procedures: four eventually had orthotopic cardiac transplantation for biventricular failure; six had an arterial switch procedure (atrial arrhythmias were treated concomitantly in two patients with cryoablation techniques). There were two early deaths (33%) and no late deaths in the six patients who underwent arterial switch operation. There were no early deaths in the transplanted patients and one late death 7 years after transplant from chronic rejection. The two deaths in the arterial switch group were related to an untransferred paracommissural coronary artery in one patient with resultant myocardial infarction and unanticipated postoperative left ventricular dysfunction in another patient secondary to presumed inadequate left ventricular hypertrophy. Postmortem examination revealed the left ventricular posterior wall had 7 mm of muscle and 3 mm of fibrous tissue, not 10 mm of muscle. One patient awaits arterial switch conversion.

Staged conversion from atrial baffle to arterial switch begins with the pulmonary artery banding to achieve proximal pulmonary artery pressure equal to 75% of the aortic or right ventricular pressure. Pressor support and mechanical ventilation usually are required for the first few days. Postoperative surveillance is performed by serial echocardiography and cardiac catheterization to determine left ventricular volume, pressure, and muscle mass. When these parameters are close to normal for the child's age, the child undergoes an arterial switch. The arterial switch technique is performed in the usual manner after atrial baffle takedown (Figures 26.22–26.24) [88], pulmonary artery band removal, and proper coronary artery identification.

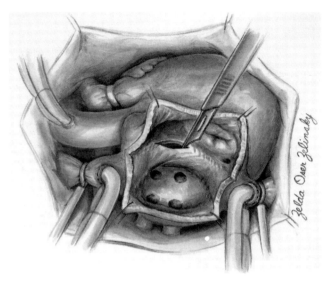

Figure 26.22 Atrial view of the Mustard pericardial baffle. Lines of incision and scalpel show the technique at baffle excision. (Reproduced with permission from Mavroudis *et al.* [88].)

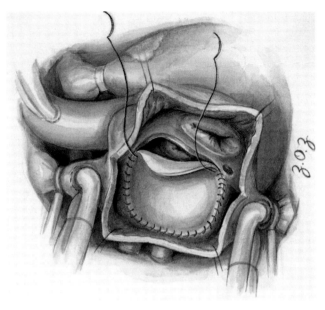

Figure 26.24 Atrial septation with polytetrafluoroethylene to reconstruct the right and left atria anatomically and physiologically. (Reproduced with permission from Mavroudis *et al.* [88].)

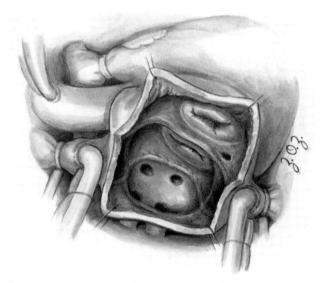

Figure 26.23 Diagrammatic representation of the common atrium after pericardial baffle excision. (Reproduced with permission from Mavroudis *et al.* [88].)

We found that an extension graft is necessary to provide continuity between the proximal neopulmonary artery and the distal pulmonary artery because of inadequate pulmonary artery length caused by dense scarring from the multiple procedures. Severe right ventricular dysfunction after an atrial baffle procedure for TGA does not improve after tricuspid valve replacement. Staged conversion to the arterial switch can improve right ventricular function and provide anatomic repair with left ventricle-to-aorta continuity. Orthotopic cardiac transplantation may be the only

alternative if the left ventricle does not respond to pulmonary artery banding.

Late Complications and Reoperations Following the Arterial Switch Operation

Acquired Supravalvar Pulmonary Stenosis

Theoretical long-term complications after successful arterial switch include great vessel anastomotic constriction, neoaortic valvar insufficiency, and coronary insufficiency. These complications have manifest over time, requiring interventions in a small percentage of patients [165,188,232]. The most common cause for reoperation early on in the collective experience has been supravalvar pulmonic stenosis. Yacoub *et al.* [110] first recognized this problem (1982), which has since been confirmed by others [104,110,233,234]. Several groups [104,110,234] have documented residual right ventricular-to-pulmonary artery pressure gradients mostly caused by constrictions at the supravalvar anastomotic site, presumably resulting from pericardial patch constriction, anastomotic tension, or suture purse-string. Supravalvar pulmonary artery stenosis can also occur more peripherally owing to inadequate dissection or unfavorable anatomy as a result of the maneuver of Lecompte [91]. With increasing experience [130,233,235] acquired pulmonary artery stenosis has been quite low (<10%) and does not appreciably change over time. A single pantaloon patch of fresh autologous pericardium is the preferred method of neopulmonary artery reconstruction [84] and in contrast to earlier reports [104,235] side-by-side great vessel anatomic configuration did not affect coronary transfer or future incidence of pulmonary stenosis. The Congenital Heart Surgeons Society Transposition Study has underlined these findings, showing a low incidence of supravalvar pulmonary stenosis (6%).

We have reoperated on only six patients for pulmonary stenosis in our combined series of patients [165,188]. We attribute these results to the use of large pericardial patches (early in the series) and a single large pantaloon pericardial patch (later in the series) to fill out the dissected sinuses of Valsalva of the neopulmonary artery. When required, reoperation should be uncomplicated (Figure 26.25) [34]. The multiple refinements with neopulmonary artery reconstruction have fulfilled their theoretical expectations. More information will become available as these children grow into adulthood.

Postoperative Arrhythmias

It was initially thought that atrial and ventricular arrhythmias, which were frequently seen with the atrial baffle operations, would not occur in patients who had arterial switch. Longer follow-up and critical review, however, have uncovered several physiologic and anatomic problems leading many authors to recommend lifelong surveillance. Hayashi and associates [236] noted a small but measurable incidence of late-onset atrial and ventricular arrhythmias in TGA patients treated with arterial switch, especially in those who had associated VSD closure. Angeli et al. [237] identified RVOT obstruction, coronary artery obstructions, and neoaortic root dilation with neoaortic insufficiency as rare causes for reoperation. These same themes have been highlighted by others involving coronary obstructions and neoaortic regurgitation [238–241]. It is clear that patients who have had arterial switch for TGA will require lifelong follow-up for rare but identifiable complications [125].

Neoaortic Insufficiency and Neoaortic Anastomotic Stenosis

Early angiographic and echocardiographic evaluation [127,130,234,242] has not demonstrated significant supravalvar neoaortic stenosis. There is also a low incidence of

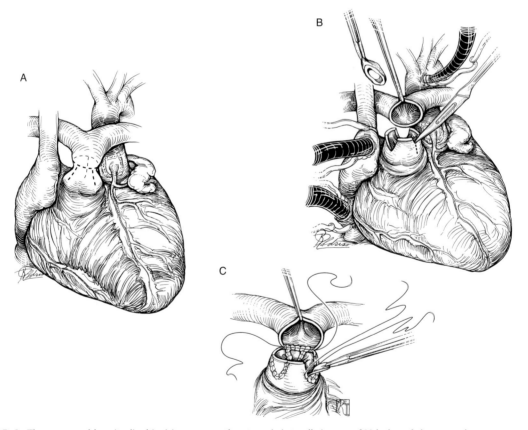

Figure 26.25 A, The proposed longitudinal incisions across the stenosis into all sinuses of Valsalva of the neopulmonary artery are shown. **B,** The supravalvar stenotic area is excised and incisions are made into the respective sinuses of Valsalva. **C,** Pericardial or synthetic patches are sutured into the enlarged sinuses of Valsalva; this is followed by neopulmonary artery reconstruction.

neoaortic valvar insufficiency, which when present usually does not progress [78,243]. We also have found a low incidence of neoaortic valvar insufficiency in our patients, resulting in 12 patients who had neoaortic valvuloplasty or replacement. Some of these patients required further reoperations resulting from failed valvuloplasty procedures or somatic growth [165]. Many of these patients had a pulmonary artery band before the arterial switch or complex arterial switch associated with VSD, aortic interruption, or Taussig-Bing anomaly. The speculation is strong that pulmonary artery banding under these circumstances causes proximal pulmonary artery and annular dilatation that can lead to neoaortic insufficiency after arterial switch [237–241]. The trend away from the use of pulmonary artery banding should help to minimize this problem in the future. However there will be patients who require pulmonary artery banding such as those born with low birthweight, those with low left ventricular mass, and those with right ventricular failure after atrial baffle. Care must be taken to minimize the time between the pulmonary artery banding and the arterial switch to avoid the annular dilatation effects of the pulmonary artery band. Technical aspects of neoaortic valve operations require extensive exposure of the neoaorta, which can be quite challenging in light of the preexisting Lecompte maneuver. We have found that proximal right pulmonary artery transection and main neopulmonary artery retraction results in excellent exposure of both the neoaortic valve and transferred coronary arteries. Figure 26.26 [165] demonstrates the exposure for neoaortic valvuloplasty (David operation). Because the neoaortic valve repair/replacement occupies more space, an interposition graft is placed between the main neopulmonary trunk and the distal right pulmonary artery (Figure 26.26E) [165].

Coronary Artery Problems

The most common cause of acute failure of the arterial switch operation is coronary artery obstruction caused by anastomotic problems, anatomic subtypes, and intramural courses. With increasing experience involving thorough coronary dissection, mobilization, and accurate coronary button transfer to the neoaorta, the incidence of acute coronary insufficiency has decreased. Long-term ischemic complications, however, have been reported [125,165], which have required proximal aortacoronary artery patch arterioplasty (using pericardium or a harvested pulmonary artery wall graft) and/or internal thoracic to coronary artery bypass grafts (Figure 26.27) [165]. It is not always known, preoperatively, whether proximal arterioplasty will treat the problem, leaving authors [125] to use both strategies to ensure revascularization.

Recently, we had experience [165] with an 18-year-old male patient who had an uncomplicated neonatal switch operation for TGA and intact ventricular septum. At the time of the arterial switch operation, an intramural coronary was transferred without being unroofed. Eighteen years later, he suffered an ischemic cardiac arrest, resuscitation using ECMO, and eventual reoperation to unroof the intramural course of the coronary artery (Figure 26.28) [165]. Postoperative CT scan (Figure 26.29) [165] reveals an excellent result; moreover he retained neurologic and myocardial function despite undergoing a below-the-knee amputation as a result of ECMO. This experience further underlines the idea that coronary unroofing should be performed at the initial operation.

Damus-Stansel-Kaye Procedure

As noted previously, an alternative anatomic and physiologic correction for patients with TGA was suggested by Damus [244], Stansel [216], and Kaye [217] and subsequently successfully applied by Danielson and colleagues [245] and Damus *et al.* [215]. Unlike the arterial switch operation the coronary arteries are not transferred to a neoaorta. Instead flow from the left ventricle to the aorta is established by connecting the proximal cut-end portion of the pulmonary artery end-to-side into the ascending aorta. The right ventricle is connected to the distal pulmonary artery by a valved conduit. The VSD, if present, can be closed through the right ventriculotomy in the usual fashion without an internal baffle. The aortic valve, which still arises from the right ventricle, is kept closed by the aortic pressure, which is greater than the right ventricular pressure. This procedure has been especially useful in patients who are undergoing staged conversion from atrial baffle procedure to systemic correction because dense adhesions after multiple operations may prohibit coronary transfer and arterial switch [246]. Others have used this approach for patients with Taussig-Bing anomaly with good results. The disadvantages of this operation are 1) the fate of the aortic valve, which is situated over the right ventricle in a static closed position and is subject to leaking and clot formation; and 2) the obvious need for periodic conduit changes as the child grows.

TGA, VSD, and Pulmonary Stenosis

The therapeutic alternatives for patients with TGA, VSD, and pulmonary stenosis are dependent on the severity and type of pulmonary stenosis and the size and location of the VSD. The more severe the pulmonary stenosis and the smaller the VSD, the earlier in life that cyanosis is detected. Several treatment options for these patients center on the initial palliative options and the corrective operations are generally performed later in life. If the patients show symptoms of severe cyanosis, a systemic-to-pulmonary artery shunt and balloon or surgical septectomy may be

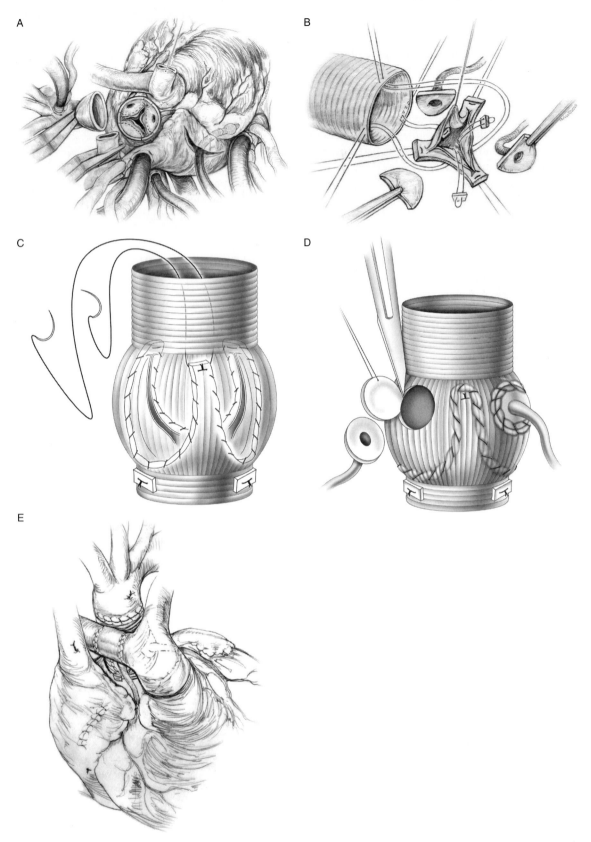

Figure 26.26 Neoaortic valve-sparing operation as modified after the David procedure. **A,** Neoaortic exposure after right pulmonary artery transection, main neopulmonary artery retraction, cardioplegic arrest, and neoaortic transection. The dotted lines represent incisions that allow dissection of the coronary artery buttons and the noncoronary sinus of Valsalva neoaortic wall. **B,** Pledgeted sutures placed at the neoaortic annulus equidistant between the commissures and passed through the Dacron graft, which allow seating over the neoaorta. Coronary artery buttons are liberally dissected for later implantation. **C,** The seated Dacron graft. Hemostatic sutures within the graft are used to complete the reconstruction. **D,** The creation of orifices in the Dacron graft with coronary artery reimplantation. **E,** The operation is completed with a Gore-Tex interposition tube graft to reconstruct the right pulmonary artery. (Reproduced with permission from Mavroudis *et al.* [165].)

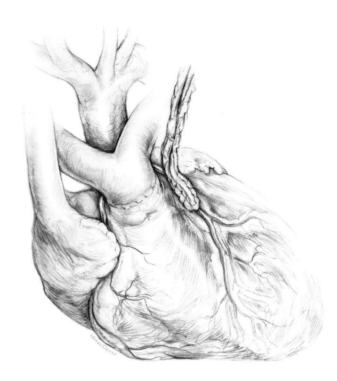

Figure 26.27 Internal thoracic artery (ITA) to left anterior descending coronary artery (LAD) bypass in a patient who had an arterial switch operation and Lecompte maneuver. The bypass graft is placed in the proximal third of the LAD where the luminal diameter of the artery is most likely to be larger. (Reproduced with permission from Mavroudis *et al.* [165].)

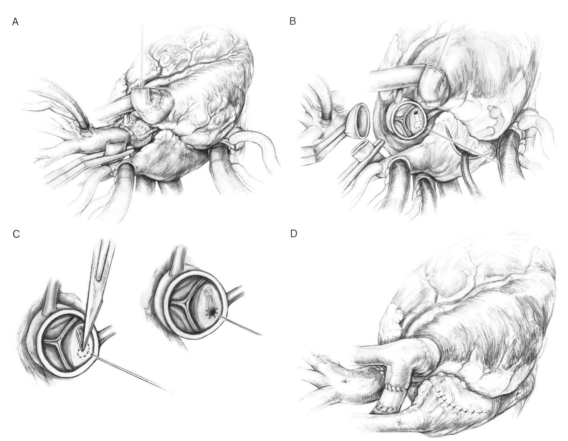

A

B

C

D

Figure 26.28 A, Aortic root exposure by right pulmonary artery transection and proximal neopulmonary artery retraction in a patient who had transfer of an intramural coronary artery and presented 18 years postoperatively with acute myocardial infarction and cardiac arrest. The dotted line represents the intramural course. **B,** After antegrade and retrograde cardioplegic arrest, the neoaorta is transected and the intramural coronary artery is visualized. **C,** A scalpel unroofs the intramural coronary artery and individual sutures are placed to reapproximate the coronary and neoaortic intimal layers. **D,** The operation is completed with a Gore-Tex interposition tube graft to reconstruct the right pulmonary artery, thereby avoiding proximal neoaortic constriction and right pulmonary artery tension. (Reproduced with permission from Mavroudis *et al.* [165].)

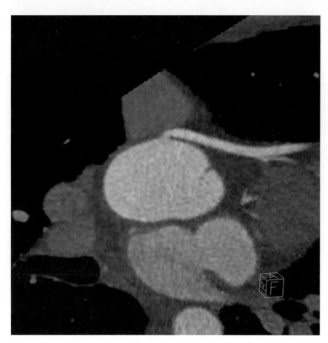

Figure 26.29 Computed tomographic scan showing postoperative unroofing of the previously transferred intramural coronary artery of an 18-year-old patient. (Reproduced with permission from Mavroudis *et al.* [165].)

necessary to increase mixing. Others with a more balanced combination of defects may do well for months without palliation.

The classic corrective procedure for these patients has been the Rastelli operation (Figure 26.30) [34,51], which diverts left ventricular flow via an intraventricular baffle to the aorta and establishes right ventricular-to-pulmonary artery continuity by a valved conduit. Ideally the VSD should be large and doubly committed to avoid the development of baffle-induced subaortic stenosis. Occasionally intraventricular alterations must be performed to ensure adequate left ventricular-to-aortic flow, including 1) enlargement of the VSD; 2) subaortic muscle resection; and 3) reattachment of obstructive tricuspid papillary muscles. Because of these possibilities most surgeons prefer to delay this procedure until after 6–12 months of life, performing palliative procedures as necessary in the early stages of life. Mortality rates between 10% and 29% [247–249] have been reported for the initial procedure. However, statistics for long-term survival show a continued risk of death owing to reoperations for conduit stenosis and left ventricular dysfunction in some patients.

In an effort to decrease the subsequent operations required for conduit replacements, Lecompte introduced a method to reconstruct the pulmonary outflow tract without a prosthetic conduit [52], which he termed the REV proce-

dure [250]. The procedure is comprised of 1) infundibular resection to enlarge the VSD; 2) intraventricular baffle to direct left ventricular flow to the aorta; 3) aortic transection in order to perform the maneuver of Lecompte; and 4) direct pulmonary artery to right ventricular reconstruction using an anterior patch (Figures 26.31 and 26.32) [34]. Lecompte reported on 50 patients (4 months to 15 years, mean 3.8 years) who had this operation with an 18% operative mortality rate and no late death [250]. Six patients had reoperations: two for recurrent pulmonary stenosis and the other four for residual VSDs. The long-term results of this operation were recently reported by DiCarlo and associates [251]. They reviewed 205 patients who underwent the REV procedure between 1980 and 2003. Hospital mortality was 12%. Overall survival and freedom from any reoperation at 25 years were 85% and 45%, respectively. They concluded that their results were more favorable than those reported for the Rastelli operation in terms of survival and need for reoperation for left or right outflow tract obstruction [251].

Another option for patients with TGA, VSD, and pulmonary stenosis is the arterial switch. There are selected patients who have well developed pulmonary valves and annuli, based on data from echocardiography and angiography, with subpulmonic obstruction owing to prolapsed tricuspid valvar tissue through the VSD (Figure 26.33) [34]. Under these circumstances it is possible to reduce the accessory valvar tissue back through the VSD into the right ventricle, close the VSD, and complete the arterial switch. We have successfully performed an arterial switch in three such patients, each time reducing the accessory tricuspid tissue through the VSD and out of the left ventricular outflow tract. The decision to progress with the arterial switch was based on favorable transpulmonary artery left ventricular outflow tract evaluation at the time of operation before aortic transection. This way the Rastelli operation can still be performed in the event of unfavorable left ventricular outflow tract evaluation. Careful preoperative consideration must be given to both arterial switch and Rastelli operations to maximize the probability of a successful outcome.

The Nikaidoh procedure and the various manifestations relating thereto [252–257] have offered surgeons a new approach to TGA, VSD, and pulmonary stenosis. The rationale for this operation is based on the shortcomings of the Rastelli procedure. While the Rastelli operation is a reasonable option, it is not ideal because the left ventricular to aortic tunnel will 1) often require septal resection; 2) often result in subaortic/tunnel stenosis; and 3) reduce the size of the right ventricular cavity. The aortic translocation repair (Nikaidoh operation), on the other hand, provides an unobstructed pathway from the left ventricle to the neoaorta while limiting the need for septal resection and the large right ventriculotomy necessary for the Rastelli

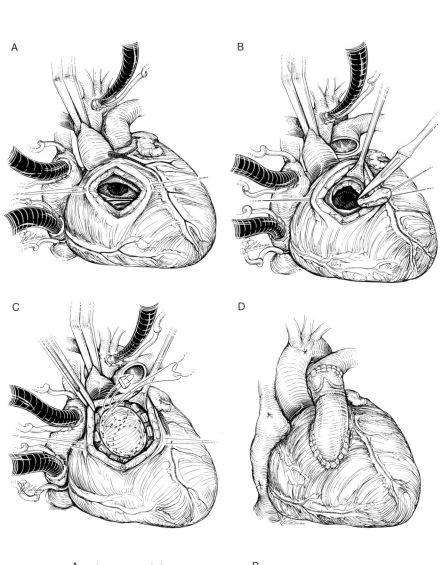

Figure 26.30 The Rastelli operation. **A**, A right ventricular incision is made with due regard to the tricuspid valve attachments, the ventricular septal defect anatomy, coronary artery distribution, and intended position of the conduit. **B**, A comprehensive infundibular resection is performed to maximize left ventricular-to-aortic continuity. **C**, The ventricular septal defect is closed with a large patch, creating an ample tunnel to the aorta. The distal pulmonary artery is opened at the most appropriate site for the distal conduit anastomosis. **D**, The valved conduit is in place after separation from cardiopulmonary bypass.

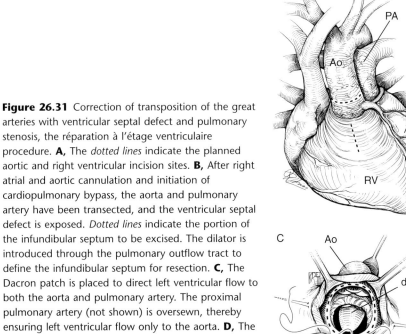

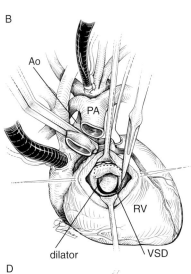

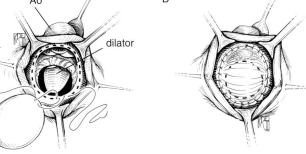

Figure 26.31 Correction of transposition of the great arteries with ventricular septal defect and pulmonary stenosis, the réparation à l'étage ventriculaire procedure. **A**, The *dotted lines* indicate the planned aortic and right ventricular incision sites. **B**, After right atrial and aortic cannulation and initiation of cardiopulmonary bypass, the aorta and pulmonary artery have been transected, and the ventricular septal defect is exposed. *Dotted lines* indicate the portion of the infundibular septum to be excised. The dilator is introduced through the pulmonary outflow tract to define the infundibular septum for resection. **C**, The Dacron patch is placed to direct left ventricular flow to both the aorta and pulmonary artery. The proximal pulmonary artery (not shown) is oversewn, thereby ensuring left ventricular flow only to the aorta. **D**, The left ventricle-to-aorta internal baffle is shown completed. (Ao, aorta; LV, left ventricle; PA, pulmonary artery; RV, right ventricle; VSD, ventricular septal defect.)

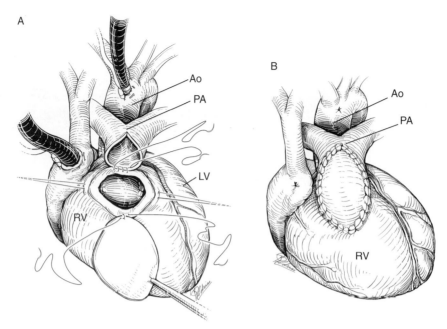

Figure 26.32 A, The superior portion of the right ventriculotomy is sutured directly to the posterior portion of the main pulmonary artery. **B,** A pericardial or synthetic patch is used to complete the right ventricle-to-pulmonary artery reconstruction. Sometimes a monocusp is placed within this reconstruction to create pulmonary valvar competence. (Ao, aorta; LV, left ventricle; PA, pulmonary artery; RV, right ventricle; VSD, ventricular septal defect.)

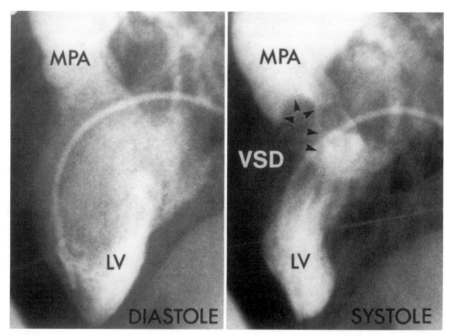

Figure 26.33 Cine cardioangiogram in diastole (left) and systole (right) of a patient with transposition of the great arteries, ventricular septal defect, and subpulmonic stenosis caused by a prolapsed tricuspid valve pouch through the ventricular septal defect. Arrowheads show the extent of prolapse of the tricuspid pouch causing left ventricular outflow obstruction. The pouch was reduced through the ventricular septal defect into the right ventricle, thereby relieving the subpulmonic obstruction. Successful arterial switch and ventricular septal defect closure was accomplished. (MPA, main pulmonary artery; VSD, ventricular septal defect; LV, left ventricle.)

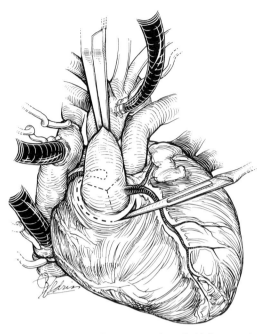

Figure 26.34 Aortic translocation or the Nikaidoh procedure involves aortic root immobilization. The aortic cannula above the cross-clamp is shown. The subaortic right ventricular space is entered through the transverse incision. Coronary arteries can be probed via the coronary ostia to localize the trunks and major branches of the coronary arteries, if necessary.

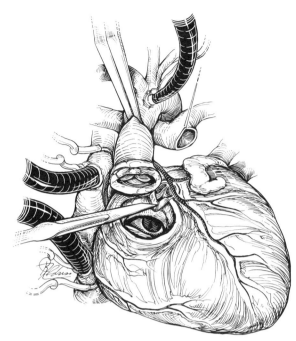

Figure 26.35 The ventricular septal defect is visualized. On completion of the aortic root mobilization, the main pulmonary artery is transected. The left ventricular outflow tract is opened and the subpulmonic stenosis is resected. Simple anterior division of the pulmonary annulus opens the left ventricular outflow tract widely, because there is often no separating muscular structure between the two semilunar valves.

operation (Figures 26.34–26.39) [34]. To date, experience with this surgical strategy is impressive but limited [252–257]. Significant potential long-term complications include neoaortic insufficiency, coronary obstructions, and pulmonary regurgitation.

TGA-VSD-Coarctation/Interrupted Aortic Arch

Perhaps the most challenging form of TGA is that which is associated with VSD and coarctation or interrupted aortic arch (see also Chapter 15, *Interrupted Aortic Arch*). The anatomic proportions are particularly vexing because the ascending aorta is often 50% smaller than the pulmonary artery trunk, the transverse arch is small, and the VSD is often malaligned. Early on in the collective surgical experience, surgeons applied a two-staged repair, preferring to address the coarctational interrupted aortic arch through a left thoracotomy, which was often combined with a pulmonary artery band [258,259]. After somatic growth, a complete repair through a median sternotomy was accomplished. Subsequent authors [260,261] found that a one-stage approach through a median sternotomy could be performed with acceptable mortality without the intervening problems that were associated with staged repair such as

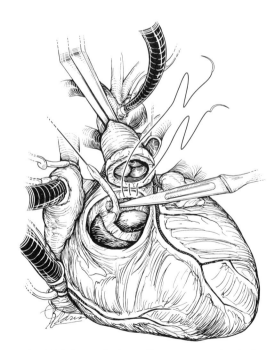

Figure 26.36 Left ventricular outflow reconstruction is shown by repositioning of the aortic root posteriorly and by resection of the infundibulum.

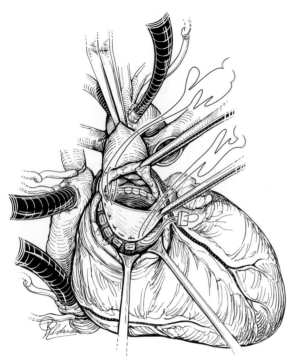

Figure 26.37 Closure of the ventricular septal defect by a patch. The posterior wall of the aortic root is sutured in two layers to the open orifice of the pulmonary annulus. The retractor is in the wide opening of the right ventricular outlet.

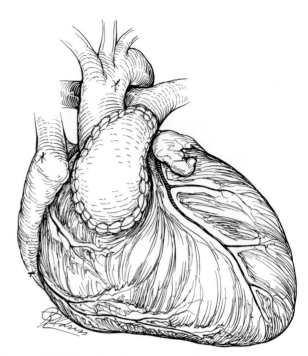

Figure 26.39 Completed reconstruction is shown.

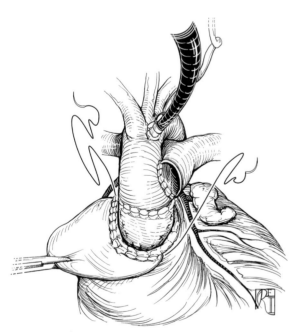

Figure 26.38 The distal segment of the main pulmonary artery is fixed to the aorta. The right ventricular outflow tract is reconstructed with a pericardial gusset. The atrial septal defect is closed through a right atriotomy (not shown).

neoaortic insufficiency caused by the preexisting pulmonary artery band and left ventricular outflow tract obstruction [260]. During the refinement of the operation, special attention was paid to neoaortic-aortic mismatch, neoaortic insufficiency, and transverse arch-descending aorta restenosis. In particular, Mohammadi and colleagues [260] reviewed 109 survivors out of 120 patients with TGA, VSD, coarctation/interrupted aortic arch in three groups of patients: 1) those who had a two-stage repair; 2) those who had a one-stage repair using extended end-to-end repair for the coarctation/interrupted aortic arch; and 3) those who had pulmonary homograft arch patch augmentation to more accurately size match the neoaortic reconstruction. Not surprisingly, the group that had aortic patch augmentation had the highest short- and long-term survival, the lowest incidence of recoarctation, and the lowest incidence of neoaortic regurgitation, leading the authors to extol the virtues of neoaortic patch augmentation for these patients in association with arterial switch and VSD closure.

The conduct of cardiopulmonary bypass is usually performed with double arterial cannulation (ascending aorta and ductus arteriosus). Alternatively, the ascending aorta can be perfused through a Gore-Tex graft that is anastomosed into the side of the innominate artery in concert with the ductal arterial catheter. This allows regional perfusion techniques to be used in the event that the surgical team wants to avoid deep hypothermia and circulatory arrest.

The descending, transverse, and ascending aortic arch can be augmented with a pulmonary homograft, which will ensure adequate outflow and a better anatomic match to the proximally reconstructed neoaorta. These techniques have been shown to increase survival and decrease the need for future reoperations in these infants.

References

1. Talner CN. (1998) Report of the New England Regional Infant Cardiac Program, by Donald C Fyler, MD, Pediatrics, 1980, 65(suppl), 375–461. Pediatrics, 102, 258–259.
2. Baillie M. (1793) *Morbid Anatomy of Some of the Most Important Parts of the Human Body*, 2nd ed. London: J Johnson and G Nicol.
3. De La Cruz MV, Da Rocha JP. (1956) An ontogenetic theory for the explanation of congenital malformations involving the truncus and conus. Am Heart J 51, 782–805.
4. Peacock TB. (1858) *On Malformations of the Human Heart, With Original Cases*. London: J Churchill.
5. Peacock TB. (1866) *On Malformations of the Human Heart*, 2nd ed. London: J Churchill.
6. Shaner RF. (1949) Malformation of the atrio-ventricular endocardial cushions of the embryo pig and its relation to defects of the conus and truncus arteriosus. Am J Anat 84, 431–455.
7. Shaner RF. (1951) Complete and corrected transposition of the aorta, pulmonary artery and ventricles in pig embryos, and a case of corrected transposition in a child. Am J Anat 88, 35–62.
8. Shaner RF. (1962) Comparative development of the bulbus and ventricles of the vertebrate heart with special reference to Spitzer's theory of heart malformations. Anat Rec 142, 519–529.
9. Shaner RF. (1962) Anomalies of the heart bulbus. J Pediatr 61, 233–241.
10. Grant RP. (1962) The morphogenesis of transposition of the great vessels. Circulation 26, 819–840.
11. Grant RP. (1962) The embryology of ventricular flow pathways in man. Circulation 25, 756–779.
12. Bremer JL. (1928) Part I. An interpretation of the development of the heart. Part II. The left aorta of reptiles. Am J Anat 42, 307–369.
13. Bremer JL. (1931) The presence and influence of two spiral streams in the heart of the chick embryo. Am J Anat 49, 409–440.
14. Bremer JL. (1942) Transposition of the aorta and the pulmonary artery: an embryologic study of its cause. Arch Pathol 34, 1016–1030.
15. de Vries PA, Saunders JB. (1962) Development of the ventricles and spiral outflow tract in the human heart. Contrib Embryol 37, 89–114.
16. Goerttler K. (1955) [Effect of blood flow as a factor on the form of the heart during development]. Beitr Pathol Anat 115, 33–56.
17. Goerttler K. (1956) [Hemodynamic research on the origin of malformations of the arterial cardiac end]. Virchows Arch 328, 391–420.
18. Jaffee OC. (1970) Comparative and experimental studies of the development of blood flow patterns in embryonic hearts. In: *Cardiac Development with Special Reference to Congenital Heart Disease*. Dayton, OH: University of Dayton Press.
19. Vanmierop LH, Alley RD, Kausel HW, *et al.* (1963) Pathogenesis of transposition complexes. I. Embryology of the ventricles and great arteries. Am J Cardiol 12, 216–225.
20. Vanmierop LH, Wiglesworth FW. (1963) Pathogenesis of transposition complexes. III. True transposition of the great vessels. Am J Cardiol 12, 233–239.
21. Vanmierop LH, Wiglesworth FW. (1963) Pathogenesis of transposition complexes. II. Anomalies due to faulty transfer of the posterior great artery. Am J Cardiol 12, 226–232.
22. Van Praagh R, Van Praagh S. (1966) Isolated ventricular inversion. A consideration of the morphogenesis, definition and diagnosis of nontransposed and transposed great arteries. Am J Cardiol 17, 395–406.
23. Van Praagh R, Van Praagh S, Vlad P, *et al.* (1964) Anatomic types of congenital dextrocardia: diagnostic and embryologic implications. Am J Cardiol 13, 510–531.
24. Rowe RD, Freedom RM, Mehrizi A. (1981) *The Neonate with Congenital Heart Disease*. Philadelphia, PA: WB Saunders.
25. Wood AE, Freedom RM, Williams WG, *et al.* (1983) The Mustard procedure in transposition of the great arteries associated with juxtaposition of the atrial appendages with and without dextrocardia. J Thorac Cardiovasc Surg 85, 451–456.
26. Mathew R, Rosenthal A, Fellows K. (1974) The significance of right aortic arch in D-transposition of the great arteries. Am Heart J 87, 314–317.
27. Idriss FS, DeLeon SY, Nikaidoh H, *et al.* (1977) Resection of left ventricular outflow obstruction in D-transposition of the great arteries. J Thorac Cardiovasc Surg 74, 343–351.
28. Jex RK, Puga FJ, Julsrud PR, *et al.* (1990) Repair of transposition of the great arteries with intact ventricular septum and left ventricular outflow tract obstruction. J Thorac Cardiovasc Surg 100, 682–686.
29. Sohn YS, Brizard CP, Cochrane AD, *et al.* (1998) Arterial switch in hearts with left ventricular outflow and pulmonary valve abnormalities. Ann Thorac Surg 66, 842–848.
30. Moene RJ, Oppenheimer-Dekker A, Wenink AC, *et al.* (1985) Morphology of ventricular septal defect in complete transposition of the great arteries. Am J Cardiol 55, 1566–1570.
31. Penkoske PA, Westerman GR, Marx GR, *et al.* (1983) Transposition of the great arteries and ventricular septal defect: results with the Senning operation and closure of the ventricular septal defect in infants. Ann Thorac Surg 36, 281–288.
32. Moene RJ, Oppenheimer-Dekker A, Bartelings MM. (1983) Anatomic obstruction of the right ventricular outflow tract in transposition of the great arteries. Am J Cardiol 51, 1701–1704.
33. Trusler GA, Freedom RM. (1985) Complete transposition of the great arteries. In: Arciniegas E, ed. *Pediatric Cardiac Surgery*. Chicago, Ill: Year Book.
34. Mavroudis C, Backer CL. (2003) Transposition of the great arteries. In: Mavroudis C, Backer CL, eds. *Pediatric Cardiac Surgery*, 3rd ed. Philadelphia, PA: Mosby, Inc.

35. Gittenberger-de Groot AC, Sauer U, Oppenheimer-Dekker A, *et al.* (1983) Coronary arterial anatomy in transposition of the great arteries: a morphologic study. Pediatr Cardiol 4(suppl 1), 15–24.

36. Gittenberger-de Groot AC, Sauer U, Quaegebeur J. (1986) Aortic intramural coronary artery in three hearts with transposition of the great arteries. J Thorac Cardiovasc Surg 91, 566–571.

37. Jatene AD, Fontes VF, Souza LC, *et al.* (1982) Anatomic correction of transposition of the great arteries. J Thorac Cardiovasc Surg 83, 20–26.

38. Kurosawa H, Imai Y, Kawada M. (1991) Coronary arterial anatomy in regard to the arterial switch procedure. Cardiol Young 1, 54–62.

39. Smith A, Arnold R, Wilkinson JL, *et al.* (1986) An anatomical study of the patterns of the coronary arteries and sinus nodal artery in complete transposition. Int J Cardiol 12, 295–307.

40. Deal BJ, Chin AJ, Sanders SP, *et al.* (1985) Subxiphoid two-dimensional echocardiographic identification of tricuspid valve abnormalities in transposition of the great arteries with ventricular septal defect. Am J Cardiol 55, 1146–1151.

41. Huhta JC, Edwards WD, Danielson GK, *et al.* (1982) Abnormalities of the tricuspid valve in complete transposition of the great arteries with ventricular septal defect. J Thorac Cardiovasc Surg 83, 569–576.

42. Moene RJ, Oppenheimer-Dekker A. (1982) Congenital mitral valve anomalies in transposition of the great arteries. Am J Cardiol 49, 1972–1978.

43. Fyler DC. (1992) D-transposition of the great arteries. In: Fyler DC, ed. *Nadas' Pediatric Cardiology*. Philadelphia, PA: Hanley & Belfus.

44. Serraf A, Nakamura T, Lacour-Gayet F, *et al.* (1996) Surgical approaches for double-outlet right ventricle or transposition of the great arteries associated with straddling atrioventricular valves. J Thorac Cardiovasc Surg 111, 527–535.

45. Aziz KU, Paul MH, Rowe RD. (1977) Bronchopulmonary circulation in d-transposition of the great arteries: possible role in genesis of accelerated pulmonary vascular disease. Am J Cardiol 39, 432–438.

46. Paul MH. (1983) Transposition of the great arteries. In: Adams FH, Emmanouilides GC, eds. *Moss' Heart Disease in Infants, Children and Adolescents*. Baltimore, MD: Williams & Wilkins.

47. Freed MD, Heymann MA, Lewis AB, *et al.* (1981) Prostaglandin E1 infants with ductus arteriosus-dependent congenital heart disease. Circulation 64, 899–905.

48. Lang P, Freed MD, Bierman FZ, *et al.* (1979) Use of prostaglandin E1 in infants with D-transposition of the great arteries and intact ventricular septum. Am J Cardiol 44, 76–81.

49. Chiu IS, Anderson RH, Macartney FJ, *et al.* (1984) Morphologic features of an intact ventricular septum susceptible to subpulmonary obstruction in complete transposition. Am J Cardiol 53, 1633–1638.

50. Silove ED, Taylor JF. (1973) Angiographic and anatomical features of subvalvar left ventricular outflow obstruction in transposition of the great arteries. The possible role of the anterior mitral valve leaflet. Pediatr Radiol 1, 87–91.

51. Rastelli GC, Wallace RB, Ongley PA. (1969) Complete repair of transposition of the great arteries with pulmonary stenosis. A review and report of a case corrected by using a new surgical technique. Circulation 39, 83–95.

52. Lecompte Y, Neveux JY, Leca F, *et al.* (1982) Reconstruction of the pulmonary outflow tract without prosthetic conduit. J Thorac Cardiovasc Surg 84, 727–733.

53. Vouhe PR, Tamisier D, Leca F, *et al.* (1992) Transposition of the great arteries, ventricular septal defect, and pulmonary outflow tract obstruction. Rastelli or Lecompte procedure? J Thorac Cardiovasc Surg 103, 428–436.

54. Haworth SG, Radley-Smith R, Yacoub M. (1987) Lung biopsy findings in transposition of the great arteries with ventricular septal defect: potentially reversible pulmonary vascular disease is not always synonymous with operability. J Am Coll Cardiol 9, 327–333.

55. Newfeld EA, Paul MM, Muster AJ, *et al.* (1974) Pulmonary vascular disease in complete transposition of the great arteries: a study of 200 patients. Am J Cardiol 34, 75–82.

56. Bartlett JM, Wypij D, Bellinger DC, *et al.* (2004) Effect of prenatal diagnosis on outcomes in D-transposition of the great arteries. Pediatrics 113, e335–e340.

57. Jouannic JM, Gavard L, Fermont L, *et al.* (2004) Sensitivity and specificity of prenatal features of physiological shunts to predict neonatal clinical status in transposition of the great arteries. Circulation 110, 1743–1746.

58. Kumar RK, Newburger JW, Gauvreau K, *et al.* (1999) Comparison of outcome when hypoplastic left heart syndrome and transposition of the great arteries are diagnosed prenatally versus when diagnosis of these two conditions is made only postnatally. Am J Cardiol 83, 1649–1653.

59. Skinner J, Hornung T, Rumball E. (2008) Transposition of the great arteries: from fetus to adult. Heart 94, 1227–1235.

60. Chew C, Stone S, Donath SM, *et al.* (2006) Impact of antenatal screening on the presentation of infants with congenital heart disease to a cardiology unit. J Paediatr Child Health 42, 704–708.

61. Stoll C, Garne E, Clementi M. (2001) Evaluation of prenatal diagnosis of associated congenital heart diseases by fetal ultrasonographic examination in Europe. Prenat Diagn 21, 243–252.

62. Garne E, Stoll C, Clementi M. (2001) Evaluation of prenatal diagnosis of congenital heart diseases by ultrasound: experience from 20 European registries. Ultrasound Obstet Gynecol 17, 386–391.

63. Khoshnood B, De Vigan C, Vodovar V, *et al.* (2005) Trends in prenatal diagnosis, pregnancy termination, and perinatal mortality of newborns with congenital heart disease in France, 1983–2000: a population-based evaluation. Pediatrics 115, 95–101.

64. Park IS, Yoon SY, Min JY, *et al.* (2006) Metabolic alterations and neurodevelopmental outcome of infants with transposition of the great arteries. Pediatr Cardiol 27, 569–576.

65. Pasquini L, Sanders SP, Parness IA, *et al.* (1987) Diagnosis of coronary artery anatomy by two-dimensional echocardiography in patients with transposition of the great arteries. Circulation 75, 557–564.

66. Pasquini L, Sanders SP, Parness IA, *et al.* (1994) Coronary echocardiography in 406 patients with d-loop transposition of the great arteries. J Am Coll Cardiol 24, 763–768.

67. Rashkind WJ, Miller WW. (1966) Creation of an atrial septal defect without thoracotomy. A palliative approach to complete transposition of the great arteries. JAMA 196, 991–992.

68. Frank L, Dillman JR, Parish V, *et al.* (2010) Cardiovascular MR imaging of conotruncal anomalies. Radiographics 30, 1069–1094.

69. Chantepie A, Schleich JM, Gournay V, *et al.* (2000) [Preoperative mortality in transposition of the great vessels]. Arch Pediatr 7, 34–39.

70. Blalock A, Hanlon CR. (1950) The surgical treatment of complete transposition of the aorta and the pulmonary artery. Surg Gynecol Obstet 90, 1–15.

71. Conte S, Jensen T, Ramsoe Jacobsen J, *et al.* (1999) Arterial switch with internal pulmonary artery banding. A new palliation for TGA and VSD in complex cases. J Cardiovasc Surg (Torino) 40, 313–316.

72. Mustard WT. (1964) Successful two-stage correction of transposition of the great vessels. Surgery 55, 469–472.

73. Senning A. (1959) Surgical correction of transposition of the great vessels. Surgery 45, 966–980.

74. Trusler GA, Freedom RM. (1983) Transposition of the great arteries: the Mustard procedure. In: Sabiston DC, Spencer FC, eds. *Gibbon's Surgery of the Chest*. Philadelphia, PA: WB Saunders.

75. Horer J, Herrmann F, Schreiber C, *et al.* (2007) How well are patients doing up to 30 years after a Mustard operation? Thorac Cardiovasc Surg 55, 359–364.

76. Horer J, Karl E, Theodoratou G, *et al.* (2008) Incidence and results of reoperations following the Senning operation: 27 years of follow-up in 314 patients at a single center. Eur J Cardiothorac Surg 33, 1061–1067; discussion 1067–1068.

77. Abe T, Kuribayashi R, Sato M, *et al.* (1978) Successful Jatene operation for transposition of the great arteries with intact ventricular septum. A case report. J Thorac Cardiovasc Surg 75, 64–67.

78. Backer CL, Ilbawi MN, Ohtake S, *et al.* (1989) Transposition of the great arteries: a comparison of results of the mustard procedure versus the arterial switch. Ann Thorac Surg 48, 10–14.

79. Bove EL. (1989) Current technique of the arterial switch procedure for transposition of the great arteries. J Card Surg 4, 193–199.

80. Castaneda AR, Norwood WI, Jonas RA, *et al.* (1984) Transposition of the great arteries and intact ventricular septum: anatomical repair in the neonate. Ann Thorac Surg 38, 438–443.

81. Castaneda AR, Trusler GA, Paul MH, *et al.* (1988) The early results of treatment of simple transposition in the current era. J Thorac Cardiovasc Surg 95, 14–28.

82. Freedom RM, Culham JA, Olley PM, *et al.* (1981) Anatomic correction of transposition of the great arteries: pre- and postoperative cardiac catheterization, with angiocardiography in five patients. Circulation 63, 905–914.

83. Harinck E, Van Mill GJ, Ross D, *et al.* (1980) Anatomical correction of transposition of great arteries with persistent ductus arteriosus. One year after operation. Br Heart J 43, 95–98.

84. Idriss FS, Ilbawi MN, DeLeon SY, *et al.* (1988) Transposition of the great arteries with intact ventricular septum. Arterial switch in the first month of life. J Thorac Cardiovasc Surg 95, 255–262.

85. Idriss FS, Ilbawi MN, DeLeon SY, *et al.* (1988) Arterial switch in simple and complex transposition of the great arteries. J Thorac Cardiovasc Surg 95, 29–36.

86. Ilbawi MN, Idriss FS, DeLeon SY, *et al.* (1987) Preparation of the left ventricle for anatomical correction in patients with simple transposition of the great arteries. Surgical guidelines. J Thorac Cardiovasc Surg 94, 87–94.

87. Kreutzer G, Neirotti R, Galindez E, *et al.* (1977) Anatomic correction of transposition of the great arteries. J Thorac Cardiovasc Surg 73, 538–542.

88. Mavroudis C, Backer CL, Idriss FS. (1991) Special considerations for and reoperations after the arterial switch operation. In: Mavroudis C, Backer CL, eds. *Arterial Switch Cardiac Surgery: State of the Art Review*, vol 5. Philadelphia, PA: Hanley & Belfus.

89. Backer CL, Idriss FS, Mavroudis C. (1991) Surgical techniques and intraoperative judgments to facilitate the arterial switch operation in transposition with intact ventricular septum. In: Mavroudis C, Backer CL, eds *Arterial Switch Cardiac Surgery: State of the Art Review*, vol 5. Philadelphia, PA: Hanley & Belfus.

90. Kurosawa H, Imai Y, Takanashi Y, *et al.* (1986) Infundibular septum and coronary anatomy in Jatene operation. J Thorac Cardiovasc Surg 91, 572–583.

91. Lecompte Y, Zannini L, Hazan E, *et al.* (1981) Anatomic correction of transposition of the great arteries. J Thorac Cardiovasc Surg 82, 629–631.

92. Mamiya RT, Moreno-Cabral RJ, Nakamura FT, *et al.* (1977) Retransposition of the great vessels for transposition with ventricular septal defect and pulmonary hypertension. J Thorac Cardiovasc Surg 73, 340–344.

93. Mavroudis C. (1987) Anatomical repair of transposition of the great arteries with intact ventricular septum in the neonate: guidelines to avoid complications. Ann Thorac Surg 43, 495–501.

94. Mavroudis C, Arensman FW, Rees AH. (1989) Anatomical repair of transposition of the great arteries with intact ventricular septum in the neonate. In: Kron IL, Mavroudis C, eds *Innovations in Congential Heart Surgery Cardiac Surgery: State of the Art Review*, vol 3. Philadelphia, PA: Hanley & Belfus.

95. Muster AJ, Berry TE, Ilbawi MN, *et al.* (1987) Development of neo-coarctation in patients with transposed great arteries and hypoplastic aortic arch after Lecompte modification of anatomical correction. J Thorac Cardiovasc Surg 93, 276–280.

96. Blume ED, Altmann K, Mayer JE, *et al.* (1999) Evolution of risk factors influencing early mortality of the arterial switch operation. J Am Coll Cardiol 33, 1702–1709.

97. Kirklin JW, Blackstone EH, Tchervenkov CI, *et al.* (1992) Clinical outcomes after the arterial switch operation for transposition. Patient, support, procedural, and institutional risk factors. Congenital Heart Surgeons Society. Circulation 86, 1501–1515.

98. Lupinetti FM, Bove EL, Minich LL, *et al.* (1992) Intermediate-term survival and functional results after arterial repair for transposition of the great arteries. J Thorac Cardiovasc Surg 103, 421–427.

99. Norwood WI, Dobell AR, Freed MD, *et al.* (1988) Intermediate results of the arterial switch repair. A 20-institution study. J Thorac Cardiovasc Surg 96, 854–863.

100. Pacifico AD, Stewart RW, Bargeron LM Jr. (1983) Repair of transposition of the great arteries with ventricular septal defect by an arterial switch operation. Circulation 68, II49–II55.

101. Pigott JD, Chin AJ, Weinberg PM, *et al.* (1987) Transposition of the great arteries with aortic arch obstruction. Anatomical review and report of surgical management. J Thorac Cardiovasc Surg 94, 82–86.

102. Planche C, Bruniaux J, Lacour-Gayet F, *et al.* (1988) Switch operation for transposition of the great arteries in neonates. A study of 120 patients. J Thorac Cardiovasc Surg 96, 354–363.

103. Planche C, Lacour-Gayet F, Serraf A, *et al.* (1998) [Anatomical repair in transposition of great vessels]. Bull Acad Natl Med 182, 1739–1753; discussion 1753–1755.

104. Quaegebeur JM, Rohmer J, Ottenkamp J, *et al.* (1986) The arterial switch operation. An eight-year experience. J Thorac Cardiovasc Surg 92, 361–384.

105. Ross D, Rickards A, Somerville J. (1976) Transposition of the great arteries: logical anatomical arterial correction. Br Med J 1, 1109–1111.

106. Serraf A, Lacour-Gayet F, Bruniaux J, *et al.* (1993) Anatomic correction of transposition of the great arteries in neonates. J Am Coll Cardiol 22, 193–200.

107. Sidi D, Heurtematte Y, Kachaner J, *et al.* (1983) [Problems posed by preparation of the left ventricle for anatomical correction in simple transposition of the great vessels]. Arch Mal Coeur Vaiss 76, 575–583.

108. Wernovsky G, Mayer JE Jr, Jonas RA, *et al.* (1995) Factors influencing early and late outcome of the arterial switch operation for transposition of the great arteries. J Thorac Cardiovasc Surg 109, 289–301; discussion 302.

109. Williams WG, Freedom RM, Culham G, *et al.* (1981) Early experience with arterial repair of transposition. Ann Thorac Surg 32, 8–15.

110. Yacoub M, Bernhard A, Lange P, *et al.* (1980) Clinical and hemodynamic results of the two-stage anatomic correction of simple transposition of the great arteries. Circulation 62, I190–I196.

111. Yacoub MH, Radley-Smith R, Hilton CJ. (1976) Anatomical correction of complete transposition of the great arteries and ventricular septal defect in infancy. Br Med J 1, 1112–1114.

112. Yacoub MH, Radley-Smith R, Maclaurin R. (1977) Two-stage operation for anatomical correction of transposition of the great arteries with intact interventricular septum. Lancet 1, 1275–1278.

113. Fleming WH. (1979) Why switch? J Thorac Cardiovasc Surg 78, 1–2.

114. Laks H. (1989) The arterial switch procedure for the neonate: coming of age. Ann Thorac Surg 48, 3–4.

115. Lincoln CR, Lima R, Rigby ML. (1983) Anatomical correction of simple transposition of great arteries during neonatal transition. Lancet 2, 39.

116. Rubay J, de Leval M, Bull C. (1988) To switch or not to switch? The Senning alternative. Circulation 78, III1–III4.

117. Stark J. (1984) Transposition of the great arteries: which operation? Ann Thorac Surg 38, 429–431.

118. Yacoub MH. (1979) The case for anatomic correction of transposition of the great arteries. J Thorac Cardiovasc Surg 78, 3–6.

119. Boyadjiev K, Ho SY, Anderson RH, *et al.* (1990) The potential for subpulmonary obstruction in complete transposition after the arterial switch procedure. An anatomic study. Eur J Cardiothorac Surg 4, 214–218.

120. Haas F, Wottke M, Poppert H, *et al.* (1999) Long-term survival and functional follow-up in patients after the arterial switch operation. Ann Thorac Surg 68, 1692–1697.

121. Serraf A, Roux D, Lacour-Gayet F, *et al.* (1995) Reoperation after the arterial switch operation for transposition of the great arteries. J Thorac Cardiovasc Surg 110, 892–899.

122. Tamisier D, Ouaknine R, Pouard P, *et al.* (1997) Neonatal arterial switch operation: coronary artery patterns and coronary events. Eur J Cardiothorac Surg 11, 810–817.

123. Williams WG, Quaegebeur JM, Kirklin JW, *et al.* (1997) Outflow obstruction after the arterial switch operation: a multiinstitutional study. Congenital Heart Surgeons Society. J Thorac Cardiovasc Surg 114, 975–87; discussion 987–990.

124. Akiba T, Neirotti R, Becker AE. (1993) Is there an anatomic basis for subvalvular right ventricular outflow tract obstruction after an arterial switch repair for complete transposition? A morphometric study and review. J Thorac Cardiovasc Surg 105, 142–146.

125. Mavroudis C, Backer CL, Duffy CE, *et al.* (1999) Pediatric coronary artery bypass for Kawasaki congenital, post arterial switch, and iatrogenic lesions. Ann Thorac Surg 68, 506–512.

126. Tanel RE, Wernovsky G, Landzberg MJ, *et al.* (1995) Coronary artery abnormalities detected at cardiac catheterization following the arterial switch operation for transposition of the great arteries. Am J Cardiol 76, 153–157.

127. Arensman FW, Sievers HH, Lange P, *et al.* (1985) Assessment of coronary and aortic anastomoses after anatomic correction of transposition of the great arteries. J Thorac Cardiovasc Surg 90, 597–604.

128. Goor DA, Shem-Tov A, Neufeld HN. (1982) Impeded coronary flow in anatomic correction of transposition of the great arteries: prevention, detection, and management. J Thorac Cardiovasc Surg 83, 747–754.

129. Rowlatt UF. (1962) Coronary artery distribution in complete transposition. JAMA 179, 269–278.

130. Yacoub MH, Radley-Smith R. (1978) Anatomy of the coronary arteries in transposition of the great arteries and methods for their transfer in anatomical correction. Thorax 33, 418–424.

131. Ebels T, Meuzelaar K, Gallandat Huet RC, *et al.* (1989) Neonatal arterial switch operation complicated by intramural left coronary artery and treated by left internal

mammary artery bypass graft. J Thorac Cardiovasc Surg 97, 473–475.

132. Mariani MA, Waterbolk TW, Ebels T. (1998) Transposition of the great arteries and isolated origin of the sinus node artery. Ann Thorac Surg 66, 2087–2089.

133. Mayer JE Jr, Sanders SP, Jonas RA, *et al.* (1990) Coronary artery pattern and outcome of arterial switch operation for transposition of the great arteries. Circulation 82(5 Suppl), IV139–IV145.

134. Bergouignan M, Fontan F, Trarieux M, *et al.* (1961) [Choreiform syndromes in children during cardiosurgical operations under deep hypothermia]. Rev Obstet Ginecol Venez 105, 48–60.

135. Clarkson PM, MacArthur BA, Barratt-Boyes BG, *et al.* (1980) Developmental progress after cardiac surgery in infancy using hypothermia and circulatory arrest. Circulation 62, 855–861.

136. Ehyai A, Fenichel GM, Bender HW Jr. (1984) Incidence and prognosis of seizures in infants after cardiac surgery with profound hypothermia and circulatory arrest. JAMA 252, 3165–3167.

137. Mavroudis C, Greene MA. (1992) Cardiopulmonary bypass and hypothermic circulatory arrest in infants. In: Jacobs ML, Norwood WI, eds. *Pediatric Cardiac Surgery: Current Issues.* Stoneham, MA: Butterworth-Heinemann.

138. Molina JE, Einzig S, Mastri AR, *et al.* (1984) Brain damage in profound hypothermia. Perfusion versus circulatory arrest. J Thorac Cardiovasc Surg 87, 596–604.

139. Treasure T, Naftel DC, Conger KA, *et al.* (1983) The effect of hypothermic circulatory arrest time on cerebral function, morphology, and biochemistry. An experimental study. J Thorac Cardiovasc Surg 86, 761–770.

140. Greeley WJ, Kern FH, Ungerleider RM, *et al.* (1991) The effect of hypothermic cardiopulmonary bypass and total circulatory arrest on cerebral metabolism in neonates, infants, and children. J Thorac Cardiovasc Surg 101, 783–794.

141. Swain JA, McDonald TJ Jr, Griffith PK, *et al.* (1991) Low-flow hypothermic cardiopulmonary bypass protects the brain. J Thorac Cardiovasc Surg 102, 76–83; discussion 84.

142. Bellinger DC, Wypij D, Kuban KC, *et al.* (1999) Developmental and neurological status of children at 4 years of age after heart surgery with hypothermic circulatory arrest or low-flow cardiopulmonary bypass. Circulation 100, 526–532.

143. Jonas RA, Bellinger DC, Rappaport LA, *et al.* (1993) Relation of pH strategy and developmental outcome after hypothermic circulatory arrest. J Thorac Cardiovasc Surg 106, 362–368.

144. Newburger JW, Jonas RA, Wernovsky G, *et al.* (1993) A comparison of the perioperative neurologic effects of hypothermic circulatory arrest versus low-flow cardiopulmonary bypass in infant heart surgery. N Engl J Med 329, 1057–1064.

145. Rappaport LA, Wypij D, Bellinger DC, *et al.* (1998) Relation of seizures after cardiac surgery in early infancy to neurodevelopmental outcome. Boston Circulatory Arrest Study Group. Circulation 97, 773–779.

146. Wernovsky G, Wypij D, Jonas RA, *et al.* (1995) Postoperative course and hemodynamic profile after the arterial switch operation in neonates and infants. A comparison of low-flow cardiopulmonary bypass and circulatory arrest. Circulation 92, 2226–2235.

147. Aoshima M, Yokota M, Shiraishi Y, *et al.* (1988) Prolonged aortic cross-clamping in early infancy and method of myocardial preservation. J Cardiovasc Surg (Torino) 29, 591–595.

148. Corno AF, Bethencourt DM, Laks H, *et al.* (1987) Myocardial protection in the neonatal heart. A comparison of topical hypothermia and crystalloid and blood cardioplegic solutions. J Thorac Cardiovasc Surg 93, 163–172.

149. DeLeon SY, Idriss FS, Ilbawi MN, *et al.* (1988) Comparison of single versus multidose blood cardioplegia in arterial switch procedures. Ann Thorac Surg 45, 548–553.

150. Ganzel BL, Katzmark SL, Mavroudis C. (1988) Myocardial preservation in the neonate. Beneficial effects of cardioplegia and systemic hypothermia on piglets undergoing cardiopulmonary bypass and myocardial ischemia. J Thorac Cardiovasc Surg 96, 414–422.

151. Yonenaga K, Yasui H, Kado H, *et al.* (1990) Myocardial protection by retrograde cardioplegia in arterial switch operation. Ann Thorac Surg 50, 238–242.

152. Lamberti JJ, Cohn LH, Laks H, *et al.* (1975) Local cardiac hypothermia for myocardial protection during correction of congenital heart disease. Ann Thorac Surg 20, 446–455.

153. Brown JW, Park HJ, Turrentine MW. (2001) Arterial switch operation: factors impacting survival in the current era. Ann Thorac Surg 71, 1978–1984.

154. Chiu IS, Chu SH, Wang JK, *et al.* (1995) Evolution of coronary artery pattern according to short-axis aortopulmonary rotation: a new categorization for complete transposition of the great arteries. J Am Coll Cardiol 26, 250–258.

155. Shukla V, Freedom RM, Black MD. (2000) Single coronary artery and complete transposition of the great arteries: a technical challenge resolved? Ann Thorac Surg 69, 568–571.

156. Sim EK, van Son JA, Edwards WD, *et al.* (1994) Coronary artery anatomy in complete transposition of the great arteries. Ann Thorac Surg 57, 890–894.

157. van Son JA. (1996) Classification of origin and proximal epicardial course of coronary arteries in transposition of the great arteries. J Cardiovasc Surg (Torino) 37, 251–254.

158. Laks H. (1994) Single ventricle with double inlet atrioventricular connection. In: Mavroudis C, Backer CL, eds. *Pediatric Cardiac Surgery*, 2nd ed. St Louis, MO: Mosby.

159. Rossi MB, Ho SY, Anderson RH, *et al.* (1986) Coronary arteries in complete transposition: the significance of the sinus node artery. Ann Thorac Surg 42, 573–577.

160. Chang YH, Sung SC, Lee HD, *et al.* (2005) Coronary reimplantation after neoaortic reconstruction can yield better result in arterial switch operation: comparison with open trap door technique. Ann Thorac Surg 80, 1634–1640.

161. Zheng JH, Xu ZW, Liu JF, *et al.* (2008) Arterial switch operation with coronary arteries from a single sinus in infants. J Card Surg 23, 606–610.

162. Asou T, Karl TR, Pawade A, *et al.* (1994) Arterial switch: translocation of the intramural coronary artery. Ann Thorac Surg 57, 461–465.

163. Li J, Tulloh RM, Cook A, et al. (2000) Coronary arterial origins in transposition of the great arteries: factors that affect outcome. A morphological and clinical study. Heart 83, 320–325.

164. Cleuziou J, Horer J, Henze R, et al. (2008) Surgical management of single intramural coronary artery in Taussig-Bing anomaly detected at arterial switch operation. Thorac Cardiovasc Surg 56, 170–172.

165. Mavroudis C, Stewart RD, Backer CL, et al. (2011) Reoperative techniques for complications following arterial switch. Ann Thorac Surg 92, 1747–1755.

166. Parry AJ, Thurm M, Hanley FL. (1999) The use of 'pericardial hoods' for maintaining exact coronary artery geometry in the arterial switch operation with complex coronary anatomy. Eur J Cardiothorac Surg 15, 159–164; discussion 164–165.

167. Murthy KS, Cherian KM. (1996) A new technique of arterial switch operation with in situ coronary reallocation for transposition of great arteries. J Thorac Cardiovasc Surg 112, 27–32.

168. Moat NE, Pawade A, Lamb RK. (1992) Complex coronary arterial anatomy in transposition of the great arteries. Arterial switch procedure without coronary relocation. J Thorac Cardiovasc Surg 103, 872–876.

169. Hirata Y, Chen JM, Quaegebeur JM, et al. (2008) Should we address the neopulmonic valve? Significance of right-sided obstruction after surgery for transposition of the great arteries and coarctation. Ann Thorac Surg 86, 1293–1298; discussion 1298.

170. Sinzobahamvya N, Blaschczok HC, Asfour B, et al. (2007) Right ventricular outflow tract obstruction after arterial switch operation for the Taussig-Bing heart. Eur J Cardiothorac Surg 31, 873–878.

171. Rheuban KS, Kron IL, Bulatovic A. (1990) Internal mammary artery bypass after the arterial switch operation. Ann Thorac Surg 50, 125–126.

172. Anderson HL 3rd, Attorri RJ, Custer JR, et al. (1990) Extracorporeal membrane oxygenation for pediatric cardiopulmonary failure. J Thorac Cardiovasc Surg 99, 1011–1019; discussion 1019–1021.

173. Atkins BZ, Danielson DS, Fitzpatrick CM, et al. (2010) Modified ultrafiltration attenuates pulmonary-derived inflammatory mediators in response to cardiopulmonary bypass. Interact Cardiovasc Thorac Surg 11, 599–603.

174. Davies MJ, Nguyen K, Gaynor JW, et al. (1998) Modified ultrafiltration improves left ventricular systolic function in infants after cardiopulmonary bypass. J Thorac Cardiovasc Surg 115, 361–369; discussion 369–370.

175. Williams WG, McCrindle BW, Ashburn DA, et al. (2003) Outcomes of 829 neonates with complete transposition of the great arteries 12–17 years after repair. Eur J Cardiothorac Surg 24, 1–9; discussion 10.

176. Cohen MS, Wernovsky G. (2006) Is the arterial switch operation as good over the long term as we thought it would be? Cardiol Young 16(Suppl 3), 117–124.

177. Dibardino DJ, Allison AE, Vaughn WK, et al. (2004) Current expectations for newborns undergoing the arterial switch operation. Ann Surg 239, 588–96; discussion 596–598.

178. Freed DH, Robertson CM, Sauve RS, et al. (2006) Intermediate-term outcomes of the arterial switch operation for transposition of great arteries in neonates: alive but well? J Thorac Cardiovasc Surg 132, 845–852.

179. Prandstetter C, Hofer A, Lechner E, et al. (2007) Early and mid-term outcome of the arterial switch operation in 114 consecutive patients : A single centre experience. Clin Res Cardiol 96, 723–729.

180. Qamar ZA, Goldberg CS, Devaney EJ, et al. (2007) Current risk factors and outcomes for the arterial switch operation. Ann Thorac Surg 84, 871–878; discussion 878–879.

181. Rastan AJ, Walther T, Alam NA, et al. (2008) Moderate versus deep hypothermia for the arterial switch operation–experience with 100 consecutive patients. Eur J Cardiothorac Surg 33, 619–625.

182. Sarris GE, Chatzis AC, Giannopoulos NM, et al. (2006) The arterial switch operation in Europe for transposition of the great arteries: a multi-institutional study from the European Congenital Heart Surgeons Association. J Thorac Cardiovasc Surg 132, 633–639.

183. Wernovsky G, Hougen TJ, Walsh EP, et al. (1988) Midterm results after the arterial switch operation for transposition of the great arteries with intact ventricular septum: clinical, hemodynamic, echocardiographic, and electrophysiologic data. Circulation 77, 1333–1344.

184. Wong SH, Finucane K, Kerr AR, et al. (2008) Cardiac outcome up to 15 years after the arterial switch operation. Heart Lung Circ 17, 48–53.

185. Yamazaki A, Yamamoto N, Sakamoto T, et al. (2008) Long-term outcomes and social independence level after arterial switch operation. Eur J Cardiothorac Surg 33, 239–243.

186. McGoon DC. (1972) Surgery for transposition of the great arteries. Circulation 45, 1147–1149.

187. Bove EL, Beekman RH, Snider AR, et al. (1988) Arterial repair for transposition of the great arteries and large ventricular septal defect in early infancy. Circulation 78, III26–III31.

188. Rudra HS, Mavroudis C, Backer CL, et al. (2011) The arterial switch operation: 25-year experience with 258 patients. Ann Thorac Surg 92, 1742–1746.

189. Salerno TA, Chiong MA. (1983) The hemodynamic and metabolic effects of cardioplegic rearrest in the pig. Ann Thorac Surg 35, 280–287.

190. Wright RN, Levitsky S, Holland C, et al. (1978) Beneficial effects of potassium cardioplegia during intermittent aortic cross-clamping and reperfusion. J Surg Res 24, 201–209.

191. Yamaguchi M, Hosokawa Y, Imai Y, et al. (1990) Early and midterm results of the arterial switch operation for transposition of the great arteries in Japan. J Thorac Cardiovasc Surg 100, 261–269.

192. Serraf A, Bruniaux J, Lacour-Gayet F, et al. (1991) Anatomic correction of transposition of the great arteries with ventricular septal defect. Experience with 118 cases. J Thorac Cardiovasc Surg 102, 140–147.

193. Mavroudis C, Gevitz M, Ring WS, et al. (1999) The Society of Thoracic Surgeons National Congenital Heart Surgery Database Report: analysis of the first harvest (1994–1997). Ann Thorac Surg 68, 601–624.

194. Major WK Jr, Matsuda H, Subramanian S. (1976) Failure of the Jatene procedure in a patient with D-transposition and intact ventricular septum. Ann Thorac Surg 22, 386–388.

195. de Leval MR, McKay R, Jones M, *et al.* (1981) Modified Blalock-Taussig shunt. Use of subclavian artery orifice as flow regulator in prosthetic systemic-pulmonary artery shunts. J Thorac Cardiovasc Surg 81, 112–119.

196. Duncan BW, Poirier NC, Mee RB, *et al.* (2004) Selective timing for the arterial switch operation. Ann Thorac Surg 77, 1691–1696; discussion 1697.

197. Kang N, de Leval MR, Elliott M, *et al.* (2004) Extending the boundaries of the primary arterial switch operation in patients with transposition of the great arteries and intact ventricular septum. Circulation 110(11 Suppl 1), II123–II127.

198. Bisoi AK, Sharma P, Chauhan S, *et al.* (2010) Primary arterial switch operation in children presenting late with d-transposition of great arteries and intact ventricular septum. When is it too late for a primary arterial switch operation? Eur J Cardiothorac Surg 38, 707–713.

199. Van Praagh R. (1968) What is the Taussig-Bing malformation? Circulation 38, 445–449.

200. Lev M, Rimoldi HJ, Eckner FA, *et al.* (1966) The Taussig-Bing heart. Qualitative and quantitative anatomy. Arch Pathol 81, 24–35.

201. Patrick DL, McGoon DC. (1968) An operation for double-outlet right ventricle with transposition of the great arteries. J Cardiovasc Surg (Torino) 9, 537–542.

202. Kawashima Y, Fujita T, Miyamoto T, *et al.* (1971) Intraventricular rerouting of blood for the correction of Taussig-Bing malformation. J Thorac Cardiovasc Surg 62, 825–829.

203. Snoddy JW, Parr EL, Robertson LW, *et al.* (1978) Successful intracardiac repair of the Taussig-Bing malformation in 2 children. Ann Thorac Surg 25, 158–163.

204. Harvey JC, Sondheimer HM, Williams WG, *et al.* (1977) Repair of double-outlet right ventricle. J Thorac Cardiovasc Surg 73, 611–615.

205. Kirklin JW, Pacifico AD, Blackstone EH, *et al.* (1986) Current risks and protocols for operations for double-outlet right ventricle. Derivation from an 18 year experience. J Thorac Cardiovasc Surg 92, 913–930.

206. Yacoub MH, Radley-Smith R. (1984) Anatomic correction of the Taussig-Bing anomaly. J Thorac Cardiovasc Surg 88, 380–388.

207. Mavroudis C, Backer CL, Muster AJ, *et al.* (1996) Taussig-Bing anomaly: arterial switch versus Kawashima intraventricular repair. Ann Thorac Surg 61, 1330–1338.

208. Van Praagh R. (1984) Discussion of: Yacoub MH, Radley-Smith R. Anatomic correction of the Taussig-Bing anomaly. J Thorac Cardiovasc Surg 88, 387–388.

209. Hightower BM, Barcia A, Bargeron LM Jr, *et al.* (1969) Double-outlet right ventricle with transposed great arteries and subpulmonary ventricular septal defect. The Taussig-Bing malformation. Circulation 39(5 Suppl 1), I207–I213.

210. Abe T, Komatsu S, Chiba M, *et al.* (1982) Successful modified Senning operation for the repair of Taussig-Bing malformation. J Cardiovasc Surg (Torino) 23, 1–5.

211. Luber JM, Castaneda AR, Lang P, *et al.* (1983) Repair of double-outlet right ventricle: early and late results. Circulation 68, II144–II147.

212. Ottino G, Kugler JD, McNamara DG, *et al.* (1980) Taussig-Bing anomaly: total repair with closure of ventricular septal defect through the pulmonary artery. Ann Thorac Surg 29, 170–176.

213. Wedemeyer AL, Lucas RV Jr, Castaneda AR. (1970) Taussig-Bing malformation, coarctation of the aorta, and reversed patent ductus arteriosus. Operative correction in an infant. Circulation 42, 1021–1027.

214. Muster AJ, Bharati S, Aziz KU, *et al.* (1979) Taussig-Bing anomaly with straddling mitral valve. J Thorac Cardiovasc Surg 77, 832–842.

215. Damus PS, Thomson NB Jr, McLoughlin TG. (1982) Arterial repair without coronary relocation for complete transposition of the great vessels with ventricular septal defect. Report of a case. J Thorac Cardiovasc Surg 83, 316–318.

216. Stansel HC Jr. (1975) A new operation for d-loop transposition of the great vessels. Ann Thorac Surg 19, 565–567.

217. Kaye MP. (1975) Anatomic correction of transposition of great arteries. Mayo Clin Proc 50, 638–640.

218. Binet JP, Lacour-Gayet F, Conso JF, *et al.* (1983) Complete repair of the Taussig-Bing type of double-outlet right ventricle using the arterial switch operation without coronary translocation. Report of one successful case. J Thorac Cardiovasc Surg 85, 272–275.

219. Smith EE, Pucci JJ, Walesby RK, *et al.* (1982) A new technique for correction of the Taussig-Bing anomaly. J Thorac Cardiovasc Surg 83, 901–904.

220. Ceithaml EL, Puga FJ, Danielson GK, *et al.* (1984) Results of the Damus-Stansel-Kaye procedure for transposition of the great arteries and for double-outlet right ventricle with subpulmonary ventricular septal defect. Ann Thorac Surg 38, 433–437.

221. Kanter K, Anderson R, Lincoln C, *et al.* (1986) Anatomic correction of double-outlet right ventricle with subpulmonary ventricular septal defect (the "Taussig-Bing" anomaly). Ann Thorac Surg 41, 287–292.

222. Parr GV, Waldhausen JA, Bharati S, *et al.* (1983) Coarctation in Taussig-Bing malformation of the heart. Surgical significance. J Thorac Cardiovasc Surg 86, 280–287.

223. Quaegebeur JM. (1983) The optimal repair for the Taussig-Bing heart. J Thorac Cardiovasc Surg 85, 276–277.

224. Rodefeld MD, Ruzmetov M, Vijay P, *et al.* (2007) Surgical results of arterial switch operation for Taussig-Bing anomaly: is position of the great arteries a risk factor? Ann Thorac Surg 83, 1451–1457.

225. Ohtake S, Idriss FS, Ilbawi MN, *et al.* (1989) Severe systemic right ventricular dysfunction after Mustard operation for transposition. Circulation 80(suppl ll), 70.

226. Ohtake S, Idriss FS, Backer CL, *et al.* (1990) Fate of tricuspid valve as a systemic atrioventricular valve: a 20 year follow-up of TGA with Mustard repair. J Am Coll Cardiol 15, 79A (abstr).

227. Mee RB. (1986) Severe right ventricular failure after Mustard or Senning operation. Two-stage repair: pulmonary artery banding and switch. J Thorac Cardiovasc Surg 92, 385–390.

228. Helvind MH, McCarthy JF, Imamura M, *et al.* (1998) Ventriculo-arterial discordance: switching the morphologically left ventricle into the systemic circulation after 3 months of age. Eur J Cardiothorac Surg 14, 173–178.

229. de Jong PL, Bogers AJ, Witsenburg M, *et al.* (1995) Arterial switch for pulmonary venous obstruction complicating Mustard procedure. Ann Thorac Surg 59, 1005–1007.

230. Reisman M, Rosengart RM, Degner TL, *et al.* (1999) Post-Mustard procedure pulmonary venous obstruction: An opportunity for anatomic correction with a one-stage arterial switch. Pediatr Cardiol 20, 301–303.

231. Shinebourne EA, Jahangiri M, Carvalho JS, *et al.* (1994) Anatomic correction for post-mustard pulmonary venous obstruction. Ann Thorac Surg 57, 1655–1656.

232. Mavroudis C, Backer CL. (2000) Arterial switch after failed atrial baffle procedures for transposition of the great arteries. Ann Thorac Surg 69, 851–857.

233. Paillole C, Sidi D, Kachaner J, *et al.* (1988) Fate of pulmonary artery after anatomic correction of simple transposition of great arteries in newborn infants. Circulation 78, 870–876.

234. Rees A, Solinger R, Eibl F, *et al.* (1989) Conventional Doppler echocardiography and Doppler color flow mapping in the evaluation of the arterial switch operation. Clin Res 37, 42.

235. Kanter KR, Anderson RH, Lincoln C, *et al.* (1985) Anatomic correction for complete transposition and double-outlet right ventricle. J Thorac Cardiovasc Surg 90, 690–699.

236. Hayashi G, Kurosaki K, Echigo S, *et al.* (2006) Prevalence of arrhythmias and their risk factors mid- and long-term after the arterial switch operation. Pediatr Cardiol 27, 689–694.

237. Angeli E, Raisky O, Bonnet D, *et al.* (2008) Late reoperations after neonatal arterial switch operation for transposition of the great arteries. Eur J Cardiothorac Surg 34, 32–36.

238. Agnoletti G, Ou P, Celermajer DS, *et al.* (2008) Acute angulation of the aortic arch predisposes a patient to ascending aortic dilatation and aortic regurgitation late after the arterial switch operation for transposition of the great arteries. J Thorac Cardiovasc Surg 135, 568–572.

239. Hayashi Y, Cochrane AD, Menahem S, *et al.* (2007) Neoaortic root dilatation with saccular aneurysm formation after the arterial switch operation for Taussig-Bing anomaly. J Thorac Cardiovasc Surg 133, 569–572.

240. Losay J, Touchot A, Capderou A, *et al.* (2006) Aortic valve regurgitation after arterial switch operation for transposition of the great arteries: incidence, risk factors, and outcome. J Am Coll Cardiol 47, 2057–2062.

241. Marino BS, Wernovsky G, McElhinney DB, *et al.* (2006) Neo-aortic valvar function after the arterial switch. Cardiol Young 16, 481–489.

242. Martin MM, Snider AR, Bove EL, *et al.* (1989) Two-dimensional and Doppler echocardiographic evaluation after arterial switch repair in infancy for complete transposition of the great arteries. Am J Cardiol 63, 332–336.

243. Martin RP, Ettedgui JA, Qureshi SA, *et al.* (1988) A quantitative evaluation of aortic regurgitation after anatomic correction of transposition of the great arteries. J Am Coll Cardiol 12, 1281–1284.

244. Damus PS. (1975) Letter to the editor. Ann Thorac Surg 20, 724–725.

245. Danielson GK, Tabry IF, Mair DD, *et al.* (1978) Great-vessel switch operation without coronary relocation for transposition of great arteries. Mayo Clin Proc 53, 675–682.

246. Mavroudis C, Backer CL, Idriss FS. (1992) Arterial switch for transposition of the great arteries and associated malposition anomalies. In: Karp RB, Laks H, Wechsler AS, eds. *Advances in Cardiac Surgery*. St Louis, MO: Mosby.

247. Imamura E, Morikawa T, Tatsuno K, *et al.* (1977) Conduit repairs of transposition complexes. A report of 14 cases. J Thorac Cardiovasc Surg 73, 570–577.

248. Marcelletti C, Mair DD, McGoon DC, *et al.* (1976) The Rastelli operation for transposition of the great arteries. Early and late results. J Thorac Cardiovasc Surg 72, 427–434.

249. Moulton AL, de Leval MR, Macartney FJ, *et al.* (1981) Rastelli procedure for transposition of the great arteries, ventricular septal defect, and left ventricular outflow tract obstruction. Early and late results in 41 patients (1971 to 1978). Br Heart J 45, 20–28.

250. Lecompte Y. (1991) Reparation a l'etage ventriculaire – the REV procedure: technique and clinical results. Cardiol Young 1, 63–70.

251. Di Carlo D, Tomasco B, Cohen L, *et al.* (2011) Long-term results of the REV (reparation a l'etage ventriculaire) operation. J Thorac Cardiovasc Surg 142, 336–343.

252. Bautista-Hernandez V, Marx GR, Bacha EA, *et al.* (2007) Aortic root translocation plus arterial switch for transposition of the great arteries with left ventricular outflow tract obstruction: intermediate-term results. J Am Coll Cardiol 49, 485–490.

253. Hazekamp M, Portela F, Bartelings M. (2007) The optimal procedure for the great arteries and left ventricular outflow tract obstruction. An anatomical study. Eur J Cardiothorac Surg 31, 879–887.

254. Morell VO. Aortic translocation for TGA with VSD and PS. Cardiothoracic Surgery Network, Expert Techniques, Congenital Cardiac, November 2005.

255. Morell VO, Wearden PD. (2007) Aortic translocation for the management of transposition of the great arteries with a ventricular septal defect, pulmonary stenosis, and hypoplasia of the right ventricle. Eur J Cardiothorac Surg 31, 552–554.

256. Nikaidoh H. (1984) Aortic translocation and biventricular outflow tract reconstruction. A new surgical repair for transposition of the great arteries associated with ventricular septal defect and pulmonary stenosis. J Thorac Cardiovasc Surg 88, 365–372.

257. Sayin OA, Ugurlucan M, Saltik L, *et al.* (2006) Modified Nikaidoh procedure for transposition of great arteries, ventricular septal defect and left ventricular outflow tract obstruction. Thorac Cardiovasc Surg 54, 558–560.

258. Bove EL, Byrum CJ, Kavey RE, *et al.* (1987) Arterial repair for simple and complex forms of transposition of the great arteries. J Cardiovasc Surg (Torino) 28, 54–60.

259. Gontijo Filho B, Fantini FA, Lopes RM, *et al*. (2007) Surgical strategy in transposition of the great arteries with aortic arch obstruction. Rev Bras Cir Cardiovasc 22, 176–183.

260. Mohammadi S, Serraf A, Belli E, *et al*. (2004) Left-sided lesions after anatomic repair of transposition of the great arteries, ventricular septal defect, and coarctation: surgical factors. J Thorac Cardiovasc Surg 128, 44–52.

261. Planche C, Serraf A, Comas JV, *et al*. (1993) Anatomic repair of transposition of great arteries with ventricular septal defect and aortic arch obstruction. One-stage versus two-stage procedure. J Thorac Cardiovasc Surg 105, 925–933.

27

Congenitally Corrected Transposition of the Great Arteries

Eric J. Devaney[1] and Edward L. Bove[2]

[1]Rady Children's Hospital at the University of California, San Diego, CA, USA
[2]C.S. Mott Children's Hospital at the University of Michigan, Ann Arbor, MI, USA

Congenitally corrected transposition of the great arteries (CCTGA) is a complex congenital heart defect characterized by both atrioventricular and ventriculoarterial discordance (Figure 27.1) [1]. In other words, the morphologic right atrium receiving the systemic venous return is connected to the morphologic left ventricle via a mitral valve while the morphologic left atrium which receives pulmonary venous return is connected to the morphologic right ventricle via a tricuspid valve; concurrently, the connections between the ventricles and great arteries are transposed with the left ventricle connected to the pulmonary artery and the right ventricle connected to the aorta. The end result is a physiologically "normal" circulation with deoxygenated systemic venous blood flowing to the lungs and oxygenated pulmonary venous blood being delivered to the systemic circulation.

Although some cases of CCTGA may remain clinically silent, the majority of cases present with symptoms, usually due to the nearly universal occurrence of associated defects, principally ventricular septal defects (VSDs), pulmonary stenosis or atresia, and tricuspid valve abnormalities. The conduction system in CCTGA is notably abnormal, and there is a high incidence of spontaneous heart block. Congenitally corrected transposition may occur with situs solitus (normal atrial situs) or situs inversus. Due to the anatomic complexities associated with CCTGA, it is important to adhere to strict terminology in describing the cardiac chambers and their connections. For example, we will describe the morphologic right or left ventricle based upon its pure anatomic characteristics and not simply by its location in the thoracic cavity. A segmental nomenclature has also been proposed which uses a three letter code to describe the three cardiac segments, respectively, the atrial situs (S, situs solitus; I, situs inversus; or A, situs ambigu-

ous), the ventricular looping (D, dextro-transposed; L, levo-transposed), and the great artery position (S, normally related great arteries; D, dextro-transposed; or L, levo-transposed). Using this system, a normal heart is coded (S,D,S), while CCTGA in situs solitus is described as (S,L,L) and in situs inversus as (I,D,D). The limitation of the segmental system is the absence of an explicit description of chamber connections. Other terms used to describe CCTGA include corrected transposition, L-transposition, and atrioventricular discordance with transposition. As noted, the clinical presentation of CCTGA is dictated by the associated cardiovascular abnormalities, and, in turn, these will determine the progression of symptoms and the surgical management of this complex lesion.

History

Congenitally corrected transposition is a rare defect which represents less than 1% of all forms of congenital heart disease. The pathologist von Rokitansky first described this lesion in 1875 [2]. He recognized its physiologic significance and described it as "corrected transposition." A number of anatomists including Anderson, Lev, and van Praagh have since characterized the anatomic features of CCTGA including the anomalous conduction system [3–12]. Classical surgical repair of CCTGA was first reported in a series from the University of Minnesota in 1957 [3]. The anatomic repair of CCTGA was introduced by Imai and colleagues in 1989 [13] and subsequently by Mee et al. [14] and Ilbawi and coworkers [15].

Anatomy

Congenitally corrected transposition occurs in situs solitus in about 90% of cases and situs inversus in the remainder

Pediatric Cardiac Surgery, Fourth Edition. Edited by Constantine Mavroudis and Carl L. Backer.
© 2013 Blackwell Publishing Ltd. Published 2013 by Blackwell Publishing Ltd.

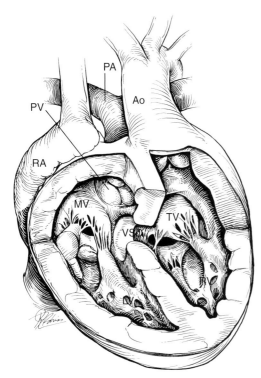

Figure 27.1 The typical anatomy of congenitally corrected transposition of the great arteries with VSD is demonstrated in this cut-away view of a heart in situs solitus. Note the anterior and leftward position of the aorta. The discordant atrioventricular and ventriculoarterial connections are clearly demonstrated. (Ao, aorta; LV, left ventricle; MV, mitral valve; PA, pulmonary artery; PV, pulmonary valve; RA, right atrium; RV, right ventricle; TV, tricuspid valve; VSD, ventricular septal defect.)

[16]. In situs solitus, the morphologic right ventricle is anatomically positioned to the left of the morphologic right ventricle. Levocardia is usually present, but occasionally, the apex of the heart is directed to the right, resulting in dextrocardia. In situs inversus, the relationships are inverted in a mirror image fashion and dextrocardia is typically present.

Associated defects occur in 98% of cases [16]. Ventricular septal defect is the most common anomaly, found in over 75% of cases. The VSD is usually perimembranous and nonrestrictive in nature. Most commonly, the VSD is subpulmonic. Occasionally, multiple VSDs are present. The left ventricular (pulmonary) outflow tract is stenotic or atretic in 50% of cases, and the obstruction may occur at a valvar or subvalvar level. Tricuspid valve abnormalities, including Ebstein's malformation, are common, occurring in over 50% of cases. These are especially significant as the tricuspid valve is the systemic atrioventricular valve in CCTGA. Straddling of either the mitral or tricuspid valve across a VSD may occur, and this may result in right or left ven-

tricular hypoplasia preventing the performance of a biventricular repair. Left ventricular hypoplasia may also occur as a result of the combination of pulmonary atresia with an intact ventricular septum (or restrictive VSD).

The aorta is typically positioned anterior and to the left of the pulmonary artery in cases of CCTGA with situs solitus. The coronary artery anatomy is usually a mirror image pattern of normal with the morphologic left coronary artery arising from the right facing sinus and giving rise to the left anterior descending and circumflex branches and the morphologic right coronary artery arising from the left facing sinus. The pattern is reversed in situs inversus. In situs solitus, the conduction system is abnormally positioned due to abnormal ventricular looping with resultant malalignment of the atrial and ventricular septa (Figure 27.2) [1,4–6,8,9]. This results in a superiorly displaced AV node which is positioned anteriorly on the atrial septum near the junction of the superior limbus and the atrioventricular (mitral) valve. The bundle of His leaves the node and travels anterior to the pulmonary valve. The bundle travels in the subendocardium of the morphologic (right-sided) left ventricle. It has been postulated that heart block may result from the long course of the bundle of His which predisposes it to damage from ischemia or stretch. Interestingly, in cases of CCTGA with situs inversus (with associated D-looping of the ventricles), the anatomy of the conduction tissue is normal, albeit in mirror image orientation.

Natural History and Physiology

Even in the absence of associated defects, the life expectancy of patients with isolated CCTGA is diminished [17]. Natural history studies have shown that any dysfunction of the systemic (morphologic right) ventricle or systemic atrioventricular (tricuspid) valve tends to develop and worsen over time, leading to significant morbidity and mortality [17–20]. Tricuspid valve regurgitation is an important determinant of long-term outcome. Prieto and colleagues found tricuspid valve regurgitation to be an independent risk factor for death [20]. Survival at 20 years was 93% in the absence of significant regurgitation, but only 49% when regurgitation was present. Tricuspid valve regurgitation may result from anatomic malformation of the valve, including Ebstein's malformation, or it may occur as a result of annular dilation from progressive right ventricular dysfunction. More recently, it has been recognized that shift of the ventricular septum to the right (towards the morphologic left ventricle), results in tricuspid regurgitation. In fact, tricuspid regurgitation has been shown to improve after pulmonary artery banding which increases left ventricular pressure and shifts the ventricular septum back to the left (towards the morphologic right ventricle) [21]. In a longitudinal study of adult patients with isolated CCTGA, Presbitero found that significant tricuspid insufficiency occurred in 50% of patients and tended to appear in the third decade of life [17]. Graham and colleagues authored a multi-institutional study which assessed the long-term outcomes of adults with CCTGA [18]. This study reported that by the age of 45, congestive heart failure was much more common in patients having associated defects in comparison to those with the isolated form of the defect. Moreover, congestive heart failure was noted to become more prevalent in all patients with advancing age. Although some authors have found normal right ventricular function in patients with CCTGA [22,23], others have documented defects under stressed conditions. Using exercise radionuclide stress testing, Hornung et al. [24] found that right ventricular dysfunction and perfusion abnormalities were common findings in patients with CCTGA. Fredriksen et al. evaluated exercise capacity in adults with CCTGA and found reduced aerobic capacity and impaired right ventricular function with exercise despite normal function at rest [25].

Most patients with CCTGA will present as a result of an associated defect. Patients with significant obstruction of the left ventricular outflow tract (pulmonary stenosis or atresia) will present early in life with cyanosis. Those with significant tricuspid regurgitation or a large VSD will develop early congestive heart failure. Bradycardia from spontaneous heart block can occur early or late and lead to symptoms including heart failure [26–28]. The incidence of

heart block has been estimated at 2% per year following the diagnosis of CCTGA, and the rate is higher in patients with an intact ventricular septum [29]. Late tricuspid insufficiency and right ventricular dysfunction occur with increasing frequency throughout life [18].

Diagnosis

The diagnosis of CCTGA is usually made by echocardiography. Assessment of the left ventricular outflow tract and the atrioventricular valves can be performed and the anatomic location of any VSD may be characterized. It is important to identify any straddling of atrioventricular valves, as this will have an impact on the subsequent surgical repair. Cardiac catheterization may provide additional anatomic information as well as hemodynamic data. Magnetic resonance imaging is an emerging modality which can provide valuable complementary data.

Surgical Management

The traditional approach to the repair of CCTGA has been directed at the treatment of the associated defects, e.g. VSD closure (Figure 27.2) [1], tricuspid valve repair or replacement, or placement of a conduit between the left ventricle and pulmonary artery to bypass left ventricular outflow tract obstruction (Figure 27.3) [1]. This approach leaves the right ventricle as the systemic ventricle and the tricuspid valve as the systemic atrioventricular valve. Although the

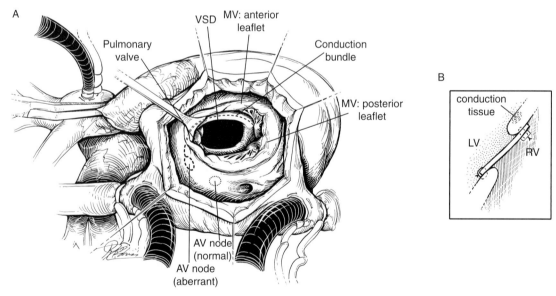

Figure 27.2 Transatrial closure of the ventricular septal defect. This technique may be used for both classic and anatomic repairs. **A,** Right atriotomy exposes the mitral valve which can be retracted to reveal the VSD which is usually perimembranous in location. Note the abnormal location of the AV node and the pathway of the bundle of His passing anterior to the pulmonary annulus and

along the morphologic left ventricular side of the crest of the ventricular septum. **B,** Sutures must be taken on the opposite side of the septum in the area of the conduction tissue. (AV, atrioventricular; LV, left ventricle; MV, mitral valve; RV, right ventricle; VSD, ventricular septal defect.)

A

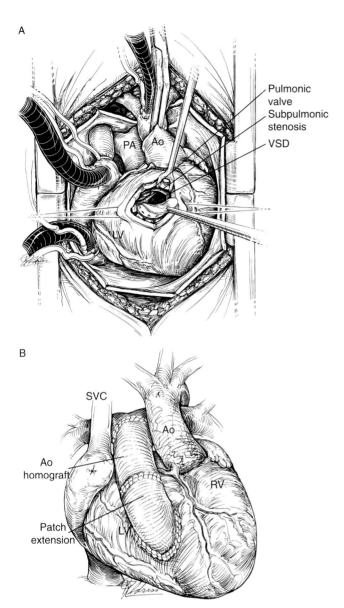

Pulmonic
valve
Subpulmonic
stenosis

VSD

PA   Ao

LV

B

SVC

Ao

Ao
homograft

RV

Patch
extension   LV

Figure 27.3 Classic repair of congenitally corrected transposition of the great arteries with left ventricular outflow tract obstruction. **A,** The ventricular septal defect (VSD) may be closed transatrially or through a left ventriculotomy as shown here. Again, sutures must be taken on the morphologic right ventricular side of the septum in the area of the conduction tissue to avoid heart block. **B,** A valved conduit is then implanted between the left ventricle and the pulmonary artery, while the native pulmonary artery is oversewn. When an allograft is used, a patch extension or hood is frequently utilized to allow a better fit. (Ao, aorta; PA, pulmonary artery; RV, right ventricle SVC, superior vena cava.)

early results associated with this classic approach have improved, the late results are associated with significant morbidity and mortality, primarily due to complications related to failure of the right ventricle and the systemic atrioventricular valve.

Recently, an alternative surgical approach of anatomic repair has been developed, with the goal of restoring the left ventricle as the systemic ventricle and the right ventricle as the pulmonary ventricle. This can be accomplished by performing a double switch operation which combines an atrial switch (Figure 27.4) and arterial switch procedure (Figure 27.5) for patients with CCTGA without pulmonary stenosis. Patients with a large VSD are excellent candidates for this approach as the left ventricle is already at systemic pressure and can tolerate the arterial switch. Patients with CCTGA and intact ventricular septum who have significant tricuspid regurgitation or right ventricular dysfunction are also candidates for the double switch, but these patients will require a period of left ventricular retraining which can be accomplished by placement of a pulmonary artery band in a fashion completely analogous to patients with classic transposition and intact ventricular septum. When initially placing the band, a reasonable goal is to achieve a left ventricular pressure of 50% systemic. This is frequently accompanied by a shift of the ventricular septum to the left with an associated improvement in tricuspid valve function. Typically it is not possible to achieve higher left ventricular pressures at the initial banding due to the development of left ventricular dysfunction. Repeat band tightening will be required for sufficient left ventricular retraining. Anatomic repair can be carried out when the left ventricular pressure equals or exceeds 80% systemic and left ventricular function is normal. Alternatively, for patients with CCTGA with VSD and left ventricular outflow tract obstruction, an atrial switch is combined with a Rastelli procedure (baffling the VSD to the aorta and placement of a right ventricle to pulmonary artery conduit) (Figure 27.6) [1]. In these cases, left ventricular retraining is usually not necessary. In some cases, the VSD may need to be enlarged to allow unobstructed left ventricular outflow.

Classic Repair

VSD Closure

Repair is performed via median sternotomy (Figure 27.2) [1]. Cannulation of the distal ascending aorta and both vena cavae is accomplished. Cardiopulmonary bypass with mild hypothermia is established, followed by cardioplegic arrest. A conventional right atriotomy is performed, and the ventricular septum is exposed through the mitral valve. The VSD is usually located in a perimembranous position, although it can be elsewhere. The key anatomic feature to remember is that the conduction tissue passes along the anterior and superior margin of the defect in the subendocardium of the morphologic left ventricle. The implication of this anatomic fact is that sutures must be taken on the opposite side of the septum (from the surgeon's point of view) to avoid injury to this region [30,31].

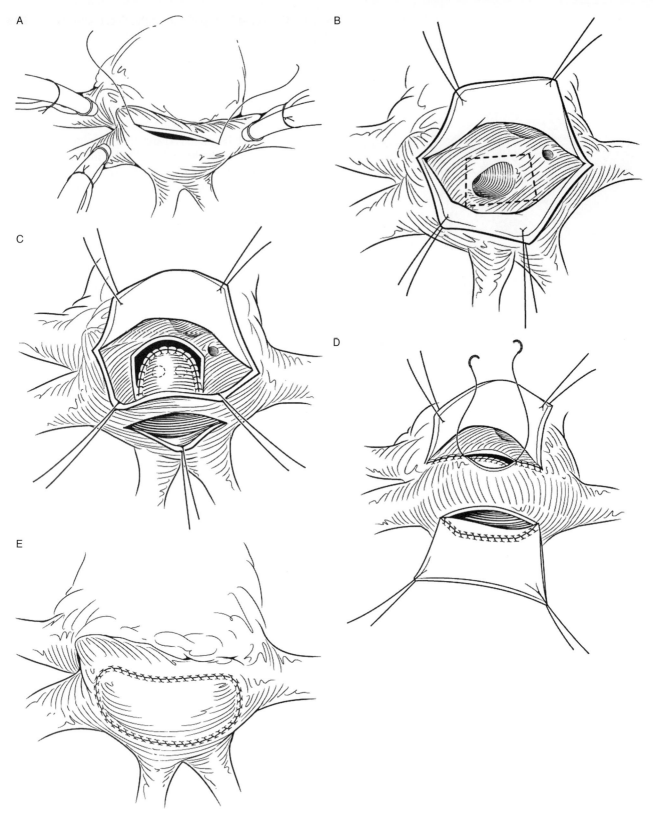

Figure 27.4 The Senning operation in CCTGA. **A,** Right atriotomy is made. In this technique, the precise location of the atriotomy is not critical since the pulmonary venous pathway will be patch augmented. **B,** The atrial septum is mobilized on a lateral (posterior) pedicle. **C,** The atrial septum is sutured to the floor of the left atrium around the pulmonary veins, and a longitudinal left atriotomy is made. **D,** The posterior edge of the right atriotomy is then folded into the right atrium and sewn along the inner atrial wall and along the divided edge of the atrial septum. This redirects the caval flow across the atrial septum. The pulmonary venous pathway is augmented using a patch (preferably homograft tissue) which is sewn posteriorly to the lateral edge of the left atriotomy. **E,** The patch is then sewn along the outer wall of the right atrium to connect with the anterior edge of the original right atriotomy.

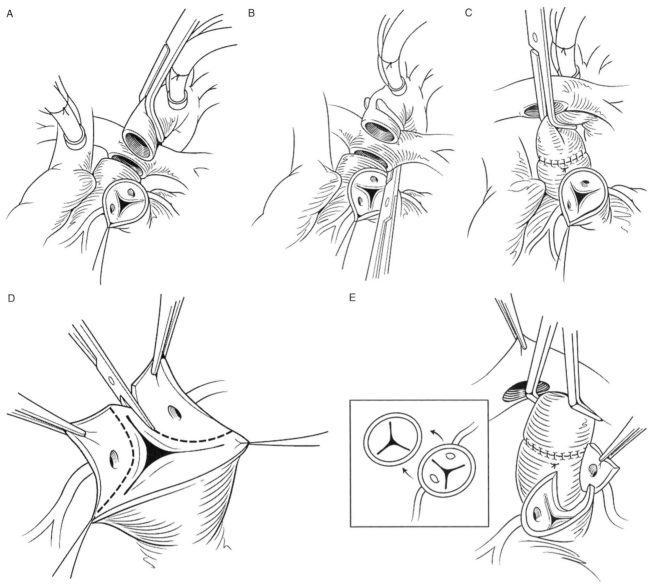

Figure 27.5 The arterial switch procedure in anatomic repair of CCTGA. **A,** The pulmonary artery is transected at its bifurcation and the aorta is divided several millimeters beyond this point. Note the morphologic left coronary artery arising from the right facing sinus and the morphologic right coronary from the left. **B,** The Lecompte maneuver is performed. **C,** The neoaortic anastomosis is performed. The superior extents of the neoaortic valve commissures are marked externally with sutures to identify the valve. **D,E,** Coronary buttons are mobilized for coronary transfer. **F,** Using the closed technique, the neoaorta is briefly pressurized, and the optimal site for coronary implantation is identified. In most cases, direct coronary transfer is possible, but when tension or distortion is likely, a trapdoor technique can be used using a pericardial patch. **G,** The defects created by removal of the coronary buttons are reconstructed using an autologous pericardial patch which is cut into a trouser shape. In order to avoid distortion, the orifice of the pulmonary bifurcation is shifted to the left as shown. **H,** The completed arterial switch.

Once the posterior and inferior margin of the defect is reached, sutures may be taken on the morphologic left ventricular side as this area is free of all conduction tissue. The suture line can be completed along the base of the posterior mitral leaflet. The defect is usually closed using a polytetrafluoroethylene patch and a running polypropyl-ene suture, although an interrupted suture technique may also be used.

Left Ventricular Outflow Tract Repair
The nature of left ventricular outflow tract obstruction is usually valvar or subvalvar. In CCTGA, the pulmonary

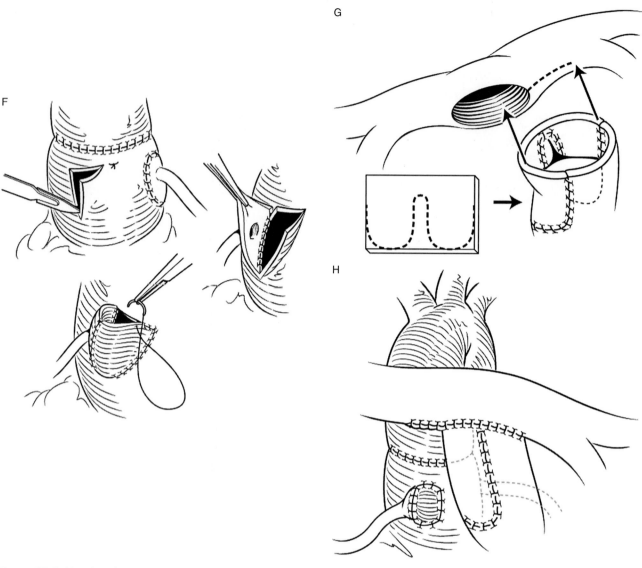

Figure 27.5 (*Continued*)

valve occupies a posterior wedged position between the mitral and tricuspid valves. This limits exposure of this area. In addition, the presence of conduction tissue traveling along the anterior border of the pulmonary valve limits any attempts to directly enlarge this area without creating heart block. In some cases it is possible to relieve the obstruction by simply resecting some subvalvar muscle or extraneous chordal tissue. In general, however, the area of obstruction must be bypassed using a conduit placed between the left ventricle and the pulmonary artery (Figure 27.3) [1]. Care must be taken in making the ventriculotomy to avoid injury to the coronaries or the mitral valve apparatus. In these cases, the VSD may optionally be closed via the ventriculotomy. The procedure is performed under cardioplegic arrest. The choice of conduit is a matter of personal choice, but the most common options include the use of a heterograft, pulmonary homograft, or bovine jugular venous graft.

Tricuspid Valve Procedures

Patients with significant tricuspid valve abnormalities are candidates for tricuspid valve repair or replacement. Exposure of the tricuspid valve is analogous to exposure of the mitral valve in the normal heart. The interatrial groove is widely developed before cardioplegic arrest of the heart. The left atrium is entered and the use of a dedicated retractor aids in exposure of the tricuspid valve. Due to abnormal ventricular looping, it may still be difficult to visualize the tricuspid valve, and in some cases, transection of the superior vena cava will allow for improved expo-

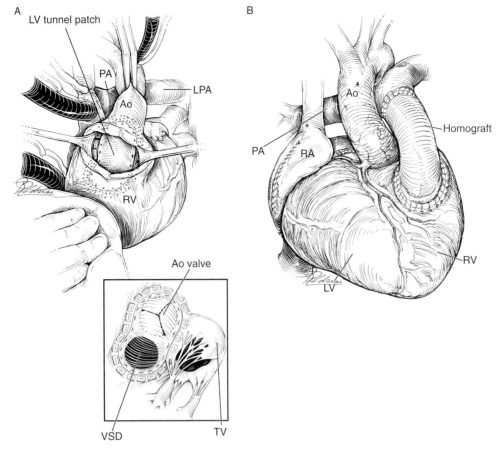

A   LV tunnel patch

PA

Ao

LPA

RV

Ao valve

VSD   TV

B

Ao

Homograft

PA

RA

RV

LV

Figure 27.6 The Rastelli procedure in anatomic repair of CCTGA. **A,** With the apex of the heart elevated, a right ventriculotomy is made and an intraventricular baffle is created to connect the VSD to the aortic valve. The inset provides more detail illustrating the intraventricular baffle. **B,** A valved conduit is then implanted between the right ventriculotomy and the pulmonary artery. (Ao, aorta; LPA, left pulmonary artery; LV, left ventricle; PA, pulmonary artery; RA, right atrium; RV, right ventricle; TV, tricuspid valve; VSD, ventricular septal defect.)

sure. Valvuloplasty may be considered when the mechanism of insufficiency is clear, but it should be noted that the repair of Ebstenoid valves is very difficult in this setting, and tricuspid valve replacement using a bioprosthetic or mechanical valve may be preferred.

Anatomic Repair

Senning and Arterial Switch Procedure (Double Switch)

In the absence of significant left ventricular outflow tract obstruction, a double switch procedure may be performed. Candidates for this procedure include patients with CCTGA and concurrent VSD, right ventricular dysfunction, or tricuspid valve insufficiency. In addition, patients must have adequate left ventricular hemodynamics to tolerate the arterial switch. Exclusion criteria include ventricular hypoplasia and straddling atrioventricular valves. Due to the complexity of the procedure, the double switch is usually

performed at 6–8 months of age, although it can be accomplished in the neonate. When a large VSD is present, pulmonary artery banding may be necessary as an initial intervention to limit congestive heart failure while waiting for definitive repair.

The double switch is performed with bicaval venous cannulation (taking care to cannulate each vena cava quite distally) and cardiopulmonary bypass with moderate hypothermia. A patch of autologous pericardium is harvested and treated with glutaraldehyde for later use. The Senning operation is the preferred atrial switch procedure (Figure 27.4). This technique uses a flap of autologous atrial tissue to redirect venous return at the atrial level. The interatrial groove is extensively developed. Following cardioplegic arrest, a conventional right atriotomy is performed, and the VSD (if present) can be closed as previously described. The atriotomy is extended superiorly and inferiorly to within 1 cm of each cavoatrial junction. The atrial septum is then mobilized as a laterally based flap which is then dropped into the left atrium and sewn around the origins of the pulmonary veins. If the atrial septum is deficient, it can be augmented using a polytetrafluoroethylene patch. The coronary sinus is usually cut back for a length of 1–2 cm. Next, a longitudinal left atriotomy is made. The systemic venous pathway is completed by folding the posterior edge of the previous right atriotomy over the caval orifices and along the original line of the atrial septal attachment. This maneuver redirects systemic venous return across the atrial septum to the tricuspid valve. The pulmonary venous pathway is then routinely augmented using a generous patch of pulmonary allograft tissue which is sewn along the posterior edge of the left atriotomy, along the outer wall of the right atrium, and terminating along the anterior edge of the original right atriotomy. More recently, the pulmonary venous pathway has been augmented using a posteriorly based autologous flap of pericardium, either alone or in combination with a patch of pulmonary allograft. The Senning procedure can be performed even in the presence of dextrocardia. When dextrocardia is present, the heart is completely mobilized and the left pleural space is widely opened. The heart may then be displaced into the left chest to improve exposure.

The arterial switch operation is performed using standard techniques employed for patients with classic transposition (Figure 27.5). The aorta and pulmonary arteries are transected around the level of the pulmonary bifurcation. The coronaries are mobilized with generous buttons of arterial wall. In most cases, a Lecompte maneuver is performed with translocation of the distal pulmonary artery anterior to the aorta. The neoaortic anastomosis is then accomplished and coronary implantation is performed using the closed technique. The resected sinuses of the neopulmonary artery are reconstructed using the previously harvested autologous pericardium. Next, it is usually necessary to shift the orifice of the distal pulmonary artery towards the left to prevent distortion in the neopulmonary artery and provide an easier fit. This is readily accomplished by incising the pulmonary artery orifice well onto the left pulmonary artery and simply oversewing the original orifice. The operation is completed with the performance of the neopulmonary anastomosis.

Senning and Rastelli Procedure

Patients with significant, unresectable left ventricular outflow tract obstruction or pulmonary atresia are not candidates for an arterial switch. For these patients, a combined Senning and Rastelli procedure is employed (Figure 27.6) [1]. When significant cyanosis is present, an initial shunt procedure is usually performed. Definitive repair is then deferred until 6–8 months of age. The Senning procedure is performed as previously described. A right ventriculotomy is created and an intraventricular baffle (polytetrafluoroethylene) is inserted to channel the VSD (and left ventricular outflow) to the aorta. A right ventricle

to pulmonary artery conduit is then implanted. As always, care must be taken to avoid injury to the conduction tissue. In some cases enlargement of the VSD must be performed to allow unobstructed left ventricular outflow. To avoid heart block, the VSD is enlarged along its posterior and inferior margin.

Results

Classic Repair

The reported mortality for classic repair of defects associated with CCTGA ranges widely, largely dependent on the era of each study [32–37]. The Mayo Clinic found that during the 1970s and early 1980s early mortality varied from 18% to 26%, while for more recent cohorts of patients, the mortality was 3% [32]. Long-term follow up of survivors revealed an overall survival of 77% at 5 years and 67% at 10 years. Yeh *et al.* from Toronto reported a large series of CCTGA patients undergoing surgical repair and reported an operative mortality of 6% [38]. At 20-year follow-up of these patients, survival was 48%. For tricuspid valve insufficiency, repair can be performed with a low mortality, but a recurrence rate of up to 50% has been reported [21,33]. The results of tricuspid valve replacement have been reviewed by van Son and colleagues who found an early mortality of 10% and a 10-year survival of 68% [36]. In this series, all early and late deaths were secondary to right ventricular failure. Other reports have similarly documented a substantial late mortality from systemic ventricular failure [35,39]. Despite the recognition of the anatomy of the anomalous conduction tissue, the complication of postsurgical heart block remains as high as 20% [34,35].

Patients who have undergone an atrial switch repair of classic transposition also have a right ventricle in the systemic position. This large historical cohort of patients provides an opportunity to evaluate the long-term functional status of the systemic right ventricle. A number of studies have demonstrated that adult survivors remain at risk for premature death due to late systemic ventricular failure which occurs in over 10% of patients and is responsible for nearly half of all late deaths [40–44]. Interestingly, the incidence of late tricuspid insufficiency appears to be much lower than in corrected transposition, probably due to the absence of intrinsic valvar abnormalities which are common in corrected transposition.

Anatomic Repair

Anatomic repair of CCTGA has been pursued by a number of large centers, and the results have been encouraging [14,45–52]. The largest reported series to date comes from the Birmingham group, which has performed anatomic repair in 51 patients with CCTGA [50]. In this group, 29 patients underwent a Senning/arterial switch while 22 had a Senning/Rastelli. The early mortality was 5.6%, and actuarial survival at 9 years was 95% (excluding early mortality) with 94% of the survivors in New York Heart Association (NYHA) functional class I. Left ventricular retraining was required in 31%. Outcomes for this group were comparable to the group not requiring retraining, although the need for retraining remained a statistically significant risk factor for late cardiac failure [53]. Other groups have reported large series of patients with no early mortality [46,48,51]. Jahangiri and colleagues [21] examined tricuspid valve function following various surgical procedures for CCTGA and observed that tricuspid insufficiency decreased postoperatively following pulmonary artery banding and following anatomic repair. On the contrary, tricuspid insufficiency typically worsened following placement of a systemic to pulmonary artery shunt. Following classic repair techniques, early tricuspid valve function was unchanged but late reintervention for tricuspid valve intervention was frequent and was associated with a high mortality. In a contemporary series, Shin'oka et al. reported similar early results for both classic and anatomic repair of CCTGA in the absence of significant tricuspid valve insufficiency [54]. When CCTGA was accompanied by tricuspid insufficiency, patients undergoing anatomic repair demonstrated superior results over those having classic repair.

At the University of Michigan, a total of 55 patients have undergone anatomic repair of CCTGA (Senning and arterial switch, n = 30; Senning and Rastelli, n = 25). A previous report summarizes the results of an earlier cohort [45]. The overall hospital survival was 95% with one death following the Senning/arterial switch and two deaths following Senning/Rastelli. There were no new cases of complete heart block although four patients had preoperative heart block. One 7-year-old patient who underwent left ventricular retraining developed left ventricular dysfunction following double switch. This resulted from pure diastolic dysfunction, and the patient ultimately required cardiac transplantation. Late reoperations have included conduit replacement (n = 1), relief of superior vena cava obstruction (n = 1), and relief of pulmonary venous obstruction (n = 1). Neoaortic insufficiency, coronary obstruction, and left ventricular outflow tract obstruction have not been seen in this patient cohort. Tricuspid valve insufficiency, when present, was noted to significantly improve following anatomic repair ($p = 0.001$).

Conclusion

Corrected transposition of the great arteries is a rare defect and frequently accompanied by associated cardiac defects, which modify its physiology, mode of presentation, and natural history. Even in the absence of associated defects, corrected transposition is associated with a poor survival resulting from the development of right (systemic) ventricular failure and tricuspid (systemic atrioventricular)

valve insufficiency. Corrected transposition of the great arteries presents a challenge for surgical repair. Classic repair strategies address the associated defects and leave the right ventricle and tricuspid valve on the systemic side of the circulation. As a result, classic repair is complicated by early and late right ventricular and tricuspid valve dysfunction. Anatomic repair restores the right and left ventricles (and their atrioventricular valves) to the pulmonary and systemic circulations, respectively, and, despite its early risk, may improve long-term outcomes for these patients, although longer-term follow up will be necessary to confirm this hypothesis.

References

1. Karl TR, Cochrane AD. (2003) Congenitally corrected transposition of the great arteries. In: Mavroudis C, Backer CL, eds. *Pediatric Cardiac Surgery*, 3rd ed. Philadelphia, PA: Mosby, Inc.
2. von Rokitansky C. (1875) *Die Defecte der Scheidwande des Herzens*. Vienna: Wilhelm Braumuller.
3. Anderson RC, Lillehei CW, Lester RG. (1957) Corrected transposition of the great vessels of the heart: a review of 17 cases. Pediatrics 20, 626–646.
4. Anderson RH. (2004) The conduction tissues in congenitally corrected transposition. Ann Thorac Surg 77, 1881–1882.
5. Anderson RH, Arnold R, Wilkinson JL. (1973) The conducting system in congenitally corrected transposition. Lancet 1, 1286–1288.
6. Anderson RH, Becker AE, Arnold R, et al. (1974) The conducting tissues in congenitally corrected transposition. Circulation 50, 911–923.
7. Anderson RH, Becker AE, Gerlis LM. (1975) The pulmonary outflow tract in classically corrected transposition. J Thorac Cardiovasc Surg 69, 747–757.
8. Anderson RH, Danielson GK, Maloney JD, et al. (1978) Atrioventricular bundle in corrected transposition. Ann Thorac Surg 26, 95–97.
9. Lev M, Licata RH, May RC. (1963) The conduction system in mixed levocardia with ventricular inversion (corrected transposition). Circulation 28, 232–237.
10. Lev M, Rowlatt UF. (1961) The pathologic anatomy of mixed levocardia. A review of thirteen cases of atrial or ventricular inversion with or without corrected transposition. Am J Cardiol 8, 216–263.
11. Van Praagh R, Papagiannis J, Grunenfelder J, et al. (1998) Pathologic anatomy of corrected transposition of the great arteries: medical and surgical implications. Am Heart J 135, 772–785.
12. Van Praagh R, Van Praagh S. (1967) Anatomically corrected transposition of the great arteries. Br Heart J 29, 112–119.
13. Yamagishi M, Imai Y, Hoshino S, et al. (1993) Anatomic correction of atrioventricular discordance. J Thorac Cardiovasc Surg 105, 1067–1076.
14. Karl TR, Weintraub RG, Brizard CP, et al. (1997) Senning plus arterial switch operation for discordant (congenitally corrected) transposition. Ann Thorac Surg 64, 495–502.
15. Ilbawi MN, DeLeon SY, Backer CL, et al. (1990) An alternative approach to the surgical management of physiologically

corrected transposition with ventricular septal defect and pulmonary stenosis or atresia. J Thorac Cardiovasc Surg 100, 410–415.

16. Allwork SP, Bentall HH, Becker AE, *et al.* (1976) Congenitally corrected transposition of the great arteries: morphologic study of 32 cases. Am J Cardiol 38, 910–923.

17. Presbitero P, Somerville J, Rabajoli F, *et al.* (1995) Corrected transposition of the great arteries without associated defects in adult patients: clinical profile and follow up. Br Heart J 74, 57–59.

18. Graham TP Jr, Bernard YD, Mellen BG, *et al.* (2000) Long-term outcome in congenitally corrected transposition of the great arteries: a multi-institutional study. J Am Coll Cardiol 36, 255–261.

19. Huhta JC, Danielson GK, Ritter DG, *et al.* (1985) Survival in atrioventricular discordance. Pediatr Cardiol 6, 57–60.

20. Prieto LR, Hordof AJ, Secic M, *et al.* (1998) Progressive tricuspid valve disease in patients with congenitally corrected transposition of the great arteries. Circulation 98, 997–1005.

21. Jahangiri M, Redington AN, Elliott MJ, *et al.* (2001) A case for anatomic correction in atrioventricular discordance? Effects of surgery on tricuspid valve function. J Thorac Cardiovasc Surg 121, 1040–1045.

22. Benson LN, Burns R, Schwaiger M, *et al.* (1986) Radionuclide angiographic evaluation of ventricular function in isolated congenitally corrected transposition of the great arteries. Am J Cardiol 58, 319–324.

23. Dimas AP, Moodie DS, Sterba R, *et al.* (1989) Long-term function of the morphologic right ventricle in adult patients with corrected transposition of the great arteries. Am Heart J 118, 526–530.

24. Hornung TS, Bernard EJ, Celermajer DS, *et al.* (1999) Right ventricular dysfunction in congenitally corrected transposition of the great arteries. Am J Cardiol 84, 1116–1119, A10.

25. Fredriksen PM, Chen A, Veldtman G, *et al.* (2001) Exercise capacity in adult patients with congenitally corrected transposition of the great arteries. Heart 85, 191–195.

26. Dick M 2nd, Van Praagh R, Rudd M, *et al.* (1977) Electrophysiologic delineation of the specialized atrioventricular conduction system in two patients with corrected transposition of the great arteries in situs inversus (I,D,D). Circulation 55, 896–900.

27. Ikeda U, Yamamoto K, Hasegawa H, *et al.* (1992) Conduction disturbance and pacemaker therapy in patients with corrected transposition of the great arteries. Cardiology 81, 325–329.

28. Wilkinson JL, Smith A, Lincoln C, *et al.* (1978) Conducting tissues in congenitally corrected transposition with situs inversus. Br Heart J 40, 41–48.

29. Huhta JC, Maloney JD, Ritter DG, *et al.* (1983) Complete atrioventricular block in patients with atrioventricular discordance. Circulation 67, 1374–1377.

30. de Leval MR, Bastos P, Stark J, *et al.* (1979) Surgical technique to reduce the risks of heart block following closure of ventricular septal defect in atrioventricular discordance. J Thorac Cardiovasc Surg 78, 515–526.

31. Doty DB, Truesdell SC, Marvin WJ Jr. (1983) Techniques to avoid injury of the conduction tissue during the surgical

treatment of corrected transposition. Circulation 68, II63–II69.

32. Biliciler-Denktas G, Feldt RH, Connolly HM, *et al.* (2001) Early and late results of operations for defects associated with corrected transposition and other anomalies with atrioventricular discordance in a pediatric population. J Thorac Cardiovasc Surg 122, 234–241.

33. Scherptong RW, Vliegen HW, Winter MM, *et al.* (2009) Tricuspid valve surgery in adults with a dysfunctional systemic right ventricle: repair or replace? Circulation 119, 1467–1472.

34. Szufladowicz M, Horvath P, de Leval M, *et al.* (1996) Intracardiac repair of lesions associated with atrioventricular discordance. Eur J Cardiothorac Surg 10, 443–448.

35. Termignon JL, Leca F, Vouhe PR, *et al.* (1996) "Classic" repair of congenitally corrected transposition and ventricular septal defect. Ann Thorac Surg 62, 199–206.

36. van Son JA, Danielson GK, Huhta JC, *et al.* (1995) Late results of systemic atrioventricular valve replacement in corrected transposition. J Thorac Cardiovasc Surg 109, 642–652; discussion 652–653.

37. Voskuil M, Hazekamp MG, Kroft LJ, *et al.* (1999) Postsurgical course of patients with congenitally corrected transposition of the great arteries. Am J Cardiol 83, 558–662.

38. Yeh T Jr, Connelly MS, Coles JG, *et al.* (1999) Atrioventricular discordance: results of repair in 127 patients. J Thorac Cardiovasc Surg 117, 1190–1203.

39. McGrath LB, Kirklin JW, Blackstone EH, *et al.* (1985) Death and other events after cardiac repair in discordant atrioventricular connection. J Thorac Cardiovasc Surg 90, 711–728.

40. Graham TP, Jr., Atwood GF, Boucek RJ Jr, *et al.* (1975) Abnormalities of right ventricular function following Mustard's operation for transposition of the great arteries. Circulation 52, 678–684.

41. Kirjavainen M, Happonen JM, Louhimo I. (1999) Late results of Senning operation. J Thorac Cardiovasc Surg 117, 488–495.

42. Puley G, Siu S, Connelly M, *et al.* (1999) Arrhythmia and survival in patients >18 years of age after the Mustard procedure for complete transposition of the great arteries. Am J Cardiol 83, 1080–1084.

43. Siebenmann R, von Segesser L, Schneider K, *et al.* (1989) Late failure of systemic ventricle after atrial correction for transposition of great arteries. Eur J Cardiothorac Surg 3, 119–123; discussion 123–124.

44. Turina MI, Siebenmann R, von Segesser L, *et al.* (1989) Late functional deterioration after atrial correction for transposition of the great arteries. Circulation 80, I162–I167.

45. Devaney EJ, Charpie JR, Ohye RG, *et al.* (2003) Combined arterial switch and Senning operation for congenitally corrected transposition of the great arteries: patient selection and intermediate results. J Thorac Cardiovasc Surg 125, 500–507.

46. Duncan BW, Mee RB, Mesia CI, *et al.* (2003) Results of the double switch operation for congenitally corrected transposition of the great arteries. Eur J Cardiothorac Surg 24, 11–19; discussion 19–20.

47. Ilbawi MN, Ocampo CB, Allen BS, *et al.* (2002) Intermediate results of the anatomic repair for congenitally corrected

transposition. Ann Thorac Surg 73, 594–599; discussion 599–600.

48. Imamura M, Drummond-Webb JJ, Murphy DJ Jr, *et al.* (2000) Results of the double switch operation in the current era. Ann Thorac Surg 70, 100–105.

49. Koh M, Yagihara T, Uemura H, *et al.* (2006) Intermediate results of the double-switch operations for atrioventricular discordance. Ann Thorac Surg 81, 671–677; discussion 677.

50. Langley SM, Winlaw DS, Stumper O, *et al.* (2003) Midterm results after restoration of the morphologically left ventricle to the systemic circulation in patients with congenitally corrected transposition of the great arteries. J Thorac Cardiovasc Surg 125, 1229–1241.

51. Ly M, Belli E, Leobon B, *et al.* (2009) Results of the double switch operation for congenitally corrected transposition of the great arteries. Eur J Cardiothorac Surg 35, 879–883; discussion 883–884.

52. Sano T, Riesenfeld T, Karl TR, *et al.* (1995) Intermediate-term outcome after intracardiac repair of associated cardiac defects in patients with atrioventricular and ventriculoarterial discordance. Circulation 92(9 Suppl), II272–II278.

53. Quinn DW, McGuirk SP, Metha C, *et al.* (2008) The morphologic left ventricle that requires training by means of pulmonary artery banding before the double-switch procedure for congenitally corrected transposition of the great arteries is at risk of late dysfunction. J Thorac Cardiovasc Surg 135, 1137–1144, 44 e1–e2.

54. Shin'oka T, Kurosawa H, Imai Y, *et al.* (2007) Outcomes of definitive surgical repair for congenitally corrected transposition of the great arteries or double outlet right ventricle with discordant atrioventricular connections: risk analyses in 189 patients. J Thorac Cardiovasc Surg 133, 1318–1328, 28 e1–e4.

CHAPTER **28**

The Functionally Univentricular Heart and Fontan's Operation

Marshall L. Jacobs

Cleveland Clinic Children's Hospital, Cleveland, OH, USA

Background

Among the most challenging of congenital cardiac anomalies is the broad category of hearts that lack two well developed ventricles. As challenging as they are to manage medically and surgically, they are at least as difficult to describe and classify. The most commonly applied terms *single ventricle* and *univentricular heart* are imprecise and spark heated debate among morphologists and embryologists. Only rarely do hearts posses a true solitary ventricle. Yet there is a variety of circumstances where a single, well developed ventricle is associated with an additional incomplete, rudimentary or hypoplastic ventricle. Ultimately, the principles that have evolved for the medical and surgical management of hearts that are not septatable are consistent with the idea of a functionally univentricular heart.

As opposed to the common circumstance where there are two atria, and each atrium is connected to its own ventricle, the hearts considered in this chapter are those in which the atrial chambers connect to only one ventricle that is well developed and dominant. The features of a well developed ventricle include an inlet portion, supporting the subvalvar tensor apparatus, a trabecular zone, and an outlet portion to a great artery. Most often in functionally univentricular hearts, there is an additional incomplete, rudimentary or hypoplastic ventricle that lacks an atrioventricular connection. The obligatory physiology in the setting of a functionally univentricular heart is that the systemic and pulmonary circulations are arranged in parallel fashion, rather than in series as in the normal heart. This results in a drastically altered natural history, which without surgical intervention most often culminates in death of the patient, anywhere from the first days of life to the second decade of life. The evolution of palliative and reconstructive cardiac operations has impacted enormously

on the life expectancy and quality of life of such individuals. It has therefore become increasingly important to precisely and thoroughly describe and classify these anomalies. In this chapter, we consider the functionally univentricular heart to encompass those anomalies that are characterized by the lack of two completely well developed ventricles. Hypoplastic left heart syndrome, which is the most common of the functionally univentricular cardiac malformations, is considered separately in Chapter 31, *Hypoplastic Left Heart Syndrome*. Also covered elsewhere in this text are those cardiac anomalies where, even in the presence of two well developed ventricles, the heart may be considered nonseptatable and thus lend itself to treatment strategies that are described here.

Nomenclature and Classification

Before the era of surgical therapy for these complicated malformations, the study of incomplete hearts was largely descriptive. Pathologists and anatomists debated the questions of what constitutes a *single ventricle*, or a univentricular heart, and the debate continues today. There is no one system of nomenclature that has been accepted by all practitioners in the field. Historically, the terms *single ventricle* and *common ventricle* were employed interchangeably by Abbott [1], Taussig [2], and Edwards [3]. Lev [4] used the designation *single ventricle* when an outlet chamber was present and the term *common ventricle* when an outlet chamber was absent. Most often, there is an incomplete or rudimentary outlet chamber. The connection between the main ventricular chamber and the outlet chamber has been given a variety of names: ventricular septal defect, bulboventricular foramen, outlet foramen, trabecular septal defect, and interventricular communication.

Pediatric Cardiac Surgery, Fourth Edition. Edited by Constantine Mavroudis and Carl L. Backer.
© 2013 Blackwell Publishing Ltd. Published 2013 by Blackwell Publishing Ltd.

Most single ventricle anomalies are currently described using Van Praagh's segmental anatomy approach [5] or Anderson's system of sequential chamber localization [6]. There are important and fundamental differences. According to Van Praagh and colleagues [7], a single or common ventricle is one ventricular chamber that receives both the tricuspid and mitral valves or a common atrioventricular valve. Thus, this system excludes tricuspid and mitral atresia from single ventricle anomalies. Anderson *et al.* also emphasize the nature of the connections between the atrial and ventricular structures but assert that the unifying criteria for univentricular hearts is that the entire atrioventricular junction is connected to only one chamber in the ventricular mass [6]. A second ventricular chamber, if present, will lack any atrioventricular connection and be rudimentary. Hence the term *univentricular atrioventricular connection* is used by Anderson to describe the functionally single ventricle. The acknowledgement that in the vast majority of cases a single, well developed ventricle exists in association with a second hypoplastic or rudimentary ventricle, calls for terminology that is descriptively accurate but does not deny ventricular status to the chamber, which is not completely developed. Thus, in 2006, Jacobs and Anderson applied the term "functionally univentricular," which is applicable whenever one or the other ventricle is incapable, for whatever reason, of supporting either the systemic or the pulmonary circulation [8].

In 2000, a consensus was reached by the Society of Thoracic Surgeons International Congenital Heart Surgery Nomenclature and Database Project [9] that the nomenclature proposed for functionally univentricular hearts would encompass hearts with double-inlet atrioventricular connection (both double-inlet left ventricle [DILV] and double-inlet right ventricle [DIRV]), hearts with absence of one atrioventricular connection (including tricuspid atresia and mitral atresia), hearts with a common atrioventricular valve and only one completely well developed ventricle (unbalanced common atrioventricular canal defect), hearts with only one fully developed ventricle and heterotaxy syndrome, and finally other rare forms of univentricular hearts that do not fit in one of the specified major categories. As in the organization of this textbook, separate status was accorded to hypoplastic left heart syndrome, while still acknowledging that it is a common form of functionally univentricular heart.

Anatomy

Double-Inlet Ventricle

Double-inlet ventricle (DIV) is a congenital cardiac malformation in which both atria connect to only one ventricular chamber by either two separate atrioventricular valves or a common atrioventricular valve. Rarely does the ventricular mass consist only of a solitary ventricle. In addition to one fully developed ventricle there is usually an additional ventricle, which is incomplete (rudimentary) in addition to being hypoplastic. There may be no atrioventricular connection to the incomplete ventricle, or the incomplete ventricle may be connected to an atrium by way of overriding of one of the atrioventricular valves. The term DIV applies if more than 50% of the overriding valve lies over the dominant ventricle.

The dominant ventricle in DIV may have left ventricular internal architecture, right ventricle internal architecture, or indeterminate architecture (rare). The hypoplastic rudimentary chamber, when present, is always of the opposite architecture to the dominant ventricle. The nondominant chamber is referred to as rudimentary (incomplete) because it lacks one or more of its component parts. Generally the inlet portion is absent. Occasionally the outlet portion is lacking as well, leaving only the trabeculated part. The rudimentary chamber is connected to the dominant chamber by an interventricular communication (ventricular septal defect or bulboventricular foramen) of size which may vary from small and physiologically restrictive of flow to large and nonrestrictive. Occasionally, both ventricles are incomplete, as for example where there is double inlet to one chamber and double outlet from the other.

Atrial arrangement is variable, though in DILV atrial situs solitus predominates. In DIRV or indeterminate ventricle, about half have situs solitus, and half have atrial isomerism, predominantly right isomerism. There are usually two atrioventricular valves, both opening into the dominant ventricle. In about 20% of cases one of the two atrioventricular valves overrides the remnant of ventricular septum, or the tensor apparatus of one of the atrioventricular valves may straddle the septum. The anatomy of the atrioventricular valves and conduction system is abnormal in DIV. The atrioventricular node can be anywhere around the perimeter of the right-sided atrioventricular valve. In general, two separate coronary arteries arise from the two aortic sinuses facing the pulmonary trunk. There are usually prominent epicardial branches, which delineate the points of attachment of the septum to the ventricular free wall, and therefore indicate the boundaries of the rudimentary ventricular chamber.

Double-inlet left ventricle is the most common anatomic subtype. The dominant ventricle is of left ventricular morphology. The rudimentary chamber is of right ventricular morphology, with coarse apical trabeculations and frequently a septal band (trabecula septomarginalis) bordering the ventricular septal defect anteriorly. When the rudimentary chamber gives rise to one or both great vessels, a smooth-walled infundibulum is present. The rudimentary chamber is usually situated anterosuperiorly with respect to the dominant ventricle and is more often to the left but may be to the right. Of DILVs, the largest subtype is DILV with ventricular

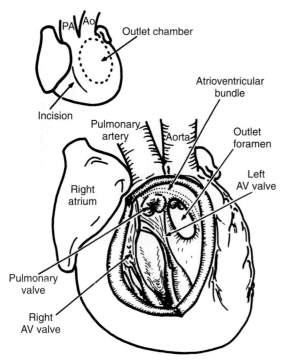

Figure 28.1 The relationships of the intracardiac structures and the disposition of the conduction tissue in double-inlet left ventricle with left-sided rudimentary right ventricle. (Ao, aorta; AV, atrioventricular; PA, pulmonary artery.) (Reproduced with permission from L. H. S. Van Mierop *et al.* [143].)

L-loop, left-sided rudimentary right ventricle, and ventriculoarterial discordance (single left ventricle {S, L, L}) (Figure 28.1) [10]. As the descriptive nomenclature implies, there is a right-sided dominant morphologic left ventricle, which receives right-sided and left-sided atrioventricular valves. The aorta arises from the rudimentary left-sided right ventricle. The pulmonary trunk arises from the base of the left ventricle. Uncommonly, there may be valvar or subvalvar pulmonary stenosis and rarely pulmonary atresia. The ventricular septal defect, or bulboventricular foramen, lies beneath the infundibular septum and may be of any size. When it is large, the aorta is usually well developed. When the ventricular septal defect is restrictive it produces subaortic stenosis, and there is commonly hypoplasia of the aortic arch, coarctation or interrupted aortic arch. Double-inlet left ventricle with ventricular D-loop, right-sided rudimentary right ventricle, and ventriculoarterial concordance occurs in about 10% of cases. Also known as Holmes heart, this type of functional single ventricle consists of a large left ventricle, which is leftward and posterior, and a small rudimentary right ventricle, which is situated to the right, anteriorly and superiorly. There are generally two atrioventricular valves, often with the right-sided valve straddling. Pulmonary stenosis is common.

In DIRV both atria connect to a morphologically right ventricle. The rudimentary left ventricular chamber lies posteriorly and inferiorly (in the hip pocket) with relation to the dominant right ventricle. Most often the hypoplastic ventricle communicates with the main chamber by a very small ventricular septal defect and lacks an outflow to any great vessel. In these cases the ventriculoarterial connection is either double-outlet right ventricle or right ventricular aorta with pulmonary atresia. There may be two atrioventricular valves entering the right ventricle, with or without the left one straddling, or there may be a common atrioventricular valve. Double-inlet indeterminate ventricle refers to the rare instance of a primitive ventricular heart without an outlet chamber [11].

Tricuspid Atresia

The term tricuspid atresia refers to univentricular hearts with absent right atrioventricular connection. The anatomic hallmark is the lack of a direct connection between the right atrium and right ventricle. Most often the tricuspid valve is totally absent, the floor of the right atrium being constituted of muscular tissue. Less often there is membranous atresia of the right atrioventricular connection, with the floor of the right atrium occupied by a primitive or vestigial valve-like structure that is imperforate, though there may be rudimentary chordae on the right ventricular side. Still less commonly, an Ebstein's type of tricuspid valve is present with complete fusion of leaflets.

In tricuspid atresia, the right atrium may be moderately enlarged, and is thickened in comparison to normal. The only outlet from the right atrium is the atrial septal defect, which is almost always of the ostium secundum type and is generally large (the exception being the presence of a restrictive atrial septal defect in about one half of cases of tricuspid atresia with transposition of the great arteries [TGA]). Occasionally a redundant aneurysm of septum primum may prolapse into the left atrium, with theoretical potential to obstruct mitral inflow. Rarely, the atrial septal defect may be restrictive. The Eustachian valve of the inferior vena cava may be very prominent and occasionally appears to subdivide the right atrium (cor triatriatum dexter). The left atrium is dilated but is usually morphologically normal. There is univentricular atrioventricular connection consisting of a left-sided mitral valve between the morphologically left atrium and left ventricle. There is nearly always atrial situs solitus with ventricular D-loop. While the left ventricle is large and well developed, Becker and Anderson [12] argue that it is not a normal ventricle. The septum separating it from the right ventricular chamber does not extend to the crux of the heart, and because the right atrioventricular connection is absent, there is no inlet septum. There is a crevice in the posterior part of the left ventricular chamber into which a dimple, generally present in the muscular floor of the right atrium, points. The right ventricular chamber in tricuspid atresia has no inlet portion and is connected to the dominant left ventricle by a ventricular septal defect with entirely muscular rims. The size of the trabecular portion and the outlet portion of the rudimentary right ventricle is determined by the size of the ventricular septal defect and the nature of the ventriculoarterial connections.

In tricuspid atresia, coronary artery patterns are usually normal. Systemic venous connections are generally normal, though a persistent left superior vena cava is present in 10–15% of cases. The sinoatrial node is in the normal position. The atrioventricular node is situated to the right of the central fibrous body, and the course of the atrioventricular conduction system depends on the location of the ventricular septal defect; it is generally inferior and posterior to the defect.

Anatomic subtypes of tricuspid atresia are generally classified based on morphology and physiology as originally proposed in 1906 by Kühne [13] and later modified by Edwards and Burchell in 1949 [14]. Tandon *et al.* [15] further refined the system of classification in 1974 to encompass rarer types of ventriculoarterial connection. The fundamental categories are type I: those with normally related great arteries (approximately 70%); type II: those with D-TGA (approximately 30%); and type III: those with L-TGA (rare). Each of these groups is further subdivided based on the degree of obstruction to pulmonary blood flow: type A pulmonary atresia, type B pulmonary stenosis or hypoplasia (moderate pulmonary blood flow), and type C pulmonary artery and valve with no obstruction (increased pulmonary blood flow) (Figure 28.2) [16].

Mitral Atresia

As with absence of the right atrioventricular connection, absent left atrioventricular connection can occur with any of the morphologies possible in univentricular heart. The classical example of mitral atresia is univentricular heart of right ventricular type with absent left atrioventricular connection. As in tricuspid atresia, the atretic valve may be imperforate with immature chordal apparatus beneath, but more commonly the atrioventricular connection is truly absent, the floor of the atrium being separated from the ventricle by fibro-fatty tissue [17]. When mitral atresia and aortic atresia are both present, those hearts are considered a category of hypoplastic left heart syndrome. Mitral atresia with a patent aortic outlet is generally characterized by atrial situs solitus, ventricular D-loop, a dominant right ventricle connected to the right atrium by a patent right-sided (generally tricuspid) valve and a hypoplastic left ventricle situated posteriorly and to the left. Various conotruncal arrangements are possible. The two most common are (1) double-outlet right ventricle in which case

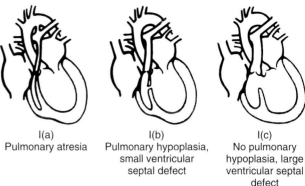

Tricuspid atresia with no transposition (69% - 83%)

I(a)
Pulmonary atresia

I(b)
Pulmonary hypoplasia, small ventricular septal defect

I(c)
No pulmonary hypoplasia, large ventricular septal defect

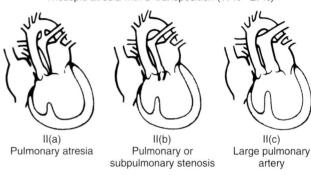

Tricuspid atresia with D-transposition (17% - 27%)

II(a)
Pulmonary atresia

II(b)
Pulmonary or subpulmonary stenosis

II(c)
Large pulmonary artery

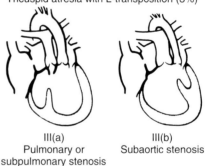

Tricuspid atresia with L-transposition (3%)

III(a)
Pulmonary or subpulmonary stenosis

III(b)
Subaortic stenosis

Figure 28.2 The anatomic classification of tricuspid atresia, as suggested by Tandon and Edwards in 1974. (Reproduced with permission from Pearl *et al.* [16].)

the small left ventricle is a blind chamber connected to the right ventricle by a ventricular septal defect but with no outlet to a great vessel; or (2) concordant ventriculoarterial connection in which case the hypoplastic left ventricle functions as an outlet chamber giving rise to the aorta. Frequently the ventricular septal defect is restrictive, causing subaortic obstruction, and the hypoplastic left ventricle gives rise to a small aorta with aortic arch hypoplasia, coarctation, or rarely, interruption. The interatrial communication is frequently restrictive. Mitral atresia with ventriculoarterial discordance and patent aortic root is a rare entity but has been described.

Another, less common arrangement with left atrioventricular valve atresia (but not mitral atresia) is that of atrial situs solitus, ventricular L-loop with a patent right-sided atrioventricular valve emptying into a right-sided dominant left ventricle, with a rudimentary left-sided right ventricle above which is an atretic left-sided atrioventricular valve. The conotruncal anatomy is either ventriculoarterial discordance (aorta from rudimentary right ventricle), or double-outlet left ventricle. The ventricular septal defect may be restrictive.

Unbalanced Common Atrioventricular Canal Defect

This is a rare subset of hearts with common atrioventricular junction in which there is clear dominance of one ventricular chamber and hypoplasia of the other. Unlike most other functionally univentricular hearts, the less developed hypoplastic ventricle in unbalanced common atrioventricular canal defect is generally not rudimentary, but rather hypoplastic, as a consequence of inflow from the atria being directed preferentially to the dominant ventricle. The anatomy is thought to be the consequence of malalignment of the common atrioventricular valve with respect to the ventricular mass. This may occur in either the complete form of common atrioventricular canal defect with a large nonrestrictive ventricular septal defect, or in the intermediate form, with a restrictive ventricular septal defect. The position of the common atrioventricular valve in relation to the plane of the ventricular septum determines the degree of imbalance and thus the degree of hypoplasia of one ventricle. In the right dominant form of common atrioventricular canal defect the right ventricle is large, the left ventricle is smaller than normal, and the position of the common atrioventricular valve in relation to the septum is rightward. In the left dominant form, the left ventricle is larger than normal, the right ventricle is smaller than normal, and the position of the common atrioventricular valve is leftward. In this form, right ventricular hypoplasia is readily apparent. In the right dominant form it may be difficult to distinguish right ventricular dominance and left ventricular hypoplasia from the common scenario of flow-related right ventricular enlargement seen in balanced or nonmaligned common atrioventricular canal defects. Several diagnostic tools or measurements have been advanced to accurately predict the inadequacy of one ventricle, of which the most useful is probably the atrioventricular valve index proposed by Cohen and Rychik and colleagues [18]. While abnormal development of the aortic outflow (aortic arch hypoplasia, coarctation) is a common accompaniment of unbalanced common atrioventricular canal defect with right ventricular dominance, the converse is not necessarily true, and one does not predictably observe pulmonary stenosis or hypoplasia in the left ventricular dominant form of unbalanced common atrioventricular canal defect.

Functionally Univentricular Heart in Heterotaxy Syndrome

Atriovisceral heterotaxy refers to those anatomic circumstances where failure of normal right-left differentiation results in ambiguities of visceral and atrial situs, together with a variety of characteristic anomalies of systemic and pulmonary venous connections, abnormalities of abdominal organs, and heart malformations, which fall into readily recognizable patterns. Becker and Anderson [19] provide the useful description: "a particular arrangement of the thoracoabdominal viscera characterized by isomerism of the paired organs such as the lungs and atria together with a tendency for the unpaired organs to be midline in position." They, therefore, refer to this family of anomalies as atrial isomerism. Others have emphasized that there are two basic subdivisions [20,21], associated on the one hand with absence of the spleen (asplenia, bilateral right-sidedness [21]), and on the other with multiple spleens, (polysplenia, bilateral left-sidedness [20]). Thus, the more commonly used terminology *asplenia* and *polysplenia syndrome*. The majority of heterotaxy syndrome patients have a functionally univentricular heart. In addition to anomalies of systemic and pulmonary venous return, the cardiac abnormalities are characterized by endocardial cushion defect (atrioventricular canal type common atrioventricular valve) and frequently pulmonary stenosis or atresia.

Of asplenia patients, more than half have functionally univentricular heart, and typically they have a single right ventricle (42%) with double-outlet right ventricle (82%), pulmonary stenosis or atresia (96%), bilateral superior vena cava (71%), and a form of common atrioventricular valve (93%). Systemic arterial outflow obstruction is rare. Total anomalous pulmonary venous connection is typically to an extracardiac vein (64%) (Figure 28.3) [22]. There are bilateral sinoatrial nodes. The coronary sinus is almost always absent. Bilateral hepatic veins connect isomerically to the atria. Pulmonary anatomy is typically bilateral trilobed lungs with bilateral epiarterial bronchi.

Fewer than one half of polysplenia syndrome patients have functionally univentricular heart, but of those with single ventricles, two thirds have single (dominant) right ventricle. Not infrequently, ventricular morphology is indeterminate, without there being a rudimentary chamber. Interruption of the inferior vena cava and azygous continuation is common (80%). Bilateral hepatic veins are frequently present. Anomalous pulmonary venous drainage is typically to the right atrium, though isomeric or ipsilateral pulmonary venous connections (not truly anomalous) are common. Ventriculoarterial connection is concordant or

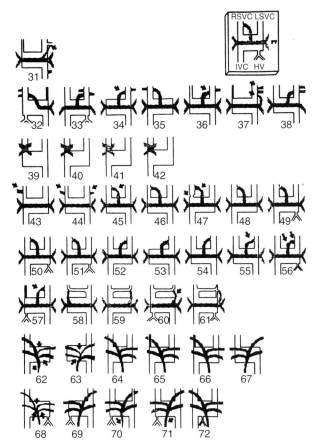

Figure 28.3 Diagrammatic representation of systemic and pulmonary venous connections in 42 cases of visceral heterotaxy with asplenia associated with extracardiac pulmonary venous connections. (HV, hepatic veins; IVC, inferior vena cava; LSVC, left superior vena cava; PV, pulmonary veins; RSVC, right superior vena cava.) (Reproduced with permission from Rubino *et al.* [22].)

DORV (30%). Pulmonary atresia is significantly less frequent than in asplenia. The sinoatrial node may be hypoplastic and misplaced or may be absent. Bilateral superior vena cavae are common, and a persistent left superior vena cava may drain to the coronary sinus. Pulmonary anatomy is typically bilateral bilobed lungs with bilateral hyparterial bronchi.

Natural History

The natural history of patients with functionally univentricular heart is determined by the adequacy, at any point in time, of systemic blood flow and pulmonary blood flow and the effect of the combined volume load on ventricular function. In the current era, it is challenging to determine the true natural history of these malformations because of the influence of surgical interventions. Since the 1950s, surgical interventions to augment pulmonary blood flow (aor-

topulmonary shunts) and to decrease pulmonary blood flow (pulmonary artery banding) have drastically altered the outlook for survival of patients with functionally univentricular heart.

Moodie *et al.* [23] did study a population of unoperated patients with single ventricle hearts and described mortality of 50% 14 years after diagnosis. Deaths were most commonly attributed to congestive heart failure (20%), arrhythmia (20%), or unidentified causes (10%). More recently, Franklin [24] studied survival *without definitive repair* in 191 patients presenting in infancy (first year of life) with DIV. Some of the patients had undergone palliative procedures, but none had undergone complete separation of the pulmonary and systemic circulations. Actuarial survival was 57% at 1 year, 43% at 5 years, and 42% at 10 years [24].

Certain anatomic substrates have important impacts on the natural history. Atresia of the left atrioventricular valve (mitral atresia or left-sided atrioventricular valve atresia with ventricular L-loop) often coexists with a restrictive interatrial communication. This combination, which results in pulmonary venous obstruction, frequently causes death owing to hypoxia and acidosis in the early days or weeks of life. Even when the interatrial communication is not restrictive at birth, there is a strong tendency for it to become restrictive over time.

One of the most important anatomic factors which impacts negatively on survival in patients with functionally univentricular heart is the presence or development of systemic ventricular outflow obstruction or subaortic stenosis, which occurs when the aorta arises from the rudimentary chamber. This includes patients with DILV and discordant ventriculoarterial connection, those with tricuspid atresia and discordant ventriculoarterial connection, and those with mitral atresia and concordant ventriculoarterial connection. Systemic ventricular outflow obstruction is generally caused by small size of the interventricular communication, which is the only pathway for blood flow into the rudimentary subaortic outlet chamber. In circumstances where the ventricular septal defect is small at birth, there is generally aortic hypoplasia, frequently with coarctation, and occasionally with interrupted aortic arch. Even when the ventricular septal defect is nonrestrictive at birth, it often significantly narrows over time, and subaortic obstruction then becomes apparent [25]. The tendency for subaortic obstruction to progress after some forms of palliation, notably pulmonary artery banding, has been well described [26]. More recently it has been clearly documented that any operative strategy that reduces the total volume work of a single ventricle heart is accompanied by geometric changes characterized by increased wall thickness and mass to volume ratio and diminution in the size of the bulboventricular foramen or subaortic ventricular septal defect, if present [27]. This can occur at any stage of palliation, or following a Fontan operation.

In tricuspid atresia, the natural history is quite variable, but it is predicted by the underlying pathophysiology as in all functionally univentricular hearts. Most patients with tricuspid atresia and normally related great arteries have some degree of obstruction to pulmonary blood flow. This generally progresses as the ventricular septal defect becomes more obstructive or infundibular obstruction increases, and as a result there is increasing cyanosis. Without surgical intervention, over 90% of patients will die by one year of age from complications of hypoxia. Patients with normal or increased pulmonary blood flow at birth will show early symptoms of congestive heart failure and may succumb to this in the first months of life. If they survive the period of increased pulmonary blood flow they may gradually develop intracardiac obstruction to pulmonary blood flow, but are otherwise at risk for the development of pulmonary vascular obstructive disease. In either case, a falsely reassuring period of clinical improvement may occur as their circulation becomes more balanced [28] before their course progresses to either cyanosis, pulmonary vascular obstructive disease, or ventricular dysfunction owing to chronic volume overload.

Patients with tricuspid atresia and ventriculoarterial discordance (associated TGA) have, in general, a worse prognosis. Unobstructed pulmonary blood flow results in congestive heart failure and death within the first year of life. Subaortic obstruction complicates the scenario, further shortening survival time. In the extreme case, there is ductal dependency of the systemic circulation in the newborn. The rare patient with tricuspid atresia and TGA who has no subaortic obstruction and some degree of pulmonary stenosis may survive for a few years without surgical intervention. As in all patients with functionally univentricular heart without definitive surgical intervention, the left ventricle in patients with tricuspid atresia will, over time, develop progressive dysfunction resulting from chronic volume overload and chronic hypoxia. Patients who survive beyond the first few years of life often develop severe left ventricular dysfunction with low ejection fraction and mitral regurgitation.

Finally, the discussion of the natural history of functionally univentricular heart is incomplete without consideration of the impact of anomalies of pulmonary venous connection. While total anomalous pulmonary venous connection in functionally univentricular heart occurs most commonly in the setting of heterotaxy syndrome (and then most commonly in asplenia patients), it can occur in any of the anatomies covered in this chapter, as well as in cases of hypoplastic left heart syndrome. The natural history without surgery depends on the adequacy of pulmonary blood flow, which is influenced both by the presence of pulmonary stenosis and by the degree of obstruction of the pulmonary venous connection. Early mortality is very high among infants with single ventricle and total anomalous pulmonary venous connection [29], and late death is a continuing risk.

Evolution of Surgery for Functionally Univentricular Hearts

The development in the 1940s of the Blalock-Taussig shunt [30] and the original description in 1952 of pulmonary artery banding [31] ushered in an era of palliation for selected patients with single ventricle hearts who suffered from either a shortage or an excess of pulmonary blood flow. Of course, these early palliative efforts were undertaken, not as elements of a planned staged approach to definitive reconstruction but rather in an effort to salvage fragile patients severely compromised by either cyanosis or congestive heart failure.

Septation of the Single Ventricle

The first instance of definitive therapy for a single ventricle by means of septation of the main chamber and complete separation of the pulmonary and systemic circulations occurred in 1956 at the Mayo Clinic. A patient believed preoperatively to have congenitally corrected TGA with ventricular septal defect, was found intraoperatively to have a single ventricle. Septation was performed, and the patient lived 6 months. According to Kirklin and Barratt-Boyes [32] the concept of septation lay dormant for several years, and was revisited later by the Mayo Clinic group and by others including in 1972 by Sakakibara and associates [33] and in 1973 Edie and associates [34]. Additional cases from the Mayo Clinic were reported by McGoon *et al.* [35]. These early efforts at septation all involved opening the ventricle. Doty and colleagues in 1979 [36] described the right atrial approach to septation. In general the surgical mortality associated with septation was high, heart block was a frequent complication, and less than one third of patients were said to enjoy satisfactory late results. Not surprisingly, enthusiasm for this form of treatment was limited, although at the time the alternatives were few. Among a few others, Kirklin and colleagues at the University of Alabama in Birmingham pursued efforts at septation (Figure 28.4) [37] and in 1982 published their experience, focusing on 16 patients with univentricular heart with left anterior subaortic outlet chamber, the anatomical arrangement they believed to be most satisfactorily suited for septation of the dominant ventricle [38]. Hospital mortality was 44%. Five of the seven patients with outlet foramen obstruction died despite surgical enlargement of the outlet foramen. Of the remaining patients with unobstructed outlet foramen, there were two hospital deaths (18%), both in patients with small ventricular size. Reviewing this experience, McKay and associates [38] reported that at intermediate follow-up the majority of survivors were

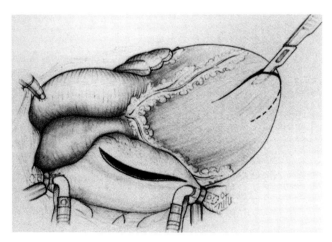

Figure 28.4 The positions of the atrial and ventricular incisions used in the combined approach for ventricular septation. (Reproduced with permission from Pacifico *et al.* [37].)

without symptoms, but the patients subjected to exercise testing performed well below normals for age and size. This important study identified the presence of outlet foramen obstruction, and small ventricular size, as incremental risk factors for hospital death. The authors drew the following inferences: that a shunt should be advised prior to septation in all patients with small heart size and pulmonary stenosis (either naturally occurring or secondary to pulmonary artery banding), regardless of their degree of cyanosis. This, they anticipated, would result in enlargement of the ventricular cavity and increase the probability of successful septation. For patients without pulmonary stenosis they suggested a protocol of septation early in life.

Despite such careful analyses, the morbidity and mortality associated with septation have remained high [39]. Frequently encountered complications include heart block requiring permanent pacemakers, late residual ventricular septal defect, atrioventricular valve incompetence requiring reoperation, and a high incidence of sudden death [40]. Careful selection of candidates excludes the majority of functional single ventricle patients from this form of definitive therapy. Important selection criteria include the anatomy and function of the atrioventricular valves and the presence or absence of pulmonary or subaortic stenosis. Atrioventricular valve repair, if necessary, is associated with increased rates of mortality. Pulmonary valve or subvalvar stenosis not amenable to direct relief requires an extracardiac conduit, which is also associated with increased morbidity and mortality [37].

As other forms of definitive surgical therapy for functional single ventricle have evolved, the application of septation became quite limited. Nonetheless, improvements in technique continued to be made. Importantly, Ebert in 1984 [41] proposed a two-staged approach to ventricular septa-

tion. He reported favorable results in five patients. At the first stage, a small patch was placed in the apex and a second patch between the atrioventricular and semilunar valves. The central section was left open. A pulmonary artery band was placed at this time if one had not been placed previously. Six to 18 months later the second stage of the repair was undertaken. This consisted of closure of the central portion of the ventricular septal defect with additional patch material. None of the patients acquired heart block in association with surgery. Ebert suggested that the procedure seemed to allow the apical and base patches to stiffen and heal to the endocardium, with fewer sutures required because the central area was open and no pressure differential existed across the patch. Despite Ebert's very encouraging initial report, subsequent applications of this innovative technique have been limited. Despite the relative rarity of ventricular septation as a primary approach to functionally univentricular heart, there continue to appear, from around the world, isolated reports of satisfactory functional status of patients subjected to septation with follow-up of one to three decades [42–44].

The Cavopulmonary Shunt

The superior vena cava to ipsilateral pulmonary artery anastomosis is generally known by the name Glenn shunt. In fact, the concept of the superior cavopulmonary anastomosis was developed concurrently and independently by several surgical teams. Years before the first clinical application of cavopulmonary shunting, several investigators studied the concept of the *dispensable right ventricle*. Rodbard and Wagner [45] in Chicago in 1949 experimentally anastomosed the right atrial appendage to the pulmonary artery and ligated the main pulmonary artery in dogs, demonstrating the feasibility of right ventricular exclusion. The first report of experimental cavopulmonary connection was published in 1950 in Italy by Carlo Carlon and coworkers of Padua [46] who advanced the notion that an "advantage would be received if the blood of the superior vena cava should reach the capillary region of the right lung by way of a convenient anastomosis between the great venous trunk and the arterial system of the right lung." The experimental canine preparation was an end-to-end anastomosis between the proximal end of the divided azygous vein and the right pulmonary artery with preatrial ligation of the superior vena cava. Carlon's first clinical experience was not reported until 1964. In the meantime, Glenn and colleagues at Yale published their first report of experimental cavopulmonary shunts in 1956—a large study of 59 operated dogs, with six long-term survivors [47]. The first clinical report by Glenn was published in 1958 [48]. It is following this report, and subsequent series by the same authors, that the superior cavopulmonary anastomosis has become widely known as the Glenn shunt. Interestingly however, a fundamentally similar operation was at the same time being developed and evaluated in Budapest (and later North Carolina) by Frances Robicsek and associates [49], in Russia by Darbinian and Galankin [50] and by Meshalkin [51], in Italy by Carlon and others [46], and in the United States by Shumacher [52]. In retrospect, it appears likely that the first attempts at clinical cavopulmonary shunts were by Harris B Shumacher in 1954. His two young patients, one with truncus arteriosus and one with TGA, both had markedly elevated pulmonary vascular resistance and both died within hours of operation.

The Glenn shunt found a unique and important place in the management of cyanotic heart disease in general, and functionally univentricular hearts in particular, in that it differed in an important physiologic way from systemic to pulmonary artery shunts. The cavopulmonary anastomosis was capable of increasing pulmonary blood flow and thus systemic arterial saturation without increasing the volume load on the systemic ventricle. It also proved the feasibility of transpulmonary flow without complete dependence on a subpulmonary ventricle. During the 1960s and early 1970s, the classic Glenn shunt was used extensively with good results to palliate patients with tricuspid atresia and to a lesser extent other forms of functional single ventricle, although cyanosis eventually recurred in a high proportion of patients [53]. The unidirectional Glenn shunt was eventually modified by Dogliotti and colleagues [54], Haller *et al.* [55], and Azzolina and coworkers [56] to allow the flow of superior vena cava blood into both pulmonary arteries with an end-to-side superior vena cava to pulmonary artery anastomosis. This technique preserves the confluence and integrity of the central pulmonary arteries and eventually supplanted the classic Glenn anastomosis as preferred palliation for functional single ventricles. Currently, without particularly good reason, the bidirectional superior cavopulmonary anastomosis is generally and widely referred to as the bidirectional Glenn shunt.

Fontan's and Kreutzer's Operations

The first successful complete physiologic repair of tricuspid atresia, with separation of the pulmonary and systemic circulations, was accomplished in 1968 by Frances Fontan and colleagues and was reported in 1971 [57]. This followed the experimental work of Isaac Starr and colleagues [58] who had shown that functional destruction of a dog's right ventricle did not result in systemic venous hypertension, the previously described experiments in 1949 by Rodbard and Wagner [45] and by Warden, De Wall, and Varco in 1954 [52], which demonstrated the feasibility of bypassing the right ventricle by means of a right atrial to pulmonary artery anastomosis. Hurwitt and associates [59] reported an unsuccessful attempt to treat tricuspid atresia by right atrium to pulmonary artery anastomosis in 1955. Fontan's

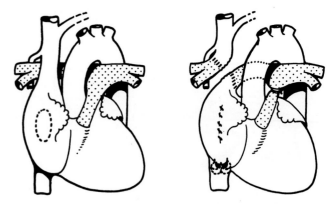

Figure 28.5 Artist's drawing of Fontan's original repair for tricuspid atresia type Ib. Case 1. (Reproduced with permission from Fontan *et al.* [57].)

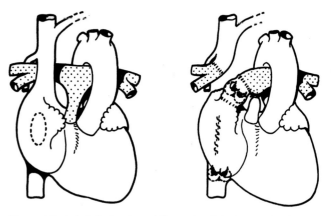

Figure 28.6 Artist's drawing of Fontan's original operation for repair of tricuspid atresia type IIb. (Reproduced with permission from Fontan *et al.* [57].)

first corrective operation for tricuspid atresia involved the construction of a Glenn anastomosis and anastomosis of the right atrial appendage to the proximal end of the divided right pulmonary artery (Figure 28.5) [57]. In the subsequent two patients, an aortic homograft valved conduit was placed between the right atrium and the proximal right pulmonary artery (Figure 28.6) [57]. In all three patients, an additional homograft valve was placed at the junction of the inferior vena cava with the right atrium. The atrial septal defect was closed, and the main pulmonary artery was ligated or divided. The utilization of inflow and outflow valves, together with the strict inclusion criteria suggested by Choussat, Fontan, and colleagues [60], suggest a belief on their part that the right atrium of patients with tricuspid atresia could, to some extent, assume the pumping function of a subpulmonary ventricle.

Kreutzer in 1973 reported a modification of Fontan's operation in which the patient's own main pulmonary artery with its intact pulmonary valve was excised from

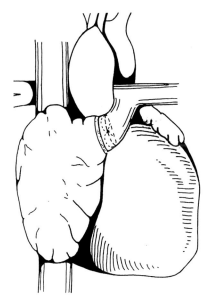

Figure 28.7 Artist's original drawing of Kreutzer's operative repair of tricuspid atresia, incorporating direct anastomosis of the patient's own pulmonary annulus with the right atrial appendage. (Reproduced with permission from Kreutzer *et al.* [61].)

the right ventricle and anastomosed to the right atrial appendage (Figure 28.7) [61]. The atrial septal defect and ventricular septal defect were closed. A Glenn anastomosis was not performed, and no inferior vena caval valve was used. At the 2009 meeting of the American Association for Thoracic Surgery, Kreutzer reported that one of his earliest patients was well 38 years after initial atriopulmonary anastomosis (and 3 years following conversion to total cavopulmonary connection [TCPC]) [62].

During the decade following Fontan and Kreutzer's pioneering work, a variety of modifications of their original operations were used to treat patients with tricuspid atresia. The value of maintaining the confluence of the pulmonary arteries became evident, and direct connection of the pulmonary arteries to the posterosuperior portion of the right atrium (as opposed to the right atrial appendage) emerged as the favored style of atrial pulmonary connection. Of course for tricuspid atresia, the operation was completed by closure of the atrial septal defect and of the main pulmonary artery. In most cases, the selection criteria espoused by Fontan's group were applied, so that patients did not undergo definitive operation until they were at least 4 years old, and often much older. Failure rates were high, and significant postoperative morbidity was common. In hopes of improving the hemodynamic status of these patients, several surgeons proposed the incorporation of the hypoplastic right ventricle into the pulmonary circulation, reasoning that the pump function contributed by a small right ventricle was better than none at all. In 1978, Bowman [63] introduced the use of porcine valved syn-

thetic conduits to establish antegrade flow from the right atrium to the right ventricle and described significant subsequent increase in the volume of the right ventricular cavity. Others accomplished similar arrangements using homograft valved conduits. The operations for tricuspid atresia were completed by closure of both the atrial septal defect and the ventricular septal defect and relief of pulmonary stenosis if present. Recognizing the inherent long-term problems associated with valved conduits, Björk and colleagues [64] in 1979 described an anterior right atrium to right ventricle communication using as its inferior wall a flap of right atrial tissue, roofed over with autologous pericardium. The utility of these atrioventricular reconstructions was limited by the potential for sternal compression of the conduit or pathway constructed between the right atrium and the right ventricle. Efforts to document the utility of incorporation of the hypoplastic right ventricle into the pulmonary circulation yielded inconsistent results [65,66], though some authors, such as Ilbawi *et al.* [67] were convinced that incorporation of a right ventricle of greater than 30% normal size contributed to increased stroke volume, lower systemic venous pressure, and better systemic ventricular function.

As experience with modifications of Fontan's operation increased, there was considerable impetus to extend the concept of *right ventricular exclusion* beyond tricuspid atresia to other forms of functionally single ventricle. Yacoub and Radley-Smith [68] were among the first to use an atrial pulmonary connection (with valved conduit in their initial case) for correction of single ventricle. The challenge of applying the principles of Fontan's and Kreutzer's operations to single ventricle hearts with atrioventricular connections other than right atrioventricular valve atresia, eventually led numerous investigators to pursue technical solutions. Among the problems faced were the difficulty of reliably closing a patent right-sided atrioventricular valve (without creating heart block) in hearts with a dominant or single left ventricle and normal left-sided atrioventricular valve, and the even more vexing challenge of creating an unobstructed pathway for pulmonary venous return from the left atrium, through an atrial septal defect, and into the right-sided atrioventricular valve in hearts with left atrioventricular valve atresia. Initial efforts, which involved the placement of a large contoured patch over both the atrial septal defect and the opening of the right-sided atrioventricular valve, were met with high rates of failure as the patch was frequently displaced toward the atrial septal defect and atrioventricular valve (obstructing pulmonary venous inflow) by the higher pressure on the systemic venous right atrial side of the patch. To address these challenges, elaborate means of atrial partitioning were devised [69,70] to ensure unobstructed caval flow to the pulmonary arteries and unobstructed pulmonary venous flow to the functional atrioventricular valve(s) of the systemic ventricle. Atrial partitioning was accomplished with either a pericardial or synthetic patch, a flap of atrial wall (reminiscent of Senning's operation for TGA), or even an intra-atrial tube graft.

By the middle of the 1980s, experience with modified Fontan operations for treatment of tricuspid atresia and other forms of functional single ventricle was becoming widespread. Several important lessons had been learned. Contrary to earlier notions, the pumping function of the right atrium was of little or no importance. Similarly, the notion that valves were required in the pathway between the caval veins and the pulmonary circulation had been dispelled. It was apparent that the principal determinants of success of a Fontan type connection were 1) unobstructed pathways with generous connections between the systemic veins and the pulmonary arteries; 2) preservation of the anatomic and functional integrity of the pulmonary vasculature (low pulmonary vascular resistance and minimal distortion); and 3) adequate function of the systemic ventricle. The feasibility of extracardiac TCPC in complex forms of heterotaxy syndrome with interrupted inferior vena cava and azygous or hemiazygous continuation of the inferior vena cava had been demonstrated by Kawashima and associates [71], who accomplished TCPC by means of anastomosis of the superior vena cava to the pulmonary arteries. This left only the return from the coronary circulation and the hepatic veins draining to the right atrium. At the 1988 meeting of the American Association for Thoracic Surgery, de Leval described elegant hydrodynamic studies, which led him and his colleagues to a modified approach to Fontan reconstructions that entailed exclusion of most or all of the right atrium from the systemic venous to pulmonary artery pathway [72]. The operation he described consisted of 1) end-to-side anastomosis of the superior vena cava to the undivided right pulmonary artery; 2) construction of a composite intra-atrial tunnel with use of the posterolateral wall of the right atrium; and 3) use of a prosthetic patch to channel the inferior vena cava to the enlarged orifice of the transected superior vena cava that is anastomosed to the main pulmonary artery. The operation, referred to as TCPC was touted as having the following advantages: 1) technical ease and reproducibility regardless of type of atrioventricular connection; 2) avoidance of injury to the atrioventricular node and minimizing the amount of atrial tissue subjected to elevated venous pressure in order to reduce the risk of early or late arrhythmias; and 3) reduction of turbulence with subsequent diminution of energy loss and lessened risk of thrombosis. As was the case two decades earlier with the evolution of the unidirectional cavopulmonary anastomosis, numerous surgical teams devised and described operations fundamentally similar to de Leval's TCPC roughly contemporaneously (Figure 28.8) [73,74].

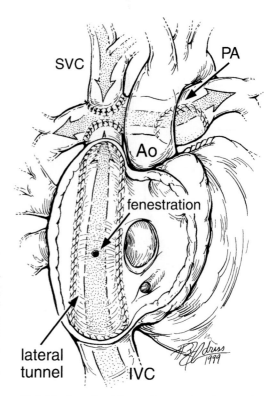

Figure 28.8 The lateral atrial tunnel type of total cavopulmonary connection. The lateral atrial tunnel is comprised of a gusset of polytetrafluoroethylene (PTFE) and of right atrial wall. In this instance, a single fenestration has been created in the polytetrafluoroethylene baffle. (Ao, aorta; IVC, inferior vena cava; PA, pulmonary artery; SVC, superior vena cava.) (Reproduced with permission from Backer *et al.* [74].)

de Leval's unique contribution was the analysis of in vitro studies, which demonstrated that the previously popular atrial pulmonary connection was a poor hydrodynamic design. These studies showed that the stream lines of superior and inferior vena caval blood collided within the atrial chamber, creating turbulence. Interestingly, the flow disturbances, demonstrated in the atrial cavity and at its inlets and outlet, were exaggerated by pulsation. While the technique presented by de Leval and associates at that time was essentially the lateral atrial tunnel combined with superior cavopulmonary connection, they also alluded to the possibility of interposition of a circumferential tube graft between the caval orifices as another means of TCPC. A fundamentally similar technique had already been described separately by Danielson and Norwood (personal communications) using an intra-atrial tube graft, and was proposed shortly thereafter by Marcelletti using an extracardiac tube graft [75]. de Leval, and the other early proponents of these techniques cited the theoretical advantages of having the entire right atrial wall at low pressure if a tube graft was used, and having a minimal amount of right

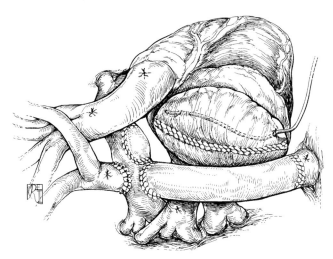

Figure 28.9 The total extracardiac conduit type of total cavopulmonary connection. In this instance, a right-sided superior cavopulmonary anastomosis is combined with the interposition of a polytetrafluoroethylene graft conduit between the divided inferior vena cava and the underside of the pulmonary artery confluence. (Reproduced with permission from Mavroudis *et al.* [76].)

atrial wall (the sinus venarum) at elevated central venous pressure when the lateral atrial tunnel was used.

For a period of time, the lateral atrial tunnel became the most widely used type of TCPC. However, over the latter half of the 1990s, the technique of using an extracardiac conduit to complete the TCPC (Figure 28.9) [76] met with increasing popularity [77,78]. In this operation, the divided superior vena cava is anastomosed to the ipsilateral pulmonary artery in end-to-side fashion. The inferior vena cava is transected and the cardiac end is oversewn. A conduit is interposed between the opened inferior vena cava and the underside of the pulmonary artery. Both homograft and prosthetic tube grafts (most often polytetrafluoroethylene [PTFE]) have been used to accomplish the so-called "extracardiac TCPC." The main theoretical advantages suggested by proponents of this method include the avoidance of atrial suture lines and the fact that none of the atrial wall is subjected to high venous pressures. An additional theoretical advantage rests in the possibility of accomplishing the extracardiac conduit Fontan procedure using normothermic or minimally hypothermic cardiopulmonary bypass without aortic cross-clamping in patients with a previously established superior cavopulmonary connection. In some instances, in fact, the conduit operation can be accomplished without the use of cardiopulmonary bypass [79]. The principle potential disadvantage, of course, is related to the use of a circumferential conduit without growth potential. Given this consideration, proponents of TCPC

using a circumferential extracardiac conduit generally postpone the procedure until the patient has grown large enough to accept a conduit size not likely to be outgrown when full somatic growth is achieved.

Staging Fontan's Operation

Refinement of the technical aspects of modified Fontan operations led to a significant decrement in the overall mortality associated with these procedures. Nonetheless, nearly two decades after Fontan's pioneering work and despite concerted efforts to identify those factors that would allow Fontan operations to be undertaken with minimal risk, there persisted throughout the 1980s a troublesome degree of morbidity and early mortality following modified Fontan procedures. Too often, in carefully selected patients with adequate preoperative ventricular function and pulmonary vascular anatomy and resistance, the postoperative course was characterized by elevation of central venous pressure, tachycardia, sequestration of fluid in the pleural and peritoneal spaces, and hypotension, which was only transiently responsive to volume administration at the expense of further increases in venous pressure. Little improvement was seen with administration of inotropic agents and vasodilators and with external compressive devices to promote venous return while minimizing volume administration. Echocardiography frequently showed a strikingly high ventricular wall thickness to cavity volume ratio, regardless of the contractile state of the myocardium.

It became evident that the conversion from the unoperated or palliated state to the post-Fontan circulation was associated with rapid removal of a chronic volume load, but that regression of myocardial mass proceeds slowly. This results in a maladaptive response to removal of the ventricular volume load characterized by a markedly increased ventricular myocardial mass-to-volume ratio [27]. The persistence of increased muscle mass in the setting of acutely diminished ventricular volume results in increased ventricular wall thickness and decreased cavity dimensions. This significant change in mass-to-volume relationship of the ventricle, can result in significant alterations in both systolic and diastolic properties of the ventricle. This realization shed light on earlier observations that older age and increased ventricular mass (hypertrophy) were risk factors for mortality in association with the Fontan operation [80]. More importantly, it lead to the hypothesis that dividing Fontan's operation into two procedures could accomplish early reduction of the volume work of the single ventricle and might minimize the impact of changes in ventricular geometry on outcome and survival.

At the end of the decade of the 1980s and in the early 1990s, several groups investigated the merits of a staged approach to Fontan's operation. For some, the protocol of performance of an early bidirectional superior caval pulmonary anastomosis followed later by a completion Fontan procedure was a pathway selected specifically for high-risk Fontan candidates [81], while others [82] pursued a two-staged approach to Fontan's operation for virtually all patients. They postulated that some of the morbidity and mortality associated with Fontan's operation would be eliminated by staging. As importantly, they suggested that the duration of the palliated state could be minimized and that the volume load on the single ventricle should be reduced as early in life as is practical. Thus in 1989, Norwood introduced the hemi-Fontan procedure, as the first step in a two-stage process of achieving TCPC. Obligating superior vena caval return to pass through the lungs before returning to the functional single ventricle, the hemi-Fontan operation is the physiologic equivalent of the bidirectional Glenn anastomosis. Because it is planned as an intermediate step before an anticipated completion Fontan procedure, it differs technically from a bidirectional Glenn anastomosis in ways that simplify the eventual completion Fontan. At the time of association of the pulmonary arteries with the superior vena cava, the natural connection of the right atrium with the superior vena cava is maintained, but the caval orifice is first enlarged (to be as large as the inferior vena caval right atrial connection) and then closed with a patch that is easily removed at the final stage. Other sources of pulmonary blood flow including systemic to pulmonary shunts and antegrade flow to the pulmonary arteries are eliminated. Pulmonary artery architecture is optimized by augmentation of the central confluence with homograft vascular patch material. Other potential hemodynamic burdens such as systemic ventricular outflow tract obstruction or atrioventricular valve regurgitation are addressed as part of the hemi-Fontan procedure. Bove and associates later modified Norwood's operative technique, avoiding an incision across the cavoatrial junction, with the theoretical goal of preserving the integrity of the sinoatrial node and its blood supply, with the hope that this would enhance the likelihood of preserving sinus rhythm [83].

For patients who have undergone a hemi-Fontan procedure, the final stage or completion Fontan procedure is technically very straightforward. The patch which had been used to occlude the opening of the right atrium into the superior vena cava is excised, and a lateral atrial tunnel is constructed, directing flow from the inferior vena cava to the previously created amalgamation of the superior vena cava with the pulmonary arteries. A majority of surgeons have persisted in using the technically more straightforward bidirectional Glenn anastomosis rather then the hemi-Fontan operation as the first of two stages. In these circumstances, the completion Fontan by lateral atrial tunnel requires re-establishment of the connection between the right atrium and the superior cavopulmonary amalgamation. Alternatively, after a bidirectional Glenn anastomosis, the completion Fontan may be easily accomplished using an extracardiac conduit.

The Incomplete Fontan Operation

Some of the same issues that are addressed by staging Fontan's operation led others to pursue the concept of a Fontan operation with deliberately incomplete atrial partitioning. One of the earliest and most enthusiastic proponents of this approach was Laks and colleagues [84] who advocated incorporation of an adjustable (snare controlled) atrial septal defect. While first applied with respect to the naturally occurring atrial septal defect at the time of atriopulmonary connection in hearts with atretic right-sided atrioventricular connection, this concept was subsequently applied to the more widely used TCPC. When constructing the lateral atrial tunnel, the suture line is interrupted on one edge of the tunnel patch. The subsequent gap at the edge of the patch may be enlarged by excision of a small amount of material, and this gap is then encircled with a snaring suture of polypropylene, both ends of which are brought out through the atrial wall and passed through a small piece of tubing, which is used as a tourniquet to adjust the size of the opening (Figure 28.10) [16]. The atrial septal defect may be closed after separation from bypass, or the tourniquet may be positioned under the linea alba at the lower end of the incision to be used at

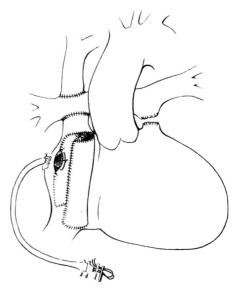

Figure 28.10 The lateral atrial tunnel type of Fontan connection with incomplete atrial partitioning (adjustable interatrial communication with snaring suture of polypropylene and exteriorized tourniquet) as advocated by Laks. (Reproduced with permission from Pearl *et al.* [16].)

a later time. The advantage claimed for the adjustable atrial septal defect is that it facilitates decompression of the systemic venous system and improves ventricular filling during an early postoperative course that may be characterized by transient elevation of pulmonary vascular resistance and altered ventricular function, but it can be closed following a period of recovery, thus eliminating the secondary problems associated with persistence of a right-to-left shunt.

Others have advocated simple fenestration of the prosthetic portion of the lateral atrial tunnel [85]. This is generally accomplished using the kind of aortic punch device that is used in aortocoronary bypass surgery. A simple round hole (of 4, 5, or 6 mm diameter depending on patient body size) is made in the synthetic patch. This is most easily accomplished when the lateral atrial tunnel is made of PTFE. Often the patient will undergo cardiac catheterization following complete recovery from the Fontan procedure, and the fenestration may be closed using a catheter-deployed device if satisfactory hemodynamics are observed during a period of trial occlusion of the fenestration with a balloon-tipped catheter [86]. Hemodynamic changes observed during fenestration occlusion most often include an increase in systemic venous pressure, increase in systemic arterial oxygen saturation, and slight decrease in measured cardiac output [87]. If the increase in systemic venous pressure or decrease in cardiac output is dramatic, then closure of the fenestration is not advisable. Early reports of the *fenestrated Fontan procedure* showed decreased operative mortality in high-risk patients. Fenestration has been applied for all Fontan patients by many surgical teams, as it also appears to be associated with a diminution of morbidity in the form of pleural effusions and ascites [88].

Surgical Methods

We routinely perform Fontan's operation in two stages. In the current era, most surgeons and centers do. The first stage has the important goal of reducing the volume load of the single ventricle, which in the unoperated or palliated state must pump blood to both the pulmonary and systemic vascular beds. This is accomplished by means of a superior cavopulmonary connection—either a bidirectional Glenn anastomosis or hemi-Fontan procedure. Many surgeons choose the bidirectional Glenn anastomosis because of technical simplicity, and because it can be performed on a beating heart with cardiopulmonary bypass or without cardiopulmonary bypass using a superior vena cava to right atrial shunt. In the latter case, the patient is dependent on preexisting antegrade pulmonary blood flow during construction of the superior vena cava to pulmonary artery anastomosis. Whether or not to completely eliminate other sources of pulmonary blood flow at the

time of a bidirectional Glenn anastomosis is controversial. Proponents of maintaining an additional source of antegrade pulmonary blood flow claim higher systemic oxygen saturation and pulsatility of pulmonary blood flow as advantages. Proponents of eliminating all sources of pulmonary blood flow other than the cavopulmonary connection emphasize the important physiologic goal of minimizing the volume load on the ventricle, and cite higher superior vena cava pressures and a higher incidence of pleural effusions and chylothorax, as complications associated with failure to eliminate other sources.

We prefer the hemi-Fontan operation [89], because it does minimize the volume work of the systemic ventricle and because of its preparatory nature, which significantly simplifies the completion Fontan procedure. It is usually undertaken at 4–8 months of age but may be accomplished as soon as the pulmonary vasculature has matured sufficiently to allow superior vena caval blood to flow through the lungs without resulting in an undesirably high superior vena caval pressure. In practice, this is often true before 4 months of age (the author's earliest successful hemi-Fontan operation was performed at 9 weeks of age).

The Hemi-Fontan Procedure

The hemi-Fontan procedure is performed with the infant positioned supine. A radial or femoral artery line is inserted for monitoring pressure and blood gases. Central venous lines are not used. Surface cooling is begun following tracheal intubation. This includes the use of a cooling blanket beneath the patient, the application of ice bags to the head, and cooling of the operating room. The operative approach is by median sternotomy. Sufficient dissection to afford access to the aorta and the right atrium is accomplished before heparinization. Bypass is established with ascending aortic perfusion and drainage via a single cannula in the systemic venous atrium. All systemic to pulmonary artery shunts are occluded at initiation of bypass, and flow is adjusted to 150 mL/kg/min. The perfusate is gradually cooled to approximately 16 °C. During the cooling phase of cardiopulmonary bypass the remainder of the dissection is accomplished, with particular attention to freeing the pulmonary artery confluence behind the ascending aorta. When nasopharyngeal and esophageal temperatures have both reached 18 °C, the aortic cross-clamp is applied and circulation is temporarily discontinued. Blood is drained via the venous cannula into the cardiotomy reservoir, and the cannula is then removed. Cold crystalloid cardioplegia (30 mL/kg) is infused into the aortic root and is scavenged from the right atrium. An incision is made in the most superior portion of the right atrium and carried superiorly onto the medial aspect of the right superior vena cava (Figure 28.11) [89]. Through this incision the atrial septal defect is inspected, and if necessary it is enlarged. The

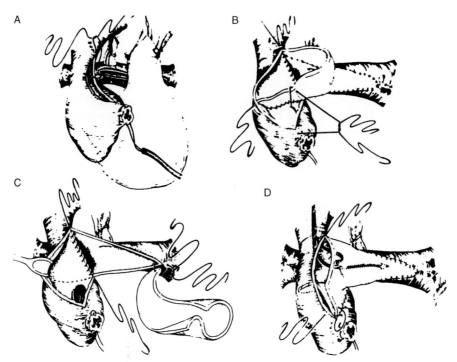

Figure 28.11 Artist's drawing of the hemi-Fontan procedure. **A,** The systemic-to-pulmonary artery shunt is occluded during the initial phase of cardiopulmonary bypass. During hypothermic circulatory arrest, the confluence of the pulmonary arteries is opened anteriorly. An incision is made in the superior portion of the right atrium and extended onto the medial aspect of the superior vena cava. The right pulmonary artery is anastomosed to the superior vena cava. **B,** A gusset of cryopreserved pulmonary artery homograft material is used for anterior augmentation of the confluence of the pulmonary arteries. **C,** This same homograft material is used to occlude the enlarged junction of the right atrium with the superior vena cava. **D,** The same homograft patch creates a roof over the patulous amalgamation of the superior vena cava with the pulmonary arteries. (Reproduced with permission from Norwood *et al.* [89].)

confluence of the right and left branch pulmonary arteries is opened anteriorly to a point just medial to the upper lobe branch on each side. In the absence of naturally occurring or surgically created pulmonary atresia, the main pulmonary artery is transected and oversewn proximally at the level of the pulmonary valve. (Simple ligation of the main pulmonary artery is ill advised, as it results in a cul-de-sac beyond the valve where stasis may predispose to thrombus formation). The posterior lip of the opened right superior vena cava is anastomosed in side-to-side fashion to the right pulmonary artery. If a left superior vena cava is present, it too is opened along its medial aspect, occluded at its cardiac end, and anastomosed in side-to-side fashion to the ipsilateral branch pulmonary artery. A single patch of cryopreserved pulmonary artery homograft tissue is used to augment the confluence of the pulmonary arteries anteriorly, to create a roof over each anastomosis of the vena cava(e) to the branch pulmonary arteries and to occlude the inflow of the right superior vena cava into the right atrium. The incision through, and subsequent patching of the junction of the right superior vena cava with the right atrium effectively enlarges this connection to a caliber equivalent to that of the junction of the inferior vena cava

with the right atrium, but temporarily occludes this connection until it is reopened at the time of the completion Fontan procedure. Bypass is resumed and the cross-clamp is removed. In general the reconstruction can be accomplished during a period of hypothermic circulatory arrest of about 30 minutes duration.

During rewarming, the lungs are ventilated to minimize impedance to transpulmonary flow. After rewarming, separation from bypass is generally accomplished with minimal inotropic support. Following decannulation, catheters inserted through the cannulation purse string in the morphologic right atrium are used for infusions and to monitor cardiac filling pressure. Early in our experience we also placed catheters in the cavopulmonary amalgamation for pressure monitoring but no longer feel this is necessary. Sternal closure is accomplished routinely. Postoperative management includes judicious administration of fluids guided by cardiac filling pressures and early extubation, which can usually be accomplished 5–8 hours after completion of surgery. Diuretics are generally administered beginning on the first postoperative day. Hospitalization usually lasts a week or less. Facial swelling and irritability (which we suspect is attributable to headache from transiently elevated venous pressure) often persist for a few days, and are more common in younger infants. Pleural effusion and chylothorax are extremely rare. Oxygen saturation in room air at discharge from the hospital is generally in the range of 80–84%.

Because it is intended specifically to be preparatory to an eventual completion Fontan procedure, concomitant procedures to address adverse hemodynamic circumstances should always be accomplished at the time of the hemi-Fontan procedure. Thus among 400 consecutive patients undergoing hemi-Fontan procedures by Norwood and Jacobs between May 1989 and August 1995 [90], 61 concomitant procedures were performed including atrial septectomy (17), relief of aortic arch obstruction (13), proximal main pulmonary artery to aortic anastomosis (6), repair or revision of previous repair of anomalous pulmonary venous connection (6), atrial ventricular valvuloplasty (6), and others (13). While the construction of a large side-to-side amalgamation of the superior vena cava and the confluence of the pulmonary arteries is facilitated by the absence of a drainage cannula from the superior vena cava, the same surgical result can be achieved using continuous cardiopulmonary bypass with venous drainage via the right atrium and via a small cannula placed high in the superior vena cava near its junction with the innominate vein if the surgeon wishes to avoid using hypothermic circulatory arrest.

The Completion Fontan Procedure

The completion Fontan procedure is usually performed 12–24 months after the hemi-Fontan operation. In theory, it should be undertaken whenever ventricular remodeling is complete and the mass to volume relationship of the systemic ventricle has normalized. Electively waiting longer than this prolongs the period during which systemic arterial oxygen saturation is at lower than normal levels and may increase the likelihood of the development of intrapulmonary shunting secondary to development of pulmonary arteriovenous fistulae. In practice, the completion Fontan by lateral atrial tunnel technique is generally undertaken when the patient is about 2 years old. If the plan for completion Fontan includes use of an extracardiac conduit, the procedure may be postponed to allow the patient to become somewhat larger and is usually undertaken at about 3 years of age.

Preparation and intraoperative monitoring are the same as for the hemi-Fontan procedure. Use of central venous lines is avoided in order to minimize the likelihood of thrombus formation within venous pathways. After repeat median sternotomy, minimal dissection is required to make preparations for cardiopulmonary bypass, which again is established with ascending aortic perfusion and drainage via a single cannula in the right atrium. Direct caval cannulation is avoided to minimize distortion and narrowing of these vessels, and caval tourniquets are unnecessary, eliminating the likelihood of caval or phrenic nerve injury. Bypass is established at flows of 120–150 mL/kg/min, and the patient is cooled until esophageal and nasopharyngeal temperatures reach 18 °C. During cooling, enough of the ascending aorta is mobilized to afford access for cross-clamping. The free wall of the right atrium is carefully dissected from the adjacent pericardium. When the desired temperature is reached, the aorta is cross-clamped and cold cardioplegic solution is infused. The venous cannula is removed. An incision is made in the free wall of the right atrium, parallel and slightly anterior to the sulcus terminalis. This incision extends inferiorly to the level of the Eustachian valve of the inferior vena cava and superiorly to within a few millimeters of the patched junction of the right atrium with the superior vena cava. The patch of homograft tissue that was previously placed to separate the right atrium from the confluence of the superior vena cava and pulmonary arteries is widely excised (Figure 28.12) [91]. Lateral tunnel cavopulmonary connection is performed using a gusset of PTFE. In our practice, this is generally trimmed from a 10 mm tube graft that has been split longitudinally. The gusset is sewn inferiorly around the opening of the inferior vena cava into the right atrium and along the interior atrial wall just posterior to the edge of the atrial septal defect. Superiorly the gusset is sewn to the edges of the opening of the right atrium into the superior vena cava and pulmonary arteries. The lateral tunnel is then completed by incorporating the anterior edge of the PTFE gusset in the closure of the atriotomy incision. Two important features of this type of lateral atrial tunnel Fontan are 1) insuring that the opening of the right atrium into the superior vena cava and pulmonary arteries is as large as the inferior vena caval opening; and 2) avoidance of suturing directly to the sulcus terminalis, which is believed to be important in the development of postoperative tachyarrhythmias. In most instances we choose to fenestrate the lateral tunnel and usually accomplish this by creating three separate holes in the PTFE gusset using a 2.5- or 2.7-mm punch device. Fenestrations of this size promote decompression of the venous pathway and enhance ventricular filling postoperatively, but generally go on to spontaneous closure, avoiding the need for devices in the venous pathway [92]. The completion Fontan procedure as described here can generally be completed with a period of hypothermic circulatory arrest of about 20 minutes duration.

As with the hemi-Fontan procedure, resumption of cardiopulmonary bypass is accompanied by ventilation of the lungs to optimize transpulmonary flow during rewarming. Low-dose inotropic support is used routinely, though it is often not necessary. Following decannulation, lines are inserted through the atrial purse string for infusion and

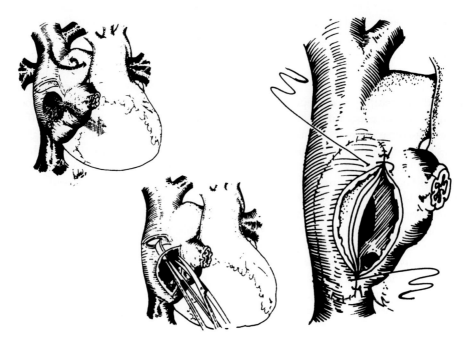

Figure 28.12 Completion of Fontan's procedure in a patient with previous hemi-Fontan operation. Through a lateral atriotomy incision, the homograft dam occluding the junction of the right atrium with the superior vena cava is excised widely. Atrial partitioning is accomplished using the lateral atrial tunnel technique. A gusset of polytetrafluoroethylene is used, with incorporation of the lateral edge of the polytetrafluoroethylene graft into the atriotomy closure. (Reproduced with permission from Jacobs *et al.* [91].)

monitoring of the cardiac filling pressure. We no longer monitor pressure in the cavopulmonary pathway, though we did so in earlier patients managed this way. One mediastinal chest tube is placed. The pleural spaces are opened to communicate with the pericardial space. Rather than inserting chest tubes in the pleural spaces at operation, we drain them later with 7 French polyvinyl catheters, only if significant pleural effusions occur. This method enhances early mobilization of the patient. Most patients can be extubated 5–8 hours after completion of surgery. We routinely administer baby aspirin, angiotensin converting enzyme inhibitors, and diuretics postoperatively. Intravenous inotropic support is generally continued for 2–3 days. The average duration of hospitalization using this scheme of management has been 10 days.

In certain patients, the extracardiac conduit type of completion Fontan is preferred. This is true when there is concern that an intracardiac lateral atrial tunnel may obstruct abnormal pathways of pulmonary venous drainage or when there are abnormalities of cardiac position and the ventricular apex is directed to the same side as the principle systemic venous connections. As mentioned, the operation may be performed at a slightly later age in order to optimize the size of the extracardiac conduit. Preparation and management of cardiopulmonary bypass are the same as for the lateral tunnel completion Fontan procedure. During the period of hypothermic circulatory arrest, the

inferior vena cava is transected approximately 1 cm above the diaphragm and the cardiac end is oversewn. With the circulation arrested, a conduit of PTFE is anastomosed in end-to-end fashion to the inferior vena cava. The conduit is trimmed to an appropriate length and the superior end of the conduit is anastomosed to the pulmonary arteries. In patients with a prior bidirectional Glenn shunt, the anastomosis is performed between the conduit and the underside of the right pulmonary artery. The ideal alignment or offset between the anastomoses of the superior vena cava and the inferior caval conduit to the pulmonary artery are the subject of considerable controversy [93,94]. Many surgeons prefer to place the conduit-to-pulmonary artery anastomosis somewhat centrally, in the belief that this may increase the chances of achieving a favorable distribution of inferior vena cava blood flow to the right and left lungs. In patients with a prior hemi-Fontan, the superior end of the conduit may be anastomosed anteriorly to an opening created in the homograft roof over the amalgamation of the superior vena cava with the pulmonary arteries. As a general principle, most surgeons attempt to implant a conduit of such a size that it is unlikely that the patient will outgrow it. In practice, this translates into frequent use of conduits of 20–22 mm diameter, in patients with body weight of 10–15 kg. While such conduits certainly look large in children of this size, it is not clear that they are sufficiently large that they will not be associated with pressure gradients or restriction of flow in adult size patients. On the other hand, there is evidence from computational flow dynamic modeling studies that 16 and 18 mm conduits are ideal for children 2–3 years old and that larger conduit sizes are associated with more stagnation volume in the lateral aspect of conduits larger than 20 mm and backflow in the expiratory phase of respiration at the lateral portion of conduits larger than 18 mm [95].

Numerous methods of fenestration of the extracardiac TCPC have been devised. In patients with a hemi-Fontan connection, a fenestration can be created in the patch which occludes the right atrium to superior vena caval junction. Alternatively, in any patient, fenestration may be accomplished by creation of a small window between the conduit and the adjacent wall of the right atrium by side-to-side anastomosis. Some authors have recommended the interposition of a small PTFE graft or shunt between the extracardiac conduit and the right atrium. This seems unnecessarily complicated. A very reliable and straightforward approach to fenestration of the extracardiac conduit type of Fontan connection involves suturing of the atrial orifice of the divided inferior vena cava to the leftward aspect of the conduit, in an end-to-side fashion. The circumferential suture line surrounds the fenestration, but remains away from the actual edge of the fenestration [96]. Following the extracardiac conduit completion Fontan procedure, postoperative monitoring and management are the same as described above for the lateral tunnel completion Fontan.

The techniques described above, including the conduct of bypass using a single cannula in the right-sided atrium and the use of hypothermic circulatory arrest to complete the TCPC, are elements of a strategy for Fontan operations that the author has used with considerable success. In fact, these techniques form the basis for a protocol associated with no mortality among 100 consecutive patients subjected to completion Fontan operations, including many with multiple risk factors [97]. It must be acknowledged, however, that a majority of surgeons currently perform the completion Fontan procedure using continuous cardiopulmonary bypass with mild or moderate hypothermia and that many reserve aortic cross-clamping for instances when associated repairs (such as valvuloplasty) are indicated [98]. Still others complete an extracardiac total cavopulmonary bypass without using bypass support, when technically feasible.

Results of Surgery

Mortality

Over the first two decades of the history of Fontan's operation and its modifications, the predominant influences on operative survival were appropriate patient selection and evolution and refinement of surgical techniques. It has become apparent that good health of the pulmonary vascular bed and satisfactory function of the systemic ventricle are essential ingredients for survival. Ventricular hypertrophy, pulmonary artery distortion, elevated pulmonary vascular resistance, atrioventricular valve regurgitation, and systemic ventricular outflow obstruction consistently emerged as incremental risk factors for suboptimal outcome. Early on, patients at both extremes of age seemed to be at higher risk with respect to operative mortality. Over time, the operations themselves became simpler rather than more complex, and eventually the TCPC (in one of a very few forms) could be applied more or less generically, usually without modifications necessitated by the details of atrioventricular and ventriculoarterial connections or ventricular morphology. In the last decade, the importance of patient selection has given way to the more powerful influence of patient preparation. Thus with more thoughtful palliation in neonates, and with staging procedures performed early in life to minimize the duration over which ventricular myocardium must adapt to excessive volume work, it has now become the case that most infants with functional single ventricles have a high likelihood of eventually undergoing a modified Fontan procedure with relatively low risk of operative mortality. These observations are born out by reports of steadily improving results of Fontan operations at many centers.

A 1996 report from the Mayo Clinic [99] compared the early morbidity and mortality as well as predictors of outcome for two consecutive cohorts of patients who underwent Fontan operations at that institution. The recent cohort of 339 patients (1987–1992) was compared with an earlier cohort of 500 patients (1973–1986). Overall mortality was considerably lower for the recent cohort (9% vs 16%, $p = 0.002$) despite increased anatomic complexity of patients. One year survival improved to 88% from 79%, and 5-year survival to 81% from 73%. The authors attributed the improved outcomes to patient selection, younger age at time of operation, and refinements in surgical technique and postoperative management.

A 1997 report from the Children's Hospital Boston reviewed their experience with the first 500 consecutive patients who underwent modified Fontan procedures there [100]. The incidence of early failure decreased from 27.1% in the first quartile to 7.5% in the last quartile. In a multivariate model, factors associated with an increased probability of early failure include a mean preoperative pulmonary artery pressure of 19 mmHg or more, younger age at operation, heterotaxy syndrome, a right-sided tricuspid valve as the only systemic atrioventricular valve, pulmonary artery distortion, an atrial pulmonary connection originating at the right atrial body or appendage, the absence of a baffle fenestration, and longer cardiopulmonary bypass time. An increased probability of late failure was associated with the presence of a pacemaker before the Fontan operation. More recently the Children's Hospital Boston group reported the results of 220 patients who underwent lateral tunnel Fontan procedures with 10-year follow-up [101]. There were 12 early deaths, seven late deaths, four successful takedown operations, and four heart transplantations. Kaplan-Meier estimated survival was 93% at 5 years and 91% at 10 years, and freedom from failure was 90% at 5 years and 87% at 10 years. Freedom from new supraventricular tachyarrhythmia was 96% at 5 years and 91% at 10 years; freedom from new bradyrhythmia was 88% at 5 years and 79% at 10 years.

Similar improved outcomes have been reported by other institutions, paralleling the experience at those two very large centers. The impact of staging on the outcome of Fontan procedures is difficult to analyze, as most consecutive series are influenced by several additional factors that have contributed to reduced mortality. Jacobs and Norwood [91] in 1994 reported a significant improvement in survival with a two-staged approach to Fontan's operation (8% mortality for completion Fontan vs. 16% mortality for primary Fontan operation). While there are mortalities associated with the hemi-Fontan or bidirectional Glenn procedures, it is difficult to compare outcomes between groups that had early staging versus those with later primary Fontan operations, because information concerning nonsurgical mortality of single ventricle patients that occurs in the palliated or unoperated state is less readily available. Whether an early first-stage procedure (hemi-Fontan or bidirectional Glenn) selects out poorer candidates by means of operative mortality at that early stage, or alternatively enables more single ventricle patients to ultimately reach a Fontan completion, is debated. Increasing evidence suggests that the latter is true. In 1996 the author reported on 400 patients who had undergone hemi-Fontan operations at the Children's Hospital of Philadelphia between 1989 and 1995, revealing an overall mortality of 8%, which was reduced to 4% in the latter half of the series and 0% in the most recent quartile [90].

Contemporary results are represented by the authors' experience between 1996 and 2006, which includes 113 superior cavopulmonary anastomoses with three operative deaths and one late death and 100 completion Fontan procedures with no operative deaths and one late death. Each of the 100 Fontan procedures had been preceded by either a hemi-Fontan or bidirectional Glenn anastomosis. Eighty-four completion Fontans were of the lateral atrial tunnel type, and 16 were of the extracardiac conduit type. Patient age ranged from 1.5 to 15 years, with 98 patients less than 4 years old and median age 26 months [97].

As mentioned above, many surgeons perform Fontan's operation with bicaval cannulation and continuous cardi-

opulmonary bypass at mild to moderate hypothermia. Still others, in selected cases, accomplish completion Fontan procedures of the extracardiac conduit type without any extracorporeal bypass support. In the author's series, the hemi-Fontan procedure and all completion Fontan procedures were accomplished using hypothermic cardiopulmonary bypass and limited circulatory arrest as described above. This technique avoids potential problems of caval stenosis and phrenic nerve injury that may be related to cannulation, and minimizes the need for dissection and thus the potential for bleeding. Similar techniques used by Spray and associates at the Children's Hospital of Philadelphia [102] and by Mosca and Bove and associates at the University of Michigan [103] have yielded comparable results with operative mortality in the range of 1–2%. The report by Mosca and associates [103] of 100 consecutive Fontan operations for hypoplastic left heart syndrome revealed improved survival from 79% to 98% in consecutive cohorts and attributed much of the improvement in survival to evolution of the operative strategy from cardiopulmonary bypass and moderate systemic hypothermia in the earlier cohort, to profound hypothermia and circulatory arrest in the later cohort.

A more recent report from the same institution summarized their 15-year experience with 636 primary Fontan operations between 1992 and 2007 [104]. Total cavopulmonary connection was by lateral atrial tunnel in 92% and by extracardiac conduit in 8%. Hospital survival was 96%. Long-term survival was 97% at a mean follow-up of 50 months (range, 0–173 months). Ventricular anatomy and preoperative hemodynamics did not predict early or late survival. Longer aortic cross-clamp time was associated with decreased late survival ($p = 0.01$). Fontan takedown was required in 3%. The majority of recent cases were accomplished using continuous cardiopulmonary bypass support.

The progressive reduction of the operative mortality associated with modified Fontan procedures is clearly multifactorial. Clearer understanding of the fundamental physiologic and anatomic issues have led to refinements in operative technique, early neutralization of potential risk factors, widespread use of a staged approach, and selective application of the concept of fenestration or incomplete partitioning. While further reduction of operative mortality is important and may be anticipated in the future, major emphasis now must be placed on optimizing functional outcome and understanding and managing the late complications associated with Fontan operations and the unique circulatory physiology that results from them.

Late Considerations

In 1990, Kirklin and Blackstone and colleagues in collaboration with Professor Fontan [105] applied the meticulous

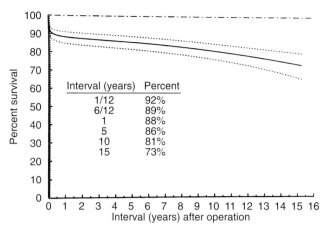

Figure 28.13 Fontan and Kirklin's predictive survival after a "perfect Fontan operation" performed under ideal circumstances. The multivariable risk factor equation for survival was derived from analysis of a heterogeneous group of patients (n = 334; deaths = 110) who underwent Fontan operations. To derive the survival curve shown in this figure, optimal values were entered for each of the risk factors. (Reproduced with permission from Fontan *et al.* [105].)

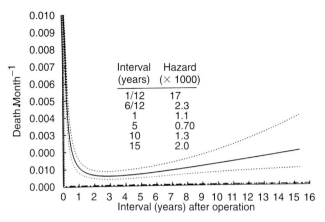

Figure 28.14 Nomogram of the predicted hazard function for death after a "perfect Fontan operation" performed under ideal conditions. Note the gradually rising late phase of hazard. (Reproduced with permission from Fontan *et al.* [105].)

statistical methods that characterize their analyses of outcomes following cardiac surgery to a heterogenous group of patients undergoing an initially complete (nonstaged, nonfenestrated) Fontan operation. The hazard function for such patients had three phases: an early phase of about one year duration with rapidly declining risk of death, a relatively flat period of very low constant risk of death, and a gradually rising late phase of hazard, which becomes evident about 8 years after operation. They reasoned that many deaths after the Fontan operation may have been owing to circumstances that, based on lessons learned, could be avoided. To address the question of whether the persisting and rising hazard function for death years after the Fontan operation could be a result of these now avoidable circumstances, they undertook an analysis of survival under circumstances that could be considered ideal (Figure 28.13) [105]. Into the multivariable risk factor equation derived from the analysis of the above group of patients, they entered optimal values (within the realm of realism) for each of the risk factors. Under these ideal circumstances, the 15-year survival was predicted to be 73%, and the gradually rising late phase of hazard was still present (Figure 28.14) [105]. The only risk factor identified for the late phase of hazard was older age at operation. Is it then the case that the late phase of hazard for premature death is an inevitable accompaniment of the circulatory state after the Fontan operation? The answer is unknown. Many of the issues and events that complicate the course of survivors of Fontan operations are only now beginning to be understood.

Functional Status

Numerous studies of patients following Fontan-type repairs have found that resting cardiac indices were not different from those of healthy children. Some but not all achieve exercise cardiac indices similar to controls. The predominant mechanism for achieving high cardiac output during exercise is increased heart rate, with low-normal resting ejection fraction and smaller increments in ejection fraction with exercise than in normals. One recent study [106] demonstrated an inverse relationship between peak oxygen uptake and age at Fontan operation (particularly in patients with single ventricle of right ventricular morphology). Mahle and associates at the Children's Hospital of Philadelphia undertook an evaluation of the impact of early ventricular unloading on exercise performance in preadolescents with single ventricle and Fontan physiology [107]. Evaluating the exercise stress test results of 46 patients, they concluded that volume unloading at younger age was associated with increased aerobic capacity ($p = 0.003$). Patients who had reduction of ventricular volume work by hemi-Fontan or Fontan procedures before 2 years of age were compared with a group that had successful Fontan operations, but in whom the volume loaded state of the single ventricle had persisted for more than two years. The authors observed better peak exercise capacity in the group which had undergone early volume unloading. Recently, 147 patients (ages 7–18 years) at a median of 8.1 years after Fontan, were evaluated as part of the Pediatric Heart Network cross-sectional study of Fontan survivors. Findings included the observation that physical activity levels were reduced in this patient group, independent of exercise capacity, and were associated with lower perceived general health but not other aspects of functional status [108].

Neurologic Status

As operative survival has improved, emphasis has been appropriately placed on assessment of neurodevelopmental outcome. Uzark and colleagues [109] in San Diego tested 32 patients who had undergone the Fontan procedure and found, on average, normal developmental indices. Goldberg and colleagues [110] at the University of Michigan studied a group of 51 patients who had undergone Fontan operations. They undertook developmental testing, behavior evaluation, and central nervous system imaging. Most of the Fontan survivors evaluated in the study demonstrated intelligence scores within or above the normal range. These patients performed significantly better in areas of verbal intelligence than in nonverbal areas. The diagnosis of hypoplastic left heart syndrome and a history of perioperative seizures were independent risk factors for lower developmental scores. Nearly half the patients who underwent imaging of the central nervous system (magnetic resonance imaging [MRI] or computed tomography [CT]) were demonstrated to have acquired abnormalities, but the authors did not find that significant developmental abnormalities appeared to be related to evidence of central nervous systemic ischemia. An evaluation of 133 patients who had undergone Fontan procedures at Children's Hospital Boston in the 1970s and 1980s [111] revealed that most individual patients had cognitive outcomes and academic function within the normal range, but the performance of the cohort was lower than that of the general population. Importantly, in a review of 645 patients who underwent the Fontan procedures at the same institution, du Plessis and associates [112] found a 2.6% incidence of stroke following the Fontan operation. The risk period for stroke extended from the first postoperative day to 32 months after the Fontan procedure.

Thromboembolic Complications

Thromboembolic events account for significant morbidity and mortality following Fontan procedures. Retrospective studies have reported the incidence of thromboembolic events after Fontan operations ranging from 3% to 20% [113,114]. The time course of these events ranges from 24 hours after surgery to as late as 16 years (Figure 28.15) [115]. Efforts have been made to characterize abnormalities of coagulation that are associated with the post-Fontan state [116,117] but they are hampered in part by lack of age-specific controls. There is general agreement that ligation of the main pulmonary artery leaving a blind pouch or cul-de-sac distal to the pulmonic valve is a worrisome substrate for the occurrence of thromboembolism. Almost every other assertion with regard to thromboembolic events after Fontan's operation is the subject of controversy. As yet, there is a lack of evidence from randomized controlled

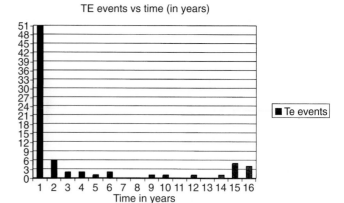

Figure 28.15 Graphic representation of the frequency, over time in years, of thromboembolic events occurring in patients who have undergone Fontan operations. These data are derived from a review by the author of the English language literature on the subject. (TE, thromboembolic.) (Reproduced with permission from Jacobs *et al.* [115].)

trials to support the use of any specific strategy for post-Fontan anticoagulation therapy. In the absence of any compelling evidence to support the routine use of warfarin therapy, the author gives aspirin (81 mg daily) to all Fontan patients beginning on postoperative day one and continuing indefinitely. This strategy combined with operative techniques described above, has resulted in freedom from clinically apparent thromboembolic complications [115]. A recent retrospective study from the University of Michigan found that anticoagulation with aspirin was associated with a statistically significantly decreased risk for cerebrovascular events in Fontan patients [118]. Notwithstanding the lack of evidence of a consistent benefit of warfarin therapy in patients who have undergone Fontan procedures, there are circumstances in which this type of more aggressive anticoagulation is probably warranted in individual patients. These certainly would include instances where there is evidence of pathway obstruction, low cardiac output, and chronic or recurrent arrhythmias [119].

Systemic Ventricular Outflow Tract Obstruction

Subaortic obstruction is a frequent accompaniment of single ventricle anatomy. It occurs most often when the aorta arises from an outlet chamber that is connected to the dominant ventricle by a bulboventricular foramen or ventricular septal defect. This connection may be restrictive of flow at birth, or may become obstructive after surgical procedures that reduce the volume work of the ventricle [27]. This phenomenon impacts on the management of patients with functional single ventricle at many stages. In neonates, significant systemic ventricular outflow obstruction is often associated with aortic arch hypoplasia. With

Figure 28.16 Artist's illustration of the surgical management of subaortic stenosis (systemic ventricular outflow tract obstruction) in a neonate with functional single ventricle. The case illustrated is of double-inlet left ventricle with L-transposition of the great arteries and significant aortic arch hypoplasia. Under hypothermic circulatory arrest, the aortic arch is augmented with a gusset of cryopreserved pulmonary artery homograft tissue. A separate homograft patch is used to augment the side-to-side amalgamation of the transected main pulmonary trunk with the ascending aorta. A systemic-to-pulmonary artery shunt is constructed (not shown in the illustration), completing a stage I Norwood palliative procedure. (Reproduced with permission from Jacobs *et al.* [122].)

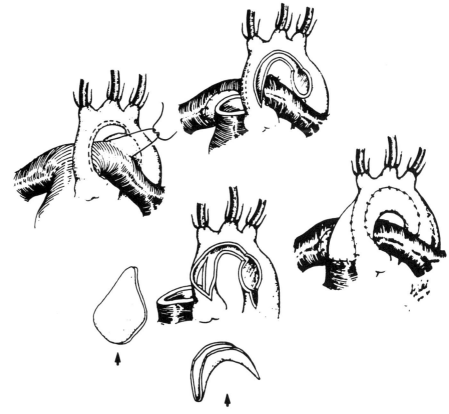

parallel pulmonary and systemic circulations, and particularly when there is a patent arterial duct, it is difficult to quantitate subaortic obstruction. In the setting of ventriculoarterial discordance, the potential for development of systemic ventricular outflow obstruction must be presumed, even if it is not readily apparent. Thus it must be considered in planning initial palliation. For some time, it has been recognized that pulmonary artery banding is associated with a tendency for subaortic obstruction to progress [120]. Thus, this technically simple means of palliation must be considered carefully when there is anatomic substrate for systemic ventricular outflow obstruction. Appropriate alternatives are the performance of a stage 1 Norwood procedure or palliative arterial switch as the initial operation. Apical ventricular to aortic conduits or direct relief of subaortic obstruction are less desirable strategies. If systemic ventricular outflow obstruction is not addressed definitively at the time of initial palliation, it may progress with important consequences at any stage during the sequence of reconstructive procedures or may develop after a completed Fontan operation [121]. This fact, together with the known deleterious effects of systemic ventricular outflow obstruction and the associated secondary myocardial changes on the function of the single ventricle, suggests that an optimal strategy for dealing with subaortic obstruction in single ventricle

hearts is simply to prevent it. Thus, if present in the neonate, subaortic stenosis is best managed by amalgamation of the proximal main pulmonary artery with the ascending aorta and relief of arch obstruction (Figure 28.16) [122–124]. Alternatively, the same goal can be achieved by a palliative arterial switch operation and arch repair (Figure 28.17) [125–127]. In hearts where subaortic obstruction was not important or apparent at initial presentation but where the potential for its development exists (i.e. ventriculoarterial discordance or subaortic conus), it is advisable to address the issue by means of a pulmonary artery to aortic anastomosis (Damus-Kaye-Stansel procedure) at the time of the hemi-Fontan or bidirectional Glenn anastomosis. If these guidelines are followed, only rarely will a direct ventricular approach to relief of subaortic stenosis be required, and the adverse impact of myocardial hypertrophy on outcome of Fontan's operation should be effectively neutralized by prevention.

Rhythm Disturbances

Both tachyarrhythmias and bradyrhythmias complicate the course and management of patients who undergo Fontan operations. Though not completely understood, they are thought to be consequences of 1) injury to the sinoatrial node or its blood supply, 2) extensive atrial incisions and

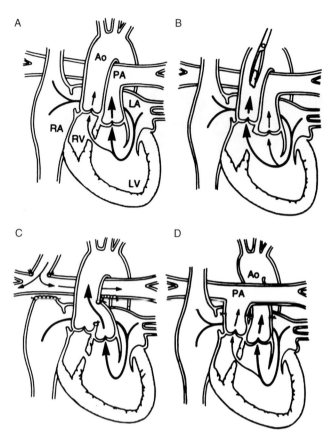

Figure 28.17 Methods of treatment of subaortic stenosis in hearts with functional single ventricle. **A,** Anatomy of type IIc tricuspid atresia with significant subaortic stenosis. **B,** Direct resection of myocardium with ventricular septal defect enlargement. **C,** Damus-Kaye-Stansel operation, main pulmonary artery-to-ascending aortic anastomosis. **D,** Palliative arterial switch operation. (Ao, aorta; LA, left atrium; LV, left ventricle; PA, pulmonary artery; RA, right atrium; RV, right ventricle.)

sutures lines, and 3) chronic exposure of atrial myocardium to elevated pressure. In some instances, they are directly related to the underlying anatomic substrate (as in hearts with atrioventricular discordance or heterotaxy with intrinsic abnormalities of the conduction system) or to hemodynamic factors such as atrioventricular valve regurgitation. Analysis of risk factors for the development of tachyarrhythmias after Fontan operations support these hypotheses. A study of nearly 500 patients who underwent modified Fontan operations at the Mayo Clinic between 1985 and 1993 [128] revealed the following risk factors for supraventricular tachyarrhythmias: atrioventricular valve regurgitation, abnormal atrioventricular valve, preoperative supraventricular tachyarrhythmias, and age at operation. The type of Fontan connection was not strongly predictive, though the frequency of supraventricular tachyarrhyth-

mias was slightly lower in patients with an atrial pulmonary connection with lateral tunnel then those with TCPC. In a study from the Children's Hospital Boston of 334 early survivors of Fontan operations done between 1973 and 1991 [129], atrial flutter was identified in 54 patients (16%) at a mean 5.3 ± 4.7 years (range 0–19.7 years). Atrial flutter developed sooner and was more likely to occur in patients who were older at the time of Fontan operation. The presence of sinus node dysfunction was associated with a higher incidence of atrial flutter. While there was a lower prevalence of atrial flutter in patients with a TCPC, the follow-up for that group was shorter. Analysis of a smaller series of Fontan patients by Paul and associates [130] in Hannover, Germany also revealed a lower risk of supraventricular tachyarrhythmias with TCPC as compared with atrial pulmonary connection.

Strategies to minimize the risk of post-Fontan arrhythmias include technical modifications that minimize the likelihood of injury to the sinus node and its blood supply, minimization of atrial incisions and sutures line (particularly in the region of the sulcus terminalis), and early interventions against atrioventricular valve regurgitation. It is not yet absolutely clear whether the TCPC using lateral atrial tunnel technique is superior to atrial pulmonary connection with regard to the risk of arrhythmias, though increasing evidence suggests that this is the case. Proponents of the extracardiac conduit type of TCPC suggested the potential advantage of avoiding incisions and suture lines in the region of the sinus node and its blood supply and predicted a lower frequency of postoperative arrhythmias. However, at least one study comparing the incidence of early sinus node dysfunction between groups of Fontan patients who had either lateral atrial tunnel or extracardiac conduit types of completion Fontan procedures, found no discernible difference in the incidence of early postoperative sinus node dysfunction [131]. Options for management of recurrent or persistent postoperative arrhythmias following Fontan procedures include 1) pharmacologic antiarrhythmic therapy, 2) permanent pacing to address sinus node dysfunction and potentially minimize the likelihood of tachyarrhythmias, and 3) in selected instances conversion from atrial pulmonary connections to TCPC of the lateral tunnel or extracardiac Fontan type [132]. The most aggressive and most productive approach has combined conversion to TCPC, atrial reduction, modified maze-type procedure, and permanent pacing (Figure 28.18) [76, 133,134]. At the 2007 meeting of the Society of Thoracic Surgeons, Mavroudis *et al.* presented a series of 111 consecutive Fontan conversions with arrhythmia surgery and pacemaker therapy [135]. There were one early (0.9%) and six late deaths (5.4%); six patients required cardiac transplantation (5.4%). Two late deaths occurred after transplantation. Four risk factors for death or transplantation were identified: presence of a right or ambiguous ventricle, pre-

A

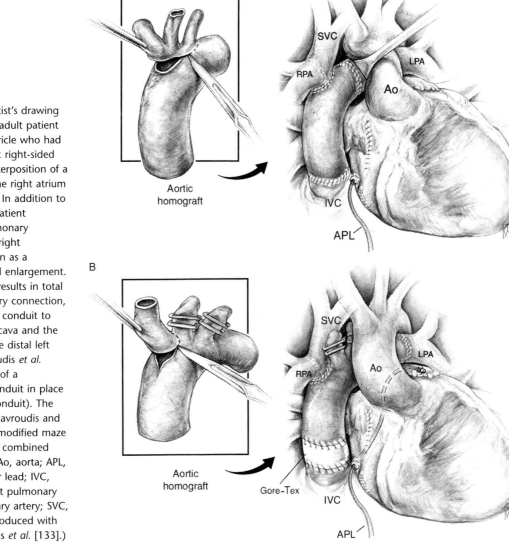

Figure 28.18 Original artist's drawing of a Fontan revision in an adult patient with double-inlet left ventricle who had undergone previous classic right-sided Glenn anastomosis and interposition of a valved conduit between the right atrium and left pulmonary artery. In addition to conduit obstruction, the patient developed right lung pulmonary arteriovenous fistulas and right pulmonary vein obstruction as a consequence of right atrial enlargement. The operative conversion results in total extracardiac cavopulmonary connection, using an aortic homograft conduit to connect the inferior vena cava and the Glenn anastomosis and the distal left pulmonary artery. (Mavroudis *et al.* currently recommend use of a polytetrafluoroethylene conduit in place of the aortic homograft conduit). The procedure described by Mavroudis and associates also includes a modified maze antiarrhythmic procedure, combined with permanent pacing. (Ao, aorta; APL, antitachycardia pacemaker lead; IVC, inferior vena cava; LPA, left pulmonary artery; RPA, right pulmonary artery; SVC, superior vena cava.) (Reproduced with permission from Mavroudis *et al.* [133].)

operative protein-losing enteropathy (PLE), preoperative moderate-to-severe atrioventricular valve regurgitation, and long (>239 minutes) cardiopulmonary bypass time. Evidence supported performance of biatrial maze procedures in patients with history of left atrial re-entry tachycardia or atrial fibrillation.

Protein-Losing Enteropathy

Protein-losing enteropathy is a syndrome characterized by excessive loss of serum proteins into the intestinal lumen. Manifestations include edema, immunodeficiency from hypogammaglobulinemia, malabsorption of fat, intestinal lymphocyte loss, hypercoagulopathy from loss of clotting factors, and electrolyte disorders including hypocalcemia

and hypomagnesemia. Protein-losing enteropathy is known to occur with certain primary gastrointestinal disorders, abnormalities of gut lymphatic drainage, and certain cardiovascular disorders. After Fontan operations, the incidence of PLE has been estimated to be as high as 13.4% [136] though the prevalence in an international multicenter study was 3.7% [137]. The time to onset after Fontan operation is quite variable. Survival after the diagnosis of PLE is poor, with 50% of patients dying within 5 years of diagnosis and 80% within 10 years.

The pathophysiology of PLE is not clear. While Fontan patients share the common feature of elevated central venous pressure with other cardiac patients known to be at risk for PLE (constrictive pericarditis, tricuspid regurgitation, inferior vena caval obstruction), PLE has been known to occur in Fontan patients with generally very satisfactory hemodynamics (low venous pressure) and is not an invariable accompaniment of failing Fontan circulation with markedly elevated venous pressure. A relationship between PLE and altered portal venous blood flow after the Fontan operation has also been proposed [138]. A general hypothesis holds that PLE after Fontan operation is related to low cardiac output and low flow states, which may result in increased mesenteric vascular resistance leading to altered intestinal mucosal function. A similar process with a break in mucosal integrity to protein loss can occur at the bronchial mucosal level, with leakage of proteinaceous material into the airways resulting in bronchial casts or plastic bronchitis. This rare complication also occurs in a small number of patients after the Fontan operation. While PLE is associated with a high rate of mortality, certain interventions appear to have merit in selected cases. All Fontan patients with PLE or plastic bronchitis should undergo full hemodynamic evaluation including catheterization. Adverse anatomic and hemodynamic factors including pathway obstruction, atrioventricular valve regurgitation, and systemic ventricular outflow obstruction must be addressed. Beyond this, fenestration of the atrial septum or venous pathway by surgical means [139] or catheter techniques [140] has been reported to result in resolution of some cases of PLE, though at the expense of arterial desaturation. When PLE has occurred in patients with significant sinus node dysfunction, pacing has reportedly been associated with improvement [141]. Medical therapy with either corticosteroids or heparin has been used with some success. Currently, there is cautious optimism that another form of medical therapy may benefit Fontan patients with PLE. The drug sildenafil, a phosphodiesterase 5 inhibitor, leads to increased cellular levels of cyclic guanosine monophosphate and causes vasodilation. Extensive experience has proven sildenafil to be effective treatment in children and adults with pulmonary hypertension. Although experience in the single ventricle population is limited, it has been postulated that sildenafil may lower pulmonary vascular resistance and improve forward flow through the pulmonary circuit, thus increasing cardiac output in Fontan patients. Thus far sildenafil has been shown to contribute to the resolution of PLE and plastic bronchitis in case reports and to improve exercise performance in patients after Fontan operation following a single dose [142]. Ultimately, in patients with PLE refractory to all of these measures, heart transplantation may represent the only therapeutic alternative.

Conclusion

For the vast majority of patients with functionally univentricular hearts, some modification of Fontan's operation represents, at the present time, the best form of surgical reconstruction. The role of septation is difficult to assess, particularly because it is applicable to a select minority of patients. The evolution over three decades from Fontan's and Kreutzer's initial corrective operations for tricuspid atresia to the current forms of surgical management has been associated with progressive decline in the risk of operative mortality. Though the body of knowledge concerning functionally univentricular heart patients and strategies for management culminating in a Fontan connection has become vast, many questions remain unanswered. Perhaps most important of these is the issue of whether or not the late phase risk of premature death after an "ideal Fontan operation" identified two decades ago by Fontan and Kirklin is in fact inevitable. Current research is focused on means of increasing the durability and extending the longevity of the Fontan circulation for patients with functionally univentricular hearts and physiology.

References

1. Abbott ME. (1936) *Atlas of Congenital Cardiac Disease*. New York, NY: American Heart Association, pp. 50–52.
2. Taussig H. (1939) Cardiovascular anomalies: a single ventricle with a diminutive outlet chamber. J Tech Methods 19, 120.
3. Edwards JE. (1960) Congenital malformations of the heart and great vessels. In: Gould SE, ed. *Pathology of the Heart*. Springfield, IL: Charles C Thomas.
4. Lev M. (1953) *Autopsy Diagnosis of Congenitally Malformed Hearts*. Springfield, IL: Charles C. Thomas.
5. van Praagh R, Plett JA, van Praagh S. (1979) Single ventricle. Pathology, embryology, terminology and classification. Herz 4, 113–150.
6. Anderson RH, Becker AE, Wilkinson JL. (1975) Proceedings: Morphogenesis and nomenclature of univentricular hearts. Br Heart J 37, 781–782.
7. Vanpraagh R, Ongley PA, Swan HJ. (1964) Anatomic types of single or common ventricle in man. Morphologic and geometric aspects of 60 necropsied cases. Am J Cardiol 13, 367–386.
8. Jacobs ML, Anderson RH. (2006) Nomenclature of the functionally univentricular heart. Cardiol Young 16(Suppl 1), 3–8.
9. Jacobs ML, Mayer JE Jr. (2000) Congenital Heart Surgery Nomenclature and Database Project: single ventricle. Ann Thorac Surg 69(4 Suppl), S197–S204.
10. Becker AE, Wilkinson JL, Anderson RH. (1979) Atrioventricular conduction tissues in univentricular hearts of left ventricular type. Herz 4, 166–175.
11. Becker AE, Anderson RH. (1981) Double inlet ventricles. In: *Pathology of Congenital Heart Disease*. London: Butterworths, pp. 241–256.
12. Becker AE, Anderson RH. (1981) Absence of an atrioventricular connection (AV valve atresia). In: *Pathology of Congenital Heart Disease*. London: Butterworths, pp. 257–278.
13. Kühne M. (1906) Uber zwei fälle kongenitaler atresie des ostium venosum dextrum. Jahrbuch fur Kinderheilkunde und Physiche Erziehung 63, 235–249.

14. Edwards JE, Burchell HB. (1949) Congenital tricuspid atresia; a classification. Med Clin North Am 33, 1177–1196.

15. Tandon R, Edwards JE. (1974) Tricuspid atresia. A reevaluation and classification. J Thorac Cardiovasc Surg 67, 530–542.

16. Pearl MJ, Permut LC, Laks H. (1996) Tricuspid atresia. In: Baue AE, Geha AS, Hammond GL, et al., eds. *Glenn's Thoracic and Cardiovascular Surgery*, 6th ed. Stamford, CO: Appleton & Lange.

17. Thien G, Daliento L, Fresura C, et al. (1981) Atresia of left atrioventricular orifice. Anatomical investigation in 62 cases. Br Heart J 45, 393.

18. Cohen MS, Jacobs ML, Weinberg PM, et al. (1996) Morphometric analysis of unbalanced common atrioventricular canal using two-dimensional echocardiography. J Am Coll Cardiol 28, 1017–1023.

19. Becker AE, Anderson RH. (1981) Atrial isomerism ("Situs Ambiguous"). *Pathology of Congenital Heart Disease*. London: Butterworths, pp. 211–224.

20. Moller JH, Nakib A, Anderson RC, et al. (1967) Congenital cardiac disease associated with polysplenia. A developmental complex of bilateral "left-sidedness". Circulation 36, 789–799.

21. Van Mierop LH, Wiglesworth FW. (1962) Isomerism of the cardiac atria in the asplenia syndrome. Lab Invest 11, 1303–1315.

22. Rubino M, Van Praagh S, Kadoba K, et al. (1995) Systemic and pulmonary venous connections in visceral heterotaxy with asplenia. Diagnostic and surgical considerations based on seventy-two autopsied cases. J Thorac Cardiovasc Surg 110, 641–650.

23. Moodie DS, Ritter DG, Tajik AJ, et al. (1984) Long-term follow-up in the unoperated univentricular heart. Am J Cardiol 53, 1124–1128.

24. Franklin RC, Spiegelhalter DJ, Anderson RH, et al. (1991) Double-inlet ventricle presenting in infancy. I. Survival without definitive repair. J Thorac Cardiovasc Surg 101, 767–776.

25. Rao PS. (1983) Further observations on the spontaneous closure of physiologically advantageous ventricular septal defects in tricuspid atresia: surgical implications. Ann Thorac Surg 35, 121–131.

26. Freedom RM, Benson LN, Smallhorn JF, et al. (1986) Subaortic stenosis, the univentricular heart, and banding of the pulmonary artery: an analysis of the courses of 43 patients with univentricular heart palliated by pulmonary artery banding. Circulation 73, 758–764.

27. Donofrio MT, Jacobs ML, Norwood WI, et al. (1995) Early changes in ventricular septal defect size and ventricular geometry in the single left ventricle after volume-unloading surgery. J Am Coll Cardiol 26, 1008–1015.

28. Dick M, Fyler DC, Nadas AS. (1975) Tricuspid atresia: clinical course in 101 patients. Am J Cardiol 36, 327–337.

29. Gaynor JW, Collins MH, Rychik J, et al. (1999) Long-term outcome of infants with single ventricle and total anomalous pulmonary venous connection. J Thorac Cardiovasc Surg 117, 506–513; discussion 513–514.

30. Blalock A, Taussig HB. (1945) The surgical treatment of malformations of the heart in which there is pulmonary stenosis or pulmonary atresia. JAMA 128, 189.

31. Muller WH Jr, Dammann JF Jr. (1952) The treatment of certain congenital malformations of the heart by the creation of pulmonic stenosis to reduce pulmonary hypertension and excessive pulmonary blood flow; a preliminary report. Surg Gynecol Obstet 95, 213–219.

32. Kirklin JW, Barratt-Boyes BG. (1993) Double inlet ventricle and atretic atrioventricular valve. *Cardiac Surgery*, 2nd ed. New York: Churchill Livingstone, pp. 1549–1580.

33. Sakakibara S, Tominaga S, Imai Y, et al. (1972) Successful total correction of common ventricle. Chest 61, 192–194.

34. Edie RN, Ellis K, Gersony WM, et al. (1973) Surgical repair of single ventricle. J Thorac Cardiovasc Surg 66, 350–360.

35. McGoon DC, Kanielson GK, Ritter DG, et al. (1977) Correction of the univentricular heart having two atrioventricular valves. J Thorac Cardiovasc Surg 74, 218–226.

36. Doty DB, Schieken RM, Lauer RM. (1979) Septation of the univentricular heart. Transatrial approach. J Thorac Cardiovasc Surg 78, 423–430.

37. Pacifico AD, Kirklin JK, Kirklin JW. (1985) Surgical management of double inlet ventricle. World J Surg 9, 579–589.

38. McKay R, Pacifico AD, Blackstone EH, et al. (1982) Septation of the univentricular heart with left anterior subaortic outlet chamber. J Thorac Cardiovasc Surg 84, 77–87.

39. Stefanelli G, Kirklin JW, Naftel DC, et al. (1984) Early and intermediate-term (10-year) results of surgery for univentricular atrioventricular connection ("single ventricle"). Am J Cardiol 54, 811–821.

40. Feldt RH, Mair DD, Danielson GK, et al. (1981) Current status of the septation procedure for univentricular heart. J Thorac Cardiovasc Surg 82, 93–97.

41. Ebert PA. (1984) Staged partitioning of single ventricle. J Thorac Cardiovasc Surg 88, 908–913.

42. Naito Y, Fujiwara K, Komai H, et al. (2001) Midterm results after ventricular septation for double-inlet left ventricle in early infancy. Ann Thorac Surg 71, 1344–1346.

43. Nomura K, Kurosawa H, Arai T. (2002) A 30-year follow-up after ventricular septation: the first and the present patient. Ann Thorac Surg 74, 1237–1238.

44. Ottenkamp J, Hazekamp MG. (2002) Double-inlet left ventricle: successfully staged ventricular septation with 12.5 years follow-up. Ann Thorac Surg 73, 699.

45. Rodbard S, Wagner D. (1949) By-passing the right ventricle. Proc Soc Exp Biol Med 71, 69.

46. Carlon CA, Mondini PG, De Marchi R. (1950) [A new vascular anastomosis for the surgical therapy of various cardiovascular defects]. G Ital Chir 6, 760–774.

47. Fenn JE, Glenn WW, Guilfoil PH, et al. (1956) Circulatory bypass of the right heart. II. Further observations on vena caval-pulmonary artery shunts. Surg Forum 6, 189–193.

48. Glenn WW. (1958) Circulatory bypass of the right side of the heart. IV. Shunt between superior vena cava and distal right pulmonary artery; report of clinical application. N Engl J Med 259, 117–120.

49. Robicsek F, Temesvari A, Kadar RL. (1956) A new method for the treatment of congenital heart disease associated with impaired pulmonary circulation; an experimental study. Acta Med Scand 154, 151–161.

50. Darbinian TM, Galankin NK. (1956) [Anastomosis between superior venoa cava and the right pulmonary artery]. Eksp Khirurgiia 1, 54–57.

51. Meshalkin EN. (1956) [Anastomosis of the upper vena cava with the pulmonary artery in patients with congenital heart disease with blood flow insufficiency in the lesser circulation]. Eksp Khirurgiia 1, 3–12.

52. Warden HE, De Wall RA, Varco RL. (1955) Use of the right auricle as a pump for the pulmonary circuit. Surg Forum 5, 16–22.

53. Kopf GS, Laks H, Stansel HC, et al. (1990) Thirty-year follow-up of superior vena cava-pulmonary artery (Glenn) shunts. J Thorac Cardiovasc Surg 100, 662–670; discussion 670–671.

54. Dogliotti AM, Actis-Dato A, Venere G, et al. (1961) [The operation of vena cava-pulmonary artery anastomosis in Fallot's tetralogy and in other heart diseases]. Minerva Cardioangiol 9, 577–593.

55. Haller JA, Jr., Adkins JC, Worthington M, et al. (1966) Experimental studies on permanent bypass of the right heart. Surgery 59, 1128–1132.

56. Azzolina G, Eufrate S, Pensa P. (1972) Tricuspid atresia: experience in surgical management with a modified cavopulmonary anastomosis. Thorax 27, 111–115.

57. Fontan F, Baudet E. (1971) Surgical repair of tricuspid atresia. Thorax 26, 240–248.

58. Starr I, Jeffers WA, Meade RH. (1943) The absence of conspicuous increments of venous pressure after severe damage to the right ventricle of the dog, with a discussion of the relation between clinical congestive heart failure and heart disease. Am Heart J 26, 291.

59. Hurwitt ES, Young D, Escher DJ. (1955) The rationale of anastomosis of the right auricular appendage to the pulmonary artery in the treatment of tricuspid atresia; application of the procedure to a case of cor triloculare. J Thorac Surg 30, 503–512.

60. Choussat A, Fontan I, Besse P, et al. (1978) Selection criteria for Fontan's procedure. In: Anderson RH, Shinebourne EA, eds. Paediatric Cardiology. Edinburgh: Churchill Livingstone.

61. Kreutzer G, Galindez E, Bono H, et al. (1973) An operation for the correction of tricuspid atresia. J Thorac Cardiovasc Surg 66, 613–621.

62. Kreutzer GO, Schlichter AJ, Kreutzer C. (2010) The Fontan/Kreutzer procedure at 40: an operation for the correction of tricuspid atresia. Semin Thorac Cardiovasc Surg Pediatr Card Surg Annu 13, 84–90.

63. Bowman FO Jr, Malm JR, Hayes CJ, et al. (1978) Physiological approach to surgery for tricuspid atresia. Circulation 58, I83–I86.

64. Björk VO, Olin CL, Bjarke BB, et al. (1979) Right atrial-right ventricular anastomosis for correction of tricuspid atresia. J Thorac Cardiovasc Surg 77, 452–458.

65. Coles JG, Leung M, Kielmanowicz S, et al. (1988) Repair of tricuspid atresia: utility of right ventricular incorporation. Ann Thorac Surg 45, 384–389.

66. Lee CN, Schaff HV, Danielson GK, et al. (1986) Comparison of atriopulmonary versus atrioventricular connections for modified Fontan/Kreutzer repair of tricuspid valve atresia. J Thorac Cardiovasc Surg 92, 1038–1043.

67. Ilbawi MN, Idriss FS, DeLeon SY, et al. (1989) When should the hypoplastic right ventricle be used in a Fontan operation? An experimental and clinical correlation. Ann Thorac Surg 47, 533–538.

68. Yacoub MH, Radley-Smith R. (1976) Use of a valved conduit from right atrium to pulmonary artery for "correction" of single ventricle. Circulation 54(6 Suppl), III63–III70.

69. DeLeon SY, Ilbawi MN, Idriss FS, et al. (1989) Direct tricuspid closure versus atrial partitioning in Fontan operation for complex lesions. Ann Thorac Surg 47, 761–764.

70. Puga FJ, Chiavarelli M, Hagler DJ. (1987) Modifications of the Fontan operation applicable to patients with left atrioventricular valve atresia or single atrioventricular valve. Circulation 76, III53–III60.

71. Kawashima Y, Kitamura S, Matsuda H, et al. (1984) Total cavopulmonary shunt operation in complex cardiac anomalies. A new operation. J Thorac Cardiovasc Surg 87, 74–81.

72. de Leval MR, Kilner P, Gewillig M, et al. (1988) Total cavopulmonary connection: a logical alternative to atriopulmonary connection for complex Fontan operations. Experimental studies and early clinical experience. J Thorac Cardiovasc Surg 96, 682–695.

73. Jonas RA, Castaneda AR. (1988) Modified Fontan procedure: atrial baffle and systemic venous to pulmonary artery anastomotic techniques. J Card Surg 3, 91–96.

74. Backer CL, Mavroudis C. (2008) Congenital heart disease. In: Norton JA, Bollinger RR, Chang AE, et al., eds. Surgery: Basic Science and Clinical Evidence. New York: Springer Verlag.

75. Marcelletti C, Corno A, Giannico S, et al. (1990) Inferior vena cava-pulmonary artery extracardiac conduit. A new form of right heart bypass. J Thorac Cardiovasc Surg 100, 228–232.

76. Mavroudis C, Deal BJ, Backer CL, et al. (1999) The favorable impact of arrhythmia surgery on total cavopulmonary artery Fontan conversion. Semin Thorac Cardiovasc Surg Pediatr Card Surg Annu 2, 143–156.

77. Burke RP, Jacobs JP, Ashraf MH, et al. (1997) Extracardiac Fontan operation without cardiopulmonary bypass. Ann Thorac Surg 63, 1175–1177.

78. Mavroudis C, Backer CL, Deal BJ. (1997) The total cavopulmonary artery Fontan connection using lateral tunnel and extracardiac techniques. Oper Tech Card Thorac Surg 2, 180–195.

79. Petrossian E, Reddy VM, Collins KK, et al. (2006) The extracardiac conduit Fontan operation using minimal approach extracorporeal circulation: early and midterm outcomes. J Thorac Cardiovasc Surg 132, 1054–1063.

80. Kirklin JK, Blackstone EH, Kirklin JW, et al. (1986) The Fontan operation. Ventricular hypertrophy, age, and date of operation as risk factors. J Thorac Cardiovasc Surg 92, 1049–1064.

81. Bridges ND, Jonas RA, Mayer JE, et al. (1990) Bidirectional cavopulmonary anastomosis as interim palliation for high-risk Fontan candidates. Early results. Circulation 82 (5 Suppl), IV170–IV176.

82. Norwood WI, Jacobs ML. (1993) Fontan's procedure in two stages. Am J Surg 166, 548–551.

83. Douglas WI, Goldberg CS, Mosca RS, *et al.* (1999) Hemi-Fontan procedure for hypoplastic left heart syndrome: outcome and suitability for Fontan. Ann Thorac Surg 68, 1361–1367; discussion 1368.

84. Laks H, Haas GS, Pearl MJ, *et al.* (1988) The use of an adjustable intraatrial communication in patients undergoing the Fontan and other definitive heart procedures. Circulation 78(suppl 2), 357 (abstr).

85. Bridges ND, Mayer JE Jr, Lock JE, *et al.* (1992) Effect of baffle fenestration on outcome of the modified Fontan operation. Circulation 86, 1762–1769.

86. Hijazi ZM, Fahey JT, Kleinman CS, *et al.* (1992) Hemodynamic evaluation before and after closure of fenestrated Fontan. An acute study of changes in oxygen delivery. Circulation 86, 196–202.

87. Mavroudis C, Zales VR, Backer CL, *et al.* (1992) Fenestrated Fontan with delayed catheter closure. Effects of volume loading and baffle fenestration on cardiac index and oxygen delivery. Circulation 86(5 Suppl), II85–II92.

88. Castaneda AR. (1992) From Glenn to Fontan. A continuing evolution. Circulation 86(5 Suppl), II80–II84.

89. Norwood WI Jr, Jacobs ML, Murphy JD. (1992) Fontan procedure for hypoplastic left heart syndrome. Ann Thorac Surg 54, 1025–1029; discussion 1029–1030.

90. Jacobs ML, Rychik J, Rome JJ, *et al.* (1996) Early reduction of the volume work of the single ventricle: the hemi-Fontan operation. Ann Thorac Surg 62, 456–461; discussion 461–462.

91. Jacobs ML, Norwood WI Jr. (1994) Fontan operation: influence of modifications on morbidity and mortality. Ann Thorac Surg 58, 945–951; discussion 951–952.

92. Jacobs ML, Rychik J, Zales VR, *et al.* (1998) Modification of the fenestrated Fontan operation: spontaneous closure of multiple small fenestrations. Proceedings of the Second World Congress of Pediatric Cardiology and Cardiac Surgery. pp. 357–359.

93. Sharma S, Goudy S, Walker P, *et al.* (1996) In vitro flow experiments for determination of optimal geometry of total cavopulmonary connection for surgical repair of children with functional single ventricle. J Am Coll Cardiol 27, 1264–1269.

94. Van Haesdonck JM, Mertens L, Sizaire R, *et al.* (1995) Comparison by computerized numeric modeling of energy losses in different Fontan connections. Circulation 92(9 Suppl), II322–II326.

95. Itatani K, Miyaji K, Tomoyasu T, *et al.* (2009) Optimal conduit size of the extracardiac Fontan operation based on energy loss and flow stagnation. Ann Thorac Surg 88, 565–572; discussion 572–573.

96. Ruiz E, Guerrero R, d'Udekem Y, *et al.* (2009) A technique of fenestration for extracardiac Fontan with long-term patency. Eur J Cardiothorac Surg 36, 200–202; discussion 202.

97. Jacobs ML, Pelletier GJ, Pourmoghadam KK, *et al.* (2008) Protocols associated with no mortality in 100 consecutive Fontan procedures. Eur J Cardiothorac Surg 33, 626–632.

98. Schreiber C, Kostolny M, Weipert J, *et al.* (2004) What was the impact of the introduction of extracardiac completion

99. for a single center performing total cavopulmonary connections? Cardiol Young 14, 140–147.

99. Cetta F, Feldt RH, O'Leary PW, *et al.* (1996) Improved early morbidity and mortality after Fontan operation: the Mayo Clinic experience, 1987 to 1992. J Am Coll Cardiol 28, 480–486.

100. Gentles TL, Mayer JE Jr, Gauvreau K, *et al.* (1997) Fontan operation in five hundred consecutive patients: factors influencing early and late outcome. J Thorac Cardiovasc Surg 114, 376–391.

101. Stamm C, Friehs I, Mayer JE Jr, *et al.* (2001) Long-term results of the lateral tunnel Fontan operation. J Thorac Cardiovasc Surg 121, 28–41.

102. Mott AR, Spray TL, Gaynor JW, *et al.* (2001) Improved early results with cavopulmonary connections. Cardiol Young 11, 3–11.

103. Mosca RS, Kulik TJ, Goldberg CS, *et al.* (2000) Early results of the Fontan procedure in one hundred consecutive patients with hypoplastic left heart syndrome. J Thorac Cardiovasc Surg 119, 1110–1118.

104. Hirsch JC, Goldberg C, Bove EL, *et al.* (2008) Fontan operation in the current era: a 15-year single institution experience. Ann Surg 248, 402–410.

105. Fontan F, Kirklin JW, Fernandez G, *et al.* (1990) Outcome after a "perfect" Fontan operation. Circulation 81, 1520–1536.

106. Ohuchi H, Yasuda K, Hasegawa S, *et al.* (2001) Influence of ventricular morphology on aerobic exercise capacity in patients after the Fontan operation. J Am Coll Cardiol 37, 1967–1974.

107. Mahle WT, Wernovsky G, Bridges ND, *et al.* (1999) Impact of early ventricular unloading on exercise performance in preadolescents with single ventricle Fontan physiology. J Am Coll Cardiol 34, 1637–1643.

108. Blaufox AD, Sleeper LA, Bradley DJ, *et al.* (2008) Functional status, heart rate, and rhythm abnormalities in 521 Fontan patients 6 to 18 years of age. J Thorac Cardiovasc Surg 136, 100–107, 7e.

109. Uzark K, Lincoln A, Lamberti JJ, *et al.* (1998) Neurodevelopmental outcomes in children with Fontan repair of functional single ventricle. Pediatrics 101, 630–633.

110. Goldberg CS, Schwartz EM, Brunberg JA, *et al.* (2000) Neurodevelopmental outcome of patients after the Fontan operation: A comparison between children with hypoplastic left heart syndrome and other functional single ventricle lesions. J Pediatr 137, 646–652.

111. Wernovsky G, Stiles KM, Gauvreau K, *et al.* (2000) Cognitive development after the Fontan operation. Circulation 102, 883–889.

112. du Plessis AJ, Chang AC, Wessel DL, *et al.* (1995) Cerebrovascular accidents following the Fontan operation. Pediatr Neurol 12, 230–236.

113. Jahangiri M, Ross DB, Redington AN, *et al.* (1994) Thromboembolism after the Fontan procedure and its modifications. Ann Thorac Surg 58, 1409–1413; discussion 1413–1414.

114. Monagle P, Cochrane A, McCrindle B, *et al.* (1998) Thromboembolic complications after fontan procedures– the role of prophylactic anticoagulation. J Thorac Cardiovasc Surg 115, 493–498.

115. Jacobs ML, Pourmoghadam KK, Geary EM, *et al.* (2002) Fontan's operation: is aspirin enough? Is coumadin too much? Ann Thorac Surg 73, 64–68.

116. Monagle P, Andrew M. (1998) Coagulation abnormalities after Fontan procedures. J Thorac Cardiovasc Surg 115, 732–733.

117. Rauch R, Ries M, Hofbeck M, *et al.* (2000) Hemostatic changes following the modified Fontan operation (total cavopulmonary connection). Thromb Haemost 83, 678–682.

118. Barker PC, Nowak C, King K, *et al.* (2005) Risk factors for cerebrovascular events following Fontan palliation in patients with a functional single ventricle. Am J Cardiol 96, 587–591.

119. Jacobs ML, Pourmoghadam KK. (2007) Thromboembolism and the role of anticoagulation in the Fontan patient. Pediatr Cardiol 28, 457–464.

120. Freedom RM, Sondheimer H, Sische R, *et al.* (1977) Development of "subaortic stenosis" after pulmonary arterial banding for common ventricle. Am J Cardiol 39, 78–83.

121. Finta KM, Beekman RH, Lupinetti FM, *et al.* (1994) Systemic ventricular outflow obstruction progresses after the Fontan operation. Ann Thorac Surg 58, 1108–1112; discussion 1112–1113.

122. Jacobs ML, Rychik J, Murphy JD, *et al.* (1995) Results of Norwood's operation for lesions other than hypoplastic left heart syndrome. J Thorac Cardiovasc Surg 110, 1555–1561; discussion 1561–1562.

123. Jacobs ML, Rychik J, Donofrio MT, *et al.* (1995) Avoidance of subaortic obstruction in staged management of single ventricle. Ann Thorac Surg 60(6 Suppl), S543–S545.

124. Jonas RA, Castaneda AR, Lang P. (1985) Single ventricle (single- or double-inlet) complicated by subaortic stenosis: surgical options in infancy. Ann Thorac Surg 39, 361–366.

125. Kopf GS. (1994) Tricuspid atresia. In: Mavroudis C, Backer CL, eds. *Pediatric Cardiac Surgery*, 2nd ed. St Louis, MO: Mosby.

126. Karl TR, Watterson KG, Sano S, *et al.* (1991) Operations for subaortic stenosis in univentricular hearts. Ann Thorac Surg 52, 420–427; discussion 427–428.

127. Lacour-Gayet F, Serraf A, Fermont L, *et al.* (1992) Early palliation of univentricular hearts with subaortic stenosis and ventriculoarterial discordance. The arterial switch option. J Thorac Cardiovasc Surg 104, 1238–1245.

128. Durongpisitkul K, Porter CJ, Cetta F, *et al.* (1998) Predictors of early- and late-onset supraventricular tachyarrhythmias after Fontan operation. Circulation 98, 1099–1107.

129. Fishberger SB, Wernovsky G, Gentles TL, *et al.* (1997) Factors that influence the development of atrial flutter after the Fontan operation. J Thorac Cardiovasc Surg 113, 80–86.

130. Paul T, Ziemer G, Luhmer L, *et al.* (1998) Early and late atrial dysrhythmias after modified Fontan operation. Pediatr Med Chir 20, 9–11.

131. Cohen MI, Bridges ND, Gaynor JW, *et al.* (2000) Modifications to the cavopulmonary anastomosis do not eliminate early sinus node dysfunction. J Thorac Cardiovasc Surg 120, 891–900.

132. Marcelletti CF, Hanley FL, Mavroudis C, *et al.* (2000) Revision of previous Fontan connections to total extracardiac cavopulmonary anastomosis: A multicenter experience. J Thorac Cardiovasc Surg 119, 340–346.

133. Mavroudis C, Backer CL, Deal BJ, *et al.* (1998) Fontan conversion to cavopulmonary connection and arrhythmia circuit cryoblation. J Thorac Cardiovasc Surg 115, 547–556.

134. Kawahira Y, Uemura H, Yagihara T, *et al.* (2001) Renewal of the Fontan circulation with concomitant surgical intervention for atrial arrhythmia. Ann Thorac Surg 71, 919–921.

135. Mavroudis C, Deal BJ, Backer CL, *et al.* (2007) J. Maxwell Chamberlain Memorial Paper for congenital heart surgery. 111 Fontan conversions with arrhythmia surgery: surgical lessons and outcomes. Ann Thorac Surg 84, 1457–1465; discussion 1465–1466.

136. Feldt RH, Driscoll DJ, Offord KP, *et al.* (1996) Protein-losing enteropathy after the Fontan operation. J Thorac Cardiovasc Surg 112, 672–680.

137. Mertens L, Hagler DJ, Sauer U, *et al.* (1998) Protein-losing enteropathy after the Fontan operation: an international multicentric study. In: Yasuharu I, Kazuo M, eds. *Proceedings of the Second World Congress of Pediatric Cardiology and Cardiac Surgery*, 2nd ed. New York: Futura Publishing Co, pp. 34–36.

138. Rychik J, Gui-Yang S. (2002) Relation of mesenteric vascular resistance after Fontan operation and protein-losing enteropathy. Am J Cardiol 90, 672–674.

139. Jacobs ML, Rychik J, Byrum CJ, *et al.* (1996) Protein-losing enteropathy after Fontan operation: resolution after baffle fenestration. Ann Thorac Surg 61, 206–208.

140. Warnes CA, Feldt RH, Hagler DJ. (1996) Protein-losing enteropathy after the Fontan operation: successful treatment by percutaneous fenestration of the atrial septum. Mayo Clin Proc 71, 378–379.

141. Cohen MI, Rhodes LA, Wernovsky G, *et al.* (2001) Atrial pacing: an alternative treatment for protein-losing enteropathy after the Fontan operation. J Thorac Cardiovasc Surg 121, 582–583.

142. Rychik J. (2010) Forty years of the Fontan operation: a failed strategy. Semin Thorac Cardiovasc Surg Pediatr Card Surg Annu 13, 96–100.

143. Van Mierop LHS, Oppenheimer-Dekker A, Bruins CLDCH, eds. (1978) *Embryology and Teratology of the Heart and the Great Arteries Conducting System; Transposition of the Great Arteries; Ductus Arteriosus*. The Hague: Leiden University Press.

CHAPTER 29

Ebstein Anomaly

Morgan L. Brown and Joseph A. Dearani

Mayo Clinic, Rochester, MN, USA

Anatomy

Dr. Wilhelm Ebstein, a young Polish physician, described the cardiac findings of a 19-year-old man who had died of cyanotic heart disease in 1866 [1]. Ebstein described the characteristic anatomical findings in this anomaly, as well as the hemodynamic abnormalities, and correctly correlated them with the patient's signs and symptoms.

Ebstein anomaly is a malformation of the tricuspid valve and right ventricle that is characterized by a spectrum of several features (Table 29.1). Ebstein anomaly is a myopathy of the right ventricle that results in variable degrees of "failure of delamination" of the tricuspid valve leaflets from the underlying endocardium. The tricuspid leaflets are usually bizarre, dysplastic, and may be muscularized. The abnormal leaflets are often tethered by shortened chordae, and papillary muscle(s) may directly insert into the leading edge of the leaflet(s). Chordae may be few to absent, and leaflet fenestrations are common. As the severity of Ebstein anomaly increases, the fibrous transformation of leaflets from their muscular precursors remains incomplete, with the septal leaflet being the most severely involved (i.e., most nondelaminated) and the anterior leaflet being the least severely involved (i.e., most delaminated, having greatest mobility). This results in a downward displacement of the hinge point (functional annulus) of the posterior and septal leaflets in a spiral fashion below the true tricuspid annulus. There are varying degrees of delamination of all three leaflets, resulting in infinite variability from one patient to another. Although the anterior leaflet is most likely to have the greatest degree of delamination, it can also be severely deformed so that the only mobile leaflet tissue is displaced toward the right ventricular outflow tract. The malformed tricuspid valve is usually incompetent and rarely stenotic.

The atrialized right ventricle can vary in its thickness and in its ability to contract. Infrequently, it can have near normal thickness and show evidence of contraction by echocardiography or magnetic resonance imaging (MRI). More often, it is thinned, dyskinetic, and dilated. In general, the entire free wall of the right ventricle, both proximal and distal to the abnormal insertion of the tricuspid leaflets, including the infundibulum, is also dilated. Dilatation of the right ventricular free wall is associated not only with thinning of the wall, but also with an absolute decrease in the number of myocardial fibers [2]. The atrioventricular node is located at the apex of the triangle of Koch, and the conduction system is in its normal position. Atrial septal defect (ASD) is the most common associated anomaly and other cardiac defects (e.g., ventricular septal defect, patent ductus arteriosus, or pulmonary stenosis) anomalies may also be present.

In those congenital cardiac anomalies in which there is situs solitus and atrioventricular discordance with ventriculoarterial discordance (corrected transposition), Ebstein anomaly of the left-sided (systemic, morphologically tricuspid) atrioventricular valve may be present. The remainder of this chapter focuses on the classic right-sided Ebstein anomaly.

Physiology

Forward flow of blood through the right side of the heart is retarded because of the functional impairment of the right ventricle and the incompetence of the deformed tricuspid valve. Moreover, during contraction of the right atrium, the atrialized portion of the right ventricle that is in continuity with the right atrium, distends or acts as a passive reservoir, thus decreasing the volume of right ventricular blood ejected. During ventricular systole, the atrialized right ventricle contracts, creating a pressure wave that impedes venous filling of the right atrium, which is in the diastolic phase. In the majority of cases, there is a communication between the left and right atria, either because of

Pediatric Cardiac Surgery, Fourth Edition. Edited by Constantine Mavroudis and Carl L. Backer.
© 2013 Blackwell Publishing Ltd. Published 2013 by Blackwell Publishing Ltd.

patency of the foramen ovale or a distinct secundum ASD. The shunt of blood through the septal opening is generally from right to left but may be bidirectional. The overall effect of these structural abnormalities on the right atrium is to produce gross dilatation, which may reach enormous proportions, even in infancy. This dilatation leads to further incompetence of the tricuspid valve and further widening of the interatrial communication.

As a consequence of atrial dilatation, atrial tachyarrhythmias are common. In addition, approximately 15% of patients will have one or more accessory conduction pathways associated with Wolff-Parkinson-White syndrome, and 1–2% of patients will have atrioventricular nodal reentrant tachycardia (AVNRT) [3,4]. In end-stage heart failure, ventricular arrhythmias may be present.

Table 29.1 Anatomical features of the spectrum of Ebstein anomaly.

Adherence of the tricuspid leaflets to the underlying myocardium (failure of delamination)

Downward (apical) displacement of the functional annulus (septal > posterior > anterior)

Dilation of the "atrialized" portion of the right ventricle with variable degrees of hypertrophy and thinning of the wall

Redundancy, fenestrations, and tethering of the anterior leaflet

Dilation of the right atrioventricular junction (true tricuspid annulus)

The Neonate

Presentation and Diagnosis

In the newborn period, any degree of tricuspid regurgitation is accentuated by the normally occurring elevated pulmonary arteriolar resistance. As a result, neonates with Ebstein anomaly may develop severe right-sided heart failure and cyanosis. Severe tricuspid regurgitation results in elevated right atrial pressures and may result in profound right-to-left atrial shunt across the patent foramen ovale. Low cardiac output may also result from paradoxical motion of the septum or malposition of the interventricular septum because of the enlarged right ventricle. If the neonate survives this critical period, the degree of cyanosis and of heart failure may diminish as fetal pulmonary hypertension regresses.

In the neonatal period, decreasing pulmonary vascular resistance with pulmonary vasodilators may be helpful to unload the right ventricle, promote antegrade blood flow into the lungs, and improve right ventricular function. In some cases, a large patent ductus arteriosus may allow a circular shunt, where blood flows from the aorta into the patent ductus arteriosus, to the right ventricle, to the right atrium, to the left atrium, and then to the left ventricle [5]. If this circular shunt occurs, administration of prostaglandins should be stopped to allow ductal closure.

Chest X-ray typically demonstrates profound cardiomegaly (Figure 29.1). Echocardiography remains the standard for establishing the diagnosis. The tricuspid valve should

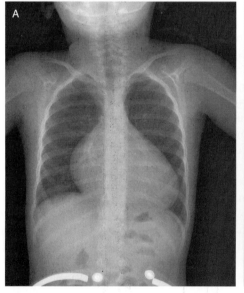 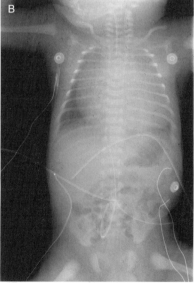

Figure 29.1 These two chest films demonstrate the characteristic cardiac silhouette in Ebstein anomaly and the extreme cardiac enlargement. **A,** Child age 4 years. This child had oxygen saturations between 50% and 90%, headaches, and episodes of supraventricular tachycardia. **B,** Neonate on the first day of life. This baby required immediate intubation, nitric oxide, and prostaglandin infusion to maintain adequate oxygenation.

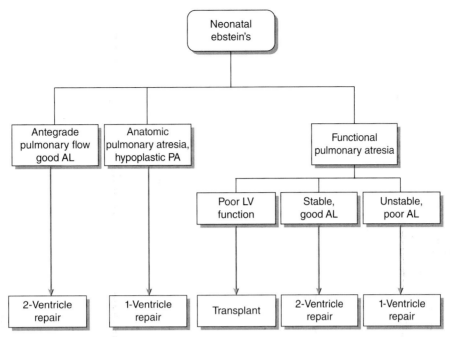

Figure 29.2 This simplified algorithm provides a guideline for decision-making with the symptomatic neonate with Ebstein anomaly. A good anterior leaflet for potential monocusp repair is large, sail-like, and mobile. (AL, anterior leaflet; LV, left ventricle; PA, pulmonary arteries.) (Reproduced with permission from Knott-Craig *et al.* [11].)

be thoroughly assessed, and the Great Ormond Street Ebstein Score (GOSE score) calculated [6]. The GOSE score, as described by Celermajer, is calculated in the four-chamber view to create a ratio of the combined areas of the right atrium and atrialized right ventricle compared to the functional right ventricle, left atrial, and the left ventricular areas.

It is important that the right ventricular outflow tract be completely visualized to ascertain whether there is "anatomic" or "functional" pulmonary atresia. Functional pulmonary atresia refers to a setting of severe tricuspid regurgitation and right ventricular dysfunction, with reduced or absent antegrade blood flow across a normal anatomic pulmonary valve. Any degree of anatomic right ventricular outflow tract obstruction (RVOTO; infundibulum, pulmonary valve, or branch pulmonary arteries) is a risk factor for both early and late mortality [7]. Differentiating functional from anatomic pulmonary atresia in the neonatal period may be difficult, and the administration of nitric oxide or sildenafil at the time of echocardiography may be useful to decrease pulmonary vascular resistance, allowing forward blood flow into the lungs in cases of functional pulmonary atresia.

Indications for Surgery

In neonates or infants who remain in congestive heart failure or profoundly cyanotic with appropriate medical therapy, surgery is required. Asymptomatic neonates who

have a GOSE score of 3 or 4 or symptomatic neonates with a GOSE score of 3 or 4, mild cyanosis, a cardiothoracic ratio of more than 0.80, or severe tricuspid regurgitation are other indications for surgery [8]. There are three potential treatment pathways that can be considered in the neonate: the biventricular repair (Knott-Craig approach), single ventricle repair (i.e., right ventricular exclusion technique [Starnes approach]), or cardiac transplantation (Figure 29.2) [9–11].

Surgical Strategies

One approach to repair of neonatal or infant Ebstein anomaly is the biventricular strategy that has been described by Knott-Craig [8,10–12]. In this method, there is subtotal closure of the ASD and repair of the tricuspid valve. Multiple tricuspid valve repair methods have been described to improve the chance of successful valve competency, but they depend on having a mobilizable anterior leaflet. The Knott-Craig technique is generally a monocusp repair based on a satisfactory anterior leaflet (Figure 29.3) [12]. The incomplete closure of the ASD allows for right-to-left shunting that may be helpful in the early postoperative period when there is high risk of right ventricular dysfunction and elevated pulmonary vascular resistance. In order to reduce the heart size and allow for lung development, generous right atrial reduction is performed routinely.

Starnes has pioneered the right ventricular exclusion approach. In this univentricular strategy, the tricuspid

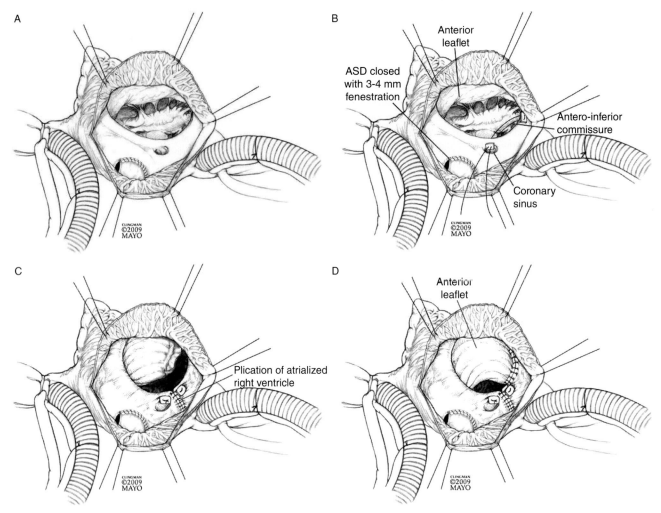

Figure 29.3 A, In the biventricular Knott-Craig repair [12], the tricuspid valve is repaired creating a monocusp valve. If the anterior leaflet leading edge is fused to the free wall of the right ventricle, it must be delaminated to allow for free movement of the anterior leaflet. A pledgeted suture may be placed through the dominant papillary muscle of the anterior leaflet and brought to the interventricular septum at the site of the laminated septal leaflet (Sebening stitch). This maneuver will maintain apposition of the free wall of the right ventricle and the anterior leaflet to the posterior aspect of the tricuspid annulus and may provide durability to the repair (not shown). **B,** When the annulus is very dilated (>20 mm), a pledgeted suture is placed at the antero-inferior commissure through the medial wall of the coronary sinus. This will reduce the size of the tricuspid valve annulus. **C,** The tricuspid valve orifice is reduced in size and the anterior leaflet is detached from its annulus. **D,** The anterior leaflet is rotated clockwise and reattached to create a monocusp repair. Plication of the atrialized right ventricle completes the tricuspid valve repair. A functional orifice of approximately 13 mm is generally considered adequate. The atrial septal defect has been subtotally closed, leaving a 3 mm residual defect or fenestration. (Copyright © 2009 Mayo Foundation for Medical Education and Research.)

valve orifice is patched closed, the interatrial communication is enlarged, and a systemic-to-pulmonary artery shunt is placed [13–16]. This approach is particularly appealing in those patients who have anatomic RVOTO or an abnormal anterior leaflet that would preclude a successful valve repair. Right ventricular decompression of thebesian venous drainage is facilitated by placing a small fenestration (4–5 mm punch) in the tricuspid valve patch (Figure 29.4) [15]. This also allows progressive involution of the enlarged, dysfunctional right ventricle, which is helpful in the long term while preparing for the eventual Fontan procedure. In patients who have a patent right ventricular outflow tract, a competent pulmonary valve is required to prevent blood from entering the right ventricle, resulting in distension. If an incompetent pulmonary valve is present, the main pulmonary artery should be ligated or oversewn. These maneuvers are important to avoid persistent dilatation of a poorly functioning right ventricle that can com-

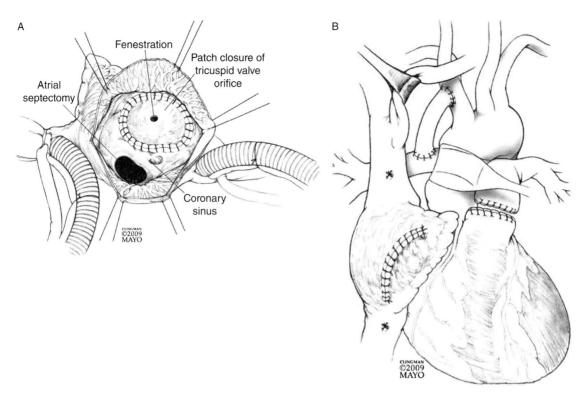

Figure 29.4 A, In the Starnes approach to neonatal Ebstein anomaly [15], fixed autologous pericardium is sewn to the anatomic annulus (at the atrioventricular groove) using a running suture. Careful examination of the surface of the right ventricular myocardium is needed to ensure no distortion of the right coronary artery. A 4-mm fenestration of the patch is performed, which allows for decompression of the right ventricle. **B,** If the pulmonary valve is competent, the pulmonary artery is divided and the valve is oversewn. If the pulmonary artery is small, a single hemoclip may be applied. Pulmonary blood flow is provided by a systemic to pulmonary artery shunt. In this illustration, a 3.5-mm Gore-Tex shunt connects the innominate artery to the right pulmonary artery. (Copyright © 2009 Mayo Foundation for Medical Education and Research.)

promise and impair left (systemic) ventricular function in the eventual Fontan circulation. Right atrial reduction is also routinely performed to allow space for the lung development.

Sano proposed a modification to the Starnes single ventricle approach. Total right ventricular exclusion is performed in which the free wall of the right ventricle is resected and closed primarily or with a polytetrafluoroethylene patch [17]. This procedure acts like a large right ventricular plication. This adaptation of the Starnes method may improve left ventricular filling, as well as provide decompression to the lungs and left ventricle.

In the most severe cases of Ebstein anomaly, heart transplantation remains an option, but is rarely necessary in the current era given the improved early results with the Knott-Craig and Starnes approaches. Limitations of heart transplantation include the scarcity of donor organs in the neonatal age group and the adverse effects of long-term immunosuppression and its associated complications in the transplant recipient. Finally, the development of smaller ventricular assist devices and advances in extracorporeal membrane oxygenation have provided mechanical support options in the perioperative period for the management of these challenging infants [18–20].

Children and Adults

Presentation and Diagnosis

In children, symptoms include fatigue, decreased exercise tolerance, dyspnea on exertion, and cyanosis. Palpitations because of paroxysmal atrial arrhythmias and premature ventricular beats are common and increase with age. A systolic murmur of tricuspid regurgitation may be heard along the left sternal border or may be absent. Low-intensity diastolic and presystolic murmurs, which result from anatomical or functional tricuspid stenosis (occurs rarely), may be present. There is wide splitting of both the first and second heart sounds. Atrial and ventricular filling sounds are relatively common and contribute to the cadence quality that is so often found in patients with Ebstein anomaly. The arterial and jugular venous pulse forms are usually normal. A large V wave may be seen in the jugular venous pulse. The liver may be palpably enlarged, but ascites and peripheral edema are generally not common; when present, advanced right-sided heart failure is present.

The electrocardiogram is usually abnormal, but it is not diagnostic. Complete or incomplete right bundle branch block and right-axis deviation are typically present; atrial arrhythmias are common, particularly in older patients. On chest X-ray, the cardiac silhouette may vary from almost normal to the typical Ebstein configuration, which consists of a globular-shaped heart with a narrow waist (pedicle), similar to that seen with pericardial effusion. This appearance is produced by enlargement of the right atrium and displacement of the right ventricular outflow tract outward and upward. Vascularity of the pulmonary fields is either normal or decreased.

Echocardiography allows an accurate evaluation of the tricuspid leaflets and its subvalvar apparatus, the right atrium, the atrialized portion of the right ventricle, and the right and left ventricles (Table 29.2). Doppler echocardiography and color-flow imaging allow detection of an ASD and the direction of shunt flow. The principle echocardiographic characteristic that differentiates Ebstein anomaly from other forms of congenital tricuspid regurgitation is the degree of apical displacement of the septal leaflet at the crux of the heart ($\geq 0.8\,cm/m^2$; Plate 29.1, see plate section opposite p. 594) [21]. Other features that are usually present are fibrous and/or muscular attachments between the body of the tricuspid leaflet(s) and the underlying myocardium (i.e., failure of delamination). The most useful view for the surgeon is the four-chamber view. This outlines the degree of delamination (amount of attachments between the annulus and apex) of the anterior, inferior (to a lesser

degree), and septal leaflets and indicates mobility of the leading edges. Echocardiographic factors that are favorable for valve repair include a large, mobile anterior leaflet with few free wall attachments and a free leading edge. Significant adherence of the edge or body of the leaflet to underlying endocardium (i.e., leaflet tethering) and tricuspid valve leaflet tissue present in the right ventricular outflow tract make successful valve repair more difficult. Any delamination of inferior leaflet tissue is helpful, and the more septal leaflet tissue present, the more likely a successful valve repair (especially a cone-type repair) can be realized. More recently, we have been using three-dimensional echocardiography to help delineate anatomic details of the abnormal tricuspid valve leaflets and the subvalvar apparatus. Further experience is required to determine the role of three-dimensional echocardiography in Ebstein anomaly.

MRI is being increasingly used in all types of patients with cardiac disease, including those with Ebstein anomaly. Quantitative assessment can be made of left and right ventricular size and function. Notably, however, there is little information available in the literature to guide therapy on the basis of this new imaging modality. We routinely perform MRI examination preoperatively and postoperatively to evaluate right ventricular size and function and also so that we can better understand what the other potential roles of MRI are in the evaluation of patients with Ebstein anomaly. At the present time, we prefer echocardiography for evaluation of tricuspid valve anatomy and MRI examination for assessment of right (and left) ventricular size and function.

Table 29.2 Echocardiographic information required by a surgeon. (AV, atrioventricular; RVOT, right ventricular outflow tract; RVOTO, right ventricular outflow tract obstruction.)

Echocardiographic variable	Description
Tricuspid valve regurgitation	Degree of tricuspid regurgitation Number of jets; location in relation to AV groove, and RVOT
Tricuspid valve leaflet anatomy	Degree of delamination – sites of adherence from AV groove to apex Fenestrations Status of leaflet edges and presence of linear attachment How much septal leaflet Unsupported segments
Tricuspid valve annulus dilatation	Size of annulus
Right ventricle and atrialized right ventricle	Size and function
Ventricular septum	Function, position, and motion
Left ventricular function	Size, function, and shape (D-shaped)
Right atrium	Size
Atrial septum	Presence of atrial septal defects and the shunt direction
Other cardiac anatomy	Rule out presence of RVOTO and left-sided valvular disease

In general, satisfactory anatomical and functional information can be obtained by echocardiography and MRI so that cardiac catheterization and angiography are usually not necessary. Hemodynamic catheterization may be occasionally required when there is left ventricular dysfunction in order to measure left- and right-sided pressures, especially if a bidirectional cavopulmonary shunt is being considered (see One-and-a-half ventricle approach), or in the case of a single ventricle pathway, before the modified Fontan procedure is performed.

Atrial and ventricular arrhythmias are common in patients with Ebstein anomaly; they often present therapeutic challenges and may experience sudden death, a common mode of late mortality. Twenty-four-hour ambulatory electrocardiographic monitoring is suggested for rhythm assessment in patients with palpitations or tachycardia. Invasive electrophysiologic study is performed for all patients with Ebstein anomaly who have pre-excitation on their electrocardiogram or who have a history of recurrent supraventricular tachycardia, undefined wide-complex tachycardia, or syncope as aspects of their clinical presentation [3,4].

Indications for Surgery

Although medical management, including diuretics and antiarrhythmic drugs, may be used to manage some of the symptoms of heart failure and arrhythmias, most patients eventually require surgery. Observation alone may be considered for asymptomatic patients with no right-to-left shunting, mild cardiomegaly, and normal exercise tolerance. Many patients in New York Heart Association (NYHA) classes I and II can be managed medically. Surgery is offered when symptoms or cyanosis are present, decreased exercise tolerance is noted on formal exercise testing, or if paradoxical embolism occurs. Surgery is also advised if there is progressive increase in heart size on chest X-ray, progressive right ventricular dilatation or reduction of systolic function by echocardiography, or appearance of atrial or ventricular arrhythmias. In borderline situations, the echocardiographic determination of high probability of tricuspid valve repair makes the decision to proceed with earlier surgery easier. When anatomy is appropriate for a cone repair, we are now advising surgery between 2 and 5 years of age, particularly when any degree of right ventricular dilatation is present. Once symptoms develop and patients progress to NYHA class III or IV, medical management has little to offer; surgery then becomes the only chance for improvement.

Surgical Strategies

A biventricular repair is possible for the vast majority of patients beyond the period of infancy. In some circumstances, a one-and-a-half ventricle (addition of a bidirectional cavopulmonary shunt) is advantageous when there is significant right ventricular dilatation or dysfunction, a leftward shift of the interventricular septum, or cyanosis. In addition, the bidirectional cavopulmonary shunt is helpful if the resultant tricuspid valve repair has a small effective orifice. Finally, the bidirectional cavopulmonary shunt may also reduce hemodynamic stress on a more complex (multiple suture lines) tricuspid valve repair, as the volume of the right ventricle can be reduced by 35–45%, depending on the patient's age. Cardiac transplantation is rarely indicated and is reserved for patients with severe biventricular dysfunction.

Our surgical management of patients with Ebstein anomaly consists of 1) closure of any atrial septal communications; 2) reconstruction of the tricuspid valve using the cone technique; 3) bioprosthetic tricuspid valve replacement when the valve cannot be successfully repaired; 4) selective plication of the atrialized right ventricle; 5) performance of any indicated antiarrhythmic procedures; 6) right reduction atrioplasty; 7) correction of associated anomalies; and 8) selective application of the bidirectional cavopulmonary shunt. Intraoperative transesophageal echocardiography is used in all cases.

Tricuspid Valve Repair

Reconstruction of the deformed tricuspid valve began in 1958 when Hunter and Lillehei attempted to create a competent valve by repositioning the displaced posterior and septal leaflets [22]. Although some good results have been reported with other early attempts at tricuspid valve repair [23,24], it has not been generally effective in establishing a competent valve in the moderate and severe forms of Ebstein anomaly, and heart block may be more frequent.

In 1972, David Danielson at the Mayo Clinic developed a repair based on the construction of a monocuspid valve by the use of the anterior leaflet of the tricuspid valve, which is usually enlarged in this anomaly; competency is obtained by coaptation of the anterior leaflet with the ventricular septum [25,26]. This repair also included posterior tricuspid annuloplasty; plication of the free wall of the atrialized right ventricle, bringing the functional tricuspid annulus up to the true annulus; and excision of redundant right atrial wall (right reduction atrioplasty). Although the basic principles of this original repair remain the same, we had subsequently incorporated various modifications in the repair because numerous anatomical variants of the anomaly have been encountered. One such modification is to repair the valve where it exists in the right ventricle (i.e., repairing the valve at the level of the displaced functional annulus) by bringing the papillary muscle(s), which are attached to the right ventricular free wall down to the ventricular septum, anchoring it with pledgeted sutures.

More recently, we have been using the cone reconstruction as described by da Silva and colleagues [27]. This technique is different from all previous valvuloplasty techniques in that it is closest to an "anatomic repair" (Figure 29.5) [28].

A

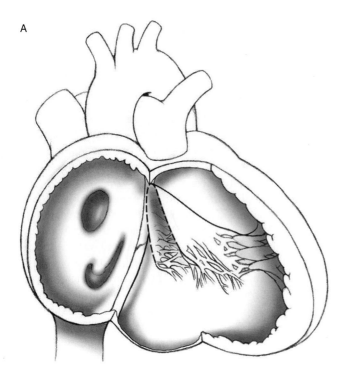
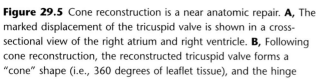

B

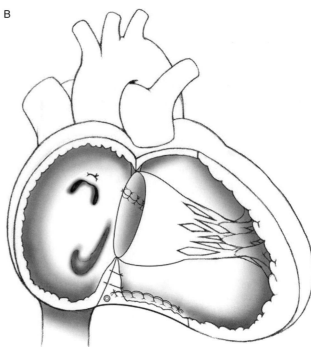

Figure 29.5 Cone reconstruction is a near anatomic repair. **A,** The marked displacement of the tricuspid valve is shown in a cross-sectional view of the right atrium and right ventricle. **B,** Following cone reconstruction, the reconstructed tricuspid valve forms a "cone" shape (i.e., 360 degrees of leaflet tissue), and the hinge point has been moved to the true tricuspid annulus. The atrialized right ventricle and true tricuspid valve annulus have been plicated to reduce the size of the tricuspid valve annulus. (Reproduced with permission from Dearani *et al.* [28]. Copyright © 2008 Mayo Foundation for Medical Education and Research.)

The end result of the cone reconstruction includes 360 degrees of tricuspid leaflet tissue surrounding the right atrioventricular junction. This allows leaflet tissue to coapt with leaflet tissue, similar to what occurs with normal tricuspid valve anatomy. In addition, the reconstructed tricuspid valve is reattached at the true tricuspid valve annulus (atrioventricular junction) so that the hinge point of the valve is now in a normal anatomical location. Thinned, transparent atrialized right ventricle is plicated so that any areas of right ventricular dyskinesis are eliminated. Right ventricular plication also helps reduce the size of the enlarged right ventricle, and it decreases tension on the numerous sutures required for the cone reconstruction. When somatic growth is complete, the final tricuspid repair is reinforced with a flexible annuloplasty band. Redundant right atrium is excised so the size of the right atrium is closer to normal. Since this technique can be applied to the wider variety of anatomical variations encountered with Ebstein anomaly, we have adopted this repair technique and have reported the details of the surgery (Figure 29.6) [28].

Relative contraindications to the cone reconstruction include the neonate, older age (>50 years), moderate pulmonary hypertension, significant left ventricular dysfunction (ejection fraction <30%), complete failure of delamination of septal and inferior leaflets with poor delamination of the anterior leaflet (i.e., <50% delamination of the anterior leaflet), severe right ventricular enlargement, and severe dilatation of the true tricuspid annulus (right atrioventricular junction).

Many others have reported their techniques and results of tricuspid repair for Ebstein anomaly in older children and adults, including Carpentier, Hetzer, Wu, Chen, and Quaegebeur [29–38]. Thus, tricuspid valve repair techniques continue to evolve to address the infinite anatomic variations present with this anomaly. Although each of the many described techniques provide value to the surgeon who is confronted with this anomaly, it is our belief that the cone reconstruction provides the most anatomic reconstruction and is preferred when the anatomy allows.

Tricuspid Valve Replacement

Prosthetic tricuspid valve replacement remains a good alternative for the treatment of Ebstein anomaly when valve repair is not feasible. Bioprosthetic (porcine) valve replacement, as opposed to mechanical valve replacement, is generally preferred because of relatively good durability of the porcine bioprosthesis in the tricuspid position and the lack of need for warfarin anticoagulation. While bioprosthetic valves do not have the thromboembolic complications of mechanical valves, they do have a limited

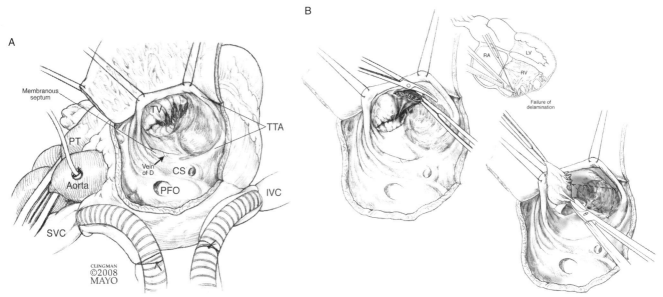

Figure 29.6 Cone reconstruction technique. **A,** Standard aortic cannulation and bicaval cannulation is performed. A right atriotomy is performed, parallel to the atrioventricular groove. Valve exposure is facilitated by stay sutures. The tricuspid valve anatomy is examined, and the atrialized right ventricle evaluated. The membranous septum and atrioventricular node are marked by a small vein (vein of D); fatty tissue is generally present in this area. **B,** The first incision is made in the anterior leaflet at 12:00; the incision is a few millimeters away from the true annulus. Using scissors, the incision is extended in a clockwise fashion, and it is common for there to be a true space between the anterior leaflet and the right ventricle in this region (i.e., a normally delaminated leaflet). It is also common for the anterior leaflet to be muscularized in this area adjacent to the annulus and for there to be degrees of failure of delamination (inset) of the medial aspect of the anterior leaflet and even more of failure of delamination of the inferior leaflet. Takedown of these fibrous and muscular attachments between the body of the leaflet(s) and the free wall of the right ventricle is called a *surgical delamination*. It is important for the surgical delamination process to include takedown of all attachments between the atrioventricular groove and leading edge of the leaflet(s), which is often close to the apex of the right ventricle. Care must be taken to keep all fibrous and occasionally muscular attachments of the leading edge of the leaflet(s) to the myocardium intact. The dotted triangle represents the atrialized right ventricle, which will be later plicated. **C,** The anterior leaflet should be examined to determine whether there are individual chordal attachments present, direct papillary muscle insertions into the leading edge, or whether the leading edge is attached directly (linear) to the myocardium. When a linear attachment is present (inset), fenestrations should be created in the distal aspect of the leaflet to create *neochordae*. This allows blood to enter the right ventricular cavity. Care must be taken not to injure the underlying thinned right ventricular myocardium when the surgical delamination process is being performed. **D,** To complete the cone reconstruction, after all tricuspid valve leaflets (anterior, septal, and inferior) are mobilized, the inferior leaflet (or most medial aspect of the anterior leaflet if no inferior leaflet is present) is rotated clockwise to meet the mobilized proximal edge of the septal leaflet. These two leaflets are approximated with interrupted fine monofilament sutures. This neotricuspid valve orifice is composed of 360 degrees of native tricuspid valve tissue. The more septal leaflet that is present, the easier and more successful this entire process is. Before reattachment of the neotricuspid valve to the true annulus, the atrialized right ventricle is examined and plicated as needed. **E,** To obliterate noncontractile, thinned portions of the atrialized right ventricle, an internal apex-to-base triangular plication of the atrialized right ventricle may be employed. We believe plication helps reduce tension on repair sutures at the level of the true annulus, helps reduce annular size, and eliminates paradoxical motion of the enlarged right ventricle. Monofilament 4-0 or 5-0 is started close to the apex of the right ventricle. This plication suture line is partial thickness and predominantly incorporates the endocardium. As the plication proceeds toward the atrioventricular groove (the base of the "triangular" plication), it is important to inspect and be sure that there is no compromise of the right coronary artery. **F,** The neotricuspid valve is reanchored at the true annulus. It is now our practice to reattach the septal leaflet to the ventricular septum just proximal (i.e., on the ventricular side of the true annulus) to the area of the conduction tissue and membranous septum. In older children and adults, the repair is completed with a flexible annuloplasty band to reinforce the neotricuspid valve annular reconstruction. We reinforce each end of the annuloplasty band with a mattress suture backed with felt pledgets; the inferior suture typically incorporates the orifice of the coronary sinus. This is particularly important when there has been a significant reduction in the size of the true annulus during the course of the neotricuspid valve reconstruction. (CS, coronary sinus; IVC, inferior vena cava; LV, left ventricle; PFO, patent foramen ovale; PT, pulmonary trunk; RA, right atrium; RV, right ventricle; SVC superior vena cava; TTA, true tricuspid valve annulus.) (Reproduced with permission from Dearani *et al.* [28]. Copyright © 2008 Mayo Foundation for Medical Education and Research.)

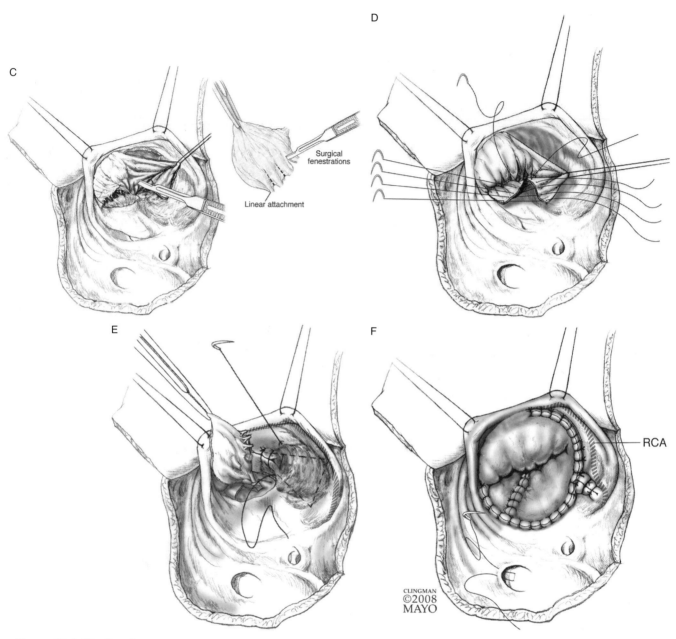

Figure 29.6 (*Continued*)

durability, particularly in infants and young children. Bioprosthetic valves are also undesirable in the small patient, because reoperation may be required for replacement of the valve because of somatic growth as well as structural valve deterioration. Mechanical valves in the tricuspid position may be associated with a higher frequency of valve malfunction and thrombotic complications than mechanical valves in other cardiac positions [39], particularly when right ventricular function is poor.

When the tricuspid valve cannot be reconstructed and replacement is necessary, valve leaflet tissue toward the right ventricular outflow tract (which can cause RVOTO) is excised and the prosthetic valve (usually a porcine bioprosthesis) is inserted. It is important to anchor the prosthesis in the right atrium, opposed to the atrioventricular groove. The suture line is deviated to the atrial side of the atrioventricular node and membranous septum to avoid injury to the conduction mechanism (Figure 29.7) [40]. A small vein (vein of D) crossing the tricuspid annulus adjacent to the membranous septum typically marks the atrioventricular node. The coronary sinus can be left to drain into the right atrium if there is sufficient room between it

A

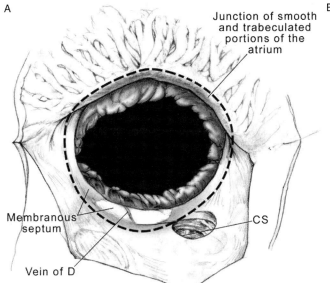

Junction of smooth and trabeculated portions of the atrium

Membranous septum

CS

Vein of D

B

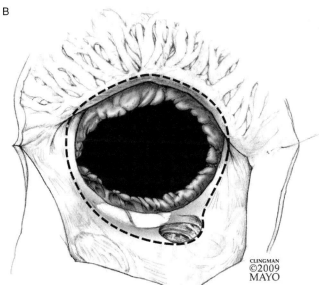

CLINGMAN
©2009
MAYO

Figure 29.7 Diagram of technique for tricuspid valve replacement in Ebstein anomaly. The valve suture line is placed on the atrial side of the membranous septum and atrioventricular node to avoid injury to the conduction system. The suture line is also deviated cephalad to the tricuspid annulus posterolaterally when the tissues are thin to avoid injury to the right coronary artery. This results in the prosthesis being mounted in an intra-atrial position. **A,** When there is sufficient distance between the coronary sinus and the atrioventricular node, the coronary sinus is left draining normally into the right atrium. **B,** If the coronary sinus and the conduction tissue are in close proximity, the suture line is deviated further into the right atrium, leaving the coronary sinus to drain into the right ventricle. The sutures are tied with the heart perfused and beating to ensure that normal atrioventricular conduction is preserved. (CS, coronary sinus.) (Reproduced with permission from Dearani *et al.* [40]. Copyright © 2009 Mayo Foundation for Medical Education and Research.)

and the atrioventricular node; if the distance is short, the coronary sinus can be left to drain into the right ventricle so that heart block can be avoided. To avoid injury to the right coronary artery, the suture line is deviated toward the atrial side of the tricuspid valve annulus anteriorly and inferiorly where the smooth and trabeculated portions of the atrium meet each other. The struts of the porcine bioprosthesis are oriented so that they straddle the area of the membranous septum and conduction tissue. The valve sutures are tied with the heart beating (after intracardiac communications are closed) to detect any disturbances in atrioventricular conduction.

In our experience of more than 800 operations for Ebstein anomaly, we make every effort to repair rather than replace the tricuspid valve. Although our experience has demonstrated excellent durability of porcine bioprostheses in older children and adults [7,41], others have shown poor durability of bioprostheses in young patients (Figure 29.8) [7,42,43]. This decreased durability in young children is related to both increased calcification and rapid somatic growth, which results in patient prosthesis mismatch. In young children, we accept repairs that reduce the degree of tricuspid regurgitation to a moderate degree to avoid tricuspid valve replacement. In our experience, tricuspid

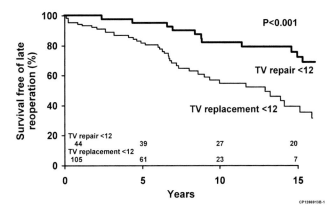

Figure 29.8 Patients less than 12 years of age were stratified into patients who had tricuspid valve repair or replacement. This cutoff was chosen because an adult-sized tricuspid valve prosthesis can generally be inserted into a 12-year-old patient with Ebstein anomaly. There was a significant advantage for young patients (<12 years) who had a tricuspid valve repair versus tricuspid valve replacement ($p < 0.001$). We prefer tricuspid valve repair whenever possible in all young patients with Ebstein anomaly. (Reproduced with permission from Brown *et al.* [7].)

bioprostheses in patients with Ebstein anomaly have greater durability in both pediatric and adult populations compared to bioprostheses in other cardiac positions and even when compared with bioprosthetic tricuspid valve replacement for other cardiac diagnoses [41]. We speculate that this favorable experience may be related to the large size of the bioprosthesis that can be implanted relative to patient somatic size and to the normal, low right ventricular systolic pressure after repair in patients with Ebstein anomaly. Both of these factors would tend to reduce turbulence and stress on the bioprosthesis. For this reason, in older adult patients (>50 years of age), we believe that a successful, durable tricuspid valve repair should have less than moderate tricuspid regurgitation; if this cannot be obtained, then we proceed with bioprosthetic replacement. For adult patients who are taking warfarin anticoagulation for other reasons and who want to potentially minimize the need for a subsequent reoperation for bioprosthetic deterioration, a mechanical valve can be considered. Mechanical valves should generally be avoided when there is significant right ventricular dysfunction since the discs may not open and close properly, resulting in a greater propensity for valve thrombosis even in the presence of therapeutic warfarin anticoagulation.

One-and-a-Half Ventricle Repair

The bidirectional cavopulmonary shunt is used selectively and more frequently in the current era. The bidirectional cavopulmonary shunt is helpful when the right ventricle is severely dilated or dysfunctional or if there is displacement of the interventricular septum toward the left ventricle (D-shaped left ventricle) [44]. This may also be advisable if there is preoperative arterial desaturation at rest or with exercise that suggests poor right ventricular function. Finally, a right-to-left atrial pressure ratio greater than 1.5 after separation from cardiopulmonary bypass also indicates poor right ventricular function and can be used as a guide for placement of a bidirectional cavopulmonary shunt [45]. The construction of a bidirectional cavopulmonary shunt may allow for less-than-perfect tricuspid valve repairs or more complex tricuspid valve repairs, since it will decrease the volume of blood traveling through the right ventricle and stress on the repair suture lines. The bidirectional cavopulmonary shunt should also be used if a tricuspid valve repair has resulted in an effective valve orifice that has mild to moderate stenosis (mean gradient >6–7 mmHg) or in more complex repairs with multiple suture lines. Finally, patients who receive a bidirectional cavopulmonary shunt may tolerate longer intervals between repeat tricuspid valve operations for progressive tricuspid regurgitation or failing tricuspid valve prostheses.

Since concomitant left ventricular dysfunction may be present when there is significant right ventricular dilata-tion and/or dysfunction, it is important to document by direct pressure measurements that the pulmonary arterial and left atrial pressures are low (which is usually the case); otherwise, the bidirectional cavopulmonary shunt will not be feasible. If the left ventricular end-diastolic pressure is less than 15 mmHg, the transpulmonary gradient is less than 10 mmHg, and the mean pulmonary arterial pressure is less than 18–20 mmHg, a bidirectional cavopulmonary shunt is permissible. Even in the presence of moderate left ventricular dysfunction (ejection fraction, 35–40%) it is usually feasible to perform a bidirectional cavopulmonary shunt in the setting of Ebstein anomaly. If the tricuspid valve requires replacement, the prosthesis should be down-sized, since the amount of flow across the tricuspid orifice is reduced.

Chauvaud [30,31], Marianeschi [46], and Quiñonez [44] have proposed that the use of a bidirectional cavopulmonary shunt may decrease operative mortality and facilitate the postoperative management of patients with severe right ventricular dysfunction. The literature suggests that the frequency of bidirectional cavopulmonary shunt application in Ebstein anomaly is increasing; in a series of 150 patients in a European registry, almost 26% underwent a one-and-a-half ventricle repair [47]. However, late results of a bidirectional cavopulmonary shunt in patients in Ebstein anomaly are unknown.

Disadvantages of the bidirectional cavopulmonary shunt may include pulsations of the head and neck veins, facial swelling, and the development of arteriovenous fistulae in the pulmonary vasculature [48]. In addition, the placement of this shunt compromises access to the heart from the internal jugular approach for electrophysiologic studies and for pacemaker lead placement. The bidirectional cavopulmonary shunt is a promising application in the management of patients with Ebstein anomaly, particularly those with severe right ventricular dysfunction, but it should be reserved for selected patients mentioned above, until the late outcomes are well described.

The need to proceed to the Fontan procedure in the older child and adult with Ebstein anomaly is rarely, if ever indicated. While many have suggested the Fontan procedure in the child or adult with Ebstein anomaly and profound right ventricular dilatation and/or dysfunction, we have experienced poor outcome in those patients with a Fontan circulation who have two ventricles, one of which is enlarged and functions poorly – this is typically the case with Ebstein anomaly. In this most difficult group, we proceed with one-and-a-half ventricle repair, and rarely resort to transplantation.

Plication of the Atrialized Right Ventricle

Whether plication (or actual excision) of the atrialized right ventricle is necessary or desirable is controversial. Potential advantages include: 1) reduction in the size of the nonfunctional portion of the right ventricle, improving transit of blood flow through the right heart; 2) reduction of compression of the left ventricle (pancake effect), improving left ventricular function; and 3) reduction of tension on the tricuspid valve repair suture lines (particularly the cone repair), providing more space for the lungs (especially important in infants). All internal forms of right ventricular plication by necessity interrupt some coronary arterial supply to right ventricular musculature, and many have the potential risk of kinking the right coronary artery, problems that may generate ventricular arrhythmias and compromise right and left ventricular function. The decision whether to plicate the atrialized right ventricle and how much to plicate are based on the anatomy encountered and the surgeon's personal philosophy. In our practice, we routinely plicate the atrialized right ventricle when it is noted to be thinned and dilated. We believe it is also important when a complex tricuspid valve repair, such as the cone repair, has been performed in order to reduce tension on the suture lines that may be present – this is more likely to occur when there is marked right ventricular and annular dilatation. It is important to emphasize that during the course of any ventricular plication technique, there should be frequent inspection of the right coronary artery and its major branches in order to minimize potential compromise of arterial blood supply to the right (and left) ventricle.

Right Reduction Atrioplasty and Surgical Treatment of Arrhythmias

A right reduction atrioplasty is performed routinely at the time of atriotomy closure because there is almost always significant right atrial dilatation. Special attention is Made to leave a small rim of tissue anterior to the crista terminalis for suture placement during the closure. In all circumstances of right atriotomy closure, we avoid placing suture lines in the crista terminalis, which can produce the substrate for atrial tachyarrhythmias [49,50].

Atrial fibrillation and atrial flutter are the most frequent atrial tachyarrhythmias that occur in Ebstein anomaly. For most patients, the lesion sets of a Cox III right-sided maze procedure have been successful [51]. With the availability of newer devices (radiofrequency ablation and cryoablation) the time taken to perform the complete biatrial Cox maze III procedure is shortened significantly. Consequently, we perform a biatrial maze procedure much more frequently at the present time for all diagnoses associated with atrial arrhythmias. This is particularly important if there is continuous atrial fibrillation, left atrial dilatation, or concomitant mitral regurgitation. It is our practice to follow the lesions in both atria that have been previously described [52,53]. In addition, if there is evidence of atrial flutter, we add a lesion to the right atrial isthmus (i.e., the posterolateral tricuspid annulus to the coronary sinus to the inferior vena cava). We make an effort to close the left atrial appendage as part of the maze procedure.

For patients with AVNRT who have had unsuccessful ablation in the electrophysiology lab preoperatively, perinodal cryoablation is performed after institution of cardiopulmonary bypass, right atriotomy, and closure of intracardiac septal defects. Multiple applications of the cryoprobe (freezes) are made around and within the coronary sinus and then carried anteriorly toward the proximal atrioventricular node until temporary complete heart block is noted, at which time rewarming is begun immediately. Normal atrioventricular conduction returns shortly thereafter. When indicated, supplemental freezes are made superior and anterior to the atrioventricular node and His bundle.

For patients with accessory conduction pathway (i.e., Wolff-Parkinson-White), mapping and ablation is performed preoperatively in all patients. Rarely is intraoperative mapping and ablation performed at the time of repair of Ebstein anomaly in the current era.

Heart Transplantation

Transplantation is an option in patients with Ebstein anomaly with severe biventricular dysfunction (i.e., a left ventricular ejection fraction <25%). In our experience, patients with severe right ventricular dysfunction and normal or mild to moderately depressed left ventricular function can be managed with a conventional two ventricle approach or a one-and-a-half ventricle approach (bidirectional cavopulmonary shunt with tricuspid repair or replacement) [54]. Other patients with Ebstein anomaly that should be considered for transplantation are those with significant left ventricular dilatation and dysfunction and those with severe mitral regurgitation with significant left ventricular dysfunction. Hemodynamic cardiac catheterization to ascertain left-sided filling pressures and pulmonary artery pressures is also helpful in this group of patients when trying to determine feasibility of conventional operation versus transplantation.

Postoperative Management

Postoperative care of the biventricular repair in a neonate can be challenging. Tolerance of early low peripheral oxygenation (from the subtotal ASD closure) is common, and inhaled nitric oxide may be necessary to decrease pulmonary vascular resistance and augment antegrade pulmonary flow. Delayed sternal closure is used liberally. Prophylactic use of a peritoneal dialysis catheter also may be used to ensure complete decompression of the abdomen and facilitate ventilation. As pulmonary pressures decrease, forward flow will gradually increase through the pulmonary valve, improving oxygenation.

Postoperative care of neonates with the single ventricular approach is similar to that of any shunt-palliated patient with a univentricular heart, as there should be a balance between optimizing systemic perfusion and obtaining adequate oxygenation. Delayed sternal closure and peritoneal drainage may also be beneficial. As with other patients with a shunt-dependent pulmonary circulation, careful surveillance is required between the first operation and second-stage procedure (bidirectional cavopulmonary shunt), which is usually performed at 4–6 months of age.

In children and adults, the postoperative period is generally straightforward when left ventricular function is normal and right ventricular dysfunction is not severe. Routinely, we separate from bypass using epinephrine and milrinone infusions. We are cautious in the administration of colloid and crystalloid and prefer a right atrial pressure of less than 10 mmHg. We maintain reasonably fast heart rates (100–120 beats/min) and use temporary atrial pacing to accomplish this if needed. Delayed sternal closure, especially in patients with severe dilatation and dysfunction of the right ventricle can be life saving. To decrease right ventricular afterload (i.e., decrease pulmonary arterial pressures), nitric oxide and mild hyperventilation may be helpful in some patients. Intra-aortic balloon placement should be considered in patients with concomitant severe left ventricular dysfunction or known elevation in pulmonary artery pressures (infrequent). Atrial and ventricular arrhythmias should be avoided or treated aggressively through the optimization of metabolic parameters and the use of amiodarone and/or lidocaine.

Medical therapy in patients who have undergone repair of Ebstein anomaly is dependent on the method of repair. In patients with tricuspid valve repair, afterload-reducing agents should be used to decrease right ventricular afterload as much as possible. Patients who receive a tricuspid valve replacement with a porcine valve are prescribed warfarin for 3 months postoperatively, followed by lifelong aspirin (81 mg). Because of the reduction of blood flow across the tricuspid valve in the one-and-a-half ventricular repair, if a patient receives tricuspid valve replacement and a bidirectional cavopulmonary shunt, anticoagulation with warfarin may extend up to 6 months or until all prosthetic valve leaflets are noted to be mobile on echocardiography [44]. If patients have any postoperative arrhythmias, amiodarone is used for a minimum of 3 months and then reassessed.

Risk Factors and Outcome

When the diagnosis of Ebstein anomaly is made prenatally or in the neonate, the prognosis is poor. Survival for patients diagnosed between birth and 2 years of age was only 68% in one series [14]. Important features to determine with echocardiography that predict outcome in neonates with Ebstein anomaly include assessing patency of the right

Table 29.3 Celermajer index and the estimated risk of mortality. (aRV, atrialized right ventricle; LA, left atrium; LV, left ventricle; RA, right atrium; RV, right ventricle.) (Reproduced with permission from Jaquiss et al. [56].)

GOSE score	Index RA + aRV / RV + LA + LV	Risk of mortality [55,57]
1	<0.5	0%
2	0.5–0.99	10%
3	1–1.49	44–100%
4	≥1.50	100%

ventricular outflow tract and the GOSE score [14]. Patients who have the most severe GOSE score (grades 3 and 4) have a very poor prognosis (Table 29.3) [13,55–57].

Although early mortality for operation in the symptomatic neonate is high (biventricular repair is ~25%), the intermediate outcome with the biventricular approach appears to be promising. In 2007, Knott-Craig published his experience with 27 neonates and young infants [11]. These patients had concomitant anatomic or functional pulmonary atresia (n = 18), ventricular septal defect (n = 3), small left ventricle (n = 3), and hypoplastic branch pulmonary arteries (n = 3). Twenty-three patients (n = 25) received a biventricular repair with tricuspid valve repair, and two received valve replacement. Survival to hospital dismissal was 74%, and there were no late deaths (median follow-up, 5.4 years; maximum, 12 years). All patients were in functional NYHA class I. Although these early results for repair of Ebstein anomaly during the neonatal period are poor compared to many other neonatal anomalies corrected in the first month of life (e.g., arterial switch procedure, Norwood stage I, etc.), they have become a benchmark for this very difficult patient population.

The early results of the single ventricle pathway in neonates with Ebstein anomaly is similarly high (operative mortality, ~25%), but results continue to improve in the current era [13]. Of 16 neonates, two patients had tricuspid valve repair, one patient had heart transplant, 10 patients had a right ventricular exclusion procedure with a fenestrated tricuspid valve patch, and three patients had a right ventricular exclusion procedure with a nonfenestrated tricuspid valve patch. The operative survival was 80% (8 of 10) in patients with a fenestration and 33% in patients with no fenestration, leading the authors to recommend fenestration of the tricuspid valve patch. Among the nine hospital survivors of right ventricular exclusion, three underwent completion of the Fontan, and all nine have had a successful bidirectional cavopulmonary shunt (second stage).

In children and adults, the early and late (more than 25 years follow-up) results of our experience at the Mayo

Clinic have been reported [7,58,59]. In our experience with children (mean age, 7.1 ± 3.9 years) who underwent tricuspid valve repair, moderate or more tricuspid regurgitation on dismissal echocardiogram was the only risk factor for late reoperation [58]. Overall early mortality was 6% (3 of 52), but none since 1984. Overall survival was 90% at 10 years and 90% at 15 years. In our larger cohort of 539 children and adults who underwent operation for Ebstein anomaly, mitral regurgitation, RVOTO, higher hematocrit (cyanosis), greater than moderate right ventricular dysfunction, and moderate or greater left ventricular dysfunction were all independently associated with late mortality [7].

In 2007, Dr da Silva published his series of 40 patients who underwent the cone tricuspid valve repair technique [27]. Patient's average age was 16.8 ± 12.3 years, and after a mean follow-up of 4 years (range, 3 months to 12 years), only one patient died, and two patients required late tricuspid valve rerepair. The cone technique has the potential to cause tricuspid valve stenosis, although no patients in this initial cohort experienced this complication. Additional follow-up is required to determine if this method of repair has long term durability.

In a recent study of our patients at Mayo Clinic, the functional outcome after operation for Ebstein anomaly was good, and reported exercise tolerance was comparable to patients' peers [60]. In a small group who had exercise testing, there was improvement in the exercise tolerance after surgery, but this improvement was believed to be a result of the elimination of the right-to-left shunt at the atrial level rather than because of improvement in ventricular function [61,62]. Late reoperation, rehospitalization, and atrial tachyarrhythmias continued to be problematic, with a freedom from rehospitalization for cardiac causes including reoperation of 91%, 79%, 68%, 53%, and 35% at 1, 5, 10, 15, and 20 years, respectively [60]. Thus, further improvements in the durability of tricuspid valve repair and replacement, as well as improved control of atrial arrhythmias should be sought to improve the quality of life in patients with Ebstein anomaly.

References

1. Ebstein W. (1866) Ueber einen sehr seltenen Fall von Insufficienz der Valvula tricuspidalis, bedingt durch eine angeborene hochgradige Missbildung derselben. Arch Anat Physiol 238–255.
2. Anderson KR, Lie JT. (1979) The right ventricular myocardium in Ebstein's anomaly: a morphometric histopathologic study. Mayo Clin Proc 54, 181–184.
3. Greason KL, Dearani JA, Theodoro DA, et al. (2003) Surgical management of atrial tachyarrhythmias associated with congenital cardiac anomalies: Mayo Clinic experience. Semin Thorac Cardiovasc Surg Pediatr Card Surg Annu 6, 59–71.
4. Khositseth A, Danielson GK, Dearani JA, et al. (2004) Supraventricular tachyarrhythmias in Ebstein anomaly: management and outcome. J Thorac Cardiovasc Surg 128, 826–833.
5. Wald RM, Adatia I, Van Arsdell GS, et al. (2005) Relation of limiting ductal patency to survival in neonatal Ebstein's anomaly. Am J Cardiol 96, 851–856.
6. Celermajer DS, Bull C, Till JA, et al. (1994) Ebstein's anomaly: presentation and outcome from fetus to adult. J Am Coll Cardiol 23, 170–176.
7. Brown ML, Dearani JA, Danielson GK, et al. (2008) The outcomes of operations for 539 patients with Ebstein anomaly. J Thorac Cardiovasc Surg 135, 1120–1136.
8. Knott-Craig CJ, Overholt ED, Ward KE, et al. (2002) Repair of Ebstein's anomaly in the symptomatic neonate: an evolution of technique with 7-year follow-up. Ann Thorac Surg 73, 1786–1792; discussion 1792–1793.
9. Brown ML, Dearani JA. (2009) Ebstein malformation of the tricuspid valve: current concepts in management and outcomes. Curr Treat Options Cardiovasc Med 11, 396–402.
10. Knott-Craig CJ, Overholt ED, Ward KE, et al. (2000) Neonatal repair of Ebstein's anomaly: indications, surgical technique, and medium-term follow-up. Ann Thorac Surg 69, 1505–1510.
11. Knott-Craig CJ, Goldberg SP, Overholt ED, et al. (2007) Repair of neonates and young infants with Ebstein's anomaly and related disorders. Ann Thorac Surg 84, 587–592; discussion 592–593.
12. Knott-Craig CJ. (2008) Management of neonatal Ebstein's anomaly. Oper Tech Thorac Cardiovasc Surg 13, 101–108.
13. Reemtsen BL, Fagan BT, Wells WJ, et al. (2006) Current surgical therapy for Ebstein anomaly in neonates. J Thorac Cardiovasc Surg 132, 1285–1290.
14. Reemtsen BL, Polimenakos AC, Fagan BT, et al. (2007) Fate of the right ventricle after fenestrated right ventricular exclusion for severe neonatal Ebstein anomaly. J Thorac Cardiovasc Surg 134, 1406–1410; discussion 1410–1412.
15. Reemtsen BL, Starnes VA. (2008) Fenestrated right ventricular exclusion (Starnes' procedure) for severe neonatal Ebstein's anomaly. Oper Tech Thorac Cardiovasc Surg 13, 91–100.
16. Starnes VA, Pitlick PT, Bernstein D, et al. (1991) Ebstein's anomaly appearing in the neonate. A new surgical approach. J Thorac Cardiovasc Surg 101, 1082–1087.
17. Sano S, Ishino K, Kawada M, et al. (2002) Total right ventricular exclusion procedure: an operation for isolated congestive right ventricular failure. J Thorac Cardiovasc Surg 123, 640–647.
18. Di Russo GB, Clark BJ, Bridges ND, et al. (2000) Prolonged extracorporeal membrane oxygenation as a bridge to cardiac transplantation. Ann Thorac Surg 69, 925–927.
19. Schmid C, Debus V, Gogarten W, et al. (2006) Pediatric assist with the Medos and Excor systems in small children. ASAIO J 52, 505–508.
20. Weyand M, Kececioglu D, Kehl HG, et al. (1998) Neonatal mechanical bridging to total orthotopic heart transplantation. Ann Thorac Surg 66, 519–522.
21. Seward JB. (1993) Ebstein's anomaly: ultrasound imaging and hemodynamic evaluation. Echocardiography 10, 641–664.

22. Hunter SW, Lillehei CW. (1958) Ebstein's malformation of the tricuspid valve; study of a case together with suggestion of a new form of surgical therapy. Dis Chest 33, 297–304.

23. Hardy KL, May IA, Webster CA, et al. (1964) Ebstein's Anomaly: a Functional Concept and Successful Definitive Repair. J Thorac Cardiovasc Surg 48, 927–940.

24. Hardy KL, Roe BB. (1969) Ebstein's anomaly. Further experience with definitive repair. J Thorac Cardiovasc Surg 58, 553–561.

25. Danielson GK, Maloney JD, Devloo RA. (1979) Surgical repair of Ebstein's anomaly. Mayo Clin Proc 54, 185–192.

26. Dearani JA, Oleary PW, Danielson GK. (2006) Surgical treatment of Ebstein's malformation: state of the art in 2006. Cardiol Young 16(Suppl 3), 12–20.

27. da Silva JP, Baumgratz JF, da Fonseca L, et al. (2007) The cone reconstruction of the tricuspid valve in Ebstein's anomaly. The operation: early and midterm results. J Thorac Cardiovasc Surg 133, 215–223.

28. Dearani JA, Bacha E, da Silva JP. (2008) Cone reconstruction of the tricuspid valve for Ebstein's anomaly: anatomic repair. Oper Tech Thorac Cardiovasc Surg 13, 109–125.

29. Carpentier A, Chauvaud S, Mace L, et al. (1988) A new reconstructive operation for Ebstein's anomaly of the tricuspid valve. J Thorac Cardiovasc Surg 96, 92–101.

30. Chauvaud S. (2000) Ebstein's malformation. surgical treatment and results. Thorac Cardiovasc Surg 48, 220–223.

31. Chauvaud S, Fuzellier JF, Berrebi A, et al. (1998) Bi-directional cavopulmonary shunt associated with ventriculo and valvuloplasty in Ebstein's anomaly: benefits in high risk patients. Eur J Cardiothorac Surg 13, 514–519.

32. Chen JM, Mosca RS, Altmann K, et al. (2004) Early and medium-term results for repair of Ebstein anomaly. J Thorac Cardiovasc Surg 127, 990–8; discussion 8–9.

33. Hancock Friesen CL, Chen R, Howlett JG, et al. (2004) Posterior annular plication: tricuspid valve repair in Ebstein's anomaly. Ann Thorac Surg 77, 2167–2171.

34. Hetzer R, Nagdyman N, Ewert P, et al. (1998) A modified repair technique for tricuspid incompetence in Ebstein's anomaly. J Thorac Cardiovasc Surg 115, 857–868.

35. Quaegebeur JM, Sreeram N, Fraser AG, et al. (1991) Surgery for Ebstein's anomaly: the clinical and echocardiographic evaluation of a new technique. J Am Coll Cardiol 17, 722–728.

36. van Son JA, Kinzel P, Mohr FW. (1998) Pericardial patch augmentation of anterior tricuspid leaflet in Ebstein's anomaly. Ann Thorac Surg 66, 1831–1832.

37. Vargas FJ, Mengo G, Granja MA, et al. (1998) Tricuspid annuloplasty and ventricular plication for Ebstein's malformation. Ann Thorac Surg 65, 1755–1757.

38. Wu Q, Huang Z. (2004) A new procedure for Ebstein's anomaly. Ann Thorac Surg 77, 470–476; discussion 476.

39. Sanfelippo PM, Giuliani ER, Danielson GK, et al. (1976) Tricuspid valve prosthetic replacement. Early and late results with the Starr-Edwards prosthesis. J Thorac Cardiovasc Surg 71, 441–445.

40. Dearani JA, Mavroudis C, Quintessenza J, et al. (2009) Surgical advances in the treatment of adults with congenital heart disease. Curr Opin Pediatr 21, 565–572.

41. Kiziltan HT, Theodoro DA, Warnes CA, et al. (1998) Late results of bioprosthetic tricuspid valve replacement in Ebstein's anomaly. Ann Thorac Surg 66, 1539–1545.

42. Geha AS, Laks H, Stansel HC Jr, et al. (1979) Late failure of porcine valve heterografts in children. J Thorac Cardiovasc Surg 78, 351–364.

43. Williams DB, Danielson GK, McGoon DC, et al. (1982) Porcine heterograft valve replacement in children. J Thorac Cardiovasc Surg 84, 446–450.

44. Quinonez LG, Dearani JA, Puga FJ, et al. (2007) Results of the 1.5-ventricle repair for Ebstein anomaly and the failing right ventricle. J Thorac Cardiovasc Surg 133, 1303–1310.

45. Malhotra SP, Reddy VM, Qiu M, et al. (2009) Right ventricular unloading promotes durability of tricuspid valve repair in Ebstein's anomaly: indications for a selective one and a half ventricle strategy. Presented at: 45th Annual Meeting of the Society of Thoracic Surgeons; January 26–26, 2009; San Francisco, CA.

46. Marianeschi SM, McElhinney DB, Reddy VM, et al. (1998) Alternative approach to the repair of Ebstein's malformation: intracardiac repair with ventricular unloading. Ann Thorac Surg 66, 1546–1550.

47. Sarris GE, Giannopoulos NM, Tsoutsinos AJ, et al. (2006) Results of surgery for Ebstein anomaly: a multicenter study from the European Congenital Heart Surgeons Association. J Thorac Cardiovasc Surg 132, 50–57.

48. Kopf GS, Laks H, Stansel HC, et al. (1990) Thirty-year follow-up of superior vena cava-pulmonary artery (Glenn) shunts. J Thorac Cardiovasc Surg 100, 662–670; discussion 670–671.

49. Durongpisitkul K, Porter CJ, Cetta F, et al. (1998) Predictors of early- and late-onset supraventricular tachyarrhythmias after Fontan operation. Circulation 98, 1099–1107.

50. Gandhi SK, Bromberg BI, Rodefeld MD, et al. (1997) Spontaneous atrial flutter in a chronic canine model of the modified Fontan operation. J Am Coll Cardiol 30, 1095–1103.

51. Theodoro DA, Danielson GK, Porter CJ, et al. (1998) Right-sided maze procedure for right atrial arrhythmias in congenital heart disease. Ann Thorac Surg 65, 149–153; discussion 153–154.

52. Cox JL, Jaquiss RD, Schuessler RB, et al. (1995) Modification of the maze procedure for atrial flutter and atrial fibrillation. II. Surgical technique of the maze III procedure. J Thorac Cardiovasc Surg 110, 485–495.

53. Mavroudis C, Deal BJ, Backer CL, et al. (2008) Arrhythmia surgery in patients with and without congenital heart disease. Ann Thorac Surg 86, 857–868; discussion 868.

54. Brown ML, Dearani JA, Danielson GK, et al. (2008) Effect of operation for Ebstein anomaly on left ventricular function. Am J Cardiol 102, 1724–1727.

55. Celermajer DS, Cullen S, Sullivan ID, et al. (1992) Outcome in neonates with Ebstein's anomaly. J Am Coll Cardiol 19, 1041–1046.

56. Jaquiss RD, Imamura M. (2007) Management of Ebstein's anomaly and pure tricuspid insufficiency in the neonate. Semin Thorac Cardiovasc Surg 19, 258–263.

57. Yetman AT, Freedom RM, McCrindle BW. (1998) Outcome in cyanotic neonates with Ebstein's anomaly. Am J Cardiol 81, 749–754.

58. Boston US, Dearani JA, O'Leary PW, *et al.* (2006) Tricuspid valve repair for Ebstein's anomaly in young children: a 30-year experience. Ann Thorac Surg 81, 690–695; discussion 695–696.

59. Theodoro DA, Danielson GK, Kiziltan HT, *et al.* (1997) Surgical management of Ebstein's anomaly: 25-year experience. Circulation 96(suppl 1), 1–507.

60. Brown ML, Dearani JA, Danielson GK, *et al.* (2008) Functional status after operation for Ebstein anomaly: the Mayo Clinic experience. J Am Coll Cardiol 52, 460–466.

61. Driscoll DJ, Mottram CD, Danielson GK. (1988) Spectrum of exercise intolerance in 45 patients with Ebstein's anomaly and observations on exercise tolerance in 11 patients after surgical repair. J Am Coll Cardiol 11, 831–836.

62. MacLellan-Tobert SG, Driscoll DJ, Mottram CD, *et al.* (1997) Exercise tolerance in patients with Ebstein's anomaly. J Am Coll Cardiol 29, 1615–1622.

CHAPTER 30

Left Ventricular Outflow Tract Obstruction

Christo I. Tchervenkov,[1] Pierre-Luc Bernier,[1] Danny Del Duca,[2] Samantha Hill,[2] Noritaka Ota,[3] and Constantine Mavroudis[4]

[1]The Montreal Children's Hospital, McGill University, Montreal, QC, Canada
[2]McGill University, Montreal, QC, Canada
[3]Mt. Fuji Shizuoka Children's Hospital, Shizuoka, Japan
[4]Florida Hospital for Children, Orlando, FL, USA

Introduction

Congenital left ventricular outflow tract obstruction (LVOTO) is defined as impedance to ventricular ejection at various levels from the left ventricle to the ascending aorta. It is caused by a relatively common group of anomalies representing approximately 3–10% of patients with congenital heart disease [1]. The obstruction most commonly occurs at the aortic valve, but it may also be subvalvar, supravalvar, or a combination of these three.

LVOTO may occur as part of a complex of congenital cardiac malformations such as Shone's complex or hypoplastic left heart complex (HLHC). In the neonate with critical aortic stenosis and left ventricular hypoplasia or with HLHC, the capacity of the left heart to adequately support the systemic circulation may be compromised. For some of these patients, survival may be higher with the Norwood operation rather than with a traditional two-ventricle approach. This discussion of LVOTO is limited to that without associated interrupted aortic arch, single ventricle, transposition of the great vessels, or other complex structural heart defects. Aortic atresia will likewise not be discussed.

The classification of LVOTO is based on the primary pathologic morphology. Valvar aortic stenosis is the most frequent form, occurring in 60–75% of cases [2,3]. Subvalvar and supravalvar aortic stenosis affect 15–20% and 5–10% of patients, respectively.

Valvar Aortic Stenosis

Aortic valve abnormalities represent one of the most common forms of congenital heart disease, at 3–6% of all congenital heart defects [4,5]. Valvar aortic stenosis is the most frequent primary lesion in children with LVOTO, accounting for nearly 75% of cases. Valvar aortic stenosis has a wide spectrum of anatomic and clinical variations [6]. In its most benign form, children with a bicuspid aortic valve and/or mild aortic stenosis will remain asymptomatic except for an incidental murmur found on routine physical examination. On the other hand, newborns with critical aortic stenosis and ductus-dependent systemic circulation will become severely ill when the ductus closes, manifesting systemic hypoperfusion, acute renal failure, and severe metabolic acidosis. Although less than 10% of children are first seen with signs of critical aortic stenosis [7], they represent a distinct and challenging group of patients, with unique pathophysiologic and therapeutic considerations.

Valvar aortic stenosis has clear gender predilection, with the incidence in males three to five times higher than in females. Many other cardiac anomalies are associated frequently with valvar aortic stenosis, including ventricular septal defect (VSD), patent ductus arteriosus (PDA), hypoplastic left ventricle, and coarctation of the aorta [2,3,7]. In the neonate, critical aortic stenosis may be associated with multiple left-sided obstructions and severe hypoplasia of the left heart structures, falling within the spectrum of hypoplastic left heart syndrome (HLHS). In the largest multicenter prospective study on critical aortic stenosis involving 320 neonates less than 30 days old at diagnosis, an initial Norwood operation was performed on 179 patients (56%) [8]. This demonstrates the high incidence of left heart hypoplasia when this lesion is diagnosed in early life.

Pediatric Cardiac Surgery, Fourth Edition. Edited by Constantine Mavroudis and Carl L. Backer.
© 2013 Blackwell Publishing Ltd. Published 2013 by Blackwell Publishing Ltd.

Aortic Stenosis in the Neonate and Infant

Pathologic Anatomy

Reduced cross-sectional area in critically stenotic aortic valves is the result of abnormalities in the number and morphology of cusps and the development of valve commissures [5,9]. When seen in the neonate and infant, these valves are most frequently bicuspid, with thickened, dysmorphic leaflets, fused commissures, and an eccentric orifice. Less commonly, one finds unicuspid valves that may be commissural, with only a stenotic central orifice, or they may be unicommissural with a single eccentrically located commissure extending to the annulus and a lateral commissural attachment to the aortic wall. A tricuspid valve with three cusps and a stenotic central orifice is the least common form of valvar aortic stenosis. In older children, bicuspid valves are seen more commonly. These valves usually consist of a right and a left leaflet of unequal size, separated by the anterior and posterior commissures. The commissures usually have some degree of fusion, and there is limited mobility of the leaflets because of the straight rather than rounded shape of the commissural opening. Some valves appear to be bicuspid at first glance, but closer inspection reveals a tricuspid valve with one commissure rudimentary and fused, giving the impression of two leaflets.

Pathophysiology

LVOTO secondary to valvar aortic stenosis is usually compatible with life during fetal development. Increased left ventricular afterload, however, leads to myocardial hypertrophy with systolic and diastolic dysfunction [10]. In critical aortic stenosis, significant left ventricular dysfunction occurs with increased left atrial pressure, resulting in left-to-right shunt flow across the foramen ovale. Systemic perfusion is maintained via right ventricular ejection and the PDA. Left ventricular hypertrophy, intracavitary hypertension, and reduced coronary perfusion pressure together predispose the left ventricle to myocardial ischemia [11], which may lead to endocardial fibroelastosis [12]. In addition, severe obstruction causes reduced flow through the left heart during fetal development, which predisposes to hypoplasia of the left-sided structures such as the mitral valve, left ventricle, left ventricular outflow tract (LVOT), aortic valve, ascending aorta, and frequently the aortic arch [12].

The postnatal course depends on the severity of valvar obstruction, the degree of left ventricular dysfunction or hypoplasia, and in cases of critical stenosis, shunt flow at the atrial and ductal levels. Neonates and infants with mild to moderate forms of valvar aortic stenosis usually have a well developed left ventricle that is sufficient to support the systemic circulation. They remain clinically asymptomatic except for a systolic ejection murmur and evidence of progressive left ventricular hypertrophy. Occasionally, exercise intolerance may be present. More severe forms of valvar aortic stenosis cause increased ventricular afterload, resulting in increased ventricular wall tension and workload. This leads to myocardial hypertrophy and ventricular dysfunction. In addition, the pressure gradient across a stenotic valve causes a mismatch between coronary perfusion pressure and myocardial perfusion pressure. Consequently, myocardial ischemia, arrhythmia, and infarction are constant concerns in such situations. The subendocardial region is the area most vulnerable to ischemia, which may lead to endocardial fibroelastosis [13], a characteristic pathologic finding of valvar aortic stenosis. Patients with severe aortic stenosis manifest exertional chest pain, easy fatigability, and/or syncope.

In many neonates, the left heart is incapable of sustaining the systemic circulation, either because of severe LVOTO, severe left ventricular hypoplasia, and/or dysfunction [8]. Both systemic and coronary perfusions become dependent on the PDA. Typically, these patients have adequate peripheral perfusion with varying degrees of cyanosis, especially to the lower body, depending on the amount of flow through the native aortic valve. As the ductus begins to close soon after birth, however, these patients develop signs of cardiovascular collapse manifested by hypotension, acute renal failure, congestive heart failure, and metabolic acidosis.

Clinical Picture and Diagnosis

The timing of presentation is related to the severity of obstruction. Patients with mild aortic stenosis may remain essentially asymptomatic. As the degree of obstruction increases, exertional chest pain, easy fatigability, and syncope are manifest. Most patients with critical aortic stenosis who are not well compensated have obvious signs of cardiovascular compromise soon after birth. Only a small number of patients are first seen after 6 months of age. In these patients, a history of irritability, poor weight gain, and poor feeding is typical. However, these systems correlate poorly with the degree of obstruction.

Physical examination in patients with isolated aortic stenosis usually shows a normally developed, acyanotic child. Although the blood pressure is usually normal, a narrow pulse pressure and signs of reduced peripheral perfusion such as diminished peripheral pulses, pale cool skin, and slow capillary refill are found in more severe cases. A systolic ejection murmur may or may not be present, depending on the left ventricular function and the amount of blood flow across the stenotic valve. When present, it is best heard at the second intercostal space with good transmission to the neck apex. In very low output states, the murmur may be absent; as cardiac output and congestive heart failure improve, the murmur increases in intensity. A systolic thrill may be palpable along the right upper sternal border, in the suprasternal notch or over the carotid arteries. An ejection click may be present and strongly suggests valvar, rather than supravalvar or subvalvar, obstruction. Lower body cyanosis may be present when there is significant right-to-left shunting through the PDA. When there is sufficient forward flow in the ascending aorta to sustain normal perfusion of the brachiocephalic vessels, differential cyanosis may be observed; the abdomen and lower extremities are perfused by desaturated blood from the PDA. Hepatomegaly suggests biventricular failure and may indicate a less favorable prognosis.

The electrocardiogram typically shows evidence of left ventricular, or biventricular, hypertrophy with or without a strain pattern. In mild cases, the electrocardiogram remains normal. However, correlation between the severity of the stenosis and the presence of electrocardiogram abnormalities is poor [14]. The chest radiograph is usually normal but may show an enlarged cardiac silhouette and evidence of pulmonary congestion in neonates with critical aortic stenosis.

Echocardiography and Doppler flow studies are extremely informative noninvasive studies that can greatly facilitate the management of congenital heart disease [15]. In addition to establishing the anatomic diagnosis, echocardiography can assess ventricular function, the presence or absence of endocardial fibroelastosis, as well as associated cardiac anomalies [12]. The severity of stenosis can be estimated by measuring the pressure gradient across the stenotic valve using Doppler studies, although such gradient may be greatly underestimated when there is ventricular dysfunction or a right-to-left shunt across the PDA. Echocardiography also defines the direction of flow across the PDA and in the ascending aorta. Such information helps to determine whether the left heart is capable of supporting the systemic circulation after biventricular repair. Prenatal diagnosis is also possible using fetal echocardiography [16].

Cardiac catheterization is performed as part of catheter-based therapeutic intervention or if there is uncertainty regarding the diagnosis or other associated anomalies. Direct measurements of left-sided and right-sided pressures, as well as the peak-to-peak systolic pressure gradient across the valve, can be taken to assess valve leaflet morphology, aortic annulus size, aortic and mitral valve competence, and ventricular performance.

Treatment

Indications for Intervention

For neonates and young infants, the development of congestive heart failure or the presence of ductal-dependant systemic circulation indicates the need for urgent intervention. Beyond the neonatal period, symptomatic valvar stenosis or a significant pressure gradient across the aortic valve (>50 mmHg) constitutes an indication for surgery. Generally, aortic valvotomy is preferred at the initial surgical intervention, with aortic valve repair or replacement strategies being reserved for future interventions.

Therapeutic strategy is based on assessment of the patient's clinical status and a complete understanding of the underlying anatomic defects. Because of the frequent association of critical valvar aortic stenosis and left heart hypoplasia, one of the key issues to be decided early on is whether the left-side structures are capable of sustaining systemic circulation. This distinction is essential in deciding whether to proceed with a Norwood-type single ventricle repair or cardiac transplantation instead of valvotomy or valve replacement procedures. Previous reports have described significantly worse results in those patients requiring a "crossover" between univentricular and biventricular strategies [17,18].

Despite numerous studies, preoperative assessment of left ventricular status as a predictor of surgical outcome is still controversial. Echocardiographic dimensions most commonly are used for such purposes. Unfavorable surgical outcome after biventricular repair has been associated with a small aortic valve, a small left ventricle, and a small mitral valve. In a retrospective study, Rhodes and associates proposed a scoring system to determine quantitatively the adequacy of the left ventricle based on the aortic root dimension indexed to the body surface area, the ratio of the long-axis dimension of the left ventricle to the long-axis dimension of the heart, and the indexed mitral valve area [19]. Others have suggested that the presence of predominant or total antegrade flow in the ascending and transverse aorta is associated with survival after two-ventricle repair [20]. However, surgical series of successful biventricular repair of HLHC and LVOTO have been reported when the above criteria would have predicted a univentricular approach [21–23]. Furthermore, the Rhodes score has been shown to lack discriminating power in neonates with multiple levels of left heart obstruction [18,22].

The Congenital Heart Surgeons' Society (CHSS) conducted a prospective multicenter study on management, outcomes, and risk factors in 320 neonates with critical aortic stenosis [8]. Of these, an initial biventricular repair consisting mainly of either surgical or balloon aortic valvotomy was performed in 116 patients, and an initial Norwood operation in 179 patients. Multiple management, survival, and risk factors were assessed for the biventricular and univentricular pathways. A multiple-regression equation was established to determine the 5-year survival benefit of Norwood versus biventricular repair for each patient. The factors found to be significant were the age of patient at entry, the size of the aortic valve at the sinuses, the grade of endocardial fibroelastosis, the diameter of the ascending aorta, the presence of moderate or severe tricuspid regurgitation, and the score of the left ventricular length. Although the CHSS study is the most detailed and sophisticated analysis involving the largest-ever number of patients, the validity of this equation to determine the optimal surgical option for each patient remains to be tested in a prospective fashion.

More recently, the CHSS has reviewed a larger cohort with critical LVOTO, including the 320 neonates with critical aortic stenosis in the previously mentioned study [24]. This new analysis underscores the critical importance of deciding which patients are better suited for a univentricular and which patients for a two-ventricle approach. On the basis of that analysis, a univentricular-repair survival tool has been developed using separate risk factor analysis for death after intended univentricular or biventricular approach. This tool remains to be validated in a prospective trial.

Preintervention Management

Although relief of mechanical obstruction is the goal, therapeutic results can be improved greatly by aggressive resuscitation of the critically ill patient before invasive interventions. This usually requires endotracheal intubation and mechanical ventilation, inotropic support, and correction of fluid and electrolyte abnormalities. If signs of circulatory collapse develop with closure of the PDA, prostaglandin E1 infusion is invaluable for maintaining systemic perfusion and correcting metabolic acidosis. Using these measures, a patient's condition usually can be stabilized to allow time for proper preoperative studies and therapies that can be performed on an urgent rather than emergent basis.

Percutaneous Balloon Valvuloplasty

Percutaneous balloon valvuloplasty is considered by many the procedure of choice for relieving obstruction from valvar aortic stenosis [25–28]. Significant improvements have been made in both the technique and instrumentation since this procedure was first introduced in 1983 [29]. The CHSS evaluated the outcomes of surgical versus transcatheter balloon valvotomy in 110 neonates with critical aortic stenosis [30]. Although the transcatheter approach was associated with a greater percentage reduction in systolic gradients ($65 \pm 17\%$ vs. $41 \pm 32\%$) and lower residual median gradients (20 mm Hg, range, 0–85 mm Hg vs. 36 mm Hg, range, 10–85 mm Hg), there was a higher incidence of significant aortic regurgitation (18% vs. 3%). However, the two approaches did not differ significantly in regards to time-related survival (82% at 1 month and 72% at 5 years), as well as estimated freedom from reintervention (91% at 1 month and 48% at 5 years).

Vascular access is an important consideration for this procedure. The umbilical artery is the preferred site in neonates, whereas the femoral artery frequently is used in older patients. Axillary cannulation, as well as antegrade venous cannulation, have also been described [31].

However, severe aortic coarctation or interrupted aortic arch preclude the use of these routes. Carotid artery cannulation has been reported, including at the bedside, for relief of critical aortic valve stenosis, obviating the need to transport ill and hemodynamically unstable neonates to the cardiac catheterization laboratory [32]. A dysplastic valve with small annulus and aortic insufficiency are generally contraindications for balloon valvuloplasty.

Fetal Intervention

Balloon dilatation of the aortic valve has been described in fetal life. The objective is to limit postnatal left ventricular hypoplasia and dysfunction [33]. Although this approach is not yet considered standard of care, it may show promise in the future, allowing more patients with a borderline left ventricle to undergo a biventricular repair. In a report from Children's Hospital Boston, Tworetzky and associates performed balloon dilatation of the aortic valve in 20 fetuses at high risk for the development of HLHS by echocardiographic evaluation [34]. Technically successful procedures were those in which the guidewire was passed across the aortic valve, a 1 cm long balloon was inflated straddling the valve, and unambiguous improvement in aortic valve flow was confirmed by color Doppler imaging. There were 14 successful interventions, and these were associated with greater left-sided cardiac growth compared to unsuccessful cases. Technically unsuccessful cases shared several features, including suboptimal fetal positioning, the inability to manipulate the wire across the aortic valve, and a cannula angle that directed the wire either posterior or toward the ventricular septum instead of toward the aortic valve. In a separate report from Boston, a series of 22 fetuses diagnosed with critical aortic stenosis underwent aortic valvuloplasty [35]. Technical success increased significantly if maternal laparotomy was an option (83.3% vs. 20.0%), and laparotomy was performed in 66.6% of cases. Factors including gestational age, body mass index, or placental location were not associated with the need for laparotomy or the chances of technical success of the intervention. Postoperatively, three fetuses died, and two required preterm delivery.

Open Surgical Valvotomy and Open Surgical Valvuloplasty

Before the development of balloon valvuloplasty, a number of approaches had been employed successfully to perform surgical valvotomy. These procedures can be performed with or without cardiopulmonary bypass and with or without cardioplegia. Controversy continues concerning the advantages and disadvantages of different surgical approaches, and their use is based largely on individual preferences. Recently, some surgeons have advocated the use of a surgical aortic valvuloplasty, including commissurotomy, leaflet thinning, and excision of nodules and tissue deposits that make the aortic valve leaflets bulky and immobile [36]. Our opinion is that the open surgical aortic valvuloplasty is far superior to the closed balloon valvotomy.

Open Valvotomy with Cardiopulmonary Bypass

Many surgeons prefer to perform open valvotomy during cardiopulmonary bypass, which offers the benefit and safety of controlled circulation (Figure 30.1) [37]. The aorta can be cross-clamped and the heart arrested using a single dose of cardioplegia solution. The aortic valve is exposed through a vertical aortotomy directed toward the noncoronary cusp. The major advantage of such an approach is that it allows a detailed inspection of the valvar anatomy and a precise valvotomy, which is critical to the success of the operation. Valvotomy should be carried out by dividing fused commissures to within 1–2 mm of the aortic wall. Because only a small increase in valve diameter is needed

to gain a significant reduction in pressure gradient, it is recommended that the valvotomy be conservative in order to avoid creating aortic insufficiency. False raphes in a bicuspid aortic valve must not be incised for the same reason. In addition, the open technique allows the resection of nodules and mesenchymal tissue deposits on the valve leaflets and leaflet thinning under direct vision.

Open Valvotomy with Inflow Occlusion

Inflow occlusion offers rapid access to the aortic valve and direct visualization without cardiopulmonary bypass. The superior and inferior vena cavae are occluded with vascular clamps, and the heart is allowed to beat five to six times before the ascending aorta is cross-clamped. The aortic valve is exposed through a vertical aortotomy, and a conservative valvotomy is performed. Afterward, the heart is cleared of air by releasing the inferior vena caval clamp and filling the heart and the ascending aorta with blood. The

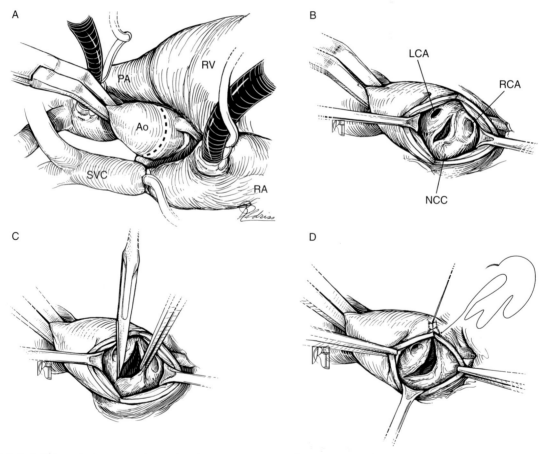

Figure 30.1 A, Initial surgical exposure for aortic valvotomy, which shows aortic cross-clamp, cardioplegia (not shown), and intended aortotomy site. **B,** Transverse aortotomy reveals a bicuspid aortic valve, which is fused at the commissures. **C,** Sharp aortic valvotomy is being performed to enlarge the left ventricular outflow tract. **D,** Valvotomy is completed and the aortotomy closure is commenced. Air maneuvers follow before cross-clamp is removed. (Ao, aorta; LCA, left coronary artery; NCC, noncoronary cusp; PA, pulmonary artery; RA, right atrium; RCA, right coronary artery; RV, right ventricle; SVC, superior vena cava.)

aortotomy is controlled with a side-biting clamp, and the cross-clamp is removed. The superior vena caval clamp is then released and the heart is resuscitated. This procedure is rarely used today because of the safety and utility of cardiopulmonary bypass and cardioplegia [38,39]. It is mentioned mostly for historical purposes.

Closed Valvotomy

Closed valvotomy is similar to balloon valvuloplasty in that the aortic valve opening is enlarged without direct visualization. This can be performed with or without cardiopulmonary bypass in a similar fashion. After a purse-string suture is placed around the left ventricular apex, a stab ventriculotomy is made in the middle of this purse string. Progressively larger Hegar dilators are inserted through the incision to enlarge the aortic valve opening to the desired diameter.

Aortic Valve Replacement

Aortic valve replacement using a pulmonary autograft with (Ross-Konno procedure) [40–42] or without aortoventriculoplasty (Ross procedure) [43–45] has been used successfully in infants who have critical aortic valve stenosis. In the Ross-Konno procedure, the LVOT is enlarged with either a synthetic patch, allograft aortic patch, or right ventricular infundibular free-wall muscular extension harvested in continuity with the autograft.

Univentricular Approach and the Norwood Operation

In patients with aortic valve stenosis that is not amenable to biventricular repair, the surgical options include staged surgical palliation and orthotopic heart transplantation. Given the limited availability of donor organs and the complications associated with long-term immunosuppression, staged surgical palliation is preferred rather than transplantation. The Norwood operation has significantly enhanced the survival of neonates with critical aortic stenosis with significant left ventricular hypoplasia.

Results

Preoperative discrimination between HLHS and isolated aortic valve stenosis has contributed to a significant reduction in operative mortality [19,46]. Although previous studies have described an operative mortality of 30–50% after aortic valvotomy in infants, more recent series [25–28,47,48] reported operative survival of 90% or higher. The major difference in the latter series is that the patients had a normal or near-normal left ventricular size. In one study, data analysis identified four morphologic variables that are predictive of death: a left ventricular long axis-to-heart long axis ratio of 0.8 or less, an indexed aortic root diameter of $3.5 \, cm/m^2$ or less, an indexed mitral valve area of

$4.75 \, cm/m^2$ or less, and a left ventricular mass index of less than $35 \, g/m^2$ [49]. The mortality rate was 100% in patients with two or more of these risk factors and 8% in patients with one or no risk factors. In the previously mentioned multicenter study on neonatal critical aortic stenosis, the 5-year survival after biventricular repair was 70% vs. 60% after the Norwood operation [8]. More important, the use of a regression equation would have provided survival benefit in favor of the Norwood operation in 50% of patients who had biventricular repair and in favor of biventricular repair in 20% of patients who had the Norwood operation. Of course, this regression equation remains to be tested in a prospective fashion as a decision-making tool.

Valvotomy for infants, whether balloon or surgical, should be considered a palliative procedure, because a large number of children eventually will require additional procedures for the aortic valve [50]. Recurrent aortic stenosis, stenosis with regurgitation, or isolated aortic regurgitation are common reasons for further interventions [51,52]. Repeat valvotomy is possible, although less effective in certain situations, and aortic valve replacement is eventually necessary.

Percutaneous Balloon Valvuloplasty

Since an initial report of successful balloon valvuloplasty for aortic valve stenosis in infancy, this modality has been used more frequently [53]. Balloon valvuloplasty during the first 60 days of life results in short-term relief of aortic stenosis in most patients. Although initially those with hypoplastic left heart structures may have worse subacute outcomes, this normalizes within 1 year [54]. Comparative studies concluded that balloon valvuloplasty and surgery for aortic stenosis provide equivalent relief as measured by ejection fraction improvement and left ventricular mass-to-volume ratio increase [55,56]. Early mortality and incidence of required additional aortic valve procedures were similar in both the balloon valvuloplasty and surgery patients [30,57]. Balloon valvuloplasty was associated with a higher incidence of important aortic regurgitation, while surgical patients had a higher incidence of residual stenosis. Long-term results are equally encouraging, with nearly two-thirds of patients being free from aortic valve surgery 10 years afterward [58], and most demonstrating catch-up growth of both the aortic valve and the left ventricle [59]. Fetal aortic valvuloplasty is demonstrating encouraging results, when technically successful. In one study, 26 out of 30 fetuses underwent a successful intrauterine angioplasty, with marked improvement in left heart physiology, including markers such as ejection fraction and antegrade flow in the transverse aortic arch [60].

Surgical Valvotomy and Surgical Valvuloplasty

Marked clinical improvement can be expected after successful valvotomy in the neonate [61–64]. This procedure, as stated previously, should be regarded as palliative rather than curative. Most patients eventually will require re-operation because of progressive aortic insufficiency, aortic stenosis, or both [52,65]. However, current evidence indicates that aortic valve replacement can be safely delayed until implantation of an adult-sized prosthesis [66]. In a report from the German Pediatric Heart Institute, a retrospective review of the early and long-term results of primary surgical aortic valvotomy in 26 neonates and 8 infants was described [36]. The operative mortality was 6%, and the risk factors for early mortality were endocardial fibroelastosis, monocuspid aortic valve, and impaired left ventricular function. The mean follow-up was 115 ± 67 months, and no late mortalities were observed. The freedom from reintervention was $85.1 \pm 6.9\%$, $78.0 \pm 9.35\%$, and $53.5 \pm 15.9\%$ at 5, 10, and 15 years, respectively.

Although mortality as high as 30–50% had been reported after aortic valvotomy in infants, this has been attributed, at least in part, to inappropriate patient selection [49,67]. Better understanding of the disease process and improved distinction between HLHS and aortic stenosis with two well developed ventricles have improved results dramatically [19,47,48,64,68]. Operative mortalities approaching zero can be achieved in neonates with isolated critical aortic stenosis [66]. A recent study demonstrated a 30-day survival after surgical commissurotomy of 95% [69]. In another multicenter study, no significant difference in survival between open and closed valvotomy was observed (87% vs. 90%, respectively) [70]. The best results are observed in patients with isolated valvar aortic stenosis [47,63]. Despite reduced early postoperative mortality, surgical repair of congenital aortic stenosis is associated with significant long-term mortality. In one study, postoperative survival gradually decreased from 93% after 30 days to 76% after 25 years [71]. More recent literature suggests that late survival has improved dramatically [66]. Complex cardiac anomalies and endocardial fibroelastosis have been associated with increased operative mortality. The quality of life for long-term survivors of congenital aortic stenosis after treatment is comparable to that of the general population [72].

Aortic Stenosis in the Older Child

Pathologic Anatomy

Compared with patients who become symptomatic early on, aortic stenosis in older children usually manifests as milder forms of valvar obstruction. Although all anatomic variants are possible, more than three-fourths of patients have a bicuspid aortic valve [73]. The etiology of bicuspid aortic valve is not known, although a genetic influence has been suggested [74]. Severely dysmorphic valves and hypoplasia of the aortic annulus are uncommon in this age group.

Pathophysiology

The predominant pathophysiology in older children with aortic stenosis is similar to that in adults, namely increased left ventricular afterload. In compensation for such pressure overload, the left ventricular muscle undergoes concentric hypertrophy. This compensatory phase may progress for a long period without being clinically apparent. Eventually, symptoms develop as ventricular hypertrophy causes decreased ventricular compliance and increased left ventricular end-diastolic pressure. Increased ventricular muscle mass is associated with increased metabolic demand, but there is no accompanied increase in the number of coronary vessels. Myocardial perfusion pressure is also reduced because of the normal or reduced aortic pressure and elevated left ventricular end-diastolic pressure [11]. The end result is a noncompliant and hypertrophied left ventricle that is susceptible to ischemia, especially at the subendocardial layer. Symptoms of volume overload may also develop if the aortic valve becomes insufficient.

Clinical Picture and Diagnosis

In sharp contrast to neonatal critical aortic stenosis, most children who are more than 1 year of age when aortic stenosis is detected show normal growth and development [75]. Typically, these patients are brought to medical attention as a result of an asymptomatic murmur detected during routine medical examinations. Symptoms of aortic stenosis develop over time. Initially, symptoms may be present only during exercise when there is increased demand on cardiac output. As the child grows, the condition of the aortic valve remains the same or worsens, and the relative stenosis becomes more severe. Symptoms of congestive heart failure, syncope, and angina become more prominent and are present even at rest. The incidence of spontaneous bacterial endocarditis is estimated to be 3 per 1000 patient-years [76]. This incidence does not correlate with either the severity of stenosis or surgery [72]. The incidence of sudden death is also increased in children with aortic stenosis and is reported to be between 1.2% and 19% per patient-year. This usually occurs in patients with severe aortic stenosis, and ischemia-induced ventricular arrhythmia is thought to be the cause.

Physical examination is most often noteworthy for a prominent apical impulse, a parasternal thrill, and a crescendo-decrescendo systolic murmur. The murmur usually is associated with a pronounced systolic ejection click. A diastolic murmur of aortic insufficiency may be noted, as well.

The electrocardiogram in children with valvar aortic stenosis demonstrates left ventricular hypertrophy, which correlates reasonably well with the magnitude of the transvalvar gradient. T-wave inversion in lead V_6 is a particularly helpful indicator of severe LVOTO. However, the

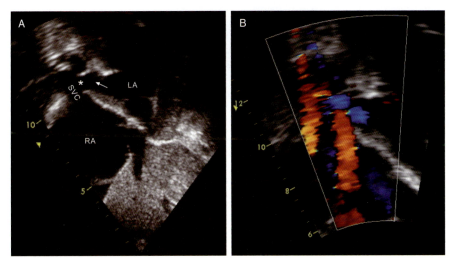

Plate 4.1 A/B, Subcostal short axis view shows a sinus venosus defect (*) with flow retrograde in the right upper pulmonary vein (arrow) directed across the defect into the superior vena cava.

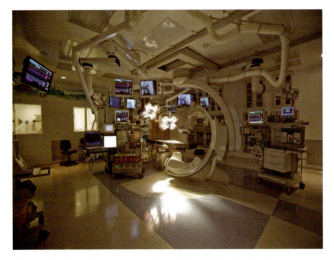

Plate 5.1 Hybrid operating suite with digital, single-plane, ceiling-mounted cardiac flat-panel detector (Toshiba America Medical Systems, Tustin, CA) at Nationwide Children's Hospital, opened October 2007 [2].

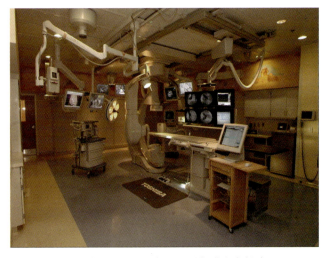

Plate 5.2 Hybrid interventional suite with digital, biplane imaging system (Toshiba America Medical Systems, Tustin, CA) at Nationwide Children's Hospital, opened June 2004.

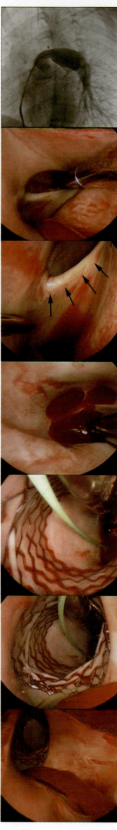

Plate 5.3 19-year-old female with a history of tetralogy of Fallot repair (including RVOT patch), who underwent pulmonary valve replacement as well as intraoperative placement of a Max LD stent to treat a proximal LPA fold, using direct vision with endoscopic guidance. The top image shows the LPA kink, identified during preprocedural cardiac catheterization. The following images document the endoscopic evaluation of the LPA intraoperatively. Notable is the ridge/fold at the LPA origin (arrows). Before stent placement, endoscopic evaluation is used to evaluate the lobar branching. After stent deployment, endoscopic evaluation documents sufficient distance of the stent from lobar branching of the LPA. The LPA appears to be wide open. After deployment, the stent was "crimped" manually over the crest between LPA and RPA. The bottom image shows the LPA origin from a distance, with the vessel being widely patent (note the difference to the preprocedural images). (RVOT, right ventricular outflow tract; LPA, left pulmonary artery; RPA, right pulmonary artery.)

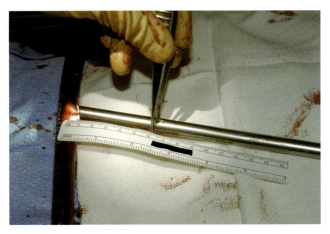

Plate 5.4 Stryker endoscope used for "hybrid" stent delivery under direct vision. The endoscope can be helpful in assessing the distance towards the origin of the pulmonary arterial side branches [2].

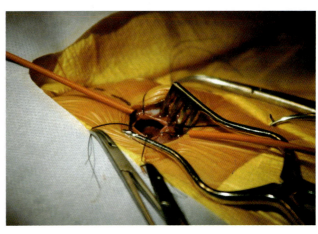

Plate 5.5 Lower midline sternotomy.

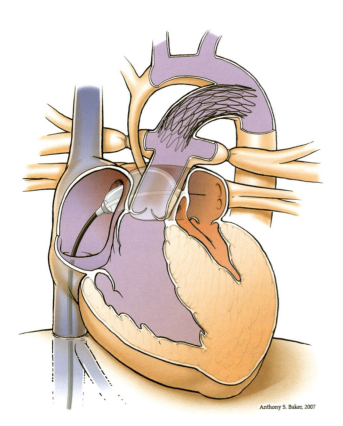

Plate 5.6 Bilateral pulmonary artery bands and a PDA stent via a median sternotomy followed by a balloon atrial septostomy several days later before discharge. (PDA, patent ductus arteriosus.) Reproduced with permission from Galantowicz et al. [71]. Hybrid approach for hypoplastic left heart syndrome: intermediate results after the learning curve. Ann Thorac Surg 85, 2063–2071. Copyright © 2008 Elsevier for Society of Thoracic Surgeons.

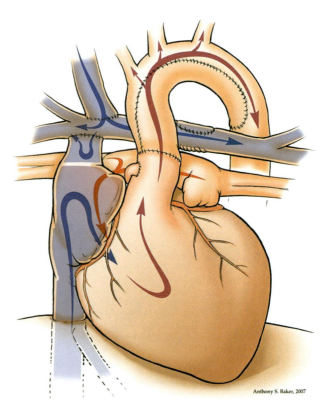

Plate 5.7 A modified cavopulmonary anastomosis. Reproduced with permission from Galantowicz et al. [71]. Hybrid approach for hypoplastic left heart syndrome: intermediate results after the learning curve. Ann Thorac Surg 85, 2063–2071. Copyright © 2008 Elsevier for Society of Thoracic Surgeons.

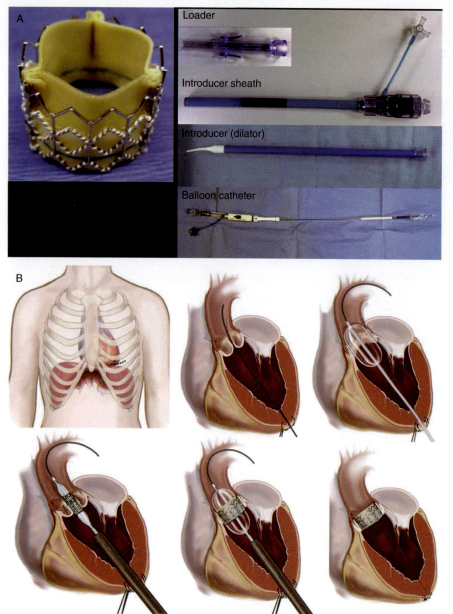

Plate 5.8 The Edwards–SAPIEN THV transapical delivery system. **A,** The bovine pericardial valve stent and short 33 Fr delivery system are labeled. **B,** Diagrams depicting the transapical puncture, balloon valvuloplasty, and delivery of the valve in the aortic position. Images courtesy of Edwards Lifesciences (Irvine, CA).

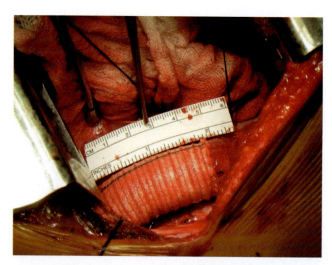

Plate 14.1 18 mm Hemashield interposition graft in a 12-year-old 40 kg child with a severe coarctation. Operation was performed with partial left heart bypass.

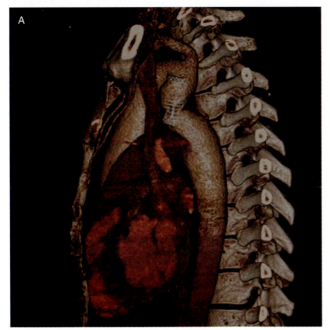

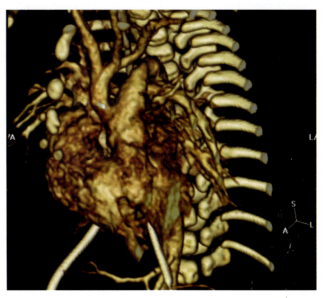

Plate 19.1 A cardiac computed tomography with three-dimensional reconstruction in a 1-day-old neonate demonstrates type A aortic arch interruption with truncus arteriosus and a patent ductus arteriosus to the descending aorta. Courtesy of Kenneth Zahka, MD.

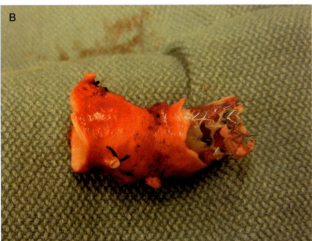

Plate 14.2 A, Three-dimensional reconstruction CT scan of a stent placed in the coarctation of a 30-year-old patient. The stent only dilated the lumen to 6mm. The coarctation and stent were resected and replaced with a #24-mm diameter graft using left heart bypass. **B,** The excised coarctation showing the stent and friable thrombus material (in the proximal position of the stent).

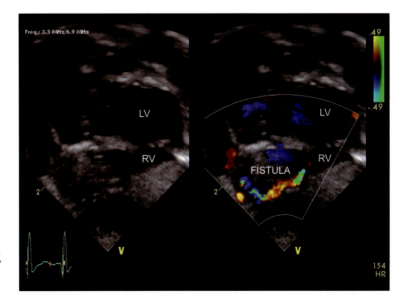

Plate 21.1 Echocardiography with color Doppler demonstration of coronary right ventricular fistula. (LV, left ventricle; RV, right ventricle.)

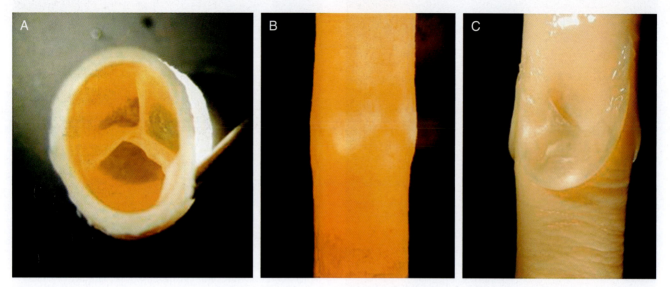

Plate 24.1 Bovine jugular venous valved conduit (Contegra). **A,** Cross-sectional view. **B,** Outside view showing sinuses. **C,** Inside-out view. Reproduced with permission from Medtronic (Minneapolis, MN).

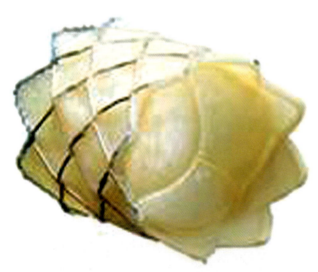

Plate 24.2 Melody® TPV. Reproduced with permission from Medtronic (Minneapolis, MN).

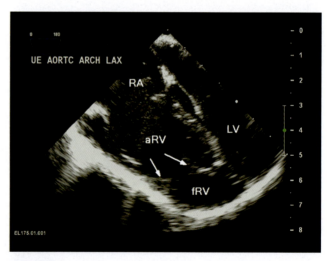

Plate 29.1 Intraoperative transthoracic echocardiogram demonstrating Ebstein anomaly. Arrows demonstrate the dysplasia and displacement of the tricuspid valve leaflets. (aRV, atrialized right ventricle; fRV, functional right ventricle; LV, left ventricle; RA, right atrium.)

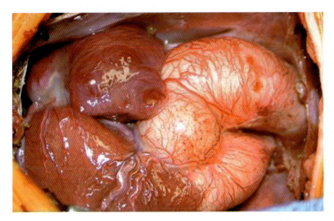

Plate 32.1 Intraoperative photograph of type II aortico-left ventricular tunnel demonstrating large aortic wall aneurysm of the tunnel.

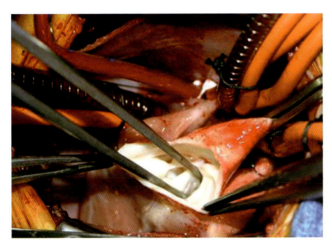

Plate 32.2 Intraoperative photograph of type II aortico-left ventricular tunnel demonstrating oval opening (with forceps passing through aortico-left ventricular tunnel) and aortic valve directly posterior. Note that the aortic valve shows central stenosis and commissural fusion.

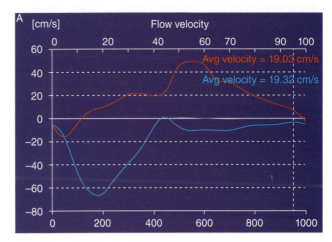

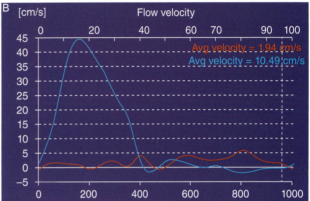

Plate 34.1 Flow velocity by magnetic resonance angiography (MRA) in an unobstructed left upper pulmonary vein (**A**) and through an obstructed right upper pulmonary vein (**B**). Note the monophasic and low-velocity flow in the obstructed vein (red line). Courtesy of Dr Shi-Joon Yoo and Mr Omar Thabit.

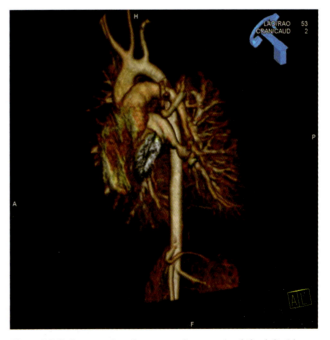

Plate 34.2 Post-repair pulmonary vein stenosis of the left side pulmonary veins at the insertion in the venous confluence. Courtesy of Dr Shi-Joon Yoo and Mr Omar Thabit.

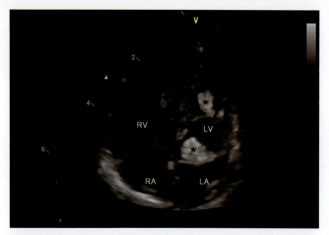

Plate 39.1 Cardiac rhabdomyoma, echocardiographic features. This four-chamber view demonstrates multiple rhabdomyomas (*) in the left and right ventricle. (LA, left atrium; LV, left ventricle; RA, right atrium; RV, right ventricle.) Courtesy of Dr Manfred Vogt, Echo Lab, Department of Pediatric Cardiology, German Heart Center, Munich, Germany.

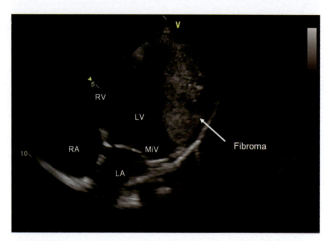

Plate 39.2 Cardiac fibroma, echocardiographic features. This four-chamber view demonstrates a large fibroma located in the left ventricle (*). (LA, left atrium; LV, left ventricle; MiV, mitral valve; RA, right atrium; RV, right ventricle.) Courtesy of Dr Manfred Vogt, Echo Lab, Department of Pediatric Cardiology, German Heart Center, Munich, Germany.

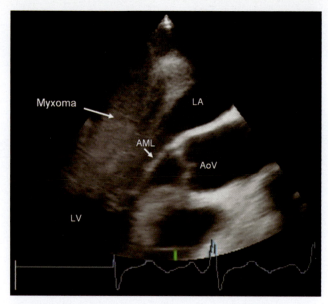

Plate 39.3 Cardiac myxoma, echocardiographic features. Transesophageal echocardiography showing a large left atrial myxoma obstructing the mitral valve during diastole. (LA, left atrium; AML, anterior mitral valve leaflet; AoV, aortic valve; LV, left ventricle.) Courtesy of Dr. Richard Henze, Echo Lab, Institute of Anesthesiology, German Heart Center, Munich, Germany.

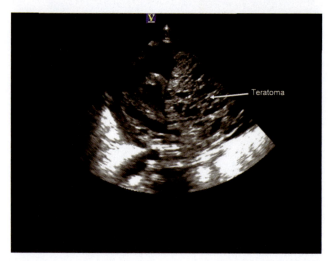

Plate 39.4 Intrapericardial teratoma, echocardiographic features. Large intrapericardial teratoma. Courtesy of Dr. Richard Henze, Echo Lab, Institute of Anesthesiology, German Heart Center, Munich, Germany.

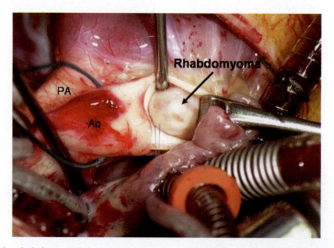

Plate 39.5 Intraoperative view of a rhabdomyoma located in the left ventricular outflow tract. (Ao, aorta; PA, pulmonary artery.)

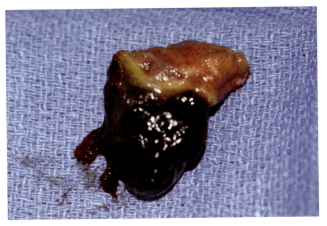

Plate 39.6 Surgically resected left atrial myxoma.

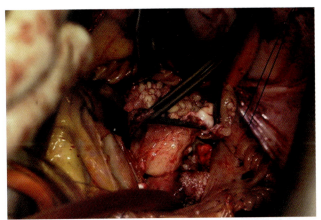

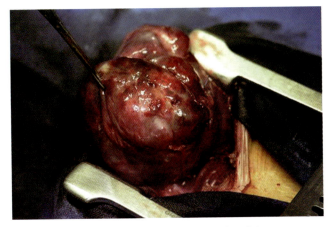

Plate 39.7 Intraoperative view of an intrapericardial teratoma.

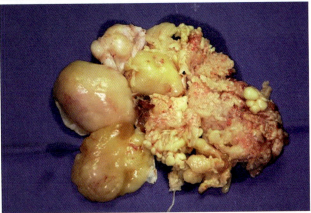

Plate 39.8 Intraoperative view of a left atrial myosarcoma (top). Surgically resected myosarcoma (bottom).

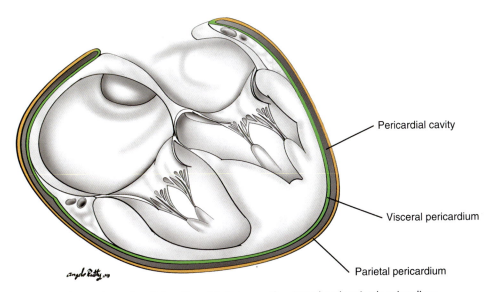

Plate 40.1 Heart and pericardium. The pericardial cavity exists between the visceral and parietal pericardium.

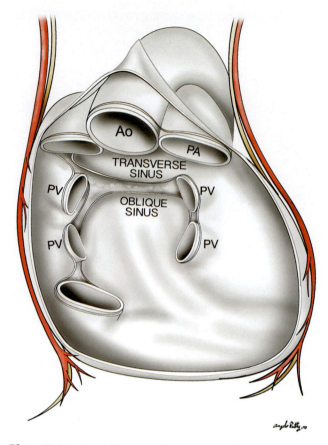

Plate 40.2 Pericardial recesses. The transverse sinus lays behind the aorta (Ao) and main pulmonary artery (PA) and the oblique sinus extends behind the left atrium in the region between all four pulmonary veins (PV).

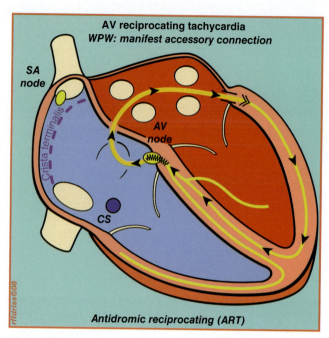

Plate 41.1 Atrioventricular (AV) reciprocating tachycardia. Wolff-Parkinson-White (WPW) syndrome or manifest accessory connection. During sinus rhythm with preexcitation, conduction from the sinus node to the ventricles proceeds simultaneously over two routes, the atrioventricular node and the accessory connection. The wave front traversing the accessory connection depolarizes ventricular tissue first, because of intrinsic slowing of conduction at the atrioventricular node. The accessory connection thus "preexcites" ventricular depolarization, giving rise to the delta wave. As depicted, there is blocked conduction in the atrioventricular node, with conduction proceeding to the ventricles via the accessory connection (preexcited). Conduction delay is encountered in ventricular muscle, allowing the wave front to proceed up the atrioventricular node (which has had time to regain conduction) to the atrium. This re-entrant circuit is termed "antidromic reciprocating tachycardia"; the "playing field" includes the atria, accessory connection, ventricles, and the atrioventricular node. Reproduced with permission from Mavroudis et al. [37,41]. Arrhythmia surgery in patients with and without congenital heart disease. Ann Thorac Surg 86, 857–868. Copyright © 2008 Elsevier for Society of Thoracic Surgeons.

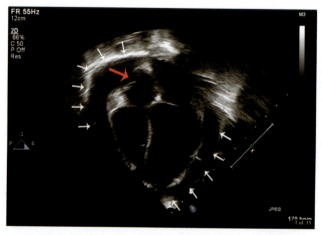

Plate 40.3 Transthoracic echocardiogram showing a large pericardial effusion with signs of tamponade. Note the large circumferential pericardial effusion (white arrows) with right atrial diastolic collapse (red arrow).

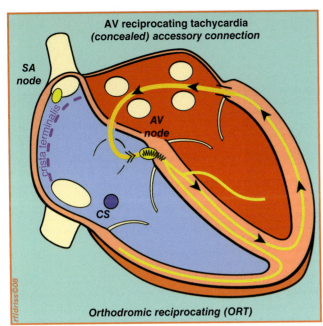

AV reciprocating tachycardia (concealed) accessory connection

SA node

Crista terminalis

AV node

CS

Orthodromic reciprocating (ORT)

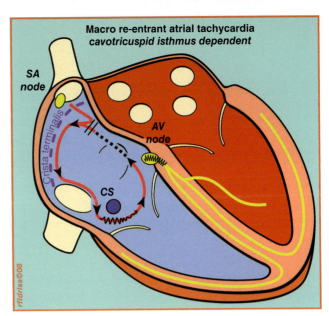

Macro re-entrant atrial tachycardia cavotricuspid isthmus dependent

SA node

Crista terminalis

AV node

CS

Plate 41.2 Atrioventricular reciprocating tachycardia depicting concealed Wolff-Parkinson-White (WPW) syndrome. Orthodromic reciprocating tachycardia, the more common form of tachycardia, utilizing an accessory connection. Conduction is blocked in the accessory connection, thus losing the delta wave (now "concealed"). Conduction proceeds normally through the AV node to the ventricle. The delay encountered in the AV node allows the accessory connection to regain electrical function, and the electrical impulse then enters the atria from the opposite direction, from ventricle to atrium, across the accessory connection. This "playing field" includes the atria, atrioventricular node, ventricles, and accessory connection. Reproduced with permission from Mavroudis *et al.* [37,41]. Arrhythmia surgery in patients with and without congenital heart disease. Ann Thorac Surg 86, 857–868. Copyright © 2008 Elsevier for Society of Thoracic Surgeons.

Plate 41.3 Cavotricuspid isthmus dependent macro re-entrant atrial tachycardia. As depicted, the "playing field" is the right atrium, where a premature atrial contraction might encounter block in the atrial septum (broken line) and proceed in an alternate route down the right atrial free wall. The wave front may encounter an area of slow conduction (squiggly arrow), in this case between the inferior vena cava, tricuspid valve, and the coronary sinus (CS). The delay encountered as the wave front traverses the area of slow conduction allows the atrial septum to recover conduction. The wave front exits the isthmus and proceeds up the atrial septum. Interruption of this circuit is targeted at the inferior isthmus owing to the clearly identified landmarks in proximity. (AV, atrioventricular; CS, coronary sinus; SA, sino-atrial.) Reproduced with permission from Mavroudis *et al.* [37,41]. Arrhythmia surgery in patients with and without congenital heart disease. Ann Thorac Surg 86, 857–868. Copyright © 2008 Elsevier for Society of Thoracic Surgeons.

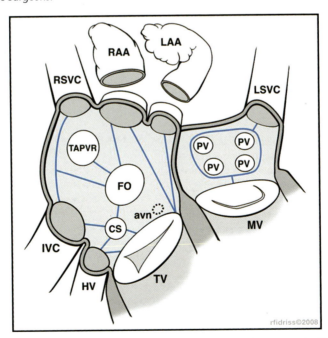

Plate 41.4 Schematic representation of the possible lines of ablation to treat macro re-entrant atrial tachycardia in the presence of various atrial anomalies associated with complex congenital heart disease. These atrial anomalies do not generally occur together, and the demonstrated lines of block are not meant to be incorporated into every operation. They are depicted only as guidelines on which to base an ablative operation when unusual anatomic obstacles are encountered in the performance of the maze procedure. (avn, atrioventricular node; CS, coronary sinus; FO, foramen ovale; HV, hepatic vein; IVC, inferior vena cava; LAA, left atrial appendage; LSVC, left superior vena cava; MV, mitral valve; PV, pulmonary veins; RAA, right atrial appendage; RSVC, right superior vena cava; TAPVR, total anomalous pulmonary venous return; TV, tricuspid valve.) Reproduced with permission from Mavroudis *et al.* [37,41]. Arrhythmia surgery in patients with and without congenital heart disease. Ann Thorac Surg 86, 857–868. Copyright © 2008 Elsevier for Society of Thoracic Surgeons.

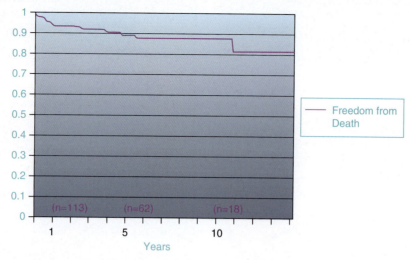

Plate 41.5 Kaplan-Meier curve showing freedom from death in 126 patients who underwent Fontan conversion with arrhythmia surgery. Reproduced with permission from Mavroudis *et al.* [37]. Late reoperations for Fontan patients: state of the art invited review. Eur J Cardiothorac Surg 34, 1034–1040. Copyright © 2008 Oxford Journals for European Association for Cardio-Thoracic Surgery and the European Society of Thoracic Surgeons.

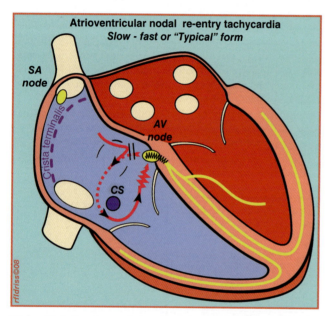

Plate 41.6 Slow-fast or "typical" form of atrioventricular (AV) nodal re-entry tachycardia. Atrioventricular conduction encounters a block in the normal fast pathway fibers superior to the compact AV node. The wave front proceeds towards the atrial isthmus, between the coronary sinus (CS) and tricuspid valve, and encounters slowing through the "slow pathway" fibers of the AV node. Exiting the isthmus, conduction is now able to reenter the fast pathway fibers, located anteriorly and superiorly, and perpetuate a reentrant circuit; simultaneously, conduction proceeds inferiorly to the ventricles. Of note, conduction to the ventricles is not relevant to the tachycardia circuit. Cryoablation of the inferior isthmus region will interrupt the circuit. (AV, atrioventricular; CS, coronary sinus; SA, sinoatrial). Reproduced with permission from Mavroudis *et al.* [41]. Arrhythmia surgery in patients with and without congenital heart disease. Ann Thorac Surg 86, 857–868. Copyright © 2008 Elsevier for Society of Thoracic Surgeons.

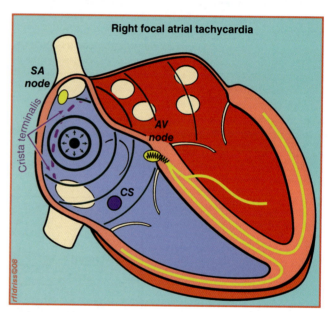

Plate 41.7 Right focal atrial tachycardia. Focal atrial tachycardia, a localized area of "impulse initiation" that is most commonly automatic in mechanism, firing repeatedly, rapidly, and independent of normal sinus function, which is inhibited. Impulse conduction is spread in a centripetal fashion across the atria, thence to the atrioventricular (AV) node and ventricles. Ablative therapy is aimed at obliteration or isolation of this localized discrete area ("hot spot"). (AV, atrioventricular; CS, coronary sinus; SA, sinoatrial; WPW, Wolff-Parkinson-White.) Reproduced with permission from Mavroudis *et al.* [41]. Arrhythmia surgery in patients with and without congenital heart disease. Ann Thorac Surg 86, 857–868. Copyright © 2008 Elsevier for Society of Thoracic Surgeons.

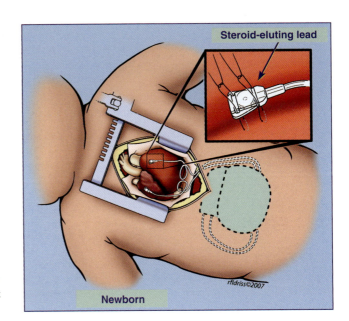

Plate 41.8 Dual-chamber pacing leads as placed through a full sternotomy in a neonate. The steroid-eluting leads are directly affixed to the epicardium with two 5-0 polypropylene sutures. Reproduced with permission from Kelle *et al.* [169]. Dual-chamber epicardial pacing in neonates with congenital heart block. J Thorac Cardiovasc Surg 134, 1188–1192.

Plate 41.9 A pocket for the pacemaker is created beneath both rectus muscles. Through a midline incision extending nearly to the umbilicus, bilateral subcutaneous flaps are created, allowing mobilization of the anterior rectus sheath. The anterior rectus sheath is entered on either side of the linea alba. This opening is extended vertically to free up the anterior rectus sheath. Next, the rectus muscle is dissected off the posterior rectus sheath. The pacemaker is implanted just above the posterior rectus sheath. The peritoneum is not entered. The rectus muscles are reapproximated in the midline with interrupted polyglactin sutures (Vicryl; Ethicon, Inc., Johnson & Johnson, New Brunswick, NJ), providing a muscular padding for the pacemaker. The subcutaneous layer is approximated with running polyglactin and the skin with subcuticular polydioxanone or interrupted nylon. Reproduced with permission from Kelle *et al.* [169]. Dual-chamber epicardial pacing in neonates with congenital heart block. J Thorac Cardiovasc Surg 134, 1188–1192.

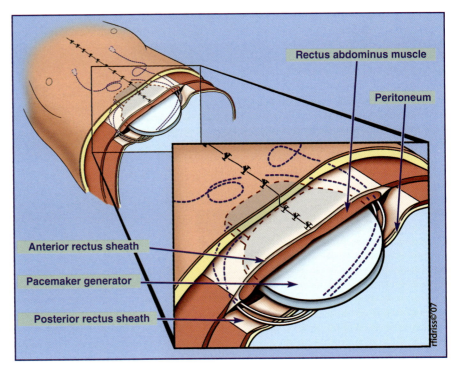

Plate 42.1 Age distribution of pediatric heart recipients for transplants from January 1996 through June 2008. Reproduced with permission from Kirk R, Edwards LB, Aurora P, *et al.* (2009) Registry of the International Society for Heart and Lung Transplantation: Twelfth Official Pediatric Heart Transplantation Report – 2009. J Heart Lung Transplant 28, 993–1006. Copyright © 2009 International Society for Heart and Lung Transplantation.

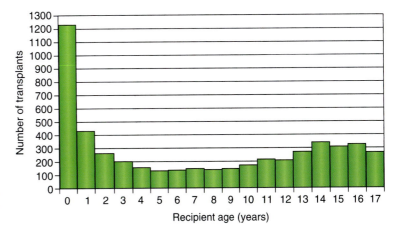

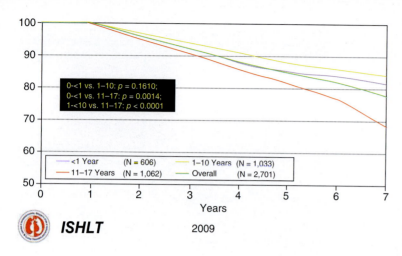

| | <1 Year | (N = 606) | | 1–10 Years | (N = 1,033) |
| 11–17 Years | (N = 1,062) | | Overall | (N = 2,701) |

Years

ISHLT   2009

Plate 42.2 Pediatric heart transplantation: conditional Kaplan-Meier survival for recent era (transplants 1/1999 to 6/2007).

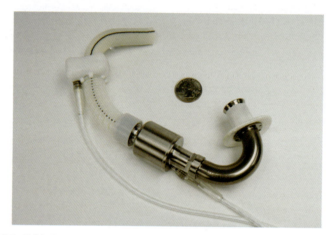

Plate 45.1 Micromed DeBakey VAD *Child*. Courtesy of micromedcv.com; Houston, Texas, USA.

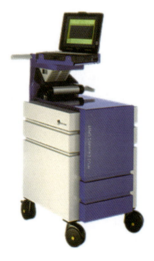

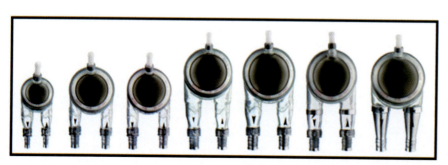

Plate 45.2 Driver controller for Berlin Heart EXCOR Pediatric VAD (top) and range of pump sizes (bottom). Courtesy of Berlin Heart, Inc. The Woodlands, Texas, USA.

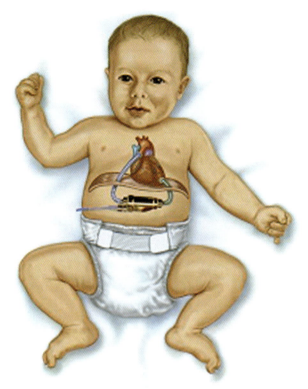

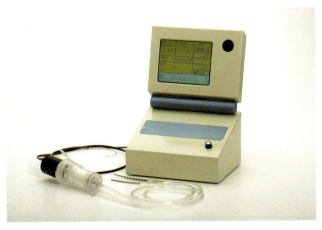

Plate 45.4 The prototype Ension Pediatric Cardiopulmonary Assist System (pCAS). The system is comprised of an integrated pump-oxygenator and a control console based on a touchscreen-driven user interface. Courtesy of Ension, Inc, Pittsburgh, Pennsylvania, USA.

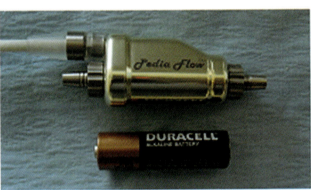

Plate 45.3 University of Pittsburgh PediaFlow Ventricular Assist System for Infants and Toddlers. Courtesy of University of Pittsburgh, Harvey Borovetz; Pittsburgh, Pennsylvania, USA.

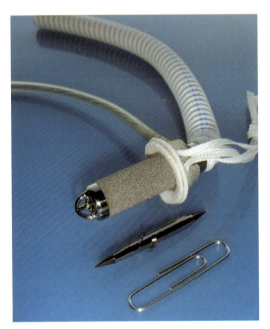

Plate 45.5 The infant Jarvik 2000 heart is 1 cm diameter, 4 cc volume, and weighs 11 g. It is positioned in the apex of the left ventricle with either a 6 mm or 8 mm outflow graft to the aorta. Pump flow ranges from 0.25 L/min up to 3 L/min, as the speed is increased from 20 000 to 45 000 RPM. Courtesy of Jarvik Heart, Inc, New York, USA.

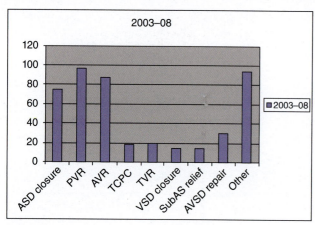

Plate 46.1 Surgical interventions performed at the Royal Brompton Hospital in adult CHD patients between 2003 and 2008. The majority of the operations were ASD closures, pulmonary valve replacements in patients with TOF or previous repair of pulmonary stenosis, and aortic valve replacements (mostly in patients with a bicuspid aortic valve). (ASD, atrial septal defect; AVR, aortic valve replacement; AVSD, atrioventricular septal defect; CHD, congenital heart disease; PVR, pulmonary valve replacement; SubAS, subaortic stenosis; TCPC, total cavopulmonary connection; TOF, tetralogy of Fallot; TVR, tricuspid valve replacement; VSD, ventricular septal defect.)

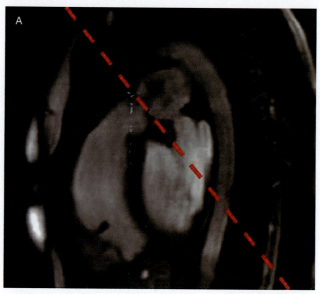

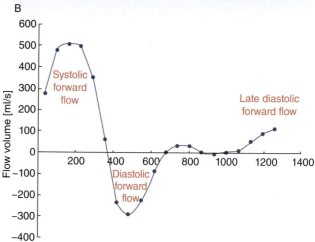

Plate 46.2 A, Right ventricular outflow tract (RVOT) cardiovascular magnetic resonance cine image obtained from a patient with repaired tetralogy of Fallot with significant late pulmonary regurgitation. The red dotted line illustrates the throughplane in which a nonbreath-hold phase encoded velocity map was acquired. **B,** Flow curve obtained from the same patient. Through integrating areas containing forward and reverse flow, a pulmonary regurgitation fraction of 34% was calculated. Reproduced with permission from Shinebourne *et al.* [168]. Tetralogy of Fallot: from fetus to adult. Heart 92, 1353–1359. Copyright © 2006 BMJ Publishing Group Ltd for British Cardiovascular Society.

correlation between the severity of aortic stenosis and the presence of electrocardiographic abnormalities is very poor [14]. Exercise electrocardiogram may further help to demonstrate physiologically important aortic stenosis as evidenced by ST segment depression and may help guide treatment strategies for patients with less well defined degrees of obstruction. Exercise tests for children with valvar aortic stenosis, in contradistinction to such examinations performed in adults with this lesion, can be performed with very low risk of untoward events.

Chest radiography findings in the child with aortic valve stenosis are often normal, although cardiomegaly or a subtle blunting of the left ventricular apex may be described. Post-stenotic dilation of the aortic root is uncommon until late childhood or early adolescence. Echocardiography and Doppler flow studies are highly reliable for valvar aortic stenosis in children and may reduce the necessity for cardiac catheterization. The correlation between the echo-Doppler and catheter measurement of cardiac gradient is usually good. Catheterization, if needed, most often is required for delineation of additional defects. In addition, therapeutic percutaneous balloon valvoplasty is being performed with encouraging results in this age group.

Treatment

Indications and Timing for Intervention
Any symptoms such as angina, syncope, or congestive heart failure with a hemodynamically significant aortic valve pressure gradient (peak-to-peak gradient >50 mmHg) constitutes an absolute indication for intervention. Severe valvar stenosis with a pressure gradient greater than 75 mmHg is also considered an indication for treatment, even without symptoms.

Mild-to-moderate stenosis (peak-to-peak gradient <40 mmHg) in asymptomatic patients is usually well tolerated. Although the nature of the disease is progressive in a large percentage of patients, it is usually safe to follow these patients with regular noninvasive studies, including electrocardiogram with exercise test and echocardiography. On average, the transvalvar gradient increases by 1 mmHg per year [77]. Echocardiographic evidence of progressive left ventricular hypertrophy, electrocardiographic evidence of left ventricular strain or ischemia, and the presence of ventricular arrhythmia are also strong indications for therapeutic intervention. Controversy exists as to the optimal treatment for asymptomatic patients with pressure gradients between 45 and 75 mmHg. Although each patient should be evaluated individually, evidence suggests that early intervention is beneficial in these patients.

Percutaneous Balloon Valvuloplasty
Percutaneous balloon valvuloplasty is often feasible in this age group. With advances in catheter techniques, balloon valvuloplasty is being applied to an increasing number of cases, even in patients who have undergone procedures for valvar aortic stenosis [78,79].

Surgical Valvotomy and Valvuloplasty
Aortic valvotomy is the standard treatment for congenital aortic stenosis for most children [61,80]. Surgical valvuloplasty is preferable to valve replacement in patients with nonregurgitant trileaflet valves [45]. In cases of recurrent valvar stenosis and regurgitation, extended aortic valvuloplasty has been described [81,82]. Aortic valve repair by multiple techniques, including pericardial leaflet extension, has been reported recently by multiple authors [83–86].

Cardiopulmonary bypass, moderate systemic hypothermia, and antegrade cold cardioplegia are used commonly for extended aortic valvuloplasty. Retrograde cardioplegia, given through the coronary sinus, may be desirable if significant aortic insufficiency is present. Exposure of the aortic valve is through a standard oblique aortotomy toward the noncoronary sinus of Valsalva. The aortic cusp is augmented by extending the commissurotomy incision into the aortic wall around the leaflet incision. The valve cusp attachment is mobilized at the commissures, and the aortic insertion of the rudimentary commissure is freed.

Most commonly, a bicuspid valve is present, with fused commissures that can be divided with a knife to within 1–2 mm of the aortic wall. Care must be taken to distinguish between true commissural fusion and a false raphe, which is frequently present in one of the bicuspid leaflets. It represents a rudimentary commissure but does not reach the wall of the aorta and offers no lateral support. An incision in a false raphe will cause valve incompetence and should be avoided. Congenitally stenotic tricuspid aortic valves are rare. Valve deformity and commissural fusion are usually present, which could make the distinction from a bicuspid valve difficult. When the diagnosis of a stenotic tricuspid aortic valve is uncertain, it should be treated as a bicuspid aortic valve to avoid creating valve insufficiency.

Unicuspid valves are less common in this age group. The technique of valvotomy is similar to that for neonates. Once again, a conservative valvotomy is advisable, because a small incision may reduce significantly the valvar stenosis, and valvar insufficiency is usually the cause of early valve replacement.

Aortic Valve Replacement in Children
It is estimated that within 10–20 years after initial valvotomy, 35% of children will require replacement of their aortic valves [47,71]. Under certain circumstances, repeat valvotomy can be performed if it is expected to relieve the stenosis, even though eventual valve replacement is

inevitable [81,87]. By delaying aortic valve replacement, it is possible to insert a larger size prosthesis and delay the need for anticoagulation and its attendant complications.

The selection of an optimal aortic prosthesis for the pediatric patient is difficult because of several limiting factors. All types of prosthetic valves have inherent drawbacks which are unique in young patients. Both porcine bioprostheses and allograft aortic valves are available in annular sizes suitable for smaller patients, but both valves suffer accelerated calcification and degeneration in the aortic position [88,89]. Such degeneration can lead to restenosis and regurgitation as early as 2 years after valve replacement. Consequently, the use of bioprosthetic and homograft aortic valves is severely limited by the prospect of frequent reoperations. The etiology of prosthetic valve degeneration in the pediatric population is unknown.

Mechanical prostheses do not suffer from limited durability [90]; however, the higher incidence of thromboembolic events associated with mechanical valve use necessitates long-term warfarin anticoagulation that is often poorly tolerated and difficult to monitor in young children.

A pulmonary autograft (Ross procedure) is another viable alternative for aortic valve replacement; this procedure was originally described by Donald Ross in 1967 [42–45,90,91]. The principle of this operation is to replace the aortic valve with the patient's own pulmonary valve, and a cryopreserved pulmonary allograft replaces the native pulmonary valve. The advantage of this operation is the placement of the patient's own pulmonary valve, which has the potential for growth, in the high-pressure aortic position to provide a durable valve, avoiding the potential for immunologic degeneration. The allograft valve, on the other hand, is placed in the low-pressure pulmonary position, which should be well tolerated even if the valve fails over time.

To perform the Ross procedure, cardiopulmonary bypass is established by aortic cannulation and bicaval venous drainage (Figure 30.2) [37]. Once cardioplegia is delivered, the aortic root is explored through a transverse incision. The technique we prefer is the root replacement. The aortic valve leaflets and sinuses are then removed, leaving only the aortic valve annulus. The coronary ostia, with a generous rim of aortic wall around them, are mobilized for coronary implantation. The pulmonary artery is opened transversely before its bifurcation, with great care taken not to damage the origin of the branch pulmonary arteries, and the pulmonary valve is inspected from above. If the pulmonary valve is acceptable, the main pulmonary artery is divided completely. With the guide of a right-angle clamp, a transverse incision is made in the anterior wall of the right ventricular outflow tract a few millimeters below the pulmonary valve. The critical part of valve har-

vesting is to leave an adequate cuff of right ventricular outflow tract muscle for suturing, without damaging the pulmonary valve, and to avoid injury to the first septal branch of the left anterior descending coronary artery. A shallower incision of the endocardial surface is made at the septum to avoid this pitfall. Once this pulmonary autograft is harvested, it is sutured to the aortic annulus using continuous or interrupted polypropylene suture. We prefer short, running sutures and a second adventitial layer over the posterior part of the circumference to decrease the risk of inaccessible hemorrhage. The coronary arteries are then implanted by continuous suture into circular openings made in the pulmonary arterial wall at the appropriate sites. Occasionally, in a small child or infant, the left coronary artery is harvested as a U-shaped button and implanted into a U-shaped defect in the pulmonary artery autograft wall. Its distal end thus becomes part of the distal aortic anastomosis. The distal pulmonary artery autograft-to-distal aorta anastomosis is then completed. A dose of cardioplegia solution is then given to assess the neoaortic valve function, to test the suture lines for leaks, and to make sure that the coronary arteries fill adequately. After reconstruction of the aorta, a cryopreserved valved pulmonary allograft is used to re-establish right ventricular-to-pulmonary artery continuity. This aortic root replacement represents the most popular surgical technique, and it can be used to deal with various aortic pathologies. Other surgical techniques of the pulmonary autograft procedure include the inclusion cylinder and scalloped subcoronary implantation, although they are technically more complicated and are less popular.

Dilatation of the pulmonary autograft is a major concern after root replacement using the Ross operation. There are some modified techniques associated with the Ross operation that may be used in order to prevent pulmonary autograft annular dilatation. Many groups have described wrapping the autograft with pericardium, Dacron, or Teflon felt at the annular level. However, none of these techniques provides support for the entire autograft with nondilatable material [92–94]. Ungerleider and colleagues have described the inclusion technique with a Dacron tube for the Ross operation [95]. However, this technique, which may limit the potential for autograft dilatation, is limited to the adult patient whose autograft growth is no longer necessary. Both techniques (conventional and inclusion) have been associated with excellent survival, as well as similar rates of long-term autograft failure, in recent reports. For root replacement, autograft dilatation was the main cause of failure. For the inclusion technique, autograft valve prolapse was the main cause of failure [96].

The technical challenge, and the potential for converting a single-valve disease into a two-valve problem, has created

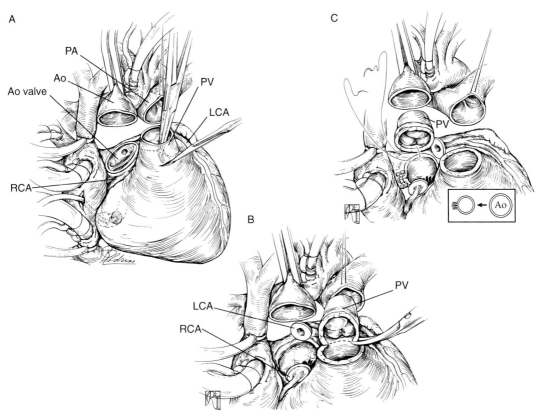

Figure 30.2 A, Conditions for the Ross procedure have been established by aortobicaval cardiopulmonary bypass, aortic cross-clamping, retrograde cardioplegia, and aortic resection. Shown here is the pulmonary autograft being harvested from the right ventricular outflow tract. The right-angle clamp ensures ventriculotomy below the pulmonary valve leaflets. Care is taken to avoid injury to the left coronary artery (LCA), the pulmonary valve structure, and the septal perforator coronary arteries. **B,** The pulmonary autograft harvest is being completed while the right and left coronary artery buttons have been formed and dissected for maximal mobilization. **C,** The pulmonary autograft is now being implanted in the left ventricular outflow tract using a running suture technique. Note that the aortic annulus has been made smaller by annular reduction using pledget-supported sutures. **D,** The neoaorta is shown in the act of reconstruction after implantation and left coronary artery anastomosis. The right coronary artery (RCA) is being anastomosed to the anterior facing sinus of Valsalva. **E,** The completed neoaortic reconstruction is shown after cross-clamp removal. The proximal homograft anastomosis has been completed and the distal connection to the confluence of pulmonary arteries is being performed. **F,** Completed Ross procedure is shown after separation from cardiopulmonary bypass. (Ao, aorta; PA, pulmonary artery; PV, pulmonary valve.)

a certain reservation toward the Ross operation as the procedure of choice in patients with valvar aortic stenosis. Although it has been shown to be safe and effective in relieving all types of LVOTO, there are concerns about the durability and the potential for growth of the pulmonary autograft in the aortic position and the fate of the pulmonary allograft in the pulmonary position [97]. However, full anticoagulation in the young child or infant, combined with the lack of growth potential of the traditional valve prostheses with the necessity of reoperation, are not small matters. This increasing appreciation of the lack of a better alternative has resulted in the renewed interest in pulmonary autograft in the pediatric population. Increasing experience with the Ross procedure has demonstrated that,

although it may be the best possible alternative at present for most pediatric patients, it is far from ideal and has its own problems.

Some type of annulus enlargement procedure usually is required with aortic valve replacement using mechanical prostheses, bioprosthetic prostheses, or autografts in the use of a small aortic annulus. Annulus-valve size mismatch is a common problem in the pediatric population; even the smallest available prosthesis (about 16–17 mm) may not fit without enlarging the annulus. In addition, prostheses larger than 16–17 mm are preferable in order to avoid or delay the need for valve replacement as these patients grow. An aortic–mitral annulus enlarging procedure (Manouguian or Nicks procedure) can be used to

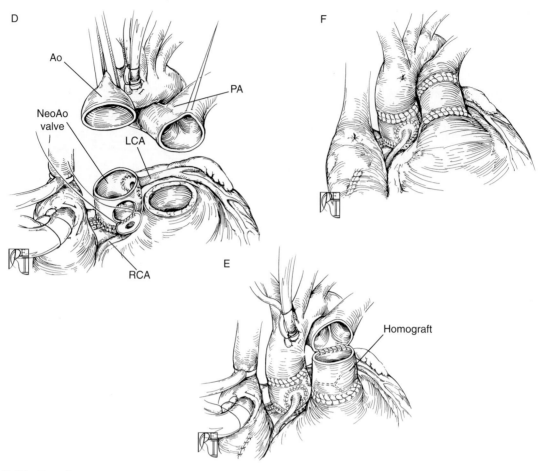

D

Ao

PA

NeoAo valve

LCA

RCA

F

E

Homograft

Figure 30.2 (*Continued*)

enlarge the aortic annulus [98,99]. Alternatively, a Konno-Rastan procedure (Figure 30.3) [37,100,101] is used commonly for annulus enlargement and has an acceptable early survival rate of 84% [98,102]. The classic Konno-Rastan procedure will enlarge the entire LVOT in addition to the aortic annulus. The modified Konno-Rastan procedure (Figure 30.4) [37] will limit the enlargement of the LVOT, exclusive of the aortic valve annulus. When significant enlargement of the LVOT is required, avoiding a prosthetic valve, a more complex anterior enlargement is useful. Combining the classic Konno-Rastan aortoventriculoplasty with the Ross procedure (Ross-Konno procedure) will relieve all subaortic, as well as valvar, stenosis (Figure 30.5) [37,41,103,104]. The Ross procedure part is essentially similar to that described earlier. The ascending aorta is transected transversely, and the aortic leaflets are resected down to the aortic annulus. A longitudinal incision is made in the aortic root toward the commissure between the left and right coronary sinuses. Anteriorly, this incision is extended in an oblique fashion into the RVOT. Posteriorly, the interventricular septum is incised leftward

to avoid the conduction system, thereby enlarging the LVOT. The incision is augmented to the desired size using an appropriately shaped Gore-Tex or Dacron patch. This allows implantation of the larger pulmonary autograft and relieves the LVOTO. The pulmonary autograft is then sutured into the enlarged LVOT as in the standard Ross procedure. The incision in the RVOT is then repaired with a prosthetic patch or bovine pericardium. In smaller children or in infants, the interventricular septum can be enlarged by using the muscle cuff of the pulmonary autograft, harvested with extra length anteriorly, although some authors caution against this practice due to residual left-to-right shunts and aneurysm formation into the RVOT [85,105]. To avoid this problem, the Ross-Konno procedure can be accomplished by excision of the small aortic annulus or a large part of it. This will result in interruption of the circular collar of the LVOT [85]. This maneuver will enlarge the LVOT and obviate the need for a large incision into the interventricular septum and RVOT (Figure 30.6) [85]. Alternatively, Mavroudis and associates [85] described a modified Ross-Konno procedure, which combines aortic

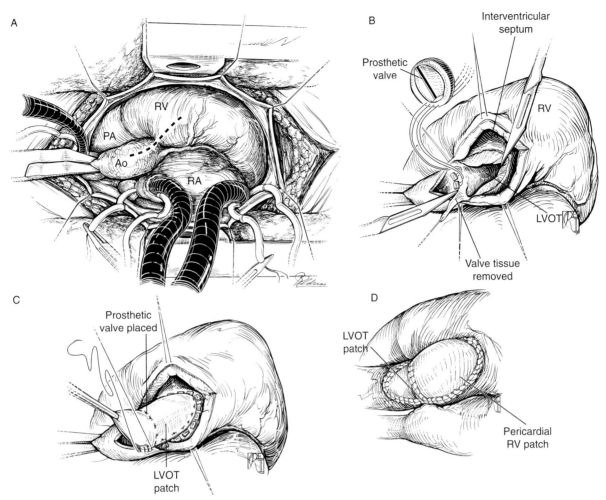

Figure 30.3 A, Operative conditions established to perform the classic Konno-Rastan operation, which involves aortic cross-clamping, cardioplegia (not shown), and the incision for aortoseptoplasty (dotted line). **B,** After the aorta is incised through the right ventricle (RV) and into the interventricular septum, the prosthetic valve can be implanted along the posterior aortic annulus. **C,** The anterior left ventricular outflow tract (LVOT) reconstruction is performed by augmenting the interventricular septum, attaching the prosthetic valve to the patch, and augmenting the ascending aorta as noted. **D,** Shown is the external reconstruction, noting the pericardial right ventricular outflow tract patch which was used to augment the subpulmonic area. (Ao, aorta; PA, pulmonary artery; RA, right atrium.)

annulus resection with an incision in the left ventricular free wall. This procedure has been associated with excellent outcomes without the attendant risk of complete heart block (Figure 30.7) [85].

Results

Balloon Valvuloplasty
Data suggest that the success rate of balloon valvuloplasty, with regard to relief of the transvalvar gradient, is comparable to that of surgical valvotomy [106,107]. Repeat balloon valvuloplasty is also possible in this age group, with good palliative results [107–109]. However, this is necessary in a minority of patients [58]. Although balloon val-

vuloplasty does incur a higher rate of aortic insufficiency than open surgical valvotomy, this appears to be less problematic in older children compared with neonates [58,108,110]. Furthermore, the excellent surgical results of the Ross operation are preserved in the context of initial balloon valvuloplasty [111].

Open Valvuloplasty and Valve Repair
Open surgical valvotomy remains the standard of care for isolated aortic stenosis in children. Recent literature demonstrates a low operative mortality (<5%) and excellent 10-year freedom from recurrent aortic stenosis or insufficiency (83% and 95%, respectively) [112]. The mortality of valvoplasty, however, is significantly higher if there is

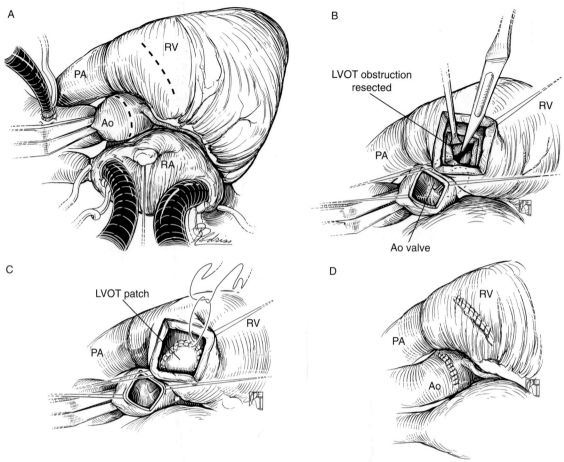

Figure 30.4 A, Operative conditions as indicated by aortic cross-clamp, cardioplegia administration (not shown), and right ventriculotomy site (dotted lines) in preparation for a modified Konno-Rastan procedure. **B,** The aortic valve is identified through the aortotomy. Shown here is sharp excision of the interventricular septum below the aortic valve annulus and away from the atrioventricular node. **C,** The subaortic left ventricular outflow tract (LVOT) is augmented by a patch which effectively closes the created ventricular septal defect. **D,** Completed right ventricular and aortic closures after the operation. (Ao, aorta, aortic; PA, pulmonary artery; RA, right atrium; RV, right ventricle.)

significant valvar regurgitation or if the valve is nontricuspid [45]. Under the latter circumstances, aortic valve replacement is preferable. The overall survival of reoperation in congenital aortic stenosis is reported to be 88.6% after 10 years [87]. Long-term results have been published, suggesting good survival (73% at 37 years), but a marked increase in the rate of intervention/death after approximately 15 years [113]. Aortic valve repair can be performed in some patients after previous balloon valvuloplasty with good intermediate-term results [114]: mean peak gradient of 32 mmHg and no more than mild regurgitation at follow-up after 22 months. Furthermore, recent results with pediatric aortic valve repair have been promising [115]. Alsoufi and associates reported their short-term and midterm results of aortic valve repair by cusp extension with autologous pericardium in 22 children who were 5–18 years of age [83]. Among these patients, 16 had previous surgical or

percutaneous intervention and 10 had a bicuspid aortic valve. The median follow-up was 1.7 years and ranged from 1 month to 5 years. Follow-up was 100% complete. No early or late mortality was observed, and the 5-year freedom from valve replacement was 75%. Although the overall cohort experienced a progression of their peak aortic gradients, those who had initial postoperative peak gradients less than 30 mmHg had stabilization of their gradients compared with those who had greater postoperative gradients.

Aortic Valve Replacement

Good clinical results, simplicity of performance, as well as the repeatability and safety of the technique, have made aortic valve replacement an important option in children. One recent report followed 45 children over the age of 1

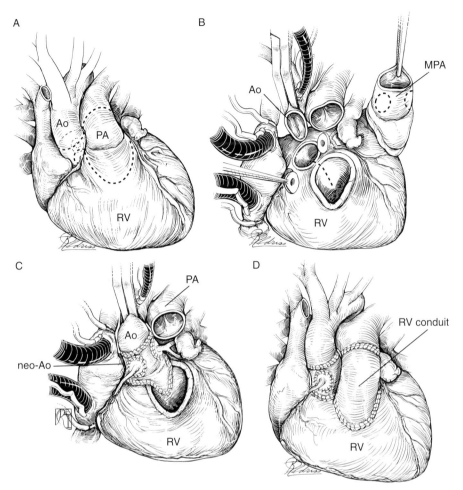

Figure 30.5 A, Intended incision and excision boundaries en route to the Ross-Konno procedure. **B,** After aortic cross-clamping, antegrade and retrograde cardioplegic arrest, aortic resection, coronary mobilization, and main pulmonary artery harvest, the interventricular septal incision is noted by the dotted line. The pulmonary autograft was harvested, with an extra portion of right ventricle to be used for the ventriculoseptoplasty part of this operation. **C,** The neoaortic left ventricular outflow reconstruction is shown using the pulmonary autograft extension into the interventricular septum ("apron extension"). **D,** The completed Ross–Konno procedure is shown after separation from cardiopulmonary bypass. (Ao, aorta, aortic; MAP, main pulmonary artery; PA, pulmonary artery; RV, right ventricle.)

year undergoing aortic valve replacement with bileaflet mechanical prostheses for an average of 9 years [116]. Over half of the patients required concomitant root enlargement procedures. Fifteen year results were excellent: survival was 92% and valve-related event-free survival was 86%. Another study confirmed the current low perioperative mortality in older patients (0%), and the normalization of left ventricular function and size [117]. However, it should be noted that at least one study showed a lower risk of complications (bleeding, thrombosis, infection) and an increased durability amongst biological valves [118].

Ross and Ross-Konno Procedure

It has been shown that the Ross procedure provides optimal hemodynamic performance with associated low valve-related complication rates, when compared with bioprosthetic and mechanical valves [119]. The Ross procedure is also associated with the regression of left ventricular dilatation and hypertrophy, and survival after pulmonary autograft replacement of the aortic valve is significantly better than with other types of valve replacement [120]. In addition, quality of life as reflected by the need for reoperation favors the Ross procedure, which has a freedom from reoperation of 87% after 9 years of follow-up [121]. A more recent study demonstrated improved results, with overall survival and freedom from reoperation of either the homograft or the autograft of 96.7% and 66.2%, respectively, at 10 years. Freedom from reoperation of the left ventricular outflow tract was 60.5% at 10 years [122].

Data on short-term and midterm follow-up of patients undergoing the pulmonary autograft procedure, including

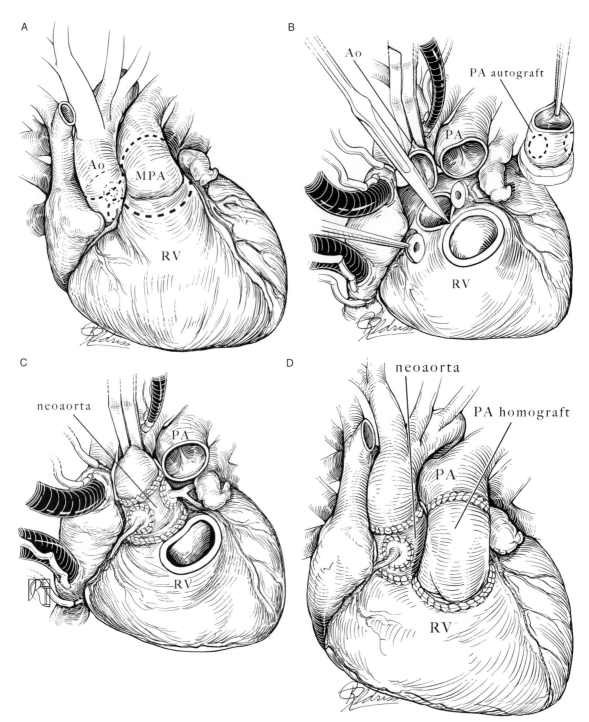

Figure 30.6 A, The intended incision and excision boundaries en route to the Ross–Konno procedure. Note that unlike Figure 30.5, no free right ventricular wall apron is included in the autograft harvest. **B,** After aortic cross-clamping, antegrade and retrograde cardioplegic arrest, aortic resection, coronary mobilization, and autograft harvest, the left ventricular outflow tract is enlarged by a localized linear incision without entry into the right ventricular cavity. **C,** The neoaortic left ventricular outflow reconstruction is shown. The right ventricular outflow is preserved without a septal incision and without the moiety that is required for the "apron extension" shown in Figure 30.5. **D,** The completed Ross–Konno procedure is shown after separation from cardiopulmonary bypass. (Ao, aorta; MPA, main pulmonary artery; PA, pulmonary artery; RV, right ventricle.) (Reproduced with permission from Mavroudis *et al.* [85].)

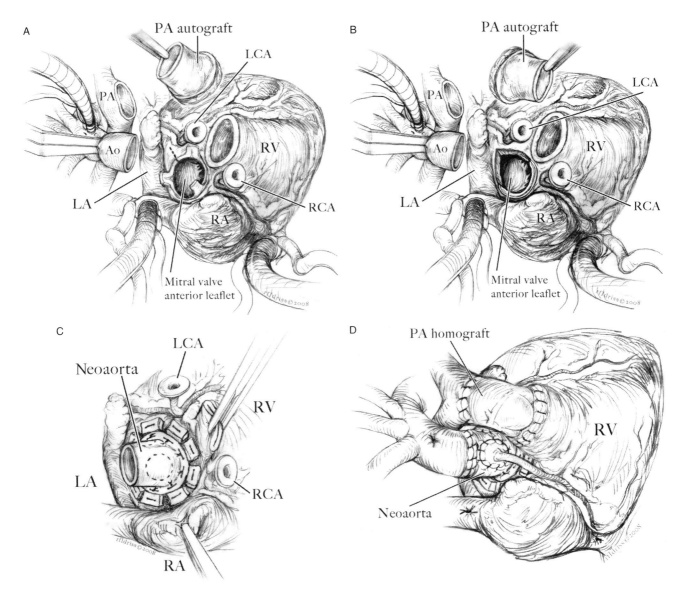

Figure 30.7 Completed modified Ross–Konno operation. **A,** The patient has been placed on aortobicaval cardiopulmonary bypass and the maneuvers involving aortic cross clamping, coronary artery mobilization, and autograft harvest from the right ventricular outflow tract are depicted. The dotted line, posterior to the course of the left main coronary artery, represents the lateral left ventricular free wall incision that will be used to enlarge the left ventricular outflow tract, which will accommodate the pulmonary autograft implantation. Careful dissection and attention to the details of anatomy to avoid injury to the pulmonary autograft, the coronary arteries and the surrounding structures is required. We employ antegrade and retrograde cold blood cardioplegia augmented by topical iced saline administered every 20 minutes for myocardial preservation. **B,** The result of circumferential resection of the aortic valve and annulus demonstrates the enlarged left ventricular outflow tract. The annulus of the aortic valve, especially when small, serves as a restrictive fibrous skeleton, which maintains the diminutive size of the left ventricular outflow.

When this fibrous skeleton is resected, the remaining muscle can stretch to accommodate the larger pulmonary autograft. The small incision at the left ventricular free wall can further open the left ventricular outflow tract in order to implant the larger pulmonary autograft. **C,** The pulmonary autograft implantation technique is depicted after annular resection and the left free wall enlarging incision. Ordinarily, a double running suture technique is used for implantation; however, the muscular neck of the left ventricular outflow tract will not hold sutures as well as the previously resected annular ring. Individual interrupted pledgeted sutures help to provide the stability that the implantation procedure requires to sustain systemic pressure. **D,** The rest of the neoaortic reconstruction and the pulmonary homograft are shown after separation from cardiopulmonary bypass. (Ao, aorta; LA, left atrium; LCA, left coronary artery; PA, pulmonary artery; RCA, right coronary artery; RA, right atrium; RV, right ventricle.) (Reproduced with permission from Mavroudis *et al.* [85].)

those with complex LVOTO, suggest that it can provide an effective means of relieving any such obstruction with a low mortality and low valve-related morbidity. The long-term results of the pulmonary autograft procedure for aortic valve disease from the original series by Ross *et al.* reported 10-year and 20-year survival of 85% and 61%, respectively [123]. Freedom from autograft replacement was 88% and 75%, while freedom from pulmonary allograft replacement was 89% and 80%, respectively. Assessment of the pulmonary autograft in children further suggested its growth potential, which is believed to be secondary to passive dilation during the early postoperative period followed by normal active growth [124,125]. The pulmonary allograft in the pulmonary position also promises to be more durable than an aortic homograft in the same position [126]. A more recent study demonstrated a hospital and 5-year survival of 100% and 98%, respectively [127]. Minimal morbidity was noted, and length of hospital stay was, on average, 6 days. Eleven percent of patients required a right ventricular to pulmonary artery conduit exchange. Freedom from significant neoaortic insufficiency at 6 years was 97%. Autograft reoperation rate secondary to aortic insufficiency or root dilation was 0%. Similarly positive results have been reported by other authors [128]. More recently, concerns have been raised that the neoaortic root growth may actually be out of proportion to somatic growth, resulting in neoaortic insufficiency [129]. Routine use of annuloplasty does not appear to reduce the rate of insufficiency [130].

The experience reported in the literature with the Ross-Konno procedure is much less than with the Ross procedure alone. However, relief of LVOTO is usually very effective [131,132]. In addition, aggressive resection of endocardial fibroelastosis and hypertrophic myocardium can be achieved with this exposure. This, in turn, results in improvement of the left ventricular stroke volume and diastolic function. Reddy and associates reported their experience with the Ross-Konno procedure in 11 patients, with median age of 12 months (range 4 days to 17 years) [41]. All patients had evidence of annular hypoplasia, and diffuse subaortic stenosis was present in five patients. The aortic root was replaced with a pulmonary autograft, and LVOT enlargement was performed using a Dacron patch (n = 2), allograft aortic patch (n = 2), or a right ventricular infundibular free wall muscular extension harvested in continuity with the autograft (n = 7). One patient died 14 days after operation. The median follow-up was 8.5 months, and there were no late deaths or reoperations.

Subvalvar Aortic Stenosis

Subvalvar aortic stenosis is defined as obstruction of the LVOT below the level of the aortic valve. This lesion has an incidence of 0.25 for every 1000 live births, and it accounts for 15–20% of all cases of LVOTO [133]. The most common form of subvalvar stenosis is a fixed obstruction due to abnormally present fibromuscular structures in the LVOT. This form is rarely apparent clinically during the first year of life, except when it is associated with other types of complex cardiac congenital lesions. Hypertrophic cardiomyopathy, which usually causes dynamic obstruction of left ventricular ejection, is much less frequently seen in the pediatric population. Other rare causes of clinically significant subvalvar stenosis include abnormal mitral valve attachments and other uncommon space-occupying lesions in the left ventricular outflow tract.

Fixed Subvalvar Stenosis and Fibromuscular Obstruction

Pathologic Anatomy

Traditionally, fixed subvalvar aortic stenosis has been classified as either discrete or diffuse, although there is probably a continuous spectrum of anatomic presentations. The discrete form of subvalvar stenosis, which represents about 70% of cases, is characterized by a thin, fibromuscular diaphragm found along the space between the base of the anterior mitral leaflet and the bottom of the aortic valve leaflets [134]. This diaphragm typically forms a crescentic or circular extension from the area of aortic-mitral fibrous continuity toward the interventricular septum. Some reports have further classified discrete subaortic stenosis into two distinct anatomic subtypes, membranous and fibromuscular [135]. On the other end of the spectrum is the diffuse form of subvalvar stenosis that is associated with a long tunnel type of fibromuscular ridge extending towards the apex of the left ventricle; about 12% of cases belong to this category [134]. In some patients, it may be difficult to distinguish diffuse subvalvar stenosis from hypertrophic cardiomyopathy.

The aortic annulus in these patients may be reduced in size but the aortic valve usually has normal trileaflet morphology. However, valvar aortic stenosis with associated left ventricular hypertrophy may also be present [136]. Subvalvar aortic stenosis may also be observed in the context of aortic valve insufficiency [137]. Turbulent flow created by the fixed anatomic obstruction is believed to be responsible for gradual thickening of the aortic valve leaflets which may, in turn, contribute to the development of aortic valve insufficiency [134,138].

Subaortic stenosis may be the result of additional structural abnormalities, including abnormal mitral valve position [139], accessory mitral valve tissue [140], anomalous insertion of mitral papillary muscles [141], anomalous muscle bundles within the LVOT [142], or posterior deviation of the infundibular septum without a ventricular septal defect [143]. Associated cardiovascular lesions in the context of subvalvar aortic stenosis are more frequent than in valvar stenosis and are found in up to 65% of cases [144,145]. Coarctation of the aorta, interrupted aortic arch, ventricular septal defect, and atrioventricular canal defects are commonly identified. Subvalvar aortic stenosis may also be a component of the Shone's complex of multilevel left-sided obstruction [146] and the hypoplastic left heart complex [23,147]. The combination of subaortic stenosis, VSD, and double-chambered right ventricle has also been described [148].

Pathophysiology

Subvalvar aortic stenosis is similar to valvar aortic stenosis in regards to pathophysiology as both lesions are associated with left ventricular pressure overload, concentric ventricular hypertrophy, and myocardial hypoperfusion [11]. For patients with similar degrees of obstruction, subvalvar stenosis is associated with more profound ventricular dysfunction compared with valvar stenosis [149]. Turbulence and jet lesions may damage aortic valve leaflets and render them susceptible to regurgitation and infections. Thick fibrous tissue may develop on the left ventricular surface of the aortic valve leaflets, a process which may deform the valve and thereby exacerbate aortic insufficiency [150].

Although the precise etiology for obstructive fibromuscular tissue in the LVOT is unknown, it is believed that anatomic or physiologic substrates for this lesion are present from birth. A discrete form of obstruction from below the level of the aortic valve develops over time as a result of abnormal contractile motion or abnormal growth and hypertrophy. In addition, the fibrous tissue which coats and tethers the leaflets of the aortic valve may impair its mobility and function, thereby contributing to the LVOTO [150]. Cape, Sigfusson, and coworkers' studies [151,152] postulated a multifactorial etiology for subaortic stenosis that included morphological abnormalities such as steepened aortoseptal angle [153], septal shear stress elevation, genetic predisposition, and cellular proliferation in response to shear stress. Septal shear stress responded markedly to changes in aortoseptal angle (from 103 dynes/cm^2 for a 150-degree angle to 150 dynes/cm^2 for a 120-degree angle) [151]. The presence and location of a ventricular septal defect enhanced this response; reduction in the distance between the ventricular septal defect and aortic annulus caused further increases in septal shear stress. Stress level increases were consistent with cellular flow studies showing growth factor stimulation and cellular proliferation. Echocardiographic studies in patients with fixed subaortic stenosis and intact ventricular septum suggest that, in addition to a steepened aortoseptal angle, these patients also have a significantly wider mitral-aortic separation, a marked aortic valve dextroposition, an increased left ventricular wall thickness, an increased septal thickness, and a smaller LVOT width [133]. A steep-ened aortoseptal angle has recently been shown to be a risk factor for the development of discrete subaortic stenosis in the adult population [154].

Clinical Picture and Diagnosis

Unlike that of valvar aortic stenosis, discrete subvalvar aortic stenosis rarely is seen as an isolated lesion in neonates and infants before 1 year of age. The progressive nature of this lesion with regard to the degree of obstruction and the development of aortic insufficiency is well documented [144,155]. Contrary to the discrete form of subaortic stenosis, the tunnel type of obstruction often is seen as a component of a complex lesion.

Children with subvalvar aortic stenosis are often found to have a systolic ejection murmur typically seen in patients with LVOTO. A diastolic murmur of aortic insufficiency is heard with increasing frequency as its prevalence increases with age. Although it is possible for the diagnosis to be made during infancy, clinically significant subvalvar aortic stenosis requiring surgery is rarely seen before a few years of age, and the incidence is highest during adolescence. Patients with subvalvar aortic stenosis most commonly show signs and symptoms of ventricular dysfunction or aortic insufficiency. Diminished exercise tolerance is a frequent finding, whereas angina and syncope are relatively uncommon.

Evidence of left ventricular hypertrophy is the most common electrocardiographic abnormality, seen in up to 85% of all children with subvalvar stenosis [155]. It is possible, however, to find normal electrocardiographic study results in patients with severe obstruction. The chest radiograph may show a mild degree of cardiomegaly, similar to that seen in patients with valvar aortic stenosis.

Echocardiography has changed significantly the approach to diagnosing complex congenital cardiac lesions. The combination of M-mode and two-dimensional echocardiography gives both anatomic measurements as well as direct visualization of the narrowed subvalvar LVOT. Continuous-wave Doppler provides estimation of the pressure gradient across the obstruction, while color Doppler study detects aortic insufficiency. With its superior ability to detect and distinguish various forms of obstructive lesions of the LVOT, echocardiography is the diagnostic method of choice.

Combined left and right heart catheterization is recommended to assess for associated cardiac anomalies, which are present in a large percentage of patients. In addition, the severity of obstruction cannot be determined accurately based on echocardiographic evaluation alone, and Doppler study may sometimes overestimate the gradient across a lesion. Cardiac catheterization provides direct measurements of peak-to-peak pressure gradient, as well as a visual road map of the lesion.

Treatment
Indications for Intervention

Surgery is indicated for any patient with symptoms attributable to subaortic stenosis, including shortness of breath, angina, syncope, or diminished exercise tolerance. In addition, evidence of progressive decompensation based on serial noninvasive studies is also an indication for surgery. In asymptomatic patients with discrete subaortic stenosis, a gradient above 30 mmHg constitutes an indication for surgery. Patients with gradients less than 30 mmHg and no significant left ventricular hypertrophy may be followed, but must be monitored for evidence of disease progression, particularly in the first years of life [156]. For asymptomatic patients with tunnel-type obstructions, a gradient higher than 50 mmHg is used. The presence of aortic insufficiency, even with a lesser gradient, is also considered an indication for surgery. Because of the progressive nature of the disease and concerns about damage to the aortic valve, some surgeons advocate surgery for subvalvar aortic stenosis at the time of diagnosis [157].

Subaortic Fibromuscular Obstruction

Subvalvar fibromuscular resection with septal myectomy is the standard surgical treatment for this form of disease. This can be achieved almost always through an aortotomy using sharp dissection. The membrane or ridge may be a complete ring or be crescent shaped, and is removed along with the appropriate amount of underlying septal muscle without creating a ventricular septal defect. Care must be taken to avoid injury to the adjacent structures, such as the mitral and aortic valves, as well as the conduction system.

In older patients with discrete subaortic fibromuscular obstruction, it is sometimes possible to enucleate the lesion by peeling away the fibrous ring from the underlying muscle, the aortic valve, or the anterior leaflet of the mitral valve, depending on the actual situation. However, it is generally recommended that myectomy be performed at the time of ring resection in order to reduce the risk of recurrence [158].

Significant reduction of left ventricle-to-aorta pressure gradient is expected after resection of subaortic fibromuscular obstruction [158]. Darcin and colleagues reported a reduction of the mean systolic gradient from 59.23 ± 35.38 mmHg preoperatively to 9.47 ± 9.91 mmHg postoperatively, with no early or late postoperative mortality [1]. Surgical intervention has also been associated with a reduced incidence of infective endocarditis [159]. It is important to have frequent and careful follow-up evaluation after surgery for subaortic stenosis, because the course of the disease is unpredictable at the time of operation, and recurrence of stenosis and progression of aortic insufficiency have been reported in as high as 55% of cases [138]. Surgery for fixed subaortic stenosis has been associated with geometric remodeling and normalization of the steepened aortoseptal angle in patients up to 10 years of age [133].

Diffuse Subaortic Stenosis

Treatment for the diffuse tunnel form of subaortic stenosis is more difficult, and the selection of procedure is dependent largely on the adequacy of the aortic valve annulus and associated lesions. When there is a well-developed aortic valve of adequate size, a septal ventriculoplasty (modified Konno-Rastan procedure) is the preferred option (Figure 30.4) [37,160,161]. The interventricular septum is exposed through an incision made in the pulmonary infundibulum. The septum is opened longitudinally in a slightly oblique fashion going from right to left, extending to just below the commissure between the left and right coronary cusps. Thickened septal muscle is then resected and the ventricular septal defect is closed using a piece of synthetic or pericardial patch to enlarge the LVOT. The right ventriculotomy can be closed primarily or with a patch. Satisfactory reduction of the LVOT gradient from 50 to 3 mmHg, and a relatively low operative mortality rate (6.2% at 2 years) have been reported [161].

If the aortic valve is damaged as a result of the subaortic stenosis, or if there is concomitant valvar hypoplasia, then an aortoventriculoplasty (classic Konno-Rastan procedure) is needed to relieve obstruction at both levels (Figure 30.3) [37,100,101]. This is similar to septal ventriculoplasty, except that the incision in the interventricular septum is extended upstream through the aortic annulus, and the aortic valve is replaced with a prosthetic valve or aortic allograft. Alternatively, root replacement with pulmonary autograft may be performed (Ross-Konno procedure) [41]. Tabatabaie and associates reported their experience with the classic Konno-Rastan procedure in diffuse subaortic stenosis [162]. Their series included 26 patients with a mean age of 12.8 ± 7 years. The mean peak systolic gradient decreased from 91.3 ± 39.3 to 28.1 ± 17.7 mmHg following surgery, the observed 30-day mortality was 11.5% (three patients), and there were no late mortalities among the 23 other patients.

Hypertrophic Cardiomyopathy

Hypertrophic cardiomyopathy, also known as idiopathic hypertrophic subaortic stenosis (IHSS), is a form of ventricular outflow tract obstruction characterized by asymmetric ventricular septal hypertrophy. The histologic hallmark of this disease is the presence of disorganized and bizarrely shaped hypertrophied myocytes. As its name implies, this condition has no known cause and it appears to follow an autosomal dominant transmission. The patient is usually asymptomatic until the second or third decade of life and the condition rarely is seen in the pediatric population.

Obstruction arising from hypertrophic cardiomyopathy can occur along the entire length of the ventricular septum. It can result from the increased bulk of the septum as a form of fixed stenosis, or in the form of dynamic obstruction as seen in systolic anterior motion of the anterior leaflet of the mitral valve. When, in rare instances, infants with hypertrophic cardiomyopathy become symptomatic, the clinical course is atypical compared with that of older patients. The diagnosis is more difficult to make, and progressive congestive heart failure, rather than sudden death, is the most common cause of demise. Risk factors associated with mortality in symptomatic pediatric patients with hypertrophic cardiomyopathy include a family history of sudden death, the presence of septal hypertrophy measuring 30 mm or greater, and a history of ventricular tachycardia and syncope [163]. Medical management includes β blockade, calcium-channel blockade, and dual-chamber ventricular pacing. A subset of patients with suspected isolated dynamic LVOTO may have isolated or concomitant fixed obstruction, and careful two-dimensional and Doppler echocardiography are needed to identify this group of patients [164]. Surgical experience in the pediatric population has been limited, but septal myectomy is safe and effective in reducing ventricular outflow obstruction. In more severe cases, a Konno-Rastan procedure may also be performed [132]. Minakata and colleagues reported their experience with septal myectomy in 56 pediatric patients with obstructive hypertrophic cardiomyopathy [165]. The mean age at the time of surgery was 11 ± 5.6 years, with a range from 2 months to 20 years. Following surgery, the mean LVOT gradient decreased from 103 ± 34 to 16 ± 12 mmHg, and there were no early deaths. Survival estimates at 5 and 10 years were 97% and 93%, respectively.

Supravalvar Aortic Stenosis

Congenital supravalvar aortic stenosis is a complex anatomical anomaly of the entire aortic root characterized by narrowing of the aortic lumen commencing immediately above the aortic valve. This represents the least common form of LVOTO and occurs in about 5–10% of patients with LVOTO [2,3] Supravalvar aortic stenosis is often part of Williams' syndrome and can also be seen in conjunction with diffuse hypoplasia of the ascending aorta, distal arterial branches, and even of the branched pulmonary arteries [166].

Pathologic Features

Great Arteries
Supravalvar aortic stenosis is broadly categorized as diffuse in 23% of cases or localized in 77% [167,168]. The main feature of this form of LVOTO is severe thickening of the sinotubular ridge creating the characteristic hourglass

appearance of the ascending aorta. This results in severe crowding of the aortic root exit, a limited space for the aortic valve leaflet expansion in systole and severe hypertension of the aortic root. On histology, the sinotubular ridge shows intimal hyperplasia, medial dysplasia and thickening with areas of necrosis and calcification. There are also areas of randomly arranged smooth muscle cells, decreased collagen content, and increased collagen deposition. Similar histological changes affecting the aorta may involve the pulmonary arterial tree, but to a much lesser degree [169,170].

Coronary Arteries
The systolic hypertension of the aortic root proximal to the obstruction exposes the coronary arteries to high pressure. Therefore, coronary artery abnormalities are frequently associated with supravalvar aortic stenosis. To varying degrees, intimal hyperplasia, fibrosis, dysplasia, disruption, and loss of internal elastic membrane with indistinct intimal-medial junction, medial hypertrophy, and adventitial fibroelastosis have been found in pathology specimens [167,168,170]. Morphologically, the coronary artery disease is more severe proximally. The coronary arteries are often markedly dilated and tortuous secondary to their exposition to a constantly very high systolic pressure proximal to the sinotubular junction [171]. High systolic pressures can also induce focal dissections and accelerated atherosclerosis of the coronary arteries. The proliferative process causing thickening of the sinotubular ridge can also extend and narrow the coronary ostia, most often the ostium of the left coronary sinus [172]. Also, the free edges of the aortic valve cusps can abnormally adhere to the intimal shelf present at the sinotubular junction. This obstructs flow to the sinuses of Valsalva and consequently entry of blood in the coronary arteries.

Valvar Abnormalities
In most cases, the aortic valve annulus is of normal size and the aortic valve leaflets are not fused and are morphologically normal. However, one should not consider abnormalities of the aortic valve to be uncommon in patients with supravalvar aortic stenosis as they are seen in 30–45% of operative or autopsy cases [168,173–175]. Thickening of the aortic cusps and aortic insufficiency due to the high systolic pressure proximal to the sinotubular junction are the most commonly described abnormalities. In most patients, they are of mild or moderate severity. These findings often will persist after relief of the supravalvar stenosis and in some surgical series, 17–40% of patients operated on for supravalvar stenosis will require reoperation for persistent stenosis [175–177]. Concomitant untreated aortic valve disease has been identified as a risk factor for reoperation and mortality. Also, as mentioned previously, the thickened aortic valve cusps tend to adhere to the

dysplastic sinotubular junction and this may isolate the coronary arteries from the aortic lumen [168,178]. In addition, supravalvar aortic stenosis can be associated with abnormalities of the mitral valve and of its apparatus; mainly fibrous thickening of the mitral leaflets and chordae tendinea [179].

Myocardial Pathology

Left ventricular hypertrophy is common with this form of LVOTO owing to the elevated pressure load on the left ventricular myocardium. The combination of this increased myocardial metabolic demand with the possible limitation of coronary blood flow secondary to the previously described anatomical abnormalities of the coronary arteries can lead to ischemic myocardial damage, which often develops during early childhood and accelerates with age [175].

Pathophysiology and Natural History

The basic pathophysiology of supravalvar aortic stenosis is similar to other forms of LVOTO. Indeed, it causes left ventricular hypertension and secondary concentric left ventricular hypertrophy and myocardial hypoperfusion. However, unlike in other forms of LVOTO, the coronary arteries are exposed to elevated systolic pressure and the coronary blood flow can be limited as described previously owing to accelerated coronary artery sclerosis. This creates the perfect substrate for myocardial hypoperfusion, ventricular fibrillation, and sudden death. Also, this form of LVOTO is often associated with involvement of the pulmonary arteries, aortic arch, and its branches. This complicates the clinical picture and the treatment. Indeed, in the diffuse form of supravalvar aortic stenosis, involvement of the main pulmonary artery and its branches, either in the form of discreet focal stenosis or, more commonly, diffuse hypoplasia, can complicate surgical intervention [180]. As mentioned before, the supravalvar form is the least common of the various types of LVOTO. Genders are equally affected. Studies show a tendency for a severe and rapid progression of supravalvar stenosis, more so than for other forms of LVOTO. On the other hand, spontaneous regression of the peripheral pulmonary stenosis is also possible [181,182]. Sudden death is also frequent if patients are left untreated due to the above-mentioned combination of left ventricular hypertrophy and premature coronary artery disease [168,175].

Clinical Picture and Diagnosis

Congenital supravalvar aortic stenosis can occur as an isolated defect or as a dominantly inherited familial arteriopathy [168]. The association of supravalvar aortic stenosis

with elfin-like facies and mental retardation is known as Williams-Beuren syndrome. The Williams-Beuren syndrome is a genomic disorder (prevalence: 1/7500 to 1/20000) caused by a hemizygous contiguous gene deletion on chromosome 7q11.23 [183]. It affects the elastin gene. Whereas supravalvar aortic stenosis associated with Williams-Beuren syndrome is associated with a complete deletion of this elastin gene and probably a disruption of adjacent genes, cases of familial non-Williams supravalvar aortic stenosis seem to result from a loss-of-function or point mutation of this same elastin gene [184–186]. The male to female ratio is 1.4:1 and patients may be seen as early as the neonatal period or in adulthood. Normally, cardiac symptoms only appear in the late stage of the syndrome [166,187–190]. Obstructive symptoms such as diminished exercise tolerance, syncope, and angina typically form the clinical picture. Systolic and diastolic murmurs may be present and may help in the diagnosis of the anomaly if the other features of Williams syndrome are not present. Signs of left ventricular hypertrophy may be noted on electrocardiography and echocardiography. Evidence of myocardial ischemia and subsequent cardiomegaly and congestive heart failure occurs progressively over time, even during childhood.

In terms of diagnostic studies, the electrocardiography may reveal signs of left ventricular hypertrophy and, if there is limited coronary flow, left ventricular strain. An echocardiography will provide the diagnosis and will delineate reliably the structural anatomy of the LVOT and other valvar abnormalities. It will also allow measurement of the gradient across the LVOT. Similar observations can be made with magnetic resonance imaging. This modality, however, will add information regarding the distal aortic arch and the great vessels that cannot be obtained from an echocardiography study. Cardiac catheterization may also be useful to better examine the status of the coronary arteries and measure precisely a pressure gradient across the LVOT. While performing coronary angiography in these patients, great care should be taken, especially if there is evidence that coronary blood flow is limited, as there is a risk of ventricular fibrillation.

Treatment

Medical and Interventional Management

Although balloon dilation has been reported anecdotally, it has not been accepted as a standard treatment for supravalvar aortic stenosis in most centers [191,192]. One exception is stenosis of the distal pulmonary arterial tree which can be amenable to balloon dilatation with or without stenting. In terms of medical management, agents reducing afterload may possibly reduce coronary perfusion in the context of a hypertrophied myocardium and should not be routinely used [193,194].

Indications for Surgery

As with other forms of LVOTO, the indication for surgery is based on the severity of the symptoms of obstruction. A LVOT gradient of 40–50 mmHg in the context of an important narrowing at the sinotubular junction is an indication to proceed with surgery. In cases where the gradient is less than 30–40 mmHg and there is no left ventricular hypertrophy, it is acceptable to follow the patients clinically and repeat biannual echocardiographic studies. However, considering the progressive nature of this disease, and in order to avoid the detrimental effect of continuously high pressures on the left ventricle, aortic valve, and coronary arteries, earlier surgical treatment may also be indicated.

Surgical Management

Surgical treatment needs to be tailored to the anatomical derangement of individual patients. Relief of all stenotic segments, restoration of normal aortic root geometry, and allowance for growth are principles determining the surgical technique chosen.

Localized Supravalvar Aortic Stenosis

In rare cases, a discrete supravalvar aortic stenosis consists only of a membrane, or localized ring, near or at the sinotubular junction. In such cases, complete excision of the stenotic segment completed by patch closure of the aortic root can be performed with satisfactory results [195]. Most commonly, however, extensive thickening of the aortic wall prevents simple local excision. A longitudinal incision in the ascending aorta across the stenosis and into the noncoronary sinus is used instead. Additionally, an endarterectomy procedure can be performed to excise a stenotic intimal ridge. The longitudinal aortotomy is closed using a teardrop-shaped single-sinus Dacron or polytetrafluoroethylene patch to create an aortoplasty including the entire stenotic segment as far in the aortic arch as is necessary [175,176]. This technique of patch enlargement was first independently reported by McGoon, Starr, and their associates in 1961 [196].

In 1976, Doty and coworkers introduced an extended aortoplasty that involves the creation of an inverted Y-shaped incision across the constricting segment and into the right and noncoronary sinuses of Valsalva (Figure 30.8) [37,197]. This operation provides a more symmetric reconstruction of the aortic root. Even if it may be difficult to achieve completely accurate restoration of the dimensions at the sinotubular junction in comparison with the aortic annulus, excellent hemodynamic results have been reported with this inverted bifurcated patch technique [175–177,198,199]. It remains our procedure of choice for surgical treatment of localized supravalvar aortic stenosis.

For more extreme cases of discrete supravalvar aortic stenosis, it may be necessary to employ a more radical

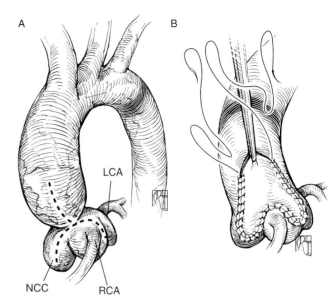

Figure 30.8 A, Projected incisions (dotted lines) for the two-sinus repair of supravalvar aortic stenosis as introduced by Doty [197]. Note that the incision in the right coronary artery (RCA) sinus is made to the left of the coronary artery orifice. **B,** A pantaloon patch is shown augmenting the two sinuses of Valsalva. (LCA, left coronary artery; NCC, noncoronary cusp.)

technique, first described by Brom (Figure 30.9) [37,200–202]. This approach, which effectively eliminates the potential stenotic segment and restores normal aortic root geometry, can be used if important narrowing of the left coronary sinus is identified. It involves complete transection of the ascending aorta just above the sinotubular junction. Longitudinal incisions are then carried out into the three sinuses of Valsalva. Three separate triangular prosthetic or pericardial patches are then used to enlarge each sinus of Valsalva. To complete the procedure, an end-to-end anastomosis is fashioned between the reconstructed aortic root and the ascending aorta. This effectively restores the aortic root geometry providing equal diameters at the aortic annulus and sinotubular junction. A modification of the above-described technique was proposed in 1993 by Myers and associates [203]. Its main advantage is to use exclusively autologous tissue for repair, thereby maintaining the potential for growth. This sliding aortoplasty is carried out by cutting out corresponding triangular patches in the ascending aorta and then suturing them into each sinus of Valsalva in an effort to restore aortic root anatomy (Figure 30.10) [37,203].

It is also important to note that abnormalities of the coronary arteries resulting in stenosis and myocardial malperfusion must be addressed at the time of surgical repair. Both coronary artery ostia should be inspected at the time of repair. Patch enlargement of coronary ostial

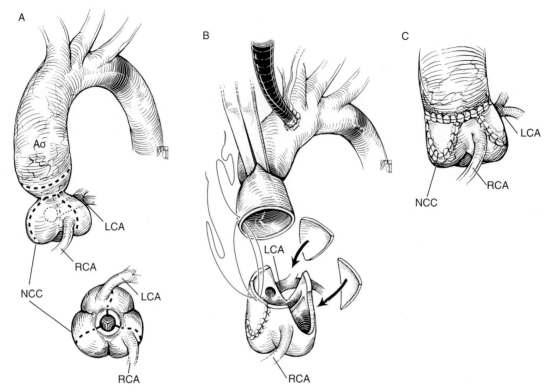

Figure 30.9 A, Projected incisions (dotted lines) for the three-patch repair of supravalvar aortic stenosis as introduced by Brom and colleagues [200]. The incisions in the coronary sinuses are performed to the left of the right coronary artery (RCA) and to the right of the left coronary artery (LCA). Care is taken to avoid any injury to the orifices. **B,** Three tailored pieces of either homograft or prosthetic material are used to augment individually the incised sinuses of Valsalva. The fibrous ring that could interfere with coronary flow is resected in all cases. **C,** The reconstructed neoaorta using the three-patch technique. (NCC, noncoronary cusp.)

obstruction has been described, as well as coronary artery bypass grafting using the internal mammary artery or other conduits [204–206].

Diffuse Supravalvar Aortic Stenosis

Surgical repair of the diffuse form of supravalvar aortic stenosis usually requires intervention at the aortic arch or beyond and, therefore, requires either deep hypothermic circulatory arrest or hypothermic low-flow bypass with direct perfusion of the brachiocephalic vessels. Experience with the diffuse form of supravalvar aortic stenosis is limited. Therefore, the operations reported in the literature are less well defined and their results less studied. Historically, a valved conduit from the left ventricular apex to the supraceliac abdominal aorta has been used for the severe form of diffuse supravalvar aortic stenosis [175,199]. This procedure, however, has been associated with high complication rates, including infective endocarditis, conduit stenosis, prosthetic valve dysfunction, and late mortality. In addition, it does not address actual or potential obstruction of the coronary arteries [207–209]. In recent years, simplification in the technique of implantation has led to a new interest in this approach for cases of very complex LVOTO [210]. However, currently, the preferred approach is the placement of an extended patch, starting from the sinus of Valsalva and extending to the aortic arch and the proximal innominate and left common carotid arteries (Figure 30.11) [37]. Good relief of the obstruction can be achieved with this technique. Indeed, any patch aortoplasty that is short of widening the entire ascending aorta and the aortic arch will be unlikely to correct the underlying anatomic abnormality and its associated physiologic derangement.

Results

Primary repair of localized supravalvar aortic stenosis has very low perioperative mortality. It also has a good late survival [211,212]. A study by Brown and associates reviewed more than 100 cases and established a 98% and 97% survival at 10 and 20 years, respectively [198]. Repair of the diffuse type of this disease is more complex and, in many studies, has a higher early mortality risk. This is thought to be due to a higher level of complexity of the

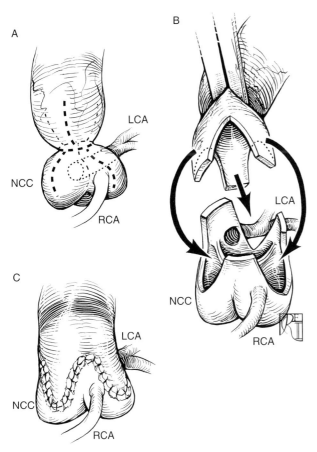

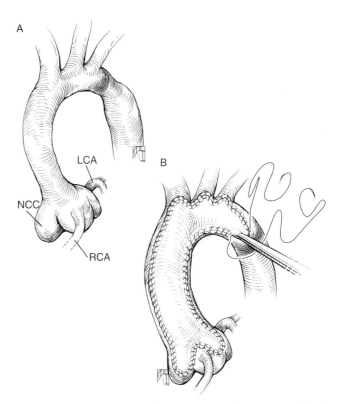

Figure 30.11 A, Shown is the narrow supravalvar area associated with hypoplasia of the ascending aorta and transverse arch. **B,** An extended patch of homograft or prosthetic material can be used to augment the entire arch of the aorta and the supravalvar area. (LCA, left coronary artery; NCC, noncoronary cusp; RCA, right coronary artery.)

Figure 30.10 A, Projected incisions (dotted lines) for the native aortic reconstruction using a three-sinus augmentation as proposed by Myers and colleagues [203]. **B,** The supravalvar incisions are made in the same manner as in Figure 30.9. Corresponding incisions are made in the ascending aorta for eventual augmentation using native tissue. **C,** The neoaortic reconstruction without prosthetic or homograft material. (LCA, left coronary artery; NCC, noncoronary cusp; RCA, right coronary artery.)

procedure, as well as the possibility for incomplete relief of the obstruction [213].

Left Ventricular Outflow Tract Obstruction as Part of Multiple Obstructions in the Heart–Aorta Complex

Although the scope of this chapter is not to discuss LVOTO when present as part of complex cardiac malformations; for completeness, two clinical entities with multiple obstructions in the left heart-aorta complex will be discussed briefly: Shone's complex and HLHC. In both of these entities, there is no valvar aortic stenosis, as the LVOTO is subvalvar. Unlike Shone's complex, patients with HLHC have as the dominant feature hypoplasia of the structures of the left heart-aorta complex. Patients with HLHC must be distinguished from those with aortic valvar stenosis with LV hypoplasia, as aortic valvotomy is not necessary in HLHC.

Shone's Complex

In 1963, Shone and associates described a developmental complex with four obstructive anomalies that had a tendency to coexist: supravalvar ring of the left atrium, "parachute" deformity of the mitral valve, subaortic stenosis, and coarctation of the aorta [146]. The report was based on eight children, of whom only two exhibited all four obstructive anomalies. The six remaining cases exhibited two or three of the lesions. Although subaortic stenosis and a supravalvar ring of the left atrium were present in all cases, they were considered functionally significant in only six of the eight cases, and in three of the six cases which did not exhibit all four components of the complex. Coarctation of the aorta and a "parachute" mitral valve were present in only four cases. Of significance, hypoplasia of the left heart was not a feature of any of these cases. The surgical treatment of these patients is challenging; the subaortic stenosis is only part of the overall problem. In many of these patients, long-term outcome is determined by the severity of the mitral valve anomaly and, to a lesser degree, by the subaortic stenosis.

Hypoplastic Left Heart Complex

The term *hypoplastic left heart complex* was first introduced by Tchervenkov and associates in 1998 to describe patients with hypoplasia of the left heart structures, without intrinsic valve stenosis or atresia [23]. Therefore, these patients have LVOTO by virtue of hypoplasia of the aortic valve and LVOT. In these critically ill neonates, there is forward flow in the ascending aorta and into the proximal branches of the aortic arch. The descending aorta circulation is via the PDA and is right-ventricle-dependent. Patients with HLHC bear some similarities to those with Shone's complex. However, hypoplasia of the structures of the left heart–aorta including hypoplasia of the left ventricle, a fundamental feature in HLHC, is not part of Shone's complex as described originally [146]. In order to clarify the terminology, the International Congenital Heart Surgery Nomenclature and Database Project considered HLHC as a subset of hypoplastic left heart syndrome [214]. Shone's complex, described in older patients and lacking the fundamental feature of hypoplasia, is considered a different entity.

The surgical treatment of patients with HLHC centers on whether the patient undergoes a two-ventricle repair or a single-ventricle palliation in the form of the Norwood operation. Although in Tchervenkov and associates' series most patients successfully underwent two-ventricle repair during the initial operation, many of these patients required reoperation for recurrent or persistent LVOTO [23].

References

1. Darcin OT, Yagdi T, Atay Y, *et al.* (2003) Discrete subaortic stenosis: surgical outcomes and follow-up results. Tex Heart Inst J 30, 286–292.
2. Kitchiner D, Jackson M, Malaiya N, *et al.* (1994) Incidence and prognosis of obstruction of the left ventricular outflow tract in Liverpool (1960–91): a study of 313 patients. Br Heart J 71, 588–595.
3. Samanek M, Slavik Z, Zborilova B, *et al.* (1989) Prevalence, treatment, and outcome of heart disease in live-born children: a prospective analysis of 91,823 live-born children. Pediatr Cardiol 10, 205–211.
4. Campbell M, Kauntze R. (1953) Congenital aortic valvular stenosis. Br Heart J 15, 179–194.
5. Roberts WC. (1973) Valvular, subvalvular and supravalvular aortic stenosis: morphologic features. Cardiovasc Clin 5, 97–126.
6. Keane JF, Driscoll DJ, Gersony WM, *et al.* (1993) Second natural history study of congenital heart defects. Results of treatment of patients with aortic valvar stenosis. Circulation 87(2 Suppl), I16–I27.
7. Kitchiner DJ, Jackson M, Walsh K, *et al.* (1993) Incidence and prognosis of congenital aortic valve stenosis in Liverpool (1960–1990). Br Heart J 69, 71–79.
8. Lofland GK, McCrindle BW, Williams WG, *et al.* (2001) Critical aortic stenosis in the neonate: a multi-institutional study of management, outcomes, and risk factors. Congenital Heart Surgeons Society. J Thorac Cardiovasc Surg 121, 10–27.
9. Maizza AF, Ho SY, Anderson RH. (1993) Obstruction of the left ventricular outflow tract: anatomical observations and surgical implications. J Heart Valve Dis 2, 66–79.
10. Pasipoularides A. (1990) Clinical assessment of ventricular ejection dynamics with and without outflow obstruction. J Am Coll Cardiol 15, 859–882.
11. Sabbah HN, Stein PD. (1988) Reduction of systolic coronary blood flow in experimental left ventricular outflow tract obstruction. Am Heart J 116, 806–811.
12. Sharland GK, Chita SK, Fagg NL, *et al.* (1991) Left ventricular dysfunction in the fetus: relation to aortic valve anomalies and endocardial fibroelastosis. Br Heart J 66, 419–424.
13. Mielke G, Mayer R, Hassberg D, *et al.* (1997) Sequential development of fetal aortic valve stenosis and endocardial fibroelastosis during the second trimester of pregnancy. Am Heart J 133, 607–610.
14. Fogel MA, Lieb DR, Seliem MA. (1995) Validity of electrocardiographic criteria for left ventricular hypertrophy in children with pressure- or volume-loaded ventricles: comparison with echocardiographic left ventricular muscle mass. Pediatr Cardiol 16, 261–269.
15. Sharma S, Anand R, Kanter KR, *et al.* (1992) The usefulness of echocardiography in the surgical management of infants with congenital heart disease. Clin Cardiol 15, 891–897.
16. Chang AC, Huhta JC, Yoon GY, *et al.* (1991) Diagnosis, transport, and outcome in fetuses with left ventricular outflow tract obstruction. J Thorac Cardiovasc Surg 102, 841–848.
17. Hammon JW Jr, Lupinetti FM, Maples MD, *et al.* (1988) Predictors of operative mortality in critical valvular aortic stenosis presenting in infancy. Ann Thorac Surg 45, 537–540.
18. Schwartz ML, Gauvreau K, Geva T. (2001) Predictors of outcome of biventricular repair in infants with multiple left heart obstructive lesions. Circulation 104, 682–687.
19. Rhodes LA, Colan SD, Perry SB, *et al.* (1991) Predictors of survival in neonates with critical aortic stenosis. Circulation 84, 2325–2335.
20. Kovalchin JP, Brook MM, Rosenthal GL, *et al.* (1998) Echocardiographic hemodynamic and morphometric predictors of survival after two-ventricle repair in infants with critical aortic stenosis. J Am Coll Cardiol 32, 237–244.
21. Blaufox AD, Lai WW, Lopez L, *et al.* (1998) Survival in neonatal biventricular repair of left-sided cardiac obstructive lesions associated with hypoplastic left ventricle. Am J Cardiol 82, 1138–1140.

22. Tani LY, Minich LL, Pagotto LT, *et al.* (1999) Left heart hypoplasia and neonatal aortic arch obstruction: is the Rhodes left ventricular adequacy score applicable? J Thorac Cardiovasc Surg 118, 81–86.

23. Tchervenkov CI, Tahta SA, Jutras LC, *et al.* (1998) Biventricular repair in neonates with hypoplastic left heart complex. Ann Thorac Surg 66, 1350–1357.

24. Hickey EJ, Caldarone CA, Blackstone EH, *et al.* (2007) Critical left ventricular outflow tract obstruction: The disproportionate impact of biventricular repair in borderline cases. J Thorac Cardiovasc Surg 134, 1429–1436; discussion 1436–1437.

25. Moore P, Egito E, Mowrey H, *et al.* (1996) Midterm results of balloon dilation of congenital aortic stenosis: predictors of success. J Am Coll Cardiol 27, 1257–1263.

26. O'Connor BK, Beekman RH, Rocchini AP, *et al.* (1991) Intermediate-term effectiveness of balloon valvuloplasty for congenital aortic stenosis. A prospective follow-up study. Circulation 84, 732–738.

27. Shaddy RE, Boucek MM, Sturtevant JE, *et al.* (1990) Gradient reduction, aortic valve regurgitation and prolapse after balloon aortic valvuloplasty in 32 consecutive patients with congenital aortic stenosis. J Am Coll Cardiol 16, 451–456.

28. Vogel M, Benson LN, Burrows P, *et al.* (1989) Balloon dilatation of congenital aortic valve stenosis in infants and children: short term and intermediate results. Br Heart J 62, 148–153.

29. Lababidi Z. (1983) Aortic balloon valvuloplasty. Am Heart J 106, 751–752.

30. McCrindle BW, Blackstone EH, Williams WG, *et al.* (2001) Are outcomes of surgical versus transcatheter balloon valvotomy equivalent in neonatal critical aortic stenosis? Circulation 104(12 Suppl 1), I152–I158.

31. Dua JS, Osborne NJ, Tometzki AJ, *et al.* (2006) Axillary artery approach for balloon valvoplasty in young infants with severe aortic valve stenosis: medium-term results. Catheter Cardiovasc Interv 68, 929–935.

32. Weber HS, Mart CR, Myers JL. (2000) Transcarotid balloon valvuloplasty for critical aortic valve stenosis at the bedside via continuous transesophageal echocardiographic guidance. Catheter Cardiovasc Interv 50, 326–329.

33. Maxwell D, Allan L, Tynan MJ. (1991) Balloon dilatation of the aortic valve in the fetus: a report of two cases. Br Heart J 65, 256–258.

34. Tworetzky W, Wilkins-Haug L, Jennings RW, *et al.* (2004) Balloon dilation of severe aortic stenosis in the fetus: potential for prevention of hypoplastic left heart syndrome: candidate selection, technique, and results of successful intervention. Circulation 110, 2125–2131.

35. Wilkins-Haug LE, Tworetzky W, Benson CB, *et al.* (2006) Factors affecting technical success of fetal aortic valve dilation. Ultrasound Obstet Gynecol 28, 47–52.

36. Miyamoto T, Sinzobahamvya N, Wetter J, *et al.* (2006) Twenty years experience of surgical aortic valvotomy for critical aortic stenosis in early infancy. Eur J Cardiothorac Surg 30, 35–40.

37. Tchervenkov CI, Chu VF, Shum-Tim D. (2003) Left ventricular outflow tract obstruction. In: Mavroudis C, Backer CL, eds. *Pediatric Cardiac Surgery*, 3rd ed. Philadelphia, PA: Mosby, Inc.

38. Jonas RA, Castaneda AR, Freed MD. (1985) Normothermic caval inflow occlusion. Application to operations for congenital heart disease. J Thorac Cardiovasc Surg 89, 780–786.

39. van Son JA, Hovaguimian H, Rao IM, *et al.* (1995) Strategies for repair of congenital heart defects in infants without the use of blood. Ann Thorac Surg 59, 384–388.

40. Calhoon JH, Bolton JW. (1995) Ross/Konno procedure for critical aortic stenosis in infancy. Ann Thorac Surg 60(6 Suppl), S597–S599.

41. Reddy VM, Rajasinghe HA, Teitel DF, *et al.* (1996) Aortoventriculoplasty with the pulmonary autograft: the "Ross-Konno" procedure. J Thorac Cardiovasc Surg 111, 158–165; discussion 165–167.

42. Starnes VA, Luciani GB, Wells WJ, *et al.* (1996) Aortic root replacement with the pulmonary autograft in children with complex left heart obstruction. Ann Thorac Surg 62, 442–448; discussion 448–449.

43. Reddy VM, Rajasinghe HA, McElhinney DB, *et al.* (1995) Extending the limits of the Ross procedure. Ann Thorac Surg 60(6 Suppl), S600–S603.

44. Sudow G, Solymar L, Berggren H, *et al.* (1996) Aortic valve replacement with a pulmonary autograft in infants with critical aortic stenosis. J Thorac Cardiovasc Surg 112, 433–436.

45. van Son JA, Reddy VM, Black MD, *et al.* (1996) Morphologic determinants favoring surgical aortic valvuloplasty versus pulmonary autograft aortic valve replacement in children. J Thorac Cardiovasc Surg 111, 1149–1156; discussion 1156–1157.

46. Bu'Lock FA, Joffe HS, Jordan SC, *et al.* (1993) Balloon dilatation (valvoplasty) as first line treatment for severe stenosis of the aortic valve in early infancy: medium term results and determinants of survival. Br Heart J 70, 546–553.

47. Brown JW, Stevens LS, Holly S, *et al.* (1988) Surgical spectrum of aortic stenosis in children: a thirty-year experience with 257 children. Ann Thorac Surg 45, 393–403.

48. Gatzoulis MA, Rigby ML, Shinebourne EA, *et al.* (1995) Contemporary results of balloon valvuloplasty and surgical valvotomy for congenital aortic stenosis. Arch Dis Child 73, 66–69.

49. Leung MP, McKay R, Smith A, *et al.* (1991) Critical aortic stenosis in early infancy. Anatomic and echocardiographic substrates of successful open valvotomy. J Thorac Cardiovasc Surg 101, 526–535.

50. Baram S, McCrindle BW, Han RK, *et al.* (2003) Outcomes of uncomplicated aortic valve stenosis presenting in infants. Am Heart J 145, 1063–1070.

51. Galal O, Rao PS, Al-Fadley F, *et al.* (1997) Follow-up results of balloon aortic valvuloplasty in children with special reference to causes of late aortic insufficiency. Am Heart J 133, 418–427.

52. Justo RN, McCrindle BW, Benson LN, *et al.* (1996) Aortic valve regurgitation after surgical versus percutaneous balloon valvotomy for congenital aortic valve stenosis. Am J Cardiol 77, 1332–1338.

53. Rupprath G, Neuhaus KL. (1985) Percutaneous balloon valvuloplasty for aortic valve stenosis in infancy. Am J Cardiol 55, 1655–1656.

54. McElhinney DB, Lock JE, Keane JF, et al. (2005) Left heart growth, function, and reintervention after balloon aortic valvuloplasty for neonatal aortic stenosis. Circulation 111, 451–458.

55. Mosca RS, Iannettoni MD, Schwartz SM, et al. (1995) Critical aortic stenosis in the neonate. A comparison of balloon valvuloplasty and transventricular dilation. J Thorac Cardiovasc Surg 109, 147–154.

56. Weber HS, Mart CR, Kupferschmid J, et al. (1998) Transcarotid balloon valvuloplasty with continuous transesophageal echocardiographic guidance for neonatal critical aortic valve stenosis: an alternative to surgical palliation. Pediatr Cardiol 19, 212–217.

57. Piechaud JF. (2001) Issues in transcatheter treatment of critical aortic stenosis in the newborn infant. J Interv Cardiol 14, 351–355.

58. Fratz S, Gildein HP, Balling G, et al. (2008) Aortic valvuloplasty in pediatric patients substantially postpones the need for aortic valve surgery: a single-center experience of 188 patients after up to 17.5 years of follow-up. Circulation 117, 1201–1206.

59. Han RK, Gurofsky RC, Lee KJ, et al. (2007) Outcome and growth potential of left heart structures after neonatal intervention for aortic valve stenosis. J Am Coll Cardiol 50, 2406–2414.

60. Selamet Tierney ES, Wald RM, McElhinney DB, et al. (2007) Changes in left heart hemodynamics after technically successful in-utero aortic valvuloplasty. Ultrasound Obstet Gynecol 30, 715–720.

61. DeBoer DA, Robbins RC, Maron BJ, et al. (1990) Late results of aortic valvotomy for congenital valvar aortic stenosis. Ann Thorac Surg 50, 69–73.

62. Gildein HP, Kleinert S, Weintraub RG, et al. (1996) Surgical commissurotomy of the aortic valve: outcome of open valvotomy in neonates with critical aortic stenosis. Am Heart J 131, 754–759.

63. Karl TR, Sano S, Brawn WJ, et al. (1990) Critical aortic stenosis in the first month of life: surgical results in 26 infants. Ann Thorac Surg 50, 105–109.

64. Messmer BJ, Hofstetter R, von Bernuth G. (1991) Surgery for critical congenital aortic stenosis during the first three months of life. Eur J Cardiothorac Surg 5, 378–382.

65. Ettedgui JA, Tallman-Eddy T, Neches WH, et al. (1992) Long-term results of survivors of surgical valvotomy for severe aortic stenosis in early infancy. J Thorac Cardiovasc Surg 104, 1714–1720.

66. Alexiou C, Chen Q, Langley SM, et al. (2001) Is there still a place for open surgical valvotomy in the management of aortic stenosis in children? The view from Southampton. Eur J Cardiothorac Surg 20, 239–246.

67. Duncan K, Sullivan I, Robinson P, et al. (1987) Transventricular aortic valvotomy for critical aortic stenosis in infants. J Thorac Cardiovasc Surg 93, 546–550.

68. Hawkins JA, Minich LL, Tani LY, et al. (1998) Late results and reintervention after aortic valvotomy for critical aortic stenosis in neonates and infants. Ann Thorac Surg 65, 1758–1762; discussion 1763.

69. Rehnstrom P, Malm T, Jogi P, et al. (2007) Outcome of surgical commissurotomy for aortic valve stenosis in early infancy. Ann Thorac Surg 84, 594–598.

70. Turley K, Bove EL, Amato JJ, et al. (1990) Neonatal aortic stenosis. J Thorac Cardiovasc Surg 99, 679–683; discussion 683–684.

71. Morris CD, Menashe VD. (1991) 25-year mortality after surgical repair of congenital heart defect in childhood. A population-based cohort study. JAMA 266, 3447–3452.

72. Gersony WM, Hayes CJ, Driscoll DJ, et al. (1993) Second natural history study of congenital heart defects. Quality of life of patients with aortic stenosis, pulmonary stenosis, or ventricular septal defect. Circulation 87(2 Suppl), I52–I65.

73. Tveter KJ, Foker JE, Moller JH, et al. (1987) Long-term evaluation of aortic valvotomy for congenital aortic stenosis. Ann Surg 206, 496–503.

74. McDonald K, Maurer BJ. (1989) Familial aortic valve disease: evidence for a genetic influence? Eur Heart J 10, 676–677.

75. Cohen LS, Friedman WF, Braunwald E. (1972) Natural history of mild congenital aortic stenosis elucidated by serial hemodynamic studies. Am J Cardiol 30, 1–5.

76. Hossack KF, Neutze JM, Lowe JB, et al. (1980) Congenital valvar aortic stenosis. Natural history and assessment for operation. Br Heart J 43, 561–573.

77. Davis CK, Cummings MW, Gurka MJ, et al. (2008) Frequency and degree of change of peak transvalvular pressure gradient determined by two Doppler echocardiographic examinations in newborns and children with valvular congenital aortic stenosis. Am J Cardiol 101, 393–395.

78. Rosenfeld HM, Landzberg MJ, Perry SB, et al. (1994) Balloon aortic valvuloplasty in the young adult with congenital aortic stenosis. Am J Cardio 73, 1112–1117.

79. Sullivan ID, Wren C, Bain H, et al. (1989) Balloon dilatation of the aortic valve for congenital aortic stenosis in childhood. Br Heart J 61, 186–191.

80. Hsieh KS, Keane JF, Nadas AS, et al. (1986) Long-term follow-up of valvotomy before 1968 for congenital aortic stenosis. Am J Cardiol 58, 338–341.

81. Caspi J, Ilbawi MN, Roberson DA, et al. (1994) Extended aortic valvuloplasty for recurrent valvular stenosis and regurgitation in children. J Thorac Cardiovasc Surg 107, 1114–1120.

82. Ilbawi MN, DeLeon SY, Wilson WR Jr, et al. (1991) Extended aortic valvuloplasty: a new approach for the management of congenital valvar aortic stenosis. Ann Thorac Surg 52, 663–668.

83. Alsoufi B, Karamlou T, Bradley T, et al. (2006) Short and midterm results of aortic valve cusp extension in the treatment of children with congenital aortic valve disease. Ann Thorac Surg 82, 1292–1299; discussion 1300.

84. Bacha EA, McElhinney DB, Guleserian KJ, et al. (2008) Surgical aortic valvuloplasty in children and adolescents with aortic regurgitation: acute and intermediate effects on aortic valve function and left ventricular dimensions. J Thorac Cardiovasc Surg 135, 552–559.

85. Mavroudis C, Backer CL, Kaushal S. (2009) Aortic stenosis and aortic insufficiency in children: impact of valvuloplasty and modified Ross-Konno procedure. Semin Thorac Cardiovasc Surg Pediatr Card Surg Annu 76–86.

86. McMullan DM, Oppido G, Davies B, et al. (2007) Surgical strategy for the bicuspid aortic valve: tricuspidization with cusp extension versus pulmonary autograft. J Thorac Cardiovasc Surg 134, 90–98.

87. Johnson RG, Williams GR, Razook JD, et al. (1985) Reoperation in congenital aortic stenosis. Ann Thorac Surg 40, 156–162.

88. Clarke DR, Bishop DA. (1993) Allograft degeneration in infant pulmonary valve allograft recipients. Eur J Cardiothorac Surg 7, 365–370.

89. Gallo I, Nistal F, Blasquez R, et al. (1988) Incidence of primary tissue valve failure in porcine bioprosthetic heart valves. Ann Thorac Surg 45, 66–70.

90. Mazzitelli D, Guenther T, Schreiber C, et al. (1998) Aortic valve replacement in children: are we on the right track? Eur J Cardiothorac Surg 13, 565–571.

91. Ross DN. (1967) Replacement of aortic and mitral valves with a pulmonary autograft. Lancet 2, 956–958.

92. Elkins RC. (1999) The Ross operation: a 12-year experience. Ann Thorac Surg 68(3 Suppl), S14–S18.

93. Sievers H, Dahmen G, Graf B, et al. (2003) Midterm results of the Ross procedure preserving the patient's aortic root. Circulation 108(Suppl 1), II55–II60.

94. Skillington PD, Fuller JA, Grigg LE, et al. (1999) Ross procedure. Inserting the autograft using a fully supported root replacement method; techniques and results. J Heart Valve Dis 8, 593–600.

95. Slater M, Shen I, Welke K, et al. (2005) Modification to the Ross procedure to prevent autograft dilatation. Semin Thorac Cardiovasc Surg Pediatr Card Surg Annu 8, 181–184.

96. de Kerchove L, Rubay J, Pasquet A, et al. (2009) Ross operation in the adult: long-term outcomes after root replacement and inclusion techniques. Ann Thorac Surg 87, 95–102.

97. Walters HL 3rd, Lobdell KW, Tantengco V, et al. (1997) The Ross procedure in children and young adults with congenital aortic valve disease. J Heart Valve Dis 6, 335–342.

98. Jonas RA. (1994) Radical aortic root enlargement in the infant and child. J Card Surg 9(2 Suppl), 165–169.

99. Kawachi Y, Tominaga R, Tokunaga K. (1992) Eleven-year follow-up study of aortic or aortic-mitral anulus-enlarging procedure by Manouguian's technique. J Thorac Cardiovasc Surg 104, 1259–1263.

100. Konno S, Imai Y, Iida Y, et al. (1975) A new method for prosthetic valve replacement in congenital aortic stenosis associated with hypoplasia of the aortic valve ring. J Thorac Cardiovasc Surg 70, 909–917.

101. Rastan H, Koncz J. (1976) Aortoventriculoplasty: a new technique for the treatment of left ventricular outflow tract obstruction. J Thorac Cardiovasc Surg 71, 920–927.

102. Frommelt PC, Lupinetti FM, Bove EL. (1992) Aortoventriculoplasty in infants and children. Circulation 86(5 Suppl), II176–II180.

103. Clarke DR. (1987) Extended aortic root replacement for treatment of left ventricular outflow tract obstruction. J Card Surg 2(1 Suppl), 121–128.

104. Sardari F, Gundry SR, Razzouk AJ, et al. (1996) The use of larger size pulmonary homografts for the Ross operation in children. J Heart Valve Dis 5, 410–413.

105. Shahid MS, Al-Halees Z, Khan SM, et al. (1999) Aneurysms complicating pulmonary autograft procedure for aortic valve replacement. Ann Thorac Surg 68, 1842–1843.

106. Rocchini AP, Beekman RH, Ben Shachar G, et al. (1990) Balloon aortic valvuloplasty: results of the Valvuloplasty and Angioplasty of Congenital Anomalies Registry Am J Cardiol 65, 784–789.

107. Sreeram N, Kitchiner D, Williams D, et al. (1994) Balloon dilatation of the aortic valve after previous surgical valvotomy: immediate and follow up results. Br Heart J 71, 558–560.

108. Knirsch W, Berger F, Harpes P, et al. (2008) Balloon valvuloplasty of aortic valve stenosis in childhood: early and medium term results. Clin Res Cardiol 97, 587–593.

109. Shim D, Lloyd TR, Beekman RH 3rd. (1997) Usefulness of repeat balloon aortic valvuloplasty in children. Am J Cardiol 79, 1141–1143.

110. Monro JL. (2008) Balloon valvuloplasty of the aortic valve in children: a surgical view. Nat Clin Pract Cardiovasc Med 5, 524–525.

111. Vida VL, Bottio T, Milanesi O, et al. (2005) Critical aortic stenosis in early infancy: surgical treatment for residual lesions after balloon dilation. Ann Thorac Surg 79, 47–51; discussion 52.

112. Alexiou C, Langley SM, Dalrymple-Hay MJ, et al. (2001) Open commissurotomy for critical isolated aortic stenosis in neonates. Ann Thorac Surg 71, 489–493.

113. Detter C, Fischlein T, Feldmeier C, et al. (2001) Aortic valvotomy for congenital valvular aortic stenosis: a 37-year experience. Ann Thorac Surg 71, 1564–1571.

114. Hawkins JA, Minich LL, Shaddy RE, et al. (1996) Aortic valve repair and replacement after balloon aortic valvuloplasty in children. Ann Thorac Surg 61, 1355–1358.

115. Cohen O, De La Zerda DJ, Odim J, et al. (2007) Aortic valve-sparing repair with autologous pericardial leaflet extension has low long-term mortality and reoperation rates in children and adults. Heart Surg Forum 10, E288–E291.

116. Masuda M, Kado H, Ando Y, et al. (2008) Intermediate-term results after the aortic valve replacement using bileaflet mechanical prosthetic valve in children. Eur J Cardiothorac Surg 34, 42–47.

117. Arnold R, Ley-Zaporozhan J, Ley S, et al. (2008) Outcome after mechanical aortic valve replacement in children and young adults. Ann Thorac Surg 85, 604–610.

118. Burczynski P, Mozol K, Mirkowicz-Malek M, et al. (2007) Evolving approach to aortic valve replacement in children and adolescents – a preliminary report. Kardiol Pol 65, 654–661; discussion 662–663.

119. Moidl R, Simon P, Aschauer C, et al. (2000) Does the Ross operation fulfil the objective performance criteria established for new prosthetic heart valves? J Heart Valve Dis 9, 190–194.

120. Brown JW, Ruzmetov M, Vijay P, *et al.* (2001) Clinical outcomes and indicators of normalization of left ventricular dimensions after Ross procedure in children. Semin Thorac Cardiovasc Surg. 13(4 Suppl 1), 28–34.

121. Elkins RC, Knott-Craig CJ, McCue C, *et al.* (1997) Congenital aortic valve disease. Improved survival and quality of life. Ann Surg 225, 503–510; discussion 510–511.

122. Kirkpatrick E, Hurwitz R, Brown J. (2008) A single center's experience with the Ross procedure in pediatrics. Pediatr Cardiol 29, 894–900.

123. Chambers JC, Somerville J, Stone S, *et al.* (1997) Pulmonary autograft procedure for aortic valve disease: long-term results of the pioneer series. Circulation 96, 2206–2214.

124. Elkins RC, Knott-Craig CJ, Ward KE, *et al.* (1994) Pulmonary autograft in children: realized growth potential. Ann Thorac Surg 57, 1387–1393; discussion 1393–1394.

125. Solymar L, Sudow G, Holmgren D. (2000) Increase in size of the pulmonary autograft after the Ross operation in children: growth or dilation? J Thorac Cardiovasc Surg 119, 4–9.

126. Niwaya K, Knott-Craig CJ, Lane MM, *et al.* (1999) Cryopreserved homograft valves in the pulmonary position: risk analysis for intermediate-term failure. J Thorac Cardiovasc Surg 117, 141–146; discussion 146–147.

127. Morales DL, Carberry KE, Balentine C, *et al.* (2008) Selective application of the pediatric Ross procedure minimizes autograft failure. Congenit Heart Dis 3, 404–410.

128. Bohm JO, Hemmer W, Rein JG, *et al.* (2009) A single-institution experience with the Ross operation over 11 years. Ann Thorac Surg 87, 514–520.

129. Pasquali SK, Cohen MS, Shera D, *et al.* (2007) The relationship between neo-aortic root dilation, insufficiency, and reintervention following the Ross procedure in infants, children, and young adults. J Am Coll Cardiol 49, 1806–1812.

130. Stewart RD, Backer CL, Hillman ND, *et al.* (2007) The Ross operation in children: effects of aortic annuloplasty. Ann Thorac Surg 84, 1326–1330.

131. van Son JA, Falk V, Mohr FW. (1997) Ross-Konno operation with resection of endocardial fibroelastosis for critical aortic stenosis with borderline-sized left ventricle in neonates. Ann Thorac Surg 63, 112–116.

132. van Son JA, Hambsch J, Bossert T, *et al.* (1999) Operative treatment of hypertrophic obstructive cardiomyopathy and aortic valve disease in infants. J Card Surg 14, 273–278.

133. Barkhordarian R, Wen-Hong D, Li W, *et al.* (2007) Geometry of the left ventricular outflow tract in fixed subaortic stenosis and intact ventricular septum: an echocardiographic study in children and adults. J Thorac Cardiovasc Surg 133, 196–203.

134. Choi JY, Sullivan ID. (1991) Fixed subaortic stenosis: anatomical spectrum and nature of progression. Br Heart J 65, 280–286.

135. Kelly DT, Wulfsberg E, Rowe RD. (1972) Discrete subaortic stenosis. Circulation 46, 309–322.

136. Serraf A, Zoghby J, Lacour-Gayet F, *et al.* (1999) Surgical treatment of subaortic stenosis: a seventeen-year experience. J Thorac Cardiovasc Surg 117, 669–678.

137. Patane S, Patane F, Marte F, *et al.* (2009) Subvalvular aortic stenosis associated with valvular aortic regurgitation in young child. Int J Cardiol 133, e81–e83.

138. de Vries AG, Hess J, Witsenburg M, *et al.* (1992) Management of fixed subaortic stenosis: a retrospective study of 57 cases. J Am Coll Cardiol 19, 1013–1017.

139. Rosenquist GC, Clark EB, McAllister HA, *et al.* (1979) Increased mitral-aortic separation in discrete subaortic stenosis. Circulation 60, 70–74.

140. Hartyanszky IL, Kadar K, Bojeldein S, *et al.* (1997) Mitral valve anomalies obstructing left ventricular outflow. Eur J Cardiothorac Surg 12, 504–506.

141. Imoto Y, Kado H, Yasuda H, *et al.* (1996) Subaortic stenosis caused by anomalous papillary muscle of the mitral valve. Ann Thorac Surg 62, 1858–1860.

142. Moulaert AJ, Oppenheimer-Dekker A. (1976) Anterolateral muscle bundle of the left ventricle, bulboventricular flange and subaortic stenosis. Am J Cardiol 37, 78–81.

143. Ozkutlu S, Tokel NK, Saraclar M, *et al.* (1997) Posterior deviation of left ventricular outflow tract septal components without ventricular septal defect. Heart. 77, 242–246.

144. Freedom RM, Pelech A, Brand A, *et al.* (1985) The progressive nature of subaortic stenosis in congenital heart disease. Int J Cardiol 8, 137–148.

145. Newfeld EA, Muster AJ, Paul MH, *et al.* (1976) Discrete subvalvular aortic stenosis in childhood. Study of 51 patients. Am J Cardiol 38, 53–61.

146. Shone JD, Sellers RD, Anderson RC, *et al.* (1963) The developmental complex of "parachute mitral valve," supravalvular ring of left atrium, subaortic stenosis, and coarctation of aorta. Am J Cardiol 11, 714–725.

147. Tchervenkov CI, Jacobs JP, Weinberg PM, *et al.* (2006) The nomenclature, definition and classification of hypoplastic left heart syndrome. Cardiol Young 16, 339–368.

148. Baumstark A, Fellows KE, Rosenthal A. (1978) Combined double chambered right ventricle and discrete subaortic stenosis. Circulation 57, 299–303.

149. Cyran SE, James FW, Daniels S, *et al.* (1988) Comparison of the cardiac output and stroke volume response to upright exercise in children with valvular and subvalvular aortic stenosis. J Am Coll Cardiol 11, 651–658.

150. Parry AJ, Kovalchin JP, Suda K, *et al.* (1999) Resection of subaortic stenosis; can a more aggressive approach be justified? Eur J Cardiothorac Surg 15, 631–638.

151. Cape EG, Vanauker MD, Sigfusson G, *et al.* (1997) Potential role of mechanical stress in the etiology of pediatric heart disease: septal shear stress in subaortic stenosis. J Am Coll Cardiol 30, 247–254.

152. Sigfusson G, Tacy TA, Vanauker MD, *et al.* (1997) Abnormalities of the left ventricular outflow tract associated with discrete subaortic stenosis in children: an echocardiographic study. J Am Coll Cardiol 30, 255–259.

153. Gross-Sawicka EM, Nagi HM, Lever HM, *et al.* (1991) Aortoseptal angulation and left ventricular hypertrophy pattern: an echocardiographic study in patients with aortic valvular stenosis. J Am Soc Echocardiogr 4, 583–588.

154. Yap SC, Roos-Hesselink JW, Bogers AJ, *et al.* (2008) Steepened aortoseptal angle may be a risk factor for

discrete subaortic stenosis in adults. Int J Cardiol 126, 138–139.

155. Shem-Tov A, Schneeweiss A, Motro M, *et al.* (1982) Clinical presentation and natural history of mild discrete subaortic stenosis. Follow-up of 1–17 years. Circulation 66, 509–512.

156. Gersony WM. (2001) Natural history of discrete subvalvar aortic stenosis: management implications. J Am Coll Cardiol 38, 843–845.

157. Brauner R, Laks H, Drinkwater DC Jr, *et al.* (1997) Benefits of early surgical repair in fixed subaortic stenosis. J Am Coll Cardiol 30, 1835–1842.

158. Rayburn ST, Netherland DE, Heath BJ. (1997) Discrete membranous subaortic stenosis: improved results after resection and myectomy. Ann Thorac Surg 64, 105–109.

159. Wright GB, Keane JF, Nadas AS, *et al.* (1983) Fixed subaortic stenosis in the young: medical and surgical course in 83 patients. Am J Cardiol 52, 830–835.

160. Erentug V, Bozbuga N, Kirali K, *et al.* (2005) Surgical treatment of subaortic obstruction in adolescent and adults: long-term follow-up. J Card Surg 20, 16–21.

161. Roughneen PT, DeLeon SY, Cetta F, *et al.* (1998) Modified Konno-Rastan procedure for subaortic stenosis: indications, operative techniques, and results. Ann Thorac Surg 65, 1368–1375; discussion 1375–1376.

162. Tabatabaie MB, Ghavidel AA, Yousefnia MA, *et al.* (2006) Classic Konno-Rastan procedure: indications and results in the current era. Asian Cardiovasc Thorac Ann 14, 377–381.

163. Borisov KV, Bockeria LA, Sinyov AF. (2008) Surgical treatment of hypertrophic obstructive cardiomyopathy in pediatric patients with severe hypertrophy. Artif Organs 32, 856–863.

164. Bruce CJ, Nishimura RA, Tajik AJ, *et al.* (1999) Fixed left ventricular outflow tract obstruction in presumed hypertrophic obstructive cardiomyopathy: implications for therapy. Ann Thorac Surg 68, 100–104.

165. Minakata K, Dearani JA, O'Leary PW, *et al.* (2005) Septal myectomy for obstructive hypertrophic cardiomyopathy in pediatric patients: early and late results. Ann Thorac Surg 80, 1424–1429; discussion 1429–1430.

166. Williams JC, Barratt-Boyes BG, Lowe JB. (1961) Supravalvular aortic stenosis. Circulation 24, 1311–1318.

167. Kim YM, Yoo SJ, Choi JY, *et al.* (1999) Natural course of supravalvar aortic stenosis and peripheral pulmonary arterial stenosis in Williams' syndrome. Cardiol Young 9, 37–41.

168. Stamm C, Li J, Ho SY, *et al.* (1997) The aortic root in supravalvular aortic stenosis: the potential surgical relevance of morphologic findings. J Thorac Cardiovasc Surg 114, 16–24.

169. Perou ML. (1961) Congenital supravalvular aortic stenosis. A morphological study with attempt at classification. Arch Pathol 71, 453–466.

170. van Son JA, Edwards WD, Danielson GK. (1994) Pathology of coronary arteries, myocardium, and great arteries in supravalvular aortic stenosis. Report of five cases with implications for surgical treatment. J Thorac Cardiovasc Surg 108, 21–28.

171. Yilmaz AT, Arslan M, Ozal E, *et al.* (1996) Coronary artery aneurysm associated with adult supravalvular aortic stenosis. Ann Thorac Surg 62, 1205–1207.

172. Meairs S, Weihe E, Mittmann U, *et al.* (1984) Morphologic investigation of coronary arteries subjected to hypertension by experimental supravalvular aortic stenosis in dogs. Lab Invest 50, 469–479.

173. Peterson TA, Todd DB, Edwards JE. (1965) Supravalvular aortic stenosis. J Thorac Cardiovasc Surg 50, 734–741.

174. Rastelli GC, McGoon DC, Ongley PA, *et al.* (1966) Surgical treatment of supravalvular aortic stenosis. Report of 16 cases and review of literature. J Thorac Cardiovasc Surg 51, 873–882.

175. van Son JA, Danielson GK, Puga FJ, *et al.* (1994) Supravalvular aortic stenosis. Long-term results of surgical treatment. J Thorac Cardiovasc Surg 107, 103–114; discussion 114–115.

176. Braunstein PW Jr, Sade RM, Crawford FA Jr, *et al.* (1990) Repair of supravalvar aortic stenosis: cardiovascular morphometric and hemodynamic results. Ann Thorac Surg 50, 700–707.

177. Delius RE, Steinberg JB, L'Ecuyer T, *et al.* (1995) Long-term follow-up of extended aortoplasty for supravalvular aortic stenosis. J Thorac Cardiovasc Surg 109, 155–162; discussion 162–163.

178. Flaker G, Teske D, Kilman J, *et al.* (1983) Supravalvular aortic stenosis. A 20-year clinical perspective and experience with patch aortoplasty. Am J Cardiol 51, 256–260.

179. Becker AE, Becker MJ, Edwards JE. (1972) Mitral valvular abnormalities associated with supravalvular aortic stenosis. Observations in 3 cases. Am J Cardiol 29, 90–94.

180. Stamm C, Friehs I, Ho SY, *et al.* (2001) Congenital supravalvar aortic stenosis: a simple lesion? Eur J Cardiothorac Surg 19, 195–202.

181. Giddins NG, Finley JP, Nanton MA, *et al.* (1989) The natural course of supravalvar aortic stenosis and peripheral pulmonary artery stenosis in Williams's syndrome. Br Heart J 62, 315–319.

182. Wren C, Oslizlok P, Bull C. (1990) Natural history of supravalvular aortic stenosis and pulmonary artery stenosis. J Am Coll Cardiol 15, 1625–1630.

183. Schubert C. (2009) The genomic basis of the Williams-Beuren syndrome. Cell Mol Life Sci 66, 1178–1197.

184. Boeckel T, Dierks A, Vergopoulos A, *et al.* (1999) A new mutation in the elastin gene causing supravalvular aortic stenosis. Am J Cardiol 83, 1141–1143.

185. Chowdhury T, Reardon W. (1999) Elastin mutation and cardiac disease. Pediatr Cardiol 20, 103–107.

186. Li DY, Toland AE, Boak BB, *et al.* (1997) Elastin point mutations cause an obstructive vascular disease, supravalvular aortic stenosis. Hum Mol Genet 6, 1021–1028.

187. Beuren AJ, Apitz J, Harmjanz D. (1962) Supravalvular aortic stenosis in association with mental retardation and a certain facial appearance. Circulation 26, 1235–1240.

188. Beuren AJ, Schulze C, Eberle P, *et al.* (1964) The Syndrome of Supravalvular Aortic Stenosis, Peripheral Pulmonary Stenosis, Mental Retardation and Similar Facial Appearance. Am J Cardiol 13, 471–483.

189. Dutly F, Schinzel A. (1996) Unequal interchromosomal rearrangements may result in elastin gene deletions causing the Williams-Beuren syndrome. Hum Mol Genet 5, 1893–1898.

190. Keating MT. (1995) Genetic approaches to cardiovascular disease. Supravalvular aortic stenosis, Williams syndrome, and long-QT syndrome. Circulation 92, 142–147.

191. Jacob JL, Coelho WM, Machado NC, et al. (1993) Initial experience with balloon dilatation of supravalvar aortic stenosis. Br Heart J 70, 476–478.

192. Pinto RJ, Loya Y, Bhagwat A, et al. (1994) Balloon dilatation of supravalvular aortic stenosis: a report of two cases. Int J Cardiol 46, 179–181.

193. Abadir S, Dauphin C, Lecompte Y, et al. (2007) [The Williams-Beuren syndrome: reconstruction of the thoracic aorta combining surgery and endovascular treatment]. Arch Mal Coeur Vaiss 100, 466–469.

194. Geggel RL, Gauvreau K, Lock JE. (2001) Balloon dilation angioplasty of peripheral pulmonary stenosis associated with Williams syndrome. Circulation 103, 2165–2170.

195. Chard RB, Cartmill TB. (1993) Localized supravalvar aortic stenosis: a new technique for repair. Ann Thorac Surg 55, 782–784.

196. McGoon DC, Mankin HT, Vlad P, et al. (1961) The surgical treatment of supravalvular aortic stenosis. J Thorac Cardiovasc Surg 41, 125–133.

197. Doty DB, Polansky DB, Jenson CB. (1977) Supravalvular aortic stenosis. Repair by extended aortoplasty. J Thorac Cardiovasc Surg 74, 362–371.

198. Brown JW, Ruzmetov M, Vijay P, et al. (2002) Surgical repair of congenital supravalvular aortic stenosis in children. Eur J Cardiothorac Surg 21, 50–56.

199. Sharma BK, Fujiwara H, Hallman GL, et al. (1991) Supravalvar aortic stenosis: a 29-year review of surgical experience. Ann Thorac Surg 51, 1031–1039.

200. Brom AG. (1988) Obstruction of the left ventricular outflow tract. In: Khonsari S, ed. Cardiac Surgery: Safeguards and Pitfalls in Operative Technique, 1st ed. Rockville, MD: Aspen Publishers.

201. Khonsari S. (1997) Left ventricular outflow tract obstruction. In: Khonsari S, ed. Cardiac Surgery: Safeguards and Pitfalls in Operative Technique, 2nd ed. Philadelphia, PA: Lippincott-Raven, pp. 257–268.

202. Kaushal S, Backer CL, Patel S, et al. (2010) Midterm outcomes in supravalvular aortic stenosis demonstrate the superiority of multisinus aortoplasty. Ann Thorac Surg 89, 1371–1377.

203. Myers JL, Waldhausen JA, Cyran SE, et al. (1993) Results of surgical repair of congenital supravalvular aortic stenosis. J Thorac Cardiovasc Surg 105, 281–287; discussion 287–288.

204. Matsuda H, Miyamoto Y, Takahashi T, et al. (1991) Extended aortic and left main coronary angioplasty with a single pericardial patch in a patient with Williams syndrome. Ann Thorac Surg 52, 1331–1333.

205. Rosenkranz ER, Murphy DJ Jr, Cosgrove DM 3rd. (1992) Surgical management of left coronary artery ostial atresia and supravalvar aortic stenosis. Ann Thorac Surg 54, 779–781.

206. Shin H, Katogi T, Yozu R, et al. (1999) Surgical angioplasty of left main coronary stenosis complicating supravalvular aortic stenosis. Ann Thorac Surg 67, 1147–1148.

207. Brown JW, Ruzmetov M, Fiore AC, et al. (2005) Long-term results of apical aortic conduits in children with complex left ventricular outflow tract obstruction. Ann Thorac Surg 80, 2301–2308.

208. DiDonato RM, Danielson GK, McGoon DC, et al. (1984) Left ventricle-aortic conduits in pediatric patients. J Thorac Cardiovasc Surg 88, 82–91.

209. Sweeney MS, Walker WE, Cooley DA, et al. (1986) Apicoaortic conduits for complex left ventricular outflow obstruction: 10-year experience. Ann Thorac Surg 42, 609–611.

210. Cooley DA, Lopez RM, Absi TS. (2000) Apicoaortic conduit for left ventricular outflow tract obstruction: revisited. Ann Thorac Surg 69, 1511–1514.

211. Hickey EJ, Jung G, Williams WG, et al. (2008) Congenital supravalvular aortic stenosis: defining surgical and nonsurgical outcomes. Ann Thorac Surg 86, 1919–1927; discussion 1927.

212. Kitchiner D, Jackson M, Walsh K, et al. (1996) Prognosis of supravalve aortic stenosis in 81 patients in Liverpool (1960–1993). Heart 75, 396–402.

213. Keane JF, Fellows KE, LaFarge CG, et al. (1976) The surgical management of discrete and diffuse supravalvar aortic stenosis. Circulation 54, 112–117.

214. Tchervenkov CI, Jacobs ML, Tahta SA. (2000) Congenital Heart Surgery Nomenclature and Database Project: hypoplastic left heart syndrome. Ann Thorac Surg 69(4 Suppl), S170–S179.

CHAPTER 31

Hypoplastic Left Heart Syndrome

Jennifer C. Hirsch,[1] Eric J. Devaney,[2] Richard G. Ohye,[1] and Edward L. Bove[1]

[1]C.S. Mott Children's Hospital at the University of Michigan, Ann Arbor, MI, USA
[2]Rady Children's Hospital at the University of California, San Diego, CA, USA

Hypoplastic left heart syndrome (HLHS) refers to a constellation of congenital cardiac anomalies characterized by marked hypoplasia or absence of the left ventricle and severe hypoplasia of the ascending aorta. The systemic circulation is dependent on the right ventricle via a patent ductus arteriosus, and there is obligatory mixing of pulmonary and systemic venous blood in the right atrium. The term hypoplastic left heart syndrome was introduced by Noonan and Nadas [1] in 1958 to describe the morphologic features of combined aortic and mitral atresia. This followed Lev's [2] description in 1952 of congenital cardiac malformations associated with underdevelopment of the left-sided chambers and a small ascending aorta and aortic arch.

Hypoplastic left heart syndrome is a relatively common form of congenital heart disease, occurring in 7–9% of neonates diagnosed with heart disease in the first year of life [3]. Without surgical intervention, HLHS is a fatal lesion, accounting for 25% of cardiac deaths in the first week of life [4]. The first successful palliation of HLHS was reported by Norwood and colleagues [5] in a series of infants operated on between 1979 and 1981. This procedure has been technically refined over the years but the essential components remain 1) atrial septectomy, 2) anastomosis of the proximal pulmonary artery to the aorta with homograft augmentation of the aortic arch, and 3) aortopulmonary shunt or a right ventricle to pulmonary artery conduit. Staged palliation of HLHS with a Fontan operation using the right ventricle as the systemic ventricle was first reported in 1983 [6], and more recent reviews describe continued improvement in short- and long-term survival [7–13].

An alternative approach to staged reconstructive surgery is orthotopic cardiac transplantation. This was first performed successfully by Leonard Bailey and colleagues in November 1985 when he transplanted the heart and ascending aorta of an 8-day-old neonate into a 4-day-old, 2.8-kg infant [14]. This followed years of research, including experimentation with xenotransplantation [15]. The advantage of cardiac transplantation is replacement of an abnormal circulation with a normal four-chambered heart in one operation. The chief disadvantages of this approach are the limited availability of donor hearts, the requirement for lifelong immunosuppression, and late graft failure.

Dramatic improvements in both staged reconstructive approaches and transplantation have been achieved in recent years [16–19]. Currently, both staged reconstruction and transplantation have a role in the management of HLHS [20,21]. The surgical techniques and results of the two methods will be reviewed in this chapter.

Pathology

Pathologic findings in a series of 230 cases of HLHS included 105 with aortic atresia and mitral stenosis (45%), 95 with aortic and mitral atresia (41%), and 30 with severe aortic and mitral stenosis (13%) [22]. The dilated and hypertrophied right ventricle is the dominant ventricle and forms the apex of the heart. The tricuspid valve annulus is invariably dilated and significant anomalies in valve morphology have been described in 5–7% of patients [22,23]. Clinically significant tricuspid regurgitation has been reported in 8–10% of patients studied and has been identified as a significant risk factor in short- and long-term survival [24,25]. In 95% of these infants, the ventricular septum is intact and the left ventricular cavity is only a small slit with thick endocardial fibroelastosis [26]. The ascending aorta is usually very small, ranging in size by two-dimensional echocardiography from 1 to 8 mm, with a mean diameter of 3.8 mm and is less than 3 mm in 55% of cases. The portion of ascending aorta between the atretic

Pediatric Cardiac Surgery, Fourth Edition. Edited by Constantine Mavroudis and Carl L. Backer.
© 2013 Blackwell Publishing Ltd. Published 2013 by Blackwell Publishing Ltd.

valve and the innominate artery serves only as a conduit for the retrograde flow of blood into the coronary arteries. The main pulmonary artery is very large and is the origin for the large ductus arteriosus carrying blood from the right ventricle into the aorta. A localized coarctation of the aorta is present in 80% of patients [25,27].

Lev had postulated that premature narrowing of the foramen ovale leads to a faulty transfer of blood from the inferior vena cava to the left atrium during fetal life in infants with HLHS [28]. Thus, altered intrauterine hemodynamics may be the physiologic cause of HLHS. Other authors have postulated that the embryologic cause is severe underdevelopment of the left ventricular outflow in the form of isolated aortic valve atresia. This aortic atresia results in the abnormal development of the remaining cardiac structures resulting from the associated blood flow patterns [29]. It is now recognized that in a subset of patients, midgestation fetal aortic stenosis will progress to HLHS. Fetal intervention with aortic valvuloplasty is now offered at select centers for this lesion in an effort to prevent progression to HLHS [30,31].

Although it was initially believed that infants with HLHS had a low incidence of associated genetic and extracardiac developmental abnormalities, recent studies have demonstrated that 28% have a genetic disorder and/or major extracardiac anomalies [32]. A detailed genetic evaluation should be performed in all infants with HLHS. Several studies have reported higher mortality rates with staged palliation for HLHS when associated with extracardiac anomalies and genetic syndromes [31,33,34].

Clinical Picture and Medical Treatment

Increasingly, the diagnosis of HLHS is being made with fetal echocardiography and there is evidence that prenatal diagnosis improves preoperative clinical status and may even improve survival after first-stage palliation [35]. For patients not diagnosed prenatally, the diagnosis is made in the newborn period because of tachypnea and cyanosis within 24–48 hours of birth. When the ductus arteriosus begins to close, diminished systemic perfusion with pallor, lethargy, and diminished pulses rapidly occurs. Cardiac examination reveals a dominant right ventricular impulse, a single second heart sound, and a nonspecific soft systolic murmur at the left sternal border. Electrocardiogram demonstrates right atrial enlargement and right ventricular hypertrophy. Chest radiograph shows cardiomegaly and increased pulmonary vascular markings. In 2% of patients a reticular pattern of obstructed pulmonary venous return is seen because of a restrictive atrial septal defect. Ductal closure results in diminished systemic perfusion with the development of metabolic acidosis, renal failure, and hemodynamic collapse.

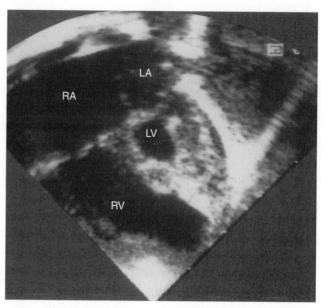

Figure 31.1 Apical four-chamber view (two-dimensional echocardiogram) demonstrating severe hypoplasia of the left ventricular cavity (LV) in an infant with aortic and mitral atresia. Right atrium (RA) and right ventricle (RV) are enlarged. The RV makes up the apex of the heart. (LA, left atrium.)

Diagnosis is by two-dimensional and color Doppler echocardiography for determination of cardiac morphology (Figure 31.1) [36] and evaluation of the arch hypoplasia (Figure 31.2) [36]. Doppler color flow shows that the blood flow in the ascending aorta is typically retrograde. Cardiac catheterization (Figure 31.3) [36] is rarely necessary, except to gain additional information in those patients with borderline left ventricular size in order to assist in decision making for the optimal method of treatment. Although initially believed to be deleterious by virtue of acutely decreasing resistance to pulmonary blood flow, current data supports the use of static balloon atrial septostomy to improve hospital survival in HLHS patients with highly restrictive atrial septal defects [37].

The initial support of these infants requires a very specific medical regimen [38]. The goals of preoperative management are to maintain ductal patency and provide the appropriate balance between the systemic and pulmonary vascular resistances. Intravenous prostaglandin E is infused at 0.03–0.1 µg/kg/minute to maintain patency of the ductus arteriosus. This dose may be titrated to keep the ductus arteriosus open, while minimizing the risk of apnea. Oxygen saturations are monitored by pulse oximetry. Acidosis is reversed with sodium bicarbonate and resuscitative efforts. The FiO_2 is adjusted to maintain relative hypoxemia (oxygen saturation, 75–80%), which aids in

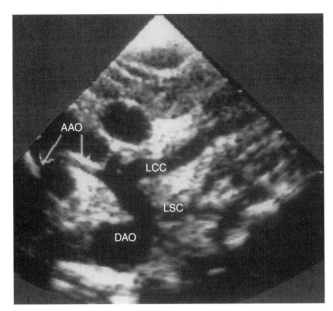

Figure 31.2 Suprasternal aortic arch view (two-dimensional echocardiogram) demonstrating severe hypoplasia of the ascending aorta (AAO), which is 3 mm in diameter in a patient with aortic valve atresia. The aortic arch flow is retrograde from the descending aorta (DAO) from the patent ductus arteriosus (not shown) into the left subclavian artery (LSC), left common carotid artery (LCC), right innominate artery (not shown), and AAO.

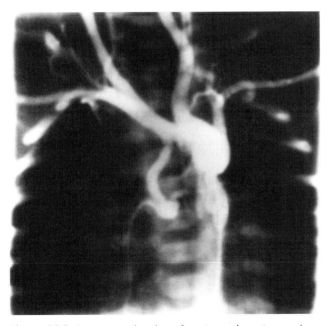

Figure 31.3 Anteroposterior view of a retrograde aortogram in a patient with HLHS showing the diminutive ascending aorta supplying the two coronary arteries and the normal caliber postductal descending aorta with coarctation.

preventing the pulmonary vasodilatation associated with high oxygen concentration. Even in the neonate who is being resuscitated from circulatory collapse, ventilation with a high concentration of oxygen is avoided, as it may only further decrease pulmonary vascular resistance and systemic blood flow. Blood transfusion should be performed to maintain hematocrit greater than 40%. Mechanical ventilation is avoided when possible, but ventilated infants may need to be sedated with intravenous fentanyl or morphine to prevent tachypnea. In cases of significant pulmonary overcirculation, hypoventilation to maintain a mild respiratory acidosis (pCO_2 45–55 mmHg) and elevate pulmonary vascular resistance may be employed. Occasionally, inhaled nitrogen can be added to reduce the FiO_2 to between 16% and 18% to further increase pulmonary vascular resistance. Inotropic support is advantageous in patients with depressed right ventricular function. Nourishment generally is provided via intravenous hyperalimentation, avoiding the added risk of necrotizing enterocolitis before surgery. Diuretics are added, as necessary when pulmonary congestion becomes apparent. This regimen balances the pulmonary and systemic vascular resistance, stabilizing the infant while therapeutic options are reviewed.

Therapy

Parents of these children are presented with three options: 1) supportive therapy only (leading usually to a rapid demise); 2) staged reconstruction; and 3) orthotopic cardiac transplantation. Each institution must assess its results with the various modes of therapy and parents must be counseled accordingly. As the results of palliative procedures and heart transplantation for HLHS have improved, in some cases even surpassing those of other complex forms of congenital heart disease, supportive therapy has been challenged [39,40]. The rest of this chapter reviews the techniques and results of staged reconstruction and cardiac transplantation.

Staged Reconstruction

The goal of staged reconstruction is a Fontan procedure, creating separate pulmonary and systemic circulations supported by a single (right) ventricle. The initial stage must provide unobstructed systemic blood flow from the right ventricle to the aorta and coronary arteries, relieve any obstruction to pulmonary venous return, and limit pulmonary blood flow by virtue of an appropriately sized systemic to pulmonary artery shunt. Owing to the relatively high pulmonary vascular resistance present in the newborn period, an arterial shunt is necessary, and the right ventricle is called upon to perform the increased volume work of both the pulmonary and systemic circulations. Preservation of right ventricular function has been aided by using smaller initial aortopulmonary or right ventricle to pulmonary artery shunts to limit right ventricular volume overload and by an interim procedure between the Norwood and Fontan operations. This staging procedure, either a bidirectional Glenn anastomosis or a hemi-Fontan procedure is usually performed at 4–6 months of age [41]. These procedures provide adequate pulmonary blood flow while decreasing volume overload on the right ventricle, improving effective pulmonary blood flow until the patient can undergo a completion Fontan procedure [42]. As described in detail later in this chapter in the section Second-stage palliation: hemi-Fontan or bidirectional Glenn anastomosis, the hemi-Fontan is a modification of the bidirectional Glenn procedure. The latter is an anastomosis between the transected superior vena cava and the pulmonary artery (the shunt is taken down). The hemi-Fontan involves a side-to-side connection between the superior vena cava/right atrial junction and the pulmonary arteries, routine augmentation of the branch pulmonary arteries, and temporary patch closure between the pulmonary arteries and the right atrium. The current stages of reconstructive surgery are shown in Table 31.1 [36].

First-Stage Palliation: Norwood Procedure

Through a midline sternotomy, the thymus is excised to gain exposure of the aortic arch. Cardiopulmonary bypass is established by arterial cannulation of the distal main pulmonary artery and venous cannulation of the right atrial appendage. A snare is engaged around the arterial cannula after it is advanced into the ductus arteriosus to exclude the pulmonary arteries. A minimum of 20 minutes of cooling to a core temperature of 18 °C begins. During this cooling phase, the ascending, transverse, and proximal

descending segments of the aorta are mobilized, and tourniquets are placed around each head vessel (Figure 31.4) [36]. The main pulmonary artery is then divided just proximal to the branch pulmonary arteries, and the opening closed with a polytetrafluoroethylene patch, pericardium, or homograft (Figure 31.5) [36]. The circulation is then arrested, the head vessels are occluded with snares, and a dose of 40 mL/kg of blood cardioplegia is administered. This can be given through a side port on the aortic cannula by clamping the descending aorta. The arterial and venous cannulae are removed. Alternatively, some groups have reported the use of regional low-flow cerebral perfusion in lieu of deep hypothermic circulatory arrest [43]. For this technique, the proximal anastomosis of the modified Blalock-Taussig shunt is performed before arresting the heart. The arterial cannula is placed into the shunt and perfusion given into the innominate artery. A vent is placed in the right atrium to scavenge venous return. The descending aorta is clamped with this technique. To date, there is no evidence in the literature to support any clinical superiority between deep hypothermic circulatory arrest and regional low-flow cerebral perfusion. The choice of perfusion strategy is largely based on center preference and surgeon facility with either technique.

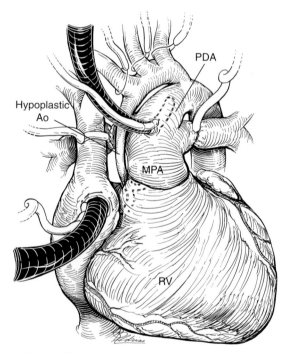

Figure 31.4 Initial steps during stage I reconstruction for hypoplastic left heart syndrome. Arterial cannulation is accomplished through the distal main pulmonary artery and venous cannulation in the right atrial appendage. The arch vessels are exposed and snares placed for occlusion during arch reconstruction. (AO, aorta; MPA, main pulmonary artery; PDA, patent ductus arteriosus; RV, right ventricle.)

Table 31.1 Staged reconstruction for hypoplastic left heart syndrome.

Procedure	Age
Stage one	**1–30 days**
Atrial septectomy	
Anastomosis proximal pulmonary artery to aorta with homograft aortic arch augmentation	
Aortopulmonary shunt	
Stage two	**4–10 months**
Bidirectional Glenn or hemi-Fontan	
Stage three	**18–24 months**
Completion Fontan	

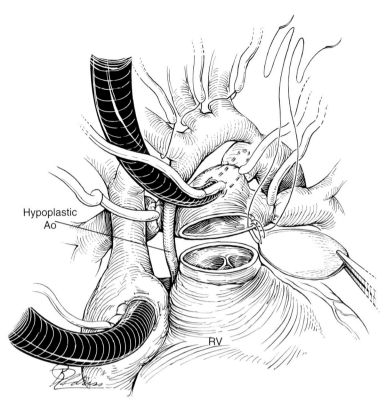

Figure 31.5 The main pulmonary artery is divided and the distal portion closed with a polytetrafluoroethylene patch. (AO, aorta; RV, right ventricle.)

Regardless of which perfusion technique is employed, the septum primum is then completely excised (atrial septectomy). This can be performed through a right atriotomy or, in some cases, through the atrial cannulation site. The ductus is ligated and divided. The remaining ductal tissue (on the undersurface of the aortic arch) is excised completely and the incision is extended at least 10 mm further down the descending aorta onto normal appearing and normal caliber aorta (Figure 31.6) [36]. This incision is then extended proximally under the transverse arch and down the diminutive ascending aorta until the level of the previously divided main pulmonary trunk is reached (Figure 31.7) [36]. Care must be taken to avoid spiraling this incision. A cryopreserved pulmonary allograft is trimmed to fashion a patch that will serve to enlarge the aorta and allow anastomosis to the proximal main pulmonary trunk (inset, Figure 31.7) [36]. Pulmonary homograft material is used for this gusset because it is pliable and relatively hemostatic. Augmentation of the aorta then begins by attaching the ascending aorta to the main pulmonary artery with interrupted monofilament sutures in the proximal corner near the coronary arteries. It is important to maintain a posterior orientation of the ascending aorta relative to the main pulmonary artery. The aorta is then patch augmented with the pulmonary allograft incorporating the

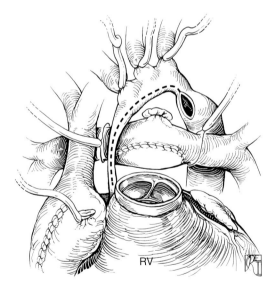

Figure 31.6 After establishing circulatory arrest and excising the atrial septum, the main pulmonary trunk is divided proximal to the bifurcation and the ductus is ligated. The remaining ductal tissue is completely excised from the aorta and the resulting opening is extended both proximally and distally as shown. (RV, right ventricle.)

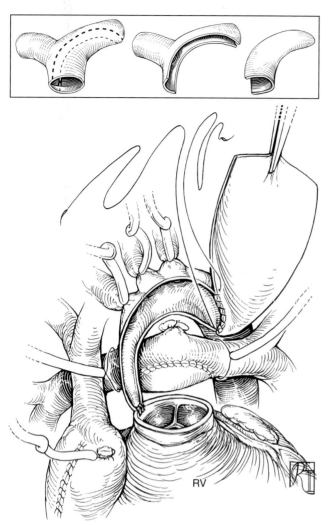

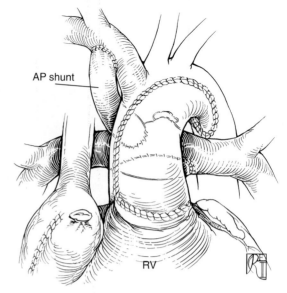

Figure 31.8 The final appearance of the Norwood reconstruction is shown. (AP, aortopulmonary; RV, right ventricle.)

Figure 31.7 The appearance after completion of the aortic incisions. The proximal aorta is anastomosed to the adjacent pulmonary trunk with interrupted fine monofilament sutures. A patch of pulmonary allograft is trimmed and used to augment the remaining ascending, transverse, and proximal descending aortic segments (inset). (RV, right ventricle.)

main pulmonary trunk proximally. The heart is flushed with saline to displace air and the cannulae are replaced to begin bypass and commence systemic rewarming to 37 °C. Warming the patient to greater than 37.5 °C is avoided as this has been correlated with neurological complications following deep hypothermic circulatory arrest. A poly-tetrafluoroethylene shunt is placed from the innominate artery to the central pulmonary artery during rewarming (Figure 31.8) [36]. A 4-mm shunt is used for patients weighing over 4 kg; smaller patients receive a 3.5-mm shunt. The proximal portion of the shunt can be attached before cardiopulmonary bypass initiation and the shunt temporarily

occluded or used to provide regional low-flow cerebral perfusion, as mentioned previously. The distal end of the shunt is placed centrally on the pulmonary arteries rather than onto the right pulmonary artery itself to promote even distribution of blood flow to both lungs. Fraser and Mee [44] have reported a modification of the Norwood technique that does not use homograft for the arch reconstruction.

Some groups have described improved survival in patients undergoing a Norwood procedure with the use of a right ventricle to pulmonary artery (RV-to-PA) conduit to provide pulmonary blood flow rather than the modified Blalock-Taussig shunt [45,46]. The modified Blalock-Taussig shunt results in significant diastolic run-off from the aorta, seen on Doppler/echocardiography as reversal of antegrade flow within the descending aorta during diastole. Since 70–80% of coronary blood flow occurs during diastole, this diastolic "steal" may significantly contribute to the decreased coronary flow seen after the Norwood procedure [47–49]. The RV-to-PA conduit has the theoretical advantage of eliminating the aortic diastolic run-off and coronary steal. The authors using the RV-to-PA conduit have noted a less complex postoperative course, in addition to improved survival. The clinically smoother course may be the result of the direct benefit of decreased diastolic run-off to other end organs, as well as indirectly from improved cardiac output. A 5- or 6-mm ringed poly-tetrafluoroethylene shunt is used if a RV-to-PA conduit is being used. The Single Ventricle Reconstruction trial (SVR), sponsored by the Pediatric Heart Network, is a multi-institutional randomized surgical trial evaluating the modified Blalock-Taussig shunt versus the RV-to-PA conduit. Results of this trial are forthcoming and should help define any potential superiority between shunt types.

A hybrid approach to the Norwood procedure has been proposed in an attempt to improve early survival by shifting the major surgical intervention until the second stage when the patient is older and end organ function has matured [50,51]. This approach involves stenting the ductus arteriosus to ensure unobstructed systemic outflow, placing bilateral pulmonary artery bands to restrict pulmonary blood flow, and a balloon atrial septostomy to alleviate any restriction to pulmonary venous return at the atrial septum. A comprehensive stage II procedure is performed at 4–6 months of age, which includes removal of the ductal stent, aortic arch reconstruction with Damus-Kaye-Stansel, and bidirectional Glenn or hemi-Fontan. Nationwide Children's Hospital has championed this procedure and reported a 97.5% survival rate with the hybrid stage I palliation and a 92% survival for patients who underwent a comprehensive stage II procedure [52]. For some centers, this is the routine procedure offered, whereas for most, the hybrid Norwood is reserved for select and often high-risk patients [51].

Postoperative Management

After weaning from cardiopulmonary bypass, an atrial monitoring catheter is placed to measure central venous pressure and an infusion of inotropes begins. At the University of Michigan, we routinely employ continuous infusions of milrinone and low-dose dopamine, adding epinephrine in doses of 0.02–0.06 µg/kg per minute if hypotension is significant. Ventilation with an initial FiO$_2$ of 100% to achieve a pCO2 of approximately 35 mmHg is initiated and adjusted depending on the systemic arterial oxygen saturation and the systemic perfusion. If poor peripheral perfusion with systemic saturations in excess of 80–85% is noted, the FiO$_2$ and minute ventilation are decreased to avoid excess pulmonary vasodilatation. The opposite maneuvers are used if the systemic oxygen saturation is less than 70–75%. Postoperative management is aimed at maintaining the delicate balance between the systemic and pulmonary vascular resistances, and therefore relative systemic and pulmonary blood flow. Many regimens of ventilation, inotropic and vasodilatory support have been employed, and multiple indicators of the adequacy of perfusion (e.g., mixed venous O$_2$ saturations, lactate, near infrared spectroscopy) have been used with varying degrees of success [18,53–57]. Ideally, the systemic arterial saturation should be maintained at 70–80%, which generally indicates that an optimal pulmonary-to-systemic blood flow ratio of less than 1 has been achieved. However, measurement of mixed venous and even pulmonary venous O$_2$ saturations is necessary to accurately assess Qp/Qs. In practice, we have found that serial lactate measurements provide an excellent indication of low cardiac output and

have come to rely on these determinations rather than mixed venous O$_2$ saturations. Some centers have reported the use of phenoxybenzamine (an α blocker) to improve systemic oxygen delivery after the Norwood procedure [18,58].

Despite these measures, most centers continue to report a significant percentage of early deaths following neonatal palliation. This has stimulated investigation into the physiology of single-ventricle patients using mathematical, experimental, and clinical models [59–64]. Many of these efforts have been flawed by the inability to create an analogous animal model that accurately measures pulmonary, systemic, and coronary blood flow. Further studies will help to delineate the relationship between O$_2$ delivery, O$_2$ demand, and coronary blood flow critical to survival in this challenging subset of patients.

Results of First-Stage Palliation

At the University of Michigan, the experience with first-stage palliation of HLHS from January 1990 to August 1995 included 158 patients [65]. All patients had classic HLHS, defined as a right ventricular dependent circulation, in association with atresia or severe hypoplasia of the aortic valve. Patients were subdivided into "standard risk" (n = 127) and "high-risk" (n = 31) populations. High-risk patients included those undergoing the Norwood procedure beyond the first month of life, patients with severe obstruction to pulmonary venous return, and those with significant noncardiac congenital conditions (e.g., prematurity, low birthweight, and chromosomal anomalies). There were 120 hospital survivors (76%). Hospital survival was significantly better among the 127 standard risk patients (86%) when compared with those in the high-risk group (42%). The risk factor analysis failed to reveal any effect on outcome of morphologic subgroup, ascending aorta size, shunt size, initial pH at hospital presentation, or duration of circulatory arrest. These findings have been supported by a recent analysis of patients with single ventricle malformations undergoing a Norwood procedure at the University of Michigan from May 2001 to April 2003 (n = 111) [33]. Noncardiac abnormalities ($p = 0.0018$), gestational age ($p = 0.03$), and weight less than 2.5 kg ($p = 0.0072$) again correlated with decreased survival [33].

At the Children's Hospital of Philadelphia, 840 patients underwent stage I surgery for HLHS between 1984 and 1999 [66]. Hospital survival steadily improved from 56% (1984–1988) to 71% (1995–1998). In that series, age over 14 days at the time of surgery and weight less than 2.5 kg at stage I were associated with increased mortality. There was no association between anatomic subtype and mortality in that series, except for patients with an intact atrial septum [67]. In the subgroup of infants with HLHS and an intact atrial septum (18 out of 316 infants over a 6.5-year period), there were only three long-term survivors (83% mortality).

At Boston Children's Hospital, 78 neonates underwent palliative reconstructive surgery between 1983 and 1991. There were 29 hospital deaths (37% mortality) [68]. Analysis of deaths revealed a greater risk of hospital death for infants with aortic atresia and mitral atresia, especially those with ascending aortic dimensions of less than 2mm. However, these morphologic subtypes have not been associated with increased risk in our experience. A risk assessment scoring system has been devised to predict survival following the Norwood procedure and includes ventricular function, tricuspid regurgitation, ascending aortic diameter, restriction at the atrial septal defect, blood type, and age at time of surgery [69]. Within a single institution, this scoring system had an area under the receiver operator curve of 0.8534 demonstrating a very high predictive value for mortality within the first 48 hours following surgery [69]. Despite excellent predictive characteristics, this scoring system has not been widely accepted.

The most recent data reflect a trend toward continuing improvement in survival for the Norwood operation. Hospital survival for 100 consecutive patients with HLHS undergoing first-stage palliation with a modified Blalock-Taussig shunt at the University of Michigan from April 2000 to April 2002 was analyzed. Overall hospital survival for the entire group was 85% (85/100). For standard-risk patients, as described above, the survival to hospital discharge was 92% (76/83) and for high-risk patients survival was 53% (9/17). Tweddell and colleagues reported a series of 81 consecutive patients (77% with HLHS) undergoing a Norwood operation with a modified Blalock-Taussig shunt with a 93% (75/81) hospital survival [70]. Sano and associates described a hospital survival of 88% (77/88) for patients with HLHS undergoing a Norwood procedure using a right ventricle-to-pulmonary artery conduit [45].

After discharge from the hospital, regular cardiovascular evaluations are important. The infant should be carefully observed for aortic arch obstruction, tricuspid insufficiency, and increasing cyanosis secondary to a limited atrial septal defect, shunt stenosis, or pulmonary artery distortion. Most centers have maintained these patients on aspirin to prevent shunt thrombosis [58]. Aspirin resistance has been identified in 26% of patients with congenital heart disease [71]. The use of clopidogrel should be considered in this subset of patients.

Second-Stage Palliation: Hemi-Fontan or Bidirectional Glenn Anastomosis

To minimize the time during which the right ventricle is subject to volume overload, the hemi-Fontan operation or a bidirectional Glenn anastomosis is typically performed between 4 and 6 months of age [41,42,72,73]. Cardiac catheterization and echocardiography are obtained before this procedure to evaluate pulmonary vascular resistance, pulmonary artery anatomy, tricuspid valve regurgitation, and right ventricular function. Both the hemi-Fontan and the bidirectional Glenn shunt are performed through a median sternotomy. To perform a bidirectional Glenn procedure, cardiopulmonary bypass is achieved with neoaortic arch cannulation and separate right-angle inferior and superior vena cavae cannulas. Alternatively, a single cannula is placed in the right atrium, and the superior vena cava is vented and occluded during the anastomosis. The aortopulmonary shunt is ligated and divided at the time of initiation of cardiopulmonary bypass. If there is any stenosis of the pulmonary artery secondary to the prior shunt or patch, it is repaired with patch augmentation. The azygous vein is ligated and divided. The superior vena caval flow is controlled with a snare, and a vascular clamp is placed at the junction of the superior vena cava and right atrium. The superior vena cava is transected and anastomosed in an end-to-side fashion to the superior aspect of the right pulmonary artery. The cardiac end of the transected superior vena cava is then oversewn.

The hemi-Fontan procedure has the same physiology as a bidirectional Glenn anastomosis but includes an anastomosis of the pulmonary arteries to an incision in the atriocaval junction. Cannulation for cardiopulmonary bypass is accomplished with arterial cannulation in the distal ascending aorta (allograft tissue) and venous cannulation through the mid portion of the right atrial wall. The patient is cooled to 25 °C, and the intraatrial portion of the cavopulmonary connection is performed under a brief period of low-flow bypass. Alternatively, cannulation of the inferior vena cava and high on the superior vena cava can be used to perform the procedure entirely on cardiopulmonary bypass. The aortopulmonary shunt is divided and the pulmonary arteries mobilized from right to left upper lobe (Figure 31.9) [36]. A patch of pulmonary allograft tissue is fashioned for augmentation of the pulmonary arteries (inset, Figure 31.10) [36]. The azygous vein is ligated. The allograft patch is begun at the left upper lobe, incorporating a separate end-to-side anastomosis for a left superior cava, if necessary (Figure 31.10) [36]. The inferior aspect of the right pulmonary arteriotomy is sewn to a separate incision in the right atriocaval junction (Figure 31.11) [36]. The incision is limited to proximal to the atriocaval junction to avoid possible injury to the sinoatrial nodal artery. A patch is placed within the right atrium, which will isolate superior vena caval return into the pulmonary arteries and provide an unobstructed pathway for connection of inferior vena caval return at the time of the Fontan procedure (Figure 31.12) [36]. The atrial septal defect is inspected and enlarged if necessary. This is best done by cutting back the coronary sinus into the left atrium. Tricuspid valve repair is also performed as needed.

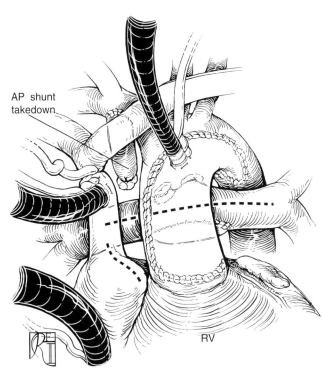

Figure 31.9 The lines of incision in the right atrial appendage and pulmonary artery confluence for the hemi-Fontan procedure are indicated. The systemic-to-pulmonary artery shunt has been ligated and divided. (AP, aortopulmonary; RV, right ventricle.)

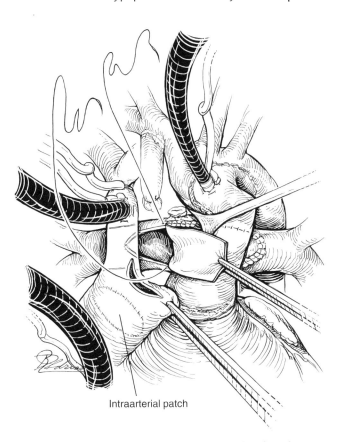

Figure 31.10 A patch of homograft is fashioned and used to augment the left pulmonary artery.

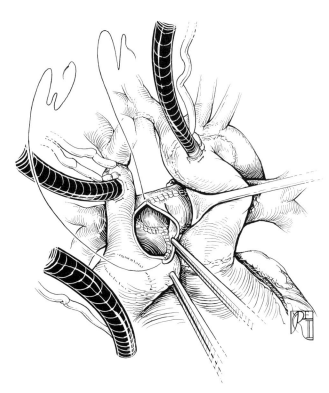

Figure 31.11 The posterior aspect of the right atriotomy is anastomosed to the inferior wall of the right pulmonary artery. The homograft patch is then used to roof the cavopulmonary connection.

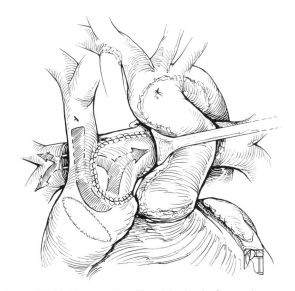

Figure 31.12 The completed hemi-Fontan is shown. A polytetrafluoroethylene patch is in place to prevent the superior vena caval return from entering the right atrium.

The advantage of the hemi-Fontan is that it shortens the time on cardiopulmonary bypass and dissection required for the completion Fontan, requiring only the removal of the intraatrial patch and placement of a lateral tunnel in the right atrium from inferior vena cava to superior vena cava. In addition, the routine augmentation of the branch pulmonary arteries helps to optimize the anatomy for the completion Fontan procedure.

The hospital records of 114 patients undergoing the hemi-Fontan procedure for HLHS between August 1993 and April 1998 at the University of Michigan Medical Center were reviewed [74]. The overall hospital survival was 98% (112/114). Sinus rhythm was present in 92%. At the time of publication, 79 of these patients had undergone the completion Fontan procedure with 74 survivors (94%). A similar study from the Children's Hospital of Boston also revealed that a cavopulmonary anastomosis done as a second-stage procedure for HLHS reduced mortality and improved intermediate survival [75]. At the Children's Hospital of Philadelphia, where this strategy was first employed, overall survival after the bidirectional cavopulmonary anastomosis (1989–1999) was 90%, and there was 100% survival of patients having a bidirectional cavopulmonary anastomosis between 1995 and 1998 [66].

Third-Stage Palliation: the Fontan Procedure

The completion Fontan procedure usually is performed at 18–24 months of age. The child is evaluated with cardiac catheterization before surgery. The Fontan technique that we have employed for HLHS anatomy is the total cavopulmonary connection with a lateral tunnel (Figures 31.13, 31.14) [36,76]. This technique minimizes the possibility of obstruction of the pulmonary venous return, which can be caused by an atriopulmonary anastomosis. Fenestration of the baffle may help prevent complications in high-risk patients and shorten the period of pleural drainage [77,78]. Technical details are reviewed in Chapter 28, *The Functionally Univentricular Heart and Fontan's Operation.* One hundred consecutive patients with classic HLHS underwent a Fontan procedure at the University of Michigan between June 2000 and August 2004 [12]. Hospital survival was excellent at 97% with durable intermediate survival of 96% at median follow up of 34 months. All patients are in New York Heart Association class I or II. Prolonged pleural drainage (greater than 2 weeks) was associated with the late development of protein-losing enteropathy ($p = 0.035$) [12]. In the largest reported series of the Fontan procedure from the University of Michigan (n = 636), 52% (n = 330) of patients had HLHS [13]. In this series, long-term survival was excellent at 97%. The association between prolonged chest tube drainage (greater than 2 weeks) was again associated with the development of protein-losing enteropathy ($p < 0.0001$) as well as dimin-

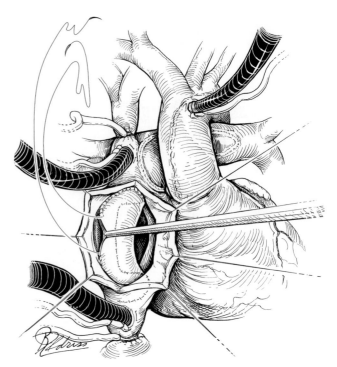

Figure 31.13 A polytetrafluoroethylene (PTFE) tunnel is shown being constructed for a lateral tunnel Fontan. The PTFE patch separating the cavopulmonary connection and the right atrium has been removed.

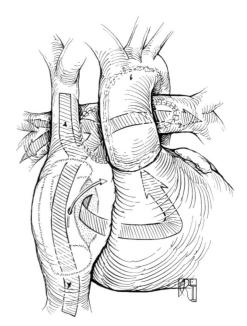

Figure 31.14 The completed Fontan procedure showing the systemic venous return from the superior and inferior vena cavae directed to the pulmonary artery. The smaller arrow illustrates the fenestration.

ished short-term ($p = 0.026$) and long-term (<0.0001) survival [13]. At the Children's Hospital of Philadelphia, overall survival after the Fontan procedure for stage III was 87%, and hospital survival after the Fontan operation has improved from 76% (1984–1988) to 100% (1995–1998) [66]. Most of these patients had a lateral tunnel with fenestration. In that series, 61 of the patients are now over 10 years of age. Several other centers have also reported significant improvements in survival following the Fontan procedure for HLHS [7,9,79,80]. A number of groups are now advocating the use of an extracardiac conduit to complete the Fontan procedure [10,81–83]. This technique may offer significant advantages, concerns include the risk of thromboembolic complications inherent to prosthetic conduits in the venous system as well as issues with somatic growth. Superiority has not been established between the extracardiac and the lateral tunnel Fontan.

Detailed computational fluid dynamic methods have been applied to the study of cavopulmonary connections [84,85]. This data has placed a greater emphasis on streamlining the cavopulmonary anastomotic design to optimize clinical results, limit energy loss, and equalize the distribution of inferior vena cava return into the branch pulmonary arteries. The lateral tunnel Fontan performed after the hemi-Fontan has been shown to be the most energy-efficient cavopulmonary connection with equal distribution of inferior vena cava return [85]. The turbulence within the cavopulmonary connection is magnified at increasing flow rates, which may contribute to the decreased exercise tolerance seen in many patients following the Fontan procedure [84].

Ongoing considerations for the Fontan procedure in this subgroup of patients include minimization of thromboembolic events, preservation of right ventricular and tricuspid valve function, and prevention of arrhythmias.

Neurodevelopmental Outcomes

Patients with HLHS, like any patient with cyanotic congenital heart disease, are at risk for neurodevelopmental delay for multiple reasons. Cyanosis, congestive heart failure, and central nervous system abnormalities are associated with HLHS and can contribute to developmental delay. In addition, cardiopulmonary bypass and hypothermic circulatory arrest at the time of repair can cause neurologic injury. In a study from our institution, Goldberg and colleagues evaluated 51 patients with single ventricle physiology, 26 patients with HLHS, and 25 patients with other cardiac anomalies [86]. The primary testing methods were the Wechsler Preschool and Primary Scale of Intelligence—revised for children 34–87 months of age and the Weschler Intelligence Scale—third edition for children 72 months to 17 years of age. Additional tests included the Bayley Scales of Infant Development, the Vineland Adaptive Behavior Scales, and the Child Behavior Checklist. The results showed that children with HLHS scored statistically lower than non-HLHS children with single ventricles. However, neither group scored significantly different from the population standards. As has been seen in children with congenital heart disease in general, patients in this study scored significantly better on tests of verbal intelligence when compared with motor skills assessments. Socioeconomic status, hypothermic circulatory arrest, and perioperative seizures were significant risk factors for impaired neurodevelopmental outcome. Duration of cardiopulmonary bypass, cardiac arrest requiring resuscitation, and clinical shock or pH less than 7.10 did not correlate with a poor neurodevelopmental result.

Orthotopic Cardiac Transplantation

Despite improving results following staged palliation of HLHS, the mortality of the reconstructive surgical approach has remained high in many centers. Because of this high mortality, interest in neonatal heart transplantation for HLHS continues in select centers and for high-risk patients. Heart transplantation provides a structurally and physiologically normal heart in one operative procedure. All results of neonatal cardiac transplantation must be analyzed realizing that 10–25% of infants listed for transplantation will die awaiting a donor heart [87]. Immunosuppression techniques and postoperative rejection surveillance with treatment of rejection and infection are discussed in Chapter 42, *Heart Transplantation*. This section will concentrate on techniques specific to neonates and their results.

Surgical Technique

Most donor hearts for neonates come from infants who have been the victims of birth asphyxia, sudden infant death syndrome, or trauma. Currently, all donor procurements are performed at the donor site of origin. Cardiopulmonary resuscitation and aggressive use of inotropic support in neonatal donors are not considered contraindications for cardiac transplantation. A donor-to-recipient weight ratio of up to 4.0 has been successful [87]. The donor cardiectomy is modified in that the entire aortic arch is harvested, well beyond the insertion of the ligamentum arteriosum.

The surgical technique of heart transplantation for infants with HLHS was originally described by Bailey and coworkers [88]. The implant is performed with cardiopulmonary bypass and profound hypothermia to 20 °C. The technique originally described by Bailey and colleagues used deep hypothermia and circulatory arrest for the entire implant and averaged circulatory arrest times of 56 minutes [89]. Since that time, technical refinements have been

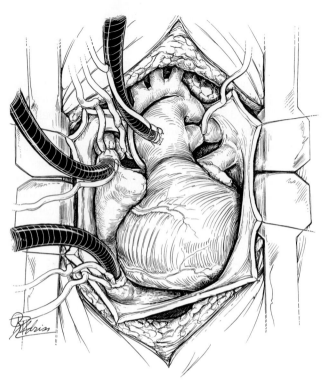

Figure 31.15 Cannulation for orthotopic cardiac transplantation in an infant with hypoplastic left heart syndrome. Arterial perfusion is via the main pulmonary artery (MPA). Note snares around right and left pulmonary arteries to prevent flow to the lungs. Venous return is with bicaval cannulation.

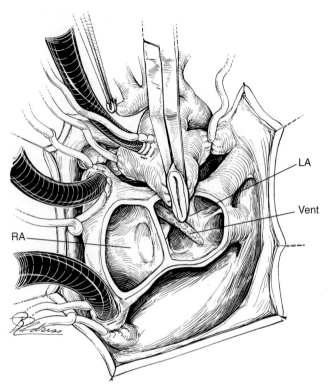

Figure 31.16 The hypoplastic heart has been excised after placement of a cross-clamp on the main pulmonary artery (MPA) and ligation and division of the tiny ascending aorta (Ao). Snares around the superior and inferior venae cavae have been engaged. Excision of the donor heart is performed with extracorporeal circulation continuing. (LA, left atrium; RA, right atrium.)

described, which help to minimize circulatory arrest and myocardial ischemia [38,90] (Figures 31.15–31.19) [36]. The decrease in donor myocardial ischemic time allows acceptance of donors from a wider geographical area.

Postoperative Support

In the current era, most transplant programs treat infant transplant recipients with triple therapy immunosuppression using corticosteroids, tacrolimus, and mycophenolate mofetil (MMF). Methylprednisolone is given at a dosage of 10 mg/kg intravenously at the start of cardiopulmonary bypass and again when circulation is resumed after arch reconstruction. A tapering dosage of methylprednisolone is used until the child tolerates oral feedings and then switched to prednisone with a target prednisone dose of 0.5 mg/kg/day. With no evident rejection (by echocardiography or biopsy), the steroids may be weaned to 0.2 mg/kg/day over the next several months, and some centers discontinue it completely.

In the absence of prohibitive renal dysfunction and oliguria, infants are initially started on tacrolimus, which can be administered intravenously at 0.5 µg/kg per hour

or orally (usually NG) at 0.05 mg/kg per dose twice daily. Perioperative blood levels of 12–15 ng/mL (by whole blood high-pressure liquid chromatography) are attained. Alternatively, if the initial postoperative renal function is poor, antithymocyte globulin (ATG) therapy can be used for induction, until the renal function normalizes.

Mycophenolate mofetil is an antiproliferative agent and potent inhibitor of de novo purine biosynthesis. Mycophenolate mofetil, as a component of triple therapy, has been shown to increase the 1-year survival and decrease the incidence of significant (≥ grade 3A) rejection in heart transplant recipients. However, reports indicate that opportunistic infections, particularly herpes simplex, are more common in patients treated with MMF [91]. The starting dose for MMF is 1200 mg/m² in divided doses twice per day, to a maximum total dosage of 3000 mg/day but titrated to maintain a white blood cell count greater than 4000 k/mm³. Many transplant centers now use therapeutic MMF monitoring based on recent evidence that levels of 2.0–2.5 µg/mL during the first post-transplant year are associated with fewer episodes of significant (≥ grade 3A) rejection [92]. Azathioprine and antithymocyte globulin are

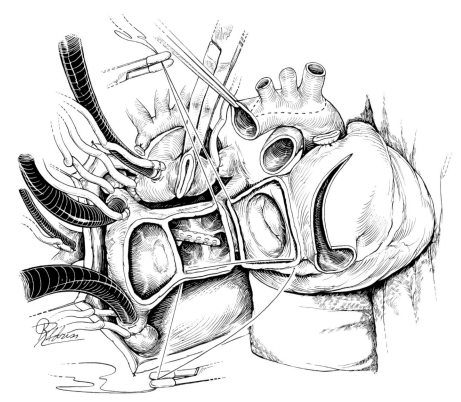

Figure 31.17 The donor heart is brought into the field, and the left atrial anastomosis is performed while extracorporeal circulation is maintained. The donor arch is tailored as indicated by the dotted lines.

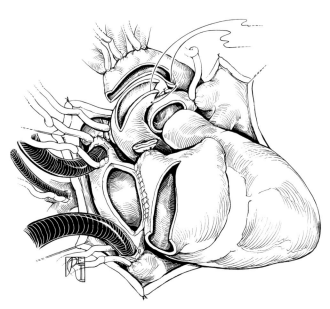

Figure 31.18 Circulatory arrest is initiated after the head vessels have been controlled by temporary occlusion. The ductus arteriosus is ligated and divided. The recipient aortic arch is prepared by aortotomy across the transverse arch and coarctation site (distal to the divided patent ductus arteriosus).

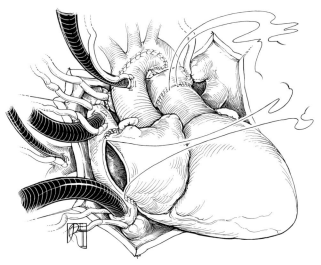

Figure 31.19 The aortic arch reconstruction is completed, procedures to remove air are performed, and the arch is cannulated, reinstituting cardiopulmonary bypass. The right atrial and the pulmonary artery anastomoses are performed with the heart perfused while the infant is rewarmed. The catheter in the left ventricle is now used as a vent.

major risk factors for increased Ebstein-Barr viral load and the development of post-transplant lymphoproliferative disease. Based on these findings, regimens incorporating MMF are preferred in the pediatric population over azathioprine-based protocols [93].

Rejection surveillance is based on clinical signs (appetite, activity, and heart rate), serial echocardiography, electrocardiography, and endomyocardial biopsy [39]. Noninvasive monitoring with serial echocardiograms is used more frequently than invasive techniques because of the limited intravenous access in small babies [94,95]. Rejection is usually treated with intravenous methylprednisolone, but rejection associated with hemodynamic compromise is treated with more aggressive therapy including steroids, ATG, and use of mechanical support as needed to maintain adequate cardiac output until myocardial function recovers. Prophylactic immunizations, including diphtheria-pertussis-tetanus and inactivated polio vaccine, begin 2 months after transplantation and are re-dosed according to the American Academy of Pediatrics recommendations, while live-attentuated viruses such as measles-mumps-rubella are withheld. More detailed information on immunosuppression and rejection surveillance is outlined in Chapter 42, *Heart Transplantation*.

Results

A multi-institutional study from the Pediatric Heart Transplant Study Group evaluating outcomes for patients with HLHS for transplantation from January 1993 to December 1998 demonstrated a decreased percentage of unpalliated HLHS patients being listed for transplantation (27% in 1993 vs. 14% in 1998) [96]. Overall, 25% of infants with HLHS die on the waiting list. Of the 175 (67%) patients who ultimately received a transplant, the 5-year actuarial survival was 72% with 76% of deaths occurring within 3 months of transplant. Overall survival including waiting list and post-transplant mortality was 68% at 3 months and 54% at 5 years [96]. The Registry of the International Society of Heart and Lung Transplantation reported the actuarial survival following heart transplantation in infants with the diagnosis of congenital heart disease to be approximately 70% at 1 year and 60% at 5 years [97]. Although the infant age group had a significantly higher early mortality compared with older infants and children with congenital heart disease, late survival for all age groups reached the same level as for infants. The major causes of death in the infant population are rejection and nonspecific graft failure. Infection accounted for a minority of the deaths. The prevalence of chronic rejection, often taking the form of coronary vasculopathy, is growing in the pediatric population. Beyond 3 years post-transplant, chronic rejection coronary artery disease was the leading cause of death. Improving immunosuppressive therapies, developing noninvasive methods of predicting cardiac rejection, and understanding the nature and treatment of coronary graft vasculopathy are challenges for the future of pediatric cardiac transplantation.

Conclusion

Hypoplastic left heart syndrome is a congenital cardiac lesion considered lethal until 1980. Now there are clearly two surgical options, staged reconstruction and cardiac transplantation. Staged reconstruction entails three procedures with an overall 5-year survival of approximately 75% for patients without significant non-cardiac anomalies or genetic syndromes. Long-term durability of the tricuspid valve and right ventricle at systemic workloads remains to be determined. Cardiac transplantation offers a single operation with perhaps a lower operative mortality, yet 25% of neonates listed for transplantation do not receive donor hearts. In addition, neonates post-transplant face a lifetime of immunosuppression with the attendant risks of rejection and infection. Both options have shown remarkable improvements in results with ongoing evolution of surgical techniques and improvements in perioperative care. Supportive care only, without intervention, is rarely offered for neonates with HLHS unless multiple noncardiac anomalies or genetic syndromes are present. The recommendations of any clinician in a given pediatric cardiac surgical unit must take into consideration that center's results and expertise with the two approaches.

References

1. Noonan JA, Nadas AS. (1958) The hypoplastic left heart syndrome; an analysis of 101 cases. Pediatr Clin North Am 5, 1029–1056.
2. Lev M. (1952) Pathologic anatomy and interrelationship of hypoplasia of the aortic tract complexes. Lab Invest 1, 61–70.
3. Fyler D, Buckley LP, Nadas AS, *et al.* (1980) New England regional infant cardiac program. Pediatrics 65, 377–461.
4. Watson DG, Rowe RD. (1962) Aortic-valve atresia. Report of 43 cases. JAMA 179, 14–18.
5. Norwood WI, Lang P, Casteneda AR, *et al.* (1981) Experience with operations for hypoplastic left heart syndrome. J Thorac Cardiovasc Surg 82, 511–519.
6. Norwood WI, Lang P, Hansen DD. (1983) Physiologic repair of aortic atresia hypoplastic left heart syndrome. N Engl J Med 308, 23–26.
7. Kaulitz R, Ziemer G, Luhmer I, *et al.* (1996) Modified Fontan operation in functionally univentricular hearts: preoperative risk factors and intermediate results. J Thorac Cardiovasc Surg 112, 658–664.
8. Gentles TL, Gauvreau K, Mayer JE Jr, *et al.* (1997) Functional outcome after the Fontan operation: factors influencing late morbidity. J Thorac Cardiovasc Surg 114, 392–405.

9. Gentles TL, Mayer JE Jr, Gauvreau K, *et al.* (1997) Fontan operation in five hundred consecutive patients: factors influencing early and late outcome. J Thorac Cardiovasc Surg 114, 376–391.

10. Petrossian E, Reddy VM, McElhinney DB, *et al.* (1999) Early results of the extracardiac conduit Fontan operation. J Thorac Cardiovasc Surg 117, 688–696.

11. Mosca RS, Kulik TJ, Goldberg CS, *et al.* (2000) Early results of the Fontan procedure in one hundred consecutive patients with hypoplastic left heart syndrome. J Thorac Cardiovasc Surg 119, 1110–1118.

12. Hirsch JC, Ohye RG, Devaney EJ, *et al.* (2007) The lateral tunnel Fontan procedure for hypoplastic left heart syndrome: results of 100 consecutive patients. Pediatr Cardiol 28, 426–432.

13. Hirsch JC, Goldberg C, Bove EL, *et al.* (2008) Fontan operation in the current era: a 15-year single institution experience. Ann Surg 248, 402–410.

14. Bailey LL, Nehlsen-Cannarella SL, Doroshow RW, *et al.* (1986) Cardiac allotransplantation in newborns as therapy for hypoplastic left heart syndrome. N Engl J Med 315, 949–951.

15. Bailey LL, Nehlsen-Cannarella SL, Concepcion W, *et al.* (1985) Baboon-to-human cardiac xenotransplantation in a neonate. JAMA 254, 3321–3329.

16. Razzouk AJ, Chinnock RE, Gundry SR, *et al.* (1996) Transplantation as a primary treatment for hypoplastic left heart syndrome: intermediate-term results. Ann Thorac Surg 62, 1–8.

17. Iannettoni MD, Bove EL, Mosca RS, *et al.* (1994) Improving results with first-stage palliation for hypoplastic left heart syndrome. J Thorac Cardiovasc Surg 107, 934–940.

18. Tweddell JS, Hoffman GM, Fedderly RT, *et al.* (1999) Phenoxybenzamine improves systemic oxygen delivery after the Norwood procedure. Ann Thorac Surg 67, 161–168.

19. Ishino K, Stumper O, De Giovanni JJ, *et al.* (1999) The modified Norwood procedure for hypoplastic left heart syndrome: early to intermediate results of 120 patients with particular reference to aortic arch repair. J Thorac Cardiovasc Surg 117, 920–930.

20. Bando K, Turrentine MW, Sun K, *et al.* (1996) Surgical management of hypoplastic left heart syndrome. Ann Thorac Surg 62, 70–77.

21. Hehrlein FW, Yamamoto T, Orime Y, *et al.* (1998) Hypoplastic left heart syndrome: "Which is the best operative strategy?" Ann Thorac Cardiovasc Surg 4, 125–132.

22. Bharati S, Lev M. (1984) The surgical anatomy of hypoplasia of aortic tract complex. J Thorac Cardiovasc Surg 88, 97–101.

23. Stamm C, Anderson RH, Ho SY. (1997) The morphologically tricuspid valve in hypoplastic left heart syndrome. Eur J Cardiothorac Surg 12, 587–592.

24. Barber G, Helton JG, Aglira BA, *et al.* (1988) The significance of tricuspid regurgitation in hypoplastic left-heart syndrome. Am Heart J 116(6 Pt 1), 1563–1567.

25. Chang AC, Farrell PE Jr, Murdison KA, *et al.* (1991) Hypoplastic left heart syndrome: hemodynamic and angiographic assessment after initial reconstructive surgery and relevance to modified Fontan procedure. J Am Coll Cardiol 17, 1143–1149.

26. Sinha SN, Rusnak SL, Sommers HM, *et al.* (1968) Hypoplastic left ventricle syndrome. Analysis of thirty autopsy cases in infants with surgical considerations. Am J Cardiol 21, 166–173.

27. Meliones JN, Snider AR, Bove EL, *et al.* (1990) Longitudinal results after first-stage palliation for hypoplastic left heart syndrome. Circulation 82(5 Suppl), IV151–IV156.

28. Lev M, Arcilla R, Rimoldi HJ, *et al.* (1963) Premature narrowing or closure of the foramen ovale. Am Heart J 65, 638–647.

29. Jacobs ML, Norwood WI. (1991) Hypoplastic left heart syndrome. In: Baue A, Geha A, Hammond G, eds. *Glenn's Thoracic and Cardiovascular Surgery*. Stanford, CT: Appleton & Lange.

30. Makikallio K, McElhinney DB, Levine JC, *et al.* (2006) Fetal aortic valve stenosis and the evolution of hypoplastic left heart syndrome: patient selection for fetal intervention. Circulation 113, 1401–1405.

31. Patel A, Hickey E, Mavroudis C, *et al.* (2010) Impact of noncardiac congenital and genetic abnormalities on outcomes in hypoplastic left heart syndrome. Ann Thorac Surg 89, 1805–1814.

32. Natowicz M, Chatten J, Clancy R, *et al.* (1988) Genetic disorders and major extracardiac anomalies associated with the hypoplastic left heart syndrome. Pediatrics 82, 698–706.

33. Stasik CN, Gelehrter S, Goldberg CS, *et al.* (2006) Current outcomes and risk factors for the Norwood procedure. J Thorac Cardiovasc Surg 131, 412–417.

34. Jacobs JP, O'Brien SM, Chai PJ, *et al.* (2008) Management of 239 patients with hypoplastic left heart syndrome and related malformations from 1993 to 2007. Ann Thorac Surg 85, 1691–1697.

35. Tworetzky W, McElhinney DB, Reddy VM, *et al.* (2001) Improved surgical outcome after fetal diagnosis of hypoplastic left heart syndrome. Circulation 103, 1269–1273.

36. Ohye RG, Mosca RS, Bove EL, *et al.* (2003) Hypoplastic left heart syndrome. In: Mavroudis M, Backer CL (eds) *Pediatric Cardiac Surgery*, 3rd ed. Philadelphia, PA: Mosby Inc.

37. Cheatham JP. (2001) Intervention in the critically ill neonate and infant with hypoplastic left heart syndrome and intact atrial septum. J Interv Cardiol 14, 357–366.

38. Backer CL, Idriss FS, Zales VR, *et al.* (1990) Cardiac transplantation for hypoplastic left heart syndrome: a modified technique. Ann Thorac Surg 50, 894–898.

39. Starnes VA, Griffin ML, Pitlick PT, *et al.* (1992) Current approach to hypoplastic left heart syndrome. Palliation, transplantation, or both? J Thorac Cardiovasc Surg 104, 189–195.

40. O'Kelly SW, Bove EL. (1997) Hypoplastic left heart syndrome. BMJ 314, 87–88.

41. Lamberti JJ, Spicer RL, Waldman JD, *et al.* (1990) The bidirectional cavopulmonary shunt. J Thorac Cardiovasc Surg 100, 22–30.

42. Douville EC, Sade RM, Fyfe DA. (1991) Hemi-Fontan operation in surgery for single ventricle: a preliminary report. Ann Thorac Surg 51, 893–900.

43. Pigula FA, Nemoto EM, Griffith BP, *et al.* (2000) Regional low-flow perfusion provides cerebral circulatory support during neonatal aortic arch reconstruction. J Thorac Cardiovasc Surg 119, 331–339.

44. Fraser CD Jr, Mee RB. (1995) Modified Norwood procedure for hypoplastic left heart syndrome. Ann Thorac Surg 60(6 Suppl), S546–S549.

45. Sano S, Ishino K, Kawada M, et al. (2003) Right ventricle-pulmonary artery shunt in first-stage palliation of hypoplastic left heart syndrome. J Thorac Cardiovasc Surg; 126, 504–510.

46. Pizarro C, Norwood WI. (2003) Right ventricle to pulmonary artery conduit has a favorable impact on postoperative physiology after Stage I Norwood: preliminary results. Eur J Cardiothorac Surg 23, 991–995.

47. Gregg DE, Khouri EM, Rayford CR. (1965) Systemic and coronary energetics in the resting unanesthetized dog. Circ Res, 16, 102–113.

48. Khouri EM, Gregg DE, Rayford CR. (1965) Effect of exercise on cardiac output, left coronary flow and myocardial metabolism in the unanesthetized dog. Circ Res 17, 427–437.

49. Donnelly JP, Raffel DM, Shulkin BL, et al. (1998) Resting coronary flow and coronary flow reserve in human infants after repair or palliation of congenital heart defects as measured by positron emission tomography. J Thorac Cardiovasc Surg 115, 103–110.

50. Galantowicz M, Cheatham JP. (2005) Lessons learned from the development of a new hybrid strategy for the management of hypoplastic left heart syndrome. Pediatr Cardiol 26, 190–199.

51. Pizarro C, Derby CD, Baffa JM, et al. (2008) Improving the outcome of high-risk neonates with hypoplastic left heart syndrome: hybrid procedure or conventional surgical palliation? Eur J Cardiothorac Surg 33, 613–618.

52. Galantowicz M, Cheatham JP, Phillips A, et al. (2008) Hybrid approach for hypoplastic left heart syndrome: intermediate results after the learning curve. Ann Thorac Surg 85, 2063–2071.

53. Mosca RS, Bove EL, Crowley DC, et al. (1995) Hemodynamic characteristics of neonates following first stage palliation for hypoplastic left heart syndrome. Circulation 92(9 Suppl), II267–II271.

54. Charpie JR, Dekeon MK, Goldberg CS, et al. (2000) Serial blood lactate measurements predict early outcome after neonatal repair or palliation for complex congenital heart disease. J Thorac Cardiovasc Surg 120, 73–80.

55. Charpie JR, Dekeon MK, Goldberg CS, et al. (2001) Postoperative hemodynamics after Norwood palliation for hypoplastic left heart syndrome. Am J Cardiol 87, 198–202.

56. Rossi AF, Sommer RJ, Lotvin A, et al. (1994) Usefulness of intermittent monitoring of mixed venous oxygen saturation after stage I palliation for hypoplastic left heart syndrome. Am J Cardiol 73, 1118–1123.

57. Hoffman GM, Stuth EA, Jaquiss RD, et al. (2004) Changes in cerebral and somatic oxygenation during stage 1 palliation of hypoplastic left heart syndrome using continuous regional cerebral perfusion. J Thorac Cardiovasc Surg 127, 223–233.

58. Poirier NC, Drummond-Webb JJ, Hisamochi K, et al. (2000) Modified Norwood procedure with a high-flow cardiopulmonary bypass strategy results in low mortality without late arch obstruction. J Thorac Cardiovasc Surg 120, 875–884.

59. Barnea O, Santamore WP, Rossi A, et al. (1998) Estimation of oxygen delivery in newborns with a univentricular circulation. Circulation 98, 1407–1413.

60. Reddy VM, Liddicoat JR, Fineman JR, et al. (1996) Fetal model of single ventricle physiology: hemodynamic effects of oxygen, nitric oxide, carbon dioxide, and hypoxia in the early postnatal period. J Thorac Cardiovasc Surg 112, 437–449.

61. Mora GA, Pizarro C, Jacobs ML, et al. (1994) Experimental model of single ventricle. Influence of carbon dioxide on pulmonary vascular dynamics. Circulation; 90(5 Pt 2), II43–II46.

62. Reddy VM, Liddicoat JR, McElhinney DB, et al. (1996) Hemodynamic effects of epinephrine, bicarbonate and calcium in the early postnatal period in a lamb model of single-ventricle physiology created in utero. J Am Coll Cardiol 28, 1877–1883.

63. Riordan CJ, Randsbaek F, Storey JH, et al. (1996) Inotropes in the hypoplastic left heart syndrome: effects in an animal model. Ann Thorac Surg 62, 83–90.

64. Riordan CJ, Randsbeck F, Storey JH, et al. (1996) Effects of oxygen, positive end-expiratory pressure, and carbon dioxide on oxygen delivery in an animal model of the univentricular heart. J Thorac Cardiovasc Surg 112, 644–654.

65. Bove EL, Lloyd TR. (1996) Staged reconstruction for hypoplastic left heart syndrome. Contemporary results. Ann Surg 224, 387–395.

66. Mahle WT, Spray TL, Wernovsky G, et al. (2000) Survival after reconstructive surgery for hypoplastic left heart syndrome: A 15-year experience from a single institution. Circulation 102(Suppl 3), III136–III141.

67. Rychik J, Rome JJ, Collins MH, et al. (1999) The hypoplastic left heart syndrome with intact atrial septum: atrial morphology, pulmonary vascular histopathology and outcome. J Am Coll Cardiol 34, 554–560.

68. Jonas RA, Hansen DD, Cook N, et al. (1994) Anatomic subtype and survival after reconstructive operation for hypoplastic left heart syndrome. J Thorac Cardiovasc Surg 107, 1121–1128.

69. Checchia PA, McGuire JK, Morrow S, et al. (2006) A risk assessment scoring system predicts survival following the Norwood procedure. Pediatr Cardiol 27, 62–66.

70. Tweddell JS, Hoffman GM, Mussatto KA, et al. (2002) Improved survival of patients undergoing palliation of hypoplastic left heart syndrome: lessons learned from 115 consecutive patients. Circulation 106(12 Suppl 1), I82–I89.

71. Heistein LC, Scott WA, Zellers TM, et al. (2008) Aspirin resistance in children with heart disease at risk for thromboembolism: prevalence and possible mechanisms. Pediatr Cardiol 29, 285–291.

72. Norwood WI Jr. (1991) Hypoplastic left heart syndrome. Ann Thorac Surg 52, 688–695.

73. MacIver RH, Stewart RD, Backer CL, et al. (2008) Results with continuous cardiopulmonary bypass for the bidirectional cavopulmonary anastomosis. Cardiol Young 18, 147–152.

74. Douglas WI, Goldberg CS, Mosca RS, et al. (1999) Hemi-Fontan procedure for hypoplastic left heart syndrome:

outcome and suitability for Fontan. Ann Thorac Surg 68, 1361–1368.

75. Forbess JM, Cook N, Serraf A, *et al.* (1997) An institutional experience with second- and third-stage palliative procedures for hypoplastic left heart syndrome: the impact of the bidirectional cavopulmonary shunt. J Am Coll Cardiol 29, 665–670.

76. de Leval MR, Kilner P, Gewillig M, *et al.* (1988) Total cavopulmonary connection: a logical alternative to atriopulmonary connection for complex Fontan operations. Experimental studies and early clinical experience. J Thorac Cardiovasc Surg 96, 682–695.

77. Mavroudis C, Zales VR, Backer CL, *et al.* (1992) Fenestrated Fontan with delayed catheter closure. Effects of volume loading and baffle fenestration on cardiac index and oxygen delivery. Circulation 86(5 Suppl), II85–II92.

78. Lemler MS, Scott WA, Leonard SR, *et al.* (2002) Fenestration improves clinical outcome of the Fontan procedure: a prospective, randomized study. Circulation 105, 207–212.

79. Koutlas TC, Gaynor JW, Nicolson SC, *et al.* (1997) Modified ultrafiltration reduces postoperative morbidity after cavopulmonary connection. Ann Thorac Surg 64, 37–43.

80. Hsu DT, Quaegebeur JM, Ing FF, *et al.* (1997) Outcome after the single-stage, nonfenestrated Fontan procedure. Circulation 96(9 Suppl), II335–II340.

81. Amodeo A, Galletti L, Marianeschi S, *et al.* (1997) Extracardiac Fontan operation for complex cardiac anomalies: seven years' experience. J Thorac Cardiovasc Surg 114, 1020–1031.

82. Gundry SR, Razzouk AJ, del Rio MJ, *et al.* (1997) The optimal Fontan connection: a growing extracardiac lateral tunnel with pedicled pericardium. J Thorac Cardiovasc Surg 114, 552–559.

83. Lardo AC, Webber SA, Friehs I, *et al.* (1999) Fluid dynamic comparison of intra-atrial and extracardiac total cavopulmonary connections. J Thorac Cardiovasc Surg 117, 697–704.

84. Sievers HH, Gerdes A, Kunze J, *et al.* (1998) Superior hydrodynamics of a modified cavopulmonary connection for the Norwood operation. Ann Thorac Surg 65, 1741–1745.

85. Bove EL, de Leval MR, Migliavacca F, *et al.* (2007) Toward optimal hemodynamics: computer modeling of the Fontan circuit. Pediatr Cardiol 28, 477–481.

86. Goldberg CS, Schwartz EM, Brunberg JA, *et al.* (2000) Neurodevelopmental outcome of patients after the Fontan operation: A comparison between children with hypoplastic left heart syndrome and other functional single ventricle lesions. J Pediatr 137, 646–652.

87. Bailey LL, Gundry SR, Razzouk AJ, *et al.* (1993) Bless the babies: one hundred fifteen late survivors of heart transplantation during the first year of life. The Loma Linda University Pediatric Heart Transplant Group. J Thorac Cardiovasc Surg 105, 805–815.

88. Bailey L, Concepcion W, Shattuck H, *et al.* (1986) Method of heart transplantation for treatment of hypoplastic left heart syndrome. J Thorac Cardiovasc Surg 92, 1–5.

89. Bailey LL, Assaad AN, Trimm RF, *et al.* (1988) Orthotopic transplantation during early infancy as therapy for incurable congenital heart disease. Ann Surg 208, 279–286.

90. Vricella LA, Razzouk AJ, Gundry SR, *et al.* (1998) Heart transplantation in infants and children with situs inversus. J Thorac Cardiovasc Surg 116, 82–89.

91. Kobashigawa J, Miller L, Renlund D, *et al.* (1998) A randomized active-controlled trial of mycophenolate mofetil in heart transplant recipients. Mycophenolate Mofetil Investigators. Transplantation 66, 507–515.

92. Yamani MH, Starling RC, Goormastic M, *et al.* (2000) The impact of routine mycophenolate mofetil drug monitoring on the treatment of cardiac allograft rejection. Transplantation 69, 2326–2330.

93. Schubert S, Renner C, Hammer M, *et al.* (2008) Relationship of immunosuppression to Epstein-Barr viral load and lymphoproliferative disease in pediatric heart transplant patients. J Heart Lung Transplant 27, 100–105.

94. Boucek MM, Mathis CM, Boucek RJ Jr, *et al.* (1994) Prospective evaluation of echocardiography for primary rejection surveillance after infant heart transplantation: comparison with endomyocardial biopsy. J Heart Lung Transplant 13(1 Pt 1), 66–73.

95. Loker J, Darragh R, Ensing G, *et al.* (1994) Echocardiographic analysis of rejection in the infant heart transplant recipient. J Heart Lung Transplant 13, 1014–1018.

96. Chrisant MR, Naftel DC, Drummond-Webb J, *et al.* (2005) Fate of infants with hypoplastic left heart syndrome listed for cardiac transplantation: a multicenter study. J Heart Lung Transplant 24, 576–582.

97. Boucek MM, Faro A, Novick RJ, *et al.* (2001) The Registry of the International Society for Heart and Lung Transplantation: Fourth Official Pediatric Report-2000. J Heart Lung Transplant 20, 39–52.

CHAPTER 32

Aortico-Left Ventricular Tunnel

Stephanie Fuller and Thomas L. Spray

The Children's Hospital of Philadelphia; University of Pennsylvania School of Medicine, Philadelphia, PA, USA

Aortico-left ventricular tunnel is a rare congenital communication between the ascending aorta and the left ventricle (LV). The incidence is estimated at 1 in 1000 infants born with congenital heart disease [1]. In 1963, Levy and colleagues [2] described three cases of aortico-left ventricular tunnel. Affected patients usually present with symptoms of congestive heart failure and dilation of the ascending aorta within the first year of life. The prognosis is good following surgical repair, although long-term progressive aortic insufficiency exists in some patients.

Pathophysiology and Anatomy

The aortico-left ventricular tunnel is an abnormal, paravalvular, endothelialized communication between the ascending aorta and the left ventricle which creates a bidirectional flow of blood from the aorta to the left ventricle. The paravalvular aortico-left ventricular tunnel typically originates from an aortic orifice cephalad to the sinotubular junction and the right coronary cusp and follows a descending path along the aortopulmonary window before entering the fibrous trigone immediately below the left-right commissure of the aortic valve. Most cases arise from the right coronary sinus. Origin from the left coronary sinus is rare [3–5]. In a postmortem series of 37 patients, the aortic opening was reported to be above the right coronary artery ostium in 14 (38%) of the patients, below the right coronary artery in 9 (25%) and at the level of the right coronary artery in 6 (16%) [6].

On gross inspection, a visible bulge is apparent along the anterolateral aspect of the aorta, which represents the fibromuscular tunnel wall that lies in direct histologic continuity with the aorta. The posterior wall contains the true aortic wall with the inferomedial aspect or the floor of the tunnel involving the muscle of the right ventricular outflow

tract [7]. Hovaguimian and colleagues [4] classified aortico-left ventricular tunnels into four types: those with a slit-like aortic orifice with no valvular distortion (type I); those with a larger, oval-shaped aortic orifice with an aneurysmal extracardiac component with or without valvar distortion (type II); those with an oval aortic orifice and an aneurysmal septal (intracardiac) component with or without right ventricular outflow tract obstruction (type III); and those with a combination of type II and III (classified as type IV) (Figure 32.1) [8].

Interestingly, careful analysis of several pathologic specimens by Ho and colleagues [7] suggests that despite this classification scheme, the tunnels never actually engage or cross the interventricular septum. Rather, the tunnels travel downward in the fibrofatty plane between the aortic root and the subpulmonary infundibulum to enter the left ventricular outflow tract in the immediate subcommissural triangle below the right and left valvar cusps just superficial to the intracardiac myocardium and immediately above the actual aorticoventricular junction (Figure 32.2) [7]. The anatomic relations of the tunnel have both pathophysiologic and therapeutic implications. Consideration must be given to the etiology of aortic valvar insufficiency as well as coronary flow, particularly when the right coronary artery arises within the tunnel.

Pathogenesis

Although the exact pathogenesis of aortico-left ventricular tunnel is not determined, proposed etiologic events to explain formation of the aortico-left ventricular tissue include an *in utero* rupture of a sinus of Valsalva aneurysm [3,8–10], degeneration of the true aortic wall analogous to *in utero* cystic medial necrosis [11], dissection of an aberrant or anomalous coronary artery [1], and malformation of the

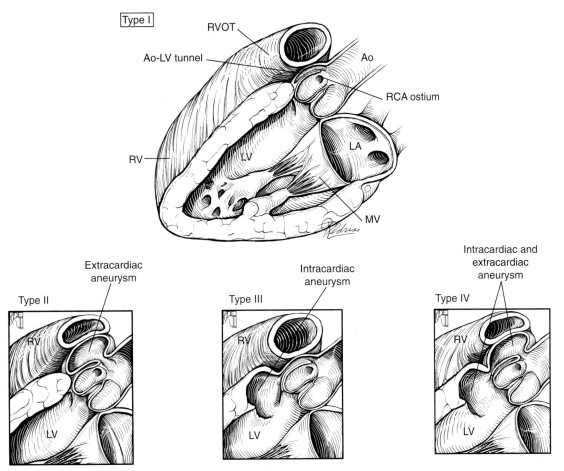

Figure 32.1 The four types of aortico-left ventricular tunnel: type I, type II, type III, and type IV. (Ao, aorta; LA, left atrium; LV, left ventricle; MV, mitral valve; RCA, right coronary artery; RV, right ventricle; RVOT, right ventricular outflow tract.)

bulbus cordis [1,3,12]. The bulbus cordis matures into components of both the subpulmonary infundibulum and the aortic vestibule and comprises the territory through which the developing coronary arteries move to attach to the sinus segment. Aberrant maturation of the bulbus cordis may account for the association between aortico-left ventricular tunnel and valvar pulmonary stenosis, valvar aortic stenosis, and proximal coronary artery anomalies [12]. Aortico-left ventricular tunnel typically originates from an aortic orifice cephalad to the sinus segment of the aorta and it is unlikely that a rupture of a sinus of Valsalva aneurysm could account for the typical appearance of this anomaly. Myers and colleagues [9] suggest instead that sinus aneurysm rupture occurs only in the rare occurrence of aortic to right ventricle fistulization. Although the suggestion of Myers *et al.* is an attractive hypothesis, Vargas and colleagues [13] clearly document an aortic origin of an aortic-right ventricular tunnel cephalad to the left sinotubular junction, which would make antecedent sinus rupture equally unlikely.

Presentation and Diagnosis

The age at presentation and severity of symptoms depend on the size of the tunnel. Neonatal and infant presentation reflects a large communication with severe left ventricular volume overload. Correct prenatal diagnosis of aortico-left ventricular tunnel has been difficult and only two known series have been reported. In the first, prenatal diagnoses were correct in only one of four presumed cases [13], and in the second, the diagnosis was correct in two of three cases [3]. Two additional single case reports have been published [14,15]. Although several fetuses were electively aborted, only three prenatally diagnosed patients survived until correction. The earliest survivor was detected at 28 weeks gestation. Prenatal echocardiography usually demonstrated preserved general cardiac architecture with valvar aortic insufficiency and/or stenosis with dysplastic valve leaflets and severe left ventricular hypertrophy and dilatation. A distinct paravalvular tunnel with regurgitant diastolic flow could be identified in three cases. Overall

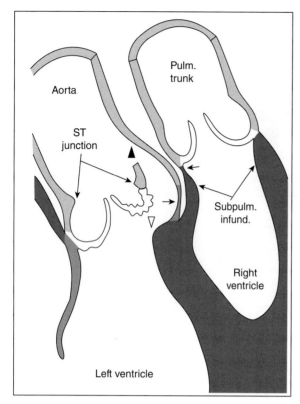

Figure 32.2 Longitudinal section of aortico-left ventricular tunnel. The tunnel originates above the sinotubular ridge (closed triangle). The ventricular orifice (open triangle) is in the area normally occupied by the interleaflet triangle. The tunnel is in an extracardiac tissue plane between the pulmonary trunk and aorta. The fine hatching (indicated by small arrows) represents fibrous areas, and stippled areas are the arterial walls. (ST junction, sino-tubular junction.) (Reproduced with permission from Ho *et al.* [7].)

survival was rare; patients with sufficient regurgitant flow to allow early prenatal diagnosis may represent the most severe end of the clinical spectrum. Reported postmortem examination of these pathologic hearts invariably demonstrated extensive myocardial fibrosis and severe aortic valve dysplasia.

Postnatally diagnosed aortico-left ventricular tunnel has been well documented in the literature, with presentation dependent on the amount of regurgitant paravalvular flow and the significance of associated coexistent anomalies such as valvar aortic regurgitation, aortic stenosis, pulmonary stenosis, and subpulmonary right ventricular outflow tract obstruction. Typical patients present with a "to and fro" murmur and congestive heart failure of varying severity. Differential diagnosis includes ventricular septal defect with aortic insufficiency, ruptured sinus of Valsalva aneurysm, coronary artery fistula, and tetralogy of Fallot with absent pulmonary valve syndrome.

Physical examination reveals pathognomonic systolic and diastolic murmurs and wide pulse pressure with bounding peripheral pulses. Although right ventricular outflow tract obstruction with or without valvar pulmonary stenosis can be the result of aneurysmal dilation of the intracardiac portion of the tunnel, cyanosis is an uncommon sign. Characteristics attributable to chronic volume overload dominate including left ventricle hypertrophy, left ventricle dilatation, and diminished ventricular function. Echocardiography is the diagnostic modality of choice, although cardiac catheterization has been recommended to detail associated lesions [16]. Color Doppler by echocardiography may be useful if it is able to differentiate the direction of blood flow in the aortic root and the tunnel. Demonstration of a paravalvular aorticoventricular communication with regurgitant diastolic flow confirms the diagnosis and demonstration of aortic insufficiency in a neonate should raise suspicion of an aortico-left ventricular tunnel.

Treatment

Surgical correction remains the mainstay of therapy. Medical management alone is thought to be ineffective, although rare patients have presented as late as 31 years of age without surgical treatment [17]. Spontaneous closure of an aortico-left ventricular tunnel has also been documented, raising the question of whether small asymptomatic lesions could be serially observed [1]. The natural progression is congestive heart failure and sudden death.

Current practice dictates surgical closure of the aortic orifice at the time of diagnosis either directly, via patch aortoplasty, or with combined closure of the aortic and the ventricular openings (Plates 32.1, 32.2, see plate section opposite p. 594). Although durable results can be achieved with direct closure alone [1], this would appear most cogent to type I aortico-left ventricular tunnels with a slit-like aortic orifice. Further, pathologic examination of autopsy specimens suggests that the ventricular orifice is not surrounded by firm muscular margins and may not be amenable to direct closure [7].

Patch aortoplasty has been advocated by most authors for all types of aortico-left ventricular tunnel to avoid distortion of the aortic valve and to obtain a long-term tension-free closure [16,18]. In performing patch closure, care must be undertaken to avoid impingement of the left-right aortic valve commissure because the orifice is usually located just above the right sinotubular junction. Similarly, the location of the ventricular end within the left-right interleaflet triangle requires great care to be undertaken when closing the ventricular orifice to avoid distortion of the hingeline of the right coronary leaflet. Although distant from the noncoronary-right coronary interleaflet triangle, anterior extensions of the left bundle branch may be jeopardized by sutures placed through the ventricular wall leading some surgeons to close the ventricular orifice through the incised tunnel itself [4,7].

Regardless of initial technique, progressive aortic regurgitation is a primary concern. Fifty percent of patients eventually require aortic valve replacement [18]. Early repair may prevent the late consequences of chronic volume overload, premature deterioration of the valve leaflets secondary to turbulent flow and subsequent dilatation of the aortic annulus and ascending aorta [8,12,18]. There may be a further theoretical advantage to closure of the ventricular orifice by buttressing the right-left commissure and supporting the lateral margin of the right coronary cusp left unsupported by the ventricular tunnel opening [7].

Conclusion

Aortico-left ventricular tunnel is a rare cardiac malformation of unclear etiology that results in the clinical syndrome of aortic insufficiency and left ventricular volume overload. Most infants will require repair in the neonatal period before hospital discharge. Treatment is surgical closure, although recently transcatheter closure has been reported in an adolescent [19]. Short-term prognosis is excellent, although some patients may eventually require valve replacement because of progressive valvar insufficiency.

References

1. Martins JD, Sherwood MC, Mayer JE Jr, *et al.* (2004) Aortico-left ventricular tunnel: 35-year experience. J Am Coll Cardiol 44, 446–450.
2. Levy MJ, Lillehei CW, Anderson RC, *et al.* (1963) Aortico-left ventricular tunnel. Circulation 27, 841–853.
3. Michielon G, Sorbara C, Casarotto DC. (1998) Repair of aortico-left ventricular tunnel originating from the left aortic sinus. Ann Thorac Surg 65, 1780–1783.
4. Hovaguimian H, Cobanoglu A, Starr A. (1988) Aortico-left ventricular tunnel: a clinical review and new surgical classification. Ann Thorac Surg 45, 106–112.
5. Grant P, Abrams LD, De Giovanni JV, *et al.* (1985) Aortico-left ventricular tunnel arising from the left aortic sinus. Am J Cardiol 55, 1657–1658.
6. Morgan T, Mazur H. (1963) Congenital aneurysm of aortic root with fistula to the left ventricle: a case report with autopsy findings. Circulation 28, 589–594.
7. Ho SY, Muriago M, Cook AC, *et al.* (1998) Surgical anatomy of aorto-left ventricular tunnel. Ann Thorac Surg 65, 509–514.
8. Shum-Tim D, Tchervenkov C. (2003) Aortico-left ventricular tunnel. In: Mavroudis C, Backer CL, eds. *Pediatric Cardiac Surgery*, 3rd ed. St. Louis, MO: Mosby, Inc.
9. Myers JL, Mehta SM. (2000) Congenital heart surgery nomenclature and database project: aortico-left ventricular tunnel. Ann Thorac Surg (Suppl) 69, 164–169.
10. Sousa-Uva M, Touchot A, Fermont L, *et al.* (1996) Aortico-left ventricular tunnel in fetuses and infants. Ann Thorac Surg 61, 1805–1810.
11. Turley K, Silverman NH, Teitel D, *et al.* (1982) Repair of aortico-left ventricular tunnel in the neonate: surgical, anatomic and echocardiographic considerations. Circulation 65, 1015–1020.
12. Llorens R, Arcas R, Herreros J, *et al.* (1982) Aortico-left ventricular tunnel: a case report and review of the literature. Texas Heart Institute J 9, 169–175.
13. Vargas FJ, Molina A, Martinez JC, *et al.* (1998) Aortico-right ventricular tunnel. Ann Thorac Surg 66, 1793–1795.
14. Cook A, Fagg N, Ho S, *et al.* (1995) Echocardiographic-anatomical correlations in aorto-left ventricular tunnel. Br Heart J 74, 443–448.
15. Grab D, Paulus WE, Terinde R, *et al.* (2000) Prenatal diagnosis of an aortico-left ventricular tunnel. Ultrasound Obstet Gynecol 15, 435–438.
16. Napoleone C, Gargiulo G, Pierangeli A. (2001) Aortico-left ventricular tunnel: Two new cases with a long-term follow-up. Ital Heart J 2, 624–626.
17. Weldner P, Dhillon R, Taylor JF, *et al.* (1996) An alternative method for repair of aortico-left ventricular tunnel associated with severe aortic stenosis presenting in a newborn. Eur J Cardiothorac Surg 10, 380–382.
18. Ando M, Igari T, Ando S, *et al.* (2004) Repair of the aortico-left ventricular tunnel originating from the right aortic sinus with severe aortic valve regurgitation. Ann Thorac Cardiovasc Surg 10, 47–50.
19. Chessa M, Chaudhari M, De Giovanni J. (2000) Aorto-left ventricular tunnel: transcatheter closure using an amplatzer duct occluder device. Am J Cardiol 86, 253–254.

33

Congenital Anomalies of the Mitral Valve

Richard D. Mainwaring[1] and John J. Lamberti[2]

[1]Stanford University School of Medicine, Stanford, CA, USA
[2]Rady Children's Hospital, San Diego, CA, USA

The mitral valve is the inlet valve to the anatomic left ventricle [1]. As a consequence of this embryologic relationship, the mitral valve is the inlet valve to the systemic ventricle when there is ventriculoarterial concordance. Isolated congenital abnormalities of the mitral valve are relatively rare [2]. Congenital mitral valve lesions are often associated with other cardiac anomalies such as the Shone complex. The anatomic mitral valve may be abnormal in a variety of connective tissue disorders. Abnormalities of the inlet valve to the systemic ventricle may also occur when it is not an anatomic "mitral valve," but rather is a trileaflet valve (derived from a common atrioventricular orifice) or has Ebstein's malformation. The anatomic mitral valve may be congenitally stenotic, or insufficient, or a mixture of both. This chapter discusses the treatment of congenital mitral stenosis and insufficiency in patients when the mitral valve is the systemic atrioventricular valve. Our goal is to describe the modalities of therapy useful in the treatment of congenital mitral stenosis and all forms of mitral insufficiency occurring in infants and children.

Historical Notes

The surgical treatment of mitral valve disease began in 1923 when Cutler operated on an 11-year-old girl with rheumatic mitral stenosis who survived for an additional 4½ years following this intervention [3]. Starkey reported his experience with closed and open techniques for repair of congenital mitral stenosis and insufficiency in 1959 [4]. In 1962, Creech and colleagues reported the successful operation in a 2-year-old with congenital mitral insufficiency [5]. Young and Robinson replaced the mitral valve in a 10-month-old infant successfully in 1964 [6]. Over the subsequent decades, improved techniques for the diagnosis and treatment of congenital mitral valve disease have

resulted in reproducible and excellent clinical results, with the overwhelming majority of patients now amenable to valve repair techniques [7–10].

Normal Mitral Valve Anatomy

The normal mitral valve is a complex apparatus composed of an annulus, leaflets, chordae tendineae, and papillary muscles [1]. The function of the mitral valve is dependent on the integrity of its components and the performance of the left ventricle. Figure 33.1 is a cross-sectional drawing of the heart showing the anatomic relationships of the normal mitral valve [11]. A fibrous annulus separates the atrium and the ventricle. The leaflets are attached to the annulus and are related to important adjacent structures. The mitral valve annulus extends along the left atrioventricular (AV) sulcus and is fixed medially to the central cardiac skeleton at the aortic root. The mitral valve is a bileaflet valve, with two well defined commissures in the anterolateral and posteromedial positions. The posterior (or mural) leaflet is longer and narrower and is usually divided into three scallops. It subtends an arc of 210 degrees. The anterior (or septal) leaflet is larger and wider and is trapezoidal in shape. The anterior leaflet attaches to the annulus along an arc of approximately 150 degrees. The surface of the leaflet is rough in appearance at the site where the leaflets oppose each other during systole. Each leaflet has a more proximal clear zone and then a thicker basal zone at the region of attachment to the annulus.

The chordae tendineae arise from two papillary muscles that are attached to the anterolateral and posteromedial ventricular wall. The posterior muscle is supplied by branches of the posterior descending coronary artery while the anterolateral papillary muscle is supplied by branches of the circumflex coronary artery. Each papillary muscle

Pediatric Cardiac Surgery, Fourth Edition. Edited by Constantine Mavroudis and Carl L. Backer.
© 2013 Blackwell Publishing Ltd. Published 2013 by Blackwell Publishing Ltd.

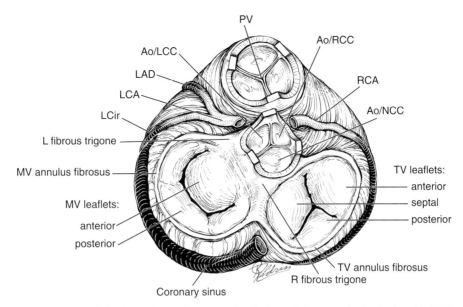

Figure 33.1 Cross-sectional drawing of the heart shows the anatomic relations of the normal mitral valve. (Ao/LCC, aortic valve left coronary cusp; Ao/NCC, aortic valve noncoronary cusp; Ao/RCC, aortic valve right coronary cusp; L, left; LAD, left anterior descending coronary artery; LCA, left coronary artery; LCir, left circumflex coronary artery; MV, mitral valve; PV, pulmonary valve; R, right; RCA, right coronary artery; TV, tricuspid valve.)

anchors chordae tendineae from both leaflets. Three varieties of chordae tendineae are recognized: first-order chordae tendineae, which originate at or near the apices of the papillary muscles and insert into the free edges of the leaflet as a fine strand; second-order chordae tendineae, which also originate at or near the apices of the papillary muscles and insert into the ventricular surface of the leaflet a short distance from the free edge and are usually thicker and less numerous than the first-order group; and third-order chordae tendineae, which are cordlike or fold-like structures sometimes containing muscle that originate from the ventricular wall and insert near the line of closure or along the basal area of the leaflet. Third-order chordae are more common along the posterior leaflet. The chordae are composed of collagen covered with a layer of endocardium. At the junction with the valvar leaflet the chordae merge imperceptibly with the leaflet tissue. The anatomy of the papillary muscles varies considerably between individuals. Some papillary muscles are broad-based, others are fingerlike. A third type is a combination of broad-based and fingerlike attachments.

The size and shape of the papillary muscles have important implications for patients with congenital heart disease. Experimental studies in animals have elegantly defined the functions of the mitral valve leaflets and mitral apparatus in both normal and pathologic states [12–14]. Two-dimensional and three-dimensional echocardiographic techniques have further refined our knowledge with regard to the function of the leaflets in normal and pathologic

states [15]. Proper closure of the mitral valve during systole is dependent on sequential contraction of the atria and then ventricles and is also interdependent on the performance of the left ventricle. An in-depth understanding of the normal anatomy and function of the mitral valve is necessary to optimize the chances for a successful repair.

Pathologic Anatomy, Classification, and Analysis

Abnormalities of the mitral valve may involve one or more components of the valve and may result in stenosis, insufficiency, or a combination of both. A segmental approach is useful from an anatomic point of view, but surgical treatment requires a more functionally oriented classification. This chapter focuses on abnormalities of the mitral valve associated with an adequate-sized left ventricle. Marked hypoplasia of the annulus or left ventricle represents a form of hypoplastic left heart syndrome (see Chapter 31, *Hypoplastic Left Heart Syndrome* for further review). We focus first on lesions primarily associated with mitral stenosis then on those associated with mitral insufficiency. It should be noted that most congenital anomalies of the mitral valve will have elements of both stenosis and insufficiency.

Mitral Stenosis Lesions

Segmental analysis of stenotic lesions begins with the supravalvar region (Figures 33.2, 33.3) [9,11]. Supravalvar

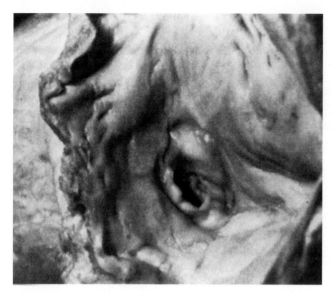

Figure 33.2 Supravalvar mitral fibrous ring viewed from the left atrium.

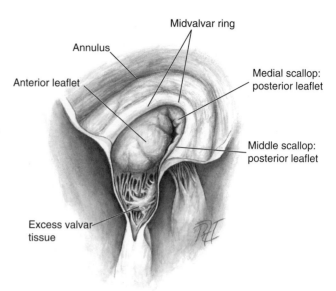

Figure 33.4 In rare instances a fibrous mitral ring within the substance of the mitral valve leaflets causes valvar stenosis (midvalvar ring) and leaflet restriction. Associated obstructive lesions often can be identified that necessitate therapy, such as excess valvar tissue and fused papillary muscles. (Reproduced with permission from Zias *et al.* [9].)

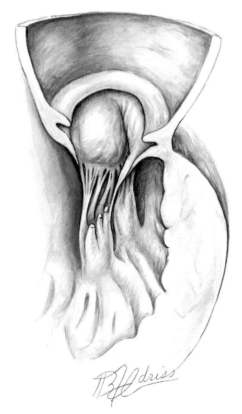

Figure 33.3 Lateral cutaway view shows mitral stenosis caused by supravalvar fibrous ring. The plane between the ring and the mitral orifice has been exaggerated for emphasis. The mitral valve itself is relatively normal with normal chordal architecture. (Reproduced with permission from Zias *et al.* [9].)

mitral stenosis is not the same as cor triatriatum and should not be confused with that entity. The "membrane" in cor triatriatum separates the atrium into two chambers. The atrial appendage originates downstream from the membrane in cor triatriatum, whereas the left atrial appendage is upstream from a supravalvar stenosing ring. In supravalvar mitral stenosis a ridge of endocardial thickening is present just above the mitral annulus [16]. This thick fibrous plate of tissue may resemble a membrane in its central portion. It may be attached at the level of the annulus or just above the annulus. This lesion is associated with congenital mitral valve stenosis and may occur in association with the Shone complex [17]. The membrane usually has a single central opening that may be eccentric in position. The size of the opening determines the degree of obstruction, and the area of the opening correlates well with the onset and degree of symptomatology. The underlying mitral valve may be functionally normal, but typically the valve is small and in some patients may be anatomically abnormal. Zias *et al.* [9] described a case of mid-valvar mitral ring (Figure 33.4) [9,11].

Congenital mitral valve stenosis may be associated with a supravalvar ring, or it may occur as an isolated lesion. Hypoplasia of the valve and its annulus can also result in significant obstruction. When hypoplasia of the valve and annulus is associated with an inadequate left ventricle, the patient must be treated as having a single ventricle. A

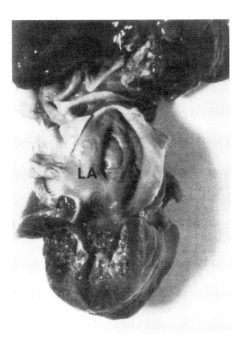

Figure 33.5 Severe mitral stenosis due to funnel valve. The left atrium (LA), funnel valve, and left ventricle are open through a sagittal cut. The commissures are fused. Thick, short chordae insert into stubby, conglomerated papillary muscles. The secondary orifices are slit like and minute. The left ventricular cavity is moderately hypoplastic, and the left atrium is markedly enlarged.

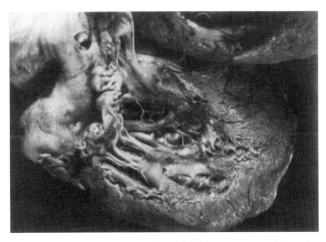

Figure 33.6 Severe congenital mitral valve stenosis involving all components of the mitral valve. The left ventricle is opened through a cut in the posterior aspect of the lateral wall. Both mitral valve leaflets are deformed, thickened, and redundant with many accessory folds. The commissures are poorly developed. Short and thick chordae insert to gigantic papillary muscles (P) and reduce the secondary orifice.

hypoplastic valve and annulus can be associated with a functionally adequate left ventricle, particularly if a ventricular septal defect is present. The hypoplastic valve may appear quite similar to a "normal" mitral valve with two leaflets and appropriate-appearing chordae tendineae. The leaflets may have reasonable function and nonfused commissures. Often the leaflets are thickened and the commissures fused. The chordae tendineae may be thick and short with inadequate development of interchordal spaces. If the chordae are shortened, a funnel-like appearance may occur (Figure 33.5) [11]. There are cases in which fusion of the leaflets will result in two orifices, a central orifice and an accessory orifice [18]. In the arcade mitral valve the anterior and posterior group of papillary muscles join together and fuse with the entire edge of the leaflet without the presence of well formed chordae. Only one papillary muscle may participate in the arcade in some cases. The arcade anatomy can produce mitral stenosis or insufficiency or a mixed lesion and may be associated with a parachute valve. The term hammock valve has been used by Carpentier to describe a valve that has fused commissures and a central orifice that is obstructed by numerous intermixed short chordae attached to abnormal hypertrophied papillary muscles [19].

Parachute mitral valve is an extreme form of congenital mitral stenosis. In this abnormality, all chordae attach to a single papillary muscle [20]. In most circumstances, the entire leaflet is connected to the posterior papillary muscle, with an absence of the anterior papillary muscle. On rare occasions the situation is reversed and the entire leaflet is connected to an anterior papillary muscle. Figure 33.6 depicts a severe case of congenital mitral stenosis involving all elements of the valve apparatus [11]. A valve that is functionally stenotic in infancy due to hypoplastic leaflets and shortened chordae may become centrally insufficient later when the left ventricle dilates. Congenital mitral stenosis may be associated with tetralogy of Fallot, ventricular septal defect, and multiple other congenital heart lesions.

Mitral Insufficiency Lesions

Congenital mitral insufficiency may be associated with many of the previously described abnormalities for congenital mitral valve stenosis. Dilatation of the mitral annulus will result in mitral insufficiency even if the valve is relatively normal in its anatomic appearance. Secondary annular dilatation can occur due to cardiomyopathy, both acquired and familial, and in association with lesions producing dilatation of the left ventricle, such as aortic insufficiency. Patients presenting with an anomalous left coronary artery may have impressive mitral regurgitation. The common AV valve found in a complete AV canal defect is often associated with insufficiency of the left AV orifice. However, this trileaflet valve is not an anatomic mitral valve. An isolated cleft of the anterior leaflet may produce important mitral insufficiency [21,22]. In Marfan's disease, the mitral valve can be quite abnormal with billowing

A

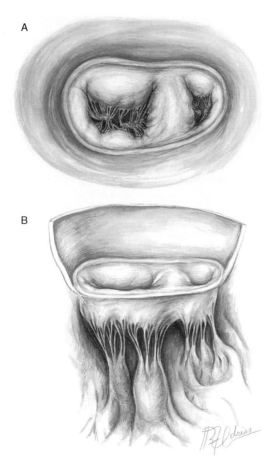

B

Figure 33.7 Left atrial (**A**) and cutaway atrioventricular (**B**) views of double-orifice mitral valve. More commonly, the smaller of the two orifices is in the right lateral position. The degree of stenosis is variable. Effective orifice-enlarging reparative techniques have not been developed. (Reproduced with permission from Zias *et al.* [9].)

leaflets and elongated chordae. In addition, Marfan patients may also have a markedly dilated annulus [23,24]. "Double-orifice mitral valve" refers to a valve with two separate orifices, each supported by its own tensor apparatus (Figure 33.7) [9,11,25]. This entity most commonly occurs in the setting of an AV canal defect [18], but it has been described with intact atrial and ventricular septae [8]. Double-orifice mitral valve may or may not result in insufficiency.

Mitral valve prolapse occurs in infants and children but is generally a benign condition [26]. The leaflets are redundant and thickened. The posterior leaflet is more commonly involved, and the excess valvar tissue balloons into the left atrial cavity. Often this valvar elongation is associated with annular dilatation. The architecture of the valve is abnormal in addition to the elongation of the valve structures. Carpentier has described chordal agenesis as a rare cause of congenital mitral insufficiency. Some patients presenting

with predominant mitral insufficiency will have anatomic findings similar to a hammock or arcade valve. In these patients there is also a deficiency of leaflet and chordal tissue.

The Carpentier classification of congenital mitral valve disease was first reported in 1976 and has been the most commonly used descriptive system [27]. This classification is predicated on analysis of the mitral valve leaflet at operation. Type 1 lesions have normal leaflet motion but produce valvar insufficiency from a dilated or deformed annulus, or by a defect or cleft in the leaflet. These lesions are subdivided into annular dilatation, cleft leaflet, and partial leaflet agenesis. Type 2 lesions involve leaflet prolapse and result from the absence or elongation of the chordae or papillary muscles producing insufficiency. Type 2 defects are subdivided into chordal elongation, papillary muscle elongation, and chordal agenesis. Type 3 lesions involve restricted leaflet motion and mitral stenosis (although valvar insufficiency can also be observed with certain lesions). Stenosis results from commissural fusion, imperforation, thickening, or shortening of the subvalvar apparatus.

There are two practical limitations to the Carpentier classification. Pure stenosis and pure insufficiency are infrequently observed, and leaflet function does not always correlate with the physiologic alterations. It is worth noting that this system was developed before the advent of routine two-dimensional echocardiography and, thus, was the only methodology available. Evaluation of the leaflets in the operating room by direct vision may be difficult despite saline irrigation of the flaccid left ventricle. Preoperative echocardiography now provides a significant enhancement in the information available to evaluate the valve and allow planning of the repair. The intraoperative transesophageal echocardiogram sometimes provides another increment of information regarding the pre-repair physiologic and functional performance of the valve. In this era, preoperative catheterization and angiography add little to the data base and are only necessary if other lesions are present or if there is severe pulmonary hypertension.

Mitruka and Lamberti [28] proposed a classification system for congenital abnormalities of the mitral valve based on the presence of stenosis or insufficiency. This classification system is directed at the physiologic consequences of altered valve anatomy and permits a systematic and segmental approach to diagnosis and treatment. In this classification scheme, type I lesions are supravalvar and type 2 lesions are valvar. In type 2 lesions, group A are annular defects and group B are leaflet abnormalities. Type 3 lesions are subvalvar with group A involving abnormalities of the chordae tendineae and group B involving defects of the papillary muscles. Type 4 are mixed lesions. When numerous defects of the valve apparatus exist, the predominant defect causing the abnormal function will direct the classification of the lesion. Multiple types of mitral valve pathology can be coded in the hierarchical system by selecting the predominant lesion as the first diagnosis and each additional lesion as a subsequent diagnosis in decreasing order of importance. A detailed explanation of the defects and the classification are provided in the reference [28].

Pathophysiology

Mitral valve abnormalities may have markedly different symptoms depending on the age of the patient. In older children and teenagers, significant mitral valve abnormalities present with symptoms including dyspnea on exertion, limited exercise tolerance, orthopnea, or paroxysmal nocturnal dyspnea. This age group may have limited exercise capacity because of the inability to increase cardiac output. The degree of impairment can be quantified using exercise testing. In some older children and teenagers, the onset of exercise limitation may be so insidious that the patient and/or family minimizes the degree of impairment. In contrast, infants and small children with significant mitral valve disease may be completely asymptomatic at rest. Fatigue and tachypnea with feeding or exertion may be signs of progressive mitral valve disease. Infants with associated pulmonary hypertension may have failure to thrive or recurrent pulmonary infections.

The physical findings may be subtle in early, isolated congenital mitral valve disease. Later, when there is heart failure and pulmonary hypertension, the physical exam becomes more characteristic of mitral valve disease in older patients. Mitral stenosis produces an apical mid-diastolic murmur. There may be presystolic accentuation of the murmur, and an opening snap may be audible. The morphology of congenital mitral stenosis is different from that seen in rheumatic heart disease and, thus, the opening snap is less predictable. Mitral regurgitation produces an apical pansystolic murmur that radiates to the axilla. When regurgitation is severe, a mid-diastolic rumble may also be heard. The second heart sound is accentuated in the presence of significant pulmonary hypertension and the precordium will be active with a right ventricular lift.

The diagnosis can usually be established by noninvasive techniques. In isolated mitral valve disease the chest X-ray will reflect left atrial dilatation and enlargement of the right ventricle. In more severe cases, the left main-stem bronchus is elevated and the left lower lobe may be collapsed. Radiologic signs of pulmonary venous congestion are present. Abnormalities on the chest X-ray may be obscured by the increased pulmonary vascularity and gross cardiomegaly. Left ventricular enlargement develops when mitral regurgitation progresses. Left ventricular failure may occur when the regurgitation fraction is greater than 50% and the end-diastolic volume is markedly increased. Important electrocardiographic findings include left atrial hypertrophy and right ventricular hypertrophy. When

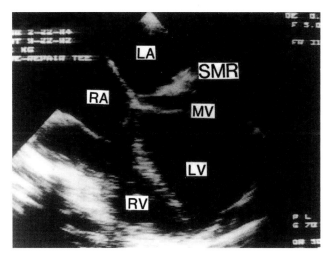

Figure 33.8 Transesophageal two-dimensional echocardiogram of an 8-year-old girl with recurrent supra-annular stenosing ring. The patient has a hypoplastic mitral annulus with a normal-sized left ventricle and an aneurysm of the membranous septum. (LA, left atrium; LV, left ventricle; MV, mitral valve; RA, right atrium; SMR, supra-annular mitral ring.)

additional lesions are present, the electrocardiogram will reflect the consequences of this physiology. Atrial fibrillation is rare in infants and children, although other atrial arrhythmias may occur.

Two-dimensional echocardiography in combination with color-flow studies and Doppler interrogation can provide precise information regarding the anatomy and function of the mitral valve. However, surface echocardiograms may not always provide the exact nature or extent of the mitral valve abnormality. A supravalvar ring may be difficult to detect by surface echocardiography, whereas transesophageal echocardiography (TEE) is particularly useful in evaluating the mitral valve. Figure 33.8 depicts a recurrent supravalvar ring detected by TEE in an 8-year-old girl [11].

Principles of Treatment

Infants and children with signs or symptoms due to congenital mitral valve disease may present a challenge in management. Most infants and children with mitral valve disease are treated medically for as long as feasible. Digoxin therapy has traditionally been instituted, although the utility of digoxin is debatable, particularly when the lesion is predominantly mitral stenosis. Diuretics and unloading therapy are useful in treating patients with significant mitral regurgitation. Afterload reduction is optimized using an angiotensin-converting enzyme (ACE) inhibitor. The purpose of medical therapy is to alleviate symptoms and to permit continued growth and development. Careful monitoring of ongoing medical management is necessary because medical treatment may mask the development of deteriorating ventricular function or worsening pulmonary artery hypertension. It is well established that chronic left atrial and pulmonary artery hypertension may eventually result in atrial dysrhythmia and chronic right heart failure.

Medical management is the first line of therapy for mitral valve disease because surgical options may be limited in younger, smaller patients [29,30]. There is no "ideal" medical device for mitral valve replacement in this patient population [31,32]. Traditionally, surgical intervention is contemplated when symptoms become severe or when exercise limitations are unacceptable. Valve repair techniques have evolved to the point that nearly all pediatric patients with favorable anatomy can undergo a successful repair. The dilemma remains for younger patients when the anatomy is not favorable for valve repair. At present, mechanical valves are the only suitable replacement option for the mitral valve in an infant, child, or young adult. The "unnatural" history following mechanical valve replacement for the mitral position is guarded in an infant or small child, making this an unattractive solution for the pediatric population [31–35].

Surgical intervention is indicated when symptoms severely compromise the lifestyle of the patient or when it is obvious that growth and development are failing. An earlier operation may be indicated when the mitral valve lesion is associated with other "correctable" defects. Relief of associated obstructing lesions, such as coarctation of the aorta or aortic stenosis, and repair of lesions producing a volume load, such as patent ductus arteriosus and ventricular septal defect, in combination with mitral valve repair may improve mitral valve function and delay the need for mitral valve replacement. When an associated congenital heart defect requires surgery, the abnormal mitral valve should always be inspected and repaired at the same time unless the mitral valve abnormality is deemed minor. Evaluation by two- and three-dimensional echocardiography usually permits an accurate assessment of the potential for valve repair. We recommend "prophylactic" surgery for relatively asymptomatic patients if the underlying mitral valve physiology is moderately or more severe and the anatomy is favorable for valve repair.

Balloon dilatation of rheumatic mitral valve stenosis is a safe and effective treatment in adults [36]. A number of centers have extrapolated this data and proposed that balloon dilatation might be effective for congenital mitral stenosis. The results for balloon dilatation of the congenitally obstructed mitral valve have not been satisfactory compared with rheumatic valves [37,38]. This should not be surprising because the pathology is quite different. We strongly discourage the use of balloon dilatation for congenital mitral stenosis based on the risk/benefit analysis

versus surgery. Complications such as acute massive mitral regurgitation and residual atrial septal defect [39] rarely occur following surgical mitral valvuloplasty.

When repair is not possible, mitral valve replacement is necessary. Bileaflet mechanical prostheses are the valve of choice for infants and small children. There is now strong evidence that all mechanical valves require the indefinite use of anticoagulation. Despite the use of anticoagulation, thromboembolic events and late valve entrapment by pannus formation can occur [40]. Coumadin anticoagulation in infants and children carries its own long-term risk, and smaller patients will eventually outgrow the prosthesis and require reoperation [41,42]. In general, mitral valve replacement in infants and children should be avoided if at all possible.

A variety of bioprosthetic valves have been tried in the mitral position in an attempt to avoid long-term coumadin anticoagulation. Several reports document the poor short- to mid-term results obtained when porcine valves are implanted in the left heart of children. If the problem of early calcific degeneration can be solved, bioprosthetic valves might become useful in infants and children. There are a few reports of the successful use of an extracardiac conduit between the left atrium and the left ventricle [43]. When a porcine valve is placed in an extracardiac conduit, it seems to be protected from accelerated degeneration. Homograft valves do not perform well when implanted on rigid stents in the mitral position. Donald Ross proposed the "top-hat" technique for replacement of the mitral valve with a pulmonary autograft [44]. Brown [45] and others [46,47] have suggested that the top-hat pulmonary autograft may be a viable solution for some young patients requiring mitral valve replacement early in life. Wider application and additional follow-up are necessary before routine consideration can be given to use of the top-hat technique. The mitral homograft [48] was suggested as a possibility for replacement without the need for anticoagulation. Unfortunately, the mitral homograft procedure has not been demonstrated to be a durable substitute for the mitral valve. In summary, the current surgical approach to mitral valve pathology should entail an aggressive effort at valve repair because there is no satisfactory long-term substitute in infants, children, and young adults with mitral valve disease.

Surgical Technique

The surgeon should carefully review all preoperative imaging studies in advance of the operation. We utilize TEE whenever possible, and it is important to be present to visualize the pre-repair TEE. At that time, the surgeon and cardiologist can review these findings and compare them with the preoperative data base. The surgeon will subsequently have the opportunity to corroborate the noninvasive findings with the intraoperative ones. In addition, changes in valve and ventricular function related to anesthesia can be noted and integrated with the preoperative analysis.

An operation on the mitral valve requires excellent exposure and considerable attention to detail. We use continuous cardiopulmonary bypass. Myocardial protection consists of repetitive doses of antegrade blood cardioplegia in conjunction with systemic hypothermia (28–30 °C). Retrograde cardioplegia may be useful in certain specific situations such as the presence of significant aortic valve insufficiency or coronary artery obstruction. Retrograde cardioplegia is relatively straightforward to use because the right atrium is often open and the coronary sinus is readily visualized. We use a purse-string suture around the coronary sinus to maximize right ventricular protection (the balloon of the catheter can sit at the ostium of the coronary sinus). Systemic hypothermia is important for two reasons. First, pulmonary venous return can interfere with visualization of the posterior aspect of the mitral valve in infants and small children. Moderate hypothermic bypass allows reduction of pump flow and control of pulmonary venous return, especially in patients with pulmonary hypertension. Hypothermia also reduces rewarming of the heart through contact with the descending aorta or by coronary collateral flow from bronchial artery connections.

The cannulation techniques are adapted to the size of the patient and the associated surgical procedures. In all patients, direct cannulation of the venae cavae permits optimal exposure. We use a right-angle cannula for this purpose. Aortic cannulation is performed in a standard fashion. The mitral valve can be approached through the dome of the left atrium, in the traditional fashion posterior to the intra-atrial groove, or through the atrial septum. A combination of incisions may be necessary in very small patients. Mobilization of the inferior and superior venae cavae and dissection of the intra-atrial groove usually permits excellent exposure with the traditional incision between the pulmonary veins and the intra-atrial groove in larger patients. In reoperations, we favor the transseptal approach if there is a prior right atriotomy scar. We do not usually extend the septal incision into the dome of the left atrium unless the left atrium is small and exposure is difficult [49]. In small infants, the superior-septal approach can be very useful. Blood cardioplegia is administered and repeated at 20–30-minute intervals. In reoperations we do not dissect the heart completely if adhesions are dense on the left side. Instead, widely opening the pleura allows the heart to fall posteriorly into the left chest.

Careful inspection of the valve is extremely important before beginning the surgical repair. A variety of atrial retractors can be used. A deep retractor may push the mitral annulus away from the surgeon and interfere with proper visualization. In smaller patients, a combination of traction sutures and small retractors may provide optimal visualization. Inspection begins at the supravalvar region, including the orifices of the pulmonary veins and the base of the left atrial appendage. The leaflets are then assessed for size, mobility, and prolapse. A small nerve hook is useful for this portion of the procedure. The chordae and the papillary muscles are then inspected. Saline can be injected into the ventricle with a piston syringe and a small red rubber catheter. The leaflets should float up and oppose. When the anatomy is clearly defined, the repair can begin. There is no reason to hurry through this process, as good myocardial protection allows cross-clamp times up to 3 hours without long-term sequelae. It is a reasonable maxim that a "good" repair is always better than placing a mechanical valve in a child. Therefore, when in doubt about the feasibility of repair, it is prudent to attempt a repair and evaluate what can be accomplished before removing the native valve. In the event that valve repair is not feasible, then there is no choice but to proceed with valve replacement.

The basic techniques for valve repair have been well described by Carpentier and colleagues [7,8,27], Duran *et al.* [50], and others [29,51,52]. A supravalvar mitral ring can be excised, but care should be taken at the periphery of the ring not to cut through the endocardium (Figure 33.9) [11]. If an endocardial opening is created, repair can be performed with fine interrupted monofilament sutures. After removal of the supravalvar ring, the mitral valve is inspected. The orifice size should be calibrated. We use Amato dilators in infants and small children and standard valve sizers in larger children to calibrate the orifice before, during, and after the repair. Our goal is to achieve competence with an orifice at the lower limits of normal size. Commissural fusion is addressed next, followed by appropriate treatment of fused subvalvar chordal attachments. In some cases incision of the commissure entails splitting fused chordal structures. Incision of the chordae can be carried down into the papillary muscles (Figure 33.10) [9,11]. When the leaflets are mobilized, an assessment of the functional orifice size is carried out. If the orifice is adequate for this size patient, we then test for insufficiency. Injection of saline into the ventricle permits gross assessment of leaflet function. Repeat cardioplegia with manual distortion of the aortic annulus can produce aortic regurgitation to fill the left ventricle and allow excellent visualization of the competence of mitral leaflet apposition.

Evaluation of a primarily regurgitant valve consists of assessment of annulus size followed by the standard stepwise assessment of the commissures, leaflets, and chordal structures. Repair consists of ensuring that the leaflets are adequately mobilized, repairing the leaflets if necessary, and closing any clefts that may be present. If inadequate leaflet tissue is present, advancement of the leaflet edge can be carried out with an autologous pericardial patch at the

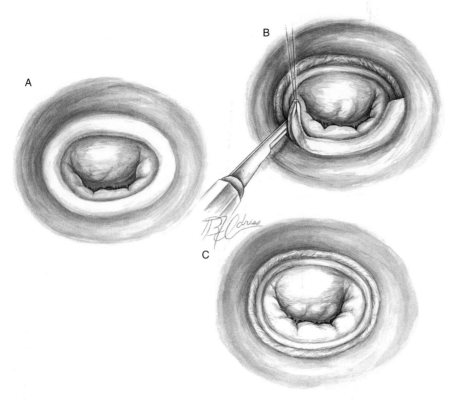

Figure 33.9 Technique for resection of a supravalvar mitral ring in the setting of a relatively normal mitral valve. **A,** Surgeon's view of supravalvar mitral ring. **B,** Sharp resection of the ring is performed under direct vision. A traction suture placed through the ring may facilitate exposure of the plane. **C,** Final result.

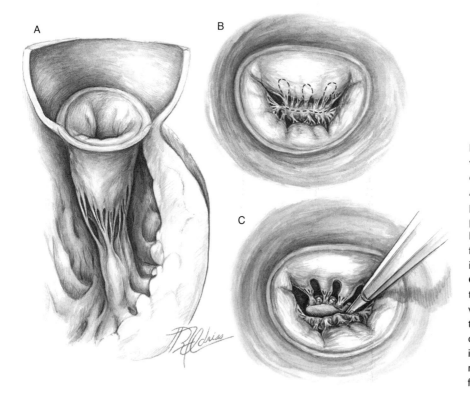

Figure 33.10 Cutaway atrioventricular view (**A**) and left atrial views (**B** and **C**) of stenotic parachute mitral valve. **A,** Single papillary muscle or fused papillary muscles usually arise from the posterior left ventricular wall. **B,** Dotted lines show the areas of proposed leaflet fenestrations and papillary muscle incision to open the ventricular inlet. **C,** Leaflet fenestrations are accomplished to maximize blood flow into the left ventricle during diastole while valvar tissue is preserved for effective coaptation during systole. The fused papillary muscle is being incised to facilitate valvar mobility. (Reproduced with permission from Zias et al. [9].)

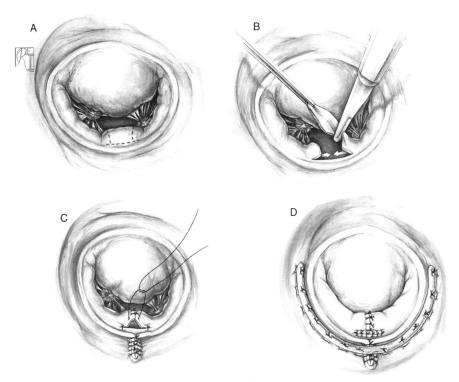

Figure 33.11 A, Artist's representation of insufficient mitral valve due to annular dilatation. Dotted lines represent the proposed posterior leaflet quadrangular resection and valvar incisions. **B,** After quadrangular resection, linear incisions are made in the posterior leaflet to accomplish sliding valvuloplasty (arrows). **C,** Posterior annulus is brought together with care not to injure the circumflex coronary artery. Resultant tightening of the annulus brings the remaining scallops of the posterior leaflet in position for valvar repair. **D,** The repair is strengthened by a semicircular Gore-Tex strip. The anterior annulus was not included in the annuloplasty technique owing to somatic growth considerations. (Reproduced with permission from Zias *et al.* [9].)

base of the leaflet [7]. We do not use pledgeted sutures along the clefts in the leaflet since we believe that pledgets reduce the mobility of the leaflet and may provide a nidus for calcification. There is ample evidence to suggest that leaflet repair can be carried out with interrupted monofilament sutures. Chordal repair or replacement can be accomplished by a variety of techniques. When posterior leaflet chordal rupture has occurred, resection of the middle third or more of the posterior leaflet can be accomplished (Figure 33.11) [9,11]. Following such a quadrangular resection, an annuloplasty can be performed. In older patients chordal transfer by leaflet flip may be useful in the treatment of anterior leaflet chordal rupture. Successful Gore-Tex replacement of chordae has been reported in adults [53] and Gore-Tex chordal replacement in children has shown promise [54–56]. We obtained an excellent result using Gore-Tex chordae in a 2-month-old infant presenting with a flail anterior leaflet due to chordal agenesis. In general, we recommend avoidance of a ring annuloplasty unless the annulus is adult size. The Wooler commissural annuloplasty [57] is quite useful in infants and children (Figure 33.12) [11,57]. It is performed with a 2-0 or 3-0 braided suture and small Teflon pledgets. The effects of a Wooler annuloplasty stitch may not always be predictable, and we have modified our technique to place a snare on the stitch and evaluate the result before tying [40] (Figure 33.13). In the event that the desired effect is not achieved, the suture can be easily removed. The Wooler annuloplasty permits substantial reduction in regurgitation without interfering with annular growth [58,59]. If an annuloplasty ring is thought to be necessary, we prefer a flexible ring [60]. In patients that have not completed their somatic growth, a partial ring may be useful. Subaortic obstruction can occur after ring placement, and care must be taken to avoid using an oversized semirigid ring.

Reparative techniques may be quite effective in patients with mitral regurgitation from certain acquired causes. Children with a dilated cardiomyopathy may develop severe mitral valve insufficiency secondary to annular dilatation. Surgical repair of the mitral valve may be quite effective in improving hemodynamics and obviate the need for cardiac transplantation [61]. Rheumatic heart disease is infrequently seen in the United States but is still common in other parts of the world. Standard techniques of annuloplasty and chordal repair can be employed after commissurotomy and valvuloplasty have been performed.

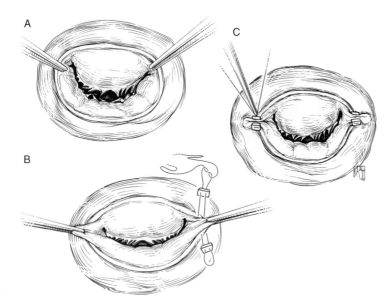

Figure 33.12 Artist's depiction of Wooler [57] or segmental annuloplasty. Variants of this technique have been described by numerous authors. **A,** The surgeon identifies the commissure and the adjacent aortic annulus. **B,** Mattress sutures of nonabsorbable material are reinforced with Teflon or pericardial pledgets. Placement of the sutures along the annulus determines the degree of annular reduction. The purpose of the sutures is to reduce the posterior annulus without disturbing leaflet coaptation. **C,** After the sutures are tied, the orifice is calibrated with a dilator, and the valve is tested with saline solution. Additional sutures may be necessary. Sometimes the annular plication distorts the leaflet coaptation, and the sutures must be removed or repositioned.

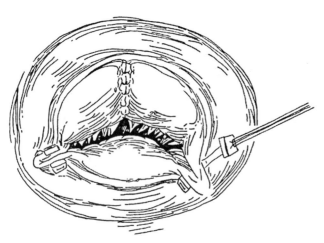

Figure 33.13 Technique for repair of left-sided atrioventricular valve regurgitation in the setting of a trileaflet valve (atrioventricular septal defect). The cleft has been closed, and a Wooler annuloplasty performed at the "anterior commissure." In the presence of residual regurgitation, a second annuloplasty stitch is placed at the posterior commissure. A snare has secured the stitch to evaluate the effectiveness of this annuloplasty. The stitch can be tied if proven effective, or easily removed if it does not achieve the desired result of improving leaflet coaptation. (Illustration courtesy of Erin Mainwaring.)

Mitral valve prolapse associated with rheumatic heart disease rarely requires operation in infants and children.

Repair of the congenitally stenotic mitral valve is quite difficult in most cases. Arcade, hammock, or parachute valves are severely abnormal, and repair is designed to facilitate the patient's somatic growth while delaying the inevitable mitral valve replacement. The leaflets are thickened and the chordae are generally thick and abnormal in number and shape. In some cases an adequate orifice can be created, but care must be taken to avoid injury to the papillary muscles and the chordal attachments with resultant severe insufficiency.

The marfanoid valve is amenable to repair in some patients using a combination of annuloplasty and chordal shortening. Chordal shortening techniques have been described by Carpentier and colleagues [7,8], Duran [50], and Oury *et al.* [51]. Most authors recommend shortening the chorda at its attachment to the papillary muscle rather than attempting to shorten the chorda itself. Figure 33.14 demonstrates this technique [11,51,54]. After the papillary muscle has been incised, the chorda is drawn down into the cleft in the muscle head. A suture is placed through the base of the chorda and then through the muscle and anchored over a pericardial strip. Another approach to chordal shortening involves the use of Gore-Tex chords of the appropriate length alongside the elongated chords (Figure 33.15) [54–56].

Reconstructive techniques can be associated with hemolysis. The preponderance of evidence would suggest that hemolysis occurs when there is a residual regurgitant jet that strikes prosthetic material such as Teflon pledgets or a Dacron ring. We do not use Teflon pledgets on the chordae but instead use small pieces of autologous pericardium. Patients with rheumatic heart disease may have progressive valvar dysfunction following placement of a Dacron ring that results in worsening of the regurgitant jet and hemolysis. Duran and colleagues [62] recommended covering the posterior aspect of the Dacron ring when performing annuloplasty for rheumatic disease in children and young adults. We would concur with this recommendation and use a thin strip of pericardium to cover the posterior portion of the ring.

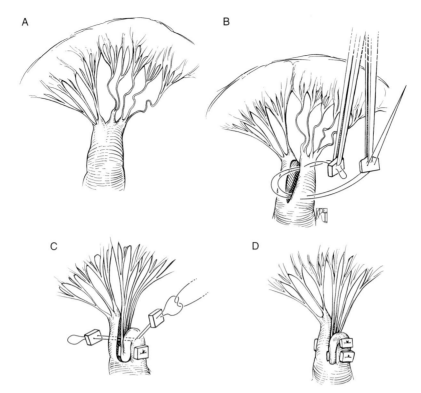

Figure 33.14 Chordal shortening technique. **A,** Elongated redundant chordae that allow prolapse of a segment of the leaflet are identified. **B,** Careful incision of the papillary head results in a trough into which the base of the chordal attachments can be drawn with a pledgeted mattress suture. **C,** Chordal shortening procedure is reinforced by a second pledget-supported mattress suture through both sides of the papillary head. **D,** Final result.

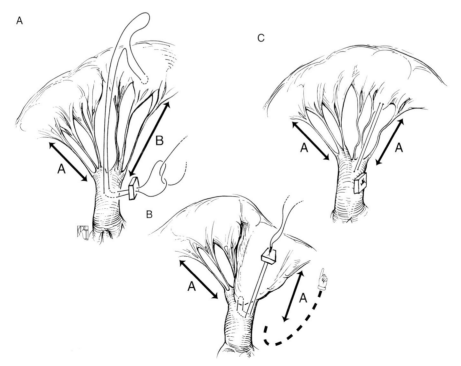

Figure 33.15 Another method for achieving chordal shortening and reinforcement involves use of polytetraflouroethylene artificial chordae. **A,** The redundant elongated chordae are characterized by solid line B. A mattress suture is placed through the free edge of the leaflet at the site where the chordae are missing or elongated. The mattress suture is then brought down to the head of the papillary muscle, and a pledget is added. **B,** Leaflet is drawn down to the papillary head. This maneuver allows the surgeon to tie the knots over the pledget at the appropriate length (solid line A). **C,** Leaflet has been elevated to its normal position, and the effect of the artificial cord on leaflet height is assessed.

Reoperation for left AV valve regurgitation following repair of AV canal defects is often very successful [40,52]. In our experience the septal cleft elongates as the leaflets grow, resulting in central insufficiency. We have seen disruption of the previous sutures as a rare cause of the "recurrent" cleft. The reoperated AV defect is a trileaflet valve that is amenable to annuloplasty at the lateral commissures and septal cleft repair by simple sutures (Figure 33.13). The same techniques can be used to repair a regurgitant tricuspid valve in a patient with corrected transposition or single ventricle. Finally, multiple annuloplasty sutures may be useful in repairing the abnormal multileaflet valve of some forms of single ventricle. We have used chordal shortening procedures in patients with single ventricle on occasion and believe there are circumstances where this is a useful and important technique. Operations for endocarditis of the mitral valve in infants and children usually require valve replacement. In some cases the leaflet can be repaired with a patch of autologous pericardium. This approach is useful when the mitral valve lesion represents extension from the aortic valve annulus.

When a complex repair is performed, the surgeon may be uncertain regarding the need for additional annuloplasty sutures or further commissural splitting. In either case, the surgeon is attempting to achieve the most competent valve possible without creating stenosis. On some occasions we will close the atrium and partially re-warm to obtain a "brief look" of the valve repair with TEE. We maintain a vent in the left atrium during the early phase of myocardial recovery to decompress the left ventricle and aid in air removal. After 20 minutes of recovery, when cardiac function is satisfactory, we wean the patient from bypass and evaluate the repair by TEE [63]. When TEE is not possible because of the size of the patient or other anatomic factors, we use epicardial echocardiography to assess the quality of the repair. A left atrial pressure line is placed, and the left atrial pressure monitoring provides additional information regarding valve function. Atrioventricular synchrony is also important in ensuring optimal function of the repaired mitral valve. We use pacing wires in valve repair cases, and AV pacing is used when appropriate during evaluation of the repair. At this time the surgeon can correlate the anatomic observations at surgery with the echocardiographic findings, left atrial trace, and other available data. Residual abnormalities detected in this fashion can then be addressed by reinstituting bypass, repeating the cardioplegia, and reopening the left atrium. On several occasions we have used this strategy to improve the repair of a congenitally stenotic valve. The brief look permits assessment of the support of the leaflets and allows a more aggressive approach to be taken if necessary. When both stenosis and insufficiency are revealed, a decision must be made, taking into account the patient's age, weight, clinical status, and ventricular function, to either accept this result or replace the valve.

The technique for mitral valve replacement in older infants and children is similar to that in adults. However, the small annulus encountered in some patients requires adjustments in technique. In adults preservation of chordal attachments is considered important in preserving ventricular function following mitral valve replacement. In infants and small children chordal preservation may not be feasible for several reasons. First, the annulus may be quite hypoplastic, and complete excision of leaflet tissue and chordae along with the tips of the papillary muscles may be necessary to allow placement of an adequate-sized prosthesis. Second, care must be taken to avoid the possibility that remnants of the native valve leaflet or chordae interfere with mechanical valve leaflet function. We routinely use small Teflon pledgets to reinforce the sutures when the annulus is thin and there is minimal tissue for suturing. In general, it is not possible to enlarge the mitral annulus. If the annulus is too small to accept a standard mechanical valve, a modified valve with a reduced sewing ring can be implanted above the annulus [35]. Supra-annular valve implantation requires placement of sutures in the wall of the atrium just below the orifices of the left lower lobe pulmonary veins and at the base of the left atrial appendage. In the anterior aspect, sutures may be placed through the true annulus at the region of aortic to mitral continuity. In some cases the supra-annular valve is tilted slightly. A tilting disk valve may be easier to orient than a bileaflet valve. Oversizing the mitral prosthesis can result in subaortic obstruction. A complete AV canal defect is one instance when the "annulus" can be enlarged. Replacement of the left AV valve early or late after repair in this circumstance often requires that the mitral prosthesis be sewn to the ventricular septal defect patch. In small patients the ventricular septal patch can be incised allowing implantation of a larger valve. The atrial septum is then reconstituted with a larger pericardial patch after valve implantation. In all valve replacement procedures, intraoperative monitoring of left atrial pressure and examination of the prosthetic valve by TEE ensures that leaflet function is unimpaired prior to decannulation.

The technique for implanting a left atrium to left ventricular apical conduit has been described [43] wherein the conduit can be implanted through a left thoracotomy or a median sternotomy. Cardiopulmonary bypass is necessary. A conduit equal in size to the diameter of the base of the left atrial appendage is selected and prepared. The conduit is attached to the apex of the left ventricle using a fishmouth ventriculotomy, which avoids obvious coronary branches. We do not use an apical stent. Monofilament polypropylene is used as a continuous suture for each anastomosis. The ventricular anastomosis is reinforced with a Teflon strip. Figure 33.16 depicts the 6-year follow-

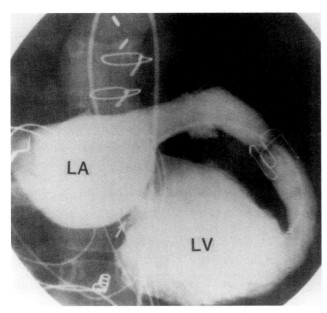

Figure 33.16 Left atrial angiogram obtained 6 years after implantation of a left atrial-to-left ventricular conduit. The conduit contains a 14-mm porcine valve. The catheter passes retrograde through the aortic valve into the left ventricle and then retrograde through the conduit to the left atrium. The hypoplastic mitral valve is indicated by the white arrow. The patient also had a recurrent supravalvar mitral ring. (LA, left atrium; LV, left ventricle.)

up angiogram of a patient born with supravalvar stenosing ring, marked hypoplasia of the mitral valve and annulus, small ventricular septal defect, normal-sized left ventricle, bicuspid aortic valve, and coarctation of the aorta [11]. The conduit was implanted in 1986 when the patient was 2.5 years old. The valve and conduit were replaced 6 years later. At each conduit operation, the native mitral valve was enlarged by resecting supravalvar fibrous tissue and cautiously opening the commissures. When the patient was 18.5 years old, the mitral valve orifice was enlarged once again and the apical conduit removed. The patient is currently functioning at New York Heart Association (NYHA) class II some 23 years after the first conduit was implanted and 7 years after the second conduit was removed.

Postoperative Care

The postoperative care of a child following repair or replacement of the mitral valve is guided by the preoperative status of the patient and the clinical condition of the patient following operation. After separation from cardiopulmonary bypass, the patient undergoes rigorous intraoperative evaluation of the repair. TEE and direct measurement of left atrial pressure (using a 20- or 22-

gauge catheter) provide important information regarding the quality of the repair. A "v" wave may be present even after a satisfactory repair, as the size and shape of the "v" wave are determined by the amount of regurgitation and compliance of the left atrium. The optimal postoperative left atrial pressure is the lowest value that still provides a satisfactory cardiac output and adequate systemic perfusion pressure. Excessive volume transfusion to provide an arbitrary left atrial filling pressure is not recommended, as this may predispose to postoperative pulmonary complications and delay in weaning from the ventilator. The left atrial pressure tracing is also useful in detecting atrial arrhythmias.

Atrial and ventricular pacing wires are placed in all patients undergoing surgery on the mitral valve. We prefer the use of two atrial electrodes placed about 8–10 mm apart. The use of two electrodes provides security if one electrode fails. In addition, the small size of the artifact produced by bipolar atrial pacing makes interpretation of the electrocardiogram simpler. In some patients we have used the left atrial appendage as well as the free wall of the right atrium for lead placement. Atrioventricular sequential pacing may be useful in optimizing cardiac output at the lowest left atrial pressure. If the patient is not in sinus rhythm, atrial pacing or AV sequential pacing is used to minimize valve regurgitation. Mild or mild-to-moderate residual regurgitation may be acceptable following repair if the alternative is implanting a prosthesis in a very small patient. Moderate residual regurgitation is indicative of an inadequate repair, and additional sutures in a cleft or another annuloplasty stitch should be pursued.

Cardiac output is assessed clinically and assumed to be adequate if the systemic arterial blood pressure is normal for the patient's age and weight and if there is adequate urinary output without acidosis. Noninvasive mixed venous cerebral and renal tissue oxygen saturation measurements (near infrared spectroscopy) may provide additional information regarding the adequacy of cardiac output. When a patient has significant pulmonary artery hypertension, we implant a pulmonary artery pressure monitoring line and measure mixed venous oxygen saturation as needed. The pulmonary artery catheter can be placed through the free wall of the right ventricle or through the right atrium and positioned in the pulmonary artery before discontinuation of cardiopulmonary bypass. In our experience the routine use of thermodilution cardiac output catheters is rarely necessary.

We routinely use dopamine at 2–5 μg/kg/min. Most patients receive vasodilator therapy, which is especially important in those with abnormal left ventricular function. Nitroprusside and/or milrinone are titrated to provide a satisfactory cardiac output. Epinephrine may be useful when significant ventricular dysfunction is present.

We do not routinely use intravenous heparin for anticoagulation during the first 36 hours after mitral valve replacement. Subcutaneous low molecular weight heparin may be useful in patients unable to take oral coumadin early after operation. Oral coumadin therapy is begun on the second postoperative day following removal of the chest tubes and pacemaker wires. Anticoagulation with coumadin is continued indefinitely in all patients following mechanical valve replacement.

The management of postoperative complications, including bleeding, low cardiac output, and multisystem organ failure, are similar to other operations requiring the use of cardiopulmonary bypass in a child with pulmonary hypertension and left ventricular dysfunction. Most complications can be prevented by meticulous attention to the details of the operation. Careful dissection in all patients, especially in reoperations, will minimize bleeding following cardiopulmonary bypass. Patients in severe biventricular failure often have hepatic dysfunction and abnormal clotting factors following operation. Multiple blood products may be necessary to achieve adequate hemostasis. Myocardial preservation and the elimination of intracardiac air before weaning from cardiopulmonary bypass should minimize postoperative cardiac dysfunction. The routine use of TEE and left atrial pressure monitoring should eliminate a poor repair or a malfunctioning prosthetic valve as a cause of a low cardiac output state following operation. Judicious fluid administration is necessary during the early postoperative interval to minimize extravascular water in the lungs.

Hemolysis can occur after extensive valve repair. Hemolysis may be associated with a peribasilar leak after prosthetic valve implantation or with mild-to-moderate regurgitation following repair. Hemoglobinuria that persists for more than a few hours following completion of operation should be carefully evaluated by standard laboratory tests. Low-grade hemolysis following valve repair may have a benign clinical course. If transfusion is necessary to maintain the hematocrit, early consideration should be given to mitral valve replacement. Beta blockade may reduce hemolysis and allow healing of the rough surfaces responsible for hemolysis. The use of β-blockade requires adequate left ventricular function.

Complete heart block can occur following mitral valve replacement in infants and small children. When the annulus is hypoplastic, the surgeon is faced with a dilemma regarding excision of leaflet tissue along the crest of the ventricular septum and suture placement in the region of the AV node and the bundle of His. If complete heart block is present at the completion of operation, permanent wires should be implanted. In select patients, biventricular pacing may improve valve function after a complex repair. We have also noted that temporary pacing from the left ventricle may improve early postoperative valve function.

Results

The operative mortality for congenital mitral valve disease is primarily related to the anatomic and physiologic abnormalities of the valve. Patients in whom the left-sided AV valve is reparable can undergo this operation with an extraordinarily low risk and favorable long-term outcomes [7–10,29,30,52,64,65]. Patients with primary mitral insufficiency have a greater likelihood of achieving a durable repair than patients with primary mitral stenosis, and thus the prognosis for the insufficiency group is far better. The need for mitral valve replacement, particularly in infants and young children, is a marker of a poorly functioning mitral valve and/or associated congenital heart defects. Other risk factors that influence outcomes include left ventricular dysfunction, the presence of severe pulmonary hypertension and chronic lung disease from recurrent infections, and the need for an emergency operation.

Oppido *et al.* recently reported their results on the surgical treatment of congenital mitral valve disease from the Royal Children's Hospital in Melbourne, Australia [64]. Their report summarized an experience with 71 patients from 1996 to 2006, of whom 70 underwent primary mitral valve repair. Figure 33.17 demonstrates the actuarial curves for this patient population [64]. At 60 months of follow-up, overall survival was 94 ± 2.8% and the freedom from reoperation was 76 ± 5.6%. A suboptimal repair was found to be a significant predictor for reoperation, with the caveat that many of the re-repairs were successful.

At the Rady Children's Hospital San Diego (RCHSD), a heterogeneous group of 216 patients have undergone an operation to treat abnormal function of the systemic AV valve. This group of patients was identified through the RCHSD database but excludes patients undergoing primary repair of an AV septal defect. The diagnoses of all patients are listed in Table 33.1. The age of the patients

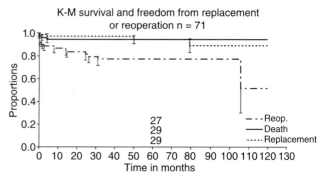

Figure 33.17 Kaplan-Meier curves showing freedom from death (solid line), reoperation (thick dashed line), and prosthesis (thin dashed line) in 71 patients undergoing mitral valve surgery. (Reproduced with permission from Oppido *et al.* [64].)

Table 33.1 Diagnoses of patients undergoing systemic AV valve repair/replacement. (AV, atrioventricular; LV, left ventricle; MR, mitral regurgitation; TGA, transposition of great arteries.)

Repair (listed in decreasing order of frequency)
Left AV valve regurgitation after repair of an AV septal defect
Systemic AV valve regurgitation in single ventricle (all forms)
Congenital mitral stenosis and or insufficiency
Rheumatic heart disease
Tricuspid valve regurgitation (late onset) after atrial switch for TGA
Mitral valve prolapse
Marfan's syndrome
Supravalvar mitral ring
Anomalous origin of left coronary from main pulmonary artery
Stent injury to mitral valve
Mitral regurgitation late after arterial switch operation

Replacement
Left AV valve regurgitation/stenosis after prior repair of an AV septal defect
Replacement of a mitral prosthesis
Cardiomyopathy with severe MR and preserved LV function
Severe AV valve regurgitation in single ventricle
Congenital mitral stenosis and/or insufficiency
Rheumatic heart disease
Corrected TGA
Hemolysis post complex repair
Mitral leaflet tumor

Table 33.2 Techniques for mitral/systemic atrioventricular valve repair.

Commisurotomy
Chordal fenestration
Papillary muscle split
Cleft repair
Annuloplasty
Segmental
Ring: partial or full
Leaflet resection
Leaflet augmentation
Chordal shortening/replacement
Alfieri stitch/create double-orifice valve

ranged from 4 months to 19 years (median age 5 years). There were 41 primary operations and 165 secondary operations. In 168 patients (78%) the AV valve could be repaired. The most common techniques used for valve repair were segmental annuloplasty and cleft closure. Each repair was tailored to the anatomic findings for that specific patient. Table 33.2 lists the repair techniques that were used in this cohort. There were two early failures (1%) in the repair group requiring valve replacement for intractable hemolysis. Forty-eight patients (22%) had valves that were deemed unsuitable for valve repair and therefore underwent valve replacement. Collectively, there were seven operative

deaths in this series (4.6%). Two deaths occurred in the valve-repair cohort (1%), both of whom were infants with single-ventricle physiology. There were five deaths in the valve-replacement group, for a cohort mortality rate of 11%. Postoperative death was related to the age of the patient at operation, the severity of illness, and the need for valve replacement at the time of surgery. Long-term follow-up revealed good-to-excellent status in most patients (NYHA class I or II). In the valve-repair group, 13 patients have required subsequent valve replacement, although there has been no late mortality in this group. There have been five late deaths in the valve-replacement cohort, of which two were directly valve related.

A review of the literature confirms that mitral valve replacement carries a higher mortality and poorer prognosis than valve repair [31,32,34,35,41,42]. For infants, the operative mortality has been reported to be as high as 33% [35]. Improved techniques of myocardial preservation and the use of low-profile valves have reduced hospital mortality in recent years to approximately 10% for infants, with a lower risk in older children. Selamet Tierney et al. have recently suggested that supra-annular placement of the mitral prosthesis is associated with worse long-term survival [42]. We have not noted a decrement in survival attributable to supra-annular placement of a mitral valve prosthesis at RCHSD. It is likely that the need for supra-annular placement is a surrogate marker for several other risk factors.

The long-term results after mechanical valve replacement do not compare favorably with valve repair [17]. Morbidity because of anticoagulation may occur, and it is now generally accepted that all patients with a mechanical valve should be anticoagulated with coumadin. Management of coumadin anticoagulation has been relatively straightforward in most patients, yet in spite of adequate levels of anticoagulation, we have seen late obstruction of mechanical valves in infants and children because of tissue overgrowth (pannus). Fibrous tissue overgrowth into the annulus results in interference of leaflet motion and has been seen in less than 2 years following implantation of a mechanical valve. Acute thrombosis occurs in some patients when clot forms at the entrapped leaflet. Thrombolytic therapy may be useful in an emergency situation, but acute thrombosis is invariably secondary to the trapped leaflet and requires surgical intervention to debride the pannus or re-replace the valve.

The functional results after valve repair are quite satisfactory. Long-term survivors of valve repair often have residual murmurs and echocardiographic evidence of mild regurgitation, but their quality of life is excellent. Mild cardiomegaly is well tolerated and afterload reduction can delay the need for late valve replacement. In our experience, 90% of patients undergoing successful valve repair have not required reoperation during a follow-up period of up to 21 years. The late results of mitral valve replacement in infants and small children are unsatisfactory, with 5-year survival rates of 50% to 80% [31–35,41,42]. Infants requiring mitral valve replacement will require re-replacement within 5 years. Porcine heterograft mitral valves fail at a rapid rate and should not be used except under unusual circumstances. Porcine valves can be expected to last 3 years in infants and perhaps 5 years in children.

The left atrium-to-left ventricular apical conduit has been successfully employed in one of our patients. This type of conduit is suitable for a patient born with a normal-sized left ventricle and a very small mitral annulus. As mitral annulus enlargement is usually not possible, the patient is faced with replacement of the mitral valve with a very small mechanical valve. When the annulus is so small that a suitable mechanical valve is not available to fit the patient, an apical conduit may be useful. We consider this a last resort because the long-term effects of the apical incision on the left ventricle are not well defined.

In summary, current surgical technique permits repair of the systemic AV valve in many infants and children requiring operation. The long-term results of successful valve repair are good to excellent. Repair avoids the short- and long-term morbidity and mortality of valve replacement as well as allowing for growth of the valve and annulus.

References

1. Wilcox BR, Anderson RH. (1985) *Surgical Anatomy of the Heart*. New York: Raven Press.
2. Freedom RM, Mawson JB, Yoo SJ, et al. (1997) Abnormalities of the mitral valve. In: Freedom RM, ed. *Congenital Heart Disease: Textbook of Angiocardiography*. Armonk NY: Futura.
3. Cutler EC, Levin SA. (1923) Cardiotomy and valvulotomy for mitral stenosis, experimental observations and clinical notes concerning an operated case with recovery. Boston Med Surg J 188, 1023.
4. Starkey GW. (1959) Surgical experiences in the treatment of congenital mitral stenosis and mitral insufficiency. J Thorac Cardiovasc Surg 38, 336–352.
5. Creech O Jr, Ledbetter MK, Reemtsma K. (1962) Congenital mitral insufficiency with cleft posterior leaflet. Circulation 25, 390–394.
6. Young D, Robinson G. (1964) Successful valve replacement in an infant with congenital mitral stenosis. N Engl J Med 270, 660–664.
7. Chauvaud S, Fuzellier JF, Houel R, et al. (1998) Reconstructive surgery in congenital mitral valve insufficiency (Carpentier's techniques): long-term results. J Thorac Cardiovasc Surg 115, 84–92; discussion 93.
8. Chauvaud SM, Mihaileanu SA, Gaer JAR, et al. (1997) Surgical treatment of congenital mitral valvar stenosis: "The Hospital Broussais" experience. Cardiol Young 7, 15.
9. Zias EA, Mavroudis C, Backer CL, et al. (1998) Surgical repair of the congenitally malformed mitral valve in infants and children. Ann Thorac Surg 66, 1551–1559.
10. Yoshimura N, Yamaguchi M, Oshima Y, et al. (1999) Surgery for mitral valve disease in the pediatric age group. J Thorac Cardiovasc Surg 118, 99–106.
11. Lamberti JJ, Mitruka SN. (2003) Congenital anomalies of the mitral valve. In: Mavroudis C, Backer CL, eds. *Pediatric Cardiac Surgery*, 3rd ed. Philadelphia PA: Mosby Inc.
12. Glasson JR, Komeda MK, Daughters GT, et al. (1996) Three-dimensional regional dynamics of the normal mitral anulus during left ventricular ejection. J Thorac Cardiovasc Surg 111, 574–585.
13. Carlhall C, Kindberg K, Wigstrom L, et al. (2007) Contribution of mitral annular dynamics to LV diastolic filling with alteration in preload and inotropic state. Am J Physiol Heart Circ Physiol 293, H1473–1479.
14. Fann JI, Ingels NBJ, Miller DC. (2007) Pathophysiology of mitral valve disease. In: Cohn LH, ed. *Cardiac Surgery in the Adult*, 3rd ed. New York: McGraw-Hill, pp. 973–1012.
15. Lamberti JJ. (2008) Mitral valve and left atrial anomalies. In: Lai W, Mertens L, Cohen L, et al., eds. *Echocardiography in Pediatric and Congenital Heart Disease. From the Fetus to the Adult*. Hoboken, NJ: Wiley-Blackwell.
16. Toscano A, Pasquini L, Iacobelli R, et al. (2009) Congenital supravalvar mitral ring: an underestimated anomaly. J Thorac Cardiovasc Surg 137, 538–542.
17. Serraf A, Zoghbi J, Belli E, et al. (2000) Congenital mitral stenosis with or without associated defects: An evolving surgical strategy. Circulation 102(19 Suppl 3), III166–171.
18. Brieger DB, Ward C, Cooper SG, et al. (1995) Double orifice left atrioventricular valve-diagnosis and management of an unexpected lesion. Cardiol Young 5, 267.
19. Carpentier A. (1983) *Congenital Malformations of the Mitral Valve*. New York: Grune & Stratton.
20. Moore P, Adatia I, Spevak PJ, et al. (1994) Severe congenital mitral stenosis in infants. Circulation 89, 2099–2106.
21. Banerjee A, Kohl T, Silverman NH. (1995) Echocardiographic evaluation of congenital mitral valve anomalies in children. Am J Cardiol 76, 1284–1291.
22. Perier P, Clausnizer B. (1995) Isolated cleft mitral valve: valve reconstruction techniques. Ann Thorac Surg 59, 56–59.
23. Cameron DE. (1996) Mitral valve surgery in children with Marfan syndrome. Progr Pediatr Cardiol 5, 205.
24. Tsang VT, Pawade A, Karl TR, et al. (1994) Surgical management of Marfan syndrome in children. J Card Surg 9, 50.
25. Honnekeri ST, Tendolkar AG, Lokhandwala YY. (1993) Double-orifice mitral and tricuspid valves in association with the Raghib complex. Ann Thorac Surg 55, 1001–1002.
26. Arfken CL, Schulman P, McLaren MJ, et al. (1993) Mitral valve prolapse and body habitus in children. Pediatr Cardiol 14, 33–36.
27. Carpentier A, Branchini B, Cour JC, et al. (1976) Congenital malformations of the mitral valve in children. Pathology and surgical treatment. J Thorac Cardiovasc Surg 72, 854–866.
28. Mitruka SN, Lamberti JJ. (2000) Congenital Heart Surgery Nomenclature and Database Project: mitral valve disease. Ann Thorac Surg 69(4 Suppl), S132–146.

29. Aharon AS, Laks H, Drinkwater DC, *et al.* (1994) Early and late results of mitral valve repair in children. J Thorac Cardiovasc Surg 107, 1262–1270; discussion 1270–1271.

30. Sugita T, Ueda Y, Matsumoto M, *et al.* (2001) Early and late results of partial plication annuloplasty for congenital mitral insufficiency. J Thorac Cardiovasc Surg 122, 229–233.

31. Ackermann K, Balling G, Eicken A, *et al.* (2007) Replacement of the systemic atrioventricular valve with a mechanical prosthesis in children aged less than 6 years: late clinical results of survival and subsequent replacement. J Thorac Cardiovasc Surg 134, 750–756.

32. Higashita R, Ichikawa S, Niinami H, *et al.* (2003) Long-term results after Starr-Edwards mitral valve replacement in children aged 5 years or younger. Ann Thorac Surg 75, 826–829.

33. Kojori F, Chen R, Caldarone CA, *et al.* (2004) Outcomes of mitral valve replacement in children: a competing-risks analysis. J Thorac Cardiovasc Surg 128, 703–709.

34. Calderone CA, Raghuveer G, Hills CB, *et al.* (2001) Long-term survival after mitral valve replacement in children aged less than five years. Circulation 104, I-143–147.

35. Kadoba K, Jonas RA, Mayer JE, *et al.* (1990) Mitral valve replacement in the first year of life. J Thorac Cardiovasc Surg 100, 762–768.

36. Abascal VM, Wilkins GT, O'Shea JP, *et al.* (1990) Prediction of successful outcome in 130 patients undergoing percutaneous balloon mitral valvotomy. Circulation 82, 448–456.

37. Fawzy ME, Ribeiro PA, Dunn B, *et al.* (1992) Percutaneous mitral valvotomy with the Inoue balloon catheter in children and adults: immediate results and early follow-up. Am Heart J 123, 462–465.

38. Spevak PJ, Bass JL, Ben-Shachar G, *et al.* (1990) Balloon angioplasty for congenital mitral stenosis. Am J Cardiol 66, 472–476.

39. McElhinney DB, Sherwood MC, Keane JF, *et al.* (2005) Current management of severe congenital mitral stenosis: outcomes of transcatheter and surgical therapy in 108 infants and children. Circulation 112, 707–714.

40. Lamberti JJ, Jensen TS, Grehl TM, *et al.* (1989) Late reoperation for systemic atrioventricular valve regurgitation after repair of congenital heart defects. Ann Thorac Surg 47, 517–522; discussion 522–523.

41. Kanter KR, Forbess JM, Kirshbom PM. (2005) Redo mitral valve replacement in children. Ann Thorac Surg 80, 642–645; discussion 645–646.

42. Selamet Tierney ES, Pigula FA, Berul CI, *et al.* (2008) Mitral valve replacement in infants and children 5 years of age or younger: evolution in practice and outcome over three decades with a focus on supra-annular prosthesis implantation. J Thorac Cardiovasc Surg 136, 954–961, 61 e1–3.

43. Amodeo A, Di Donato R, Corno A, *et al.* (1990) Systemic atrioventricular conduit for extracardiac bypass of hypoplastic systemic atrioventricular valve. Eur J Cardiothorac Surg 4, 601–603; discussion 604.

44. Ross DN, Kabbani S. (1997) Mitral valve replacement with a pulmonary autograft: the mitral top hat. J Heart Valve Dis 6, 542–545.

45. Brown JW, Ruzmetov M, Rodefeld MD, *et al.* (2006) Mitral valve replacement with Ross II technique: initial experience. Ann Thorac Surg 81, 502–507; discussion 507–508.

46. Kumar AS, Talwar S, Gupta A. (2009) Mitral valve replacement with the pulmonary autograft: midterm results. J Thorac Cardiovasc Surg 138, 359–364.

47. Kabbani S, Jamil H, Nabhani F, *et al.* (2007) Analysis of 92 mitral pulmonary autograft replacement (Ross II) operations. J Thorac Cardiovasc Surg 134, 902–908.

48. Acar C, Farge A, Ramsheyi A, *et al.* (1994) Mitral valve replacement using a cryopreserved mitral homograft. Ann Thorac Surg 57, 746–748.

49. Smith CR. (1992) Septal-superior exposure of the mitral valve. The transplant approach. J Thorac Cardiovasc Surg 103, 623–628.

50. Duran CG, Pomar JL, Revuelta JM, *et al.* (1980) Conservative operation for mitral insufficiency: critical analysis supported by postoperative hemodynamic studies of 72 patients. J Thorac Cardiovasc Surg 79, 326–337.

51. Oury JH, Grehl TM, Lamberti JJ, *et al.* (1986) Mitral valve reconstruction for mitral regurgitation. J Card Surg 1, 217–231.

52. Wood AE, Healy DG, Nolke L, *et al.* (2005) Mitral valve reconstruction in a pediatric population: late clinical results and predictors of long-term outcome. J Thorac Cardiovasc Surg 130, 66–73.

53. David TE, Omran A, Armstrong S, *et al.* (1998) Long-term results of mitral valve repair for myxomatous disease with and without chordal replacement with expanded polytetrafluoroethylene sutures. J Thorac Cardiovasc Surg 115, 1279–1285; discussion 1285–1286.

54. Matsumoto T, Kado H, Masuda M, *et al.* (1999) Clinical results of mitral valve repair by reconstructing artificial chordae tendineae in children. J Thorac Cardiovasc Surg 118, 94–98.

55. Minami K, Kado H, Sai S, *et al.* (2005) Midterm results of mitral valve repair with artificial chordae in children. J Thorac Cardiovasc Surg 129, 336–342.

56. Boon R, Hazekamp M, Hoohenkerk G, *et al.* (2007) Artificial chordae for pediatric mitral and tricuspid valve repair. Eur J Cardiothorac Surg 32, 143–148.

57. Wooler GH, Nixon PG, Grimshaw VA, *et al.* (1962) Experiences with the repair of the mitral valve in mitral incompetence. Thorax 17, 49–57.

58. Komoda T, Huebler M, Berger F, *et al.* (2009) Growth of mitral annulus in the pediatric patient after suture annuloplasty of the entire posterior mitral annulus. Interact Cardiovasc Thorac Surg 9, 354–356.

59. Fundaro P, Tartara PM, Villa E, *et al.* (2007) Mitral valve repair: is there still a place for suture annuloplasty? Asian Cardiovasc Thorac Ann 15, 351–358.

60. Gillinov AM, Tantiwongkosri K, Blackstone EH, *et al.* (2009) Is prosthetic anuloplasty necessary for durable mitral valve repair? Ann Thorac Surg 88, 76–82.

61. Walsh MA, Benson LN, Dipchand AI, *et al.* (2008) Surgical repair of the mitral valve in children with dilated cardiomyopathy and mitral regurgitation. Ann Thorac Surg 85, 2085–2088.

62. Duran CM, Gometza B, Saad E. (1994) Valve repair in rheumatic mitral disease: an unsolved problem. J Card Surg 9(2 suppl), 282–285.

63. Honjo O, Kotani Y, Osaki S, *et al.* (2006) Discrepancy between intraoperative transesophageal echocardiography and postoperative transthoracic echocardiography in assessing congenital valve surgery. Ann Thorac Surg 82, 2240–2246.

64. Oppido G, Davies B, McMullan DM, *et al.* (2008) Surgical treatment of congenital mitral valve disease: midterm results of a repair-oriented policy. J Thorac Cardiovasc Surg 135, 1313–1320; discussion 1320–1321.

65. Stulak JM, Burkhart HM, Dearani JA, *et al.* (2009) Reoperations after initial repair of complete atrioventricular septal defect. Ann Thorac Surg 87, 1872–1877; discussion 1877–1878.

CHAPTER 34

Total Anomalous Pulmonary Venous Connection

Nicola Viola[1] and Christopher A. Caldarone[2]

[1]Southampton General Hospital, Southampton, UK
[2]The Hospital for Sick Children, Toronto, ON, Canada

Overview

Total anomalous pulmonary venous connection (TAPVC) constitutes a heterogeneous group of lesions in which all of the pulmonary veins (PV) are connected to the right atrium or its tributaries. A concomitant right-to-left shunt, commonly via an interatrial communication, is required for survival after birth. Significant obstruction to pulmonary venous drainage results in pulmonary edema and cardiogenic shock which is rapidly lethal if untreated. Surgical results for the treatment of TAPVC have greatly improved over the last three decades, reducing operative mortality to less than 10% in most centers.

Embryology

Successful connection between the pulmonary venous system and the left atrium is the result of three distinct processes that involve the formation of the primitive lung and the primitive left atrium. At first, primitive lung buds originate as out-pouchings from the trachea on day 26–27 of gestation. A plexus of vessels, the splanchnic plexus, develops around the lung buds and allows the drainage of blood into the anterior cardinal veins (the primordial superior vena cava (SVC), coronary sinus, and azygous vein) and into the umbilicovitelline veins (which develop into the portal system). At approximately day 27–28 of gestation, a solitary pulmonary vein evaginates from the forming left atrium towards the venous plexus through the dorsal mesocardium. By day 28–30 of gestation fusion between the solitary vein and the pulmonary plexus is completed. Finally, between days 30 and 48 the solitary vein bridging between the left atrium and the lungs retracts back towards the posterior wall of the left atrium, a process made possible by the complete involution of the pulmonary-to-systemic vein connections. The correct axial orientation of the interatrial septum during this period is a necessary condition to enable the appropriate connections to form.

As a result of this process, four fully formed veins open into the posterior aspect of the left atrial cavity. Failure of all the pulmonary veins to divide from the splanchnic venous system and, possibly, a concomitant leftward displacement of the developing atrial septum is hypothesized to be the primary defect in embryological development responsible for TAPVC [1–4]. Unilateral lesions produced at the same stage (partial anomalous pulmonary venous connection), lesions occurring at a later stage (atresia of common pulmonary vein or cor triatriatum) or as a result of abnormal reabsorption of the common vein into the left atrium (congenital pulmonary vein stenosis and an abnormal number of pulmonary veins) are important related pulmonary venous anomalies.

Classification

Total anomalous pulmonary venous connection was classified on an embryological basis by Neill and colleagues [5], with a more recent modification proposed by Lucas [6]. Four types were identified: type one, pulmonary veins connected to right atrium; type two, pulmonary veins connected to SVC/azygous vein (right common cardinal system); type three, pulmonary veins connected to left SVC/coronary sinus (left common cardinal system); type four, pulmonary veins connected to portal vein/ductus venosus (umbilicovitelline system).

Almost contemporarily, Darling *et al.* proposed a classification, based on autopsy examinations, which has become widely recognized and is based on the level of the connection of the anomalous connecting vein [7]. In type 1, or supracardiac, the common vein connects to structures above the heart (right SVC, azygos vein, left SVC, or innominate vein). In type 2, or cardiac, the connecting vein

Pediatric Cardiac Surgery, Fourth Edition. Edited by Constantine Mavroudis and Carl L. Backer.
© 2013 Blackwell Publishing Ltd. Published 2013 by Blackwell Publishing Ltd.

is attached to cardiac structures (e.g., the right atrium or the coronary sinus). In type 3, or infracardiac, the connection is situated below the diaphragm to the inferior vena cava (IVC)/portal vein system. Type 4, or mixed, represents a combination of the above conditions [7].

Some authors have stratified these categories by the presence/absence of obstruction to pulmonary venous drainage. Obstructions can be found at the level of the connecting vein, owing to intrinsic narrowing or extrinsic compression, or at the level of the interatrial communication

Table 34.1 Mechanisms of obstruction in TAPVC.

Intrinsic stenosis	Stenosis of the individual pulmonary veins
	Stenosis of the confluence
	Stenosis of the connecting vein (single or multiple)
	Stenosis at the site of the abnormal connection drainage into a solid parenchymal organ (infracardiac type)
Extrinsic compression	Anatomical "vice" position (supracardiac type) between bronchus and pulmonary artery
	Connecting vein anterior to aortic arch (supracardiac type)
	Small esophageal hiatus (infracardiac type)
Mixed compression	Combination of intrinsic and extrinsic mechanisms
Restrictive interatrial communication	

(Table 34.1). Burroughs and Edwards defined three groups of connection between the pulmonary and the systemic veins [8]. Group I, the least obstructed, is constituted by the shortest connections as in Darling's cardiac type (type 2). Group II, with intermediate length and moderate risk of obstruction, corresponds to Darling's supracardiac type (type 1). Group III, has the longest routes of venous drainage and high risk of obstruction and corresponds to Darling's infracardiac type (type 3) [8]. Smith *et al.* tried to merge the anatomical and physiological elements into a simplified classification, based on the observation that almost all infracardiac connections are obstructed and connections above the diaphragm are seldom obstructed, and divided TAPVC into supradiaphragmatic and subdiaphragmatic types [9].

Most recently, the unified nomenclature system presented at the International Nomenclature and Database Project for Pediatric Cardiac Surgery was introduced. Using embryological principles to organize all pulmonary vein lesions into a unified classification, the Darling's classification is adopted for TAPVC because of simplicity and wide acceptance. The presence/absence of obstruction should be mentioned, and the nature and level of obstruction should be added as the last element to complete the diagnosis (Table 34.2) [2].

Cardiac Anatomy, Associated Lesions

As mentioned, a communication between the systemic and the pulmonary venous return is necessary for survival after birth. In the overwhelming majority of cases this is ensured by an interatrial communication. Rarely the communication can be represented by one or multiple ventricular

Table 34.2 Congenital Heart Surgery Nomenclature and Database Project: TAPVC.

Hierarchy Level 1 Pulmonary vein anomaly	Hierarchy Level 2 Darling's type	Hierarchy Level 3 Obstruction	Hierarchy Level 4 Type of obstruction
TAPVC	Type I (Supracardiac)	Nonobstructed	
		Obstructed	Intrinsic narrowing Extrinsic compression Obstructive interatrial septum
	Type II (Cardiac)	Nonobstructed	
		Obstructed	Intrinsic narrowing Extrinsic compression Obstructive interatrial septum
	Type III (Infracardiac)	Nonobstructed	
		Obstructed	Intrinsic narrowing Extrinsic compression Obstructive interatrial septum
	Type IV (Mixed)	Nonobstructed	
		Obstructed	Intrinsic narrowing Extrinsic compression Obstructive interatrial septum

septal defects or a patent ductus arteriosus [10,11]. Shunts at atrial level are typically of adequate size and the interatrial gradient is usually low [12,13].

The right atrium can be thick and enlarged, and Mathew *et al.* found that the left atrium is generally half the size of the expected normal, owing to a small posterior component rather than a small appendage area [14]. In most cases the left ventricle has normal size and muscular mass [15–17]. On the contrary, the right ventricle can be enlarged and hypertrophied, especially in supradiaphragmatic nonobstructive lesions [18].

Up to 90% of patients with heterotaxy and asplenia have TAPVC. Tetralogy of Fallot, double-outlet right ventricle, and interrupted aortic arch have also been reported as associated lesions [10,19–21].

Natural History

The clinical presentation of TAPVC depends on two critical elements: the degree of obstruction to the pulmonary venous drainage and the degree of obstruction to the compensatory right-to-left shunt.

At one end of the spectrum, there are neonates with completely unobstructed circulation (typically supracardiac and cardiac types). These patients present with signs and symptoms of a large left-to-right shunt. Tachypnea and arterial desaturation are present to various degrees together with signs of right ventricular volume overload. If untreated, this condition can lead to congestive heart failure. Late sequelae include pulmonary edema, pulmonary hypertension, and cyanosis.

At the other end of the neonatal clinical spectrum are neonates with severe pulmonary venous flow obstruction. In these cases, the resulting pulmonary venous and pulmonary arterial hypertension produces severe acute pulmonary edema, right ventricular antegrade flow reduction owing to the excessive increase in afterload, extreme hypoxemia, and circulatory collapse. The presence of a restrictive atrial septal defect results in reduced preload to the left ventricle, diminished systemic cardiac output, and severe cardiogenic shock. Obstructed TAPVC is rapidly lethal and presents formidable challenges to its treatment.

Diagnosis

Unobstructed TAPVC is sometimes difficult to diagnose in the first few days of life because patients may have very mild cyanosis and the absence of a murmur. After the first few months of life, infants may present with tachypnea, mild cyanosis, failure to thrive, and feeding difficulties. On examination, a loud and continuously split S2 together with a systolic ejection murmur over the pulmonary valve are common findings. Hepatomegaly, venous congestion and fine crackles on lung auscultation are possible in cases

of noncompensated cardiac failure. Neonates with an obstructed circulation become critically ill immediately after birth. In those cases hypoxia and profound cyanosis, hypotension and metabolic acidosis are commonly encountered [21,22].

Chest radiographs of unobstructed TAPVC show plethoric lungs and a large cardiac silhouette. A typical finding is the so-called snowman silhouette where the heart and the mediastinal enlargement owing to a prominent pulmonary artery, vertical vein, and SVC form an eight-shaped figure. The snowman sign is characteristic of supracardiac TAPVC, but is generally not appreciable before the age of 6 months [23]. Obstructed neonatal TAPVC shows severe pulmonary edema in the presence of a normal size and shape of the heart.

Two-dimensional and Doppler echocardiography are the primary diagnostic tools for most patients. Diagnostic findings are a distended right ventricle, a vascular confluence coupled with absent venous drainage to the left atrium on the Doppler interrogation, the presence of an accessory common vein or a dilated coronary sinus, and turbulent flow in the right atrium with a right-to-left shunt. Echocardiography has shown excellent sensitivity and specificity in fetal diagnosis and as prognostic tool [24–26]. In general, echocardiography has supplanted angiography in the vast majority of cases [22,23,27–31].

Cardiac catheterization is avoided in unstable neonates to reduce delay to treatment and contrast-related renal injury. It can be useful in nonobstructive cases to better define connections of mixed type and to identify possible associated anomalies. The site of the anomalous connection can be precisely located with a step up in oxygen saturation along the systemic vein system. Intracardiac oxygen saturation measurements characteristically demonstrate equivalent saturations in all cardiac chambers, the pulmonary artery, and the aorta.

In nonemergency cases of TAPVC, contrast-enhanced magnetic resonance angiography (MRA) can be used to provide a complete anatomic and functional diagnosis [32]. From an anatomical point of view, it allows excellent visualization of all pulmonary veins and other pulmonary-to-systemic venous connections. When compared with echocardiography, MRA has been shown to offer superior imaging of the entire pulmonary venous anatomy [33]. From a functional point of view, the amount of anomalous drainage and the resulting Qp/Qs can be calculated by using phase-contrast MRA, which depicts the velocity, volume, and pattern of blood flow of pulmonary venous flow (Plate 34.1, see plate section opposite p. 594). Moreover, a description of the secondary effects on pulmonary arterial size and blood flow, ventricular size and function are obtainable in the same study. This important information is difficult or impossible to obtain using other modalities [32,34,35].

Operative Management and Anesthetic Considerations

Despite the significant differences in physiology and clinical presentation, both obstructed and nonobstructed TAPVC pose an absolute indication for surgical repair, given the poor prognosis recorded in untreated cases. In patients with evidence of pulmonary venous obstruction, surgical repair is conducted promptly after diagnosis [36,37]. In our institution, patients with unobstructed TAPVC are electively repaired at 1–2 months of age. Alternatively, other programs choose to repair unobstructed TAPVC at the time of presentation during the neonatal period.

Medical management of patients with nonobstructed pulmonary venous connection is directed at compensating right ventricular failure, hypoxia, and congestive heart failure with mild inotropic support, diuresis, and avoidance of high levels of inspired oxygen. Assisted ventilation is rarely needed. In selected cases, alpha-blockade can be used to reduce the incidence of pulmonary hypertension.

Medical maneuvers in patients with obstructed TAPVC are limited in terms of efficacy. Neonates with obstructed TAPVC often require intubation and hyperventilation with 100% oxygen to maintain $PaCO_2$ below 30 mmHg and promote respiratory alkalosis. Sodium bicarbonate is used to correct the ensuing metabolic acidosis and enhance the action of inotropic and diuretic treatments, often necessary to support the failing ventricles. Prostaglandin E1 can be infused to maintain patency of the ductus arteriosus, which has the effect of improving systemic cardiac output through a right-to-left shunt, although this often occurs at the expense of an already reduced pulmonary circulation in conditions of severe hypoxia. Medical efforts are minimally effective in correcting the ensuing hemodynamic and meta-bolic crisis and their use is limited to provide some short-lived palliation until definitive repair is accomplished.

In some centers, cardiac catheterization has been used in critically ill patients for diagnosis and percutaneous palliation of obstructed TAPVC. A restrictive interatrial communication can be relieved with balloon septostomy. Moreover, several authors have proposed the use of percutaneous angioplasty and stenting of the obstructed common vein to palliate shock and improve preoperative optimization of the metabolic state (Figures 34.1, 34.2) [38–43]. In seven such cases reported over the last decade, four were of supracardiac type where a discrete obstruction could be identified. One patient required repeated stent implantations due to in-stent restenosis [42]. In one patient the procedure was performed with extracorporeal membrane oxygenation (ECMO) support [39]. These initial experiences have yielded promising results in obtaining hemodynamic stabilization in preparation for surgery.

Some centers have reported good result using ECMO in the critically ill neonate as preparation for surgery [44–46]. Postoperative ECMO is used in patients with severe residual pulmonary hypertension [47–49]. Once in the operating room, the anesthetic management is directed toward reducing the pulmonary vascular resistance by the use of fentanyl in high doses, aggressive correction of hypocalcemia, hypoglycemia, and lactic acidosis. Isoproterenol may be useful in normotensive patients for afterload reduction.

Surgical Repair of Supracardiac Type

Surgical repair of supracardiac TAPVC is accomplished via sternotomy with two venous cannulae (IVC and SVC) and an aortic cannula. Immediately after the initiation of cardiopulmonary bypass, the ductus arteriosus is ligated

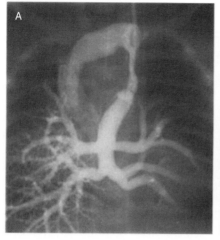 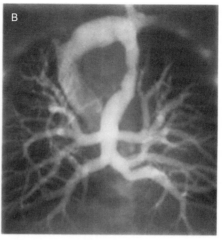

Figure 34.1 Total anomalous pulmonary venous connection of supracardiac type to the innominate vein. **A,** Both right and left pulmonary veins are unobstructed. The vertical vein, however, is severely stenotic at the junction with the innominate vein. **B,** Emergency percutaneous stent dilation was performed with acceptable short-term result. (Courtesy of Dr Shi-Joon Yoo and Mr Omar Thabit.)

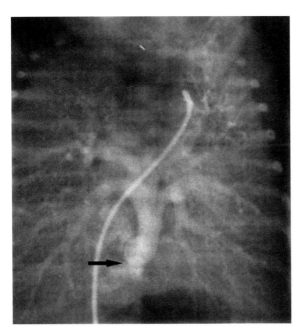

Figure 34.2 Infracardiac total anomalous pulmonary venous connection. The vertical vein is stenosed at the insertion in the venous duct (black arrow). (Courtesy of Dr Shi-Joon Yoo and Mr Omar Thabit.)

and divided. The patient is cooled to mild hypothermia at 28–30 °C or, rarely, deep hypothermia at 18–20 °C to allow deep hypothermic circulatory arrest. The aorta is cross-clamped and cardiac arrest induced with antegrade cold blood cardioplegic solution.

The heart is retracted cephalad and to the right exposing the left posterior pericardial area [50]. This maneuver is enhanced by the absent connection between the pulmonary veins and the atrium. The vertical communicating vein is ligated near its connection with the innominate vein or SVC, to avoid tethering of the vein ostia near the site of planned anastomosis. When severe preoperative obstruction is present, leaving the vertical vein patent may contribute to the relief of postoperative pulmonary vein hypertension [51], although significant residual left-to-right shunt may require reintervention [52]. A longitudinal incision is made in the confluence and the posterior wall of the left atrium. Because collateral pulmonary flow can be extensive, cardiopulmonary bypass flow rates may need to be decreased temporarily to facilitate visualization and placement of the incision. Small cardiotomy suction cannulas can then be placed in the pulmonary venous confluence and perfusion flow rates restored. Through a left atriotomy, the interatrial communication is closed primarily or with a patch of autologous pericardium. The left atrium and the confluence are then anastomosed to create the largest possible anastomosis. Some authors advocate the use of interrupted sutures, others the use of reabsorb-

able ones, with inconclusive data to support either technique. Attention must be paid to maintain adequate patency of the anastomosis without distortion of the ostium of the pulmonary veins (Figure 34.3A-C).

This approach, which involves a substantial displacement of the heart anteriorly and to the right, carries the potential for distortion of the atrium and confluence at the time of the repair and consequent postoperative stenosis. In order to avoid this problem, some centers advocate performing the posterior anastomosis across the roof of the left atrium between the SVC and the aortic root [53], so that the reciprocal position of the two chambers is left unchanged during the repair. Alternatively, the venous confluence behind the left atrium is accessed from the right following a leftward retraction of the heart. A transverse incision is conducted along the right atrium inferiorly across the Waterston groove and through the posterior wall of the left atrium. The confluence is exposed and incised longitudinally between the pulmonary vein ostia. The anastomosis is then performed starting at the leftward corner of the incision and moving rightward. The interatrial defect is closed with a patch of autologous pericardium and the repair completed [54]. This approach offers excellent visualization of the confluence without significant distortion while avoiding rightward retraction of the heart. Also this technique permits patch enlargement of the left atrium, which is usually small (Figure 34.3D-F).

Repair of the Cardiac Type

When the communicating vein is connected to the coronary sinus, access is obtained through a right atriotomy. The portion of the septum between the ostium of the coronary sinus and the fossa ovalis is incised and the Thebesian valve removed. The opening of the connecting vein is usually seen in the mid portion of the coronary sinus. The coronary sinus is then unroofed towards the left atrium. In cases in which the confluence is connected to the coronary sinus by an obstructed communication, this is also incised back to the confluence via the coronary sinus to provide unobstructed drainage of the pulmonary return. The resulting large interatrial defect is closed with a patch, normally of glutaraldehyde-treated autologous pericardium, leaving the coronary and the pulmonary venous drainage to the left of the reconstructed septum (Figure 34.4). In cases of TAPVC to the right atrium, the pulmonary drainage can be redirected into the left atrium with a baffle repair through the patent foramen ovale as in the case of a sinus venosus interatrial defect. Hiramatsu and colleagues have proposed use of posterior displacement of the interatrial septum: after its detachment from the posterior edge, the septum is reattached to the right, between the pulmonary veins and the venae cavae ostia, thus recreating the normal anatomical relationships [55].

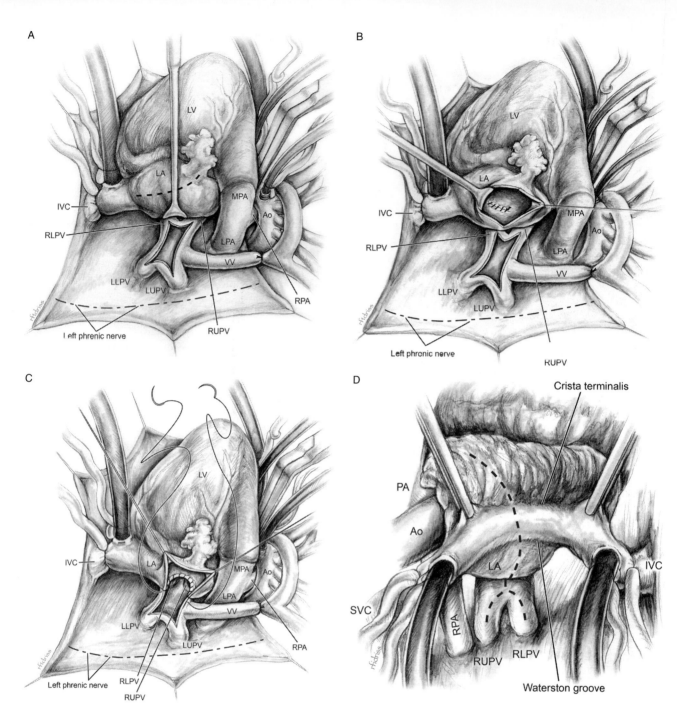

Figure 34.3 Repair of supracardiac total anomalous pulmonary venous connection with vertical vein (VV) connected to the innominate vein. **A,** The vertical vein is ligated next to its connection to the innominate, due to its accessibility in this point and the relative distance from the phrenic nerve. The incision into the confluence is extended into each of the pulmonary veins to increase the length of the anastomosis. An incision is made in the left atrial wall extending inferiorly from the base of the left atrial appendage to the inferior vena cava (IVC)-atrial junction. **B,** A secundum atrial septal defect is closed through the left atriotomy with a patch of autologous pericardium. **C,** The anastomosis between the left atrium (LA) and the venous confluence is started at the right corner and continued leftward on the superior and inferior rims as the heart is returned to its anatomic position. **D,** Alternatively, the venous confluence can be accessed from the right pericardial fossa. The LA is retracted and both atria are opened with a longitudinal incision crossing the Waterstone's groove and extending on the posterior wall of the left atrium. The pulmonary venous confluence is opened through a longitudinal incision extending from left to right. An incision is commenced in the right atrium and extended across the Waterston groove into the left atrium. **E,** The anastomosis between the left atrial wall and the venous confluence is commenced at the left corner and is brought rightward. **F,** After completion of the anastomosis the interatrial septum is augmented with the interposition of a pericardial patch to augment the left atrial cavity. **G,** The right atrial wall is finally closed with primary suture and the addition of a second pericardial patch. (LLPV, left lower pulmonary vein; LUPV, left upper pulmonary vein; LV, left ventricle; PA, pulmonary artery; RLPV, right lower pulmonary vein; RPA, right pulmonary artery; RUPV, right upper pulmonary vein; SVC, superior vena cava.)

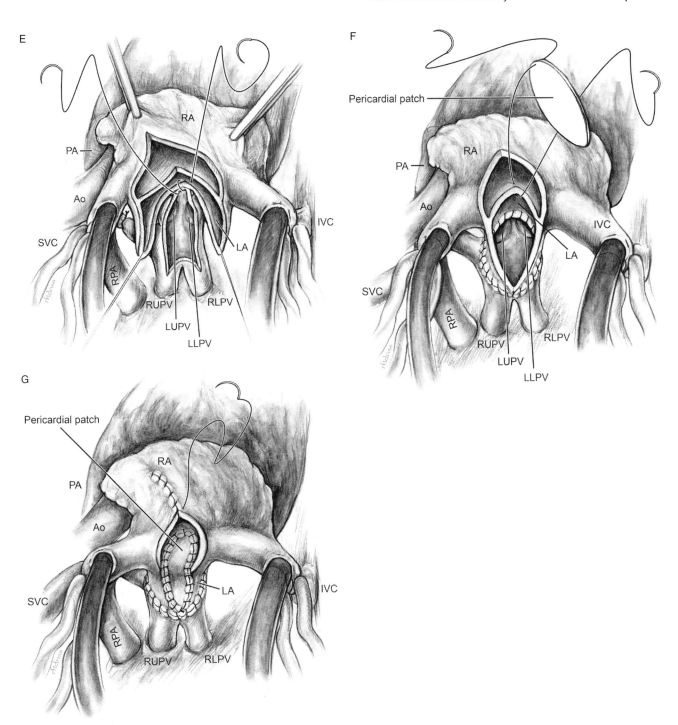

Figure 34.3 (*Continued*)

Repair of the Infracardiac Type

The vertical vein is typically extrapericardial, and descends to the abdominal cavity via the esophageal hiatus. The confluence is often aligned vertically in a Y-shape. Exposure can be obtained from a left approach retracting the heart anteriorly and to the right. Alternatively, access can be gained through a biatrial incision from the right side as described above. Once access to the confluence is obtained, the vertical vein can be ligated. As noted above, some authors recommend leaving the vertical vein intact to allow decompression of the small, non-compliant left atrium into the systemic venous system, and thereby diminish postoperative pulmonary venous hypertension [56]. Once the confluence has been opened with a vertical, Y-shaped incision, the repair is carried out as described previously

A

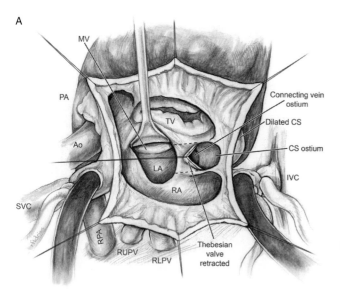

B

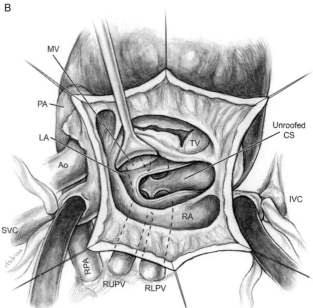

C

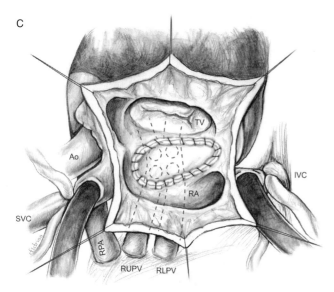

Figure 34.4 Repair of cardiac total anomalous pulmonary venous connection with connecting vein (CV) to the coronary sinus (CS). **A,** The CS is enlarged and the ostium of the CV is visualized near its ostium. A secundum atrial septal defect is retracted to permit visualization of the mitral valve (MV) in the left atrium. The pulmonary vein (PV) orifices are not present in the left atrium (LA). The CS is unroofed into the LA and the atrial septal defect thus enlarged (dotted lines). **B,** The PV confluence is inspected through the unroofed CS and all four vein ostia are inspected. **C,** The defect is then closed with a patch of autologous pericardium, leaving the unroofed CS draining to the reconstructed LA. (IVC, inferior vena cava; LLPV, left lower pulmonary vein; LUPV, left upper pulmonary vein; LV, left ventricle; PA, pulmonary artery; RLPV, right lower pulmonary vein; RPA, right pulmonary artery; RUPV, right upper pulmonary vein; SVC, superior vena cava; TV, tricuspid valve.)

(Figure 34.5). The supradiaphragmatic portion of the vertical vein can be used to augment the anastomosis to the left atrium after its division (Figure 34.5) [57].

Repair of the Mixed Type

The commonest pattern of mixed TAPVC is three veins to a posterior confluence and one separately connecting to the systemic venous system. Repair often involves an anasto-

mosis between the left atrium and the confluence as described previously and reimplantation of the fourth vein if possible. Single, unobstructed pulmonary veins can be left in situ to avoid postoperative restenosis. Imoto *et al.* have demonstrated that small residual left-to-right shunts from a single residual anomalous pulmonary vein in continuity with the systemic veins did not result in significant hemodynamic compromise [58]. More complex arrangements of the anomalous pulmonary veins may need repairs tailored to the patient's specific anatomy.

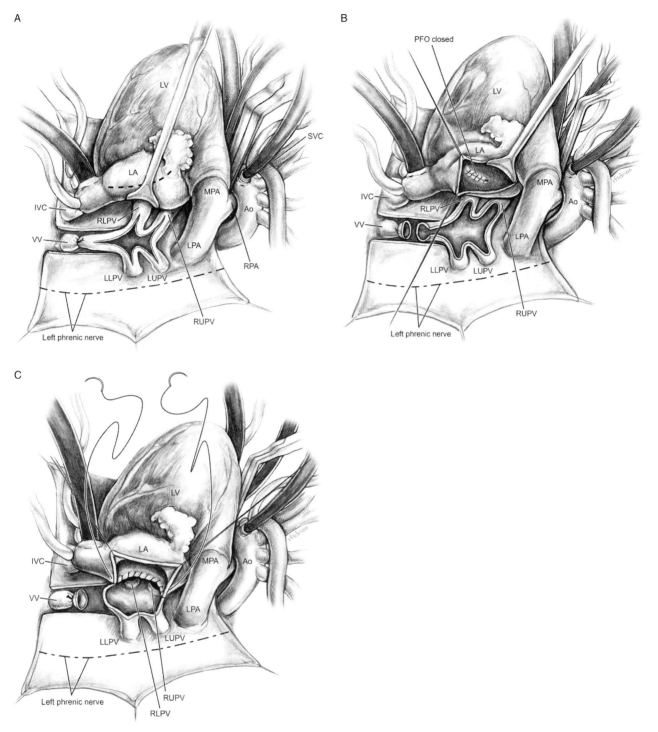

Figure 34.5 Repair of infracardiac total anomalous pulmonary venous connection with ligation of the vertical vein (VV). **A,** The VV is ligated at its emergence through the esophageal hiatus. The confluence is opened with a "Y" shaped incision. The left atrium is opened with an incision extending into the left atrial appendage (dotted line). **B,** The atrial septal defect is closed via the atriotomy. The VV is divided to increase the length of the anastomosis. **C,** The anastomosis is then completed. (IVC, inferior vena cava; LLPV, left lower pulmonary vein; LUPV, left upper pulmonary vein; LV, left ventricle; MPA, main pulmonary artery; RLPV, right lower pulmonary vein; RPA, right pulmonary artery; RUPV, right upper pulmonary vein; SVC, superior vena cava.)

Results

In a large meta-analysis reviewing the published results for repair of simple TAPVC between 1966 and 1993, Clabby *et al.* showed the perioperative mortality rates dropping from 85% in the first series to less than 5% in the last decade [59]. According to the Pediatric Cardiac Care Consortium, which reported on 437 operations for anomalous pulmonary connections performed between 1985 and 1993, supracardiac connection was seen in 40% of the cases, cardiac in 17%, infracardiac in 22%, and mixed in 10%. In 11% of the cases the type of connection was unknown. The mortality per type of connection was 14.2%, 11.6%, 32.6%, 15.8%, and 36% respectively [59]. This distribution of connection types is in accordance with most published surgical and pathology series [7,10,13,16,21]. Recently published series from the Toronto and Boston groups have confirmed the trend toward improved survival and overall good operative outcome with acceptable long-term survival rates, especially in isolated TAPVC [60,61].

In an analysis of the impact of coexisting cardiac anomalies on survival after repair of TAPVC, multivariate analysis demonstrated that single-ventricle and associated cardiac lesions adversely affected perioperative mortality and long-term survival (Figure 34.6) [36]. Moreover, when comparing survival after repair of TAPVC in the presence of two- and single-ventricle hearts, survival was 70% at 15 years in the biventricular population compared with 20% survival at 5 years in the univentricular population [36]. The type of palliation in patients with single-ventricle physiology depends on whether the pulmonary antegrade blood flow is restricted as in pulmonary stenosis or atresia, or unrestricted. In single-ventricle patients with restricted pulmonary blood flow, the presence of obstructed pul-

monary venous return may be unmasked by a palliative procedure designed to increase pulmonary perfusion (systemic-to-pulmonary shunts) [36,62]. Early palliation in single-ventricle neonates requiring repair of TAPVC and stabilization of pulmonary circulation at the same time has proven disappointing [59,62–65].

The long-term prognosis is influenced by the incidence of post-repair pulmonary vein stenosis, which occurs in 5–15% of cases. This complication has been attributed to anastomotic fibrotic stricture at the ostia of single pulmonary veins and/or to a poorly understood process of intimal hyperplasia often involving the whole length of the pulmonary veins [37,66–68]. The restenosis tends to appear within the first 6–12 months following the repair, and its hemodynamic effects can remain undetected until the degree of obstruction is severe. The occurrence of post-repair pulmonary vein stenosis is a significant risk factor for poor outcome (Figure 34.7) [37]. Several authors have found that poor prognosis is directly proportional to the number of pulmonary veins involved in the restenosis process [37,67–72]. Progressive shortness of breath has been consistently reported as the most common symptom. Chest radiographs often present congested lungs or severe pulmonary edema bilaterally or limited to the side of the obstructed veins. Lung perfusion scans show severe ventilation/perfusion mismatch with the affected side hypoperfused, but normally ventilated. Echocardiography and Doppler interrogation demonstrate turbulent or accelerated flow through the stenotic veins. However, Valsangiacomo *et al.* have shown that echocardiography was able to identify the pulmonary veins in only 89% of cases, whereas MRA visualized the central two-thirds of

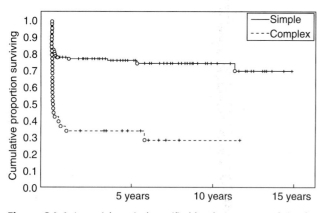

Figure 34.6 Actuarial survival stratified by the presence of simple total anomalous pulmonary venous connection (continuous line) versus total anomalous pulmonary venous connection associated with other complex cardiac anomalies (dotted line). (Reproduced with permission from Caldarone *et al.* [36].)

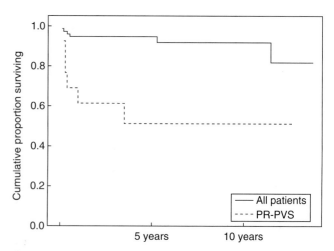

Figure 34.7 Survival after repair of total anomalous pulmonary venous drainage (<30 days mortality excluded) for all patients (continuous line) versus patients with post-repair pulmonary vein stenosis (PR-PVS; dotted line) (*p* < 0.001). (Reproduced with permission from Caldarone *et al.* [37].)

the pulmonary veins in 99% [33]. Phase-contrast MRA offers a functional evaluation and grading of the ensuing stenosis by demonstrating the type of blood flow as monophasic or biphasic. Contrast-enhanced MRA visualizes not only the stenotic lesion but also the collateral venous channels to the unobstructed pulmonary veins within the lung parenchyma [32,34]. Therefore, when pulmonary vein stenosis is suspected, we prefer to perform MRA as the initial sequence (Plate 34.2, see plate section opposite p. 594).

Almost invariably the occurrence of post-repair pulmonary vein stenosis requires surgical intervention. Conventional repair of pulmonary vein stenosis, such as resection of the anastomotic endocardial fibrotic overgrowth, patch venoplasty with or without endarterectomy, as well as percutaneous stenting techniques are associated with a high incidence of recurrent stenosis and poor prognosis [37,67,68,73].

Sutureless techniques to treat post-repair pulmonary vein stenosis have been reported by many groups. This technique avoids direct suture on the pulmonary veins, based on the assumption that this will reduce intimal hyperplasia. Cardiopulmonary bypass is instituted in the standard manner. The left atrium is incised along its posterior wall with the incision extending into the appendage to create the widest possible opening. The pulmonary veins are opened starting at the atrial junction and the incision is continued upstream until the secondary or tertiary branches are opened. The pericardium is breached below the phrenic nerve to avoid damaging it and to allow the incision of the vein below the reflection of the mediastinal pleura at the hilum of the lung. Any obstruction is then incised or resected. The atrial edge is sutured to the pericardium around the veins and to the reflection of the pericardium just below the phrenic nerve. The presence of adhesions in the posterior pericardium and hilar area contribute to hemostasis (Figure 34.8) [74]. Cine magnetic resonance imaging (MRI) studies have demonstrated favorable flow patterns and rare recurrent restenosis especially in patients with localized stenosis, and significantly lower transvenous

A

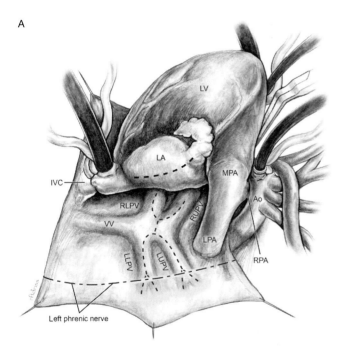

B

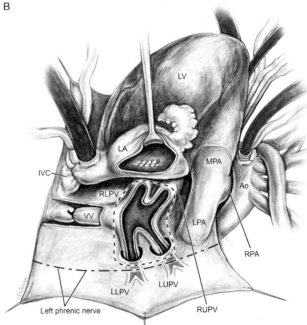

Figure 34.8 Repair of infracardiac total anomalous pulmonary venous connection with a sutureless technique. **A,** The venous confluence is retropericardial. The left atrium (LA) incision is extended into the appendage to create the widest possible opening. **B,** The posterior pericardium is breached and the descending vertical vein (VV) ligated (optional). The pulmonary veins are opened starting at the atrial junction and the incision is continued upstream until the secondary or tertiary branches are opened. **C,** The atrial edge is sutured to the pericardium along the dotted line, as indicated, avoiding direct suturing of the veins. The anastomosis is conducted from left to right. **D.** The pericardium is breached below the phrenic nerve to avoid damaging it and to

allow the incision of the vein below the reflection of the mediastinal pleura at the hilum of the lung. Any obstruction is then incised or resected. The free edge of the left atrial wall is anastomosed to the pericardium below the phrenic bundle. The integrity of the mediastinal pleura and the presence of adhesions allow drainage of pulmonary venous blood inside the newly constructed atrium. (IVC, inferior vena cava; LLPV, left lower pulmonary vein; LUPV, left upper pulmonary vein; LV, left ventricle; MPA, main pulmonary artery; RLPV, right lower pulmonary vein; RPA, right pulmonary artery; RUPV, right upper pulmonary vein; SVC, superior vena cava.)

C

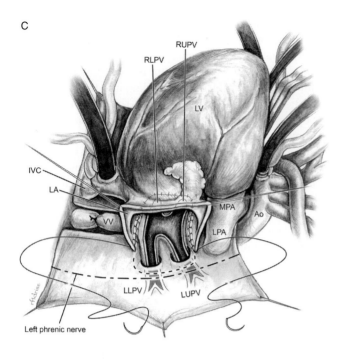

Figure 34.8 (*Continued*)

D

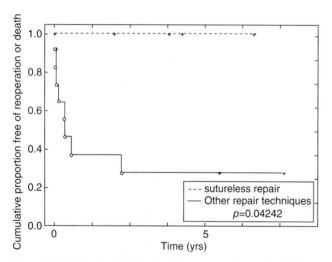

Figure 34.9 Unadjusted freedom from reoperation or death for patients with post-repair pulmonary vein stenosis stratified by sutureless technique versus other surgical techniques. (Reproduced with permission from Yun *et al.* [74].)

gradients when compared to conventional repairs. These results have promoted the use of the sutureless technique as primary repair of TAPVC (Figure 34.9) [74].

In summary, TAPVC represents a broad spectrum of anomalies that can be isolated or associated with complex cardiac anomalies. Surgical results for repair in the isolated form have steadily improved over the last three decades

and offer good long-term survival. Single ventricle circulation, severe associated anomalies, and recurrent diffuse pulmonary vein stenosis continue to represent a challenge. The sutureless technique offers significant benefit for post-repair pulmonary vein stenosis and may offer benefit for primary repair of TAPVC.

References

1. Becker AE, Anderson RH. (1981) Anomalies of pulmonary veins. In: *Pathology of Congenital Heart Disease*, 2nd ed. London: Butterworths.
2. Herlong JR, Jaggers JJ, Ungerleider RM. (2000) Congenital Heart Surgery Nomenclature and Database Project: pulmonary venous anomalies. Ann Thorac Surg 69(4 Suppl), S56–S69.
3. Kirshbom PM, Jaggers JJ, Ungerleider RM. (2003) Total anomalous pulmonary venous connection. In: Mavroudis C, Backer CL, eds. *Pediatric Cardiac Surgery*, 3rd ed. Philadelphia, PA: Mosby, Inc.
4. Moorman A, Webb S, Brown NA, *et al.* (2003) Development of the heart: (1) formation of the cardiac chambers and arterial trunks. Heart 89, 806–814.
5. Neill CA. (1956) Development of the pulmonary veins; with reference to the embryology of anomalies of pulmonary venous return. Pediatrics 18, 880–887.
6. Krabill KA, Lucas RV Jr. (1995) Abnormal pulmonary venous connections. In: Emmanouilides GC, Reimenschneider TA, Allen HD, *et al.*, eds. *Heart Disease in Infants, Children and Adolescents*. Baltimore: Williams & Wilkins.

7. Craig JM, Darling RC, Rothney WB. (1957) Total pulmonary venous drainage into the right side of the heart; report of 17 autopsied cases not associated with other major cardiovascular anomalies. Lab Invest 6, 44–64.

8. Burroughs JT, Edwards JE. (1960) Total anomalous pulmonary venous connection. Am Heart J 59, 913–931.

9. Smith B, Frye TR, Newton WA. (1961) Total anomalous pulmonary venous return: diagnostic criteria and a new classification. Am J Dis Child 101, 41.

10. Delisle G, Ando M, Calder AL, et al. (1976) Total anomalous pulmonary venous connection: Report of 93 autopsied cases with emphasis on diagnostic and surgical considerations. Am Heart J 91, 99–122.

11. Hastreiter AR, Paul MH, Molthan ME, et al. (1962) Total anomalous pulmonary venous connection with severe pulmonary venous obstruction. A clinical entity. Circulation 25, 916–928.

12. Behrendt DM, Aberdeen E, Waterson DJ, et al. (1972) Total anomalous pulmonary venous drainage in infants. I. Clinical and hemodynamic findings, methods, and results of operation in 37 cases. Circulation 46, 347–356.

13. Gathman GE, Nadas AS. (1970) Total anomalous pulmonary venous connection: clinical and physiologic observations of 75 pediatric patients. Circulation 42, 143–154.

14. Mathew R, Thilenius OG, Replogle RL, et al. (1977) Cardiac function in total anomalous pulmonary venous return before and after surgery. Circulation 55, 361–370.

15. Bharati S, Lev M. (1973) Congenital anomalies of the pulmonary veins. Cardiovasc Clin 5, 23–41.

16. Bove KE, Geiser EA, Meyer RA. (1975) The left ventricle in anomalous pulmonary venous return. Morphometric analysis of 36 fatal cases in infancy. Arch Pathol 99, 522–528.

17. Rosenquist GC, Kelly JL, Chandra R, et al. (1985) Small left atrium and change in contour of the ventricular septum in total anomalous pulmonary venous connection: a morphometric analysis of 22 infant hearts. Am J Cardiol 55, 777–782.

18. Haworth SG, Reid L. (1977) Structural study of pulmonary circulation and of heart in total anomalous pulmonary venous return in early infancy. Br Heart J 39, 80–92.

19. Barratt-Boyes BG, Simpson M, Neutze JM. (1971) Intracardiac surgery in neonates and infants using deep hypothermia with surface cooling and limited cardiopulmonary bypass. Circulation 43(5 Suppl), I25–I30.

20. DeLeon SY, Gidding SS, Ilbawi MN, et al. (1987) Surgical management of infants with complex cardiac anomalies associated with reduced pulmonary blood flow and total anomalous pulmonary venous drainage. Ann Thorac Surg 43, 207–211.

21. James CL, Keeling JW, Smith NM, et al. (1994) Total anomalous pulmonary venous drainage associated with fatal outcome in infancy and early childhood: an autopsy study of 52 cases. Pediatr Pathol 14, 665–678.

22. Murphy AM, Greeley WJ. (1995) Total anomalous pulmonary venous connection. In: Nichols DG, Cameron DE, Greeley WJ, et al., eds. Critical Heart Disease in Infants and Children. St Louis: Mosby, Inc.

23. Harris MA, Valmorida JN. (1997) Neonates with congenital heart disease, Part IV: Total anomalous pulmonary venous return. Neonatal Netw 16, 63–66.

24. Jenkins KJ, Sanders SP, Orav EJ, et al. (1993) Individual pulmonary vein size and survival in infants with totally anomalous pulmonary venous connection. J Am Coll Cardiol 22, 201–206.

25. Patel CR, Lane JR, Spector ML, et al. (2005) Totally anomalous pulmonary venous connection and complex congenital heart disease: prenatal echocardiographic diagnosis and prognosis. J Ultrasound Med 24, 1191–1198.

26. Valsangiacomo ER, Hornberger LK, Barrea C, et al. (2003) Partial and total anomalous pulmonary venous connection in the fetus: two-dimensional and Doppler echocardiographic findings. Ultrasound Obstet Gynecol 22, 257–263.

27. Brown VE, De Lange M, Dyar DA, et al. (1998) Echocardiographic spectrum of supracardiac total anomalous pulmonary venous connection. J Am Soc Echocardiogr 11, 289–293.

28. Chin AJ, Sanders SP, Sherman F, et al. (1987) Accuracy of subcostal two-dimensional echocardiography in prospective diagnosis of total anomalous pulmonary venous connection. Am Heart J 113, 1153–1159.

29. Goswami KC, Shrivastava S, Saxena A, et al. (1993) Echocardiographic diagnosis of total anomalous pulmonary venous connection. Am Heart J 126, 433–440.

30. Huhta JC, Gutgesell HP, Nihill MR. (1985) Cross sectional echocardiographic diagnosis of total anomalous pulmonary venous connection. Br Heart J 53, 525–534.

31. Krabill KA, Ring WS, Foker JE, et al. (1987) Echocardiographic versus cardiac catheterization diagnosis of infants with congenital heart disease requiring cardiac surgery. Am J Cardiol 60, 351–354.

32. Grosse-Wortmann L, Al-Otay A, Goo HW, et al. (2007) Anatomical and functional evaluation of pulmonary veins in children by magnetic resonance imaging. J Am Coll Cardiol 49, 993–1002.

33. Valsangiacomo ER, Levasseur S, McCrindle BW, et al. (2003) Contrast-enhanced MR angiography of pulmonary venous abnormalities in children. Pediatr Radiol 33, 92–98.

34. Freedom RM, Yoo SJ, Coles JG, et al. (2004) Total anomalous pulmonary venous connections. In: Freedom RM, Yoo SJ, Mikailian H, et al., eds. The Natural and Modified History of Congenital Heart Disease. Elmsford, NY: Futura/Blackwell Publishing.

35. Greil GF, Powell AJ, Gildein HP, et al. (2002) Gadolinium-enhanced three-dimensional magnetic resonance angiography of pulmonary and systemic venous anomalies. J Am Coll Cardiol 39, 335–341.

36. Caldarone CA, Najm HK, Kadletz M, et al. (1998) Surgical management of total anomalous pulmonary venous drainage: impact of coexisting cardiac anomalies. Ann Thorac Surg 66, 1521–1526.

37. Caldarone CA, Najm HK, Kadletz M, et al. (1998) Relentless pulmonary vein stenosis after repair of total anomalous pulmonary venous drainage. Ann Thorac Surg 66, 1514–1520.

38. Bu'Lock FA, Jordan SC, Martin RP. (1994) Successful balloon dilatation of ascending vein stenosis in obstructed supracardiac total anomalous pulmonary venous connection. Pediatr Cardiol 15, 78–80.

39. Kyser JP, Bengur AR, Siwik ES. (2006) Preoperative pallia- tion of newborn obstructed total anomalous pulmonary venous connection by endovascular stent placement. Catheter Cardiovasc Interv 67, 473–476.

40. Lo-A-Njoe SM, Blom NA, Bokenkamp R, et al. (2006) Stenting of the vertical vein in obstructed total anomalous pulmonary venous return as rescue procedure in a neonate. Catheter Cardiovasc Interv 67, 668–670.

41. Meadows J, Marshall AC, Lock JE, et al. (2006) A hybrid approach to stabilization and repair of obstructed total anomalous pulmonary venous connection in a critically ill newborn infant. J Thorac Cardiovasc Surg 131, e1–e2.

42. Michel-Behnke I, Luedemann M, Hagel KJ, et al. (2002) Serial stent implantation to relieve in-stent stenosis in obstructed total anomalous pulmonary venous return. Pediatr Cardiol 23, 221–223.

43. Ramakrishnan S, Kothari SS. (2004) Preoperative balloon dilatation of obstructed total anomalous pulmonary venous connection in a neonate. Catheter Cardiovasc Interv 61, 128–130.

44. Dudell GG, Evans ML, Krous HF, et al. (1993) Common pulmonary vein atresia: the role of extracorporeal mem- brane oxygenation. Pediatrics 91, 403–410.

45. Ishino K, Alexi-Meskishvili V, Hetzer R. (1999) Preoperative extracorporeal membrane oxygenation in newborns with total anomalous pulmonary venous connection. Cardiovasc Surg 7, 473–475.

46. Stewart DL, Mendoza JC, Winston S, et al. (1996) Use of extracorporeal life support in total anomalous pulmonary venous drainage. J Perinatol 16, 186–190.

47. Klein MD, Shaheen KW, Whittlesey GC, et al. (1990) Extracorporeal membrane oxygenation for the circulatory support of children after repair of congenital heart disease. J Thorac Cardiovasc Surg 100, 498–505.

48. Raisher BD, Grant JW, Martin TC, et al. (1992) Complete repair of total anomalous pulmonary venous connection in infancy. J Thorac Cardiovasc Surg 104, 443–448.

49. Weinhaus L, Canter C, Noetzel M, et al. (1989) Extracorporeal membrane oxygenation for circulatory support after repair of congenital heart defects. Ann Thorac Surg 48, 206–212.

50. Williams GR, Richardson WR, Campbell GS. (1964) Repair of total anomalous pulmonary venous drainage in infancy. J Thorac Cardiovasc Surg 47, 199–204.

51. Cope JT, Banks D, McDaniel NL, et al. (1997) Is vertical vein ligation necessary in repair of total anomalous pulmonary venous connection? Ann Thorac Surg 64, 23–28; discussion 29.

52. Cheung YF, Lun KS, Chau AK, et al. (2005) Fate of the unli- gated vertical vein after repair of supracardiac anomalous pulmonary venous connection. J Paediatr Child Health 41, 361–364.

53. Tucker BL, Lindesmith GG, Stiles QR, et al. (1976) The supe- rior approach for correction of the supracardiac type of total anomalous pulmonary venous return. Ann Thorac Surg 22, 374–377.

54. Shumacker HB, King H. (1961) A modified procedure for complete repair of total anomalous pulmonary venous drainage. Surg Gynecol Obstet 112, 763–765.

55. Hiramatsu T, Takanashi Y, Imai Y, et al. (1998) Atrial septal displacement for repair of anomalous pulmonary venous return into the right atrium. Ann Thorac Surg 65, 1110–1114.

56. Caspi J, Pettitt TW, Fontenot EE, et al. (2001) The beneficial hemodynamic effects of selective patent vertical vein follow- ing repair of obstructed total anomalous pulmonary venous drainage in infants. Eur J Cardiothorac Surg 20, 830–834.

57. Tsang VT, Stark J. (2006) Total anomalous pulmonary venous return and cor triatriatum. In: Stark JF, de Leval MR, Tsang VT, eds. Surgery for Congenital Heart Defects, 3rd ed. Chichester, England: John Wiley & Sons.

58. Imoto Y, Kado H, Asou T, et al. (1998) Mixed type of total anomalous pulmonary venous connection. Ann Thorac Surg 66, 1394–1397.

59. Clabby ML, Canter CE, Strauss AW, et al. (1998) Total anoma- lous pulmonary venous connection. In: Moller JH, ed. Surgery of Congenital Heart Disease: Pediatric Cardiac Care Consortium. Armonk, NY: Futura.

60. Hancock Friesen CL, Zurakowski D, et al. (2005) Total anom- alous pulmonary venous connection: an analysis of current management strategies in a single institution. Ann Thorac Surg 79, 596–606.

61. Karamlou T, Gurofsky R, Al Sukhni E, et al. (2007) Factors associated with mortality and reoperation in 377 children with total anomalous pulmonary venous connection. Circu- lation 115, 1591–1598.

62. Heinemann MK, Hanley FL, Van Praagh S, et al. (1994) Total anomalous pulmonary venous drainage in newborns with visceral heterotaxy. Ann Thorac Surg 57, 88–91.

63. Gaynor JW, Collins MH, Rychik J, et al. (1999) Long-term outcome of infants with single ventricle and total anomalous pulmonary venous connection. J Thorac Cardiovasc Surg 117, 506–513; discussion 513–514.

64. Hashmi A, Abu-Sulaiman R, McCrindle BW, et al. (1998) Management and outcomes of right atrial isomerism: a 26- year experience. J Am Coll Cardiol 31, 1120–1126.

65. Sadiq M, Stumper O, De Giovanni JV, et al. (1996) Management and outcome of infants and children with right atrial isomerism. Heart 75, 314–319.

66. Bando K, Turrentine MW, Ensing GJ, et al. (1996) Surgi- cal management of total anomalous pulmonary venous connection. Thirty-year trends. Circulation 94(9 Suppl), II12–II16.

67. Lacour-Gayet F, Zoghbi J, Serraf AE, et al. (1999) Surgical management of progressive pulmonary venous obstruction after repair of total anomalous pulmonary venous connec- tion. J Thorac Cardiovasc Surg 117, 679–687.

68. Najm HK, Caldarone CA, Smallhorn J, et al. (1998) A suture- less technique for the relief of pulmonary vein stenosis with the use of in situ pericardium. J Thorac Cardiovasc Surg 115, 468–470.

69. Aburawi EH, Thomson J, Van Doorn C. (2001) Late anasto- motic stenosis after correction of totally anomalous pulmo- nary venous connection. Cardiol Young 11, 320–321.

70. Korbmacher B, Buttgen S, Schulte HD, et al. (2001) Long- term results after repair of total anomalous pulmonary venous connection. Thorac Cardiovasc Surg 49, 101–106.

71. Lee ML, Wang JK, Lue HC. (1995) Visualization of pulmonary vein obstruction by pulmonary artery wedge injection and documentation by pressure tracings: report of one case with persistent wheezing following correction of total anomalous pulmonary venous connection. Int J Cardiol 49, 167–172.

72. Ricci M, Elliott M, Cohen GA, *et al.* (2003) Management of pulmonary venous obstruction after correction of TAPVC: risk factors for adverse outcome. Eur J Cardiothorac Surg 24, 28–36.

73. Coles JG, Yemets I, Najm HK, *et al.* (1995) Experience with repair of congenital heart defects using adjunctive endovascular devices. J Thorac Cardiovasc Surg 110, 1513–1519; discussion 1519–1520.

74. Yun TJ, Coles JG, Konstantinov IE, *et al.* (2005) Conventional and sutureless techniques for management of the pulmonary veins: Evolution of indications from postrepair pulmonary vein stenosis to primary pulmonary vein anomalies. J Thorac Cardiovasc Surg 129, 167–174.

CHAPTER 35

Cor Triatriatum Sinister, Pulmonary Vein Stenosis, Atresia of the Common Pulmonary Vein, and Cor Triatriatum Dexter

Ralph E. Delius[1,2] and Henry L. Walters III[1,2]
[1]Children's Hospital of Michigan, Detroit, MI, USA
[2]Wayne State University School of Medicine, Detroit, MI, USA

Cor triatriatum sinister, atresia of the common pulmonary vein, and pulmonary vein stenosis are very uncommon but related congenital lesions that share similar morphogenesis. The embryological origins of these lesions are similar to total anomalous pulmonary venous connection (TAPVC), in that each of these lesions are related to abnormal incorporation of the common pulmonary vein into the left atrium during cardiac development. The pathophysiology of these lesions, usually involving some degree of obstruction to pulmonary venous drainage or a diversion of pulmonary venous return into the right atrium, is similar as well. Not surprisingly, the clinical presentation of patients with these defects may mimic each other. Cor triatriatum dexter, also referred to as divided right atrium, is unrelated developmentally and clinically and will be considered separately.

Embryology of Pulmonary Venous System

Morphogenesis of the pulmonary venous system is well understood, and a fundamental understanding of the pulmonary venous development can elucidate the development of cor triatriatum, atresia of the common pulmonary vein, and pulmonary vein stenosis. The primordial lung buds share the splanchnic plexus with other foregut derivatives, and drainage into the systemic circulation is through the paired cardinal and umbilicovitelline veins. At about 27–29 days of gestation, a primitive pulmonary vein develops as an evagination from the posterior wall of the left atrium (Figure 35.1A) [1]. At approximately 30 days gestation the nascent pulmonary vein engages the pulmonary

portion of the splanchnic plexus and begins to drain blood from this region (Figure 35.1B) [1]. A common pulmonary vein develops, which is progressively incorporated into the posterior wall of the left atrium. After communication between the pulmonary portion of the splanchnic plexus and the heart is established, connections to the cardinal and umbilicovitelline systems involute (Figure 35.1C) [1]. Consequently, the common pulmonary vein is a transient anatomic structure. The normal left atrium is made of common pulmonary vein and primitive left atrium, with each making roughly comparable contributions to the fully developed left atrium.

Pathologic Anatomy

The morphology of pulmonary venous abnormalities is related to abnormalities of common pulmonary vein development. Timing of the development of the defect is important, as connections to systemic venous drainage are still present if the defect occurs early, while late development of common pulmonary vein abnormalities occurring after involution of the pulmonary–systemic venous connections may lead to a different congenital pulmonary venous anomaly. If the common pulmonary vein becomes atretic or fails to develop early, a connection to the splanchnic plexus and cardinal or umbilicovitelline veins is still present and can serve as collateral venous drainage, resulting in total anomalous pulmonary venous connection (TAPVC). Atresia of only the left or right portion of the common pulmonary vein leads to partial anomalous pulmonary venous return. If atresia of the common pulmonary vein occurs late, after involution of the connections to

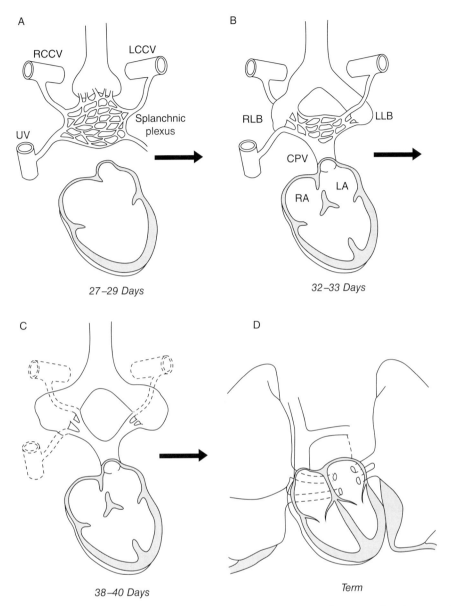

Figure 35.1 Development of the pulmonary veins. **A,** At 27–29 days of gestation, the primordial lung buds are enmeshed by the vascular plexus of the foregut (the splanchnic plexus). At this stage, there is no direct connection to the heart. Instead there are multiple connections to the umbilicovitelline and cardinal venous systems. A small evagination can be seen in the posterior wall of the left atrium (LA) to the left of the developing septum secundum. **B,** By the end of the first month of gestation, the common pulmonary vein (CPV) establishes a connection between the pulmonary venous plexus and the sinoatrial portion of the heart. At this time, the connections between the pulmonary venous plexus and the splanchnic venous plexus are still patent. **C,** Next, the connections between the pulmonary venous plexus and the splanchnic venous plexus involute. **D,** The common pulmonary vein incorporates into the left atrium so that the individual pulmonary veins connect separately and directly to the left atrium. (LCCV, left common cardinal vein; LLB, left lung bud; RA, right atrium; RCCV, right common cardinal vein; RLB, right lung bud; UV, umbilical vein.) (Reproduced with permission from Geva *et al.* [1].)

the systemic venous system, atresia of the common pulmonary vein develops, in which the pulmonary veins drain into a common pulmonary vein, which serves a blind cul-de-sac that has no connection to the left atrium or systemic venous drainage (Figure 35.2A) [1].

Stenosis of the common pulmonary vein leads to cor triatriatum sinister, giving the appearance of incomplete incorporation of the common pulmonary vein into the left atrium (Figure 35.2B) [1]. In most cases, the stenosis develops late, after involution of collateral venous connections.

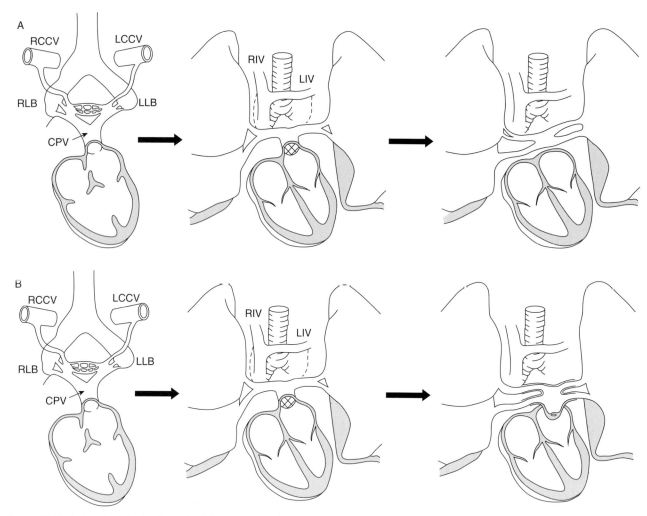

Figure 35.2 Embryologic basis of atresia of the common pulmonary vein and cor triatriatum. **A,** The common pulmonary vein (CPV) has established a connection with the left atrium and the primitive venous connections have regressed (middle panel). Normally, the connection between the common pulmonary vein and the left atrium enlarges. If the normal connection between the common pulmonary vein and the left atrium fails, the pulmonary veins drain into a blind cul de sac without a significant alternative egress for pulmonary venous blood (atresia of the common pulmonary vein). **B,** The connection between the common pulmonary vein and the left atrium is stenotic, and the common pulmonary vein dilates (cor triatriatum). (LCCV, left common cardinal vein; LIV, left innominate vein; LLB, left lung bud; RCCV, right common cardinal vein; RIV, right innominate vein; RLB, right lung bud.) (Reproduced with permission from Geva *et al.* [1].)

Early stenosis, however, can lead to cor triatriatum sinister with partial anomalous pulmonary venous connection, which suggests that collateral vessel channels were present at the time the stenosis developed.

Abnormal incorporation of the common pulmonary vein into the left atrium can lead to abnormal numbers of pulmonary veins, or stenosis of pulmonary veins at the junction with the left atrium.

Cor Triatriatum Sinister

Cor triatriatum sinister was initially described by Church in 1868, but Andral was the first to describe a heart with "three auricles" in 1829 [2,3]. This defect is rare, comprising approximately 0.1% of all congenital cardiac malformations. Males and females are equally affected. Initial surgical repair was accomplished separately in 1956 by two pioneers of early cardiac surgery, Drs John Lewis and Arthur Vineberg [4,5]. Additional cardiac defects can be seen in approximately 50% of patients with cor triatriatum sinister [6–11]. The incidence of coexisting lesions reported in postmortem series tends to be higher than the incidence seen in operative series [12].

Anatomy

The hallmark feature of cor triatriatum sinister is the drainage of pulmonary veins into an accessory chamber that is

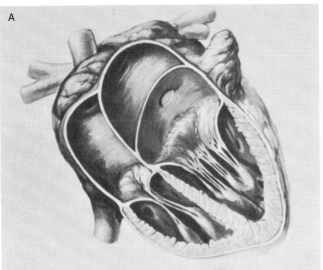

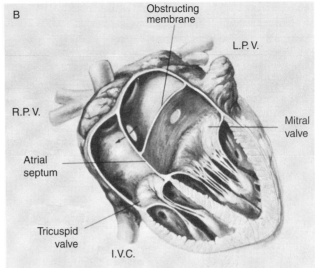

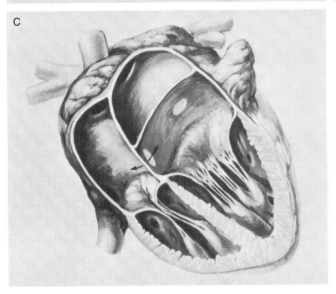

Figure 35.3 A, Cor triatriatum with intact atrial septum (type A). **B,** Cor triatriatum with atrial septal defect between the proximal left atrial chamber and the right atrium (type A₁). **C,** Triatrial heart, type A₂. The atrial septal defect connects the distal or true left atrium with the right atrium. IVC, inferior vena cava; LPV, left pulmonary vein; RPV, right pulmonary vein. (Reproduced with permission from Arciniegas *et al.* [14].)

adjacent and attached to the left atrium. This accessory chamber, in turn, drains into the left or right atrium. Failure of the common pulmonary vein to incorporate completely into the left atrium is the most commonly accepted theory of embryogenesis of cor triatriatum sinister. In most cases, the conjunction between the proximal accessory chamber and the left atrium consists of a fibromuscular membrane which is usually perforated. The size of the perforation establishes whether obstruction to pulmonary venous flow is present. In some cases, the membrane is imperforate and the accessory chamber drains directly or indirectly into the right atrium.

Several classification schemes have been developed, but none are comprehensive or universally accepted, probably due to the small number of patients in each series. The Lam classification is probably the most commonly referred to and is shown in Figure 35.3 [13,14]. Type A cor triatriatum consists of a proximal accessory chamber that receives all four pulmonary veins, with the true left atrium containing the left atrial appendage and mitral valve (Figure 35.3A) [14]. The two chambers communicate through a variable sized foramen in the membrane. Type A is further divided on the basis of the presence and location of an atrial septal defect. Subtype A1 has an atrial septal defect (ASD) communicating between the proximal chamber and the right atrium (Figure 35.3B) [14]. In Type A2 the ASD communicates between the right atrium and the true left atrium

Table 35.1 Anatomic classification of cor triatriatum. (Reproduced with permission from Geva et al. [1].)

I	Accessory atrial chamber receives all pulmonary veins and communicates with left atrium
	A. No other connections: classic cor triatriatum
	B. Other anomalous connections
	1. To right atrium directly
	2. With total anomalous pulmonary venous connection
II	Accessory atrial chamber receives all pulmonary veins and does not communicate with left atrium
	A. Anomalous connection to right atrium directly
	B. With total anomalous pulmonary venous connection
III	Subtotal cor triatriatum
	A. Accessory atrial chamber receives part of pulmonary veins and connects to left atrium
	1. Remaining pulmonary veins connect normally
	2. Remaining pulmonary veins connect anomalously
	B. Accessory atrial chamber receives part of pulmonary veins and connects to right atrium
	1. Remaining pulmonary veins connect normally

(Figure 35.3C) [14]. Type B hearts are those with coronary sinus receiving the pulmonary veins, which in fact is a form of TAPVC. Type C has no communication between the pulmonary veins and the proximal chamber. Type A is the most common, accounting for nearly two-thirds of all cases. The Lam classification scheme has many shortcomings, as type B is actually TAPVC and several anatomic variants are not included in this scheme, including unilateral cor triatriatum with partial anomalous venous return. The Lucas classification scheme, which is probably the most comprehensive nosology of cor triatriatum sinister, is outlined in Table 35.1 [1,15]. Type 1 consists of all four veins draining into the accessory chamber, which in turn communicates with the left atrium (Figure 35.4A–D) [1]. Subtypes are based on the presence or absence of other connections with the accessory chamber. Type 2 consists of the accessory chamber receiving all four pulmonary veins but does not communicate with the left atrium (Figure 35.4E) [1]. Type 3 includes subtotal cor triatriatum, with the various subtypes describing the various connections of the veins not connected to the accessory atrial chamber (Figure 35.4F–H) [1]. An even more comprehensive classification scheme including all pulmonary venous abnormalities has been proposed by Herlong et al. [16].

Pathophysiology

The pathophysiology of cor triatriatum sinister is determined by the size of the fenestration in the membrane between the accessory atrial chamber and the left atrium, by the size of communication, if present, with the right atrium, and by the effects of associated lesions. In defects in which all four veins drain into the accessory chamber, which in turn drains into the left atrium via the obstructing membrane, pulmonary venous obstruction with pulmonary hypertension will be present. A large fenestration in the membrane may be occasionally nonobstructive. The presence of an atrial septal defect between the accessory chamber and the right atrium leads to significant left-to-right shunting, with the pathophysiology being similar to TAPVC.

Clinical Presentation

The severity of symptoms and the age of presentation are dependent on the size of the communication between the pulmonary venous chamber and the left or right atrium. If the communication between the pulmonary venous chamber and left atrium is less than 3mm, and no other communications are present, the age of presentation will be in the first year of life and the clinical picture will be of pulmonary venous obstruction with low cardiac output and severe pulmonary hypertension [8]. Tachypnea, failure to thrive, and outright respiratory failure can be presenting symptoms when pulmonary venous obstruction is present. Signs of pulmonary hypertension include a long pulmonary component of the second heart sound, right ventricular heave, and pulmonary systolic ejection click. Occasionally, a diastolic murmur is heard at the apex. Electrocardiogram shows evidence of right ventricular strain. Chest radiogram shows cardiac enlargement and ground glass appearance characteristic of pulmonary venous obstruction. A nonobstructive communication between the pulmonary venous chamber and left atrium may be clinically silent and may not present until adulthood [17]. Communication to the right atrium can result in right atrial and ventricular dilatation, and the clinical presentation can mimic TAPVC.

The diagnosis of cor triatriatum sinister can be established reliably by echocardiography. A curvilinear membrane, occasionally with a windsock appearance, can be seen in the left atrial cavity. During diastole, the membrane moves toward the mitral valve. The motion and appearance of the mitral valve are normal. The relationship of the left atrial appendage to the membrane distinguishes between cor triatriatum sinister and supravalvar mitral stenosis, with the membrane superior to the left atrial appendage in cor triatriatum sinister. Transesophageal echocardiography may provide more anatomic detail, and may be a useful adjunct if transthoracic echocardiography fails to provide clear definition of the lesion. Magnetic resonance imaging (MRI) can be used as well, but as of yet, use of MRI with this lesion is sporadic [18]. Cardiac catheterization is usually not needed unless hemodynamic features are thought to be necessary prior to intervention. The presence of cor triatriatum may be masked if associated lesions

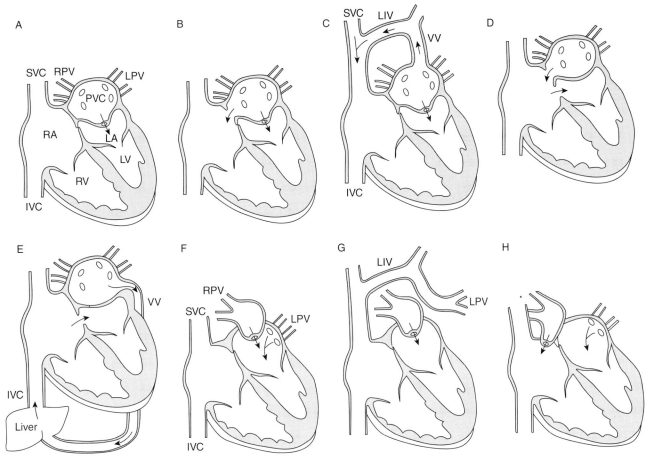

Figure 35.4 Diagram of variants of cor triatriatum. **A,** Classic cor triatriatum. The pulmonary venous chamber (PVC) receives the right and left pulmonary veins (RPV; LPV), and the only egress for pulmonary venous return is through the opening in the cor triatriatum membrane (arrow). **B,** Cor triatriatum with a communication between the PVC and the right atrium (RA). This communication allows decompression of the PVC. **C,** Cor triatriatum with an anomalous connection between the PVC and the left innominate vein (LIV). This anomalous connection (levoatrialcardinal vein) decompresses the PVC. The PVC does not communicate directly with the left atrium (LA). **D,** Pulmonary venous return reaches the right atrium (RA) through a communication between the PVC and the right atrium. Blood then reaches the left atrium via the foramen ovale. **E,** The PVC decompresses via a vertical vein to the portal vein. Subtotal cor triatriatum. **F,** The confluence of the right pulmonary veins communicates with the left atrium via a stenotic orifice. The left pulmonary veins connect normally to the left atrium. **G,** Subtotal cor triatriatum of the right pulmonary veins associated with partially anomalous pulmonary venous connection of the left pulmonary veins to the left innominate vein. **H,** Subtotal cor triatriatum of the right pulmonary veins to the right atrium via a stenotic orifice. The left pulmonary veins connect normally. This variant may be viewed as a restrictive sinus venosus defect with atresia of the orifice of the right pulmonary veins. (IVC, inferior vena cava; LV, left ventricle; RV, right ventricle.) (Reproduced with permission from Geva *et al.* [1].)

are present that feature reduced pulmonary blood flow, such as tetralogy of Fallot [19,20].

Treatment

Management of cor triatriatum sinister is surgical, although use of balloon dilation has been reported [21,22]. Experience with catheter-based intervention is limited, and long-term follow-up is lacking. The diagnosis of cor triatriatum sinister is, in itself, an indication for operation, since mortality in unoperated patients is 75%.

In virtually all cases, cardiopulmonary bypass is established through a median sternotomy, with hypothermia, aortic cross-clamping, and cardioplegia according to standard techniques. Bicaval cannulation is used for venous drainage. The cardiac exposure can be either through the right or left atrium, depending on the specific anatomic presentation and associated defects. Regardless of approach, the principles of surgical repair include complete resection of the membrane, identification of all pulmonary veins, and closure of all septal defects (Figure 35.5) [14]. Other lesions are addressed as needed.

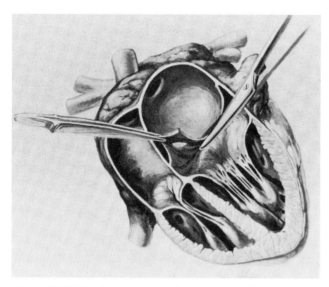

Figure 35.5 The obstructing membrane is resected; injury to the mitral valve and left atrial wall is avoided. (Reproduced with permission from Arciniegas *et al.* [14].)

Results of surgical repair of cor triatriatum sinister are good. Reported perioperative mortality is 4–25%, but mortality is largely dependent on the severity of illness at the time of presentation and associated cardiac and extracardiac anomalies [21,23–25]. The long-term prognosis after classic cor triatriatum sinister repair is excellent. The postoperative management strategy is dependent on the severity of preoperative pulmonary venous obstruction. Pulmonary vasodilators, such as nitric oxide may be necessary in patients with preoperative pulmonary hypertension. Patients who present without significant pulmonary venous obstruction typically have a benign postoperative course.

Atresia of the Common Pulmonary Vein

Atresia of the common pulmonary vein is an extremely rare malformation in which no communication exists between the pulmonary veins and left atrium. Moreover, there is no connection between the common pulmonary vein and any systemic veins. In essence, the common pulmonary vein is a blind pouch. The only drainage of common pulmonary venous flow is through small collateral connections, often bronchopulmonary veins, to the atria or systemic circulation. The clinical presentation is that of severe pulmonary venous obstruction, and patients are severely cyanotic and critically ill immediately after birth [25–27]. The differential diagnosis includes obstructed total anomalous pulmonary venous return. Diagnosis can usually be established by echocardiography; findings are similar to TAPVC, but Doppler flow studies fail to demon-strate outflow from the common pulmonary vein. Most patients are too ill for cardiac catheterizations, but if performed, they would demonstrate severe pulmonary hypertension and persistence of contrast in the pulmonary vasculature after right ventricular injection of contrast. Surgical intervention is emergent and consists of anastomosis between the posterior left atrium and the pulmonary venous confluence (Figure 35.6) [26]. Severe postoperative pulmonary hypertension can be anticipated; nitric oxide or extracorporeal membrane oxygenation (ECMO) may be needed [28]. The first successful surgical repair was reported by Khonsari in 1982 [26]. Reports of survivors have been sporadic. Long-term follow-up has not been reported to date.

Pulmonary Vein Stenosis

Stenosis of individual pulmonary veins, first reported by Reye in 1951 in an 8-year-old patient who died with severe stenosis of three veins and atresia of the fourth [29], is a rare malformation affecting one or more veins at the junction with the left atrium. Concomitant lesions are common, affecting 30–80% of patients with pulmonary venous stenosis [30]. Unilateral pulmonary vein stenosis is seen in approximately one half of patients with this diagnosis; in 30–35% all four veins are involved, with 10–15% having only a single stenotic vein. Stenosis of the pulmonary veins may appear as a relatively discrete shelf or web, as tubular hypoplasia at the junction of the pulmonary vein to the left atrium, or as diffuse hypoplasia of the pulmonary veins (Figure 35.7) [31,32]. Pulmonary vein stenosis is thought to develop from abnormal incorporation of the common pulmonary vein into the left atrium during the later stages of cardiac development. Microscopically, a fibrous intimal thickening is seen, with uniformly sized spindle cells with elongated nuclei and tapering cytoplasm [33]. The cells resemble myofibroblasts, which have the capacity to differentiate into either myocytes or fibroblasts. The rapid progression of pulmonary vein stenosis and the exuberant intimal growth and recurrent stenosis after surgical or catheter-based manipulations suggests a neoproliferative process may be responsible. Antiproliferative therapy, such as radiation or chemotherapy, has been proposed, but clinical data are lacking [33].

The clinical presentation of patients with pulmonary venous stenosis is dependent on a number of veins involved and the severity of the obstruction. Patients with bilateral involvement are more likely to present early [34]. Tachypnea and frequent respiratory infections are common presenting symptoms. Signs of pulmonary hypertension become increasingly prominent as pulmonary vein stenosis progresses. Hemoptysis can be seen in older patients. Physical examination reveals signs of pulmonary hypertension, including right ventricular lift and accentuation of

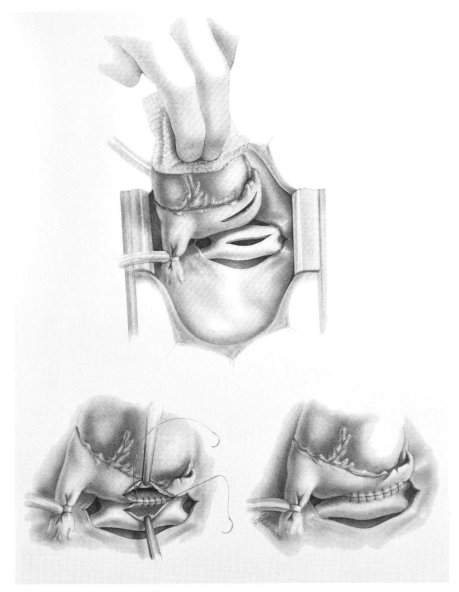

Figure 35.6 Exposure and technique of anastomosis of left atrium to common pulmonary vein channel. (Reproduced with permission from Khonsari *et al.* [26].)

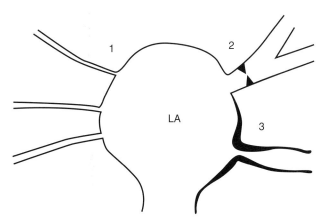

Figure 35.7 Types of pulmonary vein stenosis. 1, Long segment hypoplasia; 2, Discrete diaphragm; 3, Focal intimal fibrosis. (LA, left atrium.) (Reproduced with permission from Ward *et al.* [32].)

the pulmonary component of the second heart sound. A pulmonary systolic click may be heard. A chest X-ray shows a hazy ground glass appearance. Electrocardiogram shows right ventricular hypertrophy and strain.

Diagnosis is usually established by noninvasive imaging. All four veins can usually be identified by echocardiography if good acoustic windows are present. The presence of turbulent flow on color Doppler is suggestive of pulmonary venous stenosis. Monophasic flow or flow velocities greater than 1.6 m/s indicate potentially significant obstruction [30]. Transesophageal echocardiography can be useful and may provide better imaging of pulmonary veins. Magnetic resonance imagery and CT angiography have also been shown to be useful diagnostic techniques for imaging pulmonary veins [35].

Cardiac catheterization with angiography provides detailed views of the pulmonary veins and assessment of pulmonary hypertension. Injection of dye into the pulmonary arterial segments can selectively visualize individual pulmonary veins. Hemodynamic data show varying degrees of pulmonary hypertension, with elevated pulmonary artery wedge pressures. Left-sided obstructive lesions, such as mitral stenosis and left ventricular outflow tract obstruction can also be ruled out.

Prognosis of patients with pulmonary venous stenosis is very guarded, particularly if bilateral stenosis is present. Mortality rates of 80–100% have been reported in patients with involvement of all four veins [34,36]. Patients with only one or two veins involved have a more benign course [33]. The precise history of milder forms of pulmonary vein stenosis has not been clearly established.

Multiple surgical strategies have been applied to pulmonary venous stenosis, with varying degrees of success. Pericardial patch angioplasty is associated with a very high rate of pulmonary vein stenosis recurrence. Simple ring or web excision has had some success, but has also been associated with a high incidence of recurrence [37]. Another technique, in which surgical trauma to the pulmonary vein is minimized, has been advocated due to the notion that trauma to the veins can provide a stimulus for regrowth of obstructive tissue. An incision is made in the pulmonary vein and adjacent left atrium, and a pericardial pouch is created over these incisions, thereby avoiding suture lines in the pulmonary veins (Figure 35.8) [38]. Preliminary data are limited, but suggest improved outcomes over standard patch technique [39]. However, freedom from operation or death at 5 years is still only approximately 50% [30]. Lung transplantation has also been advocated for isolated pulmonary venous stenosis [40]. Catheter-based interventions have met with limited success. Immediate improvement is usually seen, but recurrent stenosis is nearly universal. Catheter intervention may be complementary to surgery, and can be repeated multiple times [30]. Stents have been disappointing, with a high frequency of recurrence. However, stents have been

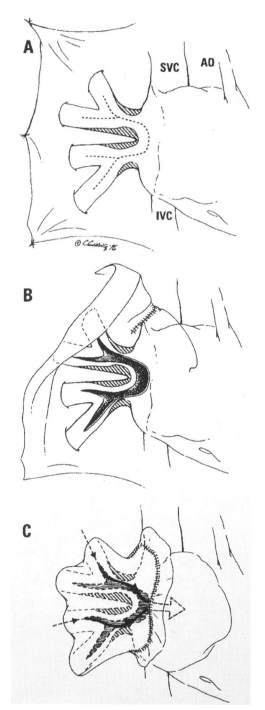

Figure 35.8 The sutureless technique for the relief of pulmonary vein (PV) stenosis. **A,** The incision is made into the left atrium and extended into both upper and lower PV ostia separately. **B,** Suturing is begun in the pericardium just above the junction of the superior PV with the left atrium. **C,** A second inferior suture is started below the inferior PV and continued in the same manner to the left atrial incision to join the superior suture line. (AO, aorta; IVC, inferior vena cava; SVC, superior vena cava.) (Reproduced with permission from Najm *et al.* [38].)

successfully used for palliation in patients listed for lung transplantation [30].

Cor Triatriatum Dexter

Cor triatriatum dexter, first described by Von Rokitansky in 1875, is an extremely rare condition in which there is abnormal partitioning of the right atrium due to persistence of the right valve of the sinus venosus [41]. During embryologic development, the right horn of the sinus venosus is gradually incorporated into the right atrium to form the nontrabeculated posterior portion of the right atrium. The embryologic right atrium forms the trabeculated portion. The embryologic right atrium and the right horn of the sinus venosus join at the sinoatrial orifice, which has two folds on either side called the right and left venous valves. The left valve becomes part of the septum secundum, and the right valve divides the right atrium into two chambers (Figure 35.9) [42]. The right valve directs oxygenated blood from the inferior vena cava across the patent foramen ovale to the left side during fetal development. Normally the right valve regresses by 12 weeks, leaving the crista terminalis superiorly and the Eustachian valve of the inferior vena cava and Thebesian valve of the coronary sinus inferiorly. Persistence of the right valve results in separation of the smooth and trabeculated portions of the right atrium, resulting in cor triatriatum dexter.

Clinical manifestations of cor triatriatum dexter are dependent on the degree of septation of the right atrium. Mild septation is usually asymptomatic, and is usually found by routine echocardiography, at necropsy, or at operation for other lesions. More severe degrees of septation can mimic right heart failure, with an elevated central venous pressure and hepatomegaly. Supraventricular tachycardia has been reported in conjunction with this lesion [43]. Cyanosis may be present if an atrial septal defect is present.

The need for intervention is based entirely on the presence of symptoms. Surgical resection or percutaneous catheter disruption of the membrane has provided symptomatic relief [43,44]. Prognosis after intervention is excellent.

References

1. Geva T, Van Praagh S. (2001) Anomalies of the pulmonary veins. In: Allen HD, Gutgesell HP, Clark EB, *et al.*, eds. *Moss and Adams' Heart Disease in Infants, Children, and Adolescents, Including the Fetus and Young Adult*, 6th ed. Philadelphia: Lippincott Williams & Wilkins, pp. 736–772.
2. Church WS. (1868) Congenital malformation of the heart: abnormal septum in the left auricle. Trans Pathol Soc London 19, 415.
3. Andral G. (1829) *Precis d'Anatomie Pathologique*. Paris.
4. Lewis FJ, Varco RL, Taufic M, *et al.* (1956) Direct vision repair of triatrial heart and total anomalous pulmonary venous drainage. Surg Gynecol Obstet 102, 713–720.
5. Vineberg A, Gialloreto O. (1956) Report of a successful operation for stenosis of common pulmonary vein (cor triatriatum). Can Med Assoc J 74, 719–723.
6. Al Qethamy HO, Aboelnazar S, Al Faraidi Y, *et al.* (2006) Cor triatriatum: operative results in 20 patients. Asian Cardiovasc Thorac Ann 14, 7–9.
7. Marin-Garcia J, Tandon R, Lucas RV Jr, *et al.* (1975) Cor triatriatum: study of 20 cases. Am J Cardiol 35, 59–66.
8. Niwayama G. (1960) Cor triatriatum. Am Heart J 59, 291–317.
9. Richardson JV, Doty DB, Siewers RD, *et al.* (1981) Cor triatriatum (subdivided left atrium). J Thorac Cardiovasc Surg 81, 232–238.
10. Van Praagh R, Corsini I. (1969) Cor triatriatum: pathologic anatomy and a consideration of morphogenesis based on 13 postmortem cases and a study of normal development of the pulmonary vein and atrial septum in 83 human embryos. Am Heart J 78, 379–405.
11. van Son JA, Danielson GK, Schaff HV, *et al.* (1993) Cor triatriatum: diagnosis, operative approach, and late results. Mayo Clin Proc 68, 854–859.
12. Krasemann Z, Scheld HH, Tjan TD, *et al.* (2007) Cor triatriatum: short review of the literature upon ten new cases. Herz 32, 506–510.
13. Lam CR, Green E, Drake E. (1962) Diagnosis and surgical correction of 2 types of triatrial heart. Surgery 51, 127–137.
14. Arciniegas E, Farooki ZQ, Hakimi M, *et al.* (1981) Surgical treatment of cor triatriatum. Ann Thorac Surg 32, 571–577.
15. Krabill KA, Lucas RV. (1995) Abnormal pulmonary venous connections. In: Emmanoulides GC, Riemenschneider TA, Allen HG, *et al.*, eds. *Heart Disease in Infants, Children, and Adolescents Including the Fetus and Young Adult*. Baltimore: Williams and Wilkins, pp. 838–874.
16. Herlong JR, Jaggers JJ, Ungerleider RM. (2000) Congenital Heart Surgery Nomenclature and Database Project: pulmonary venous anomalies. Ann Thorac Surg 69(4 Suppl), S56–S69.

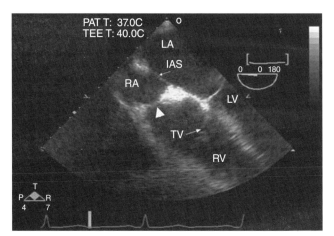

Figure 35.9 Transesophageal echocardiogram in four-chamber view shows a prominent eustachian valve (arrowhead) attached to the interatrial septum (IAS) just below the level of the fossa ovalis. (LA, left atrium; LV, left ventricle; RA, right atrium; RV, right ventricle; TV, tricuspid valve.) (Reproduced with permission from Yarrabolu *et al.* [42]. Copyright © 2007 Texas Heart Institute.)

17. Basavarajaiah S, Oxborough D, Wilson M, *et al.* (2007) Incidental finding of cor triatriatum in an asymptomatic elite athlete. J Am Soc Echocardiogr 20, 771 e9–e12.
18. Bisset GS 3rd, Kirks DR, Strife JL, *et al.* (1987) Cor triatriatum: diagnosis by MR imaging. AJR Am J Roentgenol 149, 567–568.
19. Binotto MA, Aiello VD, Ebaid M. (1991) Coexistence of divided left atrium (cor triatriatum) and tetralogy of Fallot. Int J Cardiol 31, 97–99.
20. Carroll SJ, Solowiejczyk D, Gersony WM. (2004) Preoperative diagnosis of co-existing divided left atrium and tetralogy of Fallot. Cardiol Young 14, 456–459.
21. Huang TC, Lee CL, Lin CC, *et al.* (2002) Use of Inoue balloon dilatation method for treatment of Cor triatriatum stenosis in a child. Catheter Cardiovasc Interv 57, 252–256.
22. Sivakumar K, Satish R, Tailor K, *et al.* (2008) Transcatheter management of subtotal cor triatriatum sinister: a rare anomaly. Pediatr Cardiol 29, 812–815.
23. Alkhulaifi AM, Serraf A, Lacour-Gayet F, *et al.* (2000) Congenital division of the left atrium: the influence of associated congenital lesions on the timing and mode of presentation. Cardiovasc Surg 8, 159–163.
24. Alphonso N, Norgaard MA, Newcomb A, *et al.* (2005) Cor triatriatum: presentation, diagnosis and long-term surgical results. Ann Thorac Surg 80, 1666–1671.
25. Rodefeld MD, Brown JW, Heimansohn DA, *et al.* (1990) Cor triatriatum: clinical presentation and surgical results in 12 patients. Ann Thorac Surg 50, 562–568.
26. Khonsari S, Saunders PW, Lees MH, *et al.* (1982) Common pulmonary vein atresia: Importance of immediate recognition and surgical intervention. J Thorac Cardiovasc Surg 83, 443–448.
27. Vaideeswar P, Tullu MS, Sathe PA, *et al.* (2008) Atresia of the common pulmonary vein – a rare congenital anomaly. Congenit Heart Dis 3, 431–434.
28. Dudell GG, Evans ML, Krous HF, *et al.* (1993) Common pulmonary vein atresia: the role of extracorporeal membrane oxygenation. Pediatrics 91, 403–410.
29. Reye RD. (1951) Congenital stenosis of the pulmonary veins in their extrapulmonary course. Med J Aust 1, 801–802.
30. Latson LA, Prieto LR. (2007) Congenital and acquired pulmonary vein stenosis. Circulation 115, 103–108.
31. Fong LV, Anderson RH, Park SC, *et al.* (1988) Morphologic features of stenosis of the pulmonary veins. Am J Cardiol 62, 1136–1138.
32. Ward KE, Mullins CE. (1998) Anomalous pulmonary venous connections, vein stenosis, and atresia of the common vein. In: Garson AJ, Bricker JT, Fisher DS, eds. *The Science and Practice of Pediatric Cardiology*, 2nd ed. Baltimore: Williams and Wilkins, pp. 1431–1461.
33. Sadr IM, Tan PE, Kieran MW, *et al.* (2000) Mechanism of pulmonary vein stenosis in infants with normally connected veins. Am J Cardiol 86, 577–579, A10.
34. Breinholt JP, Hawkins JA, Minich LA, *et al.* (1999) Pulmonary vein stenosis with normal connection: associated cardiac abnormalities and variable outcome. Ann Thorac Surg 68, 164–168.
35. Grosse-Wortmann L, Al-Otay A, Goo HW, *et al.* (2007) Anatomical and functional evaluation of pulmonary veins in children by magnetic resonance imaging. J Am Coll Cardiol 49, 993–1002.
36. Holt DB, Moller JH, Larson S, *et al.* (2007) Primary pulmonary vein stenosis. Am J Cardiol 99, 568–572.
37. Victor S, Nayak VM. (1995) Deringing procedure for congenital pulmonary vein stenosis. Tex Heart Inst J 22, 166–169.
38. Najm HK, Caldarone CA, Smallhorn J, *et al.* (1998) A sutureless technique for the relief of pulmonary vein stenosis with the use of in situ pericardium. J Thorac Cardiovasc Surg 115, 468–470.
39. Devaney EJ, Chang AC, Ohye RG, *et al.* (2006) Management of congenital and acquired pulmonary vein stenosis. Ann Thorac Surg 81, 992–995; discussion 995–996.
40. Mendeloff EN, Spray TL, Huddleston CB, *et al.* (1995) Lung transplantation for congenital pulmonary vein stenosis. Ann Thorac Surg 60, 903–906; discussion 907.
41. Von Rokitansky K. (1875) Die defecte der scheidewande des herzens. *Pathologisch-anatomische Abhandlung*, 2nd ed. Vienna: Wilhelm Braumuller, pp. 83–86.
42. Yarrabolu TR, Simpson L, Virani SS, *et al.* (2007) Cor triatriatum dexter. Tex Heart Inst J 34, 383–385.
43. Ott DA, Cooley DA, Angelini P, *et al.* (1979) Successful surgical correction of symptomatic cor triatriatum dexter. J Thorac Cardiovasc Surg 78, 573–575.
44. Savas V, Samyn J, Schreiber TL, *et al.* (1991) Cor triatriatum dexter: recognition and percutaneous transluminal correction. Cathet Cardiovasc Diagn 23, 183–186.

CHAPTER 36

Anomalous Systemic Venous Connections

Henry L. Walters III[1,2] and Ralph E. Delius[1,2]

[1]Children's Hospital of Michigan, Detroit, MI, USA
[2]Wayne State University School of Medicine, Detroit, MI, USA

Introduction

"Usual" systemic venous cardiac connections exist when a right-sided morphologically right atrium receives systemic venous blood from single right-sided superior and inferior vena cavae in addition to coronary venous return through the coronary sinus. The definition of "normal" systemic venous cardiac connections is more difficult and is perhaps controversial. For example, it can be argued that anatomically and physiologically "normal" connections can exist when the superior and inferior vena cavae and the coronary sinus connect to a morphologically right atrium whether this right atrium is in its usual right-sided (situs solitus) or unusual left-sided (situs inversus) position. However, cardiac surgeons consider both the mediastinal position of the superior and inferior vena cavae and the cardiac connection of these veins to be important factors in planning the conduct of surgical repair. For example, usual cannulation strategies must be altered to accommodate unusually positioned vena cavae. Hence, in this chapter, "abnormal" or "anomalous" systemic venous cardiac connections are classified as departures from the "usual" situation.

Anomalies of systemic venous connection (ASVC) are congenital disorders of the route or destination of the systemic venous return to the heart (Table 36.1) [1]. ASVC can be either partial, involving part of the systemic venous return, or total, involving all of the systemic venous return. In route abnormalities, the anomalous systemic venous return follows an abnormal pathway but eventually drains into the right-sided morphologically right atrium. Route abnormalities usually produce no physiologic sequelae. They become clinically important when they are associated with cardiac disorders requiring surgical repair. In disorders of destination, the anomalous systemic veins do not connect to the right-sided morphologically right atrium. Destination disorders, by default, must include obligatory route abnormalities as well.

While Table 36.1 [1] provides one possible classification for visualizing and categorizing ASVC, others have been proposed in the literature. One such classification is an anatomical scheme that is based upon three major categories: 1) superior vena cava (SVC); 2) inferior vena cava (IVC); and 3) hepatic veins [2]. A more physiological classification is based upon the ultimate destination of the venous drainage such as the left atrium, the right atrium, and both atria [3]. More recently the Society of Thoracic Surgeons Congenital Heart Surgery Database Committee has outlined a hierarchical scheme for classification of ASVC that is based upon abnormalities of the IVC, the SVC, and the hepatic veins [4].

History

The development of knowledge about ASVC is best illustrated by the history of its most common representative, the left superior vena cava (LSVC). In 1850, Marshall provided an embryological explanation for LSVC and he underscored its frequent association with other congenital cardiac lesions [5]. Winter [6] and Campbell's [7] descriptions of LSVC, both published in 1954, include thorough discussions of its anatomy, embryology, and relationships with other major systemic and pulmonary venous structures. While Helseth and Peterson first coined the term "unroofed coronary sinus" in 1974 [8], Raghib and colleagues made the first accurate description of the morphology of this syndrome in their classic paper of 1965 [9]. Hurwitt, in 1955, was the first to report successful ligation of an LSVC to the left atrium in a cyanotic patient [10]. In his report the LSVC was connected to the right superior

Pediatric Cardiac Surgery, Fourth Edition. Edited by Constantine Mavroudis and Carl L. Backer.

Table 36.1 Anatomic organization of anomalies of systemic venous connection.

I. Left superior vena cava connection to
   A. Coronary sinus
      1. Without coronary sinus ostial atresia
         a. Intact coronary sinus (not unroofed)
         b. Unroofed coronary sinus syndrome
            i. Complete unroofing
            ii. Partial unroofing
               a. Middle portion
               b. Distal portion
      2. With coronary sinus ostial atresia
   B. Left atrium
II. Coronary sinus connection to
   A. Left atrium (unroofed coronary sinus syndrome without left superior vena cava)
      1. Complete unroofing
      2. Partial unroofing
         a. Middle portion
         b. Distal portion
III. Right superior vena cava
   A. Absent right superior vena cava with persistent left superior vena cava
   B. Right superior vena cava to left atrium
IV. Inferior vena cava
   A. Azygos continuation to right superior vena cava
   B. Hemiazygos continuation to left superior vena cava
   C. Inferior vena cava to left atrium
   D. Inferior vena cava to coronary sinus
V. Hepatic veins
   A. Direct connection to right atrium
   B. Direct connection to left atrium
   C. Direct connection to both atria

vena cava (RSVC) by a communicating vein. The first successful anatomic repair for common atrium and LSVC to the left atrium was performed at Mayo Clinic in 1965 and reported by Rastelli and colleagues. They decided upon an intracardiac baffle repair after temporary clamp occlusion of the LSVC resulted in a rise of the left internal jugular vein pressure from 8 to 25 mmHg [11]. These same authors reported a complete intracardiac repair of a very rare form of total anomalous systemic venous connection consisting of drainage of the LSVC and inferior vena cava (IVC) directly into the left atrium in the absence of an RSVC [12].

Incidence

In one large series, 100 cases of ASVC were found among 5127 patients undergoing open heart surgery between 1955 and 1974 [13]. The 2% incidence in this older series may underestimate the true occurrence of these anomalies since patients who underwent closed heart procedures were not included and since many very complex patients likely to have ASVC may never have been offered an operation during this early era.

Anatomy

Left Superior Vena Cava to Coronary Sinus without Coronary Sinus Ostial Atresia

Embryologically, LSVC to the coronary sinus is thought to be due to the persistence of the left anterior and common cardinal veins. The LSVC descends anterior to the aortic arch and left pulmonary hilum. It enters the pericardium and contacts the heart at the left posterior atrioventricular groove where it continues into the right atrium as the coronary sinus (Figure 36.1A) [1]. The right atrial orifice of the coronary sinus is usually dilated in proportion to the size of the LSVC. While the majority of patients also have an RSVC, the size of this contralateral vessel is usually inversely proportional to the size of the LSVC. For example, when the LSVC is large the RSVC is usually small and vice versa. In 24% of cases the RSVC is hypoplastic or even atretic (Figure 36.1B) [1,13–15]. In 75% of cases the left innominate vein is absent or severely hypoplastic [6]. When an adequately sized left innominate vein is present, it provides an important alternate pathway for LSVC flow to the right atrium in addition to the coronary sinus. LSVC to the coronary sinus can coexist with azygos continuation of the IVC to the RSVC (9%), hemiazygos continuation of the IVC to the LSVC (7%), and separate entrance of the IVC and hepatic veins into the right atrium (2%) [13]. While LSVC to the coronary sinus rarely can be an isolated anomaly, it is most commonly associated with septal defects (atrial septal defect [ASD], ventricular septal defect [VSD] or common atrium), tetralogy of Fallot, atrioventricular septal defects, transposition of the great arteries, and other more complex defects [13]. While the true incidence of this anomaly is not known, it may occur in as many as 3–10% of patients with congenital heart disease. It appears to occur in 0.1–0.5% of the general population [16].

Left Superior Vena Cava with Coronary Sinus Ostial Atresia

Coronary sinus ostial atresia with persistent LSVC is a rare cardiac anomaly with 35 total cases reported in the world literature. Of these reported cases, 11 were diagnosed in living patients either by angiography or intraoperatively and the remainder were identified at autopsy [17]. Anatomically these lesions consist of a membranous occlusion of the coronary sinus ostium, thereby disconnecting the usual direct drainage of the coronary sinus (and LSVC) to the right atrium (Figure 36.1C) [1]. The gap between the blind end of the coronary sinus and the right atrium can

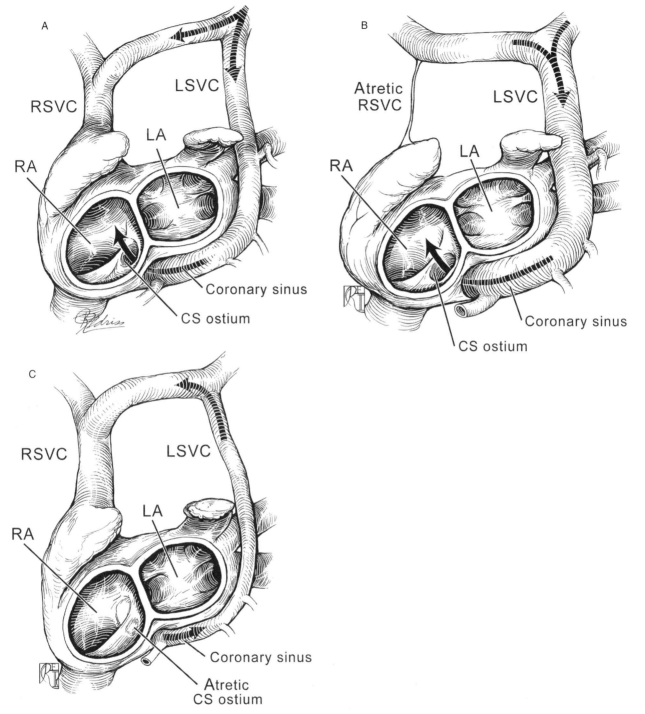

Figure 36.1 A, Left superior vena cava (LSVC) to the coronary sinus. **B,** Left superior vena cava to the coronary sinus with atretic right superior vena cava (RSVC). **C,** Coronary sinus ostial atresia with persistent LSVC. Arrows denote the retrograde flow of coronary sinus blood to the right atrium (RA). (CS, coronary sinus; LA, left atrium.)

be either a short- or a long-segment interruption [18]. The anomalous LSVC provides the major route for venous drainage from the coronary sinus; however, there can be small communicating veins between the coronary sinus and the right atrium [19]. Retrograde flow from the coro-nary sinus to the LSVC and across the innominate vein to the RSVC is most commonly found (Figure 36.1C) [1]. Other venous connections, however, can exist between the LSVC and the RSVC. For example, the LSVC can drain into the RSVC through a hemiazygos–azygos connection. Other cardiac malformations coexist in 56% of the reported cases of coronary sinus ostial atresia [17].

Unroofed Coronary Sinus Syndrome

Unroofed coronary sinus syndrome (UCSS) is a spectrum of congenital cardiac anomalies consisting of partial or complete absence of the partition between the coronary sinus and the left atrium. All patients have an interatrial communication. An LSVC is usually present but is not a requirement for UCSS. Since the coronary sinus itself is a systemic vein, UCSS should be considered a subset of ASVC regardless of whether an LSVC coexists.

Persistence of the left anterior and common cardinal veins draining into the left sinus horn with failure of the normal invagination process that separates the left sinus horn (future coronary sinus) from the left atrium is a possible embryological mechanism for development of the UCSS [9,12,20].

UCSS can consist of either complete or partial unroofing [21,22]. In complete unroofing the entire length of the partition between the coronary sinus and the left atrium is absent. An LSVC is usually present but can be absent. In partial unroofing only a segment of the partition between the coronary sinus and the left atrium is absent. This partial unroofing can occur in the midportion or the distal portion (right atrial end) of the coronary sinus.

Complete Unroofing with Left Superior Vena Cava
The LSVC forms as the confluence of the left internal jugular vein and the left subclavian vein. Its vertical descent is anterior to the distal transverse left-sided aortic arch and the left pulmonary hilum. The LSVC terminates in the superior left aspect of the left atrium (Figure 36.2A) [1]. The position of its left atrial orifice appears to be relatively constant with the left superior pulmonary vein orifice located posteriorly and inferiorly and the orifice of the left atrial appendage located anteriorly. There can be a valve like structure or a ridge near the LSVC ostium. The hemiazygos vein joins the LSVC after arching superiorly and anteriorly over the left mainstem bronchus. The left innominate vein is absent in 80–90% of cases. The RSVC is usually smaller than the LSVC, or it can be absent with the right internal jugular and subclavian veins draining into the LSVC through a right innominate vein. There may be hemiazygos continuation of the IVC to the LSVC. In this situation the hepatic veins enter the inferior right atrium separately. Occasionally the hepatic veins may enter the left atrium posterior to the interatrial septum. This, in combination with an LSVC and hemiazygos continuation of the IVC, produces total anomalous systemic venous connection.

A coronary sinus atrial septal defect (ASD) is located posteriorly and inferiorly in the interatrial septum in the position usually occupied by the right atrial orifice of the coronary sinus. When the interatrial communication is an isolated coronary sinus defect, it is separated from the atrioventricular valve annulus by an anterior remnant of interatrial septal tissue. It is also bounded superiorly and inferiorly by interatrial septal tissue and posteriorly by the posterior atrial free wall. There may be an associated secundum ASD separated from the coronary sinus ASD by interatrial septal tissue. Alternatively, the coronary sinus ASD may be confluent with a secundum and/or primum ASD. When a primum ASD coexists in confluence with the coronary sinus ASD, the anterior leaflet of the mitral valve is frequently cleft. Occasionally the complete absence of interatrial tissue creates a common atrium (Figure 36.2B) [1,9,21–24].

In the presence of complete unroofing of the coronary sinus with an LSVC, the pulmonary veins can enter the left atrium more superiorly than usual. This can create an apparent narrowing between the area of the left atrium into which the pulmonary veins enter and the portion of the left atrium to which the LSVC, left atrial appendage, and mitral valve are attached [21].

Complete Unroofing without Left Superior Vena Cava
In this case complete unroofing of the coronary sinus exists in the presence of a coronary sinus type ASD but without an LSVC (Figure 36.2C) [1].

Partially Unroofed Coronary Sinus with or without Left Superior Vena Cava
Partial absence of the partition between the coronary sinus and the left atrium can occur in the middle (Figure 36.2D) [1,25,26] or the distal [21,22] coronary sinus with or without an LSVC. Distal unroofing of the coronary sinus occurs most commonly in the presence of atrioventricular canal defects. In this situation the distal coronary sinus, including its right atrial orifice, can be unroofed resulting in a displacement of the distal opening of the coronary sinus into the left atrium (Figure 36.2E) [1].Conversely, the distal coronary sinus may be unroofed just prior to its right atrial orifice resulting in a coronary sinus ASD (Figure 36.2F) [1,22,26].

While situs solitus of the atria and viscera with levocardia are usually present, anomalies that can coexist with UCSS include dextrocardia, situs inversus, and atrial appendage isomerism with asplenia or polysplenia. UCSS has been reported in association with partial atrioventricular canal defect, complete atrioventricular canal defect, common atrium, tetralogy of Fallot, double-outlet right ventricle, pulmonary stenosis, total anomalous pulmonary venous connection, and hypoplastic left ventricle [21,22].

Right Superior Vena Cava to the Left Atrium

An RSVC draining to the left atrium is very rare as an isolated lesion, and was first reported by Kirsch and

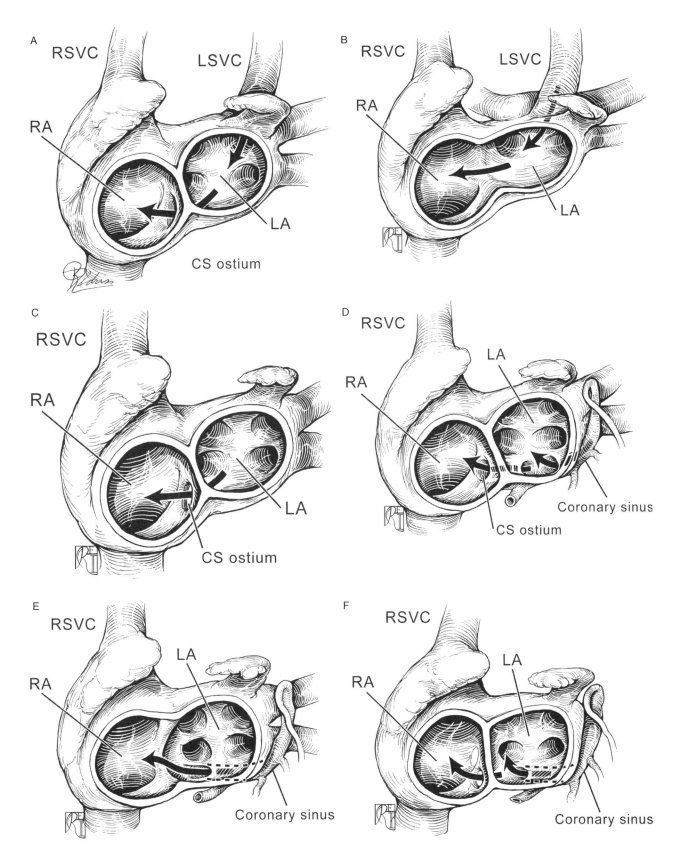

Figure 36.2 Unroofed coronary sinus syndrome. **A,** Left superior vena cava (LSVC) to the left atrium (LA) with complete unroofing of the coronary sinus and coronary sinus atrial septal defect (ASD). **B,** Left superior vena cava to the LA with complete unroofing of the coronary sinus and absence of the interatrial septum (common atrium). **C,** Complete unroofing of the coronary sinus without LSVC. **D,** Partial unroofing of the midportion of the coronary sinus with a coronary sinus ASD, absence of an LSVC. **E,** Partial unroofing of the distal portion of the coronary sinus with partial atrioventricular septal defect coexisting in confluence with coronary sinus ASD, absence of an LSVC. **F,** Partial unroofing of the distal portion of the coronary sinus with intact right atrial coronary sinus orifice with coronary sinus ASD, absence of an LSVC. (IVC, inferior vena cava; LA, left atrium; RA, right atrium; RSVC, right superior vena cava.)

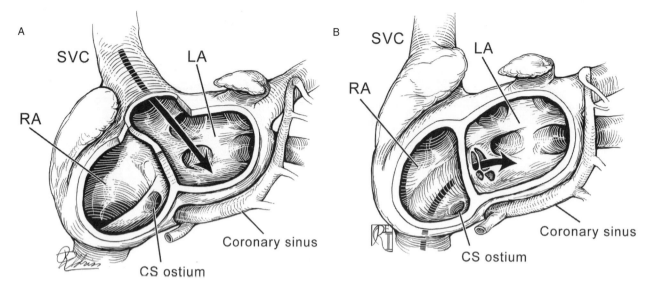

Figure 36.3 A, Right superior vena cava (SVC) to the left atrium (LA). **B,** Inferior vena cava (IVC) with fenestrated opening into the LA. (CS, coronary sinus; RA, right atrium.)

colleagues (Figure 36.3A) [1,27].True cases must be differentiated from the sinus venosus type of ASD with an SVC overriding the interatrial septum.

Direct Inferior Vena Caval Connections

The IVC normally receives the hepatic veins and then connects directly to the inferior aspect of the right-sided morphological right atrium. Very rarely the IVC connects to the right atrium through the coronary sinus. This latter anomaly has been reported in a patient with an LSVC to the coronary sinus, absent RSVC, left-sided hypoplasia (small left ventricle, parachute mitral valve, bicuspid aortic valve, hypoplastic arch, and coarctation of the aorta), primum ASD, and secundum ASD. [28] Direct connection of the IVC to the left-sided morphologically left atrium can occur either as an isolated lesion or in association with other cardiac anomalies (Figure 36.3B) [1,29–33]. One very unusual case of left-sided superior and inferior vena cavae draining into the left atrium in association with normal right superior and inferior vena cavae and an atrial septal defect has been reported [34].

Indirect Inferior Vena Caval Connections

Indirect inferior vena caval connections exist when the IVC does not connect to the atrium from below but rather "continues" as an extension of either the azygos or hemiazygos veins. In azygos continuation the IVC passes up the right paravertebral gutter and arches over to join the RSVC as a dilated azygos vein (Figure 36.4A) [1]. In hemiazygos continuation the IVC courses up the left paravertebral gutter to join the LSVC as a dilated hemiazygos vein (Figure

36.4B) [1]. Both azygos and hemiazygos continuation have been collectively referred to as "anomalous IVC with azygos continuation" or "infrahepatic interruption of the IVC" [35]. When there is azygos or hemiazygos continuation of the IVC, the hepatic veins always connect directly to the atrial mass and never via the anomalous IVC.

The incidence of indirect IVC connections is 0.6% of patients with congenital heart defects. Its incidence in patients without congenital heart defects is probably much less than the 0.3% incidence quoted for LSVC under the same circumstances [35].

Although indirect IVC connections can rarely be found in individuals with otherwise normal hearts [36], the vast majority of them occur in association with other congenital cardiac abnormalities such as atrial appendage isomerism, atrioventricular canal defect, anomalous pulmonary venous connection, double-outlet right ventricle, common atrium, pulmonary atresia, SVC anomalies (especially bilateral SVC), and others.

Atrial (Appendage) Isomerism

Heterotaxy (Greek: *heteros* – other than, and *taxis* – arrangement) is synonymous with the terms "visceral heterotaxy" and "heterotaxy syndrome." It is literally defined as a pattern of anatomic organization of the thoracic and the abdominal organs which is neither situs solitus (the usual or normal arrangement) nor complete situs inversus (the unusual or mirror image arrangement of normal) [37]. If asymmetry of the thoracic and abdominal viscera is the usual or normal situation, then the heterotaxy syndrome includes patients with an unusual degree of thoracic and abdominal visceral symmetry. Admittedly, this broad term

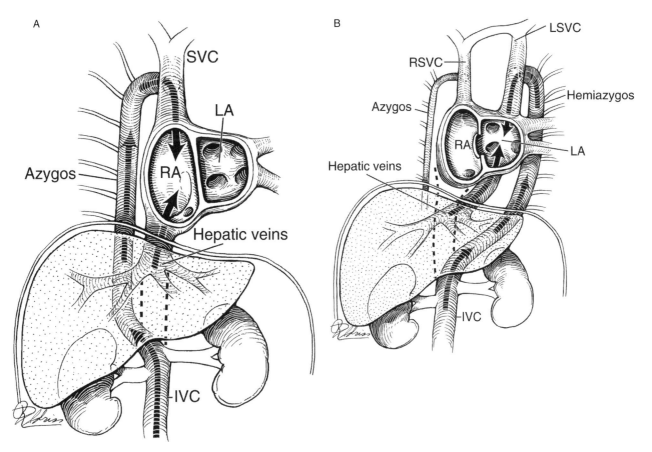

Figure 36.4 A, Azygos continuation of the inferior vena cava (IVC) to the right superior vena cava (SVC). **B,** Hemiazygos continuation of the IVC to the left superior vena cava (LSVC). Single hepatic venous trunk connects to the left atrium (LA). Secundum atrial septal defect present. (RA, right atrium; RSVC, right superior vena cava.)

includes patients with a wide variety of very complex cardiac lesions and is a term that has generated confusion and controversy in the literature. The definition of heterotaxy which currently enjoys the greatest consensus in the literature is "an abnormality where the internal thoracoabdominal organs demonstrate abnormal arrangement across the left-right axis of the body. By convention, heterotaxy does not include patients with either the expected usual or normal arrangement of the internal organs along the left-right axis, also known as 'situs solitus', nor patients with complete mirror-imaged arrangement of the internal organs along the left-right axis also known as 'situs inversus'" [38]. One way to impose order upon this diverse group of cardiac lesions is to stratify them according to the morphology of the atrial appendages [39]. This is accomplished by applying the chemistry term, isomerism, to congenital cardiac morphology. Isomerism, in the context of the congenitally malformed heart, is defined as a situation where some paired structures on opposite sides of the left–right axis of the body are, in morphologic terms, symmetrical mirror images of each other [38]. In atrial appendage isomerism, both atrial appendages are similar rather than displaying their usual distinctive right and left morphology. Right or left atrial appendage isomerism exists when both atria have right or left atrial appendage morphologic characteristics, respectively. Right atrial appendage isomerism is frequently, but not always, associated with bilaterally tri-lobed lungs (each with short bronchi) and asplenia. Left atrial appendage isomerism is frequently, but not always, associated with bilaterally bi-lobed lungs (each with long bronchi) and polysplenia.

ASVC are the rule in patients with heterotaxy syndrome. Up to 70% of patients have bilateral SVCs. In patients with right atrial appendage isomerism the superior vena cavae typically enter the atrial roof with the coronary sinus being universally absent. Also, in heterotaxy syndrome the inferior vena caval connections can be either direct or indirect. Direct communications are most commonly to the right-sided atrium but may be left-sided or, rarely, to the midline of the atrial mass. Indirect inferior vena caval connections exist when there is azygos or hemiazygos continuation. While the IVC typically connects directly to the atrium in right atrial appendage isomerism, it is usually interrupted with azygos/hemiazygos continuation in patients with left atrial appendage isomerism. Up to 30% of heterotaxy patients also have anomalous hepatic venous drainage. The hepatic veins always connect to an atrium from below, either normally, via the IVC, or by a separate and direct connection of their own. When the hepatic veins connect separately, they can do so to either atrium or to both atria. When the IVC enters the atrial mass from below, the hepatic veins can connect to the atrium either via this IVC or separately from it [40].

Diagnosis

Physical examination is neither sensitive nor specific for the diagnosis ASVC. The chest radiograph and electrocardiogram may be normal, consistent with left- and/or right-sided cardiac enlargement or characteristic of any dominant associated cardiac malformation. ASVC can be diagnosed by a number of methods. The accuracy of these methods depends upon the constant maintenance of a high index of suspicion and a high level of interest in discovering these abnormalities. Echocardiography (transthoracic and/or transesophageal) is an extremely specific and highly sensitive method for making the diagnosis of ASVC [41–43]. Prenatal echocardiography is less accurate than postnatal studies because of the limitations imposed by fetal size, movement, and position as well as shadowing by ribs or other structures. Fetal inferior vena caval anatomy is more reliably predicted than are superior vena caval connections [44]. Radionuclide angiocardiography with injection of technetium-99m pertechnetate into the left arm and the determination of differential right-to-left shunting after injection of labeled albumin microspheres into the left and right arms have been reported to accurately diagnose LSVC to the left atrium but this technique is not used currently [45]. While computer-assisted tomography with intravenous contrast administration can identify mediastinal venous anomalies [46], magnetic resonance imaging (MRI) may be more accurate without the need for the radiation and contrast exposure. Prospective studies have shown that the diagnostic yield of cardiac MRI is superior to echocardiography and, often, to cardiac angiography in defining systemic (and pulmonary) venous anatomy and its relationship to surrounding mediastinal structures [47]. Cardiac MRI is especially effective and efficient in identifying the arrangements and abnormalities of the thoracic and abdominal organs in heterotaxy syndrome, with its many visceral and cardiovascular abnormalities [40,48–50]. In the current era, noninvasive imaging, such as echocardiography and cardiac MRI, has largely replaced cardiac angiography to establish the cardiac anatomy of patients with congenital heart disease. This trend is just as apparent in patients with ASVC and heterotaxy syndrome as it is in other forms of congenital heart disease. Cardiac catheterization and angiography may need to be performed to supplement or clarify anatomical information obtained by noninvasive methods or to document hemodynamics, especially in patients with heterotaxy syndrome who may need to undergo staged Fontan palliation.

Pathophysiology and Natural History

Isolated systemic venous route abnormalities (i.e., LSVC to the coronary sinus) are asymptomatic and physiologically innocuous. When other important congenital cardiac malformations accompany systemic venous route abnormalities, the pathophysiology and natural history are determined by the associated lesion(s).

Abnormalities of systemic venous destination can produce a right-to-left shunt that results in varying degrees of cyanosis. Progressive cyanosis can produce all of the sequelae of polycythemia including cerebral embolization and abscess formation [22,51]. Since an atrial septal defect is frequently associated with ASVC, a left-to-right shunt can coexist with the right-to-left shunt producing mild-to-moderate cyanosis and right ventricular dilatation with pulmonary overcirculation. When additional important cardiac malformations are coupled with systemic venous destination anomalies, the physiologic burden of the associated cardiac lesion(s) is additive and further complicates the presentation, clinical course, and natural history.

In partially unroofed midportion of the coronary sinus there can be a left-to-right or a right-to-left shunt depending upon the relative ventricular compliances and the right atrial pressure. When this lesion is isolated, a large left-to-right shunt exists at the atrial level and dictates the clinical presentation and natural history [25,26]. When partially unroofed midportion of the coronary sinus coexists with tricuspid atresia, significant right-to-left shunting has been reported after a Fontan repair that incorporates the coronary sinus into the systemic venous pathway [52–54].

Surgical Management of Systemic Venous Route Abnormalities

Venous route abnormalities not associated with other cardiac lesions do not require surgical treatment because they are physiologically benign. When venous route abnormalities exist with associated cardiac lesions, the conduct of the cardiac surgical repair must accommodate the abnormal venous anatomy.

Left Superior Vena Cava with Coronary Sinus Ostial Atresia

Even though LSVC with coronary sinus ostial atresia is physiologically benign, this lesion can pose a grave hazard for the cardiac surgeon if it is not recognized before or at the time of cardiac surgical intervention for associated cardiac lesions. Permanent or even temporary intraoperative occlusion or vigorous manipulation of the LSVC can lead to acute obstruction of the coronary venous system causing myocardial congestion and ischemia [55]. When an LSVC (especially a small one) to the coronary sinus exists, patency of the coronary sinus orifice should be sought preoperatively or intraoperatively. If coronary sinus ostial atresia is confirmed and the only route for decompression of the LSVC is retrograde to the RSVC through the left innominate vein or through another venous connection, the LSVC should never be occluded, even temporarily. This will avoid the possibility of intraoperative or postoperative coronary venous congestion and myocardial ischemia [17].

Left Superior Vena Cava to the Coronary Sinus without Coronary Sinus Ostial Atresia

If a large left innominate vein is present between the LSVC and the RSVC, a tourniquet can be used to temporarily occlude the LSVC below the left innominate vein during the intracardiac portion of the surgical repair.

At the time of cardiac catheterization of a patient with an LSVC to the coronary sinus and a small or absent left innominate vein, an end-hole balloon catheter can be threaded retrograde through the coronary sinus into the LSVC. The balloon is inflated low in the LSVC with complete occlusion confirmed by contrast injection through the end hole. The LSVC pressure is monitored for 20 minutes [56]. Conversely, the LSVC pressure can be measured intraoperatively using an indwelling left internal jugular vein catheter or by direct venous puncture during a trial of LSVC occlusion. Occlusion pressures consistently less than 18mmHg suggest the presence of an adequately sized left innominate vein or of adequate venous collaterals. Under these circumstances the LSVC, at surgery, can be temporarily occluded with little risk of central nervous system complications. The LSVC should not be temporarily occluded if the results are equivocal or if the pressure is consistently greater than 18mmHg. These conservative guidelines are arbitrary since no rigorously derived LSVC pressure data exist upon which to formulate a strict policy.

When temporary occlusion of the LSVC is not advisable, the LSVC is cannulated directly [1]. After the institution of cardiopulmonary bypass with standard cannulation of the RSVC and IVC, a third angled venous cannula is placed directly into the LSVC. This technique affords optimal control, visualization, and ease of insertion during cannulation of the relatively inaccessible LSVC. Alternatively, a flexible venous cannula can be inserted retrograde through the coronary sinus into the LSVC after opening the right atrium [1]. This technique is relatively simple but has the disadvantage of placing a cannula in the area of the surgical repair. Barring the use of either of these cannulation techniques, the exuberant coronary sinus effluent can be recovered during the repair with a cardiotomy sucker. This technique may be associated with poor visualization due to escaped blood and the physical presence of the cardiotomy sucker in the surgical field. Furthermore, myocardial protection could be compromised by the continual flow of the relatively warm LSVC effluent through the coronary sinus.

Finally, in neonates and small infants, the use of a single right atrial venous cannula with profound hypothermia and total circulatory arrest may be advisable because of the logistical problems associated with the use of multiple cannulae in these patients.

Azygos or Hemiazygos Continuation of the Inferior Vena Cava

When azygos continuation of the IVC to a RSVC is found at the time of cardiac surgery for an associated cardiac lesion, the RSVC is typically dilated and should be directly cannulated with a large venous cannula well below the IVC (azygos) insertion. The SVC cannula should be positioned to avoid obstructing the IVC (azygos) orifice. With hemiazygos continuation of the IVC to the LSVC, the dilated LSVC is directly cannulated with a large venous cannula below the IVC (hemiazygos) entrance.

Separate Connection of Hepatic Veins into the Right Atrium

Typically, hepatic veins that connect from below to the right atrium can be directly cannulated with a small angled venous cannula as one might cannulate a small IVC. To promote optimal venous drainage, the venous cannula should not be advanced too far into the common hepatic venous trunk. If the hepatic veins enter the right atrium from below by small and separate venous branches, profound hypothermia with low flow and recovery of the hepatic venous return with the cardiotomy sucker or the use of profound hypothermia with total circulatory arrest is necessary.

Surgical Management of Systemic Venous Destination Abnormalities

Left Superior Vena Cava to the Left Atrium without a Coronary Sinus

The preoperative and intraoperative methods for determining the LSVC pressure with a trial of occlusion are the same as those described previously for LSVC to the coronary sinus. If there is a significant innominate vein between the LSVC and an RSVC and if the trial occlusion pressure is acceptable, the LSVC may be ligated below the innominate vein [57,58]. Any associated cardiac defects are then repaired.

If ligation is not an option, the LSVC to the left atrium must be routed to the correct destination (right atrium). This must be coordinated with the repair of any associated cardiac abnormalities. The cannulation strategy is identical to that for LSVC to the coronary sinus.

Repositioning the Atrial Septum

A surgical technique that is especially useful when common atrium is part of the associated cardiac pathology, is repositioning of the interatrial septum. The interatrial septum, if present, is completely excised except for the anterior limbus. A piece of autologous pericardium or other patch material is used to reposition the interatrial septum so that the systemic venous orifices lie on the right atrial side of the new interatrial septum while leaving the pulmonary venous orifices on the left atrial side (Figure 36.5) [1,59,60]. Excision of all of the native interatrial septum prior to septal repositioning allows optimal baffle placement to avoid systemic or pulmonary venous obstruction [59,60]. Repositioning of the interatrial septum can be performed in neonates with very complex forms of ASVC associated with LSVC but the operative risk and the hazard of postoperative obstructive complications is probably higher in this age group [61].

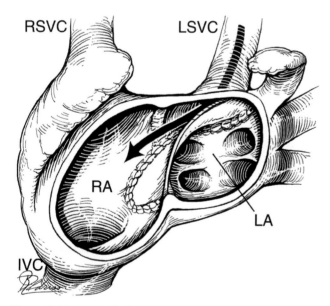

Figure 36.5 Repair of a left superior vena cava (LSVC) to the left atrium by repositioning the atrial septum. Excision of all the native interatrial septum before septal repositioning allows optimal baffle placement to avoid systemic or pulmonary venous obstruction. (IVC, inferior vena cava, RA, right atrium; RSVC, right superior vena cava.)

Superior Atrial Approach

If there is a significant amount of interatrial tissue, it is incised superiorly from the coronary sinus toward the RSVC orifice. The interatrial septum is then incised anteriorly thereby creating a medially hinged interatrial flap. Pericardium or prosthetic material is used to create a tunnel from the LSVC orifice along the superior left atrium toward the right atrium. Care is taken to avoid obstructing the left superior pulmonary vein. The remaining interatrial communication is closed with the interatrial flap. When not enough tissue exists to create an autologous interatrial flap, the interatrial communication is closed with autologous pericardium or other patch material (Figure 36.6) [1,62].

Left Superior Vena Cava Translocation with Interatrial Septal Repositioning

The placement of an interatrial baffle to separate the pulmonary and systemic venous orifices sometimes threatens to obstruct the left-sided pulmonary veins. In this circumstance, the LSVC can be detached from the left atrium and reimplanted into the roof of the left atrium closer to the plane of the native interatrial septum. The native interatrial septum is then excised and repositioned, with pericardium or other patch material, to direct all of the systemic venous flow to the pulmonary atrioventricular valve [51].

Bidirectional Cavopulmonary Connection

When the intracardiac anatomy precludes the placement of an interatrial baffle, an extracardiac repair technique can be used. The LSVC is detached from the heart and its cardiac end is oversewn. The LSVC is then sutured to an incision in the superior aspect of the left pulmonary artery [63–65]. Physiologic factors limiting the application of this technique are similar to those limiting the application of a bidirectional cavopulmonary connection to a patient with a variant of functionally single ventricle.

Roofing the Coronary Sinus

The coronary sinus can be "roofed" with autologous pericardium or by plication of the atrial wall over a stent. This roofing procedure starts at the left atrial LSVC internal orifice and continues to the level of the inferior aspect of the interatrial septum at the region normally occupied by the right atrial coronary sinus ostium [11,22]. Patch closure of the interatrial septum is performed around the new coronary sinus orifice (Figure 36.7) [1]. This technique is rarely used because of the possibility of left pulmonary vein and atrioventricular valve obstruction, injury to the conduction system, and early or late tunnel stenosis [62].

Translocation of the Left Superior Vena Cava to the Right Atrium

Although not commonly used, some have advocated detachment of the LSVC from the left atrium with implantation into the right atrium (Figure 36.8) [1]. When there

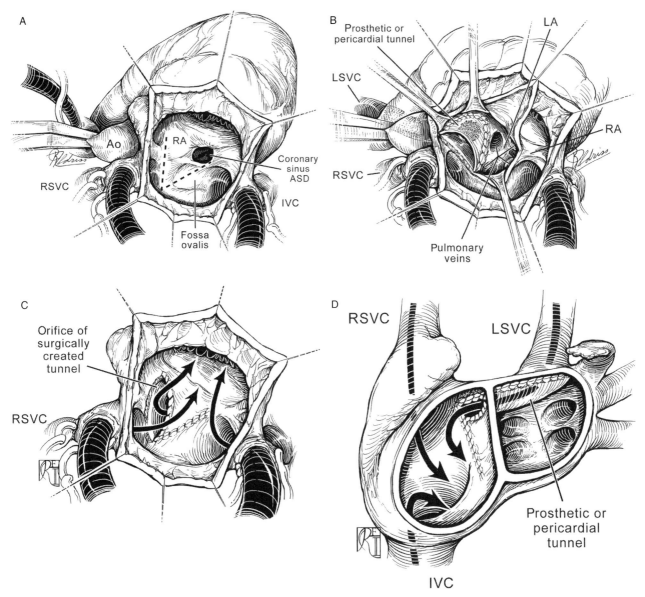

Figure 36.6 Superior atrial approach to repair a left superior vena cava (LSVC) to the left atrium (LA) with a coronary sinus atrial septal defect (ASD). **A,** Line of incision for creation of the medially hinged interatrial flap. **B,** Construction of the medially hinged interatrial flap. Pericardial or prosthetic tunnel is constructed along the superior aspect of the left atrium to connect the left superior vena caval orifice to the plane of the interatrial septum.

C, Remaining interatrial defect is closed with autologous interatrial tissue flap (pericardium or prosthetic material may be used if there is inadequate autogenous tissue). **D,** Schematic representation of a completed superior atrial repair of a left superior vena cava to the left atrium. (Ao, aorta; IVC, inferior vena cava; RSVC, right superior vena cava; RA, right atrium.)

appears to be insufficient LSVC length to achieve a tension-free anastomosis to the right atrium, the LSVC can be divided along with a generous flap of left atrial tissue. This left atrial flap is sutured into a tubular extension to lengthen the LSVC. The LSVC is then sutured to the right atrium without tension (Figure 36.9A) [1]. If further length is needed to reach the right atrium without tension, a superiorly based right atrial flap can be fashioned into a tubular

right atrial extension. This is sutured to the lengthened LSVC (Figure 36.9B) [1,24]. The technique of LSVC extension has also been adapted to implantation of the lengthened LSVC into the RSVC [66]. Successful connection of the LSVC to the right atrium with an interposition PTFE graft has also been reported [67]. The major limitation of these techniques is the possibility of stenosis or occlusion of the rerouted LSVC.

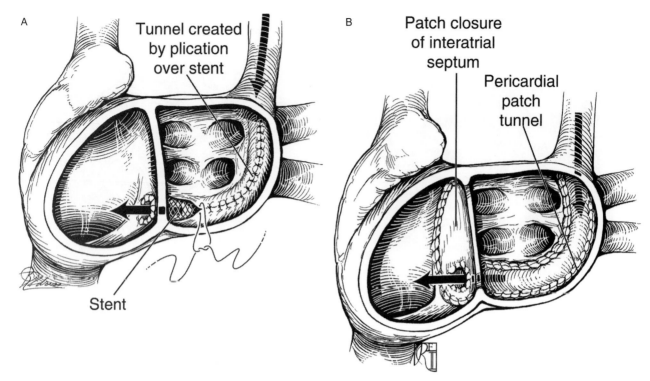

Figure 36.7 Roofing of the coronary sinus for repair of left superior vena cava to the left atrium with complete unroofing of the coronary sinus. **A,** Tunnel made by plication over stent on posterior wall of the left atrium. **B,** Tunnel made with pericardial patch: patch closure of interatrial septum.

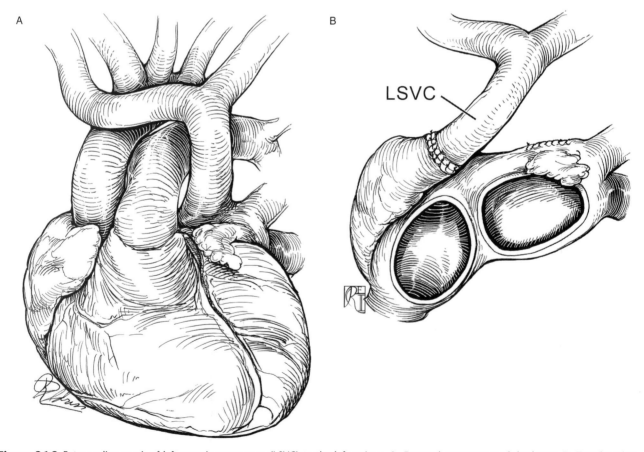

Figure 36.8 Extracardiac repair of left superior vena cava (LSVC) to the left atrium. **A,** External appearance of the heart. **B,** Translocation of the left superior vena cava to the right atrial appendage.

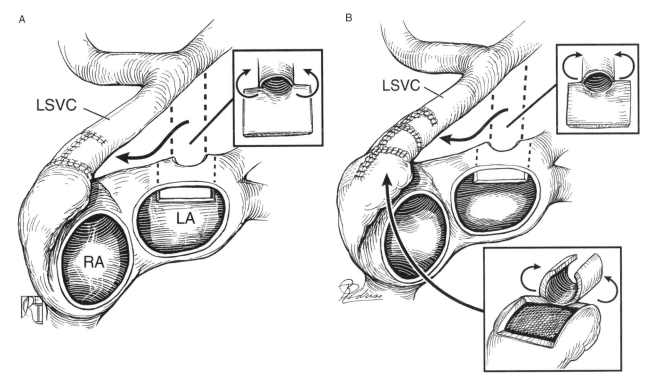

Figure 36.9 Extracardiac repair of left superior vena cava (LSVC) to the left atrium (LA). **A,** Translocation of the LSVC to the right atrium (RA) with extension of the LSVC using a tubular left atrial flap. The LSVC is detached from the LA with a flap of surrounding left atrial tissue (inset). The LSVC is lengthened by suturing the left atrial flap into a tubular extension. The lengthened LSVC is sutured to the right atrium. **B,** Translocation of the LSVC to the right atrium with right and left atrial flap extensions. The dotted lines mark the area of construction of the left atrial flap. The right atrial flap is formed into a right atrial tubular extension. The left atrial flap is formed into an LSVC extension. The lengthened LSVC is sutured to the right atrial tubular extension.

Partially Unroofed Midportion of the Coronary Sinus

If the diagnosis has not been made preoperatively, this lesion can easily be overlooked in the operating room without a high index of suspicion. The diagnosis is confirmed by passing a probe into the coronary sinus orifice, through the unroofed portion of the coronary sinus and into the left atrium. The communication with the left atrium through the defect in the roof of the coronary sinus can be confirmed by viewing the defect through a separate incision in the interatrial septum. When an LSVC is present, three potential repairs can be performed (Figure 36.10) [1]. If the LSVC can be ligated, the unroofed portion of the coronary sinus can be closed primarily or with a patch either through the mouth of the dilated coronary sinus or through an incision in the interatrial septum. A more straightforward repair consists of LSVC ligation with simple patch closure of the coronary sinus orifice. This leaves a negligible right-to-left shunt secondary to coronary sinus return to the left atrium. If the LSVC cannot be ligated, the defect in the roof of the coronary sinus must be repaired primarily or with a patch. When an LSVC is not present, the unroofed portion of the coronary sinus can be repaired or the coronary sinus orifice closed with a patch [58].

Inferior Vena Cava to the Left Atrium

Repair of drainage of the IVC to the left atrium involves excision of the interatrial septum with baffling of the IVC orifice to the right side using autologous pericardium or other patch material (Figure 36.11) [1].

Total Anomalous Systemic Venous Drainage

Repair of total anomalous systemic venous connection is accomplished by excising all of the interatrial septum, if one exists, except for the anterior limbus. The atrial mass is then partitioned with pericardium or other patch material so that the systemic venous orifices are baffled to the pulmonary atrioventricular valve and the pulmonary venous orifices are baffled to the systemic atrioventricular valve [68–71].

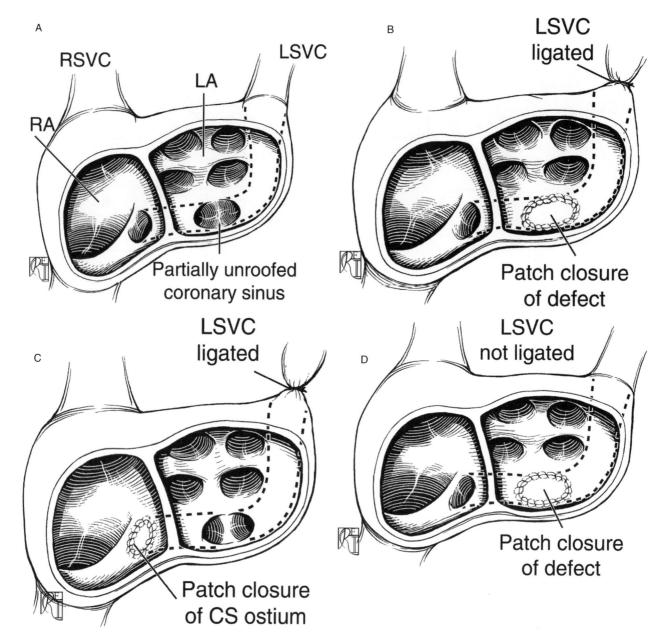

Figure 36.10 A, Repair of partially unroofed midportion of the coronary sinus with left superior vena cava (LSVC). **B,** Ligation of the LSVC and primary or patch closure of the unroofed portion of the dilated coronary sinus (CS). **C,** Ligation of the LSVC and primary or patch closure of the dilated coronary sinus right atrial orifice. **D,** Primary or patch closure of the unroofed portion of the dilated coronary sinus in a situation in which the LSVC cannot be ligated. (LA, left atrium; RA, right atrium; RSVC, right superior vena cava.)

Right Superior Vena Cava to the Left Atrium

Because of the uniqueness of this lesion nothing is known about the results of surgical treatment in the current era. Based upon one successful case report of a closed repair technique translocating the RSVC to the right atrium [27], it should be possible to improve upon this approach using cardiopulmonary bypass. Alternatively, excision of the superior interatrial septum with repositioning of the septum to the left side of the RSVC orifice using pericardium or a prosthetic patch is reasonable (Figure 36.12) [1].

Results

The mortality for repair of ASVC in isolation or associated with simple cardiac lesions is low. Survival primarily depends upon the patient's preoperative condition and the severity of the associated cardiac defects. Because these

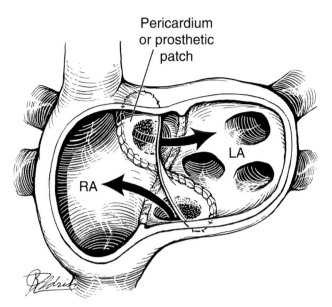

Figure 36.11 Baffle repair of inferior vena cava to the left atrium (LA) in association with partial anomalous pulmonary venous connection. The interatrial septum has been excised and pericardial or prosthetic patch is used to baffle the inferior vena cava into the right atrium (RA) and the right superior pulmonary veins into the LA.

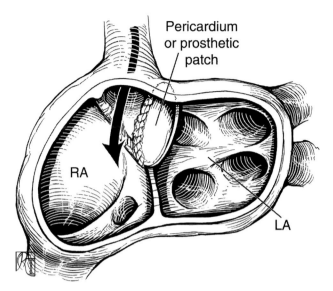

Figure 36.12 Baffle repair of right superior vena cava to the left atrium (LA). (RA, right atrium.)

anomalies are associated with a wide variety of cardiac malformations, it is difficult to determine morbidity and mortality rates directly attributable to the venous abnormalities per se.

Special Situations

Heart Transplantation in Patients with Anomalies of Systemic Venous Connection

The only absolute anatomic contraindication to heart transplantation is absence or marked hypoplasia of the central pulmonary arteries and absence or markedly diminutive pulmonary veins. ASVC increases the complexity of orthotopic cardiac transplantation and can potentially increase the operative risk. However, proper recipient selection, en bloc harvest of all donor vein and artery needed for complete reconstruction, harvesting of donor autologous pericardium, meticulous myocardial protection, and the use of profound hypothermia with low flow and intermittent total circulatory arrest are keys to a successful result [72].

During orthotopic cardiac transplantation, an LSVC to the left atrium can be reconstructed using external or internal techniques. The donor innominate vein can be harvested en bloc with the superior vena cava. The recipient LSVC is divided near its entrance into the left atrium during the recipient cardiectomy. The distal transected end of the recipient LSVC is then sutured end-to-end to the donor left innominate vein [73]. Conversely, the distal

transected end of the recipient LSVC is sutured end-to-end to a length of harvested donor descending aorta. The opposite end of this fresh, homograft interposition graft is then sutured to an incision in the roof of the donor right atrium [74]. Finally, the internal techniques of inferior or superior roofing with fresh pericardium can be used. After the recipient cardiectomy has been performed, a defect is created in the inferior aspect of the recipient interatrial septum. Inferior roofing is performed by creating a left atrial tunnel anterior to and leftward of the recipient left pulmonary veins from the LSVC orifice down to the surgically created interatrial defect (Figure 36.13) [1]. In superior roofing a defect is created in the superior aspect of the recipient interatrial septum. The superior wall of the left atrium is used as a flap to create a left atrial tunnel from the LSVC orifice to the interatrial defect (Figure 36.13) [1,75,76].

Other ASVC, such as left atrial insertion of the hepatic veins can be corrected, after recipient cardiectomy, by performing a resection of the recipient interatrial septum and creating a new interatrial septum that baffles the anomalous hepatic vein orifices to the right atrial side. This same baffle technique can be used in combination with superior or inferior roofing techniques to address transplant situations in which an LSVC and left-sided hepatic veins coexist [75,76]. In situs inversus, the left-sided morphologic right atrium can be used as a flap to construct a composite tunnel on the pericardial surface of the diaphragm from the hepatic vein orifices across the midline to the right side. The right-sided opening of this composite tunnel is sutured to the inferior vena caval orifice of the donor heart (Figure 36.14) [1,77].

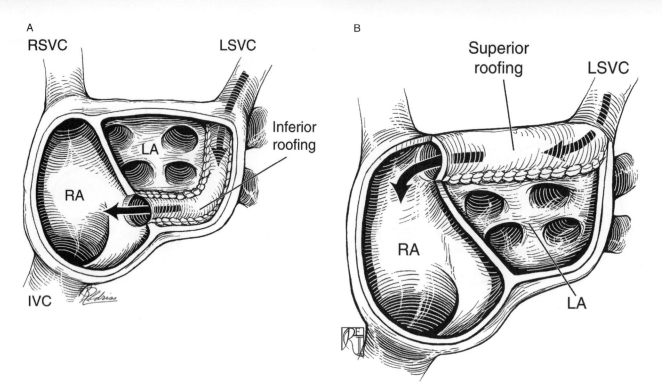

Figure 36.13 Orthotopic cardiac transplantation in a recipient with a left superior vena cava (LSVC) to the left atrium (LA) with completely unroofed coronary sinus. **A,** Pericardium or prosthetic material is used to form inferior roofing. **B,** Pericardium or prosthetic material is used to form superior roofing. (IVC, inferior vena cava; RA, right atrium; RSVC, right superior vena cava.)

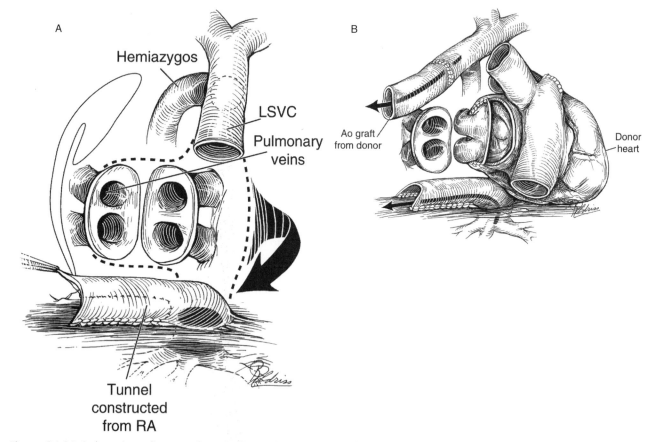

Figure 36.14 Orthotopic cardiac transplantation in a recipient with situs inversus with hemiazygos continuation of the inferior vena cava to the left superior vena cava. **A,** The left superior vena cava (LSVC) is divided. The right atrium and the left atrium are divided at the septum along the dotted line. The right and left pulmonary veins are separated and mobilized with generous cuffs of atrial tissue. The right atrium is devoted to the construction of a composite tunnel from the left-sided hepatic vein ostia, along the diaphragm and across the midline to the right side. **B,** The recipient right and left pulmonary venous cuffs are separately sutured to the donor left atrium. The ostium of the donor inferior vena cava is anastomosed to the orifice of the composite tunnel. The recipient LSVC with hemiazygos continuation is connected to the donor right atrium with donor descending thoracic aorta as an interposition graft. **C,** Completed repair. (Ao, aortic; RA, right atrium.)

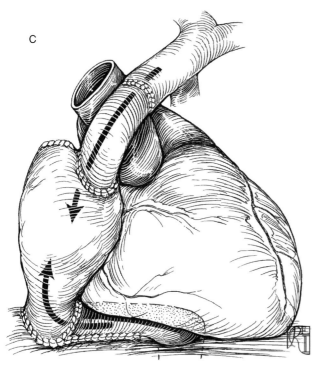

Figure 36.14 (*Continued*)

Cavopulmonary Connections in Patients with Complex Functionally Single Ventricle

Bidirectional cavopulmonary and total cavopulmonary connections are now commonly performed in patients with a variety of forms of complex functionally single ventricle. When the systemic venous return is normal, a staged approach to total cavopulmonary connection is undertaken in the usual manner. Many of these patients, however, have anomalies of systemic and pulmonary venous return. Among these patients visceral heterotaxy syndrome with atrial appendage isomerism is common. In the presence of bilateral SVCs, with or without azygos or hemiazygos continuation of the IVC, a bilateral bidirectional cavopulmonary connection is performed at 6 months of age. Intracardiac or extracardiac techniques of performing the completion total cavopulmonary connection are typically performed 1–2 years later. While the standard internal lateral tunnel technique may be used under certain circumstances, it is sometimes necessary to resort to an intracardiac tube graft to avoid pulmonary venous obstruction. In the presence of complex intracardiac anatomy and/or positional cardiac anomalies, an extracardiac tunnel or tube graft can also result in a satisfactory total cavopulmonary connection without interfering with pulmonary venous return [78–81].

References

1. Walters HL. (2003) Anomalous systemic venous connections. In: Mavroudis C, Backer CL, eds. *Pediatric Cardiac Surgery*, 3rd ed. Philadelphia, PA: Mosby, Inc.

2. Siewers RD. (1998) Anomalies of systemic venous drainage. In: Kaiser, LR, Spray TL, eds. *Mastery of Cardiothoracic Surgery*. Philadelphia, PA: Lippincott-Raven.

3. de Leval M. (1983) Anomalies of the systemic venous return. In: Stark J, de Leval MR, eds. *Surgery for Congenital Heart Defects*. London: Grune and Stratton, pp. 253–260.

4. Gaynor JW, Weinberg PM, Spray TL. (2000) Congenital Heart Surgery Nomenclature and Database Project: systemic venous anomalies. Ann Thorac Surg 69(4 Suppl), S70–S76.

5. Marshall J. (1850) On the development of the great anterior veins in man and mammalia: including an account of certain remnants of foetal structure found in the adult, a comparative view of these great veins in the different mammalia, and an analysis of their occasional peculiarities in the human subject. Philos Trans R Soc London 140, 133–169.

6. Winter FS. (1954) Persistent left superior vena cava; survey of world literature and report of thirty additional cases. Angiology 5, 90–132.

7. Campbell M, Deuchar DC. (1954) The left-sided superior vena cava. Br Heart J 16, 423–439.

8. Helseth HK, Peterson CR. (1974) Atrial septal defect with termination of left superior vena cava in the left atrium and absence of the coronary sinus. Recognition and correction. Ann Thorac Surg 17, 186–192.

9. Raghib G, Ruttenberg HD, Anderson RC, *et al.* (1965) Termination of left superior vena cava in left atrium, atrial septal defect, and absence of coronary sinus; a developmental complex. Circulation 31, 906–918.

10. Hurwitt ES, Escher DJ, Citrin LI. (1955) Surgical correction of cyanosis due to entrance of left superior vena cava into left auricle. Surgery 38, 903–914.

11. Rastelli GC, Ongley PA, Kirklin JW. (1965) Surgical correction of common atrium with anomalously connected persistent left superior vena cava: report of case. Mayo Clin Proc 40, 528–532.

12. Miller GA, Ongley PA, Rastelli GC, *et al.* (1965) Surgical correction of total anomalous systemic venous connection: report of case. Mayo Clin Proc 40, 532–538.

13. de Leval MR, Ritter DG, McGoon DC, *et al.* (1975) Anomalous systemic venous connection. Surgical considerations. Mayo Clin Proc 50, 599–610.

14. Karnegis JN, Wang Y, Winchell P, *et al.* (1964) Persistent left superior vena cava, fibrous remnant of the right superior vena cava and ventricular septal defect. Am J Cardiol 14, 573–577.

15. Lenox CC, Zuberbuhler JR, Park SC, *et al.* (1980) Absent right superior vena cava with persistent left superior vena cava: implications and management. Am J Cardiol 45, 117–122.

16. Steinberg I, Dubilier W Jr, Lukas DS. (1953) Persistence of left superior vena cava. Dis Chest 24, 479–488.

17. Santoscoy R, Walters HL 3rd, Ross RD, *et al.* (1996) Coronary sinus ostial atresia with persistent left superior vena cava. Ann Thorac Surg 61, 879–882.

18. Harris WG. (1960) A case of bilateral superior venae cavae with a closed coronary sinus. Thorax 15, 172–173.

19. Watson GH. (1985) Atresia of the coronary sinus orifice. Pediatr Cardiol 6, 99–101.

20. Lucas RV Jr, Krabill KA. (1995) Abnormal systemic venous connections. In: Emmanouilides GC, Allen HD, *et al.*, eds.

Heart Disease in Infants, Children and Adolescents, 5th ed. Baltimore: Williams & Wilkins, pp. 874–902.

21. Kirklin JW, Barratt-Boyes BG. (1993) Unroofed coronary sinus syndrome. In: Kirklin JW, Barratt-Boyes BG, eds. *Cardiac Surgery*, 2nd ed. New York: Churchill-Livingstone, pp. 683–692.

22. Quaegebeur J, Kirklin JW, Pacifico AD, *et al.* (1979) Surgical experience with unroofed coronary sinus. Ann Thorac Surg 27, 418–425.

23. Adatia I, Gittenberger-de Groot AC. (1995) Unroofed coronary sinus and coronary sinus orifice atresia. Implications for management of complex congenital heart disease. J Am Coll Cardiol 25, 948–953.

24. Shumacker HB Jr, King H, Waldhausen JA. (1967) The persistent left superior vena cava. Surgical implications, with special reference to caval drainage into the left atrium. Ann Surg 165, 797–805.

25. Allmendinger P, Dear WE, Cooley DA. (1974) Atrial septal defect with communication through the coronary sinus. Ann Thorac Surg 17, 193–196.

26. Mantini E, Grondin CM, Lillehei CW, *et al.* (1966) Congenital anomalies involving the coronary sinus. Circulation 33, 317–327.

27. Kirsch WM, Carlsson E, Hartmann AF Jr. (1961) A case of anomalous drainage of the superior vena cava into the left atrium. J Thorac Cardiovasc Surg 41, 550–556.

28. Kadletz M, Black MD, Smallhorn J, *et al.* (1997) Total anomalous systemic venous drainage to the coronary sinus in association with hypoplastic left heart disease: more than a mere coincidence. J Thorac Cardiovasc Surg 114, 282–284.

29. Black H, Smith GT, Goodale WT. (1964) Anomalous inferior vena cava draining into the left atrium associated with intact interatrial septum and multiple pulmonary arteriovenous fistulae. Circulation 29, 258–267.

30. Gardner DL, Cole L. (1955) Long survival with inferior vena cava draining into left atrium. Br Heart J 17, 93–97.

31. Gautam HP. (1968) Left atrial inferior vena cava with atrial septal defect. J Thorac Cardiovasc Surg 55, 827–829.

32. Meadows WR, Bergstrand I, Sharp JT. (1961) Isolated anomalous connection of a great vein to the left atrium. The syndrome of cyanosis and clubbing, "normal" heart, and left ventricular hypertrophy on electrocardiogram. Circulation 24, 669–676.

33. Singh A, Doyle EF, Danilowicz D, *et al.* (1976) Masked abnormal drainage of the inferior vena cava into the left atrium. Am J Cardiol 38, 261–264.

34. van Tellingen C, Verzijlbergen F, Plokker HW. (1984) A patient with bilateral superior and inferior caval veins. Int J Cardiol 5, 366–373.

35. Anderson RC, Adams P Jr, Burke B. (1961) Anomalous inferior vena cava with azygos continuation (infrahepatic interruption of the inferior vena cava). Report of 15 new cases. J Pediatr 59, 370–383.

36. Dwight T. (1901) Absence of the inferior vena cava below the diaphragm. J Anat Physiol 35, 7–20.

37. Van Praagh S, Kreutzer J, Alday L, *et al.* (1990) Systemic and pulmonary venous connections in visceral heterotaxy, with emphasis on the diagnosis of the atrial situs: a study of 109 postmortem cases. In: Clark EB, Takao A, eds. *Developmental Cardiology: Morphogenesis and Function*. Mount Kisco, NY: Futura Publishing.

38. Jacobs JP, Anderson RH, Weinberg PM, *et al.* (2007) The nomenclature, definition and classification of cardiac structures in the setting of heterotaxy. Cardiol Young 17(Suppl 2), 1–28.

39. Uemura H, Ho SY, Devine WA, *et al.* (1995) Atrial appendages and venoatrial connections in hearts from patients with visceral heterotaxy. Ann Thorac Surg 60, 561–569.

40. Cohen MS, Anderson RH, Cohen MI, *et al.* (2007) Controversies, genetics, diagnostic assessment, and outcomes relating to the heterotaxy syndrome. Cardiol Young 17(Suppl 2), 29–43.

41. Huhta JC, Smallhorn JF, Macartney FJ, *et al.* (1982) Cross-sectional echocardiographic diagnosis of systemic venous return. Br Heart J 48, 388–403.

42. Schmidt KG, Silverman NH. (1987) Cross-sectional and contrast echocardiography in the diagnosis of interatrial communications through the coronary sinus. Int J Cardiol 16, 193–199.

43. Stumper O, Vargas-Barron J, Rijlaarsdam M, *et al.* (1991) Assessment of anomalous systemic and pulmonary venous connections by transoesophageal echocardiography in infants and children. Br Heart J 66, 411–418.

44. Yeager SB, Parness IA, Spevak PJ, *et al.* (1994) Prenatal echocardiographic diagnosis of pulmonary and systemic venous anomalies. Am Heart J 128, 397–405.

45. Konstam MA, Levine BW, Strauss HW, *et al.* (1979) Left superior vena cava to left atrial communication diagnosed with radionuclide angiocardiography and with differential right to left shunting. Am J Cardiol 43, 149–153.

46. Webb RW, Gamsu G, Speckman JM, *et al.* (1982) Computed tomographic demonstration of mediastinal venous anomalies. Am J Roentgenol 139, 157–161.

47. Hong YK, Park YW, Ryu SJ, *et al.* (2000) Efficacy of MRI in complicated congenital heart disease with visceral heterotaxy syndrome. J Comput Assist Tomogr 24, 671–682.

48. Fisher MR, Hricak J, Higgins CB. (1985) Magnetic resonance imaging of developmental venous anomalies. Am J Roentgenol 145, 705–709.

49. Schultz CL, Morrison S, Bryan PJ. (1984) Azygos continuation of the inferior vena cava: demonstration by NMR imaging. J Comput Assist Tomogr 8, 774–776.

50. White CS, Baffa JM, Haney PJ, *et al.* (1997) MR imaging of congenital anomalies of the thoracic veins. Radiographics 17, 595–608.

51. Ross RD, Children's Hospital of Michigan, (Detroit, Michigan). Isolated dextrocardia with multiple systemic and pulmonary venous anomalies: a case report. Personal communication.

52. Freedom RM, Culham JA, Rowe RD. (1981) Left atrial to coronary sinus fenestration (partially unroofed coronary sinus). Morphological and angiocardiographic observations. Br Heart J 46, 63–68.

53. Rose AG, Beckman CB, Edwards JE. (1974) Communication between coronary sinus and left atrium. Br Heart J 36, 182–185.

54. Rumisek JD, Pigott JD, Weinberg PM, *et al.* (1986) Coronary sinus septal defect associated with tricuspid atresia. J Thorac Cardiovasc Surg 92, 142–145.

55. Yokota M, Kyoku I, Kitano M, *et al.* (1989) Atresia of the coronary sinus orifice. Fatal outcome after intraoperative division of the drainage left superior vena cava. J Thorac Cardiovasc Surg 98, 30–32.

56. Freed MD, Rosenthal A, Bernhard WF. (1973) Balloon occlusion of a persistent left superior vena cava in the preoperative evaluation of systemic venous return. J Thorac Cardiovasc Surg 65, 835–839.

57. Davis WH, Jordaan FR, Snyman HW. (1959) Persistent left superior vena cava draining into the left atrium, as an isolated anomaly. Am Heart J 57, 616–622.

58. Lee ME, Sade RM. (1979) Coronary sinus septal defect. Surgical considerations. J Thorac Cardiovasc Surg 78, 563–569.

59. Kabbani SS, Feldman M, Angelini P, *et al.* (1973) Single (left) superior vena cava draining into the left atrium. Surgical repair. Ann Thorac Surg 16, 518–525.

60. Sherafat M, Friedman S, Waldhausen JA. (1971) Persistent left superior vena cava draining into the left atrium with absent right superior vena cava. Ann Thorac Surg 11, 160–164.

61. Turley K, Tarnoff H, Snider R, *et al.* (1981) Repair of combined total anomalous pulmonary venous connection and anomalous systemic connection in early infancy. Ann Thorac Surg 31, 70–77.

62. Sand ME, McGrath LB, Pacifico AD, *et al.* (1986) Repair of left superior vena cava entering the left atrium. Ann Thorac Surg 42, 560–564.

63. Mavroudis C, Backer CL, Kohr LM. (1999) Bidirectional Glenn shunt in association with congenital heart repairs: the 1½ ventricular repair. Ann Thorac Surg 68, 976–981.

64. Takach TJ, Cortelli M, Lonquist JL, *et al.* (1997) Correction of anomalous systemic venous drainage: transposition of left SVC to left PA. Ann Thorac Surg 63, 228–230.

65. Van Arsdell GS, Williams WG, Freedom RM. (1998) A practical approach to 1 1/2 ventricle repairs. Ann Thorac Surg 66, 678–680.

66. Palacios-Macedo AX, Fraser CD Jr. (1997) Correction of anomalous systemic venous drainage in heterotaxy syndrome. Ann Thorac Surg 64, 235–237; discussion 237–238.

67. Gontijo B, Fantini FA, de Paula e Silva JA, *et al.* (1990) The use of PTFE graft to correct anomalous drainage of persistent left superior vena cava. J Cardiovasc Surg 31, 815–817.

68. Ghosh PK, Donnelly RJ, Hamilton DI, *et al.* (1977) Surgical correction of a case of common atrium with anomalous systemic and pulmonary venous drainage. J Thorac Cardiovasc Surg 74, 604–606.

69. Gueron M, Hirsh M, Borman J. (1969) Total anomalous systemic venous drainage into the left atrium. Report of a case of successful surgical correction. J Thorac Cardiovasc Surg 58, 570–574.

70. Krayenbuhl CU, Lincoln JC. (1977) Total anomalous systemic venous connection, common atrium, and partial atrioventricular canal. A case report of successful surgical correction. J Thorac Cardiovasc Surg 73, 686–689.

71. Roberts KD, Edwards JM, Astley R. (1972) Surgical correction of total anomalous systemic venous drainage. J Thorac Cardiovasc Surg 64, 803–810.

72. Bailey LL. (1993) Heart transplantation techniques in complex congenital heart disease. J Heart Lung Transplant 12, S168–S175.

73. Laks H, Martin SM, Grant PW. (1994) Techniques of cardiac transplantation. In: Kapoor AS, Laks H, eds. *Atlas of Heart-Lung Transplantation.* New York: McGraw-Hill.

74. Vouhe PR, Tamisier D, Le Bidois J, *et al.* (1993) Pediatric cardiac transplantation for congenital heart defects: surgical considerations and results. Ann Thorac Surg 56, 1239–1247.

75. Chartrand C. (1991) Pediatric cardiac transplantation despite atrial and venous return anomalies. Ann Thorac Surg 52, 716–721.

76. Chartrand C, Guerin R, Kangah M, *et al.* (1990) Pediatric heart transplantation: surgical considerations for congenital heart diseases. J Heart Transplant 9, 608–616; discussion 616–617.

77. Doty DB, Renlund DG, Caputo GR, *et al.* (1990) Cardiac transplantation in situs inversus. J Thorac Cardiovasc Surg 99, 493–499.

78. Marcelletti C, Corno A, Giannico S, *et al.* (1990) Inferior vena cava-pulmonary artery extracardiac conduit. A new form of right heart bypass. J Thorac Cardiovasc Surg 100, 228–232.

79. McElhinney DB, Reddy VM, Moore P, *et al.* (1997) Bidirectional cavopulmonary shunt in patients with anomalies of systemic and pulmonary venous drainage. Ann Thorac Surg 63, 1676–1684.

80. Michielon G, Gharagozloo F, Julsrud PR, *et al.* (1993) Modified Fontan operation in the presence of anomalies of systemic and pulmonary venous connection. Circulation 88, II141–II148.

81. Rosenkranz ER, Murphy DJ Jr. (1995) Modified Fontan procedure for left atrial isomerism: alternative technique. Pediatr Cardiol 16, 201–203.

CHAPTER 37

Sinus of Valsalva Aneurysm

W. Steves Ring

Children's Medical Center of Dallas, Dallas, TX, USA

Introduction

Definition

The sinus of Valsalva is defined as that portion of the aortic root bounded by the aortic cusp, the aortic valve annulus, and the sinotubular ridge. A congenital sinus of Valsalva aneurysm is a thin-walled enlargement or outpouching of the aortic wall, often appearing like a windsock that arises from the base of a single aortic sinus. Less frequently, it may appear as a simple fistulous communication between an aortic sinus and an adjacent structure. It usually originates from either the right sinus or the anterior aspect of the noncoronary sinus of Valsalva and penetrates the base of the heart into an adjacent low-pressure chamber. Rarely, it may present extracardiac or rupture freely into the pericardium. The aneurysm becomes clinically apparent when it ruptures into the adjacent low-pressure chamber creating an aortocardiac fistula, develops endocarditis, compresses or obstructs adjacent structures, or occasionally causes arrhythmias or thromboemboli. Other diseases such as endocarditis, syphilis, Marfan's syndrome, cystic medial necrosis, atherosclerosis, and trauma may involve the aortic root and cause aneurysms or fistulae of one or more sinuses of Valsalva. However, these acquired sinus of Valsalva aneurysms tend to be more evenly distributed among the three sinuses, more commonly involve multiple sinuses, are rarely associated with other congenital heart defects, and more commonly rupture outside the heart. Dilation of multiple sinuses as occurs in Marfan's syndrome or other connective tissue defects is generally considered to be an aortic root aneurysm and not an isolated sinus of Valsalva aneurysm.

History

The first description (1989) of a sinus of Valsalva aneurysm with intracardiac rupture is attributed to Hope [1]. One year later, Thurnam [2] described a series of six sinus of Valsalva aneurysms including Hope's case with five additional cases. Along with her many other anatomic descriptions of congenital heart defects, Maude Abbott [3] was one of the first to note the congenital etiology for many sinus of Valsalva aneurysms. Jones and Langley [4] also emphasized a distinction between acquired and congenital sinus of Valsalva aneurysms. In 1954, Brown [5] was the first to attempt surgical repair of a ruptured sinus of Valsalva aneurysm with endocarditis using deep hypothermia and inflow occlusion without cardiopulmonary bypass. Unfortunately, the patient expired 14 days after surgery from staphylococcal sepsis and aortic insufficiency. Lillehei [6,7] was the first to successfully use cardiopulmonary bypass to surgically correct a right sinus of Valsalva aneurysm that had ruptured into the right ventricular outflow tract. This was accomplished with primary suture closure in an 11-year-old girl on May 2, 1956 using cardiopulmonary bypass, aortic cross-clamping, and retrograde coronary sinus perfusion. Several other surgical teams accomplished and reported similar results over the next year [8–10].

Epidemiology

Congenital aneurysm of the sinus of Valsalva is a rare defect of the aortic root. The true incidence is unknown. It was reported as occurring in only 0.09% in a large autopsy series from 1914 [11], but this series did not distinguish between congenital and acquired aneurysms. The incidence of ruptured sinus of Valsalva aneurysms in large cardiac surgical series is 0.14–0.37% of western surgical series [12–16], 0.46–3.57% of surgical series in Asia [17–27], and 0.51–1.5% in Chinese series [20–22,27]. However, because the application of cardiac surgery is quite different among these regions, the relative incidence in overall cardiac surgical series may be misleading. Surgical series only of procedures for congenital heart disease may be more representative. According to this criterion, the incidence of sinus of Valsalva aneurysms was 0.26% in one western series [16], 1.37–1.5% in a series from India [23,26], and 2.0–3.57% in a series in Japan [24,25].

On the basis of collected surgical series of 361 patients, Chu *et al.* [20] estimated that the incidence of sinus of Valsalva aneurysms among Asians is up to five times higher than in western populations. Other important differences noted by Chu *et al.* include a higher incidence of right sinus of Valsalva aneurysms (86% vs. 68%), more common penetration into the right ventricle (73% vs. 60%), a higher association with ventricular septal defects (52% vs. 38%), and an equal frequency of associated aortic insufficiency (34% vs. 33%). The reason for these differences is uncertain but parallels the higher incidence of supracristal or subarterial ventricular septal defects found in Asians [28].

Congenital sinus of Valsalva aneurysms occur more frequently in men with a male to female ratio of approximately 2:1 [15,27,29–31]. There does not appear to be any familial or hereditary association [20]. Although they can occur at any age, aneurysms most commonly (50–60%) present in the third or fourth decades of life [20,30]. The mean age in most surgical series of ruptured sinus of Valsalva aneurysms is 25–40 years. Fewer than 15% of cases occur before the age of 20 years [20], although ruptured aneurysms have occurred even in neonates [32,33].

Anatomy

Knowledge of the anatomic relations between the aortic sinuses and the adjacent cardiac structures is essential for understanding the pathological anatomy, pathophysiology, and surgical treatment of sinus of Valsalva aneurysms (Figure 37.1) [34]. Aneurysms originate most commonly from the right sinus in 65–70% of western series (Figure 37.2A) [15,16,20,29–31,35], and 80–90% of Asian series (Figure 37.2B) [17,18,20,24,25,27,31]. The noncoronary sinus is less commonly involved in 20–35% of western series and 10–20% of Asian series. The left sinus is involved in fewer than 5% of western series and fewer than 1% of Asian series. Aortic pressure causes gradual enlargement of the aneurysm into an adjacent low-pressure chamber; the result is rupture with formation of an aortocardiac fistula or, less commonly, compression, obstruction, endocarditis, or free rupture into the pericardium (Figure 37.3) [20,34]. Aneurysms of the right coronary sinus tend to rupture into the right ventricle (70–90%) or right atrium (5–20%) with rare rupture into the septum, left ventricle, pulmonary artery, or pericardium (<1–2%), and never into the left

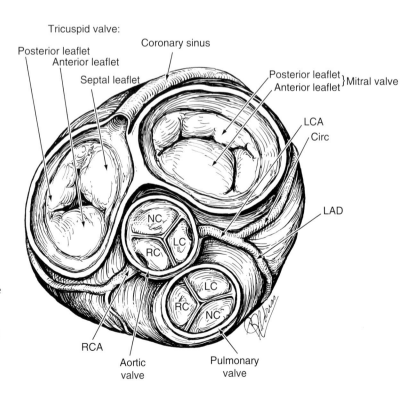

Figure 37.1 Coronal section through the base of the heart shows the aortic root, the sinuses of Valsalva, and their relations. (Circ, circumflex coronary artery; LAD, left anterior descending coronary artery; LC, left coronary cusp; LCA, left coronary artery; NC, noncoronary cusp; RC, right coronary cusp; RCA, right coronary artery.)

atrium. Noncoronary sinus of Valsalva aneurysms rupture most commonly into the right atrium (70–85%) or right ventricle (10–25%), rarely into the left atrium, left ventricle, or pericardium (<4%), and never into the pulmonary artery. Aneurysms of the left coronary sinus are rare and may rupture with variable frequencies into the right or left atrium, the right or left ventricle, the pericardium, or the pulmonary artery.

Embryology and Histology

Abbott [3] first postulated that the fundamental defect in congenital aneurysm of the sinus of Valsalva is a defective development of the bulbar septum. This concept was expanded by Jones and Langley [4] who emphasized the importance of fusion of the aortopulmonary septum with the bulboventricular septum to form the base for the right and the noncoronary sinuses, the location of most sinus of Valsalva aneurysms. They also noted the rarity of aneu-

rysms arising from the left sinus of Valsalva, which is unrelated to the bulbar septum, and the frequent association of ventricular septal defects and bicuspid aortic valves, both related to imperfect septation of the bulbus cordis. The discontinuity or lack of fusion between the annulus fibrosus and the aortic media was later confirmed histologically by Edwards and Burchell [36,37]. However, Angelini [38] has questioned this theory due to the lack of association of sinus of Valsalva aneurysms with other conotruncal defects. He has also correctly questioned the inclusion of aortic leaflet prolapse and subarterial ventricular septal defects with sinus of Valsalva aneurysms.

Classification

Sakakibara and Konno [39–42] proposed the first classification system for congenital sinus of Valsalva aneurysms. Their proposed classification includes only those aneurysms originating from the posterior, middle, or anterior third of the right sinus (types I, II, and IIIa or IIIv respectively) or the anterior third of the noncoronary sinus (type IV). The classification allows penetration of types I, II, and IIIv only into the right ventricle (v), and types IIIa and IV only into the right atrium (a). Subclassification is based on the presence or absence of a ventricular septal defect (e.g., type II VSD). Although it includes the most common types of congenital sinus of Valsalva aneurysms, this classification scheme does not account for all three possible sinuses of origin and does not account for the variety of intracardiac and extracardiac sites of penetration.

A new classification scheme based on anatomy (sinus of origin and chamber of penetration), and acuity (ruptured versus nonruptured), with a modifier added for etiology (atherosclerotic, congenital, connective tissue defects, inflammatory, infection, and trauma) has been proposed by the STS Congenital Heart Surgery Nomenclature Database

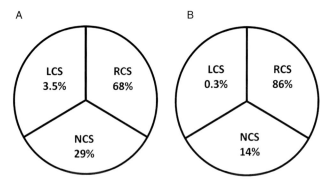

Figure 37.2 Racial differences in the location sinus of Valsalva aneurysm sites of origin. **A,** Western series (n = 395). **B,** Asian series (n = 654). (LCS, left coronary sinus; NCS, noncoronary sinus; RCS, right coronary sinus.) (Adapted from Wang [31].)

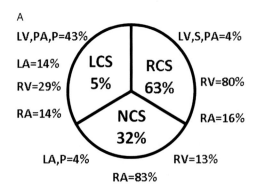
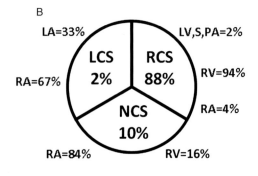

Figure 37.3 Racial differences in the location of sinus of Valsalva aneurysm chamber of penetration. **A,** Western Series (n = 151). **B,** Asian Series (n = 181). (LA, left atrium; LCS, left coronary sinuses; LV, left ventricle; P, pericardium; PA, pulmonary artery; RCS, right coronary sinuses; NCS, noncoronary sinuses; RA, right atrium; RV, right ventricle; S, ventricular septum.) (Adapted from Chu [20] and Ring [34].)

Project [43]. However, this classification scheme is new and has not yet been widely adopted.

Associated Defects

Approximately one-half of all patients with sinus of Valsalva aneurysms have associated defects. Ventricular septal defect is the most commonly associated defect, occurring in approximately 40–60% of Asian and 35–40% of western series [20,27,29–31]. These defects are found in 60–70% of cases with right sinus of Valsalva aneurysms but in only 10% of those with noncoronary sinus of Valsalva aneurysms. Aortic insufficiency occurs in 25–40% of patients, without significant differences between Asian and western series [20,31]. Other associated defects include bicuspid aortic valve (5–10%), pulmonary stenosis (5%), atrial septal defect (2–5%), patent ductus arteriosus (1–2%), and coarctation (1–2%). Rare isolated cases of associations with tetralogy of Fallot, subaortic stenosis, and other congenital defects are likely only chance occurrences, without true association.

Natural History

There is little information about the natural history of sinus of Valsalva aneurysms. However, Sakakibara and Konno [39] noted that the majority of patients with ruptured sinus of Valsalva aneurysm died within 1 year of diagnosis if not repaired surgically, with the exception of one patient followed for 17 years after the diagnosis. Adams and Sawyers [44] also reported an average survival of only 3.9 years after diagnosis, but the survival period decreased to less than 1 year when two patients who survived for 10 and 15 years were excluded. Based on these observations, most authors believe surgical repair is indicated for all patients with ruptured sinus of Valsalva aneurysm and for any patient with symptomatic nonruptured sinus of Valsalva aneurysm [45,46]. The natural history of unruptured sinus of Valsalva aneurysm is unknown because most are asymptomatic and remain undetected. Therefore, the role of surgery for asymptomatic nonruptured aneurysms remains controversial.

Diagnosis

Clinical Presentation

Unruptured sinus of Valsalva aneurysm usually is asymptomatic and often found incidentally at the time of cardiac evaluation for some other heart condition. However, when it enlarges, it may cause symptoms by distorting or compressing adjacent structures. This condition can manifest as aortic insufficiency from annular dilation or a prolapsing cusp [35,47], right ventricular outflow tract obstruction [48–55], coronary artery compression with myocardial ischemia or infarction [56–64], conduction disturbances with septal penetration [65–72], malignant arrhythmias [73,74], or a mediastinal mass [75]. Other initial manifestations include endocarditis [15,29,30] and thromboembolism [76–78].

Rupture of a sinus of Valsalva aneurysm occurs into one of the adjacent cardiac chambers, the interventricular septum, or the pericardium. Free rupture into the pericardium usually is fatal [79,80], although successful surgical repair has been reported [81,82]. Rupture or dissection into the interventricular septum results in conduction abnormalities and aortic insufficiency [83,84] or eventually free rupture into the right or left ventricle [84]. Intracardiac rupture usually occurs into one of the adjacent right cardiac chambers causing a left-to-right shunt with biventricular volume overload. Approximately 25–35% of patients with ruptured sinus of Valsalva aneurysms will develop the acute onset of dyspnea and substernal or epigastric chest pain. More commonly, about 45–50% of patients develop more gradual symptoms of congestive heart failure with dyspnea, fatigue, chest pain, and peripheral edema. Remarkably, 15–20% of patients with ruptured sinus of Valsalva aneurysms are asymptomatic [19,27,29,30].

Physical Examination

In examinations of patients who have a ruptured sinus of Valsalva aneurysm, the most notable physical finding (85–95% of cases) is a loud, continuous murmur along the left sternal border [27,30]. The differential diagnosis of this characteristic murmur includes patent ductus arteriosus, aortopulmonary window, coronary arteriovenous fistula, pulmonary arteriovenous malformation, and ventricular septal defect with associated aortic insufficiency. When the murmur is absent, pulmonary hypertension or rupture into the left ventricle should be suspected. Approximately 80% of patients have a thrill, bounding peripheral pulses, and widened pulse pressure, characteristic of aortic runoff lesions.

Diagnostic Testing

Chest radiographs usually show signs of cardiac enlargement and pulmonary overcirculation [26,27,30]. The electrocardiogram often is abnormal but nonspecific with evidence of ventricular hypertrophy, conduction disturbance, or in rare instances ischemia if a coronary artery is compromised by the aneurysm [18].

Diagnostic imaging is required in all cases with the objectives of defining: 1) the sinus of origin; 2) the chamber of penetration or perforation; 3) the presence and location of an associated ventricular septal defect; 4) the presence and degree of aortic insufficiency; and 5) the coronary

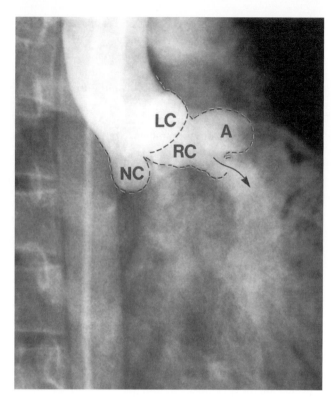

Figure 37.4 Cineangiogram in the right anterior oblique projection of a right sinus of Valsalva aneurysm ruptured into the right ventricle. (A, aneurysm; LC, left coronary sinus; NC, noncoronary sinus; RC, right coronary sinus.)

anatomy. Historically, angiography (Figure 37.4) [34] has been the "gold standard" for the evaluation of sinus of Valsalva aneurysm because it clarifies the anatomy of the root and the sinus of Valsalva aneurysm, the extent of aortic insufficiency, the coronary arteries, and most associated defects. However, angiography is not very accurate for the diagnosis of a ventricular septal defect, missing 16% of ventricular septal defects in one series [18], and nearly one-half in another [19].

Echocardiography was first used to diagnose a sinus of Valsalva aneurysm in 1974 [85,86]. Improvements in two-dimensional imaging and color flow mapping have made it the diagnostic procedure of choice [27,31,87–92]. The use of transesophageal echocardiography gives even better anatomic and functional characterization of the defect and allows better visualization when inadequate transthoracic windows compromise image quality [93–95]. However, adequate visualization of coronary anatomy may not always be achieved, and an associated ventricular septal defect may be missed because of occlusion of the ventricular septal defect by either the aneurysmal sac or the prolapsing aortic cusp [19,87]. Some authors [88,90,96] have advocated surgical correction based on echocardiography

alone, and this may be possible in many cases. However, if the surgeon is uncomfortable about any aspect of the anatomy, particularly the coronary anatomy, angiography is advised. Because an associated ventricular septal defect also is frequently missed by angiography, this is not an indication for catheterization. It is best approached by careful inspection and repair when found at the time of surgery.

The role of magnetic resonance imaging is not clearly defined [97]. However, it may provide additional anatomic information in select cases [98–102], and has even been proposed as the sole diagnostic procedure before surgical correction [100,102].

Treatment

Surgical Technique

Sinus of Valsalva aneurysms are generally repaired surgically through a median sternotomy using cardiopulmonary bypass, bicaval cannulation, and left ventricular venting (Figure 37.5) [34]. Operative transesophageal echocardiography is useful for further delineation of the relation of the aneurysm or fistula to the adjacent structures, the status of the aortic valve, and ventricular function. The aortic root is palpated for a thrill, and the external structure is inspected, looking for external evidence of aortic sinus dilation or an aortoventricular tunnel that typically arises at or above the sinotubular ridge. Hypothermic cardiopulmonary bypass is begun, and the aorta is cross-clamped before ventricular fibrillation to avoid cardiac distension either from the fistula or from aortic insufficiency. A left ventricular vent is usually placed through the right superior pulmonary vein.

Because of the degree of aortic runoff through the fistula or regurgitant aortic valve, the technique of administering cardioplegia solution must be adjusted as for cases of aortic insufficiency or ruptured sinus of Valsalva aneurysm. We believe the aorta should be opened in all cases and therefore favor direct antegrade coronary cardioplegia followed by intermittent retrograde coronary sinus cardioplegia or retrograde cardioplegia alone. Aortic root cardioplegic arrest may be used if there is no fistula or aortic insufficiency; however, aortic root cardioplegia with digital compression of the fistula is discouraged owing to unreliable occlusion of the fistula and possible impairment of delivery to the coronary artery in the compressed sinus.

Three approaches to repair of the aneurysm or fistula have been used: 1) through the chamber of origin (aorta) (Figure 37.5A) [34]; 2) through the chamber of termination (atrium [Figure 37.5B], ventricle [Figure 37.5C], or pulmonary artery [Figure 37.5D] [34]); or 3) both [34]. Although the approach in each case should be individualized, the combined approach is currently most favored [11–13,16,18,

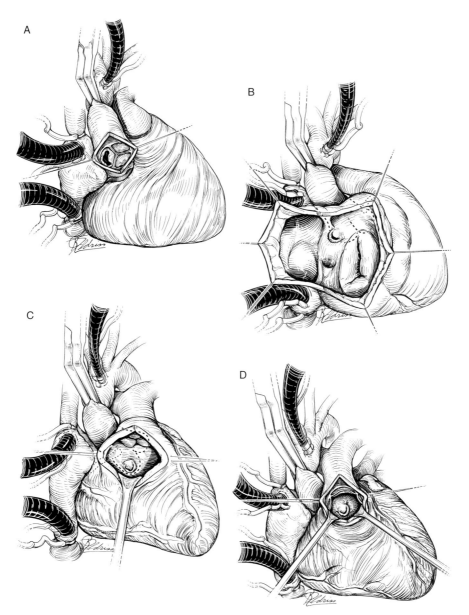

Figure 37.5 Surgical exposures for repair of sinus of Valsalva aneurysms. **A,** Initial exposure of sinus of Valsalva aneurysm through transverse aortotomy shows the relation of the aneurysm (shown here in noncoronary sinus) to the leaflets and the coronary arteries. **B,** Right atrial approach to aneurysm resection and patch repair. **C,** Presentation of aneurysm into the right ventricle exposed for repair through right ventriculotomy. **D,** Subpulmonic aneurysm with or without a ventricular septal defect exposed for repair through pulmonary arteriotomy.

23,31,35,41–43,63,103,104]. Approaching the defect only through the chamber has been advocated selectively when there is no coexisting ventricular septal defect or significant aortic insufficiency [27,105].

With either approach, the aorta is first opened for direct coronary cardioplegia delivery and to determine the anatomy of the root. This method also provides direct vision of the aneurysm orifice to prevent injury or distortion of the aortic leaflet, annulus, or coronary ostium, allows inspection for an associated ventricular septal defect,

and allows repair or replacement of the aortic valve when indicated. Careful inspection for an associated ventricular septal defect is essential, because this lesion is frequently missed at angiography or echocardiography [19,20].

Nonruptured aneurysms involving the noncoronary sinus without penetration into an adjacent chamber, the rare case involving the left sinus, or those penetrating the ventricular septum [66,67] can be repaired through an aortic approach alone. However, ruptured aneurysms involving the right or noncoronary sinus or nonruptured aneurysms with extensive penetration into an adjacent chamber are best repaired with a combined approach through the aorta and the chamber of penetration. The chamber of penetration is opened to facilitate resection of the aneurysmal sac and to reinforce the repair with a patch without injuring the conduction system. Aneurysms penetrating into the right atrium or membranous septum from the posterior third of the right sinus or from the noncoronary sinus can be approached through the right atrium. Those penetrating into the right ventricular outflow tract can usually be approached from the pulmonary artery, through the pulmonary valve. Right ventriculotomy usually is not necessary and avoided whenever possible. It is needed only for the occasional case in which the aneurysm arises from the middle third of the right sinus penetrating the region of the crista and cannot be adequately visualized through either the right atrium or the pulmonary artery.

Although a small aneurysm without associated ventricular septal defect can be closed primarily, this has been associated with a higher recurrence rate [6,8,11,16,35,39, 41,63,106,107]. Therefore, after resection of the aneurysmal sac, primary closure of the sinus defect or closure with a pericardial patch should be reinforced with a separate synthetic patch through the chamber of penetration to buttress the weakened aortic sinus and reduce the risk of recurrence. Leaving the closed neck of the aneurysm as the floor of the reconstructed sinus, and buttressing it with a nonelastic patch of Dacron, polytetrafluoroethylene, or other material forms a double layer between the aortic lumen and the right-sided chamber and reduces the risk of residual fistulous connection or recurrence. An associated ventricular septal defect may be closed through the right side either with a single patch or with a separate patch. Closure of an associated ventricular septal defect through the right side reduces the risk of conduction system injury.

Moderate or severe aortic valve insufficiency should be corrected after the sinus of Valsalva and ventricular septal defect repair to avoid distortion of the aortic valve repair. Mild aortic insufficiency rarely necessitates correction but should be carefully followed long-term, owing to a small but significant risk of progression [16,35,108]. Closure of an associated ventricular septal defect, particularly of the subarterial type below the posterior third of the right sinus, may be sufficient to prevent aortic insufficiency. However, additional aortic valvuloplasty or annuloplasty by the techniques of Trusler [109], Carpentier [110], Cosgrove [111], or Schafers [112] may be necessary. Aortic valve replacement may be necessary when there is a severely deformed insufficient or stenotic bicuspid valve, endocarditis, or failure of a repair. Complete aortic root replacement with a valved conduit and coronary reimplantation is rarely indicated unless multiple sinuses are involved. Multiple sinus involvement is rarely seen with isolated congenital sinus of Valsalva aneurysm, but is usually associated with a connective tissue abnormality (e.g., Marfan's or Ehlers–Danlos), or extensive endocarditis.

Intraoperative transesophageal echocardiography is strongly recommended for evaluation of the sinus of Valsalva aneurysm, the aortic valve, and associated anomalies such as a ventricular septal defect. More importantly, it is essential to evaluate the effectiveness of repair, including residual fistulous communications, ventricular septal defect, aortic insufficiency, tricuspid or pulmonary valve function, ventricular function, and the adequacy of de-airing.

Percutaneous transcatheter closure of a ruptured right sinus of Valsalva aneurysm was first reported in 1994 using a Rashkind umbrella device [113]. Several recent series have also reported excellent early results using an Amplatzer duct occluder device [114] or an Amplatzer septal occluder device [115] for transcatheter closure of small ruptured sinus of Valsalva aneurysms. However, follow-up has been limited, and concerns remain regarding the increased risk of endocarditis and hemolysis associated with incomplete closure. Device closure is not appropriate for cases with significant aortic insufficiency or ventricular septal defect [116].

Results

The results of surgical repair for congenital sinus of Valsalva aneurysms, without complicating factors such as endocarditis, are excellent using modern techniques of cardiopulmonary bypass and myocardial preservation. Several contemporary surgical series have had no operative mortality even when repair of a ventricular septal defect or aortic valve replacement has been necessary [18,29,31, 35,105,108]. Most other surgical series, even those extending back into the 1960s, report operative mortality of less than 5% [12,15–17,19–21,23,27,29,63,103,107,117]. The long-term results are also excellent with actuarial 10-year survival rates of 90–100% in recent western series [16,29,35], and 85–94% in Asian series [17,18,27,108]. The long-term functional results are quite acceptable with 90–100% of patients staying in New York Heart Association class I or II [19,21,27,29]. Although generally infrequent (<5%), the recurrence rate of fistula or ventricular septal defect seems to be higher when simple suture without patch repair is employed [6,8,11,16,17,35,39,41,63,106,107]. Late problems with prosthetic aortic valves or progressive native aortic insufficiency may necessitate reoperation in up to 30% of patients [16,18,27,31,35,105,108]. Progressive or recurrent native aortic insufficiency has been attributed to coexistent ventricular septal defect [16,118], coexistent bicuspid aortic valve [35], suture rather than patch repair [107,119], and the surgical approach [16,105].

The role of surgery for asymptomatic nonruptured sinus of Valsalva aneurysms remains controversial [45,46].

The wider use of echocardiography, computerized tomography, and magnetic resonance imaging for a wide variety of noncardiac conditions has resulted in more frequent detection of asymptomatic sinus of Valsalva aneurysm with unknown natural history. Rare case reports of prolonged survival [120] have prompted some authors to recommend medical follow-up evaluation of patients with asymptomatic nonruptured sinus of Valsalva aneurysms [46,121]. However, the results of repair in most experienced centers are excellent with operative mortality rates approaching zero. Meanwhile, reports of acute myocardial infarction [56,60], thromboembolism [76–78], complete heart block [65,70,83], malignant arrhythmias [74], and sudden death due to rupture [79,80] have been reported in association with previously unruptured sinus of Valsalva aneurysms. In addition, secondary bacterial endocarditis or progressive enlargement [57,122] can create a much riskier procedure at the time of repair. Therefore, we agree with most other authors that repair of a sinus of Valsalva aneurysm in adults should be undertaken at the time of diagnosis to prevent the numerous complications associated with lesions that are not repaired [29,31]. This recommendation is made with acknowledgment of the lack of good natural history studies, but these are unlikely to be performed. However, close follow-up care can be considered for children with small nonruptured aneurysms because of the risk of asymmetric distortion of the aortic valve caused by limiting growth of the affected sinus with patch material.

References

1. Hope J. (1839) *A Treatise on the Diseases of the Heart and Great Vessels*, 3rd ed. Philadelphia, PA: Lea & Blanchard.
2. Thurnam J. (1840) On aneurysms, and especially spontaneous varicose aneurysms of ascending aorta and sinus of Valsalva, with cases. Med-Chir Trans (London) 23, 323–384.
3. Abbott M. (1919) Clinical and developmental study of a case of ruptured aneurysm of the right anterior aortic sinus of Valsalva. In: Osier W, ed. *Contributions to Medical and Biological Research*. New York: Paul B Hoeber.
4. Jones A. (1949) Aortic sinus aneurysms. Br Heart J 11, 325.
5. Brown J, Heath D, Whitaker W. (1955) Cardio-aortic fistula: A case diagnosed in life and treated surgically. Circulation 12, 819–826.
6. Barragry TP, Ring WS, Moller JH, et al. (1988) 15- to 30-year follow-up of patients undergoing repair of ruptured congenital aneurysms of the sinus of Valsalva. Ann Thorac Surg 46, 515–519.
7. Lillehei CW, Stanley P, Varco RL. (1957) Surgical treatment of ruptured aneurysms of the sinus of Valsalva. Ann Surg 146, 459–472.
8. Bigelow WG, Barnes WT. (1959) Ruptured aneurysm of aortic sinus. Ann Surg 150, 117–121.
9. McGoon DC, Edwards JE, Kirklin JW. (1958) Surgical treatment of ruptured aneurysm of aortic sinus. Ann Surg 147, 387–392.
10. Morrow AG, Baker RR, Hanson HE, et al. (1957) Successful surgical repair of a ruptured aneurysm of the sinus of Valsalva. Circulation 16, 533–538.
11. Smith W. (1914) Aneurysm of the sinus of Valsalva with report of two cases. JAMA 62, 1878–1880.
12. Henze A, Huttunen H, Bjork VO. (1983) Ruptured sinus of valsalva aneurysms. Scand J Thorac Cardiovasc Surg 17, 249–253.
13. Mayer ED, Ruffmann K, Saggau W, et al. (1986) Ruptured aneurysms of the sinus of Valsalva. Ann Thorac Surg 42, 81–85.
14. Meyer J, Wukasch DC, Hallman GL, et al. (1975) Aneurysm and fistula of the sinus of Valsalva. Clinical considerations and surgical treatment in 45 patients. Ann Thorac Surg 19, 170–179.
15. Takach TJ, Reul GJ, Duncan JM, et al. (1999) Sinus of Valsalva aneurysm or fistula: management and outcome. Ann Thorac Surg 68, 1573–1577.
16. van Son JA, Danielson GK, Schaff HV, et al. (1994) Long-term outcome of surgical repair of ruptured sinus of Valsalva aneurysm. Circulation 90, II20–II29.
17. Abe T, Komatsu S. (1988) Surgical repair and long-term results in ruptured sinus of Valsalva aneurysm. Ann Thorac Surg 46, 520–525.
18. Au WK, Chiu SW, Mok CK, et al. (1998) Repair of ruptured sinus of valsalva aneurysm: determinants of long-term survival. Ann Thorac Surg 66, 1604–1610.
19. Choudhary SK, Bhan A, Sharma R, et al. (1997) Sinus of Valsalva aneurysms: 20 years' experience. J Card Surg 12, 300–308.
20. Chu SH, Hung CR, How SS, et al. (1990) Ruptured aneurysms of the sinus of Valsalva in Oriental patients. J Thorac Cardiovasc Surg 99, 288–298.
21. Dong C, Wu QY, Tang Y. (2002) Ruptured sinus of Valsalva aneurysm: a Beijing experience. Ann Thorac Surg 74, 1621–1624.
22. Lin CY, Hong GJ, Lee KC, et al. (2004) Ruptured congenital sinus of valsalva aneurysms. J Card Surg 19, 99–102.
23. Pannu HS, Shivaprakash K, Bazaz S, et al. (1995) Geographical variations in the presentation of ruptured aneurysms of sinuses of Valsalva: evaluation of surgical repair. J Card Surg 10, 316–324.
24. Taguchi K, Sasaki N, Matsuura Y, et al. (1969) Surgical correction of aneurysm of the sinus of Valsalva. A report of forty-five consecutive patients including eight with total replacement of the aortic valve. Am J Cardiol 23, 180–191.
25. Tanabe T, Yokota A, Sugie S. (1979) Surgical treatment of aneurysms of the sinus of Valsalva. Ann Thorac Surg 27, 133–136.
26. Verghese M, Jairaj PS, Babuthaman C, et al. (1986) Surgical treatment of ruptured aneurysms of the sinus of Valsalva. Ann Thorac Surg 41, 284–286.
27. Yan F, Huo Q, Qiao J, et al. (2008) Surgery for sinus of Valsalva aneurysm: 27-year experience with 100 patients. Asian Cardiovasc Thorac Ann 16, 361–365.

28. Tatsuno K, Konno S, Sakakibara S. (1973) Ventricular septal defect with aortic insufficiency. Angiocardiographic aspects and a new classification. Am Heart J 85, 13–21.

29. Moustafa S, Mookadam F, Cooper L, et al. (2007) Sinus of Valsalva aneurysms – 47 years of a single center experience and systematic overview of published reports. Am J Cardiol 99, 1159–1164.

30. Nowicki ER, Aberdeen E, Friedman S, et al. (1977) Congenital left aortic sinus-left ventricle fistula and review of aortocardiac fistulas. Ann Thorac Surg 23, 378–388.

31. Wang ZJ, Zou CW, Li DC, et al. (2007) Surgical repair of sinus of Valsalva aneurysm in Asian patients. Ann Thorac Surg 84, 156–160.

32. Breviere GM, Vaksmann G, Francart C. (1990) Rupture of a sinus of Valsalva aneurysm in a neonate. Eur J Pediatr 149, 603–604.

33. Perry LW, Martin GR, Galioto FM Jr, et al. (1991) Rupture of congenital sinus of Valsalva aneurysm in a newborn. Am J Cardiol 68, 1255–1256.

34. Ring WS. (2003) Sinus of Valsalva aneurysm. In: Mavroudis C, Backer CL, eds. Pediatric Cardiac Surgery, 3rd ed. Philadelphia, PA: Mosby, Inc.

35. Azakie A, David TE, Peniston CM, et al. (2000) Ruptured sinus of Valsalva aneurysm: early recurrence and fate of the aortic valve. Ann Thorac Surg 70, 1466–1470; discussion 1470–1471.

36. Edwards JE, Burchell HB. (1956) Specimen exhibiting the essential lesion in aneurysm of the aortic sinus. Proc Staff Meet Mayo Clin 31, 407–412.

37. Edwards JE, Burchell HB. (1957) The pathological anatomy of deficiencies between the aortic root and the heart, including aortic sinus aneurysms. Thorax 12, 125–139.

38. Angelini P. (2005) Aortic sinus aneurysm and associated defects: can we extrapolate a morphogenetic theory from pathologic findings? Tex Heart Inst J 32, 560–562.

39. Sakakibara S, Konno S. (1962) Congenital aneurysms of sinus of Valsalva. A clinical study. Am Heart J 63, 708–719.

40. Sakakibara S, Konno S. (1962) Congenital aneurysm of the sinus of Valsalva. Anatomy and classification. Am Heart J 63, 405–424.

41. Sakakibara S, Konno S. (1963) Congenital aneurysm of the sinus of Valsalva. Criteria for recommending surgery. Am J Cardiol 12, 100–106.

42. Sakakibara S, Konno S. (1968) Congenital aneurysm of the sinus of Valsalva associated with ventricular septal defect. Anatomical aspects. Am Heart J 75, 595–603.

43. Ring WS. (2000) Congenital Heart Surgery Nomenclature and Database Project: Aortic aneurysm, sinus of Valsalva aneurysm, and aortic dissection. Ann Thorac Surg 69 (Suppl), S147–S163.

44. Adams JE, Sawyers JL, Scott HW Jr. (1957) Surgical treatment of aneurysms of the aortic sinuses with aorticoatrial fistula; experimental and clinical study. Surgery 41, 26–42.

45. Holman WL. (1995) Aneurysms of the sinuses of Valsalva. In: Sabiston, DC, Spencer FC, eds. Surgery of the Chest, 6th ed. Philadelphia, PA: W.B. Saunders, pp. 1316–1326.

46. Kirklin JW, Barratt-Boyes BG. (2003) Congenital sinus of Valsalva aneurysm and aortico-left ventricular tunnel. In: Kouchoukos NT, Hanley FL, et al., eds. Kirklin/Barratt-Boyes Cardiac Surgery, 3rd ed. Philadelphia, PA: Churchill Livingstone, pp. 911–927.

47. London SB, London RE. (1961) Production of aortic regurgitation by unperforated aneurysm of the sinus of Valsalva. Circulation 24, 1403–1406.

48. Desai AG, Sharma S, Kumar A, et al. (1985) Echocardiographic diagnosis of unruptured aneurysm of right sinus of Valsalva: an unusual cause of right ventricular outflow obstruction. Am Heart J 109, 363–364.

49. Gelfand EV, Bzymek D, Johnstone MT. (2007) Images in cardiovascular medicine. Sinus of Valsalva aneurysm with right ventricular outflow tract obstruction: evaluation with Doppler, real-time 3-dimensional and contrast echocardiography. Circulation 115, e16–e17.

50. Haraphongse M, Ayudhya RK, Jugdutt B, et al. (1990) Isolated unruptured sinus of Valsalva aneurysm producing right ventricular outflow obstruction. Cathet Cardiovasc Diagn 19, 98–102.

51. Kiefaber RW, Tabakin BS, Coffin LH, et al. (1986) Unruptured sinus of Valsalva aneurysm with right ventricular outflow obstruction diagnosed by two-dimensional and Doppler echocardiography. J Am Coll Cardiol 7, 438–442.

52. Liang CD, Chang JP, Kao CL. (1996) Unruptured sinus of Valsalva aneurysm with right ventricular outflow tract obstruction associated with ventricular septal defect. Cathet Cardiovasc Diagn 37, 158–161.

53. Liau CS, Chu IT, Ho FM. (1999) Unruptured congenital aneurysm of the sinus of Valsalva presenting with pulmonary stenosis. Catheter Cardiovasc Interv 46, 210–213.

54. Shiraishi S, Watarida S, Katsuyama K, et al. (1998) Unruptured aneurysm of the sinus of Valsalva into the pulmonary artery. Ann Thorac Surg 65, 1458–1459.

55. Warnes CA, Maron BJ, Jones M, et al. (1984) Asymptomatic sinus of Valsalva aneurysm causing right ventricular outflow obstruction before and after rupture. Am J Cardiol 54, 1383–1384.

56. Brandt J, Jogi P, Luhrs C. (1985) Sinus of Valsalva aneurysm obstructing coronary arterial flow: case report and collective review of the literature. Eur Heart J 6, 1069–1073.

57. Faillace RT, Greenland P, Nanda NC. (1985) Rapid expansion of a saccular aneurysm on the left coronary sinus of Valsalva: a role for early surgical repair? Br Heart J 54, 442–444.

58. Garcia-Rinaldi R, Von Koch L, Howell JF. (1976) Aneurysm of the sinus of Valsalva producing obstruction of the left main coronary artery. J Thorac Cardiovasc Surg 72, 123–126.

59. Hiyamuta K, Ohtsuki T, Shimamatsu M, et al. (1983) Aneurysm of the left aortic sinus causing acute myocardial infarction. Circulation 67, 1151–1154.

60. Lijoi A, Parodi E, Passerone GC, et al. (2002) Unruptured aneurysm of the left sinus of valsalva causing coronary insufficiency: case report and review of the literature. Tex Heart Inst J 29, 40–44.

61. Pigula FA, Griffith BP, Kormos RL. (1997) Massive sinus of Valsalva aneurysm presenting with coronary insufficiency. Ann Thorac Surg 64, 1475–1476.

62. Takahara Y, Sudo Y, Sunazawa T, *et al.* (1998) Aneurysm of the left sinus of Valsalva producing aortic valve regurgitation and myocardial ischemia. Ann Thorac Surg 65, 535–537.

63. Trevelyan J, Patel R, Mattu R. (2000) Complications from Sinus of Valsalva aneurysm–a case of stable ischemia from compression of the left main stem and one of surgical recurrence. J Invasive Cardiol 12, 277–279.

64. Williams TG, Williams BT. (1983) Isolated unruptured aneurysm of the left coronary sinus of Valsalva. Ann Thorac Surg 35, 556–559.

65. Ahmad RA, Sturman S, Watson RD. (1989) Unruptured aneurysm of the sinus of Valsalva presenting with isolated heart block: echocardiographic diagnosis and successful surgical repair. Br Heart J 61, 375–377.

66. Bapat VN, Tendolkar AG, Khandeparkar J, *et al.* (1997) Aneurysms of sinus of Valsalva eroding into the interventricular septum: etiopathology and surgical considerations. Eur J Cardiothorac Surg 12, 759–765.

67. Choudhary SK, Bhan A, Reddy SC, *et al.* (1998) Aneurysm of sinus of Valsalva dissecting into interventricular septum. Ann Thorac Surg 65, 735–740.

68. Duras PF. (1944) Heart block with aneurysm of the aortic sinus. Br Heart J 6, 61–65.

69. Heydorn WH, Nelson WP, Fitterer JD, *et al.* (1976) Congenital aneurysm of the sinus of Valsalva protruding into the left ventricle. Review of diagnosis and treatment of the unruptured aneurysm. J Thorac Cardiovasc Surg 71, 839–845.

70. Metras D, Coulibaly AO, Ouattara K. (1982) Calcified unruptured aneurysm of sinus of Valsalva with complete heart block and aortic regurgitation. Successful repair in one case. Br Heart J 48, 507–509.

71. Raffa H, Mosieri J, Sorefan AA, *et al.* (1991) Sinus of Valsalva aneurysm eroding into the interventricular septum. Ann Thorac Surg 51, 996–998.

72. Wu Q, Xu J, Shen X, *et al.* (2002) Surgical treatment of dissecting aneurysm of the interventricular septum. Eur J Cardiothorac Surg 22, 517–520.

73. Channer KS, Hutter JA, George M. (1988) Unruptured aneurysm of the sinus of Valsalva presenting with ventricular tachycardia. Eur Heart J 9, 186–190.

74. Raizes GS, Smith HC, Vlietstra RE, *et al.* (1979) Ventricular tachycardia secondary to aneurysm of sinus of Valsalva. J Thorac Cardiovasc Surg 78, 110–115.

75. Reid PG, Goudevenos JA, Hilton CJ. (1990) Thrombosed saccular aneurysm of a sinus of Valsalva: unusual cause of a mediastinal mass. Br Heart J 63, 183–185.

76. Shahrabani RM, Jairaj PS. (1993) Unruptured aneurysm of the sinus of Valsalva: a potential source of cerebrovascular embolism. Br Heart J 69, 266–267.

77. Stollberger C, Seitelberger R, Fenninger C, *et al.* (1996) Aneurysm of the left sinus of Valsalva. An unusual source of cerebral embolism. Stroke 27, 1424–1426.

78. Wortham DC, Gorman PD, Hull RW, *et al.* (1993) Unruptured sinus of Valsalva aneurysm presenting with embolization. Am Heart J 125, 896–898.

79. Brabham KR, Roberts WC. (1990) Fatal intrapericardial rupture of sinus of Valsalva aneurysm. Am Heart J 120, 1455–1456.

80. Munk MD, Gatzoulis MA, King DE, *et al.* (1999) Cardiac tamponade and death from intrapericardial rupture corrected. of sinus of Valsalva aneurysm. Eur J Cardiothorac Surg 15, 100–102.

81. Killen DA, Wathanacharoen S, Pogson GW Jr. (1987) Repair of intrapericardial rupture of left sinus of Valsalva aneurysm. Ann Thorac Surg 44, 310–311.

82. Weijerse A, van der Schoot MJ, Maat LP, *et al.* (2008) Cardiac tamponade due to a ruptured aneurysm of the sinus of valsalva. J Card Surg 23, 256–258.

83. Walters MI, Ettles D, Guvendik L, *et al.* (1998) Interventricular septal expansion of a sinus of Valsalva aneurysm: a rare cause of complete heart block. Heart 80, 202–203.

84. Wu Q. (1997) Surgical treatment of dissecting aneurysm of the interventricular septum. Ann Thorac Surg 63, 545–547.

85. Cooperberg P, Mercer EN, Mulder DS, *et al.* (1974) Rupture of a sinus Valsalva aneurysm. Report of a case diagnosed preoperatively by echocardiography. Radiology 113, 171–172.

86. Rothbaum DA, Dillon JC, Chang S, *et al.* (1974) Echocardiographic manifestation of right sinus of Valsalva aneurysm. Circulation 49, 768–771.

87. Chiang CW, Lin FC, Fang BR, *et al.* (1988) Doppler and two-dimensional echocardiographic features of sinus of Valsalva aneurysm. Am Heart J 116, 1283–1288.

88. Dev V, Goswami KC, Shrivastava S, *et al.* (1993) Echocardiographic diagnosis of aneurysm of the sinus of Valsalva. Am Heart J 126, 930–936.

89. Engel PJ, Held JS, van der Bel-Kahn J, *et al.* (1981) Echocardiographic diagnosis of congenital sinus of Valsalva aneurysm with dissection of the interventricular septum. Circulation 63, 705–711.

90. Sahasakul Y, Panchavinnin P, Chaithiraphan S, *et al.* (1990) Echocardiographic diagnosis of a ruptured aneurysm of the sinus of Valsalva: operation without catheterisation in seven patients. Br Heart J 64, 195–198.

91. Terdjman M, Bourdarias JP, Farcot JC, *et al.* (1984) Aneurysms of sinus of Valsalva: two-dimensional echocardiographic diagnosis and recognition of rupture into the right heart cavities. J Am Coll Cardiol 3, 1227–1235.

92. Xu Q, Peng Z, Rahko PS. (1995) Doppler echocardiographic characteristics of sinus of valsalva aneurysms. Am Heart J 130, 1265–1269.

93. Blackshear JL, Safford RE, Lane GE, *et al.* (1991) Unruptured noncoronary sinus of Valsalva aneurysm: preoperative characterization by transesophageal echocardiography. J Am Soc Echocardiogr 4, 485–490.

94. McKenney PA, Shemin RJ, Wiegers SE. (1992) Role of transesophageal echocardiography in sinus of Valsalva aneurysm. Am Heart J 123, 228–229.

95. Wang KY, St John Sutton M, Ho HY, *et al.* (1997) Congenital sinus of Valsalva aneurysm: a multiplane transesophageal echocardiographic experience. J Am Soc Echocardiogr 10, 956–963.

96. Hamid IA, Jothi M, Rajan S, *et al.* (1994) Transaortic repair of ruptured aneurysm of sinus of Valsalva. Fifteen-year experience. J Thorac Cardiovasc Surg 107, 1464–1468.

97. Goldberg N, Krasnow N. (1990) Sinus of Valsalva aneurysms. Clin Cardiol 13, 831–836.

98. Dincer TC, Basarici I, Calisir C, *et al.* (2008) Ruptured aneurysm of noncoronary sinus of Valsalva: demonstration with magnetic resonance imaging. Acta Radiol 49, 889–892.

99. Ho VB, Kinney JB, Sahn DJ. (1995) Ruptured sinus of Valsalva aneurysm: cine phase-contrast MR characterization. J Comput Assist Tomogr 19, 652–656.

100. Karaaslan T, Gudinchet F, Payot M, *et al.* (1999) Congenital aneurysm of sinus of valsalva ruptured into right ventricle diagnosed by magnetic resonance imaging. Pediatr Cardiol 20, 212–214.

101. Ogawa T, Iwama Y, Hashimoto H, *et al.* (1991) Noninvasive methods in the diagnosis of ruptured aneurysm of Valsalva. Usefulness of magnetic resonance imaging and Doppler echocardiography. Chest 100, 579–581.

102. Roche KJ, Genieser NB, Ambrosino MM. (1998) Resonance imaging of a ruptured aneurysm of the sinus of Valsalva. Cardiol Young 8, 393–395.

103. Harkness JR, Fitton TP, Barreiro CJ, *et al.* (2005) A 32-year experience with surgical repair of sinus of valsalva aneurysms. J Card Surg 20, 198–204.

104. Lukacs L, Bartek I, Haan A, *et al.* (1992) Ruptured aneurysms of the sinus of Valsalva. Eur J Cardiothorac Surg 6, 15–17.

105. Jung SH, Yun TJ, Im YM, *et al.* (2008) Ruptured sinus of Valsalva aneurysm: transaortic repair may cause sinus of Valsalva distortion and aortic regurgitation. J Thorac Cardiovasc Surg 135, 1153–1158.

106. Qiang G, Dong Z, Xing X, *et al.* (1994) Surgical treatment of ruptured aneurysm of the sinus of Valsalva. Cardiol Young 4, 347–353.

107. Vural KM, Sener E, Tasdemir O, *et al.* (2001) Approach to sinus of Valsalva aneurysms: a review of 53 cases. Eur J Cardiothorac Surg 20, 71–76.

108. Murashita T, Kubota T, Kamikubo Y, *et al.* (2002) Long-term results of aortic valve regurgitation after repair of ruptured sinus of valsalva aneurysm. Ann Thorac Surg 73, 1466–1471.

109. Trusler GA, Moes CA, Kidd BS. (1973) Repair of ventricular septal defect with aortic insufficiency. J Thorac Cardiovasc Surg 66, 394–403.

110. Carpentier A. (1983) Cardiac valve surgery–the "French correction". J Thorac Cardiovasc Surg 86, 323–337.

111. Cosgrove DM, Rosenkranz ER, Hendren WG, *et al.* (1991) Valvuloplasty for aortic insufficiency. J Thorac Cardiovasc Surg 102, 571–576; discussion 576–577.

112. Schafers HJ, Langer F, Aicher D, *et al.* (2000) Remodeling of the aortic root and reconstruction of the bicuspid aortic valve. Ann Thorac Surg 70, 542–546.

113. Cullen S, Somerville J, Redington A. (1994) Transcatheter closure of a ruptured aneurysm of the sinus of Valsalva. Br Heart J 71, 479–480.

114. Zhao SH, Yan CW, Zhu XY, *et al.* (2008) Transcatheter occlusion of the ruptured sinus of Valsalva aneurysm with an Amplatzer duct occluder. Int J Cardiol 129, 81–85.

115. Arora R, Trehan V, Rangasetty UM, *et al.* (2004) Transcatheter closure of ruptured sinus of valsalva aneurysm. J Interv Cardiol 17, 53–58.

116. Rao PS, Bromberg BI, Jureidini SB, *et al.* (2003) Transcatheter occlusion of ruptured sinus of valsalva aneurysm: innovative use of available technology. Catheter Cardiovasc Interv 58, 130–134.

117. Babacan KM, Tasdemir O, Zengin M, *et al.* (1986) Fistulous communication of aortic sinuses into the cardiac chambers. Fifteen years surgical experience and a report of 23 patients. Jpn Heart J 27, 865–870.

118. Naka Y, Kadoba K, Ohtake S, *et al.* (2000) The long-term outcome of a surgical repair of sinus of valsalva aneurysm. Ann Thorac Surg 70, 727–729.

119. Pasic M, von Segesser L, Carrel T, *et al.* (1992) Ruptured congenital aneurysm of the sinus of Valsalva: surgical technique and long-term follow-up. Eur J Cardiothorac Surg 6, 542–544.

120. Martin LW, Hsu I, Schwartz H, *et al.* (1986) Congenital aneurysm of the left sinus of Valsalva. Report of a patient with 19-year survival without surgery. Chest 90, 143–145.

121. Howard RJ, Moller J, Castaneda AR, *et al.* (1973) Surgical correction of sinus of Valsalva aneurysm. J Thorac Cardiovasc Surg 66, 420–427.

122. Jebara VA, Chauvaud S, Portoghese M, *et al.* (1992) Isolated extracardiac unruptured sinus of Valsalva aneurysms. Ann Thorac Surg 54, 323–326.

38

Coronary Artery Anomalies

Constantine Mavroudis[1], Ali Dodge-Khatami[2], Carl L. Backer[3], and Richard Lorber[4]

[1]Florida Hospital for Children, Orlando, FL, USA
[2]University Heart Center, Hamburg, Germany
[3]Ann & Robert H. Lurie Children's Hospital of Chicago, formerly Children's Memorial Hospital, Chicago, IL, USA
[4]Cleveland Clinic Children's Hospital, Cleveland, OH, USA

Introduction

Congenital and acquired anomalies of the coronary arteries can be generally characterized as deviations from the standard anatomy of two patent and separately arising right and left arterial blood vessels. The arteries are the first branches of the ascending aorta, arise from their respective sinuses of Valsalva, and gradually branch distally in a gradual and centrifugal fashion. Anomalies may be schematically summarized by a lack of origin, abnormal origin, anomalous course, lack of patency, abnormal connections, and/or abnormal drainage of the coronary vessels. Congenital and acquired coronary artery anomalies are associated with significant morbidity and mortality owing to patterns of ischemia, infarction, and fistulous connections, which can lead to cardiac failure.

The spectrum of congenital coronary artery malformations includes 1) anomalous left or right coronary artery (RCA) arising from the pulmonary artery (PA); 2) anomalous aortic origin of the left main or right coronary arteries with or without obstructing intramural stenotic courses and acute angulation; 3) single coronary artery with or without anomalous course between the aorta and PA; 4) congenital atresia/stenosis of the left main coronary artery (LMCA); 5) coronary artery fistulas; and 6) coronary artery bridging. The spectrum of acquired coronary lesions includes 1) coronary artery aneurysms and stenoses associated with Kawasaki disease; 2) iatrogenic injuries caused by transcutaneous invasive procedures or surgical mishaps; and 3) the rare instances of sharp or blunt trauma.

These anomalies are described in hearts with concordant atrioventricular and ventriculoarterial connections. The multiple coronary artery variations in complex heart diseases, such as transposition of the great arteries, truncus arteriosus, and pulmonary atresia with intact ventricular septum, among others, will be discussed in the chapters dedicated to that subject.

The incidence of coronary anomalies in the general population is 0.2–1.2%. Various anomalies have been described since the 17th century, both clinically and on the basis of postmortem pathologic studies. The first landmark article, to which most authors refer, is attributed to Ogden [1], who in 1969 attempted a comprehensive classification from which the many modifications of nomenclature are derived (Table 38.1) [1]. This classification includes major, minor, and secondary anomalies, determined purely on the basis of anatomic considerations (e.g., minor is a coronary arising directly from aorta with a normal distal distribution; major is an abnormal coronary origin from the PA or abnormal communications of the coronary arteries with intracardiac structures). In light of the clinical and surgical significance of these lesions, it is debatable whether minor and major are appropriate terms in the current era. In this chapter, regarding all further classifications for coronary artery anomalies, the inclusive nomenclature system of the Society of Thoracic Surgeons (STS) Congenital Heart Surgery Nomenclature and Database Project, including all possible variations, will be referred to and used [2].

Diagnostic modalities for congenital cardiac abnormalities have evolved rapidly over the last years, and a thorough review is beyond the scope of this chapter. Although a physical examination, electrocardiogram (ECG) and chest radiograph remain integral components of the diagnostic work-up, these are undeniably complemented and almost supplanted by color flow mapping and tomographic cross-sectional imaging echocardiography. More recently,

Table 38.1 Congenital variations of the coronary artery. (Reproduced with permission from Ogden [1].)

Minor coronary variations
High take-off
Multiple ostia
Anomalous circumflex artery origin
Anomalous anterior descending artery origin
Absent proximal ostium/single ostium in other aortic sinus
Hypoplastic proximal coronary artery
Congenital proximal coronary artery
Congenital distal stenosis
Coronary artery from the posterior aortic sinus
Ventricular origin of an accessory coronary artery

Major coronary anomalies
Coronary "arteriovenous" fistula
Anomalous origin from the pulmonary artery
    Left coronary artery
    Right coronary artery
    Both coronary arteries

Secondary coronary anomalies
Secondary coronary "arteriovenous" fistula
Variations in transposition of the great vessels
Variations in truncus arteriosus
Variations in tetralogy of Fallot
Ectasia of coronary arteries in supravalvar aortic stenosis
Mural coronary artery

noninvasive magnetic resonance imaging (MRI) and computed tomography (CT) angiogram with ECG have gained increasing popularity and are the methods of choice as opposed to cardiac catheterization and coronary angiography in many leading centers [3,4], because the rate of erroneous diagnosis with conventional coronary angiography is reported to be as high as 50% in patients with coronary anomalies. Transverse sections of MRI or CT not only give the precise origin and proximal course in relation to the great vessels, but also assess the effect of coronary artery flow, with evaluation of the myocardial function, regional perfusion defects from associated ischemia, and coronary flow reserve. Indications for MR angiography include 1) uncertainty at conventional catheterization if this was performed as the primary investigation; 2) total proximal occlusion or suspicion of congenital absence of an epicardial coronary artery; 3) primary investigation for angina, arrhythmia, or syncope on exertion in young or adolescent patients; 4) evaluation before cardiac surgery to avoid intraoperative trauma, if there is an uncertain course of a known anomalous coronary; and 5) screening in highly competitive athletes to avoid increased risk of sudden death. The limitations of MR angiography are dependence on a regular heart rhythm (arrhythmias can distort the image) and the necessity for a calm and cooperative patient

with apnea during approximately 16 cardiac cycles. In babies and small children, this practically often means the need for intubation and mechanical ventilation. The usual contraindications to MRI are valid (e.g., pacemaker, intracranial clip, intraocular metal debris, claustrophobia). Compared with MRI, CT angiogram has the advantage of faster acquisition of high spatial resolution images and patient comfort. However, drawbacks of CT scanning include the exposure to radiation and iodinated contrast medium, which require strict adherence to CT voltage, amperage principles, and patient weight-adjustment to minimize radiation risk [3]. Coronary angiography is still considered by many as a first-line diagnostic tool, and certainly is useful when potential interventional measures may be anticipated (transcatheter embolization or coil occlusion). Angiography is particularly useful when diagnosing anomalies of connections to other vessels (bronchial or mediastinal), and in delineating coronary fistula [3].

Anomalous Left Coronary Artery from Pulmonary Artery

Anomalous left coronary artery originating from the pulmonary artery (ALCAPA) is a rare congenital anomaly first described by Brooks [5] in 1885. It is present in 1 of 300 000 live births (0.25–0.5%). It is the most common of the abnormal origins of coronary arteries and is the most common cause of myocardial ischemia and infarction in children [6]. This anomaly may cause myocardial ischemia or infarction, mitral insufficiency, congestive heart failure, and death in early infancy if not treated. In 1933, Bland, White, and Garland [7] described the full clinical spectrum including angina and myocardial ischemia resulting from abnormal coronary flow, and the syndrome bearing their name is synonymous to ALCAPA.

Pathophysiology

Edwards [8] is credited with the first pathophysiological explanation of coronary flow patterns in patients with ALCAPA. The onset of symptoms and the degree of myocardial ischemia depend on a balance between the rapidity of ductus closure, maintenance of pulmonary hypertension, and development of intercoronary collateral vessels to provide retrograde perfusion from the RCA to the ALCAPA [8]. This pathophysiologic concept historically led to a division of ALCAPA patients into two groups, infantile and adult, according to their coronary circulation patterns [8]. The infantile type of circulation has little or no intercoronary collateral development. The result is early onset of symptoms—days to weeks after birth. Severe myocardial ischemia, left ventricular dysfunction and dilatation, mitral regurgitation from papillary muscle ischemia, and rapid death can occur. Adult-type circulation accounts for 10–15% of cases with Bland-White-Garland syndrome and depends on intercoronary collateral vessels from the RCA that provide adequate flow into the anomalous left coronary artery. These patients may have no symptoms for decades and may have only mild to moderate myocardial damage. Survival to adulthood is conditionally possible in the presence of a large dominant RCA and a restrictive opening between the anomalous left coronary artery and the PA. This subset of patients has an estimated 80–90% incidence of sudden death at a mean age of 35 years [9]. This incidence indicates the severity of the process even in patients who do not have symptoms and thereby justifies surgical therapy as soon as the diagnosis is made. In addition to the infantile and adult categorization, a descriptive classification proposed in 1989 by Smith and associates [10] delineates various patterns of origin and their possible surgical implications. Regarding a classification, ALCAPA is an anomalous pulmonary origin of a coronary artery (APOCA) (Table 38.2) [2]; as it is the most common of all abnormal origins of coronary arteries, it is treated separately in this chapter. Incorporating Smith's classification, an inclusive nomenclature system including all possible variations of ALCAPA origin is described in the STS Congenital Heart Surgery Nomenclature and Database Project (Figure 38.1) [2].

Table 38.2 Proposed and accepted classification of anomalous pulmonary origins of coronary arteries. (Reproduced with permission from Dodge-Khatami *et al.* [2].)

Type 1 Anomalous origin of the left main coronary artery from the pulmonary artery
   From right-hand sinus (sinus 1)
   From nonfacing pulmonary sinus
   From left-hand sinus (sinus 2)
   From commissure between sinus 1 and nonfacing sinus
   From commissure between sinus 2 and nonfacing sinus
   From commissure between sinus 1 and sinus 2
   High takeoff from left or right pulmonary arteries

Type 2 Anomalous origin of the right coronary artery

Type 3 Anomalous origin of circumflex coronary artery from pulmonary artery

Type 4 Anomalous right and left coronary arteries from the pulmonary artery (both)

Convention: Sinus of pulmonary valve designated right hand (no. 1), and left hand (no. 2) as viewed from nonfacing sinus of the pulmonary trunk toward the aorta. Thus sinus 1 of the aorta faces sinus 2 of pulmonary trunk and vice versa. Both nonfacing sinuses are at the two extremities.

Clinical Features

The clinical features of ALCAPA are sweating, dyspnea, failure to thrive, and atypical angina. Most patients have moderate to severe congestive heart failure with cardiomegaly on chest radiograph, ischemic signs on ECG, and a murmur of mitral insufficiency on auscultation. Left-axis deviation on the ECG is synonymous with a significant RCA-dominant circulation [11]. The diagnosis can be made with two-dimensional echocardiography alone (Figures 38.2, 38.3) [12]. Images show the enlarged, dilated RCA and a grossly hypokinetic and dilated left ventricle. Pulsed and color-flow Doppler ultrasonography can demonstrate reversal of flow from the anomalous left coronary artery into the PA that constitutes a left-to-right shunt. When necessary, MRI, CT angiography, or cardiac catheterization are used to exclude another coronary anomaly responsible for myocardial ischemia [13,14], to define coexisting intracardiac defects or to definitely exclude ALCAPA before settling for the diagnosis of idiopathic dilated cardiomyopathy [6]. They show the coronary anatomy in full detail, including the typically enlarged RCA, delayed passage of contrast medium, and the characteristic blush from the anomalous left coronary artery into the PA, as well as associated mitral valve regurgitation (Figure 38.4) [12]. Myocardial viability studies such as dobutamine echocardiography, thallium CT myocardial perfusion imaging, or positron emission tomography (PET) scans may be used to assess hibernating myocardium. However, they are only relevant to influencing surgical strategy in patients with massive infarction or aneurysmal tissue, whereby coronary revascularization techniques would not be expected to improve myocardial function [6]. Documented absence of

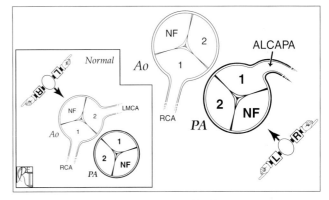

Figure 38.1 Diagram shows aortic and pulmonary artery origins of the left main coronary artery in normal and anomalous conditions. Cephalic views depict a person in the nonfacing sinus with the right hand always signifying sinus 1 and the left hand always signifying sinus 2. (Reproduced with permission from Dodge-Khatami *et al.* [2].)

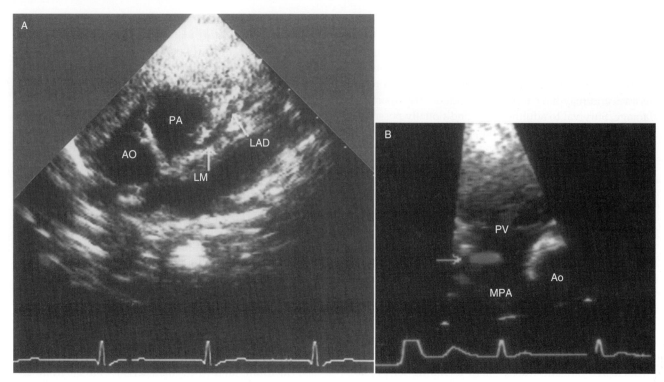

Figure 38.2 Anomalous origin of left coronary artery. **A,** Two-dimensional echocardiographic parasternal short-axis view shows origin of left main coronary artery (LM) with the left anterior descending (LAD) coronary artery from the pulmonary trunk. **B,** Color-flow Doppler echocardiogram shows turbulent flow from the left coronary artery entering the pulmonary artery trunk. (Ao, aorta; MPA, main pulmonary artery; PA, pulmonary artery; PV, pulmonary valve.)

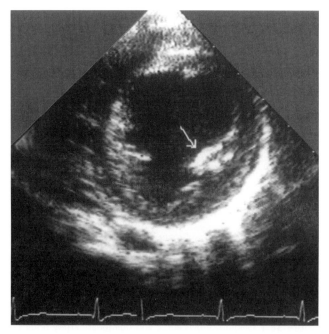

Figure 38.3 Anomalous origin of left coronary artery. Parasternal short-axis echocardiogram of the left ventricle shows bright echodensity of the papillary muscles of the mitral valve (arrow) that denotes papillary muscle ischemia.

viable tissue would be the only indication to consider heart transplantation over myocardial reperfusion [15].

Surgical Management

Attempts at medical therapy are associated with dismal survival and have no place in the current era of management for ALCAPA. Potts was the first to attempt surgical repair, creating an aortopulmonary anastomosis to increase PA blood flow and oxygen saturation in the anomalous coronary artery [16]. In 1953, Mustard [17] performed left common carotid-to-ALCAPA end-to-end anastomosis. The first successful nonpalliative operation was performed in 1959 by Sabiston [18], who ligated the ALCAPA at its origin. Cooley and associates [19] performed the first saphenous vein graft to the ALCAPA in 1960. Meyer *et al.* [20] used the left subclavian artery to bypass the origin of the ALCAPA. Already in 1974, Neches *et al.* [21] were the first to describe the direct reimplantation of the anomalous left coronary into the aorta, transferring it with a button of PA. This is the current ideal option toward achieving a definitive two-coronary artery anatomy and physiology (Figures 38.5, 38.6) [13]. In 1979, Takeuchi *et al.* [22] devised an operation for cases in which direct implantation is not

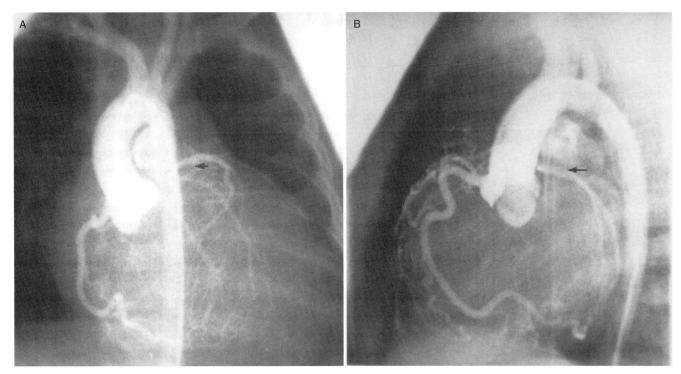

Figure 38.4 Anomalous origin of the left coronary artery. Retrograde aortogram (right [**A**] and left anterior oblique [**B**] views) shows prompt opacification of the enlarged right coronary artery and filling of the left coronary artery by collateral vessels. Arrow indicates origin of the left coronary artery from the pulmonary trunk with retrograde filling of the pulmonary artery.

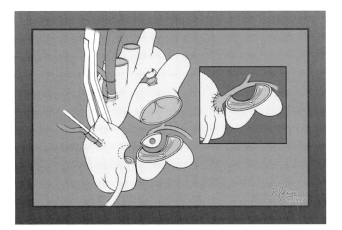

Figure 38.5 After the second dose of cardioplegia, an opening is created in the left posterolateral wall of the ascending aorta for implantation of the anomalous left coronary button. Care is taken not to injure the aortic valve. This opening is typically approximately one-third smaller in size than the button that was created. The large button of coronary artery can then act as a "conduit" for elongation of the left coronary artery. With proper mobilization of the left coronary artery, it is usually quite easy to perform this anastomosis. Once the anastomosis is created (inset), the aortic cross-clamp is removed, and now both right and left coronary arteries are directly perfused. (Reproduced with permission from Backer *et al.* [13].)

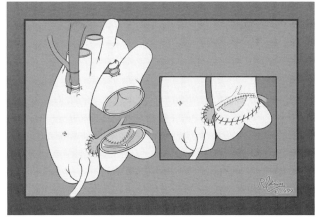

Figure 38.6 The aortic cross-clamp is off. The posterior sinus of the pulmonary artery where the button was harvested is reconstructed with a patch of fresh autologous pericardium. The pulmonary artery is reanastomosed at the site of the transection (inset). This reconstruction of the pulmonary artery with the cross-clamp off helps to minimize the aortic cross-clamp time. In almost all instances, it is possible to perform the entire procedure with two doses of cardioplegia given in the sequence described. (Reproduced with permission from Backer *et al.* [13].)

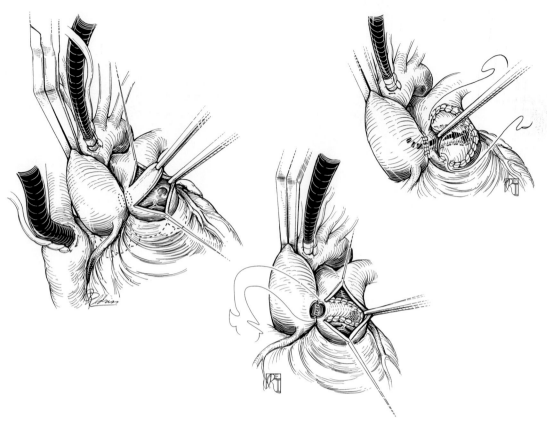

Figure 38.7 Takeuchi procedure through median sternotomy with extracorporeal circulation and cross-clamped aorta. The tunnel for coronary flow (arrow) has been made between the aorta and the anomalous left coronary artery by means of a flap of pulmonary artery wall. The pulmonary artery is then reconstructed with pericardium.

feasible, owing to unfavorable coronary artery anatomy or lack of length (Figures 38.7, 38.8) [6,12]. In the procedure bearing his name, a baffle of PA tissue is used to reroute the ALCAPA into the aorta after an intrapulmonary course. Arciniegas *et al.* [23] described interposing a segment of free subclavian artery to compensate for lack of length and reported an 80% patency rate at a maximum follow-up time of 11 months. Even in the presence of a nonfacing sinus origin of the ALCAPA or other anatomical variations, extending a cuff of pulmonary trunk tissue to elongate the coronary artery [24] or other creative surgical techniques gained through the experience from coronary transfer for arterial switch operations allows for reimplantation into the aorta [11,13–15].

Left internal thoracic arterial bypass grafting in children was described by Fortune and associates [25] in 1987. In 1988, Mavroudis *et al.* [26] proposed and performed cardiac transplantation as a last-resort solution for patients with end-stage left ventricular failure from myocardial infarction. This strategy is used only for patients with global myocardial necrosis as documented by viability studies, whereby no improvement can be expected after coronary

revascularization. In adults, direct reimplantation of the ALCAPA may be technically more difficult because of increased coronary artery friability, diminished elasticity for mobilization, the potential for tearing and catastrophic bleeding, or stenosis resulting from anastomotic tension [6,27,28]. In these patients, coronary artery bypass grafting may be more judicious, using the internal thoracic artery [29,30].

Administration of cardioplegia is a crucial point with regard to myocardial protection, common to all surgical techniques. In a review of 16 children undergoing aortic reimplantation for ALCAPA, Backer and associates [13] described a cardioplegia strategy that allows maximal myocardial protection, regardless of the degree of RCA collateralization. After ligation of the ductus and snaring of the PAs, an initial dose of antegrade blood cardioplegia into the ascending aorta is given. The PA is carefully transected and mobilized for maximum visibility, and the ALCAPA button is excised. A second dose of antegrade cardioplegia is given while the orifice of the ALCAPA is occluded with a vascular clamp, after which the coronary transfer is performed into the aorta. They report no

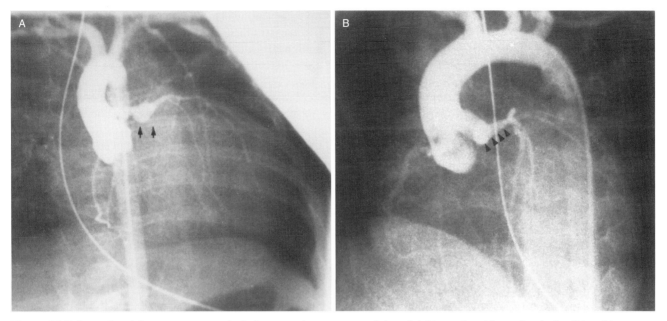

Figure 38.8 Anomalous left coronary artery. **A, B,** Postoperative aortogram (left and right anterior oblique views) after Takeuchi procedure for anomalous origin of the left coronary artery. Prompt opacification of the left coronary artery through the intrapulmonary artery tunnel is evident (arrows).

operative mortality, and no postoperative need for a left ventricular assist device or extracorporeal membrane oxygenation (ECMO) [13].

Surgical correction of ALCAPA addresses the two other structural abnormalities of the left heart that result from ischemic insult, namely global left ventricular function with or without free wall aneurysm, and the mitral valve. It is currently believed that ischemic yet viable myocardium, as assessed with stress thallium-201 or dipyridamole stress echocardiography, will recover postoperatively after reperfusion by any procedure that results in a two-coronary artery system [6,9,14,15,24,31–39]. However, scarred myocardium or its extreme aneurysmal form will not recover, and most surgeons concur in not directly addressing left ventricular aneurysms at the initial operation. Accordingly, resection of left ventricular muscle is hardly ever justified [6,15,40]. Some controversy still surrounds the issue of the mitral valve. Mitral regurgitation is related to both ischemic left ventricular dilatation and ischemic dysfunction of the papillary muscles [6,39]. Even severe mitral insufficiency fully regresses after reperfusion [6,13,15,23,24,32–34,41,42]. Although some authors advocate mitral valve annuloplasty or mitral valve replacement in cases of severe mitral regurgitation [9,31,43], most agree [6,13,15,23,24,32–34,41,42] that mitral regurgitation need not be addressed during initial surgery for reimplantation of ALCAPA. After improvement of left ventricular function, persistent significant mitral insufficiency can be repaired at a later operation. After initial ALCAPA reimplantation, Huddleston *et al.* [41] stress

the importance of following mitral valve function as an indirect sign of coronary patency. Indeed, persisting, recurring or worsening mitral valve insufficiency and left ventricular function may be a sign of coronary stenosis, warranting cardiac catheterization to document coronary patency, before reoperation for a mitral valve procedure [6,41].

Results

The combined operative mortality of all commonly used surgical techniques ranges from 0% to 23% [6,11,13–15,23,24,27–32,34,41–43]. Late death is unusual. It is now accepted that reperfusion through a two-coronary artery system with documented long-term patency should eliminate the risk of sudden death. Potential surgical complications include acute intraoperative coronary insufficiency resulting from technical error, as well as bleeding. Complications specific to the Takeuchi procedure include supravalvar pulmonary stenosis (76%), baffle leaks leading to coronary-PA fistula (52%), and aortic insufficiency [32]. Reoperations or catheter interventions are frequently necessary to correct these complications. The incidence of reoperation or reintervention is reported to be as high as 30% [9,32,43].

After successful reimplantation of ALCAPA, poor preoperative left ventricular function; stunned myocardium; or intractable ventricular arrhythmias may prohibit weaning from cardiopulmonary bypass [6]. Encouraging results have been achieved with the use of mechanical support as a bridge to recovery. Possibilities include left ventricular assist devices [44–46] and ECMO, especially when ventricular arrhythmias preclude the use of an assist device [27,41,44]. Although optimization of intraoperative cardioplegia strategies—using both antegrade and retrograde cardioplegia—combined with appropriate postoperative inotropic support should obviate the need for mechanical circulatory support [13], assist devices and ECMO play an integral part in the modern surgical treatment of patients with ALCAPA [6].

Various operative risk factors that affect survival have been identified in the management of ALCAPA. These include decreased preoperative left ventricular function [11,15,31] and young age at operation [11,32,45]. Although younger patients present with more severe left ventricular failure, early surgery results in more rapid and complete recovery of myocardial function, as assessed by echocardiography [45]. Severe mitral regurgitation has been cited as a risk factor for poor outcome after surgery [32], although not all institutions agree [11,15,31]. Sauer and associates found extreme RCA dominance (perfusion of the posterolateral left ventricle wall beyond the crux cordis) to correlate positively with operative survival ($p < 0.01$) [11]. As a corollary, left dominant or a balanced coronary circulation adversely influences operative survival ($p < 0.01$). Finally, stent thrombosis (ST) elevations on ECG in more than two chest leads or more than one standard lead indicate acute myocardial infarction and correlate with poor operative survival ($p < 0.03$) [11].

Discussion

From a nomenclature standpoint, ALCAPA is an APOCA (the most common). Keeping the sinus configuration described by Smith and colleagues [10], all variations of ALCAPA are classified according to the inclusive nomenclature system presented by the STS Congenital Heart Surgery Nomenclature and Database Project (Figure 38.1) [2].

Patients with ALCAPA may present with two types of coronary physiology that influence the onset and severity of the clinical signs and symptoms. Infantile coronary circulation is seen in most patients and is characterized by a mildly dominant RCA, fewer intercoronary collateral arteries, and no ostial stenosis of the anomalous left coronary artery. A higher "steal" phenomenon results in a more ischemic and dilated left ventricle, with earlier and more severe left ventricular failure. Early surgery is mandatory for survival of these patients. More rarely, the adult-type circulation relies on a large dominant RCA, extensive collateralization, and increased intracoronary pressure from ostial stenosis of the ALCAPA or mild pulmonary

hypertension, which results in mild to moderate left ventricular dysfunction. These patients are also at risk for malignant ventricular arrhythmia and sudden death [47], justifying surgical correction as soon as the diagnosis is made [6].

Medical treatment alone carries an unacceptably high mortality rate [9] and has no place in the current era of surgical management for ALCAPA. No difference in operative survival, late survival, or graft patency has been demonstrated for the different surgical procedures, excluding ligation of the ALCAPA, which is no longer an accepted surgical option. The current surgical goal is to achieve reperfusion through a two-coronary system, most commonly by reimplantation of the ALCAPA into the aorta, which is feasible in almost all instances despite anatomic variability [6,13,15,23,24,27–29,41–45,48].

Regardless of degree of preoperative left ventricular impairment, an aggressive early surgical approach is warranted, as it is the only possible way to salvage hibernating but viable myocardium [6,13,15,45]. Mild to moderate mitral insufficiency regresses after reperfusion and does not have to be addressed at the first operation [6,11,15,27,32,34]. Accordingly, preoperative mitral regurgitation has not been shown to increase operative mortality [6,11,15,31,34], except in one report [32] in which it was described as adversely influencing operative survival. Persistent, recurring, or worsening postoperative mitral insufficiency should warrant a cardiac catheterization to demonstrate coronary patency before reoperation on the mitral valve [41]. Left ventricular function improves substantially after restoration of a two-coronary-artery circulation, although some degree of chronic impairment from preoperative structural abnormalities may persist. Left ventricular muscle or aneurysm resection is generally unnecessary [15,39]. Documented massive infarction may be the only justification for cardiac transplantation, although this situation is generally becoming obsolete, with a higher awareness of the probable diagnosis of ALCAPA, an increased index of suspicion and immediate referral [6]. Left ventricular assist devices and ECMO improve survival in the surgical management of ALCAPA [31,41,43–46]. Although successful, cardiopulmonary bypass and cardioplegia strategies should reduce the need for postoperative mechanical circulatory support [13].

The best follow-up method for patients with ALCAPA is unknown. Electrocardiography, Holter monitoring, stress-thallium scanning, and cardiac catheterization have shown equivocal results and most often underscore any remaining left ventricular dysfunction that may be apparent only under severe stress testing. Close long-term follow-up evaluation of these patients is necessary to better understand the corrected natural history that currently constitutes the expected goal after surgical correction of ALCAPA.

Anomalous Aortic Origins of Coronary Arteries

Anomalous aortic origins of the coronary arteries (AAOCA) represent one-third of all coronary artery anomalies [49,50]. All three coronary arteries may be involved, and virtually every single combination has been reported as a case report. Most anomalous aortic origins are considered benign, except aberrant origin of the LMCA from the right aortic sinus of Valsalva (RASV) and aberrant origin of the RCA from the left aortic sinus of Valsalva (LASV), which are associated with cardiac symptoms and sudden death [3, 49–62]. The fatal potential of a minor coronary anomaly was first described by Jokl *et al.* in 1962 [58]. In 1992 Taylor *et al.* [49] proposed a classification of anomalous aortic origins (Table 38.3) [49,63–65].The inclusive nomenclature system including all possible variations of AAOCA as described in the STS Congenital Heart Surgery Nomenclature and Database Project is henceforth proposed for all further classification of AAOCA [2].

Although a chest radiograph and ECG remain a part of the standard work-up for all suspicion of AAOCA, they are most always negative. Findings at stress ECG may suggest the diagnosis of ischemia, but even standard transthoracic or transesophageal echocardiography and stress thallium are fairly unreliable [61,66]. Cardiac catheterization is in many centers still the ultimate diagnostic tool [49,50,59, 61,64,66,67] and is indicated in evaluations of young patients with unexplained exertional syncope, dizziness, or angina. Transthoracic echocardiography using contrast-enhanced, color-guided, pulse-wave Doppler-flow interrogation is a promising noninvasive imaging modality, although it is neither universally available nor easily reproducible [51].

However, for screening purposes, preferred imaging should be less invasive and avoid contrast medium or ionized radiation. Newer imaging modalities are increasingly gaining popularity and used for screening purposes, namely coronary magnetic resonance angiography, which allows three-dimensional reconstructions and multidetector CT angiography (Figures 38.9–38.12) [51].

Left Main Coronary Artery from Right Aortic Sinus of Valsalva

Left main coronary artery arising from the right aortic sinus of Valsalva (LMCA from RASV) represents the most

Table 38.3 Classification of anomalous aortic origins of coronary arteries. (CX, circumflex coronary artery; LASV, left aortic sinus of Valsalva; LMCA, left main coronary artery; RASV, right aortic sinus of Valsalva; RCA, right coronary artery.) (Reproduced with permission from Taylor *et al.* [49].)

Type	Incidence
LMCA from RASV	21% [49] of AAOC: four different courses possible in relation to great vessels
RCA from LASV	6–27% [49,64] of AAOC: can cross the aortic root anteriorly, or between the aorta and pulmonary artery
CX from RASV or RCA	10–60% [63] of AAOC (most common): courses either anterior or posterior to the great vessels, not between [63], always retroaortic [65]
Inverted coronary arteries	Rare

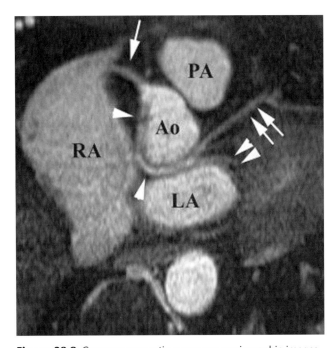

Figure 38.9 Coronary magnetic resonance angiographic images, using the "soap-bubble" reconstruction software tool, showing a common or juxtaposed origin of the left and right coronary arteries from the right sinus of Valsalva with a retroaortic course of the left main coronary artery (path no. 2). The right coronary artery has a normal course (single arrow). The left main coronary artery (single arrowhead) has a "benign" course, running posterior to the aortic root, then dividing normally into the left anterior descending (double arrows) and left circumflex (double arrowheads) coronary arteries. This view approximates a shallow left anterior oblique projection rotated 45 degrees clockwise. (Ao, aorta; LA, left atrium; PA, pulmonary artery; RA, right atrium.) (Reproduced with permission from Angelini *et al.* [51].)

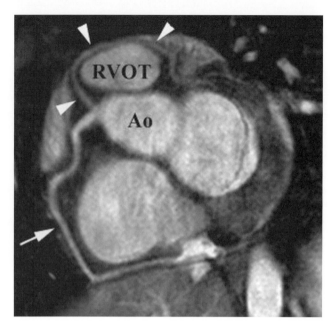

Figure 38.10 Soap-bubble reconstruction of a coronary magnetic resonance angiographic image (approximating a shallow left anterior oblique projection) revealing a common origin of both the left and right coronary arteries from the right sinus of Valsalva. The right coronary artery (RCA) has a normal course (arrow) and is visible to the crux; the left main coronary artery (arrowheads) has a "benign" course running anterior to the right ventricular outflow tract (RVOT, path no. 5), then dividing normally into the left anterior descending artery (not included in this image) and the left circumflex artery. (Ao, aorta.) (Reproduced with permission from Angelini et al. [51].)

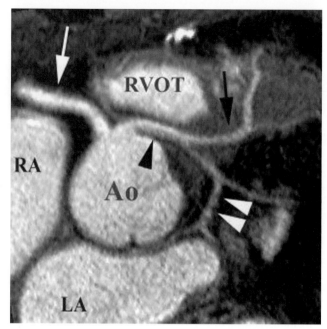

Figure 38.11 Coronary magnetic resonance angiographic image with soap-bubble reconstruction (approximating a shallow left anterior oblique projection rotated 45 degrees clockwise). The left main coronary artery (black arrowhead) originates from the right sinus of Valsalva and courses within the upper ventricular septal myocardium, between the aortic root and the right ventricular outflow tract (RVOT, path no. 4). Note that the epicardial fat is suppressed (it turns black) as a result of a fat suppression pulse used in the imaging sequence; the myocardium is gray. Both the left anterior descending (black arrow) and the left circumflex artery (double white arrowheads) also have intramyocardial courses for their proximal portions. The right coronary artery (white arrow) has a normal course within the right atrioventricular groove. (Ao, aorta; LA, left atrium, RA, right atrium.) (Reproduced with permission from Angelini et al. [51].)

serious anomaly of coronary origin and is associated with the highest incidence of symptoms and sudden death [3,49–62,66,67]. The incidence of sudden death in untreated patients reaches 57%, and up to two-thirds of these sudden deaths are related to exercise [49,61,66]. The risk of sudden death is reported as high as 82% if the LMCA courses between the great vessels [49,66,67]. Four courses of the LMCA are possible in relation to the great vessels: 1) anterior to the PA; 2) posterior to the aorta; 3) between the great vessels; and 4) septal course through the conal septum (beneath the right ventricular infundibulum) [66]. If the LMCA courses between the great vessels, the LMCA provides one or two branches to the proximal ventricular septum. Conversely, when the aberrant LMCA is posterior to the aorta, there are no septal branches from the left coronary system but branches arise from the RCA [64]. Perhaps the most important pathoanatomic element of the anomalous LMCA is the often-associated intramural (within the wall of the aorta) course that is almost always stenotic, both at its orifice and over the intramural course. The intramural

course can be above the commissure between the left and right coronary cusps or below the commissure (upstream).

The presumed pathogenesis of ischemia and sudden death include an acute origin (angle) of the anomalous vessel causing a slit-like orifice [49,50,61,64,66,67], compression of the coronary artery by aortic root distension at the onset of diastole [49,66], exercise-induced expansion of both the aortic root and the pulmonary trunk causing compression of the LMCA [49], effort-related stretching of the intramural LMCA segment adherent to the aorta along its first 1.5cm of length [61,66], and compression of the LMCA by the intercoronary commissure particularly during diastole when the aortic valve is closed [61], with resultant spasm, torsion, or kinking [49,64]. The incidence of atherosclerosis is higher among older patients with aberrant

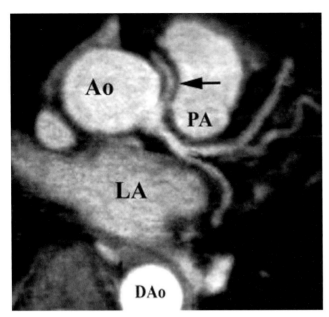

Figure 38.12 Anomalous left coronary artery originating from the opposite sinus, with an "interarterial course (path no. 3)," as seen by soap-bubble reconstruction of a coronary magnetic resonance angiographic image. This view approximates a shallow left anterior oblique projection rotated 45 degrees clockwise. The right coronary artery (black arrow) arises from the left sinus of Valsalva and courses between the aortic root and the pulmonary artery (PA). (Ao, aorta; DAo, descending aorta; LA, left atrium.) (Reproduced with permission from Angelini et al. [51].)

LMCA than among age-matched controls. The left system is congenitally small, and therefore most patients have a right dominant circulation [59,64].

Symptoms are frequent, encountered in as many as 38% of patients [49,54]. These include angina (20%), congestive heart failure (14%), syncope (14%), and myocardial infarction (6%), and their presence should alert to the increased risk of sudden death. Angina and syncope predominate among younger patients, while those older than 30 years experience angina and myocardial infarction [50]. Younger patients are more prone to sudden death, which may be their presenting symptom [49,50]. In a retrospective study of 6.3 million US military recruits (ages 17–35 years) undergoing basic military training between 1977 and 2001, 64 sudden cardiac deaths were identified [54]. Of these, the majority (61%) were owing to coronary artery pathology, among which more than half (54%) were from anomalous aortic coronary origins. Sudden cardiac deaths were more likely associated with premortem exertional chest discomfort and/or syncope, compared with deaths resulting from coronary artery disease in this same cohort.

Right Coronary Artery from Left Aortic Sinus of Valsalva

Anomalous RCA arising from the left aortic sinus of Valsalva (RCA from LASV) is reported in 0.26–0.6% of post-mortem studies [68], and 0.2% of all angiographic studies [68]. This represents 6–27% of all coronary anomalies [69]. Anomalous RCA from LASV was previously considered benign but more recently is recognized to be associated with considerable potential morbidity [49,62,68–70], with a potential risk for sudden death of up to 25%, being exercise-related in 46% of cases [49,51–57,59,61,62]. Symptoms of angina, myocardial infarction, syncope, and high-grade atrioventricular block [49,62,68–70] are believed to be related to closure of the anomalous ostium within the aortic wall during exercise or hypertensive states [52–57,69]. Proposed mechanisms of coronary ischemia and resultant left ventricular dysfunction during exertion include enlargement of the aortic root and PA, which in turn can obstruct coronary flow during diastole [62,69]. As in the case of left main coronary arising from the right coronary sinus, an RCA arising from the left coronary sinus displays the same characteristics of intramural courses, namely that the course is almost always stenotic at the orifice and along the intramural course. The anatomic configuration can be above the commissure between the right and left coronary cusps or below the commissure (upstream). No relationship is thought to exist between this coronary anomaly and atherosclerosis [62,69].

Recently there has been an increased awareness of this disease entity resulting in several retrospective studies [71–73], which have called for a prospective study to document its natural history. Kaushal et al. have noted that symptoms related to the length of the intramural course are measured by CT scans and intraoperative assessment [72]. An ongoing multi-institutional study has been organized [74] to delineate the medical and surgical outcomes of these patients over the long term.

Anomalous Circumflex Coronary Artery from Right Aortic Sinus of Valsalva or Right Coronary Artery

The reported incidence of this anomaly is 0.2–0.71% [65], which represents the most common coronary variation as reported in the Coronary Artery Surgery Study [63]. The anomalous circumflex coronary artery originates most often from the RASV (69%) [65] and commonly as a direct branch of the RCA. Symptoms and sudden death are rare, and diagnosis is incidental. The incidence of atherosclerotic coronary artery disease (ACAD) is similar to that in the control population (40%) [65], although some report a greater degree of stenosis than in controls.

Surgical Management

In the presence of symptoms, there is no debate with regard to the need for surgical correction; a coronary imaging study is performed, and surgery is planned according to standard surgical criteria for ACAD. Patients with an anomalous left coronary present more often with symptoms than those with an aberrant RCA [52]. With anomalous left coronary origin from the RASV, young patients (less than 30 years of age), regardless of symptoms or associated atherosclerosis, are recommended to undergo prophylactic corrective surgery (surgical unroofing of the intramural segment) to avoid a high risk of sudden death [49,52,55,57,60,61]. The surgical indication becomes a semi-emergency if the patient has exertional syncope, chest pain, or ventricular tachycardia [59,67]. In the asymptomatic patient with LMCA from RASV, some authors recommend delaying surgery only until 10 years of age, based on the fact that sudden death is rare in children, but would not wait longer [57,60]. If surgical repair is refused, avoidance of strenuous physical activity and competitive athletics is warranted [57,60]. In the asymptomatic young patient with an aberrant RCA from the LASV, treatment is controversial [52]. In the subgroup of asymptomatic older patients with negative results of a thallium study or absence of atherosclerotic coronary lesions, no sudden death is described [50,52,59]. Until recently, most centers have not performed prophylactic surgery on this cohort of asymptomatic patients [59]; however, this trend appears to be reversing in some centers [57].

The aim of surgery is to restore a normal anatomic position of the left coronary ostium [61] or to bypass a problematic proximal juxtacommisural or intramural course that may or may not have atherosclerotic lesions. The first attempts at surgical correction were performed using saphenous vein grafts to bypass the aberrant coronary arteries, followed shortly by internal thoracic artery bypass grafting. Although these techniques are still widely practiced [52,56,57,60] and remain unavoidable in certain circumstances, they expose the patient to the usual problems of grafted coronary artery disease and potential reintervention [57]. Furthermore, as the flow through the anomalous coronary is most often normal at rest, any type of bypass graft may have decreased postoperative patency owing to competitive flow [55,57], raising the question of whether the proximal aberrant coronary should be ligated [56]. We do not recommend this however.

In 1982, Mustafa and Yacoub and colleagues [61] were the first to propose and perform an anatomic ostial correction consisting of opening the aortic root, incising the ostium of the LMCA, and unroofing the stenotic intramural segment along its course to the midpoint of the LMCA sinus, with detachment of the intercoronary commissure. The intima of the LMCA is fixed to that of the aortic root,

and the commissure is reattached to the aortic wall, bringing the left main coronary ostium back into its natural position in the LASV (Figures 38.13–38.15) [61,75].

It is reassuring that surgical therapy is available for the specific forms of AAOCA that are potentially lethal, namely an LMCA from the RASV and an RCA from the LASV. Although the short-term follow-up of surgical repair for AAOCA seems encouraging [52,55,57] as documented by absence of ischemia on stress testing, stress echocardiography, and even exercise-perfusion scanning, the durability of the repair is still unknown [57]; subclinical changes suggestive of ischemia despite patent neocoronary ostia have been documented [52]. The long-term results of rerouting aberrant coronaries, unroofing coronary ostia, detachment of aortic valve commissures, and bypass to nondiseased vessels in the setting of AAOCA raise the respective questions of future potential ostial stenosis, aortic valve competence, and competitive graft flow. These surgical techniques are still under evaluation, and the optimal follow-up modalities and frequency of follow-up in these rare patients are still debated and await clearer guidelines.

Anomalous Pulmonary Origins of Coronary Arteries

The various APOCA are described in Table 38.2 [2], including the most common type 1, ALCAPA, already described at the beginning of this chapter. Type 2, or anomalous right coronary artery from the pulmonary artery (ARCAPA), is a very rare congenital anomaly, first described by Brooks [5], affecting 0.002% of the population [76]. Williams *et al.* [76] summarized the 70 cases ever published in the literature, including 7 of their own: 40 were children less than 18 years, and 11 were infants. Most patients were asymptomatic and presented with a murmur, but angina, congestive heart failure, cyanosis, palpitations, and even myocardial infarction with sudden death have been described [76]. Electrocardiogram findings are nonspecific, and currently, echocardiography is the most common method of diagnosis [76]. Although considered a benign lesion, the potential for sudden death as an initial and terminal presentation exists. Given the satisfactory advances achieved with standardized surgical technique and postoperative care, coronary reimplantation is indicated on diagnosis of the anomaly with expected good outcomes [76].

Single Coronary Artery

Single coronary artery is a rare anomaly frequently associated with complex congenital heart disease [77], with a reported incidence of 0.0024–0.066% [78–81]. Single coronary artery was first described by Thebesius in 1716 [82]. In 1950, Smith [83] proposed the first classification:

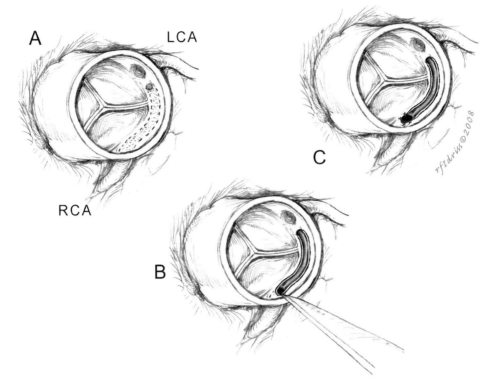

Figure 38.13 A, A transected aortic root demonstrates a normal left main coronary artery (LCA) and an abnormal intramural course of the right coronary artery (RCA), which takes its origin from the left coronary cusp, traverses intramurally (within the wall of the aorta) toward the right coronary cusp, and emerges there to perfuse the heart. **B,** The unroofing procedure is performed along the length of the intramural course. **C,** The tacking sutures are placed at the neoorifice and serve to reattach the intimal layers, thereby preventing dissection and thrombosis. We employ interrupted 8-0 Prolene. (Reproduced with permission from Mavroudis *et al.* [75].)

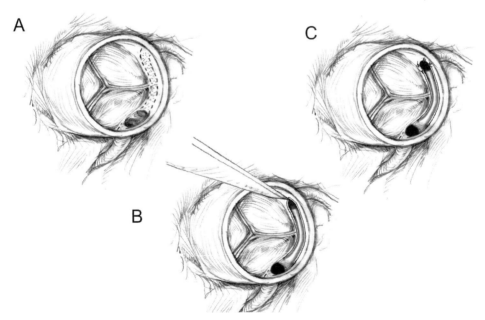

Figure 38.14 A, A transected aortic root demonstrates a normal right coronary artery and an abnormal intramural course of the left main coronary artery, which takes its origin from the right coronary cusp, traverses intramurally. **B,** The unroofing procedure is performed along the length of the intramural course. The dissection ends where the artery emerges from the aorta to supply the heart. **C,** The tacking sutures (8-0 Prolene) are placed at the neoorifice and serve to reattach the intimal layers, thereby preventing dissection and thrombosis. (LCA, left coronary artery; RCA, right coronary artery.) (Reproduced with permission from Mavroudis *et al.* [75].)

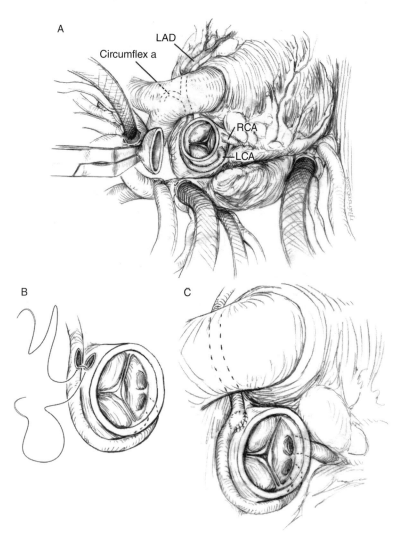

A

Circumflex a

LAD

RCA

LCA

B

C

Figure 38.15 A, The anomalous origin and pathway of the left main coronary artery is depicted. The origin is within the right coronary cusp adjacent to the takeoff of the right coronary artery. The artery is elongated and courses to the right and posterior of the aorta to emerge at the usual location and origin of the left main coronary artery near the left coronary cusp. Note that the course of the coronary artery is not intramural and the usual unroofing approach as described in the previous figures is not indicated. **B,** Instead, we have chosen to perform side-to-side anastomoses for these abnormal coronary artery courses. **C,** This procedure succeeds in a neoorifice formation more closely related to the normal coronary artery anatomy. (LAD, left anterior descending coronary artery; LCA, left coronary artery; RCA, right coronary artery.) (Reproduced with permission from Mavroudis *et al.* [75].)

• type 1: one artery supplies the entire heart, the other being truly absent; left or right in equal distribution;
• type 2: a single artery subdivides into two branches with distribution patterns corresponding to "normal" right and left coronary arteries (most common pattern) [77];
• type 3: other.

An additional subdivision of type 2 was proposed by Sharbaugh and White in 1974 [77], later modified by Lipton *et al.* in 1979 [80], and then by Yamanaka and Hobbs in 1990 [81] (Figure 38.16) [12,77]:
• type 2a: the branch that is the missing artery of origin passes anteriorly to the great vessels;
• type 2b: the branch that is the missing artery passes between the great vessels;
• type 2c: the branch that is the missing artery passes posteriorly to the great vessels.

The artery that originates from the aorta and from which the missing branch derives, is designated *L* or *R* for left or RCA, respectively. This classification (L or R and types 1, 2a, 2b, 2c, and 3) is a thorough one and has been adopted by the STS Congenital Heart Surgery Nomenclature and Database Project [2]. As mentioned previously, there exists a high incidence of associated congenital heart disease (17–40%) [78–81]. These anomalies include transposition of the great arteries, tetralogy of Fallot, truncus arteriosus, coronary arteriovenous fistula (CAVF), endocardial fibroelastosis, and bicuspid aortic valve. Type 2 is the most common form, and type 2a is more frequently associated with transposition of the great arteries and tetralogy of Fallot.

The overall survival rate is comparable with that of the general population. However, sudden death is possible (23%) [77,84] in type 2b cases in which the anomalous missing coronary artery of origin may be compressed between the great vessels. No particular ECG pattern is diagnostic, and coronary angiogram is the gold standard diagnostic tool. It remains unclear if atheromatous coronary disease is more prevalent in patients with single coronary artery [78,79]. As a corollary, the prognosis seems to be dependent on associated congenital heart defects.

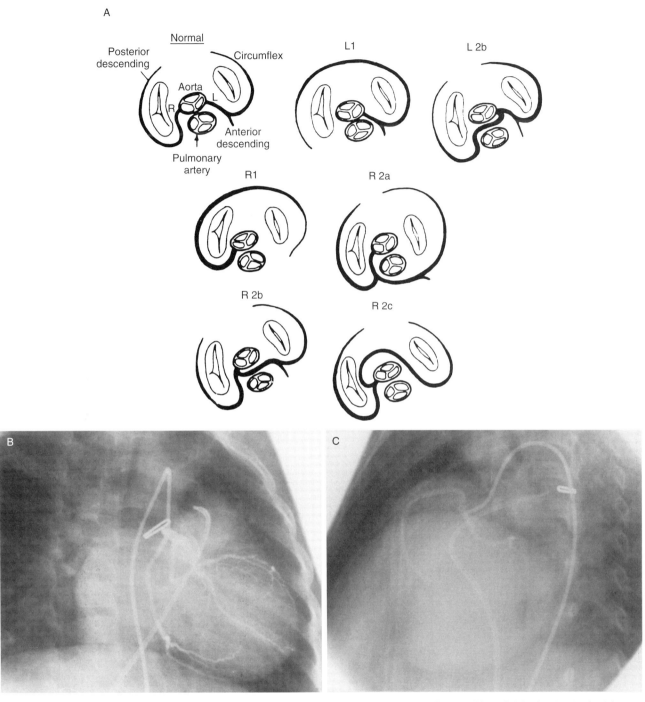

Figure 38.16 A, Single coronary artery with main patterns of distribution. Myocardial ischemia with sudden death may occur in R2b, in which the coronary artery courses between the aorta and the pulmonary artery. L, single left coronary artery; R, single right coronary artery. Frontal (**B**) and lateral (**C**) selective single right coronary arteriograms with left main coronary artery branch coursing between the great vessels. (A, Reproduced with permission from Sharbaugh *et al.* [77].)

Expectant medical management, coronary artery bypass grafting, and percutaneous coronary angioplasty have all been performed with success [78,79], although it remains unclear how these protocols potentially influenced the otherwise "natural history" of the anomaly. Currently, the extant data is insufficient to recommend optimal surgical/interventional or follow-up strategies [78,79], although some find medical treatment adequate for middle-aged or elderly patients in the absence of an ischemic coronary syndrome [78].

Congenital Atresia/Stenosis of the Left Main Coronary Artery

Congenital atresia/stenosis of the left main coronary artery (CALM) is an extremely rare minor anomaly, with approximately 60 cases described in the literature. Until the mid 1970s it was considered a single coronary artery until Lurie [85] defined it as a distinct entity with a flow pattern and physiology of its own. ALCAPA and single coronary artery are the most important differential diagnoses. In single coronary artery, a single left or RCA gives flow to the entire heart in a centrifugal anterograde pattern from the aorta to the periphery with a decreasing diameter of the vessel as it progresses distally toward the capillaries. In CALM, however, a single RCA vascularizes the entire heart, but flow in the left anterior descending (LAD) coronary artery as well as into the circumflex coronary artery is centripetal, and therefore retrograde, depending on collateral vessels from the RCA [86]. Collateral channels are through the circle of Vieussens, which includes the conal artery, intraseptals, and apical-anterior and posterior ventricular anastomoses [86,87]. There are also collaterals between the anterior interventricular branches of the right and LAD coronary arteries and between the final ramifications of the posterior descending branch of the RCA and LAD [86]. There is no left coronary ostium because the proximal left main trunk ends blindly. Most important, the LAD and circumflex coronary artery are located in their normal anatomic positions and connect in the usual way [87–90].

When excluding ALCAPA in the differential diagnosis of CALM both with regard to the clinical picture and diagnostic work-up, the ECG is unspecific and may also show evidence of ischemia or myocardial infarction in the anteroapical leads, and the chest radiograph unspecifically reveals cardiomegaly and pulmonary venous congestion. Therefore, diagnosis should be made by two-dimensional echocardiography [89], but the definitive anatomy and hence operative strategy need to be defined with coronary angiography [86–93]. The angiographic criteria common to both CALM and ALCAPA are a solitary RCA originating from the aorta with inability to inject into an obstructed left ostium and a left coronary artery filling retrograde through collateral vessels from the RCA. However, in CALM, the LAD and circumflex coronary artery are situated normally, and there is no "blush" into the PA from the proximal LMCA. Differentiating ALCAPA and CALM is not always angiographically possible, especially if the former has poor collateralization from the RCA and therefore not enough pressure to induce the characteristic "blush" in the PA [88]. Furthermore, in CALM, there is no oxygen step-up from a left-to-right shunt in the PA [88]. Evaluation for potential ischemia can be done with a stress-thallium study that typically demonstrates perfusion defects of the anteroapical segments [89,91].

The clinical manifestations strikingly resemble those of ALCAPA, and symptoms may begin in early infancy with syncope, tachyarrhythmia, dyspnea, failure to thrive, and sudden death. Survival into adulthood is rare but is possible and depends on the degree of collateralization from the RCA [86]. All patients ultimately develop ischemia on exertion, if not at rest, after the fifth decade. This condition results from left ventricular hypertrophy, increased oxygen demand, and superimposed atherosclerosis, which is estimated to be present in 15% of cases [87], similar to the frequency in a control population. Symptoms are believed to result from the delay of blood delivery to the left coronary system, as blood reaches the LAD and circumflex coronary artery in systole rather than in diastole [87]. The natural history of this disorder is poor, as patients with this anomaly have died suddenly, with or without medical treatment or while awaiting surgical correction [87,89]. An association is found with supravalvar aortic stenosis, especially in Williams-Beuren syndrome.

Surgical Management

Currently, surgery on diagnosis is the recommended therapy, consisting of bypass grafting of the LAD with saphenous vein or internal mammary artery [25]. Gay and associates [92] have performed a baffle technique using the ascending aorta to reconstruct the proximal CALM without the use of bypass grafting.

Good surgical results have been obtained with low mortality. Intermediate angiographic and clinical follow-up evaluation have demonstrated graft patency [89,91,92]. It is expected that long-term internal mammary artery graft patency will be superior to that of venous grafts.

In conclusion, CALM is an extremely rare congenital coronary anomaly that carries a serious prognosis if the patient is not treated. Ischemia, myocardial infarction, and sudden death are potential outcomes and may be prevented by surgical bypass grafting to the LAD, preferably with an internal mammary artery graft or proximal coronary arterioplasty. The clinical manifestations resemble those of ALCAPA, which is the most important differential diagnosis. The anatomic course can be confused with single coronary artery, from which CALM is clearly classified as a distinct entity. Long-term results are lacking in this very rare anomaly.

Coronary Arteriovenous Fistulas

Coronary arteriovenous fistulas represent an anomaly of termination. Coronary arteriovenous fistula was first described by Krause in 1865 [94] and is present in 1–2% of the general population [95–97]. Angiographic series report an incidence of 0.2–0.85% [98]. These fistulas represent nearly one half of all congenital coronary artery anomalies [99] and are the most common hemodynamically significant coronary anomaly [95–97,100–102]. Approximately two-thirds of fistulas are congenital, but acquired lesions are steadily increasing in number. The etiology of congenital CAVF appears to represent persistence of the embryonic intramyocardial trabecular sinusoids, with anomalous development of the intratrabecular spaces, through which blood is supplied to the myocardium during intrauterine life [98]. Acquired lesions may appear after trauma, Takayasu arteritis, cardiac surgery, in patients with indwelling transvenous pacemaker leads, postangioplasty, postendomyocardial biopsy in transplant recipients, or following interventional device closure of intracardiac defects [98,103].

Coronary arteriovenous fistulas can be isolated (55–80% of cases) [95-97,102,104] or associated with other congenital heart disease (20–45% of cases). Associated anomalies include tetralogy of Fallot, atrial septal defect, patent ductus arteriosus, ventricular septal defect, and superimposed coronary artery disease (35%) [95]. Single fistulas are most common, the frequency ranging from 74–90% [95–97,100,102,104]. Multiple fistulas are present in 10.7–16% [95,96,104] of cases, and fistulas originating from both coronaries in 4–18% [95–97,104]. Although most fistulas originate from the RCA, a recent review of large surgical series reveals both the RCA and the LAD as the most common sites of origin; coronary fistulas rarely arise from the circumflex artery [103]. The most common sites of termination are the PA and right ventricle [103]. Drainage into the right side of the heart is more prevalent (92%) owing to the lower pressures, and drainage into the left side of the heart occurs in only 8% of cases [96,100,101,103,104]. Coronary dilatation is usual, although the degree is not related to the amount of shunting [98]. Nomenclature is descriptive and includes the vessel of origin and the chamber of termination. There exists one angiographic classification by Sakakibara and associates (1966) (Table 38.4) [105].

Patients are usually asymptomatic in the first two decades of life [106]. Afterward, or in younger patients with larger fistulae, symptoms are present in 55–73% of patients and include angina (3–60%), dyspnea (34–60%), congestive heart failure (15–19%), arrhythmias (22–24%), and more rarely, dizziness, palpitations, and fatigue [95–97,100–103].

Diagnosis often can be made clinically with the finding of a continuous machinery murmur (differential diagnosis: patent ductus arteriosus, ventricular septal defect and prolapse of the aortic valve cusp, or aortopulmonary window) at the second and third right or left parasternal border. Electrocardiographic changes are present in two-thirds of patients and include ischemia, chamber overload, infarction, and arrhythmias (premature ventricular contractions [11%], atrial tachycardia [5.6%], and conduction defects [5.6%]) [95]. Cardiomegaly is present on chest radiograph in two-thirds of cases, and a left-to-right shunt may reveal itself on radiograph with increased pulmonary vascular markings in 16.5% of cases [95]. Color-flow Doppler echocardiography can define the exact anatomy in CAVF, but most surgeons agree that cardiac catheterization is needed before surgery to define multiple fistulas, hemodynamics, the eventual degree of left-to-right shunting [95], and the eventual feasibility of transcatheter device closure of solitary distal fistulous lesions [98,99,103,106]. More recently, MRI angiography and 64-slice CT allow for precise anatomical delineation of coronary fistula origins and sites of termination, thereby helping to define treatment strategy [98,106,107].

Rarely, coronary fistulas may close spontaneously [98,106]. More often, without surgery or intervention, patients with CAVF do not have a normal life expectancy [100]. The onset of symptoms and complications in untreated patients typically begins by the second or third decade of life [95,100–102,104]. These complications include myocardial infarction (3–11%), subacute bacterial endocarditis (5–20%), aneurysm formation (19–26%), and death (7–14%). Angina is caused by coronary steal, ischemia, superimposed atherosclerosis, thrombosis from turbulence and high flow, and critical coronary flow distal to the fistula. Congestive heart failure results from chronic volume overload. Aneurysmal dilatation of the coronary artery may predispose to rupture and tamponade [108]. In rare instances, sudden death may be the first manifestation of CAVF [104]. Subacute bacterial endocarditis and pulmonary hypertension are the eventual

Table 38.4 Angiographic classification. (Reproduced with permission from Sakakibara *et al.* [105].)

	Type A	Type B
Description	Proximal segment dilated to origin of fistula Distal end normal	Distal form, coronary artery dilated over entire length, terminating as a fistula in right side of the heart (end-artery type) Proximal to fistula, regular branching of coronary
Implications for surgery	Ligation of epicardial course distal to origin maintains normal branch flow No cardiopulmonary bypass required	Ligation of precapillary end by intracameral pursestring sutures at site of termination Requires cardiopulmonary bypass

results of long-standing left-to-right shunts. Pulmonary hypertension and coronary thrombosis with resultant embolization are more common in those patients older than 30 years. The risk of subacute bacterial endocarditis in unmanaged CAVF is approximately 0.002 per patient-year [104,109].

Björck and Crafoord [110] performed the first surgical correction of CAVF in 1947, while closing a patent ductus arteriosus. After a fortuitous discovery, they ligated the fistula proximally and distally [110]. Cooley and Ellis [111] performed the first tangential arteriorrhaphy in 1962, and the first successful transcatheter embolization was reported by Reidy in 1983 [112]. The goal of surgery or transcatheter device closure is to close the fistulous tract without compromising normal coronary flow. Consensus exists for surgical patients with symptoms, regardless of age [95–102,104]. In patients without symptoms however, the timing of and indications for surgery or intervention are controversial, although surgical series advocate early prophylactic closure, owing to near zero morbidity and mortality in cases of isolated fistulas [97,99,101,103,106,113]. Operative mortality ranges between 2% and 7% in cases with associated congenital heart defects, which determine the operative risk [95–102,104,105]. The various techniques described include internal cameral closure on cardiopulmonary bypass, tangential arteriorrhaphy with or without bypass, distal ligation, and proximal and distal ligation (currently abandoned) (Figures 38.17, 38.18) [12]. Other procedures include ligation and saphenous vein graft or left internal mammary artery bypass if there is compromised flow distal to the fistula and planned site of closure, closure from within the aneurysm, and finally transcatheter coil embolization [98,99,106,113]. In general, cardiopulmonary bypass is not necessary if epicardial ligation or tangential arterior-

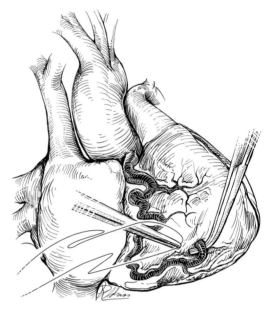

Figure 38.17 Epicardial coronary artery fistula has been dissected and is being ligated without cardiopulmonary bypass.

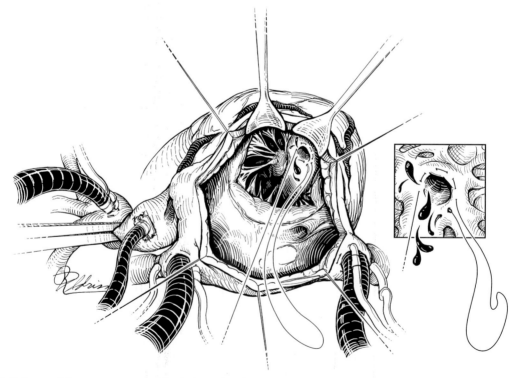

Figure 38.18 Right ventricle-to-coronary artery fistula through right atriotomy and tricuspid valve. Antegrade cardioplegia can be used to mark the effluent stream, and a purse-string suture can be used to ligate the fistula.

rhaphy [95,96,102,104,111] is performed, although it is recommended that cardiopulmonary bypass be on standby. Conversely, cardiopulmonary bypass is routinely required if there are associated congenital heart defects and ligation or purse-string closure at the intracardiac end is anticipated. Internal closure in the right heart chambers can be performed with cardiopulmonary bypass without cross-clamping or cardioplegia but on a beating or fibrillating heart [102]. Surgical techniques must be adapted to individual anatomy, and no data exist as to the superiority of one technique over another. More recently, transcatheter device or coil closure of coronary fistula has established itself as a safe alternative to surgery, when the anatomy is judged favorable. Mortality approaches zero and complications are rare [98,106]. However, no randomized studies have compared surgery with interventional techniques. No guidelines exist for a treatment algorithm depending on shunt size or anatomy, and therapeutic strategies are currently institution-dependent.

In conclusion, the nomenclature for CAVF is purely descriptive and is based on the origin and termination of the fistula. One angiographic classification (Sakakibara *et al.* [105]) has surgical implications according to type A or B. Younger patients tend to have no symptoms, but after the age of 20, symptoms develop with increased risk of complications, namely angina, myocardial infarction, congestive heart failure, fatigue, arrhythmia, aneurysm rupture and tamponade [108], subacute bacterial endocarditis, and sudden death. Surgery is recommended in all symptomatic patients at diagnosis. Operative or interventional mortality for isolated CAVF closure should be low. Consensus needs to be reached about surgical or interventional indications and timing of surgical procedure in the care of patients without symptoms. Because the natural history is not equivalent to that in the general population, many surgeons argue in favor of surgery or intervention before the onset of symptoms. This policy is advocated to avoid the increase in operative complications and death, which are more common among patients older than 20–30 years of age [97,100,101, 104,114,115]. At late follow-up, all surgically closed CAVFs remained closed, and late death was rare [103]. Improvement of functional class is the expected postoperative outcome [104]. No anatomic, clinical, or angiographic risk factors that effect operative or late survival have been defined, because most series are small. Transcatheter embolization is a relatively new technique whose long-term results remain to be evaluated [98,99,102,106,112,113].

Intramyocardial Course of Coronary Arteries (Bridging)

Intramural (intramyocardial) segments of epicardial coronary arteries, also known as *bridging*, were first described by Crainicianu in 1622 [116]. There is great discrepancy between autopsy and angiographic reports, with a wide swing of

incidence between 0.5% and 85% [116–123], as is the reported incidence in the general population, estimated between 5.4% and 85.7% [117–119,123]. Bridging is most commonly seen in the mid-segment of the LAD, although it has been described in diagonal branches, the posterior descending artery of the RCA, and in the marginal arteries of the circumflex coronary [118]. Symptoms often occur after the third or fourth decade of life [123]. There exists an association with hypertrophic cardiomyopathy, ischemic cardiomyopathy, idiopathic cardiomyopathy, mitral valve prolapse, and muscular subaortic stenosis [117,121,122]. Initial clinical reports include those by Reyman (1737) [124] and Black (1805) [125]. In 1951, Geiringer [126] reported a 23% incidence at autopsy and proposed a first classification:
• type 1: LAD coronary artery deep in the interventricular groove with a circumferential muscle bridge;
• type 2: (more common) muscle bridge from trigonum fibrosum "investing the LAD" as it passes toward the apex.

Fibrous thickening of the intima was described in both types. The first angiographic description was given in 1960 by Portsmann and Iwig [127], who coined the *milking-compression effect* of the vessel during systole. Noble *et al.* in 1976 [121] proposed the first angiographic classification according to systolic narrowing of the LAD during a stress test, as simulated by atrial pacing: group 1, less than 50% narrowing; group 2, 50–75%; and group 3, more than 75% narrowing. According to Noble *et al.* [121], only group 3 patients with severe narrowing of the LAD were at risk of myocardial ischemia at effort, which still holds true in the management algorithm in many cardiology and surgical centers. They recommended that patients avoid strenuous exercise. Furthermore, they proposed propranolol treatment to attenuate heart rate and contractility and were the first to suggest a theoretic indication for surgical relief. Kramer *et al.* in 1982 [128] proposed a variation of the Noble *et al.* classification [121] and retrospectively attempted a correlation between electrocardiographic findings and stress-thallium viability.

In 1991, Ferreira and associates [129] proposed a more detailed version of the Geiringer classification based on 50 heart specimens, taking into account the morphology of the bridge in relation to the LAD.

The mechanisms of ischemia in coronary bridging are still subject to debate. Because not all patients with ischemia have systolic bridge narrowing or fixed coronary artery disease, the ischemia-to-bridge relationship is difficult to prove [117]. Some investigators argue that muscular exercise and cardiac pacing have not consistently provoked ischemia and thereby cast further doubt on the role of myocardial bridging in ischemic heart disease. The indication for surgery is also controversial [117]. Angelini and colleagues [117] believe in the protective effect of bridges on atherosclerosis. They compare LAD bridges with peripheral intramuscular arteries of skeletal muscles that are relatively resistant to atherosclerosis.

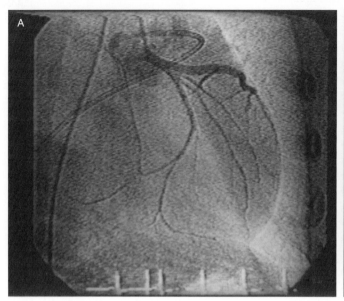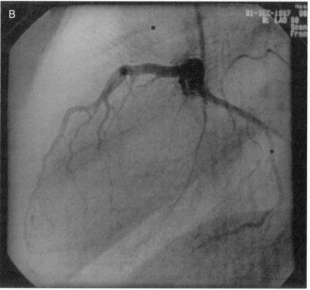

Figure 38.19 A, Coronary angiogram during systole shows constriction of the midportion of the left anterior descending coronary artery. **B,** Coronary angiogram during systole in the same patient after supra-arterial myotomy. The constrictive pattern caused by the intramural course has been alleviated.

There exists, nonetheless, angiographic evidence that systolic narrowing of coronary arteries invested by bridges does occur (Figure 38.19) [12,118,120–122,126,129–134]. Systolic coronary flow represents 5–30% of total coronary flow. There is a considerable time lag during diastole before flow in the septal coronary artery branches returns to normal. In bridging, it is estimated that one half of the flow in septal vessels is impaired during diastole [135]. Some authors postulated that turbulent flow through the bridge enhances intimal trauma and possible platelet aggregation [118,123,134]. Critical shortening of the diastolic filling time compromises local oxygen delivery, leading to ischemia, conduction abnormalities, tachyarrhythmias or syncope [118,119,123,129,131].

Currently, angiography and intravascular ultrasound (IVUS) are the gold standards for diagnosing and quantifying bridging [118]. As a rule, significant *milking* effect is present when diameter of the coronary is reduced by <70% in systole and >35% during mid-to-late diastole [118]. With IVUS, the *half moon* and early diastolic *finger tip* phenomena are highly specific for a significant bridge, depicting diameter narrowing in relation to delayed vessel relaxation, reduced antegrade systolic flow, and abrupt early diastolic flow acceleration [118]. Increased heart rate, decreased systolic blood pressure, and coronary vasospasm aggravate these phenomena [118,121–123].

Therapeutic Considerations

Initial treatment for symptomatic or asymptomatic bridging is medical [118,136]. Through their negative chrono-

tropic and inotropic effects, beta-blockers reduce tachycardia and prolong diastole, which reduces external muscle compression [118,123,130,134], and calcium channel blockers have also been used with success [118]. Nitroglycerine has been used in the symptomatic management of angina in bridging, although ischemic symptoms worsen in some patients [123]. Pacemakers are implanted if syncope and conduction disturbances exist [119]. When symptoms are refractory to medical treatment, most surgeons agree to relieve documented angiographic systolic narrowing. In 1975, Binet *et al.* were the first to perform and report surgical myotomy, thereby unroofing the supracoronary bridge over the involved vessel [137]. Later, bypass grafting distal to the bridging, using either vein or the internal thoracic artery were also performed. Both surgical myotomy and bypass grafting, with or without cardiopulmonary bypass, have met with documented good results at follow-up evaluation. This outcome is attested by disappearance of symptoms and normalization of ECG and angiographic findings [122,123,129,130,132,136,137]. Interventional percutaneous stenting of bridged vessels has been attempted, although the rate of in-stent stenosis has been relatively high, and the midterm results are still unknown [138].

In conclusion, no consensus exists for treatment of patients who have symptoms versus those who do not. There is no randomized evidence for comparing patient outcome with surgery, stenting, or medical therapy. Most reports are isolated, and there are few long-term series.

The Geiringer and Ferreira classifications are based on autopsy studies, are purely morphologic, and have no proven different clinical correlations between superficial and deep bridges. The Noble and Kramer classifications are based on angiographic studies and their relation to ischemia on ECG and stress-thallium studies. Noble's classification is chronologically the first, was developed in a controlled-study setting, and was adopted by the STS Congenital Heart Surgery Nomenclature and Database Project [2].

Coronary Aneurysms

First described by Morgagni [139] in 1761 in a patient with syphilis, and later by Bougon in 1812 [140], *coronary aneurysm* is synonymous with *ectasia* or *dilating atherosclerosis*. The first angiographic and radiologic description was documented by Munkner *et al.* in 1958 [141]. The incidence in the general population is 0.3–4.9% [142–145]. The aneurysm is more common in males (88.2%).

Aneurysm is defined as dilatations of a coronary vessel 1.5 times the adjacent normal coronary vessels. There exist two forms, fusiform and saccular, fusiforme being the more common. Fusiform aneurysms are typically poststenotic dilatations, and most occur in the setting of atherosclerosis [142]. Saccular aneurysms are more prone to rupture, thrombosis, or fistulization. Both saccular and fusiform aneurysms occur singly or in multiple patterns. They are most commonly located in the proximal and middle RCA (40–87%), followed by the LAD (25–50%), the circumflex coronary artery (24–50%), and the LMCA (7%) [142–148]. Aneurysms are caused by destruction of musculoelastic elements of the vessel wall leading to increased wall stress and dilatation [142–145,148–150]. Disease starts in the media, not in the intima, as attested by aneurysm development in the absence of atherosclerosis [141,146–149,151]. Inflammatory reactions, focal calcium, subintimal fibrosis, and lipoid material may coexist in the vessel media (Figure 38.20) [142,152].

Markis and colleagues in 1976 were the first to propose an angiographic classification [149]. Type I has diffuse ectasia of two to three vessels. Type II has diffuse ectasia of one vessel and localized ectasia in one other. Type III has diffuse ectasia in one vessel only, and type IV has localized ectasia in one vessel.

The Coronary Artery Surgery Study [148] proposed another classification of aneurysms in patients with ACAD. Group A patients have an aneurysm but no ACAD. In group B an aneurysm is present in association with atherosclerosis with less than 70% stenosis. In group C an aneurysm is present as is ACAD with more than 70% stenosis.

Most aneurysms are secondary to atherosclerosis (50%) or other conditions, including Kawasaki disease, trauma, polyarteritis nodosa, Takayasu's disease, syphilis, bacterial infection, septic embolism, dissection, scleroderma, metastatic tumor, and iatrogenic insults after angioplasty or stent placement [146,147,149–151]. Congenital aneurysms

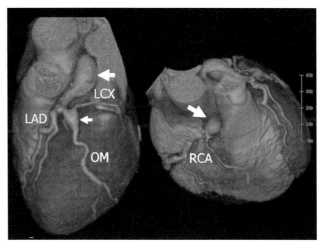

Figure 38.20 Volume rendering image from the cranial left anterior oblique view (left) showing the enormously dilated left main coronary artery (large arrow) and an aneurysm of the left circumflex artery (small arrow). Volume rendering image from the cranial right anterior oblique view (right) showing an aneurysm of the right coronary artery (arrow). (LAD, left anterior descending artery; LCX, left circumflex artery; OM, obtuse marginal artery; RCA, right coronary artery.) (Reproduced with permission from Ayusawa *et al.* [152].)

account for 20–30% of coronary aneurysms [151], associated with Ehlers-Danlos syndrome, Marfan disease, cyanotic congenital heart disease, and supravalvar aortic stenosis [141,144].

Aneurysms represent the most common manifestation of Kawasaki disease (15–20%) [146,147], and Kawasaki disease has been reported as the most frequent etiology causing aneurysms [150,153]. Some authors consider aneurysms a subset of atherosclerosis, having a prognosis no worse than that of coronary artery disease without aneurysms [141,144,147,153]. An association with abdominal aortic aneurysms and hyperlipidemia is suspected, but the true incidence is unknown [141,144,146,148,151].

Symptoms are frequent, most being indistinguishable from those of ACAD symptoms, namely angina, congestive heart failure, and myocardial infarction. The risk factors are the same as in ACAD [142,148,151]. Hypertension, abnormal ischemic ECG, and a family history of the disease [148] are more frequently encountered in patients with aneurysms [141,144,147,149] than in patients with coronary artery disease without aneurysms. The physical finding of a systolic murmur is inconsistent. Diagnosis can be made by an ECG or by echocardiography [146,147,150,151,153]. Angiography is still the standard diagnostic tool, although newer imagery with MRI and CT scanning is rapidly gaining popularity, allowing for very precise anatomic definition (Figure 38.20) [152].

The pathogenesis of ischemia and myocardial infarction is unclear if there is no associated atherosclerosis. It is postulated that local changes in flow and thrombosis in an aneurysm and subsequent embolization to the distal coronary artery could cause ischemia and left ventricular dysfunction [141,144,151]. Aneurysms are more frequently associated with three-vessel coronary artery disease (42.3%). Given the same left ventricular ejection fraction, there is a higher observed rate of myocardial infarction in those patients with aneurysms, but this finding may simply reflect a higher prevalence of three-vessel coronary artery disease.

Medical treatment has not improved the functional class of patients with aneurysms [141,144,151]. There is no difference in 5-year survival rate between medical management of aneurysms alone and that of aneurysm associated with atherosclerosis [146,148]. The short-term prognosis (24 months) after medical management of aneurysmal disease is the same as that of medically managed three-vessel coronary artery disease [149]. In patients with symptoms, prognosis is poorer and death of myocardial infarction is more probable if no surgery is performed [149].

Surgery is warranted for coronary aneurysms associated with atherosclerosis as it is for ischemic coronary artery disease without aneurysm [141,142,144–146,148,149]. In the absence of associated atherosclerosis with isolated aneurysmal disease, it is unclear if prophylactic surgery is warranted. With symptoms, bypass surgery with saphenous vein graft or left internal mammary artery (Figure 38.21) [12] carries the same low mortality and incidence of postoperative myocardial infarction at follow-up evaluation, as regular coronary artery disease surgery [148]. Accordingly, mortality 5 years after repair of aneurysms alone is similar to that for simple coronary artery disease [146,148]. Techniques for repair of saccular aneurysms include lateral aneurysmorrhaphy, thrombectomy, and endarterectomy.

In conclusion, coronary aneurysms are a surgical disease with the same operative indications and risk factors as ACAD. The approach to complicated aneurysms, that is, thrombosed, occluded, or ruptured aneurysms, is tailored according to individual findings. No current surgical consensus exists as to the superiority of thrombectomy, endarterectomy, ligation, or aneurysmorrhaphy in addition to bypass of a stenotic aneurysm.

Markis' angiographic classification (I–IV) addresses the morphology, number of lesions, and extent of aneurysmal disease. This classification appears complete and has been adopted by the STS Congenital Heart Surgery Nomenclature and Database Project [2].

Coronary Aneurysms in Kawasaki Disease

Coronary artery involvement in Kawasaki disease was first described by Kato *et al.* in 1975 [154]. Aneurysms and ectasia are present in 12.8–25% of patients with unmanaged

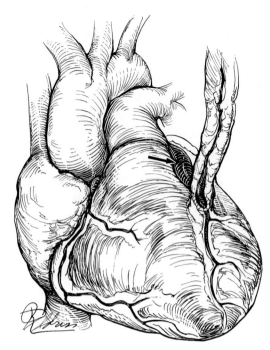

Figure 38.21 Internal thoracic artery bypass to midanterior left anterior descending coronary artery distal to saccular aneurysm.

Kawasaki disease and thus represents the most common cause of acquired coronary artery disease in children [154–169]. This consists of a vasculitis involving the arterioles, capillaries, and venules; the coronary wall undergoes focal and segmental destruction leading to aneurysm formation [154,156]. The inflammatory insult to the endothelium and coronary wall may be followed by remodeling and/or revascularization, with intimal proliferation and angiogenesis, leading to accelerated atherosclerosis [157] and stenosis [166]. Virtually all other cardiac structures may be involved, including the pericardium, myocardium, endocardium, and valves [166].

Diagnosis of cardiac lesions may be made with echocardiography and coronary angiography. Although aneurysms rarely develop before 10 days after the onset of illness, echocardiography may show perivascular brightness, ectasia, and lack of coronary tapering representing coronary arteritis in the acute stage [166]. Also, left ventricular function, mitral valve insufficiency, and pericardial effusion may be evaluated [166]. The American Heart Association (AHA) classifies aneurysms as small (<5 mm internal diameter), medium (5–8 mm), or giant (>8 mm internal diameter). The most common sites include the proximal LAD, the proximal RCA, followed by the LMCA [166]. Aneurysms of the LMCA usually do not involve the orifice unless the rare association of both LAD and circumflex artery aneurysms occurs [166]. Systemic aneurysms may occur with coronary aneurysms [162,166,168], and are associated in 0.6–11.5% of cases. These aneurysms are most commonly found in the subclavian artery, the internal mammary artery, the iliofemoral arteries, the abdominal aorta, and the renal arteries [167].

In 1982, Kato and associates [164] proposed an angiographic classification, based on anatomic and clinical findings at follow-up evaluation 4 years after acute disease. This classification divides patients into four groups. Group I represents 50% of Kawasaki patients, who have regression of aneurysm, no symptoms, no electrocardiographic changes, and a negative thallium test result. Group II Kawasaki patients (24%) have an unobstructed aneurysm. Group III patients (17%) have an obstructed aneurysm. Group IV patients (9%) have a nonstenotic irregular arterial wall.

Several scoring systems exist to predict the risk of aneurysm development in Kawasaki disease. Risk factors include male sex, age younger than 1 year, persistent fever longer than 14 days or recurrent fever, hemoglobin concentration less than 10 g/dL, white blood cell count greater than 30 000/μL, thrombocytopenia [166], erythrocyte sedimentation rate greater than 101 mm/hour, increased C-reactive protein level for more than 30 days, ischemia or myocardial infarction [170], and age older than 5 years [156]. Anemia is a strong predictor of aneurysm development and is of the normochromic normocytic type [154]. Follow-up for established aneurysms consists of a baseline echocardiographic study 6–8 weeks after acute onset, followed by echocardiographic assessment 6 and 12 months later. Coronary angiography is rarely recommended before the initial 6–12 months after onset of illness, unless clinical symptoms develop. At follow-up evaluation, the decision to perform angiography may be guided by echocardiographic findings or other noninvasive diagnostic methods suggesting ischemia [166]. Even healed vessels, as documented by angiography or echocardiography, may present with atherosclerosis, calcification, and a decreased response to vasodilators owing to depressed endothelial function [166].

Coronary aneurysms may either progress toward thrombosis of the lumen and stenosis or more rarely expand and rupture [166]. Occlusion of the coronary arteries exists in 66.1% [157,167] of cases, involving most commonly the RCA (61.5%), the LAD (53.8%), and the circumflex coronary artery (12.8%). Collateralization exists in 44.1% of cases. Giant aneurysms may evolve into life-threatening coronary lesions in 1% of patients [156,166,167] and typically do not regress [155,160,161,167]. These aneurysms progress to occlusion, myocardial infarction, and sudden death [155,160,162]. Conversely, 50% of smaller aneurysms regress within 1 year [154,156,164,165], and most of the others regress up to 2 years after initial presentation [164]. Actuarial persistence of all aneurysms combined is 72% at 1 year and 41% at 5 years [155,161,162].

High-dose intravenous gamma-globulins and aspirin have reduced the prevalence of aneurysm development to 5–10% if treatment is initiated within the first 10 days of illness [154,156,162,166,167]. Newer therapies including abciximab, a platelet glycoprotein receptor inhibitor, plasma exchange, or cyclophosphamide are still awaiting evaluation [166]. Angiographic resolution has occurred in up to two-thirds of lesions by 1 and 2 years after disease onset [166]. Factors positively associated with aneurysm regression include smaller initial size, age at onset of Kawasaki disease less than 1 year, female gender, fusiform rather than saccular, and distal segment aneurysms [155,166].

Myocardial infarction complicates the cases of 1.5% of all patients with Kawasaki disease and 11.3% of those with documented coronary disease. It is specific to patients with giant aneurysms [155], and the highest risk for infarction is within the first year after presentation [168]. Curiously, myocardial infarction is present in 35% of patients with healed coronary lesions and in 25% of those with acute coronary lesions. Mortality from myocardial infarction is high and approximates 25% [161,164].

Surgical Management

Excision or plication of coronary aneurysms have been attempted with poor results, even leading to death, and should be abandoned. Although not firmly established by clinical trials in children, indications for coronary artery bypass grafting include severe proximal stenosis (>75%), left main stenosis, proximal LAD stenosis, ischemia post-percutaneous transluminal coronary angioplasty, and proximal aneurysms [155,160,166,167]. The rationale for coronary artery bypass graft is the unacceptable rate of myocardial infarction or sudden death without surgery [155]. Furthermore, all stenotic lesions develop proximal or distal to aneurysms that are otherwise prone to rupture and/or thrombosis [30]. Saphenous vein bypass is used with good results and low mortality and has a 67% patency at 1-year angiographic follow-up evaluation [169,171]. The internal mammary artery has far better long-term patency and growth potential (86–100% at 1 year) [30,163,171]. Kitamura and associates [172] advocate the use of bilateral internal mammary artery grafts to the LAD and RCA and report no sternal infections or adverse effects on chest wall development in the pediatric population.

Patent and nonstenotic aneurysms present a particular problem, in that localized flow perturbation and stasis may be responsible for acute coronary events. If grafted, patent aneurysms can be subject to postoperative thrombosis with resulting myocardial infarction and possible death. The current recommendation is therefore to graft only stenotic vessels [166,169]. Indications for percutaneous transluminal coronary angioplasty in the management of Kawasaki disease are the same as for ACAD, namely, localized proximal stenosis [173]. A predictor of successful coronary angioplasty is the time elapsed between the onset of acute illness and the procedure, ideally within 6–8 years. Good results are obtained with a reduction in stenosis from 84% to 33% (p <0.05) [173]. Percutaneous transluminal coronary angioplasty does not seem to be indicated in the treatment of children older than 10 years or in those whose coronary arteries reveal calcification on fluoroscopy.

Transplantation has been performed for end-stage heart disease in patients with Kawasaki disease. Indications for transplantation include left ventricular dysfunction from myocardial infarction, ventricular arrhythmias and cardiac arrest, and multivessel or inoperable coronary artery disease [160]. Rejection rate is 20% with routine triple-therapy immunosuppression. At 1–6 years' follow-up evaluation, no atherosclerotic aneurysm has been documented to suggest recurrence of Kawasaki disease in the transplanted heart [160].

In summary, Kawasaki disease has become the leading cause of acquired heart disease and coronary artery involvement in the United States and Japan [166]. Coronary aneurysm and ectasia develop in 15–25% of untreated children, and high-dose intravenous immunoglobulin has decreased the incidence of late aneurysm development, with angiographic resolution in up to 50% of cases. Coronary aneurysms may develop progressive stenosis or occlusion leading to ischemia and infarction, most commonly in the first year after disease onset. The experience with angioplasty in children is limited. Surgical therapy includes coronary artery bypass grafting with good midterm results. Cardiac transplantation is feasible without documented recurrence in the graft but should become an exception in the current era of appropriate coronary follow-up evaluation.

References

1. Ogden JA. (1970) Congenital anomalies of the coronary arteries. Am J Cardiol 25, 474–479.
2. Dodge-Khatami A, Mavroudis C, Backer CL. (2000) Congenital Heart Surgery Nomenclature and Database Project: anomalies of the coronary arteries. Ann Thorac Surg 69(4 Suppl), S270–S297.
3. Friedman AH, Fogel MA, Stephens P Jr, *et al.* (2007) Identification, imaging, functional assessment and management of congenital coronary arterial abnormalities in children. Cardiol Young 17(Suppl 2), 56–67.
4. Post JC, van Rossum AC, Bronzwaer JG, *et al.* (1995) Magnetic resonance angiography of anomalous coronary arteries. A new gold standard for delineating the proximal course? Circulation 92, 3163–3171.
5. Brooks HS. (1885) Two cases of an abnormal coronary artery of the heart arising from the pulmonary artery: with some remarks upon the effect of this anomaly in producing cirsoid dilatation of the vessels. J Anat Physiol 20, 26–29.
6. Dodge-Khatami A, Mavroudis C, Backer CL. (2002) Anomalous origin of the left coronary artery from the pulmonary artery: collective review of surgical therapy. Ann Thorac Surg 74, 946–955.

7. Bland EF, White PD, Garland J. (1933) Congenital anomalies of the coronary arteries: report of an unusual case associated with cardiac hypertrophy. Am Heart J 8, 787–801.
8. Edwards JE. (1964) The direction of blood flow in coronary arteries arising from the pulmonary trunk. Circulation 29, 163–166.
9. Bunton R, Jonas RA, Lang P, *et al.* (1987) Anomalous origin of left coronary artery from pulmonary artery. Ligation versus establishment of a two coronary artery system. J Thorac Cardiovasc Surg 93, 103–108.
10. Smith A, Arnold R, Anderson RH, *et al.* (1989) Anomalous origin of the left coronary artery from the pulmonary trunk. Anatomic findings in relation to pathophysiology and surgical repair. J Thorac Cardiovasc Surg 98, 16–24.
11. Sauer U, Stern H, Meisner H, *et al.* (1992) Risk factors for perioperative mortality in children with anomalous origin of the left coronary artery from the pulmonary artery. J Thorac Cardiovasc Surg 104, 696–705.
12. Mavroudis C, Dodge-Khatami A, Backer CL. (2003) Coronary artery anomalies. In: Mavroudis C, Backer CL, eds. *Pediatric Cardiac Surgery*, 3rd ed. Philadelphia, PA: Mosby, Inc.
13. Backer CL, Hillman N, Dodge-Khatami A, *et al.* (2000) Anomalous origin of the left coronary artery from the pulmonary artery: Successful surgical strategy without assist devices. Semin Thorac Cardiovasc Surg Pediatr Card Surg Annu 3, 165–172.
14. Backer CL, Stout MJ, Zales VR, *et al.* (1992) Anomalous origin of the left coronary artery. A twenty-year review of surgical management. J Thorac Cardiovasc Surg 103, 1049–1057; discussion 1057–1058.
15. Vouhe PR, Tamisier D, Sidi D, *et al.* (1992) Anomalous left coronary artery from the pulmonary artery: results of isolated aortic reimplantation. Ann Thorac Surg 54, 621–626; discussion 627.
16. Potts WJ, quoted by Kittle CF, Diehl AM, Heilbrunn A. (1955) Anomalous left coronary artery arising from the pulmonary artery; report of a case and surgical consideration. J Pediatr 47, 198–206.
17. Mustard WT. (1962) Anomalies of the coronary artery. In: Welch KJ, ed. *Pediatric Surgery*. Chicago, IL: Year Book Medical.
18. Sabiston DC Jr, Neill CA, Taussig HB. (1960) The direction of blood flow in anomalous left coronary artery arising from the pulmonary artery. Circulation 22, 591–597.
19. Cooley DA, Hallman GL, Bloodwell RD. (1966) Definitive surgical treatment of anomalous origin of left coronary artery from pulmonary artery: indications and results. J Thorac Cardiovasc Surg 52, 798–808.
20. Meyer BW, Stefanik G, Stiles QR, *et al.* (1968) A method of definitive surgical treatment of anomalous origin of left coronary artery. A case report. J Thorac Cardiovasc Surg 56, 104–107.
21. Neches WH, Mathews RA, Park SC, *et al.* (1974) Anomalous origin of the left coronary artery from the pulmonary artery. A new method of surgical repair. Circulation 50, 582–587.
22. Takeuchi S, Imamura H, Katsumoto K, *et al.* (1979) New surgical method for repair of anomalous left coronary

artery from pulmonary artery. J Thorac Cardiovasc Surg 78, 7–11.

23. Arciniegas E, Farooki ZQ, Hakimi M, *et al.* (1980) Management of anomalous left coronary artery from the pulmonary artery. Circulation 62, I180–I189.

24. Turley K, Szarnicki RJ, Flachsbart KD, *et al.* (1995) Aortic implantation is possible in all cases of anomalous origin of the left coronary artery from the pulmonary artery. Ann Thorac Surg 60, 84–89.

25. Fortune RL, Baron PJ, Fitzgerald JW. (1987) Atresia of the left main coronary artery: repair with left internal mammary artery bypass. J Thorac Cardiovasc Surg 94, 150–151.

26. Mavroudis C, Harrison H, Klein JB, *et al.* (1988) Infant orthotopic cardiac transplantation. J Thorac Cardiovasc Surg 96, 912–924.

27. Alexi-Meskhishvili V, Berger F, Weng Y, *et al.* (1995) Anomalous origin of the left coronary artery from the pulmonary artery in adults. J Card Surg 10, 309–315.

28. Moodie DS, Fyfe D, Gill CC, *et al.* (1983) Anomalous origin of the left coronary artery from the pulmonary artery (Bland-White-Garland syndrome) in adult patients: long-term follow-up after surgery. Am Heart J 106, 381–388.

29. Kitamura S, Kawachi K, Nishii T, *et al.* (1992) Internal thoracic artery grafting for congenital coronary malformations. Ann Thorac Surg 53, 513–516.

30. Mavroudis C, Backer CL, Muster AJ, *et al.* (1996) Expanding indications for pediatric coronary artery bypass. J Thorac Cardiovasc Surg 111, 181–189.

31. Lambert V, Touchot A, Losay J, *et al.* (1996) Midterm results after surgical repair of the anomalous origin of the coronary artery. Circulation 94(9 Suppl), II38–II43.

32. Schwartz ML, Jonas RA, Colan SD. (1997) Anomalous origin of left coronary artery from pulmonary artery: recovery of left ventricular function after dual coronary repair. J Am Coll Cardiol 30, 547–553.

33. Singh TP, Di Carli MF, Sullivan NM, *et al.* (1998) Myocardial flow reserve in long-term survivors of repair of anomalous left coronary artery from pulmonary artery. J Am Coll Cardiol 31, 437–443.

34. Stern H, Sauer U, Locher D, *et al.* (1993) Left ventricular function assessed with echocardiography and myocardial perfusion assessed with scintigraphy under dipyridamole stress in pediatric patients after repair for anomalous origin of the left coronary artery from the pulmonary artery. J Thorac Cardiovasc Surg 106, 723–732.

35. Carvalho JS, Redington AN, Oldershaw PJ, *et al.* (1991) Analysis of left ventricular wall movement before and after reimplantation of anomalous left coronary artery in infancy. Br Heart J 65, 218–222.

36. Laks H, Ardehali A, Grant PW, *et al.* (1995) Aortic implantation of anomalous left coronary artery. An improved surgical approach. J Thorac Cardiovasc Surg 109, 519–523.

37. Paridon SM, Farooki ZQ, Kuhns LR, *et al.* (1990) Exercise performance after repair of anomalous origin of the left coronary artery from the pulmonary artery. Circulation 81, 1287–1292.

38. Rein AJ, Colan SD, Parness IA, *et al.* (1987) Regional and global left ventricular function in infants with anomalous origin of the left coronary artery from the pulmonary trunk: preoperative and postoperative assessment. Circulation 75, 115–123.

39. Vouhe PR, Baillot-Vernant F, Trinquet F, *et al.* (1987) Anomalous left coronary artery from the pulmonary artery in infants. Which operation? When? J Thorac Cardiovasc Surg 94, 192–199.

40. Alexi-Meskishvili V, Hetzer R, Weng Y, *et al.* (1994) Anomalous origin of the left coronary artery from the pulmonary artery. Early results with direct aortic reimplantation. J Thorac Cardiovasc Surg 108, 354–362.

41. Huddleston CB, Balzer DT, Mendeloff EN. (2001) Repair of anomalous left main coronary artery arising from the pulmonary artery in infants: long-term impact on the mitral valve. Ann Thorac Surg 71, 1985–1988; discussion 1988–1999.

42. Lange R, Vogt M, Horer J, *et al.* (2007) Long-term results of repair of anomalous origin of the left coronary artery from the pulmonary artery. Ann Thorac Surg 83, 1463–1471.

43. Isomatsu Y, Imai Y, Shin'oka T, *et al.* (2001) Surgical intervention for anomalous origin of the left coronary artery from the pulmonary artery: the Tokyo experience. J Thorac Cardiovasc Surg 121, 792–797.

44. Cochrane AD, Coleman DM, Davis AM, *et al.* (1999) Excellent long-term functional outcome after an operation for anomalous left coronary artery from the pulmonary artery. J Thorac Cardiovasc Surg 117, 332–342.

45. del Nido PJ, Duncan BW, Mayer JE Jr, *et al.* (1999) Left ventricular assist device improves survival in children with left ventricular dysfunction after repair of anomalous origin of the left coronary artery from the pulmonary artery. Ann Thorac Surg 67, 169–172.

46. Karl TR, Sano S, Horton S, *et al.* (1991) Centrifugal pump left heart assist in pediatric cardiac operations. Indication, technique, and results. J Thorac Cardiovasc Surg 102, 624–630.

47. Frapier JM, Leclercq F, Bodino M, *et al.* (1999) Malignant ventricular arrhythmias revealing anomalous origin of the left coronary artery from the pulmonary artery in two adults. Eur J Cardiothorac Surg 15, 539–541.

48. Raanani E, Abramov D, Abramov Y, *et al.* (1995) Individual anatomy demands various techniques in correction of an anomalous origin of the left coronary artery in the pulmonary artery. Thorac Cardiovasc Surg 43, 99–103.

49. Taylor AJ, Rogan KM, Virmani R. (1992) Sudden cardiac death associated with isolated congenital coronary artery anomalies. J Am Coll Cardiol 20, 640–647.

50. Cohen AJ, Grishkin BA, Helsel RA, *et al.* (1989) Surgical therapy in the management of coronary anomalies: emphasis on utility of internal mammary artery grafts. Ann Thorac Surg 47, 630–637.

51. Angelini P, Flamm SD. (2007) Newer concepts for imaging anomalous aortic origin of the coronary arteries in adults. Catheter Cardiovasc Interv 69, 942–954.

52. Brothers JA, McBride MG, Seliem MA, *et al.* (2007) Evaluation of myocardial ischemia after surgical repair of anomalous aortic origin of a coronary artery in a series of pediatric patients. J Am Coll Cardiol 50, 2078–2082.

53. Davis JA, Cecchin F, Jones TK, *et al.* (2001) Major coronary artery anomalies in a pediatric population: incidence and clinical importance. J Am Coll Cardiol 37, 593–597.

54. Eckart RE, Scoville SL, Campbell CL, *et al.* (2004) Sudden death in young adults: a 25-year review of autopsies in military recruits. Ann Intern Med 141, 829–834.

55. Erez E, Tam VK, Doublin NA, *et al.* (2006) Anomalous coronary artery with aortic origin and course between the great arteries: improved diagnosis, anatomic findings, and surgical treatment. Ann Thorac Surg 82, 973–977.

56. Fedoruk LM, Kern JA, Peeler BB, *et al.* (2007) Anomalous origin of the right coronary artery: right internal thoracic artery to right coronary artery bypass is not the answer. J Thorac Cardiovasc Surg 133, 456–460.

57. Jaggers J, Lodge AJ. (2005) Surgical therapy for anomalous aortic origin of the coronary arteries. Semin Thorac Cardiovasc Surg Pediatr Card Surg Annu 122–127.

58. Jokl E, Mc CJ, Ross GD. (1962) Congenital anomaly of left coronary artery in young athlete. JAMA 182, 572–573.

59. Liberthson RR, Dinsmore RE, Fallon JT. (1979) Aberrant coronary artery origin from the aorta. Report of 18 patients, review of literature and delineation of natural history and management. Circulation 59, 748–754.

60. Moustafa SE, Zehr K, Mookadam M, *et al.* (2008) Anomalous interarterial left coronary artery: an evidence based systematic overview. Int J Cardiol 126, 13–20.

61. Mustafa I, Gula G, Radley-Smith R, *et al.* (1981) Anomalous origin of the left coronary artery from the anterior aortic sinus: a potential cause of sudden death. Anatomic characterization and surgical treatment. J Thorac Cardiovasc Surg 82, 297–300.

62. Roberts WC, Siegel RJ, Zipes DP. (1982) Origin of the right coronary artery from the left sinus of valsalva and its functional consequences: analysis of 10 necropsy patients. Am J Cardiol 49, 863–868.

63. Click RL, Holmes DR Jr, Vlietstra RE, *et al.* (1989) Anomalous coronary arteries: location, degree of atherosclerosis and effect on survival – a report from the Coronary Artery Surgery Study. J Am Coll Cardiol 13, 531–537.

64. Kimbiris D. (1985) Anomalous origin of the left main coronary artery from the right sinus of Valsalva. Am J Cardiol 55, 765–769.

65. Ueyama K, Ramchandani M, Beall AC Jr, *et al.* (1997) Diagnosis and operation for anomalous circumflex coronary artery. Ann Thorac Surg 63, 377–381.

66. Barth CW 3rd, Roberts WC. (1986) Left main coronary artery originating from the right sinus of Valsalva and coursing between the aorta and pulmonary trunk. J Am Coll Cardiol 7, 366–373.

67. Moodie DS, Gill C, Loop FD, *et al.* (1980) Anomalous left main coronary artery originating from the right sinus of Valsalva: Pathophysiology, angiographic definition, and surgical approaches. J Thorac Cardiovasc Surg 80, 198–205.

68. Bett JH, O'Brien MF, Murray PJ. (1985) Surgery for anomalous origin of the right coronary artery. Br Heart J 53, 459–461.

69. Benge W, Martins JB, Funk DC. (1980) Morbidity associated with anomalous origin of the right coronary artery from the left sinus of Valsalva. Am Heart J 99, 96–100.

70. Bloomfield P, Erhlich C, Folland ED, *et al.* (1983) Anomalous right coronary artery: a surgically correctable cause of angina pectoris. Am J Cardiol 51, 1235–1237.

71. Brothers J, Gaynor JW, Paridon S, *et al.* (2009) Anomalous aortic origin of a coronary artery with an interarterial course: understanding current management strategies in children and young adults. Pediatr Cardiol 30, 911–921.

72. Kaushal S, Backer CL, Popescu AR, *et al.* (2011) Intramural coronary length correlates with symptoms in patients with anomalous aortic origin of the coronary artery. Ann Thorac Surg 92, 986–991, discussion 991–992.

73. Mumtaz MA, Lorber RE, Arruda J, *et al.* (2011) Surgery for anomalous aortic origin of the coronary artery. Ann Thorac Surg 91, 811–814; discussion 814–815.

74. Brothers JA, Gaynor JW, Jacobs JP, *et al.* (2010) The registry of anomalous aortic origin of the coronary artery of the Congenital Heart Surgeons' Society. Cardiol Young 20 (Suppl 3), 50–58.

75. Mavroudis C, Backer CL. (2010) Technical tips for three congenital heart operations: modified Ross-Konno procedure, optimal ventricular septal defect exposure by tricuspid valve incision, coronary unroofing and endarterectomy for anomalous aortic origin of the coronary artery. Oper Tech Thorac Cardiovasc Surg 15, 18–40.

76. Williams IA, Gersony WM, Hellenbrand WE. (2006) Anomalous right coronary artery arising from the pulmonary artery: a report of 7 cases and a review of the literature. Am Heart J 152, 1004.e9–1004.e17.

77. Sharbaugh AH, White RS. (1974) Single coronary artery. Analysis of the anatomic variation, clinical importance, and report of five cases. JAMA 230, 243–246.

78. Akcay A, Tuncer C, Batyraliev T, *et al.* (2008) Isolated single coronary artery: a series of 10 cases. Circ J 72, 1254–1258.

79. Desmet W, Vanhaecke J, Vrolix M, *et al.* (1992) Isolated single coronary artery: a review of 50,000 consecutive coronary angiographies. Eur Heart J 13, 1637–1640.

80. Lipton MJ, Barry WH, Obrez I, *et al.* (1979) Isolated single coronary artery: diagnosis, angiographic classification, and clinical significance. Radiology 130, 39–47.

81. Yamanaka O, Hobbs RE. (1990) Coronary artery anomalies in 126,595 patients undergoing coronary arteriography. Cathet Cardiovasc Diagn 21, 28–40.

82. Thebesius A. (1716) *Dissertatio Medica de Circulo Sanguinis in Cordo.* Ludg Batav, JA Langerak.

83. Smith JC. (1950) Review of single coronary artery with report of 2 cases. Circulation 1, 1168–1175.

84. Zales VR, Backer CL, Mavroudis C. (1994) Coronary artery anomalies. In: Mavroudis C, Backer CL, eds. *Pediatric Cardiac Surgery*, 2nd ed. St Louis, MO: Mosby.

85. Lurie PR. (1977) Abnormalities and diseases of the coronary vessels. In: Moss AJ, Emmanoulides GC, ed. *Heart Disease in Infants, Children, and Adolescents*, 2nd ed. Baltimore, MD: Williams & Wilkins.

86. Ghosh PK, Friedman M, Vidne BA. (1993) Isolated congenital atresia of the left main coronary artery and atherosclerosis. Ann Thorac Surg 55, 1564–1565.

87. Musiani A, Cernigliaro C, Sansa M, *et al.* (1997) Left main coronary artery atresia: literature review and therapeutical considerations. Eur J Cardiothorac Surg 11, 505–514.

88. Byrum CJ, Blackman MS, Schneider B, *et al.* (1980) Congenital atresia of the left coronary ostium and hypo-

plasia of the left main coronary artery. Am Heart J 99, 354–358.

89. Koh E, Nakagawa M, Hamaoka K, *et al.* (1989) Congenital atresia of the left coronary ostium: diagnosis and surgical treatment. Pediatr Cardiol 10, 159–162.

90. Rosenkranz ER, Murphy DJ Jr, Cosgrove DM 3rd. (1992) Surgical management of left coronary artery ostial atresia and supravalvar aortic stenosis. Ann Thorac Surg 54, 779–781.

91. Dymond D, Camm J, Stone D, *et al.* (1980) Dual isotope stress testing in congenital atresia of left coronary ostium. Applications before and after surgical treatment. Br Heart J 43, 270–275.

92. Gay F, Vouhe P, Lecompte Y, *et al.* (1989) [Atresia of the left coronary ostium. Repair in a 2-month-old infant]. Arch Mal Coeur Vaiss 82, 807–810.

93. van der Hauwaert LG, Dumoulin M, Moerman P. (1982) Congenital atresia of left coronary ostium. Br Heart J 48, 298–300.

94. Krause W. (1865) Ueber den ursprung einer accessorischen A. coronaria cordis aus der A. pulmonaris. Z Rat Med 24, 225.

95. Fernandes ED, Kadivar H, Hallman GL, *et al.* (1992) Congenital malformations of the coronary arteries: the Texas Heart Institute experience. Ann Thorac Surg 54, 732–740.

96. Olearchyk AS, Runk DM, Alavi M, *et al.* (1997) Congenital bilateral coronary-to-pulmonary artery fistulas. Ann Thorac Surg 64, 233–235.

97. Urrutia SC, Falaschi G, Ott DA, *et al.* (1983) Surgical management of 56 patients with congenital coronary artery fistulas. Ann Thorac Surg 35, 300–307.

98. Gowda RM, Vasavada BC, Khan IA. (2006) Coronary artery fistulas: clinical and therapeutic considerations. Int J Cardiol 107, 7–10.

99. Mavroudis C, Backer CL, Rocchini AP, *et al.* (1997) Coronary artery fistulas in infants and children: a surgical review and discussion of coil embolization. Ann Thorac Surg 63, 1235–1242.

100. Harris WO, Andrews JC, Nichols DA, *et al.* (1996) Percutaneous transcatheter embolization of coronary arteriovenous fistulas. Mayo Clin Proc 71, 37–42.

101. Lowe JE, Oldham HN Jr, Sabiston DC Jr. (1981) Surgical management of congenital coronary artery fistulas. Ann Surg 194, 373–380.

102. Schumacher G, Roithmaier A, Lorenz HP, *et al.* (1997) Congenital coronary artery fistula in infancy and childhood: diagnostic and therapeutic aspects. Thorac Cardiovasc Surg 45, 287–294.

103. Kamiya H, Yasuda T, Nagamine H, *et al.* (2002) Surgical treatment of congenital coronary artery fistulas: 27 years' experience and a review of the literature. J Card Surg 17, 173–177.

104. Tkebuchava T, Von Segesser LK, Vogt PR, *et al.* (1996) Congenital coronary fistulas in children and adults: diagnosis, surgical technique and results. J Cardiovasc Surg (Torino) 37, 29–34.

105. Sakakibara S, Yokoyama M, Takao A, *et al.* (1966) Coronary arteriovenous fistula. Nine operated cases. Am Heart J 72, 307–314.

106. Qureshi SA. (2006) Coronary arterial fistulas. Orphanet J Rare Dis 1, 51.

107. Dodd JD, Ferencik M, Liberthson RR, *et al.* (2008) Evaluation of efficacy of 64-slice multidetector computed tomography in patients with congenital coronary fistulas. J Comput Assist Tomogr 32, 265–270.

108. Bauer HH, Allmendinger PD, Flaherty J, *et al.* (1996) Congenital coronary arteriovenous fistula: spontaneous rupture and cardiac tamponade. Ann Thorac Surg 62, 1521–1523.

109. Liberthson RR, Sagar K, Berkoben JP, *et al.* (1979) Congenital coronary arteriovenous fistula. Report of 13 patients, review of the literature and delineation of management. Circulation 59, 849–854.

110. Biorck G, Crafoord C. (1947) Arteriovenous aneurysm on the pulmonary artery simulating patent ductus arteriosus botalli. Thorax 2, 65–74.

111. Cooley DA, Ellis PR Jr. (1962) Surgical considerations of coronary arterial fistula. Am J Cardiol 10, 467–474.

112. Reidy JF, Sowton E, Ross DN. (1983) Transcatheter occlusion of coronary to bronchial anastomosis by detachable balloon combined with coronary angioplasty at same procedure. Br Heart J 49, 284–287.

113. Alkhulaifi AM, Horner SM, Pugsley WB, *et al.* (1995) Coronary artery fistulas presenting with bacterial endocarditis. Ann Thorac Surg 60, 202–204.

114. Fetter JE, Backer CL, Muster AJ, *et al.* (1994) Successful repair of congenital left ventricle-to-coronary sinus fistulas. Ann Thorac Surg 57, 757–758.

115. Bogers AJ, Quaegebeur JM, Huysmans HA. (1987) Early and late results of surgical treatment of congenital coronary artery fistula. Thorax 42, 369–373.

116. Crainicianu A. (1622) Antomisce studien uber die coronararterien und experimentelle untersuchungen uber ihre durchgangigkeit. Virchows Arch (Pathol Anat) 238, 1.

117. Angelini P, Trivellato M, Donis J, *et al.* (1983) Myocardial bridges: a review. Prog Cardiovasc Dis 26, 75–88.

118. Bourassa MG, Butnaru A, Lesperance J, *et al.* (2003) Symptomatic myocardial bridges: overview of ischemic mechanisms and current diagnostic and treatment strategies. J Am Coll Cardiol 41, 351–359.

119. den Dulk K, Brugada P, Braat S, *et al.* (1983) Myocardial bridging as a cause of paroxysmal atrioventricular block. J Am Coll Cardiol 1, 965–969.

120. Mookadam F, Green J, Holmes D, *et al.* (2009) Clinical relevance of myocardial bridging severity: single center experience. Eur J Clin Invest 39, 110–115.

121. Noble J, Bourassa MG, Petitclerc R, *et al.* (1976) Myocardial bridging and milking effect of the left anterior descending coronary artery: normal variant or obstruction? Am J Cardiol 37, 993–999.

122. Pey J, de Dios RM, Epeldegui A. (1985) Myocardial bridging and hypertrophic cardiomyopathy: relief of ischemia by surgery. Int J Cardiol 8, 327–330.

123. Schwarz ER, Klues HG, vom Dahl J, *et al.* (1996) Functional, angiographic and intracoronary Doppler flow characteristics in symptomatic patients with myocardial bridging: effect of short-term intravenous beta-blocker medication. J Am Coll Cardiol 27, 1637–1645.

124. Reyman HC. (1737) Dissertatio de vasis cordi propriis. Haller Bibl Anat 2, 366.

125. Black S. (1805) A case of angina pectoris with a dissection. Memoirs Med Soc London. 6, 41.

126. Geiringer E. (1951) The mural coronary. Am Heart J 41, 359–368.

127. Porstmann W, Iwig J. (1960) [Intramural coronary vessels in the angiogram]. Fortschr Geb Rontgenstr Nuklearmed 92, 129–133.

128. Kramer JR, Kitazume H, Proudfit WL, et al. (1982) Clinical significance of isolated coronary bridges: benign and frequent condition involving the left anterior descending artery. Am Heart J 103, 283–288.

129. Ferreira AG Jr, Trotter SE, Konig B Jr, et al. (1991) Myocardial bridges: morphological and functional aspects. Br Heart J 66, 364–367.

130. Betriu A, Tubau J, Sanz G, et al. (1980) Relief of angina by periarterial muscle resection of myocardial bridges. Am Heart J 100, 223–226.

131. Hill RC, Chitwood WR Jr, Bashore TM, et al. (1981) Coronary flow and regional function before and after supraarterial myotomy for myocardial bridging. Ann Thorac Surg 31, 176–181.

132. Hillman ND, Mavroudis C, Backer CL, et al. (1999) Supraarterial decompression myotomy for myocardial bridging in a child. Ann Thorac Surg 68, 244–246.

133. Feld H, Guadanino V, Hollander G, et al. (1991) Exercise-induced ventricular tachycardia in association with a myocardial bridge. Chest 99, 1295–1296.

134. Vasan RS, Bahl VK, Rajani M. (1989) Myocardial infarction associated with a myocardial bridge. Int J Cardiol 25, 240–241.

135. Von Polacek P, Zechmeister A. (1968) The occurrence and significance of myocardial bridges and loops on coronary arteries. Opuscola Cardiolgica Acta Facultatis Medicae Universitatis Brunensis, Brno.

136. Huang X, Wang S, Xu J, et al. (2007) Surgical outcome and clinical follow-up in patients with symptomatic myocardial bridging. Chin Med 120, 1563–1566.

137. Binet JP, Planche C, Leriche H, et al. (1975) [Myocardial bridge compressing the anterior inter-ventricular artery. Apropos of a successfully operated case]. Arch Mal Coeur Vaiss 68, 85–90.

138. Haager PK, Schwarz ER, vom Dahl J, et al. (2000) Long term angiographic and clinical follow up in patients with stent implantation for symptomatic myocardial bridging. Heart 84, 403–408.

139. Morgagni JB. (1761) DeSedibus, et causis morbotum per anatomen indegatis. Tomus primus, Liber 11 Epist 27, Article 28, Venetiis.

140. Bougon M. (1812) Bibliot Med 37, 183.

141. Munkner T, Petersen O, Vesterdal J. (1958) Congenital aneurysm of the coronary artery with an arteriovenous fistula. Acta radiol 50, 333–340.

142. Aintablian A, Hamby RI, Hoffman I, et al. (1978) Coronary ectasia: incidence and results of coronary bypass surgery. Am Heart J 96, 309–315.

143. Anabtawi IN, de Leon JA. (1974) Arteriosclerotic aneurysms of the coronary arteries. J Thorac Cardiovasc Surg 68, 226–228.

144. Befeler B, Aranda MJ, Embi A, et al. (1977) Coronary artery aneurysms: study of the etiology, clinical course and effect on left ventricular function and prognosis. Am J Med 62, 597–607.

145. Falsetti HL, Carrol RJ. (1976) Coronary artery aneurysm. A review of the literature with a report of 11 new cases. Chest 69, 630–636.

146. Hartnell GG, Parnell BM, Pridie RB. (1985) Coronary artery ectasia. Its prevalence and clinical significance in 4993 patients. Br Heart J 54, 392–395.

147. Kosar E, Chandraratna PA. (1997) Assessment of coronary artery aneurysms with multiplane transesophageal echocardiography. Am Heart J 133, 526–533.

148. Swaye PS, Fisher LD, Litwin P, et al. (1983) Aneurysmal coronary artery disease. Circulation 67, 134–138.

149. Markis JE, Joffe CD, Cohn PF, et al. (1976) Clinical significance of coronary arterial ectasia. Am J Cardiol 37, 217–222.

150. Rab ST, King SB 3rd, Roubin GS, et al. (1991) Coronary aneurysms after stent placement: a suggestion of altered vessel wall healing in the presence of anti-inflammatory agents. J Am Coll Cardiol 18, 1524–1528.

151. Cohen P, O'Gara PT. (2008) Coronary artery aneurysms: a review of the natural history, pathophysiology, and management. Cardiol Rev 16, 301–304.

152. Ayusawa M, Sato Y, Kanamaru H, et al. (2008) Multidetector-row computed tomographic depiction of congenital coronary artery aneurysms and ectasia. Int J Cardiol 127, e172–e174.

153. Tunick PA, Slater J, Pasternack P, et al. (1989) Coronary artery aneurysms: a transesophageal echocardiographic study. Am Heart J 118, 176–179.

154. Kato H, Koike S, Yamamoto M, et al. (1975) Coronary aneurysms in infants and young children with acute febrile mucocutaneous lymph node syndrome. J Pediatr 86, 892–898.

155. Akagi T, Rose V, Benson LN, et al. (1992) Outcome of coronary artery aneurysms after Kawasaki disease. J Pediatr 121, 689–694.

156. Beiser AS, Takahashi M, Baker AL, et al. (1998) A predictive instrument for coronary artery aneurysms in Kawasaki disease. US Multicenter Kawasaki Disease Study Group. Am J Cardiol 81, 1116–1120.

157. Burns JC, Shike H, Gordon JB, et al. (1996) Sequelae of Kawasaki disease in adolescents and young adults. J Am Coll Cardiol 28, 253–257.

158. Gersony WM. (1998) Predicting coronary aneurysms in Kawasaki disease. Am J Cardiol 81, 1162–1164.

159. Suzuki A, Kamiya T, Kuwahara N, et al. (1986) Coronary arterial lesions of Kawasaki disease: cardiac catheterization findings of 1100 cases. Pediatr Cardiol 7, 3–9.

160. Checchia PA, Pahl E, Shaddy RE, et al. (1997) Cardiac transplantation for Kawasaki disease. Pediatrics 100, 695–699.

161. Dajani AS, Taubert KA, Gerber MA, et al. (1993) Diagnosis and therapy of Kawasaki disease in children. Circulation 87, 1776–1780.

162. Dajani AS, Taubert KA, Takahashi M, et al. (1994) Guidelines for long-term management of patients with Kawasaki disease. Report from the Committee on Rheumatic Fever,

Endocarditis, and Kawasaki Disease, Council on Cardiovascular Disease in the Young, American Heart Association. Circulation 89, 916–922.

163. Harada K, Yamaguchi H, Kato H. (1993) Indication for intravenous gamma globulin treatment for Kawasaki disease. In: Takahashi M, Taubert K, eds. *Proceedings of the Fourth International Symposium on Kawasaki Disease*. Dallas, TX: American Heart Association 1993, 459–462.

164. Kato H, Ichinose E, Yoshioka F, *et al.* (1982) Fate of coronary aneurysms in Kawasaki disease: serial coronary angiography and long-term follow-up study. Am J Cardiol 49, 1758–1766.

165. Nakamura Y, Yanagawa H, Ojima T, *et al.* (1998) Cardiac sequelae of Kawasaki disease among recurrent cases. Arch Dis Child 78, 163–165.

166. Newburger JW, Takahashi M, Gerber MA, *et al.* (2004) Diagnosis, treatment, and long-term management of Kawasaki disease: a statement for health professionals from the Committee on Rheumatic Fever, Endocarditis and Kawasaki Disease, Council on Cardiovascular Disease in the Young, American Heart Association. Circulation 110, 2747–2771.

167. Pahl E. (1997) Kawasaki disease: cardiac sequelae and management. Pediatr Ann 26, 112–115.

168. Satou GM, Giamelli J, Gewitz MH. (2007) Kawasaki disease: diagnosis, management, and long-term implications. Cardiol Rev 15, 163–169.

169. Suzuki A, Kamiya T, Ono Y, *et al.* (1990) Aortocoronary bypass surgery for coronary arterial lesions resulting from Kawasaki disease. J Pediatr 116, 567–573.

170. Asai T. (1983) [Evaluation method for the degree of seriousness in Kawasaki disease]. Acta Paediatr Jpn 25, 170.

171. Kitamura S, Kawachi K, Seki T, *et al.* (1990) Bilateral internal mammary artery grafts for coronary artery bypass operations in children. J Thorac Cardiovasc Surg 99, 708–715.

172. Kitamura S, Kawachi K, Harima R, *et al.* (1983) Surgery for coronary heart disease due to mucocutaneous lymph node syndrome (Kawasaki disease). Report of 6 patients. Am J Cardiol 51, 444–448.

173. Ino T, Akimoto K, Ohkubo M, *et al.* (1996) Application of percutaneous transluminal coronary angioplasty to coronary arterial stenosis in Kawasaki disease. Circulation 93, 1709–1715.

CHAPTER 39

Cardiac Tumors

Rüdiger Lange and Thomas Günther

German Heart Center, Technische Universität München, Munich, Germany

Historical Background

The first description of a primary cardiac neoplasm is credited to Matteo Realdo Colombo in 1559 [1]. During the autopsy of Cardinal Gambara, Columbo discovered a left ventricular polypus tumor. In 1666 Malpighi, in his dissertation "De polypo cordis" described for the first time a postmortem clot formation in the right and left sides of the heart [2]. The first report of a cardiac tumor in a living patient was not made until 1934, when Barnes *et al.* diagnosed a primary cardiac sarcoma with the aid of electrocardiography and biopsy of a peripheral metastatic lymph node [3]. Claude S. Beck performed the first successful resection of an intrapericardial teratoma in 1936 [4]. The first successful resection of an epicardial lipoma was performed in 1951 by Mauer [5]. In 1951 Goldberg and colleagues first diagnosed a left atrial myxoma in a 3½-year-old child by angiography but attempts at surgical removal were unsuccessful [6]. The first echocardiographic diagnosis of an intracardiac tumor was made in 1959 [7]. In 1952 Bahnson and Newman attempted to remove a large right atrial myxoma in a 54-year-old woman via right anterior thoracotomy using caval inflow occlusion, but the patient expired 24 days later [8]. Subsequently, Crafoord in 1954 employed cardiopulmonary bypass to perform the first successful resection of an atrial myxoma [9]. During the past three decades, the development and refinement of noninvasive imaging modalities as well as the technical advances in heart surgery have profoundly changed the diagnosis and treatment of cardiac tumors.

Nomenclature

Following the definitions proposed by Mehta and Myers [10], cardiac tumors are defined as an "abnormal growth of tissue in or on the heart, demonstrating partial or complete lack of structural organization, and no functional coordination with normal cardiac tissue." Cardiac tumors may be divided into two categories: primary cardiac tumors that arise from tissues of the heart and secondary cardiac tumors that arise from tissues distant from the heart, with subsequent spread to the normal tissues of the heart. Primary cardiac tumors include the following types: myxoma, papillary fibroelastoma, rhabdomyoma, fibroma, lipoma, teratoma; hemangioma; lipomatous hypertrophy of the interatrial septum, mesothelioma of atrioventricular (AV) tissue, pheochromocytoma, sarcoma, cardiac lymphoma, cardiac thrombus, and cardiac vegetation. Secondary cardiac tumors are either metastatic extensions from a remote organ system, which spread to the heart through direct hematogenous or lymphatic routes, or direct extensions of tumors originating from contiguous thoracic or infradiaphragmatic structures. The latter abdominal or pelvic tumors may spread cephalad through the inferior vena cava to the right atrium [10].

Incidence

Primary cardiac tumors are rare in all age groups. The reported incidence in autopsy series varies between 0.0017% and 0.28% [11]. Reynen analyzed the data of 22 large autopsy series to approximate the true incidence and found the frequency of primary cardiac tumors to be approximately 0.02% corresponding to 200 tumors in 1 million autopsies [12].

In the pediatric age group the incidence of primary cardiac tumors is reported to be 0.027% based on the analysis of 11 000 pediatric autopsies reviewed by Nadas and Ellison in 1968 [13]. However, with the improvement in noninvasive imaging techniques, the more intensive routine echocardiographic screening of children, and the increasing application of fetal ultrasonography in recent

Pediatric Cardiac Surgery, Fourth Edition. Edited by Constantine Mavroudis and Carl L. Backer.
© 2013 Blackwell Publishing Ltd. Published 2013 by Blackwell Publishing Ltd.

decades, pediatric cardiac tumors are diagnosed with an increasing frequency [14,15]. In a 1995 multicenter review of 14000 fetal echocardiograms, cardiac tumors were detected in 0.14% [16]. Beghetti and associates analyzed 27640 infants and children assessed for cardiac disease over a 15-year period and noticed an increase in tumor recognition from 0.06% to 0.32%. [15]. About 14% of all cardiac tumors occur in patients who are less than 16 years of age [17].

The majority of primary cardiac tumors are benign ranging between 72% and 94% in selected series [11,18–23]. The myxoma is the most common tumor type in adult patients accounting for approximately 50% of all primary tumors, followed by papillary fibroelastomas, fibromas, and lipomas [11,22,23]. In pediatric patients, more than 90% of primary cardiac tumors are benign [24]. Nearly one-half of the tumors are rhabdomyomas, followed by fibromas, intrapericardial teratomas, myxomas, and hemangiomas [18,25–29]. Rhabdomyomas, fibromas, and intrapericardial teratomas are more common in newborns and infants; myxomas predominate in older children and adolescents. Table 39.1 summarizes the approximate frequency of occurrence based on collective series [13,18,30] of primary cardiac tumors in infants and children. Approximately one-fourth of all tumors diagnosed in adults are malignant [11]. The majority (75–95%) of these tumors are sarcomas [31–33]. Primary malignant cardiac tumors in pediatric patients are exceedingly rare (<10%) [18,24,30,34].

Secondary cardiac tumors are 20–40 times more common than primary cardiac neoplasms [11,35–38]. The incidence of secondary tumor involvement in pediatric patients in autopsy series was 5.7% [30]. In adults the most common tumors causing secondary involvement of the heart are carcinomas (lung, breast, pancreas, kidney, gastrointestinal, ovary, and testes) followed by malignant melanoma, non-Hodgkin's lymphoma, and various soft tissue and

bone sarcomas [10,30,39]. In children, the most frequent primary tumors are in descending order of frequency; non-Hodgkin's lymphoma, neuroblastoma, Wilms' tumor, soft tissue and bone sarcomas, and hepatoma [30].

Clinical Appearance

Although each tumor type has its characteristic features, general comments can be made regarding the spectrum of their clinical appearance. The clinical manifestations of cardiac tumors vary considerably from asymptomatic presentations to life-threatening cardiac events [24,40]. Because various cardiac diseases may be mimicked [40,41], the presence of a cardiac tumor should always be considered in the differential diagnosis.

The symptoms are usually related to the size, location, invasiveness, number, and rate of growth of the tumor rather than the histological tumor type [15,21,42]. Symptoms are caused by tumor-related intracardiac obstruction, compression of the heart or the great vessels, embolization of tumor fragments or adherent thrombi, and tumor infiltration [29,42–45].

Cardiac tumors often remain asymptomatic until they reach an advanced stage and many tumors are discovered incidentally during routine screening. In the series of Beghetti and associates, 30 of 56 patients (54%) exhibited no symptoms and were diagnosed during routine screening for tuberous sclerosis, assessment of a cardiac murmur or even prenatally [15]. If symptoms occur, they are usually nonspecific, such as heart murmur, arrhythmia, dyspnea, and congestive heart failure [15,24,27,29,40,46].

Syncope and signs of systemic embolization (stroke, retinal, coronary mesenteric, or renal artery emboli as well as emboli to the arteries of the extremities) are also common. ElBardissi and associates reported a 25% rate of tumor embolization, most often associated with aortic valve and left atrial tumors [47]. In 30–91% of the cases, cardiac rhabdomyomas were associated with tuberous sclerosis [15,25,26,46]. These patients may present with seizures as the leading symptom. Constitutional unspecific symptoms such as fever, night sweats, arthralgia, weight loss, and fatigue are not uncommon [21,40].

Right atrial tumors may cause symptoms of right heart failure and produce the characteristic murmurs of tricuspid insufficiency or stenosis. Tumors involving the right atrium have been mistaken for congenital cardiac lesions, including Ebstein anomaly and tricuspid stenosis. Because of substantial increase in right atrial pressure, these tumors may produce cyanosis by virtue of right-to-left shunting across a patent foramen ovale [48,49]. Intracavitary tumors of the right ventricle also have been associated with right heart failure as a result of obstruction or valvar dysfunction. Tricuspid insufficiency and right ventricular outflow tract obstruction have been described [49], with the latter

Table 39.1. Benign cardiac neoplasms in children. (Reproduced with permission from McAllister *et al.* [18]. Copyright © 1978 US Government Printing Office.)

Tumor	Age 0 to 1 year n (%)	Age 1 to 15 years n (%)
Rhabdomyoma	28 (62)	35 (45)
Teratoma	9 (21)	11 (14)
Fibroma	6 (13)	12 (15.5)
Hemangioma	1 (2)	4 (5)
AV node mesothelioma	1 (2)	3 (4)
Myxoma	–	12 (15.5)
Neurofibroma	–	1 (1)
Total	**45 (100)**	**78 (100)**

mimicking pulmonary atresia with intact ventricular septum. Right heart failure may also be a consequence of extensive intramural tumor infiltration of the right ventricle. Thrombi or tissue fragments from right-sided cardiac tumors may embolize to the pulmonary circulation and cause pulmonary hypertension [48,50]. Left atrial tumors typically mimic mitral valve disease. Murmurs and hemodynamic findings consistent with mitral stenosis and insufficiency have been described. Left atrial myxomas may produce obstructive symptoms only intermittently, particularly when the patient assumes the upright position [30]. Systemic embolization of left atrial myxomas is a well documented phenomenon. The diagnosis is made by histologic examination of the embolic material or by echocardiography during a search for the embolic source. Tumors encroaching on the left ventricular cavity may produce mitral regurgitation as well as inflow or outflow tract obstruction. The differential diagnosis of such tumors includes aortic stenosis, subaortic stenosis, hypoplastic left heart syndrome [51], and hypertrophic cardiomyopathy. Extensive infiltration of a tumor into the left ventricular myocardium has resulted in cardiac failure, as well as myocardial ischemia from coronary compression [52]. In the fetus, left heart tumors can become apparent as nonimmune hydrops fetalis [53]. Rhythm disturbances are another initial feature of pediatric cardiac tumors. Virtually every type of arrhythmia has been reported [54] in patients with underlying cardiac tumors, with the type of arrhythmia primarily related to the location of the tumor. Involvement of the conduction system may yield preexcitation syndrome, bundle branch block, or various degrees of AV block [53–56]. In addition, both supraventricular and ventricular tachycardia have been described, the latter being particularly associated with fibromas, hamartomas, and rhabdomyomas [15,24,57]. Sudden death also has been reported with a variety of tumors [28]. Any child who exhibits an unexplained arrhythmia should be evaluated with echocardiography to rule out an underlying cardiac neoplasm.

Diagnostic Modalities

Chest Roentgenography

Although over 80% of patients with cardiac tumors may present with abnormalities on their chest X-ray, these abnormalities are nonspecific [58]. Cardiomegaly, mediastinal widening, pleural effusions, congestive heart failure, and pulmonary edema are common findings. Occasionally, primary cardiac tumors, particularly fibromas, may calcify and become evident on plain chest radiographs [48,59]. Any chest X-ray that reveals an irregular cardiac silhouette or suspicious mediastinal calcification should prompt further investigation for a cardiac tumor [48].

Electrocardiography

In the presence of cardiac tumors, electrocardiographic findings are not uncommon, but are also generally nonspecific. In addition to the rhythm disturbances discussed above, electrocardiographic abnormalities include various degrees of AV block, atrial enlargement, ventricular hypertrophy, and ST-T segment changes. Focal ST-T segment abnormalities may herald myocardial ischemia owing to coronary artery compression, while diffuse ST-T segment abnormalities and low voltage have been associated with extensive intramural infiltration by the tumor.

Echocardiography

Echocardiography is the primary imaging technique for the evaluation of cardiac tumors. M-mode and two-dimensional echocardiography provide a safe and effective means for the noninvasive diagnosis in the fetus and in the child [16,25,60–62]. Tumor location, extent, and characteristics (single or multiple, intramuscular or intracavitary, solid or cystic) can be evaluated accurately and rapidly (Plates 39.1–39.4, see plate section opposite p. 594). Associated pericardial effusions are identified, and timely decompression of intrapericardial fluid collections may be performed under ultrasonographic guidance. With the addition of color-flow Doppler echocardiography, the obstructive nature and hemodynamic significance of cardiac tumors can be assessed, although very small and intramurally located tumors may not be detected. In most cases echocardiography provides accurate imaging of cardiac tumors and eliminates the need for invasive imaging techniques. More intensive routine echocardiographic screening and increasing application of fetal ultrasonography leads to early diagnosis of pediatric cardiac tumors, permits prevention of life-threatening complications, and allows for better planning of postnatal care [21].

Magnetic Resonance Imaging

Echocardiography is very sensitive in predicting the etiology of most intracavitary tumors but is less reliable in determining the nature of intramural or extramyocardial neoplasms [21]. Magnetic resonance imaging (MRI) provides complementary information to echocardiography [63,64]. Magnetic resonance imaging helps to elucidate the relationship of the tumor to the normal myocardium and the great vessels [63–66]. It provides information on tumor location, size, and boundaries (Figure 39.1). Another promising attribute of MRI is its ability to characterize certain tissue types, thus enhancing its value as a noninvasive diagnostic tool. For example, a lipoma exhibits a characteristic appearance on MRI [67] (Figure 39.2). This feature is particularly valuable in planning the extent and feasibility of tumor resection [65,66]. Tumor size, location, and borders can be determined by T1-weighted standard spin echo [68]. Fast gradient cine magnetic resonance angiography sequences provide information on the hemodynamic consequences of the tumor. The addition of spatial modulation of magnetization (tagging) is helpful in the differentiation of normal myocardial motion from that of the noncontracting tumor [65]. A T2-weighted spin echo sequence is useful in distinguishing vascular tumors, such as hemangiomas, from avascular tumors, such as fibromas [68]. Generally, malignant tumors appear to be inhomogeneous, infiltrate

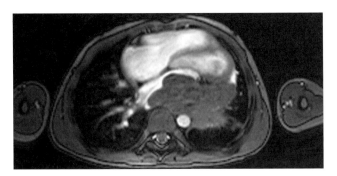

Figure 39.1 Malignant fibrous histiocytoma, magnetic resonance image. Axial T1-weighted magnetic resonance imaging demonstrating a malignant fibrous histiocytoma infiltrating the left atrium and the posterior wall of the left ventricle. (Courtesy of Dr. Albrecht Will, Department of Radiology, German Heart Center, Munich, Germany.)

the adjacent tissues, and are often associated with pericardial or pleural effusions [69]. The major shortcoming of MRI for imaging cardiac tumors in younger patients is that it requires deep sedation or even general anesthesia to eliminate artifacts caused by respiration and patient movement. Furthermore, uncontrollable tachyarrhythmias may also produce motion artifacts and thus preclude the use of MRI for cardiac imaging [70].

Angiography

Angiography once was considered the primary imaging modality for the diagnosis of cardiac tumors. Today however, cardiac catheterization is complementary in cases with associated congenital heart disease or in selected cases where hemodynamic evaluation is required. It is of particular importance in patients with suspected coronary artery disease [21]. In addition, electrophysiologic mapping at the time of angiography may identify the exact arrhythmogenic site in children with small or multiple tumors [15,24]. In the rare case in which a nonoperative tissue diagnosis is desired, transcatheter biopsy may be employed, with the inherent risk of tumor hemorrhage and tumor fragment embolization [71,72].

General Principles of Surgical Resection

Although the exact surgical management of a cardiac tumor depends largely on the site and extent of the mass,

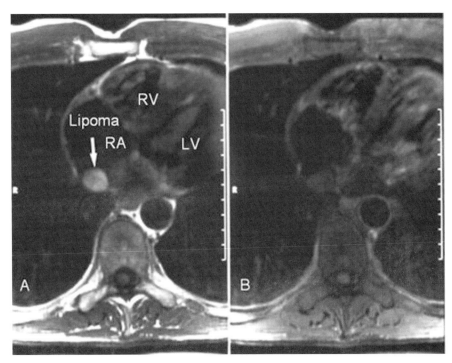

Figure 39.2 Lipoma, magnetic resonance image. Axial T1-weighted image (**A**) and with fat suppression (**B**). (LV, left ventricle; RA, right atrium; RV, right ventricle.) (Courtesy of Dr Albrecht Will, Department of Radiology, German Heart Center, Munich, Germany.)

some general comments regarding surgical resection are appropriate. Excision of virtually all intracardiac tumors requires the use of cardiopulmonary bypass, with tumor location occasionally mandating alternative cannulation sites. In contrast, most intrapericardial tumors may be excised without using cardiopulmonary bypass.

Tumors arising from the atria are approached directly through an atriotomy. A left atrial tumor can be approached through the right atrium and across the interatrial septum at the fossa ovalis.

Right ventricular tumors are usually amenable to resection via a right atriotomy and retraction of the tricuspid valve, thus obviating the need for a right ventriculotomy. Beghetti and associates report the case of a newborn with a huge right ventricular fibroma causing inflow obstruction who underwent partial resection associated with bidirectional cavopulmonary connection [73].

Surgical extirpation of left ventricular tumors, particularly those involving the outflow tract, may prove challenging [74]. In the interest of avoiding a left ventriculotomy, some tumors may be excised via a retrograde technique involving an aortotomy and retraction of the aortic valve leaflets (Plate 39.5, see plate section opposite p. 594). However, the small size of the neonatal aortic annulus may prevent complete resection via the retrograde technique, necessitating a concomitant antegrade approach via a left atriotomy and through the mitral valve. In cases of extensive left ventricular outflow tract and aortic valve involvement, the Ross procedure has proved successful [75]. A tumor mimicking hypoplastic left heart syndrome may require a variant of the Norwood operation [51,76].

General Considerations of Treatment Strategies

The vast majority of primary cardiac tumors in pediatric patients are benign. Tumor growth is slow and generally not invasive. Mechanical compromise and not the neoplastic potential should be considered [77]. Rhabdomyomas are the most common type of tumor and spontaneous regression has been reported in 50–100% of these patients [15,29,78–80]. Therefore, a conservative approach is advocated to allow the tumor to regress, and surgery is indicated only for severely symptomatic patients with hemodynamic compromise or patients with refractory dysrhythmias [15,25,27,29,41,77,79].

When an operative resection is required, the surgeon will usually attempt a complete resection [81]. Some authors even state that it should be the primary goal to remove the tumor as radically as possible in any case and to remove any potential obstruction [24,82]. Extensive myocardial involvement of the tumor or its proximity to critical structures (e.g., great vessels, coronary arteries, valves) may preclude complete excision. In many such circumstances, partial resection is appropriate [83] and can be

accomplished with satisfactory results [73,84]. Thus, total resection of the tumor is not the only therapeutic aim, and some authors argue that it is more important to restore the best possible heart function [41,77]. For malignant and unresectable benign tumor cardiac explantation, extracorporeal tumor excision and autotransplantation or orthotopic cardiac transplantation has been proposed to achieve complete resection [85–88]. The ultimate role of cardiac transplantation in treating malignant neoplastic disease in infants and children needs to be established.

The specific treatment for each type of cardiac tumor, as well as the indications for and outcome of each treatment, are discussed in more detail below.

Primary Benign Cardiac Tumors

Rhabdomyomas

The rhabdomyoma is the most common primary intracardiac tumor in the pediatric age group, found in 36–78% of pediatric clinical and autopsy series [13,15,25,29,30,34,40, 89,90]. The cardiac rhabdomyoma is a benign tumor of cardiac myocytes.

Rhabdomyoma tends to be more common in neonates and infants [18,80,91], and the majority are diagnosed within the first year of life [18,80]. In the Armed Forces Institute of Pathology series, 78% of patients with rhabdomyomas were younger than 1 year of age [18]. Males are more often affected than females [46,90].

Grossly, rhabdomyomas are white, grey, or yellow nodules that are well circumscribed and nonencapsulated (Plate 39.5, see plate section opposite p. 594). The tumors vary in size from 1 mm to 10 cm [26]. They are often located in the ventricles with equal predilection for the right and left ventricles but can also be found in the atria, at the cavoatrial junction, within the papillary muscles, within the myocardial wall and the septum, or even on the epicardial surface [18,26,29,74,90,92]. In 90% of cases, rhabdomyomas emerge from multiple sites (Plate 39.1, see plate section opposite p. 594). Although rhabdomyomas tend to reside in an intramural location, they may grow also in an intracavitary fashion and fill an entire cardiac chamber causing outflow or inflow tract obstruction. Small lesions may involve the conduction system causing dysrhythmias [26,92].

Histologically, rhabdomyomas are characterized by large, round, or polygonal cells with clear cytoplasm and abundant glycogen. Classic "spider cells" feature a central cytoplasmic mass containing the nucleus, with thin projections extending toward the cell membrane. Calcification or fibrosis is rare [26]. These tumors occur most frequently in neonates and infants, often regress over time, and are composed of cells without mitotic activity. Rhabdomyomas are believed to represent fetal hamartomas rather than true cardiac neoplasms [90].

In 1862 von Recklinghausen first described the coincidence of cardiac tumors and intracerebral sclerotic areas in a newborn baby [93]. Up to 91% of children with rhabdomyomas will have associated tuberous sclerosis [15,20,26,74,94,95]. Conversely, patients with tuberous sclerosis develop cardiac rhabdomyomas in 43–67% of cases [79,91,92,96]. Tuberous sclerosis is an autosomal dominant inherited disorder with a highly variable phenotype characterized by the development of benign tumors (hamartomas) in multiple organ systems, including skin, brain, heart, lungs, kidney, and liver [91,97]. Although it can affect virtually every organ system, the classic clinical triad of tuberous sclerosis consists of seizures secondary to cerebral cortical tubers, mental retardation, and characteristic skin lesions (adenoma sebaceum). Seizures occur in over 80% of the patients and developmental delay in over 60% [97]. However, because these clinical features may not be detected until later in life, cardiac rhabdomyomas may be the only manifestation in neonates and infants with tuberous sclerosis [98]. All newborns or fetuses with a family history of tuberous sclerosis should be evaluated for cardiac rhabdomyomas [99].

The clinical picture of rhabdomyomas depends on the number, size, and location of these tumors. The most common initial features are cardiac murmur, symptoms of cardiac obstruction, or arrhythmia. Patients with small tumors are generally asymptomatic. Jozwiak et al. analyzed 154 patients with tuberous sclerosis and found 74 patients with a cardiac rhabdomyoma. Most (61%) of these tumors were clinically silent [91]. Larger tumors may obstruct the cardiac cavity or associated valves, leading to significant hemodynamic compromise [15,25,74] (Plate 39.5, see plate section opposite p. 594). Subaortic stenosis caused by a pedunculated tumor is a common finding in infants with cardiac rhabdomyoma [26]. Tumors obstructing the right or left AV valve can simulate tricuspid or mitral valve stenosis/atresia. Obstruction of the tricuspid valve may also lead to right-to-left shunting at the level of the foramen ovale, resulting in cyanosis. Involvement of the conduction system may yield serious arrhythmias, including almost any type of atrial or ventricular dysrhythmia including pre-excitation, sinus node dysfunction, and complete AV block [24,26,92].

Many authors consider the combination of the following criteria highly suspicious for the diagnosis of a rhabdomyoma: tumor morphology and location (multiple tumors, located in the ventricles); presence of a single tumor plus involvement of other organs (central nervous system, skin, kidney); and/or a family history of tuberous sclerosis [15,25,27,79]. On echocardiography, rhabdomyomas appear as solid intramyocardial tumors, often involving multiple areas of myocardium. Their structure is homogeneous, representing echo bright densities of varying size (Plate 39.1, see plate section opposite p. 594). Large rhabdomyomas may cause right or left ventricular outflow or inflow

obstruction (Plate 39.5, see plate section opposite p. 594). Pericardial effusions have not been reported.

Spontaneous regression of rhabdomyomas is well documented and is reported to be more frequent in younger patients and in those with smaller tumors [26]. Of these patients, 50–100% show partial or complete regression [15,29,78–80]. Farooki and associates, analyzed five patients with cardiac rhabdomyoma associated with tuberous sclerosis and determined a regression rate of 0.9–6 mm/month [80].

Asymptomatic children with cardiac rhabdomyomas can be simply followed with serial echocardiographic examinations. Surgery is indicated in patients with medically refractory arrhythmias and hemodynamically significant obstruction. This is the case in up to 23% of children [15,29,74]. In the study of Beghetti et al., nine out of 44 patients exhibited a gradient in the left or right ventricular outflow tract, four with a gradient of >40 mmHg underwent surgery [15]. Critically ill neonates with severe mechanical obstruction and heart failure may be stabilized preoperatively with a prostaglandin E1 infusion to maintain patency of the ductus arteriosus. The primary goal of surgical resection is to excise the tumor. This often mandates only partial tumor excision, when a complete excision would sacrifice vital structures or a critical portion of the myocardial mass [15,24,74,83]. Typically, the remaining rhabdomyomatous tissue will regress spontaneously and cause no further sequelae. This management strategy in children with rhabdomyomas is associated with excellent short-term and long-term prognoses [15,24,29]. Tumor-related reoperations are very rare [15,29].

Fibromas

Cardiac fibromas are the second most common primary cardiac tumors in infants and children, comprising up to 20% [13,15,18,24,30]. Although most fibromas are diagnosed within the first few years of life, some remain quiescent and undiscovered until adolescence or adulthood. Fibromas are benign white, firm, well circumscribed, not encapsulated tumors predominantly located in the left ventricular free wall or the interventricular septum [13,18,20,26] (Plate 39.2, see plate section opposite p. 594). Right ventricular free wall and atrial involvement are rare [26]. In contrast to rhabdomyomas, which tend to be multiple, fibromas generally appear as single tumors [26]. These tumors infiltrate the myocardium. Fibromas may grow to a large size and cause outflow tract obstruction and compression or obliteration of cardiac chambers [24,73,100]. Pericardial effusions have not been reported. According to Freedom et al. their average size is about 5 cm in diameter [26]. Cystic degeneration and focal calcification is frequent and is an important diagnostic imaging feature [59]. Neither spontaneous regression nor malignant transformation of fibromas has been reported. A characteristic whorled appearance is featured on their cut surface and is reminiscent of a uterine leiomyoma. The histologic features of fibromas consist of relatively avascular dense connective tissue in the central portion, with fibroblasts and collagen interspersed with normal cardiac myocytes near the periphery.

As with all cardiac tumors, the initial clinical features of cardiac fibromas are largely dependent on their size and location. Because of their propensity to invade the interventricular septum and conduction system, fibromas often are associated with life-threatening arrhythmias or sudden death [15,56]. In infants with extremely large intramural tumors, severe congestive heart failure from mechanical intracavitary or valvar obstruction may be the primary mode of expression. Occasionally, fibromas may grow to great sizes in older children and yet remain clinically silent, with their presence revealed only by the incidental detection of a heart murmur or cardiomegaly on plain radiography.

On echocardiography, fibromas appear as solid intramural tumors (i.e., homogeneous, echo-bright masses) ranging from a few millimeters to several centimeters in diameter (Plate 39.2, see plate section opposite p. 594). Very large fibromas may herniate into the outflow tract of the right or left ventricle, causing severe outflow obstruction. Embolic events are rare. The indication for operative treatment of fibromas is very similar to the one described for rhabdomyomas. Even though fibromas do not apparently regress, their presence in an asymptomatic individual does not mandate surgical resection. Although complete resection is the primary surgical goal in treating symptomatic fibromas, contraindications to complete resection include situations in which the conduction system may be violated or a critical mass of ventricular myocardium would be sacrificed [24]. In such cases, partial resection has resulted in immediate clinical improvement and favorable long-term survival [24,73,77,85]. However, in some cases of massive fibroma infiltrating cardiac walls, cardiac transplantation may be the only treatment [86,101].

Myxomas

Myxoma is the most common primary benign cardiac tumor in adults and represents 50% of all benign tumors [13,18,20]. According to MacGowan and colleagues, who reviewed all patients admitted to the national cardiac surgical unit of the Republic of Ireland, the incidence is estimated to be 0.5 per 1 000 000 population per year [102]. Myxomas are rare (0–5%) in pediatric patients and are usually diagnosed in older children and adolescents [15,24,25,29,41]. However, incidental reports describe their occurrence in neonates [48].

An autosomal dominant mode of familial inheritance is discovered in approximately 10% of patients with myxomas as part of the Carney complex [103]. About 75% of myxomas originate in the left atrium and 15–20% in the right atrium [26,104]. Most myxomas arise from the endocardium of the interatrial septum at the border of the fossa ovalis. However, attachments to the posterior or anterior atrial wall and to the atrial appendage have also been described. They may arise from a broad attachment base or be pedunculated [26,104]. Only about 3–4% are located in the right or left ventricle [104]. Although myxomas are generally solitary tumors, multiple and biatrial myxomas have been identified [105]. Multiple tumors and atypical locations are more frequent in cases of familial predisposition [106]. Macroscopically, cardiac myxomas appear as polypoid, often pedunculated, round or oval, white, gray-white, yellowish, or brown masses, with a smooth or gently lobulated surface (Plate 39.6, see plate section opposite p. 594). Polypoid myxomas are compact and show little tendency toward spontaneous fragmentation. The less common villous or papillary myxomas are characterized by a surface with multiple fine villous extensions, which tend to fractionate [104]. Histologically, myxomas consist of a myxoid mucopolysaccharide matrix. Polygonal cells with eosinophilic cytoplasm are dispersed one at a time or in small clusters in the myxoid stroma [26,104]. Myxomas often contain cysts and areas of hemorrhage [104]. About 10% of the tumors show calcification with occasional foci of metaplastic bone [18,35,48,107]. Traditionally, myxomas were believed to be thrombotic in origin. However, most evidence suggests that these tumors actually arise from multipotential mesenchymal cells in the subendocardial region [108].

Although generally regarded as benign, some myxomas have been classified as malignant on the basis of local invasion or tumor recurrence at primary or embolic sites [109]. However, the true malignant potential of this neoplasm remains a controversial issue. There are two groups of patients with tumor recurrence: those with recurrent cardiac myxoma resulting from inadequate surgical excision and those with tumor recurrence at multiple sites. The latter group exhibits a poor prognosis, with a mortality of approximately 50% [26].

Most children with cardiac myxomas are symptomatic, and many suffer from the classic clinical triad of cardiac obstructive symptoms, emboli, and constitutional symptoms. Depending on their size and mobility, myxomas may obstruct the mitral or tricuspid valve during diastole (Plate 39.3, see plate section opposite p. 594) and mimic mitral or tricuspid valve stenosis with subsequent symptoms of congestive heart failure, recurrent pulmonary edema, syncope, or sudden death [110,111]. The extent of the valvar obstruction may vary with the body position [112]. In the typical situation in which a left atrial myxoma intermittently obstructs the mitral valve, symptoms may occur only in an upright position, while recumbency may cause these symptoms to subside. A mobile atrial tumor moving forward and backward across the AV valve into the ventricle can affect mitral or tricuspid valve closure and cause regurgitation. A tumor with a long pedicle may even prolapse through the AV valve and obstruct blood flow across the aortic or pulmonic valve.

Systolic or diastolic murmurs may be heard in more than half of the patients with myxomas. Diastolic murmurs result from obstructed filling of the left or right ventricle. On auscultation, a mid-diastolic murmur or characteristic "tumor plop" may be evident, the latter of which occurs during prolapse of the tumor through the mitral valve during diastole. Systolic murmurs occur when the tumor interferes with valve closure [104].

The embolic capacity of tumor fragments or thrombotic material overlying a cardiac myxoma is well described. Although most emboli originate in the left atrium and involve the systemic circulation, right-sided atrial myxomas may yield pulmonary emboli or paradoxical emboli through a patent interatrial communication [48,50]. An infant or child who sustains an unexplained embolic event must be evaluated by echocardiography for a cardiac myxoma; in such individuals it is also wise to submit the extracted embolic material for histopathologic analysis. Constitutional symptoms account for the third component of the clinical triad associated with myxomas. Such vague symptoms, which include fever, weight loss, malaise, myalgias, and arthralgias, are often attributed erroneously to a rheumatologic disorder.

An immunologic response to the tumor has been proposed as the basis for these systemic symptoms. Associated laboratory abnormalities include evidence of hemolytic anemia, thrombocytopenia, and an elevated sedimentation rate and C reactive protein level.

On echocardiography, myxomas appear as lobulated intracavitary masses attached by long pedicles to adjacent endocardium (Plate 39.3, see plate section opposite p. 594). Echocardiographic evaluation of left atrial myxomas should include careful M-mode and Doppler evaluation of the mitral valve and its potential involvement.

Right atrial myxomas exhibit corresponding symptoms to left atrial myxomas, necessitating comprehensive interrogation of the tricuspid valve and right ventricular inflow hemodynamics. In addition, because embolic events are common with myxomas, evaluation of all right heart myxomas should include Doppler echocardiographic estimation of pulmonary artery pressures to estimate pulmonary hypertension resulting from recurrent pulmonary emboli. Ventricular myxomas are rarely encountered. Myxomas in the left ventricle commonly attach to the interventricular septum or left ventricular apex by long pedicles, allowing prolapse of the tumor mass, eventually causing dynamic left ventricular outflow obstruction. Right ventricular myxomas arise from pedicles attached to the outflow tract or to the free wall and may cause right ventricular outflow tract obstruction. Broad-based attachments

to adjacent right ventricular myocardium should suggest a diagnosis other than myxoma.

The diagnosis of a cardiac myxoma is in general an indication for its surgical removal. Left untreated, many asymptomatic patients with myxomas may suffer an unexpected embolic event. Right and left atrial myxomas are approached through the right atrium via full sternotomy or right anterolateral minithoracotomy. The septum is incised at the fossa ovalis and the base of the tumor identified. Because these tumors are prone to local recurrence, it is essential to excise the tumor completely, along with a rim of normal endocardium around its base. To prevent intraoperative embolization of fragments from these friable tumors, one should avoid undue manipulation of the heart until initiation of cardiopulmonary bypass and application of the aortic cross-clamp.

Intrapericardial Teratomas

Intrapericardial teratomas are composed of multiple tissues of all three germ layers [10,18] and may contain elements of muscle, cartilage, gastrointestinal, respiratory, and neural tissue. In clinical series they represent 8–12% of all tumors [18,25,29,41] and constitute the fourth most common group of primary cardiac tumors in pediatric patients.

About two-thirds of tumors are diagnosed within the first year of life and 50% are discovered within the first month of life [18,113–115]. Approximately 20% of cardiac teratomas are malignant [116].

The majority of teratomas have an extracardiac but intrapericardial location. Intracardiac teratomas are extremely rare [18,37,117]. Teratomas are large, solitary, cystic, encapsulated tumors (Plate 39.7, see plate section opposite p. 594), which often are attached to the root of the aorta or pulmonary artery by a narrow pedicle [18]. They are usually located anteriorly and to the right side of the mediastinum, nestled between the aorta and superior vena cava [118,119]. Occasionally, intrapericardial teratomas attach to the left side of the ascending aorta, lying over the left atrium and left ventricle [114,120]. Uncommonly, these tumors may arise posterior to the aorta [120]. Older infants and children usually present with small tumors. In neonates and young infants, however, intrapericardial teratomas are rather large.

Because intrapericardial teratomas tend to be very large, they often cause obstruction of the great vessels (superior vena cava, ascending aorta, and pulmonary artery), external compression of the cardiac chambers (right atrium and right ventricle), and pulmonary parenchyma. Furthermore, as opposed to most other benign cardiac tumors, intrapericardial teratomas usually are associated with a voluminous serous pericardial effusion [119].

As a result of these features, the clinical picture is often one of neonatal respiratory distress, heart failure, and cardiac tamponade, ultimately progressing to death if timely treatment is not undertaken [114,121].

The diagnosis of intrapericardial teratomas is made easily and accurately by two-dimensional echocardiography in both the fetus [118] and infant [122–125]. These tumors appear as single, nonhomogeneous, pedunculated masses within the pericardial sac. Intrapericardial teratomas contain multiple cysts and calcifications, appearing as echolucent and echogenic foci, respectively, on two-dimensional echocardiography (Plate 39.4, see plate section opposite p. 594). Clinically significant pericardial effusions are commonly present in the critically ill neonate or infant [124,126] and are diagnosed by two-dimensional echocardiography. Ultrasonographically guided evacuation of pericardial fluid can be lifesaving for critically ill patients with evidence of cardiac tamponade. However, recurrence of pericardial effusion is the rule if the teratoma is not resected [126]. *In utero* detection of intrapericardial teratomas allows advanced planning and expeditious postnatal surgical resection before the neonate develops severe cardiorespiratory distress [127].

Because all intrapericardial teratomas eventually become symptomatic [119], complete surgical excision should be undertaken as soon as the diagnosis is made. This involves separation of the tumor from the epicardium of the cardiac chambers, as well as division of the pedicle connecting the tumor to the great vessels. Because intrapericardial teratomas normally receive their blood supply from the vasa vasorum of the aorta and pulmonary artery, one should exercise caution when dissecting the pedicle. The great majority of these tumors are completely extracardiac; therefore, cardiopulmonary bypass is rarely necessary for their removal. Early surgical excision of benign intrapericardial teratomas is considered both lifesaving and curative, because to our knowledge recurrence of these lesions has not been reported [128].

Angiomas

Tumors that form vascular channels, such as hemangiomas, lymphangiomas, and other tumors, are benign and rarely involve the heart. Hemangiomas are red, hemorrhagic tumors comprised of endothelium-lined vascular channels of various sizes and contain blood. They may occur in any chamber of the heart, visible as multiple, echolucent areas within the myocardium on two-dimensional echocardiography. Similar to the intrapericardial teratomas, these tumors are often associated with a serous pericardial effusion. Although most of these benign neoplasms are incidental findings, some may produce rhythm disturbances or obstructive symptoms. Surgical resection is indicated for small, well circumscribed, symptomatic hemangiomas [129]. In the absence of symptoms, hemangiomas of all sizes may be monitored with serial echocardiographic examinations [130,131]. However, in symptomatic patients with diffuse tumorous myocardial involvement, even cardiac transplantation may be required.

Hamartomas

The origin of myocardial hamartomas is controversial [27]. This is reflected by the various terms that have been introduced to describe this abnormality (e.g., histiocytoid cardiomyopathy, Purkinje cell tumor, foamy myocardial transformation) [27]. Myocardial hamartomas appear as grayish white nodules primarily involving the endocardial or epicardial surface of the left ventricle [24]. Histologically, the tumor cells resemble modified cardiac myocytes [57]. The individual tumor cells have large numbers of mitochondria [24]. Most of these tumors are diagnosed because the patients experience refractory life-threatening ventricular tachycardia within the first year of life [24,27,51,57,132]. A 2:1 female preponderance was reported in one series [57]. Because myocardial hamartomas are only a few cells thick, these tumors are generally below the threshold of detection by echocardiography [24]. Electrophysiologic studies and intraoperative inspection of the epicardial and endocardial surfaces are the only means of diagnosis. Intraoperative mapping, tumor excision, and cryoablation of the margins of the excision site yield cure and sustained freedom from tachyarrhythmias [24,57,132]. However, in the series of Takach et al., 3 of 16 patients required a reoperation within 24 hours because of recurrent ventricular tachycardia [24].

Other Primary Benign Cardiac Tumors

Other exceedingly rare benign pediatric cardiac tumors include lipomas, papillary fibroelastomas, mesotheliomas, and neurofibromas.

In addition, a few cases of so-called cardiac pseudotumors in pediatric patients have been described [133]. These interesting entities, which are considered a benign proliferative response to an unknown stimulus, contain a preponderance of plasma cells and are thus most aptly termed inflammatory pseudotumors. On echocardiography, these tumors appear as homogeneous intracavitary masses, often growing to fill entire cardiac chambers. Although not believed to be truly neoplastic, these lesions may form a tumor-like mass and produce cardiac symptoms identical to those caused by true cardiac tumors. As a result, surgical resection is the preferred treatment in symptomatic individuals. In asymptomatic patients monitored with serial echocardiographic examinations, spontaneous regression usually is observed.

Papillary fibroelastomas, the second most common tumor in adult patients [18,134], are very rare in the pediatric population. Gowda and colleagues reviewed the literature and identified 725 cases with histologically confirmed fibroelastoma. Only nine patients were children <10 years [134]. Familial occurrence has been reported. These tumors are benign endocardial papillomas with a characteristic flower-like appearance predominantly located on the valvar surface. The aortic valve (36.5%) is the valve most commonly involved, followed by the mitral valve (29.5%) and nonvalvar sites [134]. The tumors vary in size from 2–70 mm. Transient ischemic attack or stroke as well as angina or myocardial infarction are the most common clinical presentation. On echocardiography the tumor appears as a small, mobile, pedunculated or sessile valvar or endocardial mass [134]. The diagnosis of a fibroelastoma is in general an indication for its surgical removal. Surgery is recommended for symptomatic patients as well as asymptomatic patients with a mobile tumor.

Primary Malignant Cardiac Tumors

Primary malignant cardiac tumors are extremely rare accounting for less than 10% of primary cardiac tumors in the pediatric population [18,25,24,29,30]. The majority of these malignant neoplasms represent various types of sarcomas including angiosarcomas, rhabdomyosarcomas, leiomyosarcomas, and fibrosarcomas. Of these, angiosarcomas are the most frequently encountered (Plate 39.8, see plate section opposite p. 594) [19,22,24,33,40,135]. However, in neonates rhabdomyosarcoma seems to be more frequent [28]. Much of the literature describing malignant tumors has been limited to case reports, and there are only a limited number of studies comprising larger series of mainly adult patients [19,33,85,88].

Malignant cardiac tumors often remain asymptomatic until they reach an advanced stage [21]. About one-third of patients exhibit metastatic disease at the time of presentation [33]. Symptomatic patients complain about a variety of symptoms such as dyspnea, atypical chest pain, or congestive heart failure. Pericardial effusions are common. The tumors can arise in any part of the heart [21,33]. On echocardiography, sarcomas are single, homogenous intramural tumors, with extension into adjacent cardiac chambers generally present at the time of diagnosis (Figures 39.1, 39.3).

The prognosis of patients diagnosed with malignant cardiac tumor remains poor. Expected survival in untreated patients is less than 1 year [136]. Metastases to the lungs, liver, and brain are common [33]. In patients with unresectable tumors, a combined chemotherapy (vincristine, ifosfamide, etoposide) and radiotherapy did not improve survival [137]. Patients, who present with metastatic disease, have a median survival of 5 months compared with 15 months for patients without metastatic disease [33]. Even with complete surgical excision the median survival does not exceed 2 years [19,33,135,138].

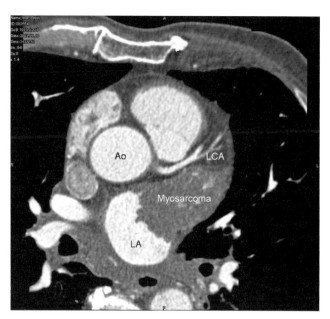

Figure 39.3 Left atrial myosarcoma, computed tomography. (LA, left atrium; Ao, aorta; LCA, left coronary artery.) (Courtesy of Dr Albrecht Will, Department of Radiology, German Heart Center, Munich, Germany.)

Tumor recurrence is frequent [33]. The role of adjuvant chemotherapy and/or radiotherapy after surgical resection remains controversial. Several studies have failed to demonstrate any benefit [33,138,139,140]. Others, however, have found chemotherapy or radiation to be efficacious in treating primary cardiac sarcomas [141,142]. In an isolated case of a 24-year-old patient with a leiomyosarcoma, Pessotto and associates could achieve complete tumor remission with combined chemotherapy and radiotherapy after surgical excision [143]. The role of cardiac transplantation for treatment of nonmetastatic cardiac sarcoma in infants and children remains controversial [87]. Talbot *et al.* performed a combined heart and lung transplantation in four patients aged 37–45 years with primary cardiac sarcoma [88]. All of these patients had tumor recurrence, and the median survival was only 31 months despite this aggressive approach [88].

Secondary Cardiac Tumors

Secondary involvement of the pediatric heart by extracardiac malignancies is more common than primary cardiac tumors [30]. Chan and associates reviewed clinical and autopsy records of 3641 infants and children with malignant solid tumors and identified 59 patients with secondary cardiac tumors [30]. Forty-five of these presented with metastases from a distant tumor site, and 14 children with a tumor extending directly into the great veins and cardiac chambers [30]. The most common malignancies in childhood with metastatic spread to the heart are lymphomas, neuroblastomas, and extracardiac sarcomas [30]. Direct tumor extension to the right atrium via the inferior vena cava may occur with primary renal (Wilms' tumor) and hepatic malignancies [30,144]. The clinical symptoms and the tumor appearance are usually dominated by the nature of the primary malignancy. Features directly attributable to cardiac involvement include hemorrhagic pericardial effusions, cardiac compression, and arrhythmias. Aside from resection of Wilms' tumors with intracaval or intracardiac extension or both, the role of surgical intervention for usually incurable malignancies with secondary cardiac invasion is limited. In patients with Wilms' tumors who have thrombus extension into the right atrium, a planned approach using cardiopulmonary bypass and intracardiac exposure has proven safe and effective [145,146]. Initial treatment with chemotherapy has resulted in complete resolution of tumor thrombus in some patients; in others, surgical management was facilitated because of reduction in the size of the tumor thrombus [145,146].

Acknowledgments

The authors wish to thank Richard Henze, MD (Institute of Anesthesiology); Manfred Vogt, MD, (Department of Pediatric Cardiology); and Albrecht Will, MD (Institute of Radiology) for their assistance in providing echocardiographic and MRIs used in this chapter.

References

1. Columbo MR. (1559) *De Re Anatomica Libri XV*. Venetiis: Ex typographia Nicolai Beuilacquae.
2. Malpighi M. (1666) *Dissertatio Eiusdem de Polypo Cordis*. Bononiae: Ex typographia iacobi montij MDCLXVI.
3. Barnes AR, Beaver DC, Snell AM. (1934) Primary sarcoma of the heart; report of a case with electrocardiographic and pathological studies. Am Heart 19, 480–491.
4. Beck CS. (1942) An intrapericardial teratoma and a tumor of the heart: both removed operatively. Ann Surg 116, 161–174.
5. Mauer ER. (1952) Successful removal of tumor of the heart. J Thorac Surg 3, 479–482.
6. Goldberg HP, Glenn F, Dotter CT, et al. (1952) Myxoma of the left atrium. Diagnosis made during life with operative and postmortem findings. Circulation 6, 762–767.
7. Effert S, Domanig E. (1959) [Diagnosis of intra-auricular tumors and large thrombi with the aid of ultrasonic echography]. Dtsch Med Wocheschr 84, 6–8.
8. Bahnson HT, Newman EV. (1953) Diagnosis and surgical removal of intracavitary myxoma of the right atrium. Bull Johns Hopkins Hosp 93, 150–163.
9. Chitwood WR Jr. (1992) Clarence Crafoord and the first successful resection of a cardiac myxoma. Ann Thorac Surg 54, 997–998.
10. Mehta SM, Myers JL. (2000) Congenital heart surgery nomenclature and database project: Cardiac tumors. Ann Thorac Surg 69, S358–S368.
11. Silverman NA. (1980) Primary cardiac tumors. Ann Surg 191, 127–138.
12. Reynen K. (1996) Frequency of primary tumors of the heart. Am J Cardiol 77, 107.
13. Nadas AS, Ellison RC. (1968) Cardiac tumors in infancy. Am J Cardiol 21, 363–366.
14. Fyke FE III, Seward JB, Edwards WD, et al. (1985) Primary cardiac tumors: experience with 30 consecutive patients since the introduction of two-dimensional echocardiography. J Am Coll Cardiol 5, 1465–1473.
15. Beghetti M, Gow RM, Haney I, et al. (1997) Pediatric primary benign cardiac tumors: a 15-year review. Am Heart J 134, 1107–1114.
16. Holley DG, Martin GR, Brenner JI, et al. (1995) Diagnosis and management of fetal cardiac tumors: a multicenter experience and review of published reports. J Am Coll Cardiol 26, 516–520.
17. Burke A, Virmani R. (1996) Tumors of the heart and great vessels. In: *Atlas of Tumor Pathology*, 3rd series. Washington DC: Armed Forces Institute of Pathology, pp. 127–170.
18. McAllister HA Jr, Fenoglio JJ Jr. (1978) Tumors of the cardiovascular system. In: *Atlas of Tumor Pathology*, 2nd series. Washington, DC: Armed Forces Institute of Pathology.
19. Blondeau P. (1990) Primary cardiac tumors – French studies of 533 cases. Thorac Cardiovasc Surg 38, 192–195.
20. Cooley DA. (1990) Surgical treatment of cardiac neoplasm: 32-year experience. Thorac Cardiovasc Surg 38, 176-82.
21. Perchinsky MJ, Lichtenstein SV, Tyers GF. (1997) Primary cardiac tumors: forty years experience with 71 patients. Cancer 79, 1809–1815.
22. Bakaeen FG, Reardon MJ, Coselli JS, et al. (2003) Surgical outcome in 85 patients with primary cardiac tumors. Am J Surg 186, 641–647.
23. ElBardissi AW, Dearani JA, Daly RC, et al. (2008) Survival after resection of primary cardiac tumors: a 48-year experience. Circulation 118(14 suppl), S7–S15.
24. Takach TJ, Reul GJ, Ott DA, et al. (1996) Primary cardiac tumors in infants and children: immediate and long-term operative results. Ann Thorac Surg 62, 559–564.
25. Sallee D, Spector ML, van Heeckeren DW, et al. (1999) Primary pediatric cardiac tumors: a 17 year experience. Cardiol Young 9, 155–162.
26. Freedom RM, Lee KJ, MacDonald C, et al. (2000) Selected aspects of cardiac tumors in infancy and childhood. Pediatr Cardiol 21, 299–316.
27. Becker AE. (2000) Primary heart tumors in the pediatric age group: a review of salient pathologic features relevant for clinicians. Pediatr Cardiol 21, 317–332.
28. Isaacs H Jr. (2004) Fetal and neonatal cardiac tumors. Pediatr Cardiol 25, 252–273.
29. Günther T, Schreiber C, Noebauer C, et al. (2008) Treatment strategies for pediatric patients with primary cardiac and pericardial tumors: a 30 year review. Pediatr Cardiol 29, 1071–1076.
30. Chan HS, Sonley MJ, Moes CA, et al. (1985) Primary and secondary tumors of childhood involving the heart, peri-

cardium, and great vessels. A report of 75 cases and review of the literature. Cancer 56, 825–836.

31. Shapiro LM. (2001) Cardiac tumours: diagnosis and management. Heart 85, 218–222.

32. Reardon MJ, Malaisrie SC, Walkes JC, et al. (2006) Cardiac autotransplantation for primary cardiac tumors. Ann Thorac Surg 82, 645–650.

33. Simpson L, Kumar SK, Okuno SH, et al. (2008) Malignant primary cardiac tumors: review of a single institution experience. Cancer 112, 2440–2446.

34. Arciniegas E, Hakimi M, Farooki ZQ, et al. (1980) Primary cardiac tumors in children. J Thorac Cardiovasc Surg 79, 582–591.

35. Prichard RW. (1951) Tumors of the heart; review of the subject and report of 150 cases. AMA Arch Pathol 51, 98–128.

36. Hanfling SM. (1960) Metastatic cancer to the heart. Review of the literature and report of 127 cases. Circulation 22, 474–483.

37. Heath D. (1968) Pathology of cardiac tumors. Am J Cardiol 21, 315–327.

38. Smith C. (1986) Tumors of the heart. Arch Pathol Lab Med 110, 371–374.

39. Chiles C, Woodard PK, Gutierrez FR, et al. (2001) Metastatic involvement of the heart and pericardium: CT and MR imaging. Radiographics 21, 439–449.

40. Butany J, Nair V, Naseemuddin A, et al. (2005) Cardiac tumours: diagnosis and management. Lancet Oncol 6, 219–228.

41. Stiller B, Hetzer R, Meyer R, et al. (2001) Primary cardiac tumors: when is surgery necessary? Eur J Cardiothoracic Surg 20, 1002–1006.

42. Pinede L, Duhaut P, Loire R. (2001) Clinical presentation of left atrial cardiac myxoma: a series of 112 consecutive cases. Medicine(Baltimore) 80, 159–172.

43. Acebo E, Val-Bernal JF, Gómez-Román JJ, et al. (2003) Clinicopathologic study and DNA analysis of 37 cardiac myxomas: a 28-year experience. Chest 123, 1379–1385.

44. Centofanti P, Di Rosa E, Deorsola L, et al. (1999) Primary cardiac tumors: early and late results of surgical treatment in 91 patients. Ann Thorac Surg 68, 1236–1241.

45. Huang Z, Sun L, Du M, et al. (2003) Primary cardiac valve tumors: early and late results of surgical treatment in 10 patients. 76, 1609–1613.

46. Verhaaren HA, Vanakker O, De Wolf D, et al. (2003) Left ventricular outflow obstruction in rhabdomyoma of infancy: meta-analysis of the literature. J Pediatr 143, 258–263.

47. ElBardissi AW, Dearani JA, Daly RC, et al. (2009) Embolic potential of cardiac tumors and outcome after resection: a case-control study. Stroke 40, 156–162.

48. Dianzumba SB, Char G. (1982) Large calcified right atrial myxoma in a newborn. Rare cause of neonatal death. Br Heart J 48, 177–179.

49. Marin-Garcia J, Fitch CW, Shenefelt RE. (1984) Primary right ventricular tumor (fibroma) simulating cyanotic heart disease in a newborn. J Am Coll Cardiol 3, 868–871.

50. Stern MJ, Cohen MV, Fish B, et al. (1981) Clinical presentation and non-invasive diagnosis of right heart masses. Br Heart J 46, 552–558.

51. Elderkin RA, Radford DJ. (2002) Primary cardiac tumours in a paediatric population. J Paediatr Child Health 38, 173–177.

52. Foster ED, Spooner EW, Farina MA, et al. (1984) Cardiac rhabdomyoma in the neonate: surgical management. Ann Thorac Surg 37, 249–253.

53. Guereta LG, Burgueros M, Elorza MD, et al. (1986) Cardiac rhabdomyoma presenting as fetal hydrops. Pediatr Cardiol 7, 171–174.

54. Mühler EG, Kienast W, Turniski-Harder V, et al. (1994) Arrhythmias in infants and children with primary cardiac tumors. Eur Heart J 15, 915–921.

55. Mehta AV. (1993) Rhabdomyoma and ventricular preexcitation syndrome. A report of two cases and review of literature. Am J Dis Child 147, 669–671.

56. Filiatrault M, Béland MJ, Neilson KA, et al. (1991) Cardiac fibroma presenting with clinically significant arrhythmias in infancy. Pediatr Cardiol 12, 118–120.

57. Garson A Jr, Smith RT Jr, Moak JP, et al. (1987) Incessant ventricular tachycardia in infants: myocardial hamartomas and surgical cure. J Am Coll Cardiol 10, 619–626.

58. Bogren HG, DeMaria AN, Mason DT. (1980) Imaging procedures in the detection of cardiac tumors, with emphasis on echocardiography: a review. Cardiovasc Intervent Radiol 3, 107–125.

59. Soler-Soler J, Romero-González R. (1975) Calcified intramural fibroma of the left ventricle. Eur J Cardiol 3, 71–73.

60. Watanabe T, Hojo Y, Kozaki T, et al. (1991) Hypoplastic left heart syndrome with rhabdomyoma of the left ventricle. Pediatr Cardiol 12, 121–122.

61. Hwa J, Ward C, Nunn G, et al. (1994) Primary intraventricular cardiac tumors in children: contemporary diagnostic and management options. Pediatr Cardiol 15, 233–237.

62. Padalino MA, Basso C, Milanesi O, et al. (2005) Surgically treated primary cardiac tumors in early infancy and childhood. J Thorac Cardiovasc Surg 129, 1358–1363.

63. Camesas AM, Lichtstein E, Kramer J, et al. (1987) Complementary use of two-dimensional echocardiography and magnetic resonance imaging in the diagnosis of ventricular myxoma. Am Heart J 114, 440–442.

64. Freedberg RS, Kronzon I, Rumancik WM, et al. (1988) The contribution of magnetic resonance imaging to the evaluation of intracardiac tumors diagnosed by echocardiography. Circulation 77, 96–103.

65. Bouton S, Yang A, McCrindle BW, et al. (1991) Differentiation of tumor from viable myocardium using cardiac tagging with MR imaging. J Comput Assist Tomogr 15, 676–678.

66. Berkenblit R, Spindola-Franco H, Frater RW, et al. (1997) MRI in the evaluation and management of a newborn infant with cardiac rhabdomyoma. Ann Thorac Surg 63, 1475–1477.

67. King SJ, Smallhorn JF, Burrows PE. (1993) Epicardial lipoma: imaging findings. AJR Am J Roentgenol 160, 261–262.

68. Kiaffas MG, Powell AJ, Geva T. (2002) Magnetic resonance imaging evaluation of cardiac tumor characteristics in infants and children. Am J Cardiol 89, 1229–1233.

69. Hoffmann U, Globits S, Schima W, et al. (2003) Usefulness of magnetic resonance imaging of cardiac and paracardiac masses. Am J Cardiol 92, 890–895.

70. Rienmuller R, Lloret JL, Tiling R, *et al.* (1989) MR imaging of pediatric cardiac tumors previously diagnosed by echocardiography. J Comput Assest Tomogr 13, 621–626.

71. Ludomirsky A, Vargo TA, Murphy DJ, *et al.* (1985) Intracardiac undifferentiated sarcoma in infancy. J Am Coll Cardiol 6, 1362–1364.

72. St John Sutton MG, Mercier LA, Giuliani ER, *et al.* (1980) Atrial myxomas: a review of clinical experience in 40 patients. Mayo Clin Proc 55, 371–376.

73. Beghetti M, Haney I, Williams WG, *et al.* (1996) Massive right ventricular fibroma treated with partial resection and cavopulmonary shunt. Ann Thorac Surg 62, 882–884.

74. Black MD, Kadletz M, Smallhorn IF, *et al.* (1998) Cardiac rhabdomyomas and obstructive left heart disease: histologically but not functionally benign. Ann Thorac Surg 65, 1388–1390.

75. Giamberti A, Giannico S, Squitieri C, *et al.* (1995) Neonatal pulmonary autograft implantation for cardiac tumor involving aortic valve. Ann Thorac Surg 59, 1219–1221.

76. Mair DD, Titus JL, Davis GD, *et al.* (1977) Cardiac rhabdomyoma simulating mitral atresia. Chest 71, 102–105.

77. Bertolini P, Meisner H, Paek SU, *et al.* (1990) Special considerations on primary cardiac tumors in infancy and childhood. Thorac Cardiovasc Surg 38, 164–167.

78. Bass JL, Breningstall GN, Swaiman KF. (1985) Echocardiographic incidence of cardiac rhabdomyoma in tuberous sclerosis. Am J Cardiol 55, 1379–1382.

79. Smythe JF, Dyck JD, Smallhorn J, *et al.* (1990) Natural history of cardiac rhabdomyomas in infancy and childhood. Am J Cardiol 66, 1247–1249.

80. Farooki ZQ, Ross RD, Paridon SM, *et al.* (1991) Spontaneous regression of cardiac rhabdomyoma. Am J Cardiol 15, 897–899.

81. Cooley DA. (1986) Surgical management of cardiac tumors. In Kapoor AS, ed. *Cancer and the Heart.* New York: Springer-Verlag.

82. Schmaltz AA, Apitz J. (1981) Primary heart tumors in infancy and childhood. Report of four cases and review of literature. Cardiology 67, 12–22.

83. McAllister HA Jr, Cooley DA. (1990) Cardiac tumors. In Cooley DA, ed. *How to Do It – Cardiac Surgery: State of the Art Reviews.* Philadelphia: Hanley and Belfus.

84. Ceithaml EL, Midgley FM, Perry LW, *et al.* (1990) Intramural ventricular fibroma in infancy: survival after partial excision in 2 patients. Ann Thorac Surg 50, 471–472.

85. Blackmon SH, Patel AR, Bruckner BA, *et al.* (2008) Cardiac autotransplantation for malignant or complex primary left-heart tumors. Tex Heart Inst J 35, 296–300.

86. Jamieson SW, Gaudiani VA, Reitz BA, *et al.* (1981) Operative treatment of an unresectable tumor of the left ventricle. J Thorac Cardiovasc Surg 81, 797–799.

87. Aravot DJ, Banner NR, Madden B, *et al.* (1989) Primary cardiac tumours – is there a place for cardiac transplantation? Eur J Cardiothorac Surg 3, 521–524.

88. Talbot SM, Taub RN, Keohan ML, *et al.* (2002) Combined heart and lung transplantation for unresectable primary cardiac sarcoma. J Thorac Cardiovasc Surg 124, 1145–1148.

89. McAllister HA Jr. (1979) Primary tumors of the heart and pericardium. Pathol Annu 14, 325–355.

90. Fenoglio JJ Jr, McAllister HA Jr, Ferrans VJ. (1976) Cardiac rhabdomyoma: a clinicopathologic and electron microscopic study. Am J Cardiol 38, 241–251.

91. Jozwiak S, Kotulska K, Kasprzyk-Obara J, *et al.* (2006) Clinical and genotype studies of cardiac tumors in 154 patients with tuberous sclerosis complex. Pediatrics 118, e1146–e1151.

92. Nir A, Tajik AJ, Freeman WK, *et al.* (1995) Tuberous sclerosis and cardiac rhabdomyoma. Am J Cardiol 76, 419–421.

93. von Recklinghausen F. (1862) Verhandlungen der gellschaft für geburtshilfe: Herr v Recklinghausen l'egt der Gesellschaft ein Herz von einem Neugeboren. Monatsschr Geburtsk 20, 1–3.

94. Harding CO, Pagon RA. (1990) Incidence of tuberous sclerosis in patients with cardiac rhabdomyoma. Am J Med Genet 37, 443–446.

95. Bosi G, Lintermans JP, Pellegrino PA, *et al.* (1996) The natural history of cardiac rhabdomyoma with and without tuberous sclerosis. Acta Paediatr 85, 928–931.

96. Smith HC, Watson GH, Patel RG, *et al.* (1989) Cardiac rhabdomyomata in tuberous sclerosis: their course and diagnostic value. Arch Dis Child 64, 196–200.

97. Tworetzky W, McElhinney DB, Margossian R, *et al.* (2003) Association between cardiac tumors and tuberous sclerosis in the fetus and neonate. Am J Cardiol 92, 487–489.

98. Simopoulos AP, Breslow A. (1966) Tuberous sclerosis in the newborn. Am J Dis Child 111, 313–316.

99. Platt LD, Devore GR, Horenstein J, *et al.* (1987) Prenatal diagnosis of tuberous sclerosis: the use of fetal echocardiography. Prenat Diagn 7, 407–411.

100. Cho JM, Danielson GK, Puga FJ, *et al.* (2003) Surgical resection of ventricular cardiac fibromas: early and late results. Ann Thorac Surg 76, 1929–1934.

101. Valente M, Cocco P, Thiene G, *et al.* (1993) Cardiac fibroma and heart transplantation. J Thorac Cardiovasc Surg 106, 1208–1212.

102. MacGowan SW, Sidhu P, Aherne T, *et al.* (1993) Atrial myxoma: national incidence, diagnosis and surgical management. Ir J Med Sci 162, 223–226.

103. Carney JA, Hruska LS, Beauchamp GD, *et al.* (1986) Dominant inheritance of the complex of myxomas, spotty pigmentation, and endocrine overactivity. Mayo Clin Proc 61, 165–172.

104. Reynen K. (1995) Cardiac myxomas. New Engl J Med 333, 1610–1617.

105. Imperio J, Summers D, Krasnow N, *et al.* (1980) The distribution patterns of biatrial myxomas. Ann Thorac Surg 29, 469–473.

106. McCarthy PM, Piehler JM, Schaff HV, *et al.* (1986) The significance of multiple, recurrent, and "complex" cardiac myxomas. J Thorac Cardiovasc Surg 91, 389–396.

107. Talley JD, Wenger NK. (1987) Atrial myxoma: overview, recognition, and management. Compr Ther 13, 12–18.

108. Govoni E, Severi B, Cenacchi G, *et al.* (1988) Ultrastructural and immunohistochemical contribution to the histogenesis of human cardiac myxoma. Ultrastruct Pathol 12, 221–233.

109. Attum AA, Johnson GS, Masri Z, *et al.* (1987) Malignant clinical behavior of cardiac myxomas and "myxoid imitators". Ann Thorac Surg 44, 217–222.

110. Arciniegas E, Hakimi M, Farooki ZQ, et al. (1980) Primary cardiac tumors in children. J Thorac Cardiovasc Surg 79, 582–591.

111. Kapoor A, Radhakrishnan S, Sinha N. (1998) Unusual presentation during childhood of left ventricular myxoma. Cardiol Young 8, 126–127.

112. Goodwin JF. (1968) The spectrum of cardiac tumors. Am J Cardiol 21, 307–314.

113. Anderson KR, Fiddler GI, Lie JT. (1977) Congenital papillary tumor of the tricuspid valve. An unusual cause of right ventricular outflow obstruction in a neonate with trisomy E. Mayo Clin Proc 52, 665–669.

114. Arciniegas E, Hakimi M, Farooki ZQ, et al. (1980) Intrapericardial teratoma in infancy. J Thorac Cardiovasc Surg 79, 306–311.

115. Dehner LP. (1983) Gonadal and extragonadal germ cell neoplasia of childhood. Hum Pathol 14, 493–511.

116. Costas C, Williams RL, Fortune RL. (1986) Intracardiac teratoma in an infant. Pediatr Cardiol 7, 179–181.

117. Cox JN, Friedli B, Mechmeche R, et al. (1983) Teratoma of the heart. A case report and review of the literature. Virchows Arch A Pathol Anat Histopathol 402, 163–174.

118. Cyr DR, Guntheroth WG, Nyberg DA, et al. (1988) Prenatal diagnosis of an intrapericardial teratoma. A cause for non-immune hydrops. J Ultrasound Med 7, 87–90.

119. Reynolds JL, Donahue JK, Pearce CW. (1969) Intrapericardial teratoma: a cause of acute pericardial effusion in infancy. Pediatrics 43, 71–78.

120. Deenadayalu RP, Tuuri D, Dewall RA, et al. (1974) Intrapericardial teratoma and bronchogenic cyst. Review of the literature and report of successful surgery in infant with intrapericardial teratoma. J Thorac Cardiovasc Surg 67, 945–952.

121. Tollens T, Casselman F, Devlieger H, et al. (1998) Fetal cardiac tamponade due to an intrapericardial teratoma. Ann Thorac Surg 66, 559–560.

122. Weber HS, Kleinman CS, Hellenbrand WE, et al. (1988) Development of a benign intrapericardial tumor between 20 and 40 weeks of gestation. Pediatr Cardiol 9, 153–156.

123. Farooki ZQ, Arciniegas E, Hakimi M, et al. (1982) Real-time echocardiographic features of intrapericardial teratoma. J Clin Ultrasound 10, 125–128.

124. Rheuban KS, McDaniel NL, Feldmau PS, et al. (1991) Intrapericardial teratoma causing nonimmune hydrops fetalis and pericardial tamponade: case report. Pediatr Cardiol 12, 54–56.

125. Farooki ZQ, Hakimi M, Arciniegas E, et al. (1978) Echocardiographic features in a case of intrapericardial teratoma. J Clin Ultrasound 6, 108–110.

126. Lintermans JP, Schoevaertds JC, Fiasse L, et al. (1973) Intrapericardial teratoma. A curable cause of cardiac tamponade in infancy. Clin Pediatr 12, 316–318.

127. Paw PT, Jamieson SW. (1997) Surgical management of intrapericardial teratoma diagnosed in utero. Ann Thorac Surg 64, 552–554.

128. Banfield F, Dick M II, Behrendt DM, et al. (1980) Intrapericardial teratoma: a new and treatable cause of hydrops fetalis. Am J Dis Child 134, 1174–1175.

129. Tabry IF, Nassar VH, Rizk G, et al. (1975) Cavernous hemangioma of the heart: case report and review of the literature. J Thorac Cardiovasc Surg 69, 415–420.

130. Grenadier E, Margulis T, Palant A, et al. (1989) Huge cavernous hemangioma of the heart: a completely evaluated case report and review of the literature. Am Heart J 117, 479–481.

131. Brizard C, Latremouille C, Jebara VA, et al. (1993) Cardiac hemangiomas. Ann Thorac Surg 56, 390–394.

132. Kearney DL, Titus JL, Hawkins EP, et al. (1987) Pathologic features of myocardial hamartomas causing childhood tachyarrhythmias. Circulation 75, 705–710.

133. Rose AG, McCormick S, Cooper K, et al. (1996) Inflammatory pseudotumor (plasma cell granuloma) of the heart. Report of two cases and literature review. Arch Pathol Lab Med 120, 549–554.

134. Gowda RM, Khan IA, Nair CK, et al. (2003) Cardiac papillary fibroelastoma: a comprehensive analysis of 725 cases. Am Heart J 146, 404–410.

135. Burke AP, Cowan D, Virmani R. (1992) Primary sarcomas of the heart. Cancer 69, 387–395.

136. Dein JR, Frist WH, Stinson EB, et al. (1987) Primary cardiac neoplasms. Early and late results of surgical treatment in 42 patients. J Thorac Cardiovasc Surg 93, 502–511.

137. Aksoylar S, Kansoy S, Bakiler AR, et al. (2002) Letter to the editor: Primary cardiac rhabdomyosarcoma. Med Pediatr Oncol 38, 146.

138. Putnam JB Jr, Sweeney MS, Colon R, et al. (1991) Primary cardiac sarcomas. Ann Thorac Surg 51, 906–910.

139. Llombart-Cussac A, Pivot X, Contesso G, et al. (1998) Adjuvant chemotherapy for primary cardiac sarcomas: the IGR experience. Br J Cancer 78, 1624–1628.

140. Donsbeck AV, Ranchere D, Coindre JM, et al. (1999) Primary cardiac sarcomas: an immunohistochemical and grading study with long-term follow up of 24 cases. Histopathology 34, 295–304.

141. Vergnon JM, Vincent M, Perinetti M, et al. (1985) Chemotherapy of metastatic primary cardiac sarcomas. Am Heart J 110, 682–684.

142. Sanoudos G, Reed GE. (1972) Primary cardiac sarcoma. J Thorac Cardiovasc Surg 63, 482–485.

143. Pessotto R, Silvestre G, Luciani GB, et al. (1997) Primary cardiac leiomyosarcoma: seven-year survival with combined surgical and adjuvant therapy. Int J Cardiol 60, 91–94.

144. Luck SR, DeLeon S, Shkolnik A, et al. (1982) Intracardiac Wilms' tumor: diagnosis and management. J Pediatr Surg 17, 551–554.

145. Ritchey ML, Kelalis PP, Haase GM, et al. (1993) Preoperative therapy for intracaval and atrial extension of Wilms' tumor. Cancer 71, 4104–4110.

146. Nakayama DK, Norkool P, deLorimier AA, et al. (1986) Intracardiac extension of Wilms' tumor. A report of the National Wilms' Tumor Study. Ann Surg 204, 693–697.

40

Diseases of the Pericardium

Victor O. Morell[1,2] and Ergin Kocyildirim[2]

[1]University of Pittsburgh Medical Center Heart and Vascular Institute, Children's Hospital of Pittsburgh, Pittsburgh, PA, USA
[2]McGowan Institute for Regenerative Medicine, University of Pittsburgh, Pittsburgh, PA, USA

Historical Perspectives

The heart is surrounded by a fibroserous sac known as the pericardium, a term derived from the Greek words *peri*, "around", and *kardia*, "heart". It was a Graeco-Roman physician, Claudius Galen, who first described and named this anatomical structure in 160 AD. He was also the first to recognize the deleterious effects of a pericardial effusion on cardiac function. In 1653 the Parisian surgeon, Jean Riolan, recommended aspiration of the pericardial fluid in patients with effusions and proposed trephining of the sternum to provide exposure to the pericardium. In 1749, when the first comprehensive book on cardiac anatomy, physiology, and pathology was published by Jean-Baptiste Senac, a French physician, there was a full chapter dedicated to the pericardium and its diseases.

One of the first clinicians to document the feasibility of surgical interventions in the heart was Louis Rhen, in Germany, who in 1913 performed the repair of a cardiac laceration with evacuation of clots from the pericardial space on a patient who was dying from cardiac tamponade after suffering a stab wound to the chest. His success stimulated other surgeons to pursue surgical approaches for the management of pericardial diseases, like French surgeon Paul Hollopeau, who in 1921 performed the first partial pericardiectomy for the management of constrictive pericarditis.

Embryology and Anatomy

In the human embryo, between week 5 and 7 of gestation, the pericardial cavity is created from the subdivision of the embryonic coelom [1]. Fusion of the pleuropericardial membranes with the foregut mesenchyme posteriorly divides the thoracic cavity into a ventral pericardial cavity and two dorsolateral pleural cavities. Abnormal development of the pleuropericardial membranes results in defects in the pericardial wall [2].

The pericardium is a bilayered sac consisting of a thick stiff outer fibrous layer and a thin inner serous layer. The fibrous outer capsule is mainly made up of collagen and elastin fibers and the serous layer of a thin elastic membrane of mesothelial cells, which envelop the inner aspect of the fibrous pericardium (serous parietal pericardium) and also the myocardium (serous visceral pericardium or epicardium). Between the two layers of the serous pericardium there is a potential space known as the pericardial cavity, which is normally lubricated by a thin layer of fluid (pericardial fluid) (Plate 40.1, see plate section opposite p. 594).

Within the pericardial cavity there are two recesses, the transverse and oblique sinuses, representing reflections of the serous pericardium between the great vessels at the base of the heart (Plate 40.2, see plate section opposite p. 594) [3]. The transverse sinus lies behind the aorta and main pulmonary artery and the oblique sinus extends behind the left atrium in the region between all four pulmonary veins. In order to provide structural support to the heart and prevent excessive cardiac motion within the thoracic cavity, the pericardium is connected to the undersurface of the sternum by the superior and inferior sternopericardial ligaments and to the posterior mediastinal structures by loose connective tissue. Also, the pericardium is attached to the central tendon of the diaphragm.

The main vascular arterial supply to the pericardium is provided by the pericardiophrenic artery, a branch of the internal mammary artery and the venous drainage is via the pericardiophrenic veins, which are tributaries of the brachiocephalic veins. The phrenic nerves provide the sensory enervation and the sympathetic trunks the vasomotor enervation.

Diseases of the Pericardium

Pericardial disease is defined as a structural or functional abnormality of the visceral or parietal pericardium that may, or may not, have a significant impact on cardiac function. The International Congenital Heart Surgery Nomenclature and Database Project described 12 types of disease processes affecting the pericardium. They were classified as effusive pericarditis (pericardial effusion), constructive pericarditis, cardiac tamponade, postoperative pericardial effusion, postoperative cardiac tamponade, postpericardiotomy syndrome, congenital defect, neoplastic process, benign mass, pericardial cyst, pneumopericardium, and chylopericardium [4,5]. Each group will be discussed briefly with common causes, diagnosis, and medical and surgical treatments.

Effusive Pericarditis

Effusive pericarditis (pericardial effusion) is defined as an inflammatory stimulation of the pericardium that results in the accumulation of appreciable amounts of pericardial fluid. It may be caused by many disorders including idiopathic, viral, uremic, tuberculous, purulent, neoplastic, traumatic, and drug induced. Pericardial effusion may be serous, purulent, or hemorrhagic.

Idiopathic pericardial effusions are quite common in the pediatric population, representing up to 37% of cases in some series [6]. In these patients there is no identifiable cause for the pericardial process. Viral effusions are often, but not always, associated with other signs and symptoms of an acute viral infection. Agents commonly responsible for the development of viral pericarditis include Coxsackie virus, adenovirus, enteric cytopathogenic human orphan (ECHO) virus, influenza virus, mumps virus, varicella virus, Epstein-Barr virus, and human immunodeficiency virus [7,8]. They are characterized by a small to large effusion occurring in children with a pericardial friction rub, which is the most common physical finding. Patients with uremic effusions commonly suffer from renal disease. Approximately 20% of uremic patients requiring chronic dialysis will develop a pericardial effusion during their lifetime [9]. The association between uremia and pericardial effusions has been well described and is recognized as one of the indicators of end-stage renal disease. However, the causes of uremic pericarditis remain uncertain [10].

Bacterial pericarditis can be primary, resulting from contiguous spread of bacteria from a mediastinal and/or pleural source, or secondary, resulting from septicemic spread from a remote source. *Staphylococcus aureus* is the most common

organism identified, followed by *Haemophilus influenza* type B. Other bacteria responsible for purulent pericarditis include *Pseudomonas aeruginosa*, *Neisseria meningitides*, *Salmonella* species, *Neisseria gonorrhoeae*, *Listeria monocytogenes*, *Escherichia coli*, *Brucella*, *Yersinia*, *Gemella morbillorum*. Tuberculosis may be associated with a serosanguineous pericardial effusion with predominance of lymphocytes. Purulent pericardial effusions can be life-threatening and occasionally require emergency interventions.

Although primary tumors of the pericardium are rare, neoplastic pericardial effusions are frequently observed in patients with neoplastic diseases and may result from local tumor invasion of the pericardium or from metastatic seeding. Occasionally, it can develop from metastatic spread to the pericardial fluid itself. Blunt or penetrating trauma, including cardiac massage during resuscitation may cause a hemorrhagic pericardial effusion. Minoxidil, anticoagulants, thrombolytics, drugs causing a lupus-like syndrome such as chlorpromazine (Thorazine), hydralazine, isoniazid, minocycline, methyldopa, procainamide and quinidine can be the causes of drug-induced pericardial effusion [11].

Pericardial effusions can be diagnosed based on the history and physical examination, electrocardiography, chest roentgenography, echocardiography, computed tomography (CT), and/or magnetic resonance imaging (MRI). The clinical presentation is determined by the primary etiology and the speed of accumulation of the pericardial fluid. If the effusion develops slowly it can be asymptomatic, while a relatively smaller but rapidly accumulating effusion can present with severe hemodynamic compromise. Large effusions may cause cough and dyspnea owing to compression of adjacent lung tissue and on auscultation distant heart sounds are present. In pericarditis there may be a friction rub, which is best heard on the left border of sternum or in the midclavicular line, between the second and the fourth intercostal space. Large effusions are usually related to neoplastic, tuberculous, or uremic processes.

On chest roentgenography an enlarged cardiac silhouette can be observed in the presence of a large effusion, but a normal cardiothoracic ratio does not rule out smaller effusions (Figure 40.1). The diagnosis is best confirmed by echocardiography, which also documents cardiac filling and ventricular function, determining the presence or absence of cardiac tamponade physiology (Plate 40.3, see plate section opposite p. 594). Computed tomography can easily detect pericardial effusions and is also useful in identifying the characteristics of the fluid (blood, chyle, transudate, etc.). Low voltage on the electrocardiogram (ECG) is a typical finding in patients with pericardial effusions.

The management of pericardial effusions includes both medical and surgical options. In the absence of hemodynamic compromise some of the pericardial effusion may

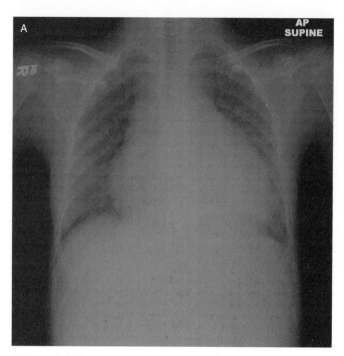
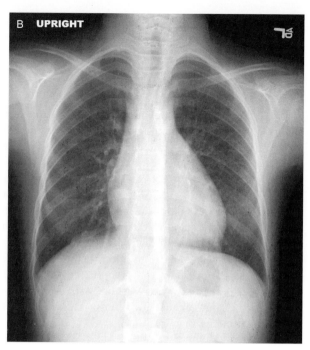

Figure 40.1 Chest roentgenography of a patient presenting with a large pericardial effusion. **A,** On admission. **B,** After pericardiocentesis.

resolve with medical management without the need for fluid analysis. Idiopathic or viral effusions usually have a benign course and tend to improve with bed rest and the use of nonsteroidal anti-inflammatory drugs such as indomethacin or salicylates. Steroids may be needed occasionally for recurrent or refractory cases.

Uremic effusions are frequently managed with nonsteroidal anti-inflammatory agents and diuretics. In these patients dialysis can also effectively treat the pericardial effusion. Uremic effusion can be quite large and may lead to cardiac tamponade requiring urgent drainage. Drainage is also indicated if the effusion persists after a 2-week course of aggressive dialysis [12,13].

Bacterial pericarditis should be managed with both antimicrobial therapy and surgical drainage, which has shown to reduced the mortality and morbidity associated with this illness [14]. Tuberculosis is the most common cause of constrictive pericarditis, therefore patients with tuberculous pericarditis may benefit from early pericardiectomy. Neoplastic pericardial effusions are often asymptomatic requiring no specific treatment but, when symptomatic, they can be managed by palliative pericardiocentesis or extended catheter drainage [15]. In recurrent cases a subxiphoid pericardiostomy and tube drainage is the preferred option. For the management of chronic recurrent malignant effusions the intrapericardial delivery of sclerosing agents (tetracycline or bleomycin) has been used with apparent success, but no controlled trials are available [16–19].

The most common surgical techniques used in the management of pericardial effusions consist of pericardiocentesis, subxyphoid pericardiostomy and video-assisted thoracoscopy. Pericardiocentesis involves placing a needle 1–2 cm below the xiphoid process, at a 45-degree angle with the skin, directed towards the tip of the left scapula and then advancing it into the pericardial space (Figure 40.2). Once the needle is in the pericardial space, a guide wire is inserted through it and a drainage catheter is advanced. The drainage catheter is then connected to a closed drainage system. The pericardial fluid should be sent for cell count, chemistry, culture, and cytology.

If the aspirated fluid is grossly bloody, it is important to rule out intracardiac placement of the needle. Therefore, an aliquot of 3–5 mL is drawn on to a clean sponge to document clotting: blood withdrawn from the pericardial space will not clot because of fibrinolysis. The risk of cardiac injury can be reduced by performing the procedure under echocardiographic guidance. Also, an ECG lead can be attached to the needle to allow for continuous ECG monitoring. As the needle is advanced, ST segment elevations suggested ventricular epicardial contact and PR segment elevation will be observed with the atrial contact. Certainly, all these patients should have normal coagulation parameters at the time of the procedure to avoid bleeding complications.

The subxiphoid pericardiostomy (pericardial window) (Figure 40.3) is usually performed under general anesthesia and requires a small vertical midline incision, extending from the xiphisternal junction to just below the xiphoid process. Then the linea alba is divided and the sternum retracted allowing for visualization of the anterior pericardium. In patients with significant effusion, immediately on pericardial entry there is a fluid outrush, which should be associated with a rise in systemic blood pressure and a decrease in the heart rate. In the event of any cardiac injury and massive bleeding, the opposite will occur [20]. An advantage to this approach is that a piece of pericardium can be excised and sent to the pathology lab for examination. A pericardial drainage tube is placed through a separate skin incision and secured at skin level. Complications of subxiphoid pericardiostomy are rare but include bleeding, infection, incisional hernia, anesthetic complications, and cardiac injury [21].

Video-assisted thoracoscopic surgery is another safe and effective technique for the creation of a pericardial window (Figure 40.4) [22]. With the patient in a lateral decubitis position and through three small incisions in the chest, the endoscopic trocars are inserted in the pleural space. Under single-lung ventilation a thoracoscope and two thoracoscopic instruments are inserted allowing for bimanual dissection. Once the phrenic nerve is visualized, the pericardium is grasped and a window is created allowing for drainage of the pericardial fluid into the pleural space.

Constrictive Pericarditis

Constrictive pericarditis is defined as an inflammatory process of the fibrous and serous layers of the pericardium

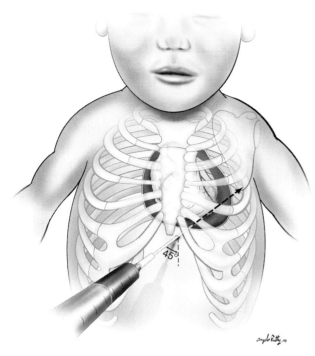

Figure 40.2 Pericardiocentesis technique. The needle is advanced at a 45-degree angle with the skin and directed towards the tip of the left scapula.

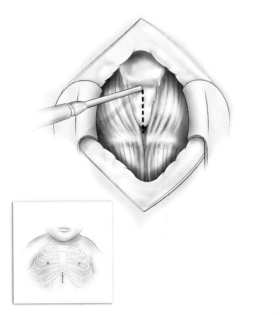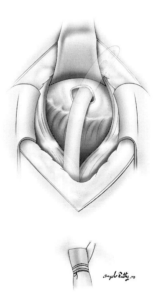

Figure 40.3 Subxiphoid pericardiostomy technique. First, an incision over the xiphoid process is made. After excising or dividing the xiphoid process and with upward retraction of the distal sternum, the pericardium is visualized and entered. This approach allows for open pericardial drainage and/or biopsy.

that leads to pericardial thickening and compression of the cardiac chambers, ultimately resulting in a significant reduction in cardiac function [5]. Although tuberculous pericarditis remains the leading cause of constrictive pericarditis worldwide, its incidence has declined in western countries [23]. Presently, idiopathic constrictive pericarditis is the most common etiology in the western world, followed by postcardiotomy and postmediastinal irradiation.

Physiologically, the thickened adherent pericardium decreases ventricular compliance and restricts cardiac filling in late diastole. Normally, the decrease in intrathoracic pressure that occurs with inspiration is transmitted to all cardiac chambers and therefore the pressure gradient between the pulmonary veins and the left-sided chambers remains unchanged. With constrictive pericarditis, the thickened pericardium isolates the cardiac chambers from intrathoracic pressure changes resulting in a decrease in the pressure gradient between the systemic and pulmonary veins and the cardiac chambers. This results in a reduction in the filling of all cardiac chambers [24].

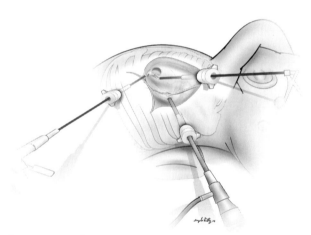

Figure 40.4 Video-assisted thoracoscopic pericardial window. After careful placement of the three trocars into the left pleural space, placement of the video camera and two endoscopic instruments allows for the creation of a pericardial window.

Symptoms and signs include fatigue, exercise intolerance, pedal edema, and in extreme cases syncope on exertion, hepatic congestion, and ascites. Jugular venous distention with inspiration (*Kussmaul's sign*) is present. On auscultation muffled heart sounds, a prominent S3 gallop, and/or a pericardial knock are common findings. The chest X-ray may show pericardial calcifications and a normal cardiac silhouette in a patient with right-sided heart failure symptoms. Echocardiography may demonstrate the pericardial thickening. Computed tomography and MRI provide excellent additional information for the diagnosis.

Cardiac catheterization remains a very useful diagnostic tool in the management of constrictive pericarditis, especially when ruling out the presence of a restrictive cardiomyopathy. The significant factor leading to altered pathophysiology is the presence of the thickened inelastic pericardium interfering with ventricular expansion during diastole, particularly the latter two-thirds of diastole. Both left and right ventricular diastolic pressure waveforms show an early diastolic dip followed by a plateau (*square root* sign). There is usually equilibration of the mean right atrial pressure, pulmonary artery wedge pressure, and the right and left ventricular end-diastolic pressures (Figure 40.5). Pulmonary arterial systolic pressure is usually normal or slightly elevated and usually not greater than 40 mmHg. Also, myocardial biopsy could be helpful in documenting findings suggestive of restrictive cardiomyopathy (myocyte hypertrophy, interstitial fibrosis, myocytolysis, and endocardial sclerosis).

The surgical management of constrictive pericarditis involves the complete removal of the pericardium, which is usually performed through a midline sternotomy approach (Figure 40.6). First, the pericardium is incised longitudinally with a scalpel and once in the correct plane it is removed first from the left ventricle and left atrium. Bleeding during dissection can be controlled by gentle compression with warm saline or fine sutures. Human fibrin glue can also be considered to stop the bleeding [25]. Extra care must be taken to mobilize and preserve the phrenic nerves. After the resection of the right atrial and

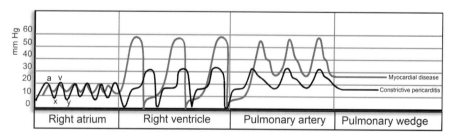

Figure 40.5 Pressure tracings in constrictive pericarditis and myocardial disease.
Note the plateaued end-diastolic pressure of the right ventricle and equalization of diastolic pressures in all cardiac chambers with constrictive pericarditis.

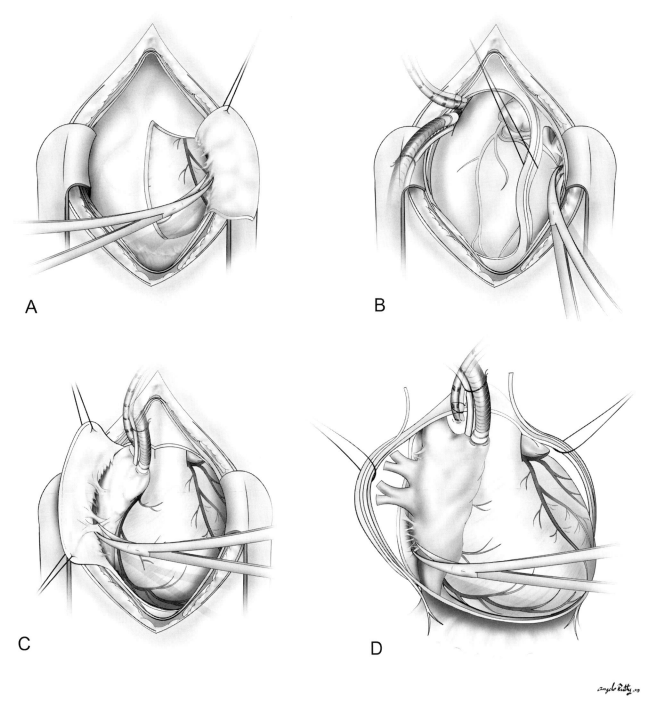

Figure 40.6 Total pericardiectomy. **A,** The pericardium over the left ventricle and left atrium is first removed, followed by the pericardium over the right ventricle. **B,** The phrenic nerves are preserved but the pericardium posterior to the nerves should also be resected. **C,** The pericardium over the right atrium and (**D**) pulmonary veins should also be resected.

right ventricular pericardium, the dissection of the pericardium around the aorta, pulmonary artery, superior vena cava and inferior vena cava is completed.

Constrictive pericarditis is a rare condition in children. Surgical treatment offers good short- and long-term results

[26]. The complete removal of the pericardium is very important because incomplete removal could result in persistent symptoms. The outcomes are not as good in patients with radiation-induced constrictive pericarditis because there is usually a component of myocardial injury. Early

surgical treatment should be considered in tuberculous constrictive pericarditis [27].

Cardiac Tamponade

Cardiac tamponade can be defined as cardiac compression [5] and it occurs when enough fluid, air, pus, or tumor accumulates in the pericardial space to cause a significant increase in the intrapericardial pressure that results in impaired cardiac filling. As a direct result of the elevated intrapericardial pressure there is a rise in the ventricular end-diastolic pressure, which equalizes with the central venous pressure. This hemodynamic abnormality results in a reduction of the ventricular diastolic filling, stroke volume, and cardiac output.

Beck's triad is a collection of physical signs frequently observed in patients with cardiac tamponade and consists of an elevated central venous pressure, a decreased arterial blood pressure, and muffled heart sounds. *Kussmaul's sign*, a rise in the central venous pressure with spontaneous inspiration, is frequently present in patients with cardiac tamponade or constrictive pericarditis. *Pulsus paradoxus*, a drop in the systolic arterial blood pressure greater than 10 mmHg with inspiration, is also commonly observed in these patients.

The diagnosis of cardiac tamponade could be challenging. A chest X-ray often shows mediastinal enlargement, but a normal cardiothoracic ratio does not rule out the diagnosis. Echocardiography is very useful because it also provides physiologic data. Echocardiographic features of the cardiac tamponade include late diastolic right atrial collapse, diastolic right ventricular collapse, and large respiratory variation of flow velocity through the heart valves [28–31]. On cardiac catheterization there is near equality of the diastolic pressures in all cardiac chambers and the pulmonary artery, with an elevated central venous pressure.

Pericardial fluid removal is the definitive treatment. If there is a suspicion of cardiac tamponade pericardiocentesis is a method of both diagnosis and treatment. Aspiration of a few milliliters of fluid in a newborn or only 10–15 mL in an adult patient can be a life-saving procedure [32]. Open surgical drainage may be necessary in some cases, especially in postoperative patients with active mediastinal bleeding.

Postoperative Pericardial Effusion

Postoperative pericardial effusions have been reported to develop in up to 85% of patients after cardiac surgery [33,34]. Pericardial effusions that present during the immediate perioperative period (less than 30 days) are considered "early" effusions. The patient's exposure to the cardiopulmonary bypass circuit, with its adverse effects (systemic inflammatory response and coagulopathy), cer-

tainly plays a role in their development. "Late" effusions present at a time removed from the immediate perioperative period (more than 30 days) and their etiology appears to be multifactorial.

The location, size, and rate of accumulation of these effusions play a significant role in the patient's clinical presentation. Most are asymptomatic and the effusions are detected in a routine follow-up examination, but postoperative pericardial effusions may lead to cardiac tamponade. Medical treatment with diuretic and nonsteroidal anti-inflammatory agents is the first option for patients with small to moderate effusions without hemodynamic instability. Steroid therapy is usually reserved for persistent or recurrent cases. Surgical intervention in the form of percutaneous or open drainage is indicated in cases of large effusions or in patients that have failed medical management.

Postoperative Cardiac Tamponade

Pericardial effusions resulting in cardiac tamponade have been reported in up to 8.8% of patients after open heart surgery [33,34]. Early cardiac tamponade is one that develops within 30 days of surgery and is usually associated with the presence of postoperative bleeding or coagulopathy. Even with an open pericardial cavity the acute accumulation of a moderate amount of blood can readily cause cardiac tamponade. On chest X-ray the presence of an enlarged cardiac silhouette is suggestive of the diagnosis. Echocardiography is very useful in documenting the size and location of the effusion and the presence of diastolic right atrial or ventricular collapse. The differential diagnosis with hemodynamic parameters is presented in Table 40.1 [32]. The management of this condition usually requires urgent mediastinal exploration with the evacuation of blood and clots and control of the bleeding. In an emergency, opening of the lower end of the sternotomy

Table 40.1 Differential diagnosis of postoperative cardiac tamponade.

	Right atrial pressure	Left atrial pressure	Pulmonary artery pressure	Systemic pressure
Hypovolemia	↓	↓	↓	↓
Acute tamponade	↑	↓	→	↓
Myocardial dysfunction	↑	↑	↑	↓
Acute pulmonary hypertension	↑	↓	↑	↓

incision with partial evacuation of the mediastinal hematoma can be life saving [25].

Late postoperative cardiac tamponade is one that presents at a time removed from the immediate perioperative period (more than 30 days) [5]. The etiology of this condition appears to be multifactorial and is related to factors like the presence of prolonged postoperative mediastinal drainage and the development of postpericardiotomy syndrome [35,36]. Because of its insidious nature patients often present with minimal symptoms and without obvious clinical signs of cardiac tamponade. Therefore, the diagnosis can be easily missed. These "late" effusions respond well to percutaneous drainage under fluoroscopic or echocardiographic guidance but occasionally open surgical drainage is required, especially for loculated posterior effusions.

Postpericardiotomy Syndrome

Postpericardiotomy syndrome is a febrile illness observed in patients after a surgical procedure that involved opening the pericardium. Symptoms tend to develop weeks to months after pericardiotomy and include fever, pericardial or pleuritic pain, friction rubs, pericardial or pleural effusions, and electrocardiographic changes. The etiology is still unclear, but the underlying mechanism is thought to be an immunologic process characterized by the development of anticardiac antibodies [37]. Approximately two-thirds of patients have been found to have a marked increase in antibody titers to a variety of viral agents including coxsackie B, adenovirus, and cytomegalovirus, suggestive of a viral etiology [38]. However, a prospective study by Webber and associates found no evidence to support this theory and concluded that the use of viral titers in the setting of cardiopulmonary bypass and recent blood transfusions is unreliable [39].

The incidence of postpericardiotomy syndrome after cardiac surgery is approximately 30%, but patients under 2 years of age seem to be less affected [38,40]. Medical management consists of the use of anti-inflammatory agents including aspirin, indomethacin, and other nonsteroidal anti-inflammatory agents. Steroid therapy is effective and dramatically hastens the recovery. Pericardiocentesis is reserved for the management of large pericardial effusions. A surgically created pericardial window may be necessary in refractory cases.

Congenital Defects of Pericardium

Congenital defects of the pericardium are rare and include complete absence of the pericardium and partial left- or right-sided defects. Most pericardial defects (86%) occur on the left side and result from premature atrophy of the left duct of Cuvier during embryologic development [2]. In 30% of cases, congenital pericardial defects are associated with cardiovascular or pulmonary congenital anomalies including atrial septal defect, tetralogy of Fallot, patent ductus arteriosus, pulmonary sequestration, bronchogenic cyst, and diaphragmatic defects [41]. Although mostly asymptomatic, congenital pericardial defects may present with syncope, chest pain, or arrhythmias [42,43]. Also, cardiac herniation through the defect could lead to incarceration of the myocardium, torsion of the great arteries, and sudden death [44]. A combination of chest X-ray, echocardiography, CT, and/or MRI is useful in establishing the diagnosis but frequently these defects are identified incidentally at autopsy or during surgery.

Asymptomatic patients with complete absence of the pericardium or with small defects require no surgical intervention. Moderate-sized defects are rarely of clinical significance and, despite the potential for cardiac chamber herniation, most authors advise leaving them untreated. Therefore surgical intervention is reserved for symptomatic patients [32]. Surgical repair consists of primary closure or pericardioplasty. During repair, care must be taken to avoid injuring the phrenic nerve, which usually runs along the anterior border of the defect.

Pericardial Neoplasia

Malignant diseases of the pericardium include lymphoma, leukemia, thymoma, mesothelioma, teratoma, angiosarcoma, rhabdomyosarcoma, or metastatic disease [5]. They are quite rare in children. The most common primary pericardial malignancy is mesothelioma, but the majority of pericardial malignant tumors are metastatic in nature. Early diagnosis is often difficult owing to the lack of symptoms. As the disease advances patients often develop signs and symptoms of cardiac tamponade owing to the presence of a large pericardial effusion or because of cardiac compression by the tumor mass. Diagnostic studies include chest X-ray, echocardiography, CT or MRI, and pericardiocentesis for cytology. A pericardial biopsy is often necessary to establish the diagnosis. Surgical resection of the primary pericardial tumor with or without chemotherapy and/or radiation is the preferred treatment. The management of malignant pericardial effusions has been previously discussed in this chapter.

Benign Pericardial Mass

Benign primary tumors of the pericardium include lipomas, fibrous polyps, hemangiomas, and dermoid tumors [5,25]. Patients are usually asymptomatic, but when symptoms develop they are usually related to cardiac compression. The diagnosis is made by chest X-ray, echocardiography, CT, and/or MRI. Surgical resection is the treatment of choice.

Pericardial Cyst

A pericardial cyst is defined as a sac enclosing fluid or semisolid matter found in close proximity to the pericardium, although rarely communicating with the pericardium, and they can be intrapericardial or extrapericardial [5]. The most common locations for these cysts are the right periphrenic angle (Figure 40.7), the left periphrenic angle, and the anterior mediastinum. Pericardial cysts are rare and usually asymptomatic, however they may cause cardiac compression, chronic inflammatory symptoms, or cardiac chamber erosion [25]. Pericardial cysts are usually discovered on a routine chest X-ray but echocardiography, CT, or MRI are useful diagnostic studies. Surgical excision is recommended to confirm the diagnosis.

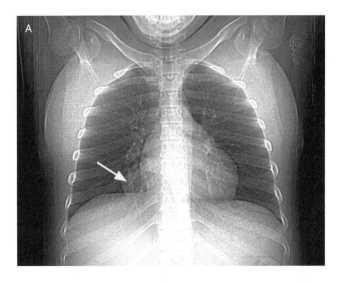

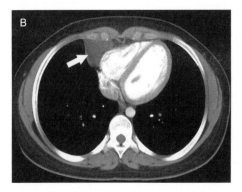

Figure 40.7 Images of a patient with a pericardial cyst. **A,** Chest roentgenography reveals an abnormal shadow in the right periphrenic angle (arrow). **B,** A chest computed tomography scan confirms the presence of a cystic mass at the right periphrenic angle (arrow).

Pneumopericardium

Pneumopericardium is defined as the presence of air within the pericardial cavity and it can be idiopathic, traumatic, or infectious in origin [5]. Idiopathic pneumopericardium is believed to result from the rupture of terminal alveoli releasing air that courses along the bronchi into the tissue planes leading into the pericardium. It is usually self-limited and resolves spontaneously. In rare cases, it can lead to the development of a tension pneumopericardium with signs and symptoms of cardiac tamponade.

Neonatal pneumopericardium is a rare clinical condition that can be life threatening and is seen in neonates with existing lung pathology requiring mechanical ventilation [45–47]. It may be associated with other air leak syndromes such as pneumomediastinum, pneumothorax, and pneumoperitoneum. Neonatal pneumopericardium can be successfully treated by the nitrogen washout technique [48].

Traumatic pneumopericardium is a rare condition, whose significance lies in the possibility of developing a tension pneumopericardium. The most common cause is penetrating chest trauma but it is also seen after blunt trauma. The presence of a pneumopericardium in a patient with a penetrating chest injury should raise concerns of the possibility of cardiac injury, and hence it should be considered a relative indication for surgical intervention. Tracheal and esophageal injuries could also be present.

Infectious pneumopericardium can be seen in patients with a secondary fistulous communication between the pericardium and an infected contiguous organ or with a primary pericardial infection with a gas-forming organism. The medical management is directed to the eradication of the infection.

Chylopericardium

Chylopericardium is defined as a chylous effusive process of the pericardium. It can be idiopathic, posttraumatic, post thoracic surgery, postcardiotomy, or neoplastic in origin [5] and may present with signs of cardiac tamponade. Patients with increased superior vena cava pressures are at risk for the development of a chylopericardium, and that includes single ventricle patients with a Fontan circulation and patients with superior vena cava obstruction or thrombosis. Neoplastic processes or surgical trauma affecting the thoracic lymphatic drainage can also result in the formation of a chylous pericardial effusion.

The initial management of a chylopericardium consists of drainage of the pericardial fluid and the institution of low-fat enteral nutrition with medium-chain triglycerides. If persistent, total parenteral nutrition is then indicated. Also, the use of octreotide has been reported with some success [49]. In the presence of caval obstruction, strong consideration should be given at re-establishing unobstructed superior vena cava flow. Surgical ligation of the thoracic duct is performed in patients in whom conservative medical management failed.

References

1. Sadler TW. (1995) *Langman's Medical Embryology*, 7th ed. Baltimore, MD: Lippincott Williams & Wilkins.
2. Southworth H, Stevenson CS. (1938) Congenital defects of the pericardium. Arch Intern Med 61, 223–240.
3. International Anatomical Nomenclature Committee (1983) *Nomina Anatomica*, 5th ed. Baltimore, MD: Lippincott Williams & Wilkins.
4. Mavroudis C, Jacobs JP. (2000) Congenital Heart Surgery Nomenclature and Database Project: overview and minimum dataset. Ann Thorac Surg 69(4 Suppl), S2–S17.
5. Mehta SM, Myers JL. (2000) Congenital Heart Surgery Nomenclature and Database Project: diseases of the pericardium. Ann Thorac Surg 69(4 Suppl), S191–S196.
6. Kuhn B, Peters J, Marx GR, *et al.* (2008) Etiology, management, and outcome of pediatric pericardial effusions. Pediatr Cardiol 29, 90–94.
7. Friman G, Fohlman J. (1993) The epidemiology of viral heart disease. Scand J Infect Dis Suppl 88, 7–10.
8. Van Reken D, Strauss A, Hernandez A, *et al.* (1974) Infectious pericarditis in children. J Pediatr 85, 165–169.
9. Gunukula SR, Spodick DH. (2001) Pericardial disease in renal patients. Semin Nephrol 21, 52–56.
10. Alpert MA, Ravenscraft MD. (2003) Pericardial involvement in end-stage renal disease. Am J Med Sci 325, 228–236.
11. Rubin RL. (1999) Etiology and mechanisms of drug-induced lupus. Curr Opin Rheumatol 11, 357–363.
12. Leehey DJ, Daugirdas JT, Ing TS. (1983) Early drainage of pericardial effusion in patients with dialysis pericarditis. Arch Intern Med 143, 1673–1675.
13. Rutsky EA, Rostand SG. (1987) Treatment of uremic pericarditis and pericardial effusion. Am J Kidney Dis 10, 2–8.
14. Hoffman JIE, Stanger P. (2003) Diseases of pericardium. In: Rudolph CD, Rudolph AM, *et al.*, eds. *Rudolph's Pediatrics*, 21st ed. New York: McGraw-Hill Medical.
15. Tsang TS, Seward JB, Barnes ME, *et al.* (2000) Outcomes of primary and secondary treatment of pericardial effusion in patients with malignancy. Mayo Clin Proc 75, 248–253.
16. Davis S, Rambotti P, Grignani F. (1984) Intrapericardial tetracycline sclerosis in the treatment of malignant pericardial effusion: an analysis of thirty-three cases. J Clin Oncol 2, 631–636.
17. Girardi LN, Ginsberg RJ, Burt ME. (1997) Pericardiocentesis and intrapericardial sclerosis: effective therapy for malignant pericardial effusions. Ann Thorac Surg 64, 1422–1427; discussion 1427–1428.
18. Shafi S, Oh JK, Jae K. (2007) Diseases of the pericardium, cardiac tumors, and cardiac trauma. In: Dale DC, Federman DD, *et al.*, eds. *ACP Medicine*, 3rd ed. Hamilton, Ontario: BC Decker Inc.
19. Shepherd FA, Morgan C, Evans WK, *et al.* (1987) Medical management of malignant pericardial effusion by tetracycline sclerosis. Am J Cardiol 60, 1161–1166.
20. Meyerson SL, D'Amico TA. (2007) Pericardial procedures. In: Souba WW, Fink MP, *et al.*, eds. *ACS Surgery: Principles and Practice*, 6th ed. New York: WebMD Professional Publishing.
21. Moores DW, Allen KB, Faber LP, *et al.* (1995) Subxiphoid pericardial drainage for pericardial tamponade. J Thorac Cardiovasc Surg 109, 546–551; discussion 551–552.
22. Nataf P, Cacoub P, Regan M, *et al.* (1998) Video-thoracoscopic pericardial window in the diagnosis and treatment of pericardial effusions. Am J Cardiol 82, 124–126.
23. Rooney JJ, Crocco JA, Lyons HA. (1970) Tuberculous pericarditis. Ann Intern Med 72, 73–81.
24. Sengupta PP, Eleid MF, Khandheria BK. (2008) Constrictive pericarditis. Circ J 72, 1555–1562.
25. Stark J, Tsang VT. (2006) Miscellaneous: Straddling atrioventricular valves, pericardium, tumours, diverticula, and ectopia cordis. In: Stark J, de Leval M, Tsang VT, eds. *Surgery for Congenital Heart Defects*, 3rd ed. Chichester: John Wiley & Sons.
26. McCaughan BC, Schaff HV, Piehler JM, *et al.* (1985) Early and late results of pericardiectomy for constrictive pericarditis. J Thorac Cardiovasc Surg 89, 340–350.
27. Bozbuga N, Erentug V, Kirali K, *et al.* (2004) Midterm results of aortic valve repair with the pericardial cusp extension technique in rheumatic valve disease. Ann Thorac Surg 77, 1272–1276.
28. Gillam LD, Guyer DE, Gibson TC, *et al.* (1983) Hydrodynamic compression of the right atrium: a new echocardiographic sign of cardiac tamponade. Circulation 68, 294–301.
29. Kronzon I, Cohen ML, Winer HE. (1983) Diastolic atrial compression: a sensitive echocardiographic sign of cardiac tamponade. J Am Coll Cardiol 2, 770–775.
30. Schiller NB, Botvinick EH. (1977) Right ventricular compression as a sign of cardiac tamponade: an analysis of echocardiographic ventricular dimensions and their clinical implications. Circulation 56, 774–779.
31. Singh S, Wann LS, Klopfenstein HS, *et al.* (1986) Usefulness of right ventricular diastolic collapse in diagnosing cardiac tamponade and comparison to pulsus paradoxus. Am J Cardiol 57, 652–656.
32. Jacobs JP. (2003) Diseases of the pericardium. In: Mavroudis C, Backer CL, eds: *Pediatric Cardiac Surgery*, 3rd ed. Philadelphia, PA: Mosby, Inc.
33. Malouf JF, Alam S, Gharzeddine W, *et al.* (1993) The role of anticoagulation in the development of pericardial effusion and late tamponade after cardiac surgery. Eur Heart J 14, 1451–1457.
34. Shabetai R. (1991) The effects of pericardial effusion on respiratory variations in hemodynamics and ventricular function. J Am Coll Cardiol 17, 249–250.
35. Hochberg MS, Merrill WH, Gruber M, *et al.* (1978) Delayed cardiac tamponade associated with prophylactic anticoagulation in patients undergoing coronary bypass grafting. Early diagnosis with two-dimensional echocardiography. J Thorac Cardiovasc Surg 75, 777–781.
36. Solem JO, Kugelberg J, Stahl E, *et al.* (1986) Late cardiac tamponade following open-heart surgery. Diagnosis and treatment. Scand J Thorac Cardiovasc Surg 20, 129–131.
37. Prince SE, Cunha BA. (1997) Postpericardiotomy syndrome. Heart Lung 26, 165–168.

38. Engle MA, Zabriskie JB, Senterfit LB, *et al.* (1980) Viral illness and the postpericardiotomy syndrome. A prospective study in children. Circulation 62, 1151–1158.

39. Webber SA, Wilson NJ, Junker AK, *et al.* (2001) Postpericardiotomy syndrome: no evidence for a viral etiology. Cardiol Young 11, 67–74.

40. Engle MA, McCabe JC, Ebert PA, *et al.* (1974) The Postpericardiotomy syndrome and antiheart antibodies. Circulation 49, 401–406.

41. Harken AH, Hammond GI, Edmunds LH Jr. (1996) Pericardial diseases. In: *Cardiac Surgery in the Adult*. New York: McGraw-Hill.

42. Chapman JE Jr, Rubin JW, Gross CM, *et al.* (1988) Congenital absence of pericardium: an unusual cause of atypical angina. Ann Thorac Surg 45, 91–93.

43. Gatzoulis MA, Munk MD, Merchant N, *et al.* (2000) Isolated congenital absence of the pericardium: clinical presentation, diagnosis, and management. Ann Thorac Surg 69, 1209–1215.

44. Saito R, Hotta F. (1980) Congenital pericardial defect associated with cardiac incarceration: case report. Am Heart J 100, 866–870.

45. Fellous L, Tourneux P, Brule-Pepin R, *et al.* (2005) [Pneumopericardium: a rare complication of meconium aspiration syndrome]. Arch Pediatr 12, 83.

46. Kumar A, Bhatnagar V. (2005) Respiratory distress in neonates. Indian J Pediatr 72, 425–428.

47. Rucker J. (1987) [Pneumopericardium in hyaline membrane syndrome in premature infants]. Padiatr Padol 22, 51–58.

48. Hummler HD, Bandstra ES, Abdenour GE. (1996) Neonatal fellowship. Neonatal pneumopericardium: successful treatment with nitrogen washout technique. J Perinatol 16, 490–493.

49. Pratap U, Slavik Z, Ofoe VD, *et al.* (2001) Octreotide to treat postoperative chylothorax after cardiac operations in children. Ann Thorac Surg 72, 1740–1742.

CHAPTER 41

Surgical Therapy of Cardiac Arrhythmias

Constantine Mavroudis,[1] Barbara J. Deal,[2] and Carl L. Backer[2]

[1]Florida Hospital for Children, Orlando, FL, USA
[2]Ann & Robert H. Lurie Children's Hospital of Chicago, formerly Children's Memorial Hospital, Chicago, IL, USA

Evolving Role of Surgical Therapy

Historical Considerations

The definitive cure of arrhythmias originated with the surgical elimination of accessory connections performed by Sealy and colleagues at Duke University in 1968 [1], culminating in the impressive surgical results by Cox *et al.* in successful elimination of accessory connection function in more than 90% of operated patients [1–3]. Success with the ablation of accessory connections led to atrioventricular node modification for atrioventricular nodal re-entry tachycardia (AVNRT) [4], atrial isolation techniques for automatic atrial tachycardia [5], and ablative surgery in association with endocardial resection for ventricular tachycardia [6,7]. The technique of surgical interruption of these arrhythmia circuits was subsequently studied extensively in the dog model and resulted in the development of the highly successful Cox-maze procedure for elimination of atrial fibrillation, again with success rates over 90% [8–16]. Guiraudon successfully performed ablation of the right atrial isthmus as treatment for right atrial flutter [17], and subsequently Josephson and colleagues developed mapping and resection techniques for ventricular tachycardia, particularly those associated with ventricular scar or aneurysms secondary to ischemic disease [18]. Williams and others [19] applied these techniques to the therapy of ventricular tachycardia complicating repaired congenital heart disease, particularly tetralogy of Fallot. These impressive surgical arrhythmia results were supplanted by the development of catheter ablation techniques in the electrophysiology laboratory beginning in the 1990s, initially for atrioventricular nodal re-entry and accessory connections, and extending to most arrhythmia substrates including atrial fibrillation, relegating surgical therapy to a largely

historical category [20–28]. Danielson and colleagues at the Mayo clinic persisted in the application of the right atrial isthmus ablation to surgical repairs of patients with atrial arrhythmias with congenital heart disease, particularly Ebstein anomaly [29]. The high success rates for the transcatheter ablation of arrhythmias largely replaced the techniques of surgical intervention as newer mapping technologies and ablation energies were refined, and defibrillator therapy supplanted ventricular arrhythmia surgery. During the first 20 years of transcatheter ablation the knowledge of arrhythmia circuits was considerably advanced, while the cumbersome custom epicardial mapping systems used in the operating room languished.

As the subset of patients with congenital heart disease gained markedly improved survival rates following surgery, the development of late postoperative arrhythmias increased and resulted in significant late morbidity and mortality. Lesions such as tetralogy of Fallot, atrial septal defects, transposition of the great arteries, Ebstein anomaly, and single-ventricle physiology were associated with the highest risk of developing late arrhythmias. The recognition of the development of arrhythmias as an "electromechanical" problem was first proposed by Gatzoulis and colleagues [30] in patients with repaired tetralogy of Fallot; isolated intervention for arrhythmias with the transcatheter approach did not address the ongoing progression of hemodynamic complications. The correlation of the need for reoperations with the high risk of arrhythmia development in certain congenital lesions emphasizes the complex interaction of hemodynamics with arrhythmia development (Table 41.1). Using the integration of knowledge gained with catheter ablation into the surgical repair of congenital lesions, Mavroudis and colleagues in Chicago re-initiated the surgical techniques of arrhythmia intervention beginning in 1994 [31–41]. Initial results with

Pediatric Cardiac Surgery, Fourth Edition. Edited by Constantine Mavroudis and Carl L. Backer.
© 2013 Blackwell Publishing Ltd. Published 2013 by Blackwell Publishing Ltd.

Table 41.1 Congenital heart disease: Incidence of reoperation and late arrhythmia development. (ASD atrial septal defect; AVSD, atrioventricular septal defect; SVT, supraventricular tachycardia; TAPVC, total anomalous pulmonary venous connection; TGA, transposition of the great arteries; VT, ventricular tachycardia.)

Lesion	% Reoperation	% SVT	% VT
Ebstein anomaly	>25	40–60	–
TGA, atrial switch	27	30–50	5–10
ASD/TAPVC/AVSD	1–9	5–15	–
Single ventricle	>27	40–60	2–5
Tetralogy of Fallot	26	35	7

Table 41.2 Indications for arrhythmia surgery.

Indication	Substrates
Failed catheter ablation	Multiple accessory connections Epicardial substrates Anatomic complexity Hemodynamic instability, severe congestive failure
Arrhythmias in patients undergoing concomitant repair of congenital heart disease	Ebstein anomaly Atriopulmonary repairs of single ventricle Revisions of prior repairs: conduit or valve replacements
Preventive arrhythmia surgery	Prophylactic atrial maze procedures Left cervicosympathetic denervation in long QT syndromes
Device therapy	Antibradycardia pacing Antitachycardia pacing Defibrillator therapy Resynchronization therapy

conversion of the atriopulmonary Fontan to an extracardiac total cavopulmonary connection associated with right and later left atrial arrhythmia surgery resulted in often dramatic improvements in hemodynamic status, and reduced the midterm recurrence of arrhythmias to less than 20% in this most difficult population. These techniques were then applied to subsequently more challenging anatomical substrates including ventricular inversion and heterotaxy syndromes, neonates, and patients with severe congestive heart failure secondary to arrhythmias. The use of arrhythmia surgery techniques was then applied to the prophylactic prevention of arrhythmia development in patients known to be at risk, such as patients undergoing re-do operations for conduit changes or late repairs of atrial septal defects. The ease of incorporation of arrhythmia surgery techniques into the operative repair of congenital heart disease emphasizes the need for a comprehensive electrical and mechanical approach to the repair of congenital heart disease, and provides a standard and a challenge for the operative repairs of the next decades.

This chapter will review the indications for arrhythmia surgery, the presently available operative techniques and results based on the mechanism of arrhythmia, the collaborative roles of the electrophysiologist and the surgeon in the planning and performance of arrhythmia surgery, the indications and techniques of pacemaker and antitachycardia device therapy, and the management of early postoperative arrhythmias. The goal is to understand the available techniques for arrhythmia surgery and current success rates based on arrhythmia substrate in order to appropriately guide patient selection and evaluation.

Indications for Arrhythmia Surgery

Table 41.2 summarizes current indications for arrhythmia surgery in our institutions. In 1983 Cox wrote "the selection of patients for the surgical treatment of cardiac arrhythmias is based on several variables. These variables include the patient's age and general condition, the nature of the presenting arrhythmia, its response to medical treatment, and the presence of associated anomalies that may require additional surgical correction" [42]. The results achieved over the last 2 decades in arrhythmia surgery indicate that age and complexity of anatomical substrate are no longer important hurdles to successful arrhythmia surgery. Rather, an awareness of preexisting arrhythmias, suitability of the arrhythmia substrate to current surgical techniques versus catheter ablation, and intervention to limit the development of later arrhythmias are important determinants of the decision to perform arrhythmia surgery. In the early phase of the current era of arrhythmia surgery, only patients who had failed multiple attempts at catheter ablation techniques with structurally normal hearts were referred for surgery as a last resort; the improvement in catheter ablation techniques has limited this occurrence to very few patients. However, in patients requiring concomitant arrhythmia surgery where catheter ablation techniques are difficult, such as Ebstein anomaly or heterotaxy syndrome, or where catheter ablation techniques require prolonged procedures with less than optimal success rates, high arrhythmia recurrences, or risk of complications, a more streamlined therapeutic approach would be to appropriately map the arrhythmia substrate and proceed to arrhythmia surgery if initial catheter attempts are unsuccessful. Arrhythmia surgery in the setting of congenital heart disease offers certain powerful advantages compared to

Table 41.3 Techniques for arrhythmia surgery.

Technique	Substrate
Resection or dissection Focal substrates	AV groove accessory connection Atrial wall tissue, appendages Endocardial fibrosis or scar Aneurysm
Ablation	Accessory connection Areas of early activation, scar Connection between anatomic barriers
Maze procedures Macro re-entrant circuits	Modified right atrial maze Left atrial maze Cox-maze IIII procedure
Denervation	Left cervical ganglion sympathectomy

Table 41.4 Mechanisms of supraventricular tachycardia commonly associated with congenital heart lesions.

Supraventricular tachycardia	Congenital heart disease
Accessory connection-mediated	Ebstein anomaly Atrial septal defect Congenitally corrected transposition of the great arteries Hypertrophic cardiomyopathy
Atrial re-entry	Atrial septal defect Single ventricle following atriopulmonary repairs Transposition of the great arteries with Mustard/Senning repairs Atrioventricular septal defects Tetralogy of Fallot Total anomalous pulmonary venous connections
Atrioventricular nodal re-entry	Mustard/Senning repairs of transposition of the great arteries Left ventricular outflow obstructive lesions
Atrial fibrillation	Mitral valve disorders Ebstein anomaly of tricuspid valve Single ventricle, especially tricuspid atresia Atrial septal defects Tetralogy of Fallot Hypertrophic cardiomyopathy Eisenmenger's syndrome

the transcatheter approach, including direct visualization of the anatomy and the ability to rapidly perform complete lines of block between difficult to access anatomic barriers. The high success rates and low risk of recurrence of tachycardia in addition to improved hemodynamic outcomes provide a standard of comparison for the optimal selection of intervention, such as atrial fibrillation in the setting of complex heart disease, or tachycardia associated with single-ventricle physiology.

The techniques we currently use for arrhythmia surgery are summarized in Table 41.3, and the operative techniques are discussed in detail in subsequent sections. Knowledge of the mechanisms of tachycardia is essential to the appropriate application of arrhythmia surgery techniques. The fundamental distinction to be made when planning a surgical approach is to identify either macro re-entrant circuits and their constituent parts, or a focal tachycardia: macro re-entry circuits are treated with either dissection or ablation of an accessory connection or a maze procedure, and focal tachycardia is approached with either resection or localized ablation; the distinction is of critical importance as a maze procedure will not effectively treat focal atrial tachycardia. Macro re-entrant circuits require a circuit with unidirectional block in one limb, and slowed conduction in the other limb allowing re-entry to occur, and may be initiated and terminated with pacing techniques, allowing elucidation of the substrate. Elimination of conduction through a critical part of the re-entrant circuit will terminate tachycardia. The keys to success in arrhythmia surgery are the accurate identification of the arrhythmia mechanism and its anatomic substrate, and the appropriate delivery of incisions, ablative lesions, or resection; the limitations are thus the accuracy of electrical mapping, anatomic exposure, and ablation techniques (Table 41.4).

Operative Planning

The success of a surgical arrhythmia strategy begins with appropriate patient selection, based on the anticipated success rates of arrhythmia surgery, the complexity of anatomic repair, and the ability of the patient to tolerate the combined surgical procedures safely. A thorough understanding of the anatomy of the congenital heart disease and prior surgical repairs provides valuable information regarding the potential arrhythmia substrates, supplemented by careful review of the tracings obtained during clinical arrhythmias. Obtaining medical records of a patient's extended history is often difficult, particularly in older patients with repaired congenital heart disease whose original surgeries were performed remotely in time and geography. Detailed review of prior operative reports is important, and may identify surgeon-specific variations in technique that will impact the surgical approach, such as the deviation of the atrial septum to the left atrium in atriopulmonary repairs of single ventricle; knowledge of these surgical variations will require modification of the standard right atrial surgery. A realistic assessment of the time and exposure required to appropriately perform arrhythmia surgery in complicated cases, and the ability of impaired ventricular function to withstand surgery, is needed.

The careful delineation of the arrhythmia mechanism and critical anatomic components usually necessitates preoperative invasive electrophysiologic study; the exception to this is isolated atrial fibrillation, as the need to perform right and left atrial maze surgery is clear. Patients with congenital heart disease may not uncommonly have more than one arrhythmia mechanism, such as accessory connection-mediated tachycardia or AVNRT in addition to atrial flutter. In these cases a stepwise approach may be employed, using transcatheter ablation preoperatively for one mechanism, and reliance on surgery for a technically more challenging arrhythmia. It has been our preference to attempt transcatheter ablation of accessory connections preoperatively whenever possible, using surgery in this situation for multiple accessory connections or in the setting of Ebstein anomaly. The presence of right atrial thrombus, right-to-left shunts, or hemodynamic instability during tachycardia will restrict the ability to perform preoperative studies. Visual reproductions of the anatomy as defined in the catheterization laboratory using angiography or three-dimensional reconstructions, with superimposition of the electrophysiologic target, are valuable to provide the surgeon with appropriate landmarks. Reliance on only intraoperative mapping of tachycardia mechanism is not optimal, as tachycardia may not be inducible under situations of anesthesia with the chest open.

Intraoperative electrophysiologic mapping is used in the following settings: to confirm anatomic landmarks important to the arrhythmia circuit, to assess efficacy of surgical techniques particularly when multiple arrhythmia mechanisms are present, mapping when vascular access is restricted, and mapping when provision of cardiopulmonary bypass for hemodynamically unstable arrhythmias is needed. Patients with atrial baffles or patches over the right-sided atrioventricular valve may have restricted access to the critical atrial isthmus between the coronary sinus and the inferior vena cava; successful ablation of the arrhythmia circuit requires baffle or patch removal in order to apply the lesions. The anatomy of Ebstein anomaly or ventricular inversion, particularly in the presence of dextrocardia, is not always readily mapped in the catheterization laboratory, and such complex anatomy may benefit from correlation of anatomic landmarks under visual inspection with the target of ablation. The ability of the operative team to cooperate with electrophysiologic mapping becomes imperative in the setting of hemodynamically unstable tachycardia, such as incessant atrial tachycardia resulting in severe congestive heart failure. In this setting, mapping and elimination of tachycardia can avoid the need for implantation of mechanical circulatory support devices and may be life saving.

Intraoperative mapping systems historically have relied on custom-developed multiple electrode arrays, which were not commercially available, and were designed to lay on the epicardial surface of the atrium or ventricle. Use of these systems also required sophisticated engineering support for the display of the electrical signals. The complexity of these systems posed a significant deterrent to widespread acceptance of surgical mapping. However, the advances of catheter ablation technology resulted in the manufacture of many configurations of multiple electrode array catheters with steerable handles, which can be adapted for use in the operating room using standard mapping display systems. In addition, placement of an esophageal electrogram at the start of the procedure provides additional anatomic information and an atrial reference electrogram throughout the surgery.

After cannulation but before commencement of bypass, a reference bipolar electrode is sutured to either the atrial or ventricular surface, and is used as a stable reference and as a pacing electrode. For mapping of accessory connections, a steerable deca-polar catheter can then be positioned along the atrioventricular groove, with sterile connectors to the electrophysiology recording computer. Atrial mapping can be performed with one or more deca-polar catheters secured to the atrial surface of interest with sutures or wet gauze. Ventricular mapping of the epicardial surface can be performed with either more than one catheter in place, or sequential positioning of a catheter. Due to ventricular wall thickness, epicardial ventricular mapping may differ from the earliest site of endocardial electrical activity by as much as 1.5 cm, limiting accuracy. Right ventricular endocardial mapping may or may not be feasible, depending on tachycardia inducibility on bypass. Some centers have developed custom-made "plunge" needle electrodes to record across the depth of the ventricular muscle to overcome this limitation.

Clarity of electrode anatomical positioning must be communicated with precision from the surgeon to the electrophysiologist, recognizing that surgical anatomic relationships are typically described with different spatial terms than the standard electrophysiology nomenclature developed using fluoroscopy. It has been our practice for the surgeon to draw a map of the anatomy, with the electrode positions delineated. Miscommunication, or misinterpretation, at this point will result in inaccurate mapping and inaccurate guidance for lesion placement. The importance of this step cannot be overstated. With electrodes in place, the quality of electrograms is verified, with catheter repositioning as necessary to obtain good contact with the epicardial surface. Before pacing is initiated to induce tachycardia, an understanding of the process for hemodynamic support and tachycardia termination must be agreed on.

Typically, tachycardia induction and electrogram recording can be performed in less than 20 minutes. Catheters may be repositioned sequentially during tachycardia to obtain sufficient electrograms to determine earliest activation and circuit delineation. After termination of tachycardia, the electrophysiologist can proceed with review of electrograms and clarification of activation sequences while surgery progresses. Once more, it is our practice to frequently produce a visual representation of the tachycardia focus or circuit superimposed on anatomic landmarks, often as a drawing, to assure that the spatial target is clearly understood by both the electrophysiologist and the surgeon.

Clear communication between the electrophysiologist and the surgeon before surgery is essential, with agreement on the proposed mapping and ablative approach and the alternatives as dictated by anatomic considerations. The need for more mapping information needs to be weighed and reassessed versus the hazards of surgical dissection and exposure of anatomy that may not be easily accessible. Certain types of arrhythmia surgery may require repeat pacing and mapping during surgery to verify efficacy of the ablative technique. Inducibility of the clinical arrhythmia following initial ablation may require additional efforts at ablation, taking into account the safety of further operative efforts. Finally, integration of device therapy needs to be considered, including the potential for resynchronization therapy or defibrillator as well as antibradycardia or antitachycardia pacing.

Acute postoperative care frequently involves atrial pacing at rates higher than the intrinsic rhythm, to maintain a stable rhythm and limit atrial ectopy. In patients undergoing surgery for atrial fibrillation, early postoperative atrial tachycardia can occur in 30–40% of patients following the left atrial maze procedure. To avoid this high incidence of recurrent atrial tachycardia, intravenous antiarrhythmic medication, amiodarone, is infused until oral medications are tolerated. Antiarrhythmic medication is continued for 3 months postoperatively in patients with atrial fibrillation, in gradually decreasing dosages. For all other patients undergoing arrhythmia surgery for re-entrant tachycardias, repeat electrophysiology testing is performed without antiarrhythmic medication prior to hospital discharge, to assess both efficacy of the procedure and potential proarrhythmic effects. Testing is performed in the baseline state and with infusion of catecholamines, usually isoproterenol. In patients with inducible arrhythmia, appropriate medication or antitachycardia pacing algorithms are instituted. Patients with inducible ventricular tachycardia undergo defibrillator implantation prior to hospital discharge. For the majority of patients without inducible postoperative arrhythmias, following electrophysiology study beta-blocking medications are administered for 3 months postoperatively.

Accessory Connection-Mediated Atrial Tachycardia

Mechanism

Wolff-Parkinson-White (WPW) syndrome is the association of episodes of tachycardia with the appearance of a delta wave on electrocardiography (pre-excitation) [37]. During sinus rhythm with pre-excitation, conduction proceeds simultaneously from the sinus node to the ventricles over two routes, the atrioventricular node and the accessory connection. The electrical wave front traverses the accessory connection and depolarizes ventricular tissue first, because of intrinsic slowing of conduction at the atrioventricular node. This is the manifest form of accessory connections (pre-excitation, or WPW). In order for a re-entrant tachycardia to occur, there must be unidirectional block in one pathway with slowed conduction in the other. Plate 41.1 (see plate section opposite p. 594) shows unidirectional block in the AV node, with conduction proceeding antegrade to the ventricles via the accessory connection [37,41]. The ventricular muscle is responsible for conduction delay, allowing the wave front to proceed retrogradely up the atrioventricular node (which has had time to regain conduction) to the atrium. This re-entrant circuit is termed antidromic reciprocating tachycardia; the re-entrant circuit includes the atria, accessory connection, ventricles, and the atrioventricular node. The more common form of tachycardia in association with an accessory connection is called orthodromic reciprocating tachycardia. Plate 41.2 (see plate section opposite p. 594) illustrates conduction block in the accessory connection, thus resulting in loss of the delta wave [37,41]. Conduction proceeds normally through the atrioventricular node to the ventricle. The delay encountered in the atrioventricular node and ventricular muscle allows the accessory connection to regain electrical conductivity, and the electrical wavefront then enters the atria from the opposite direction. This re-entrant circuit is similar to antidromic reciprocating atrial tachycardia except that the electrical pathways are reversed and pre-excitation is concealed.

Surgical Therapy of Accessory Connection-Mediated Tachycardia

Indications

Surgical ablation of accessory connections achieved success rates of 95% or greater before being supplanted by the widespread application of the radiofrequency catheter ablation technique [2,11–15]. Presently, surgical ablation of supraventricular tachycardia (SVT) is performed for patients failing both medical and catheter ablation techniques and for patients with complex congenital heart disease undergoing surgical repair. Certain accessory connections, especially in the posteroseptal region, may have an epicardial course [43], limiting the success of ablation using an endocardial catheter approach. Right-sided accessory connections in patients with Ebstein anomaly tend to be multiple, with an increased likelihood of antidromic reciprocating tachycardia posing a therapeutic challenge. Recurrence risks for pre-excitation due to right-sided accessory connections are significantly higher following ablation procedures than for accessory connections in other locations [44,45] and often require multiple ablation procedures. The decision as to whether to persist with multiple ablation procedures or opt for surgical repair is individualized.

In patients with manifest accessory connections and congenital heart disease undergoing surgical repair, current recommendations are to assess the characteristics of the accessory connection and to perform preoperative ablation in patients with inducible SVT and rapidly conducting accessory connections [46,47], owing to the risk of refractory tachycardia during the early postoperative period. With complex congenital heart disease, the ablation procedure may pose technical difficulties, which require prolonged fluoroscopy times or more than one ablation procedure [48–51]. For patients requiring surgical intervention for their structural heart disease, decisions must be made on an individual basis as to the optimal way to manage both problems, minimizing the number and extent of procedures and the risk to the patient.

Over the past decade, electrophysiologic mapping and catheter ablation have improved to the point where surgical ablation is rarely necessary. Nevertheless, for those rare occasions where concomitant cryoablation for accessory connections becomes necessary, a comprehensive review of the surgical dissections are presented herein.

Surgical Technique

Following a comprehensive preoperative electrophysiologic study [19], intraoperative epicardial or endocardial mapping, or both, are performed during surgery to confirm the preoperative electrophysiologic findings and to assess the immediate postoperative result. The technique of intraoperative mapping has been previously discussed. The general goal of surgical therapy for the WPW syndrome or concealed bypass tract is to divide or cryoablate accessory connections, which are responsible for the re-entry phenomenon and clinical tachycardia. Two surgical techniques, the endocardial and epicardial techniques, were developed (Figure 41.1) [52]. The endocardial technique [2,11,14] requires cardiopulmonary bypass and is performed within the right atrium or left atrium, depending on the anatomic location of the bypass tract. The epicardial technique [12,13,15] may or may not require cardiopulmonary bypass, depending on the location of the accessory connection and is performed on the epicardial surface of the heart at the

atrioventricular junction by dividing the atrial end of the connection. Excellent results are achieved by both techniques, the choice being surgeon dependent and institution dependent.

Left Free-Wall Accessory Connections

Ablation of left free-wall accessory connections is usually performed by the *endocardial* technique from within the left atrium using cardiopulmonary bypass and cardioplegic arrest. The exposure is through a left atriotomy, usually performed at the interatrial (Sondergaard's) groove, similar to that for mitral valve repair/replacement. After proper exposure, a curvilinear incision is made parallel to and 2 mm away from the posterior mitral annulus, extending from the left fibrous trigone to the posterior septum (Figure 41.2) [53]. A dissection plane is then developed between the fat pad of the atrioventricular groove and the superior portion of the left ventricle, extending to the epicardial reflection throughout the entire length of the initial incision (Figure 41.2) [53]. The dissection is completed by extending the ends of the incision and the dissection, "squaring off" to the mitral annulus to divide any accessory connection, which might be located at the juxta-annular area [11]. This dissection exposes the entire left free-wall space to the respective boundaries, thereby ensuring division of any or all accessory connections. The endocardial incision is then sutured to complete the procedure.

The *epicardial* approach (Figure 41.3) [53] for left free-wall accessory connections requires upward and rightward cardiac retraction for proper exposure, which frequently results in severe hemodynamic instability. As a result, most surgeons employing this technique prefer to use cardiopulmonary bypass, although no intracavitary exposure is required for this technique. Once exposure is achieved, the epicardial reflection of the atrium is entered and a plane of dissection is established between the atrioventricular groove fat pad and the atrial wall. Coronary sinus tributaries often require ligation and division, and care must be taken to avoid coronary artery injury. The dissection plane is extended to the level of the posterior mitral valve annulus and carried slightly onto the top of the posterior left ventricle. This maneuver divides the atrial end of all accessory connections in this area except for those which lie immediately adjacent to the mitral valve annulus. If present, these juxta-annular connections can be interrupted by a cryosurgical probe that is placed at the level of the mitral valve annulus. The atrial epicardial reflection is then reapproximated by suture technique. Both techniques have their respective advantages and disadvantages [11,12] and can be applied selectively, depending on the anatomic circumstances governing the operation. Anatomic variation may be especially important in simultaneous repair of congenital heart disease and ablation of accessory connections. Under these circumstances, the

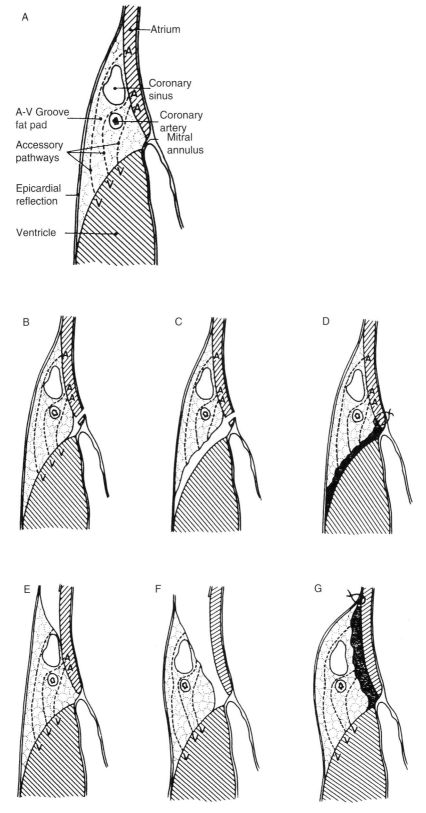

Figure 41.1 Diagrammatic representation of a cross-section of the posterior left heart. **A,** The different depths at which left free-wall connections can be located in relation to the mitral annulus and epicardial reflection are shown. **B–D,** The endocardial surgical technique. **E–G,** The epicardial technique. (Reproduced with permission from Cox [52].)

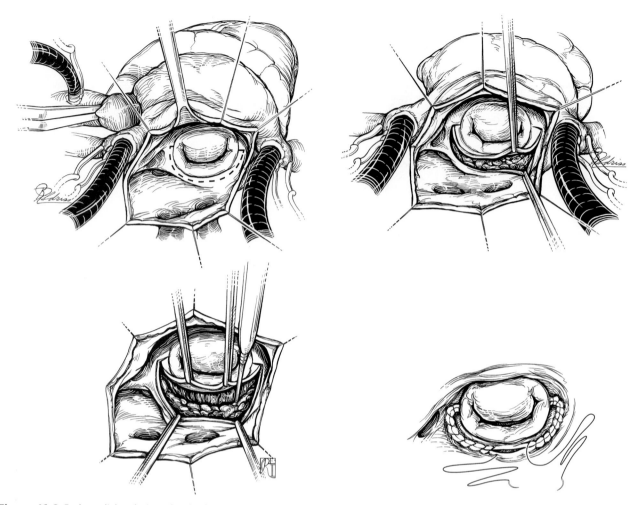

Figure 41.2 Endocardial technique for dividing left free-wall accessory connections in Wolff-Parkinson-White syndrome.

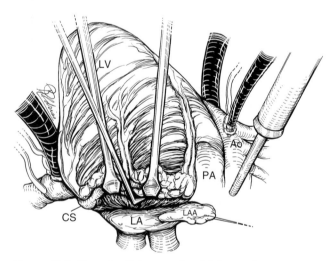

Figure 41.3 The epicardial approach to left free-wall accessory connections. A schematic of the left ventricle, viewed from an operative position. The fat pad is mobilized and the atrioventricular junction exposed. (Ao, aorta; CS, coronary sinus; LA, left atrium; LAA, left atrial appendage; LV, left ventricle; PA, pulmonary artery.)

atrioventricular anatomic connections may vary, especially when there is a subaortic muscular conus, atrioventricular discordance, and juxtaposition of the atrial appendages. The surgeon should be familiar with both techniques and be ready to alter the procedure depending on the pathoanatomy.

Posterior Septal Accessory Connections

The *endocardial* approach to posterior septal connections is through the right atrium. Normothermic cardiopulmonary bypass usually is used with certain precautions, which include closure of any intracardiac shunts before proceeding with the operation. Preoperative evaluation, particularly transthoracic echocardiography, may not always detect the presence of a patent foramen ovale. Care then is taken to fibrillate the heart shortly after cardiopulmonary bypass and before right atrial entry in order to check for, and close, a patent foramen ovale. This maneuver will ensure that no air is introduced into the left ventricle during a beating cardiac cycle. After complete patent foramen ovale closure, the heart can be defibrillated and the operation continued.

After completion of the endocardial mapping, a supra-annular incision is made 2 mm above the posterior medial tricuspid valve annulus, beginning at least 1 cm posterior to the His bundle (Figure 41.4) [2,53]. The supra-annular incision is extended counterclockwise onto the posterior right atrial free wall. This incision provides exposure to the posterior septal space near the left ventricle and the epicardial reflection at the posterior right ventricle near the crux of the heart. The posterior septal space fat pad is then dissected away from the top of the posterior ventricular septum while the heart is beating or during hypothermic cardioplegic arrest, depending on the vascularity of the dissection plane and the preference of the surgeon.

The *epicardial* approach to posterior septal accessory connections is very similar to that for the left free-wall connections except of course for the location. The posterior septal accessory connections are divided by developing a dissection plane between the fat pad and the top of the posterior ventricular septum, following the mitral annulus over to the posterior superior process of the left ventricle, and following the epicardial reflection from the posterior right ventricle, across the crux, onto the posterior left ventricle. Cryolesions are placed at regular intervals around the annulus to ensure complete division of all accessory connections.

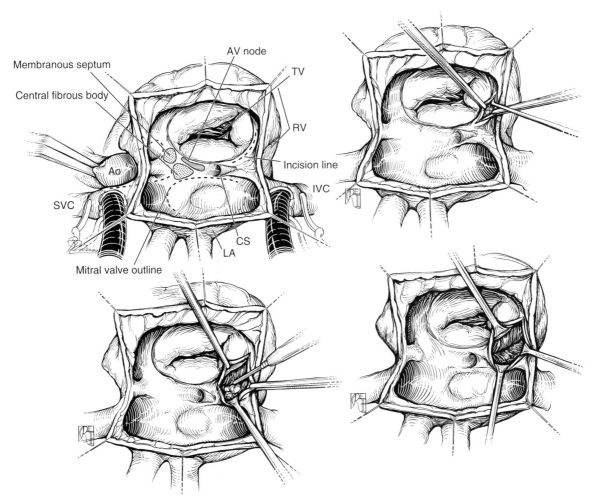

Figure 41.4 Endocardial technique for surgical division of posterior septal accessory connections in Wolff-Parkinson-White syndrome. The junction of the posterior medial mitral and tricuspid valve annuli forms an inverted V at the posterior edge of the central fibrous body, and the fat pad comes to a point at the apex of that V. The apex of the V is always posterior to the His bundle, although the distance between the apex of the V and the His bundle may vary. As long as the dissection in this region remains posterior to the central fibrous body, the His bundle will not be damaged. After the anterior point of the fat pad is gently dissected away from the apex of the V (i.e., away from the posterior edge of the central fibrous body), the mitral valve annulus comes into view at the point where it joins the tricuspid valve to form the central fibrous body. (Ao, aorta; AV, atrioventricular node; CS, coronary sinus; IVC, inferior vena cava; LA, left atrium; LV, left ventricle; RV, right ventricle; SVC, superior vena cava; TV, tricuspid valve.)

Right Free-Wall Accessory Connections

The *epicardial* dissection for right free-wall accessory connections can be performed without cardiopulmonary bypass in the majority of cases. An incision is made in the epicardium, establishing a dissection plane between the right atrial wall and the atrioventricular groove fat pad to the tricuspid valve annulus (Figure 41.5) [53] throughout the entire length of the right atrial free wall. Cryolesions at appropriate intervals can ensure complete accessory connection ablation.

The *endocardial* technique can be used if there is concern about epicardial bleeding or if a concomitant intracardiac repair is necessary. Under cardioplegic arrest, a supra-annular incision is placed 2 mm above the tricuspid valve annulus, extending around the entire right free-wall. A dissection plane is then established between the underlying atrioventricular groove fat pad and the top of the right ventricle throughout the length of the supra-annular incision. The dissection is extended to the epicardial reflection off the ventricle, thereby dividing all the penetrating fibers in this area. The incision can then be closed.

Anterior Septal Accessory Connections

The *epicardial* approach to anterior septal accessory connections was less successful than the *endocardial* approach, leading most surgeons to use the endocardial exposure for this connection [13]. The endocardial dissection is similar to that for the right free-wall lesions except for location. A supra-annular incision is made just anterior to the His bundle, 2 mm above the tricuspid annulus and extended in a clockwise direction onto the right anterior free-wall. The dissection plane is established between the fat pad occupying the anterior septal space and the top of the right ventricle and developed to the aorta medially and to the epicardial reflection off the ventricle anteriorly. Great care is required to avoid injury of the right coronary artery, which courses through the fat pad in this area, and the aortic wall at the right coronary sinus of Valsalva.

Special Considerations

Accessory connections are frequently present in patients with Ebstein anomaly of the tricuspid valve and in patients with congenitally corrected transposition of the great arteries who have associated Ebstein malformation of the systemic tricuspid valve. These connections tend to be multiple and due to the abnormal anatomy of the atrioventricular groove, are sometimes technically difficult to completely eliminate with the transcatheter approach, and have a higher risk of recurrence following an initially successful ablation. In this setting, operative dissection of the atrioventricular groove provides a technical advantage.

Macro Re-Entrant Atrial Tachycardia (Atrial Re-Entry Tachycardia, Atrial Flutter)

Mechanism

Macro re-entrant atrial tachycardia is a large tachycardia circuit present in either the right or left atrium (Plate 41.3, see plate section opposite p. 594) [37,41,54–56]. The re-entrant circuit requires unidirectional block and an area of slow conduction in order to sustain tachycardia. A premature atrial contraction can propagate an electrical wave front that encounters unidirectional block near the atrial septum and is redirected inferiorly by an alternative route, to the right atrial free-wall. The electrical wave front encounters an area of slow conduction, usually at the area between the inferior vena cava, tricuspid valve, and the coronary sinus. The electrophysiologic delay allows the area of unidirectional block to recover conduction. The electrical wave front now enters opposite the area of unidirectional block that establishes the re-entrant circuit. Cryoablation lesions are used to interrupt this circuit at the inferior isthmus, defined as the area between the coronary sinus, tricuspid annulus, and the inferior vena cava. The cryoablation lesion, therefore, transforms an area of slow conduction to an area of no conduction, thereby eliminating the circuit. Multiple areas of slow conduction may exist in patients with congenital heart disease from prior incisions, patches, or wall stress.

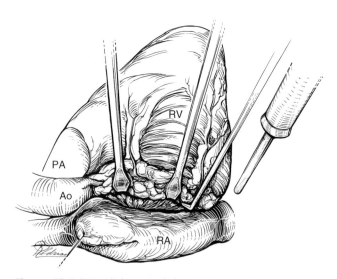

Figure 41.5 Epicardial approach for right free-wall accessory connections. A schematic view of the exposure of the right coronary fossa and anterior right ventricular atrioventricular sulcus. (AO, aorta; LV, left ventricle; PA, pulmonary artery; RA, right atrium; RV, right ventricle.)

Indications for Surgery

Patients with refractory atrial tachycardia failing catheter ablation procedures, and patients with tachycardia requiring repair of associated intracardiac defects, are considered candidates for surgical arrhythmia intervention. Success rates for eliminating right atrial macro re-entrant surgery using the modified right atrial maze procedure are over 95% [31–33,35,37,40,41,55,56]. In rare cases of tachycardia in the neonate with structural heart disease, in which the ablation procedure poses significant risk to the infant, surgical ablation may be performed safely. In patients who have had Fontan surgery, transcatheter ablation therapy has limited success because of the frequent association of coexisting hemodynamic abnormalities. Those centers that have recognized this problem have achieved excellent results with a combined approach of repair of associated lesions in combination with Fontan conversion and arrhythmia surgery [35,39,40,57].

Structurally Normal Hearts

In the structurally normal heart, atrial re-entry tachycardia is uncommon and usually is amenable to radiofrequency catheter ablation procedures. If the area of re-entry encompasses a wide area of atrial tissue, the catheter technique may not be successful, and resection coupled with cryoablation may be effective. We have operated successfully on an 11-year-old girl who had paroxysmal sinoatrial re-entry tachycardia since infancy, refractory to virtually all antiarrhythmic therapy, and failing two ablation procedures. Endocardial mapping localized tachycardia to the posterolateral right atrium; during surgery, repeat activation mapping indicated additional involvement of the posterior left atrium. Resection of the posterolateral right atrium was performed, with an encircling incision around the pulmonary veins. The child had no recurrence of the atrial re-entrant tachycardia in 4 years, but she developed late sinus bradycardia requiring an atrial pacemaker 3 years postoperatively.

Concomitant Repair of Congenital Heart Disease

A small population of patients with congenital heart disease will have atrial tachycardia identified before any surgical intervention; arrhythmia management may be incorporated into single-stage therapy at the time of surgery without limitations of patient weight or complexity of anatomy [57–59].

We have experience with a few patients with atrial re-entry tachycardia originating near the rim of an unrepaired atrial primum or secundum septal defect. Because of the need for atrial surgery, we elected not to perform catheter ablation but to ablate under direct vision intraoperatively. After mapping the tachycardia preoperatively, surgical repair includes excision of the rim of the atrial defect, with localized cryoablation of the involved perimeter of the defect. Anatomic ablation of the inferomedial right atrial isthmus, between the os of the coronary sinus and the inferior vena cava, may treat atrial flutter successfully. We have performed right atrial cryoablation for an infant with recurrent atrial flutter at the time of initial repair of tetralogy of Fallot.

More commonly, atrial tachycardia occurs as a late sequelae of intracardiac repair of congenital heart disease. Atrial re-entry tachycardia occurs in 20–50% of postoperative Mustard or Senning patients [60,61], more than 40–50% of Fontan patients [62,63], and 34% of tetralogy of Fallot patients [64]. In the absence of hemodynamic problems, particularly in the non-Fontan patient, such arrhythmias most often are treated successfully using radiofrequency catheter ablation [65,66]. However, if patients have residual hemodynamic abnormalities, or in Fontan patients with atriopulmonary repairs, consideration should be given to integration of the principles of catheter ablation into the surgical repair to minimize interventions for the patient. In contrast to nonsustained ventricular arrhythmias, which may improve after repair of residual hemodynamic problems, atrial arrhythmias tend to persist after surgery. Direct intervention for atrial arrhythmias during surgery is highly effective and relies on four techniques; inferomedial right atrial ablation for typical atrial flutter, a modified right atrial maze procedure for multiple atrial re-entrant circuits, a Cox-maze III procedure for atrial fibrillation, and atrial pacemaker implantation, either to avoid bradycardia or as an antitachycardia device.

Atrial re-entry tachycardia following the Mustard or Senning procedure is amenable to catheter ablation, although a retrograde catheter approach via the aorta and across the tricuspid valve into the pulmonary venous atrium is often necessary [50,67], with the attendant risk of creating aortic insufficiency. If the patient requires reoperation for hemodynamic problems, such as atrial baffle leak repair, direct surgical cryoablation between identified anatomic barriers can be performed successfully with minimal prolongation of the surgical repair, in contrast to lengthy fluoroscopy time. We have used this approach successfully in two patients.

Atrial Re-Entry Tachycardia in Fontan Patients

Catheter ablation of atrial re-entry tachycardia following surgical repair of congenital heart disease has acute success rates of 30–80% [68,69], with short-term recurrence rates for single-ventricle patients greater than 50% [70]. The catheter approach is more likely to fail in hearts with residual hemodynamic problems and markedly thickened atria [71]. The Fontan population is particularly problematic because significant atrial arrhythmias occur in at least 50% of patients during long-term follow-up [62,63] and because of limited success of the catheter approach with high recurrence of tachycardia [70,72]. Factors contributing to the disappointing results of the catheter approach include chronic atrial hypertension and dilation, distorted anatomy, multiple re-entrant circuits, restricted catheter access, particularly following lateral tunnel-type repairs, and the inability to deliver ablation lesions of sufficient depth to create a line of block. The ability to perform three-dimensional mapping of the multiple re-entrant circuits and to track the continuity of the ablation lines of block [73–75], coupled with newer types of energy delivery enabling deeper lesions, may improve the results of catheter ablation in patients with lateral tunnel type repairs [76].

Most atriopulmonary Fontan patients with disabling atrial arrhythmias have significant hemodynamic abnormalities, including obstruction of the right atrium-to-pulmonary artery connection, pulmonary venous obstruction, and massively dilated right atria with sluggish venous flow, predisposing to atrial thrombosis [63]. In addition, in some patients recurrent atrial re-entry tachycardia may progress to atrial fibrillation, which is not amenable to catheter ablation in this population. The loss of atrial contractility is particularly debilitating in patients with single-ventricle physiology. We and clinicians in other centers initially attempted to treat the disabling arrhythmias with surgical revision of the Fontan anastomosis, without direct intervention for the arrhythmia substrate [36,77–83]. This approach resulted in improved hemodynamics but almost uniform recurrence of atrial tachycardia [36,77–83].

The association of hemodynamic abnormalities and recurrent tachycardia following surgical repair led us to combine a surgical approach to arrhythmia therapy with revision of the Fontan hemodynamics in postoperative Fontan patients with refractory atrial tachycardia [36,39,40]. We have now performed 127 Fontan revisions in combination with arrhythmia surgery over the last 15 years. Patients with atrial macro re-entry tachycardia undergo a modified right atrial maze procedure (Figure 41.6) [59], while patients with atrial fibrillation undergo the modified right atrial maze in addition to a left atrial Cox-maze III procedure. The modified right atrial maze is designed to interrupt critical areas of re-entry specific to the Fontan patient which are: the atriotomy scar, the rim of the atrial septal defect and the lateral right atrial wall, the right atrial isthmus, and the prior atriopulmonary connection. Patients with atrial fibrillation undergo the Cox-maze III procedure involving the right and left atria (Figure 41.7) [59].

Maze Surgical Technique
The modified right atrial maze procedure and the modified Cox-maze III procedure were developed to repair re-entrant

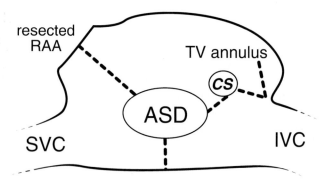

Figure 41.6 Modified right atrial maze procedure for atrial re-entry tachycardia. Large section of anterior right atrial wall is resected, including incision from SVC to IVC. Cryoablation lesions are indicated by dotted lines. (ASD, atrial septal defect; CS, coronary sinus; IVC, inferior vena cava; RAA, right atrial appendage; SVC, superior vena cava; TV, tricuspid valve.) (Reproduced with permission from Deal et al. [59].)

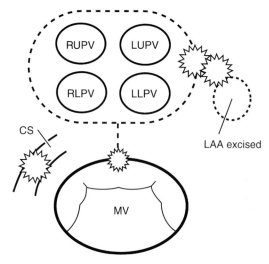

Figure 41.7 Left atrial incisions and cryoablation lesions of Cox-maze III procedure for atrial fibrillation. Incisions are indicated by dotted lines, cryoablation lesions by star. (LAA, left atrial appendage; LLPV, left lower pulmonary vein; LUPV, left upper pulmonary vein; MV, mitral valve; RLPV, right lower pulmonary vein; RUPV, right upper pulmonary vein.) (Reproduced with permission from Deal et al. [59].)

atrial circuits that tend to be multiple in patients with varying anatomy and complex congenital heart disease (Plate 41.4, see plate section opposite p. 594; Figures 41.8–41.12) [8,37,38,41,84,85]. Plate 41.4, see plate section opposite p. 594, demonstrates the possible lines of ablation that can be used to treat macro re-entrant atrial tachycardia in the presence of various atrial anomalies [37,41]. These include juxtaposition of the atrial appendages, total anomalous pulmonary venous connection, separate atrial entry of the hepatic veins, persistent left superior vena cava, and absence of the coronary sinus. The most common anatomic variances of single ventricle that require adaptation of the right-sided maze procedure are tricuspid atresia, mitral atresia, and common atrioventricular valve. Figures 41.8, 41.9, and 41.10 show the cryoablation lesions that are applied to areas of slow conduction in these patients [85]. In addition, the Cox-maze III procedure treats atrial fibrillation and has been modified for patients with single ventricle, as noted in Figures 41.11 and 41.12 [37,84,85].

Conduct of Fontan Conversion

Three basic types of existing first time anatomic connections undergoing revision are atrial compartmentalization with right atrium-to-pulmonary artery anastomosis, classic right Glenn operation and an atrium-to-left pulmonary artery anastomosis, and a total cavopulmonary artery reconstruction.

At the time of Fontan conversion, or any re-do congenital heart operation, adhesions from previous operations, dilated right atria, long-standing abnormal physiology of the atriopulmonary circuit, and right ventricular-to-pulmonary artery conduit or anterior aorta all contribute to the difficulty of sternal re-entry [37]. In rare cases, the femoral vessels can be dissected before the resternotomy for rapid cannulation and institution of cardiopulmonary bypass when there is high risk for cavitary entry. Early identification of the aorta and atrium is achieved so that rapid institution of cardiopulmonary bypass can be accomplished in the event of unwanted mishaps during dissection. To avoid injury to the phrenic nerves the dissection plane should remain medial to the pericardium and entry into the cardiac chambers is to be avoided to reduce the risk of paradoxical air embolus occurring through residual

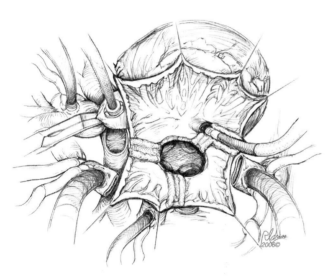

Figure 41.8 Atrial view of a patient with tricuspid atresia who had an atriopulmonary Fontan operation after aortic cross-clamping and cardioplegic arrest. The inferior and superior venae cavae have been transected, the atrial wall excision has been performed, and the atrial septal patch has been removed. No measures are taken to preserve the sinoatrial node, which is nonfunctional in a significant number of patients. Cryoablation lesions are placed in four areas to complete the modified right-sided maze procedure. The first two cryoablation lesions are standard for all anatomic substrates and are performed by connecting (1) the superior portion of the atrial septal ridge with the incised area of the right atrial appendage and (2) the posterior portion of the atrial septal ridge with the posterior cut edge of the atrial wall, which extends through the crista terminalis. The next part is the isthmus ablation. These lines of block are dependent on the anatomic substrate. In patients with tricuspid atresia, as noted here, the cryoablation lesion is placed to connect (3) the posteroinferior portion of the coronary sinus os with the transected inferior vena cava os. The last lesion (4) connects the coronary sinus os with the inferior edge of the atrial septal defect. (Reproduced with permission from Mavroudis *et al.* [85].)

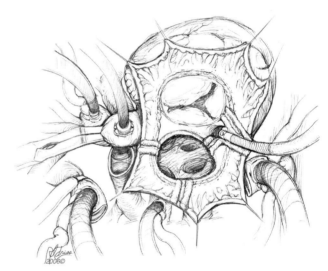

Figure 41.9 This drawing demonstrates the modified right-sided maze procedure in a patient with double-outlet right ventricle and mitral atresia. As noted in Figure 41.8, the two standard cryoablation lesions connecting the rim of the atrial septal defect with (1) the incised area of the right atrial appendage and (2) the posterior cut edge of the atrial wall, respectively, are shown. The isthmus block is accomplished by creating cryoablation lesions (3) to connect the posteroinferior portion of the coronary sinus os with the transected inferior vena cava os, and (4) to connect the tricuspid valve annulus with the transected inferior vena cava os. These isthmus block lesions are usually placed across the ridge of the resected atrial compartmentalization patch. An additional lesion (5) connects the coronary sinus os with the inferior edge of the atrial septal defect. (Reproduced with permission from Mavroudis *et al.* [85].)

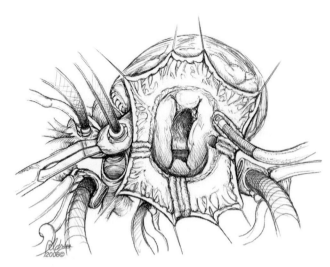

Figure 41.10 This drawing demonstrates the modified right-sided maze procedure in a patient with single-ventricle and unbalanced atrioventricular canal. As noted in Figure 41.8, the two standard cryoablation lesions connecting the rim of the atrial septal defect with (1) the incised area of the right atrial appendage and (2) the posterior cut edge of the atrial wall, respectively, are shown. The isthmus block is accomplished by creating cryoablation lesions (3) to connect the posteroinferior portion of the coronary sinus os with the transected inferior vena cava os and (4) to connect the common atrioventricular valve annulus with the transected inferior vena cava os. These isthmus block lesions are usually placed across the ridge of the resected atrial compartmentalization patch. The lesion connecting the coronary sinus os with the atrial septal defect is not performed because the anatomic ridge is not usually absent. (Reproduced with permission from Mavroudis et al. [85].)

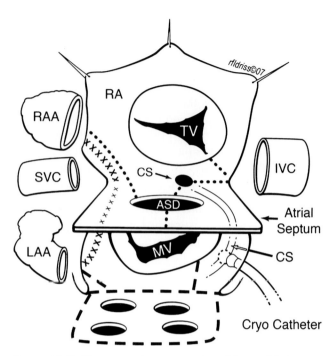

Figure 41.11 Diagrammatic representation of the modified right-sided maze procedure for right atrial re-entry tachycardia (dotted lines) and the left atrial Cox-maze procedure (dashed lines) for atrial fibrillation and left atrial re-entry tachycardia. Additional cryoablation lines are: (1) coronary sinus (CS) to atrial septal defect (ASD) for modified right-sided maze procedure, and (2) base of the right atrial appendage (RAA) to the base of the left atrial appendage (LAA) across the domes of the right and left atria for the left atrial Cox-maze procedure. The addition of the coronary sinus-to-atrial septal defect lesion did not change what we call the modified right-sided maze procedure; however, the addition of the right atrial appendage-to-left atrial appendage lesion caused us to change the name of the left-sided operation to left atrial Cox-maze procedure which infers that we use this same operation for both left atrial re-entry tachycardia and atrial fibrillation. (ASD, atrial septal defect; AVN, atrioventricular node; CS, coronary sinus; FO, foramen ovale; HV, hepatic vein; IVC, inferior vena cava; LAA, left atrial appendage; LSVC, left superior vena cava; MV, mitral valve; PV, pulmonary valve; RA, right atrium; RAA, right atrial appendage; RSVC, right superior vena cava; SVC, superior vena cava; TAPVR, total anomalous pulmonary venous return; TV, tricuspid valve.) (Reproduced with permission from Mavroudis et al. [37,84].)

intracardiac shunts. Careful preoperative planning and extreme caution during the resternotomy should insure a safe outcome for the patient [86].

Once the sternum is opened we proceed to aortic and direct vena cava cannulation using right-angled cannulas inserted high in the superior vena cava and straight cannulas in the inferior vena cava [37]. After the commencement of cardiopulmonary bypass the inferior vena cava is transected and anastomosed to a 24 mm Gore-Tex (W.L. Gore & Associates, Flagstaff, AZ) tube graft. A vent is placed in the right superior pulmonary vein, the aorta is cross-clamped, and cold blood cardioplegia is delivered. With the heart arrested, an atrial septectomy and resection of the right atrial appendage are performed. Linear cryoablation lesions for the right-sided maze procedure are placed with a Surgifrost device (CryoCath Inc., Kirkland, Quebec, Canada) applied at −160°C for 1 minute. The lesions extend from the base of the right atrial appendage to the cut edge of the atrial septal defect, across the crista terminalis from the cut edge of the atrium to the atrial

septal defect, and from the transected inferior vena cava to the coronary sinus. In addition, if a tricuspid valvar orifice is present, a lesion is created from the inferior vena cava to the annulus of the tricuspid valve. A lesion is placed to prevent macro re-entrant circuits extending from the coronary sinus to the edge of the atrial septal defect. In patients with atrial fibrillation, the Cox-maze III procedure is performed. The left atrial appendage is excised and an encircling pulmonary venous isolation is performed using

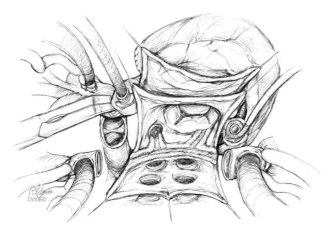

Figure 41.12 Left atrial view of a univentricular heart that shows the standard incisions, excisions, and cryoablation lesions which, when combined with the right atrial component, complete the Cox-maze III procedure. The incisions include a partial encircling pulmonary vein isolation and a left atrial appendage resection. Standard cryoablation lesions (−60 °C for 60 seconds) are placed to complete the pulmonary vein isolation, to create a cryoablation lesion from the isolated pulmonary veins toward the posterior mitral (P3 or medial mitral scallop) or tricuspid valve annulus, and to extend the pulmonary vein isolation to the cut edge of left atrial appendage base. A cryoablation lesion is placed on the coronary sinus (−60 °C for 120 seconds). (Reproduced with permission from Mavroudis *et al.* [85].)

cryoablation and/or incisional techniques. A cryoablation lesion is placed from the cut portion of the excised left atrial appendage to the confluence of the pulmonary veins. An additional lesion is placed from the encircling atriotomy lesion to the annulus of the mitral valve, directing it at the inferomedial scallop. A circular lesion, created for 2 minutes, is placed on the epicardial surface of the coronary sinus directly opposite the endocardial lesion involving the mitral valve. At the conclusion of the Cox-maze III procedure, the right atrium is closed with running polypropylene, the heart de-aired, and the cross-clamp removed. This sequence can be altered in the event that other left-sided lesions require surgical repair.

For patients with atriopulmonary anastomoses, a standard total cavopulmonary artery connection is accomplished using a lateral tunnel or an extracardiac technique [87–90]. Pulmonary artery reconstruction, when necessary, is performed at that time. In patients with a prior right Glenn procedure and an atrium-to-left pulmonary artery anastomosis, more creative pulmonary artery reconstructions are required. Left-sided (systemic circulation) procedures are performed under cardioplegic arrest; they include prosthetic atrial patch resection, valvar reconstructions, and completion of left atrial cryoablative lesions when needed.

After atriorrhaphy and removal of the aortic cross-clamp, total cavopulmonary connection is then completed, using a polytetrafluoroethylene conduit for the inferior vena cava connection to the pulmonary artery. Earlier in our experience, transmural atrial wires were implanted using the technique reported by Hoyer and associates [91,92]. Presently the epicardial approach is used for the atrial pacemaker leads. Initially, an atrial antitachycardia pacemaker was used. With subsequent use of the more extensive modified right atrial maze procedure, tachycardia recurrence is rare, and an atrial rate-responsive pacemaker is preferred. Separation from cardiopulmonary bypass is followed by transesophageal echocardiographic assessment.

Pacemaker Implantation

Achievement of acceptable pacing thresholds in the atrium may be challenging because of the extensive resection, reconstruction, and ablative lesions [37,85]. Typically, epicardial bipolar steroid eluting leads are placed on the right atrium near the atrioventricular groove anterior to the atriotomy. The technique of lead implantation is illustrated in Figures 41.13 and 41.14 [93]. It is important to find a portion of atrium relatively free of adhesions. In difficult situations, these leads can be placed on the dome of the left atrium or at the base of the left atrial appendage. Device selection has evolved over the years to the current use of epicardial dual chamber antitachycardia pacing systems. Ventricular leads are placed on the ventricular diaphragmatic surface or the anterior ventricular wall according to optimal threshold measurements. Placement of ventricular leads will minimize the effects of atrial lead far field R wave sensing, and will provide the capability of dual-chamber pacing should atrioventricular block develop with time. For the ventricular lead we have tried to use the steroid eluting bipolar epicardial leads, but when there is a large amount of scar tissue or fat on the ventricle we have used two screw-in leads attached in a "Y" configuration for bipolar sensing. Multisite ventricular pacing has been used in the setting of marked QRS prolongation to achieve ventricular synchrony and improved cardiac function [84,85]. In the rare setting of prior cardiac arrest because of ventricular arrhythmia, implantation of epicardial defibrillator patches or subcutaneous coils has been performed.

Anatomic and Electrophysiologic Variations of Fontan Conversion

Takedown of Right Atrial-to-Right Ventricular Bjork Modification

In the setting of surgical conversion of a Bjork–Fontan modification to a total cavopulmonary artery connection, the dilemma arises of what to do with the right ventricle [85]. Disconnecting the main pulmonary artery and leaving the right ventricle, however small, without an egress of

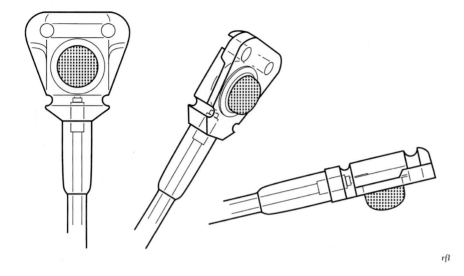

Figure 41.13 Steroid eluting lead. Medtronics model #4965. The round protruding portion is the porous-tipped electrode platinized with platinum black and coated with dexamethasone. At the proximal portion of the lead there is a groove for the retaining suture. At the distal portion of the lead there are two holes for the other retaining suture to pass through. (Reproduced with permission from Dodge-Khatami *et al.* [93].)

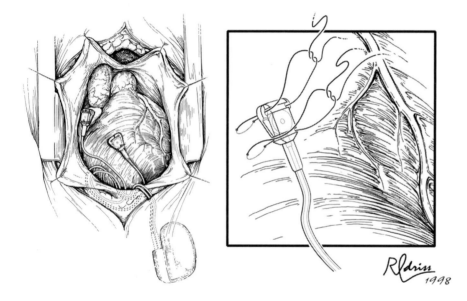

Figure 41.14 Steroid eluting lead is directly affixed to the epicardium as illustrated with two 5-0 Prolene sutures. Illustration shows dual chamber pacing leads as placed through a full sternotomy in a patient who also underwent intracardiac surgery. (Reproduced with permission from Dodge-Khatami *et al.* [93].)

blood flow has the potential problems of right ventricular dilatation and leftward interventricular septal deviation caused by accumulation of thebesian blood flow. We have performed Fontan conversion with arrhythmia surgery on 14 patients (14/109; 12.8%) with tricuspid atresia (n = 13) and unbalanced atrioventricular canal (n = 1) who had a previous right atrial to right ventricular Bjork-Fontan connection with (Figure 41.15; n = 2) [85] and without (Figure 41.16; n = 12) [85] an interposition bioprosthetic valve [85]. The distinct surgical considerations in this setting are: 1) takedown of the Bjork-Fontan anastomosis, and 2) management of the right ventricle. Most of the patients without the bioprosthetic valve interposition graft had a communication that was formed by a posterior reversed right atrial flap and an anterior prosthetic patch that formed the right

atrial to right ventricular connection. Takedown of these connections involves a careful and extensive dissection of the right atrioventricular grove to facilitate right atrial appendage amputation, right atrial wall reduction, epicardial pacemaker lead placement, and adequate right ventricular wall patch closure. The dissection of the right atrioventricular groove is commenced near the ascending aorta where an undissected plane is readily achieved (Figures 41.17, 41.18) [85]. The dissection is continued as far as possible toward the posteroseptal area as long as the dissection plane safely allows (Figure 41.19) [85]. Care must be taken not to enter the right coronary artery, which occurred in two patients in this series (1.8%). Because the injury was caused by electrocautery dissection in one, cardioplegic arrest and Gore-Tex patch (W.L. Gore & Associates,

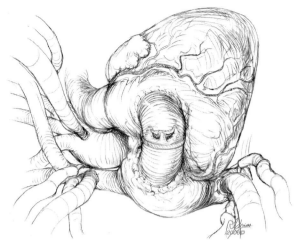

Figure 41.15 Global view of a Bjork-Fontan modification illustrating a right atrial to right ventricular valved connection using a prosthetic graft roof. The patient is undergoing aorto-bicaval cannulation for Fontan conversion and arrhythmia surgery. (Reproduced with permission from Mavroudis *et al.* [85].)

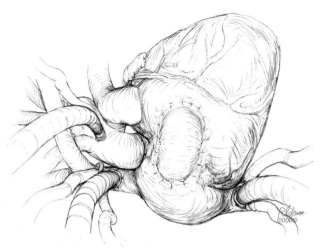

Figure 41.16 Global view of a Bjork-Fontan modification illustrating a right atrial to right ventricular nonvalved connection using a prosthetic graft roof. The patient is undergoing aorto-bicaval cannulation for Fontan conversion and arrhythmia surgery. (Reproduced with permission from Mavroudis *et al.* [85].)

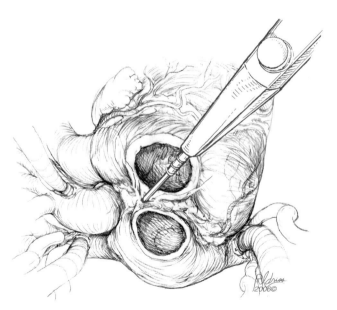

Figure 41.17 Artist's depiction of electrocautery dissection at the atrioventricular groove commencing at the base of the aorta with extension to the right ventricular free wall. Care is taken to perform this dissection with a low electrocautery setting to avoid unwanted injury to the right coronary artery. (Reproduced with permission from Mavroudis *et al.* [85].)

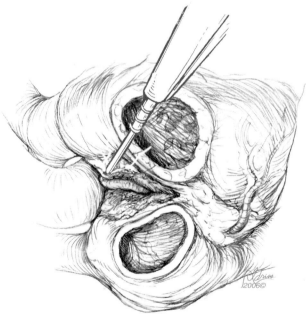

Figure 41.18 The atrioventricular dissection plane is developed with visualization of the proximal right coronary artery. These landmarks are used to complete the rest of the dissection. (Reproduced with permission from Mavroudis *et al.* [85].)

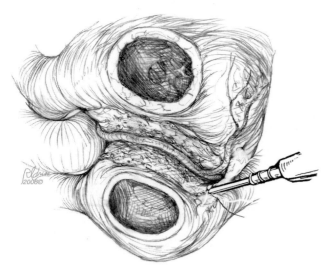

Figure 41.19 Artist's depiction of completed electrocautery dissection of the entire atrioventricular groove. The amount of atrium freed from this maneuver allows for a larger atrial reduction and provides unscarred atrial tissue for the atrial pacemaker leads that are placed at the end of the Fontan conversion. (Reproduced with permission from Mavroudis et al. [85].)

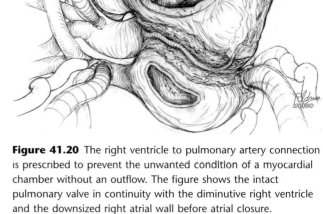

Figure 41.20 The right ventricle to pulmonary artery connection is prescribed to prevent the unwanted condition of a myocardial chamber without an outflow. The figure shows the intact pulmonary valve in continuity with the diminutive right ventricle and the downsized right atrial wall before atrial closure. (Reproduced with permission from Mavroudis et al. [85].)

Flagstaff, AZ) arterioplasty were performed without sequelae. The other injury was caused by sharp dissection and was repaired with cardioplegic arrest and interrupted suture technique without sequelae. Our approach to the remaining right ventricle is to preserve the right ventricular to main pulmonary artery connection to allow easy egress of blood into the pulmonary arteries (Figures 41.20, 41.21) [85]. We have found that the developed right ventricular pressure is low under these circumstances because of decreased right ventricular preload and does not affect the nonpulsatile blood flow established by the extracardiac total cavopulmonary connection (TCPC). Figure 41.22 shows a right ventricular patch and right atrial closure in association with the extracardiac total cavopulmonary connection [85]. The extensive atrioventricular groove dissection has aided the right atrial wall reduction and allowed for unscarred atrial wall for optimal epicardial pacemaker lead placement.

Takedown of Atrioventricular Valve Isolation Patch for Right-Sided Maze Procedure

In the developing era of Fontan procedures for complex diagnoses such as double-inlet ventricles, criss-cross hearts, and straddling atrioventricular valves, the smaller right-sided atrioventricular valve was oftentimes isolated with a patch when the left-sided atrioventricular valve was large enough and functional [37,85]. Patching of this valve accomplished separation of the circulations by performing an atriopulmonary connection together with an atrial septal

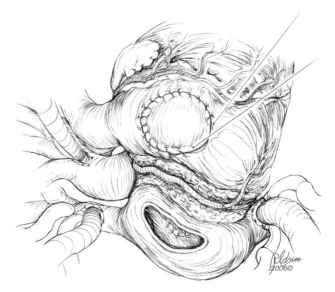

Figure 41.21 The diminutive right ventricular free wall is closed with a Gore-Tex patch allowing free egress of right ventricular blood (largely thebesian flow) to the main pulmonary artery. (Reproduced with permission from Mavroudis et al. [85].)

defect closure. The important anatomic and electrophysiologic considerations relate to the distance of the patch to the annulus and the partitioning of the coronary sinus. Oftentimes, the isolation was performed to leave the coronary sinus on the ventricular side to avoid complete heart block (Figure 41.23), which means that the right-sided

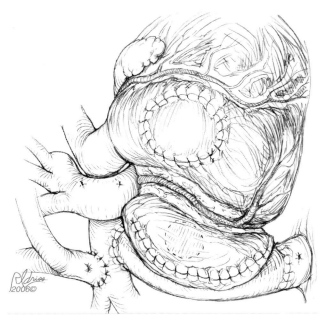

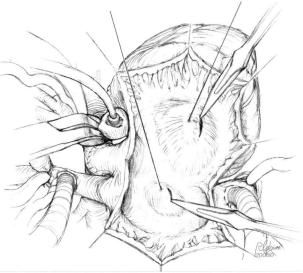

Figure 41.24 The isolation patch is sharply removed to uncover the tricuspid valve and the coronary sinus to perform the right-sided maze procedure. The atrial septal defect patch is also being removed. (Reproduced with permission from Mavroudis *et al.* [85].)

Figure 41.22 The completed extracardiac connections are shown. Right atrial wall reduction and closure is noted by the long atrial suture line. Right ventricular to main pulmonary artery continuity is maintained by a right ventricular patch, thus insuring outflow of thebesian venous flow and avoidance of right ventricular dilatation. (Reproduced with permission from Mavroudis *et al.* [85].)

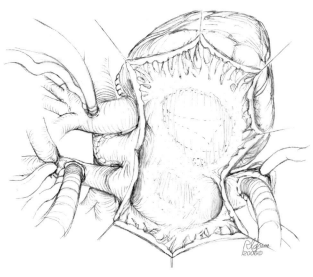

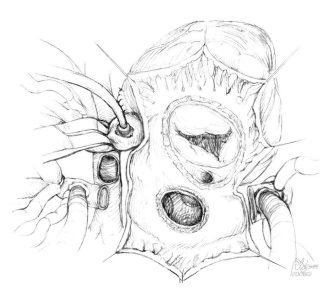

Figure 41.25 Right atrial view showing the results of isolation patch removal and atrial septal defect creation. The anatomic landmarks for application of the cryoablation lesions are now manifest. (Reproduced with permission from Mavroudis *et al.* [85].)

Figure 41.23 Right atrial view of a patient with double-inlet ventricle who had an atriopulmonary Fontan with tricuspid valve isolation and atrial septal defect closure. (Reproduced with permission from Mavroudis *et al.* [85].)

arrhythmia circuit might be partitioned to the pulmonary venous atrium. Under these circumstances, the right-sided maze cannot be safely performed because the traditional landmarks, namely the coronary sinus and the tricuspid valve, are not exposed. Therefore, the patch must be

removed to accomplish the cryoablation procedure. Figure 41.24 shows the technique of tricuspid valve and atrial septal patch removal, respectively [85]. Figure 41.25 depicts the dissection plane associated with tricuspid valve patch removal. The cryoablation lesions can now be performed with adequate landmark identification which will insure transmural cryoablation (Figure 41.26) [85]. This part of the operation would have been in question if the cryoablation

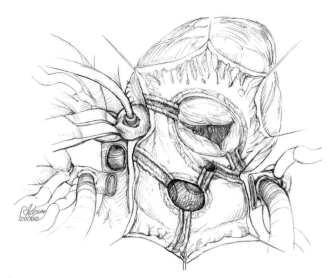

Figure 41.26 The cryoablation lesions are shown after proper identification of the tricuspid valve annulus and coronary sinus. The cryoablation lesion from the base of the right atrial appendage to the anterior tricuspid annulus is optional. (Reproduced with permission from Mavroudis *et al.* [85].)

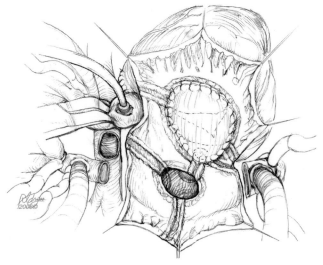

Figure 41.27 Right atrial view of Gore-Tex tricuspid valve isolation after cryoablation. The suture line for attachment is placed in the valve tissue near the annulus to avoid injury to the atrioventricular node. (Reproduced with permission from Mavroudis *et al.* [85].)

lesions were made on top of the prosthetic patch material. If the tricuspid valve is competent by bulb syringe testing, one can elect to allow the valve to function normally. If there is any question of valve competency or if there was antecedent valve dysfunction or injury, the valve can be isolated again with a Gore-Tex patch anchored to the leaflets of the tricuspid valve near the annulus (Figure 41.27) [85].

Right Atrial Cannulation in the Presence of a Right Atrial Clot

Approximately 5% of patients undergoing atriopulmonary to total cavopulmonary artery Fontan conversion can have right atrial clots, sometimes as a consequence of multiple transcatheter radiofrequency ablation attempts [94]. Fontan conversion in the setting of right atrial thrombus is fraught with hazards because of compromised cardiac output during sternotomy and dissection, the risk of clot dislodgement with cannulation, and the potential for venous catheter occlusion [85]. Preoperative evaluation using magnetic resonance imaging or computerized tomography to assess clot size and location can be complemented by epicardial echocardiography to guide safe atrial cannulation. Oftentimes, it is preferable to perform aorto-right atrial bypass to establish adequate cardiopulmonary bypass and improved perfusion while the dissection is completed which can lead to bicaval cannulation. During this time it is important to place the single atrial catheter away from the clot as shown in Figure 41.28 [85].

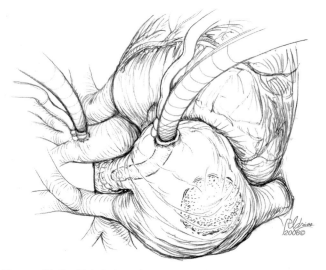

Figure 41.28 Global view of aorto-uniatrial cardiopulmonary bypass with the venous catheter placed away from the clot in the inferior portion of the right atrium where it was identified by epicardial echocardiography. Oftentimes, when the right atrium is large, single atrial cannulation for cardiopulmonary bypass can help with the completion of the dissection without causing hemodynamic instability. This can then be followed by conversion to bicaval cannulation. (Reproduced with permission from Mavroudis *et al.* [85].)

Distended Left Superior Vena Cava Causing Left Pulmonary Vein Stenosis

A distended left superior vena cava without circulatory egress may result in significant left pulmonary vein stenosis and compromise the Fontan circulation [85]. We have recognized and addressed this problem in two patients: one was caused by congenital orifice atresia in the right atrium and ill advised previous surgical ligation at the innominate vein connection, and the second was caused by coronary sinus occlusion because of lengthy radiofrequency catheter ablation. Both of these conditions resulted in an enlarging cardiac chamber caused by blood accumulation without egress anterior to the course of the left pulmonary veins, producing stenosis (Figure 41.29) [85]. During Fontan conversion and arrhythmia surgery, the coronary sinus was unroofed (Figure 41.30) in one patient and occlusive fibrous tissue/thrombus was resected in the other, relieving the pathway obstructions [85].

Discontinuous Pulmonary Arteries

Modification of the extracardiac Fontan may be used to convert patients with discontinuous pulmonary arteries resulting from the combination of a right classic Glenn procedure and a right atrial to left pulmonary artery connection [37]. Aortic homografts have a natural favorable curve to accomplish an end-to-end anastomosis between the distal homograft and left pulmonary artery, a side-to-side anastomosis between the homograft and the classic Glenn, and an end-to-end anastomosis between the proximal homograft and the inferior vena cava. Recognition of the possible need for future cardiac transplantation led us to modify our reconstructive procedures to avoid the use of allograft material, which has been shown to increase panel reactive antibody (PRA) levels and interfere with optimal immunosuppression. We now favor polytetrafluoroethylene grafts for reconstruction of discontinuous pulmonary arteries (Figure 41.31) [37,85].

Right Ventricular Hypertension and Tricuspid Regurgitation after Atriopulmonary Fontan for Pulmonary Atresia and Intact Ventricular Septum

In the setting of pulmonary atresia and intact ventricular septum, either the right ventricular to pulmonary artery connection is atretic or has been disconnected [37,85]. We have had experience with two patients with pulmonary atresia and intact ventricular septum who were treated with an atriopulmonary Fontan procedure and main pulmonary artery disconnection. Over the years, the right ventricle enlarged, became hypertrophied, and developed suprasystemic right ventricular pressure, resulting in right atrial hypertension and dilatation because of the significant tricuspid regurgitation. An extracardiac total cavopulmonary connection without addressing the tricuspid valve would increase the resultant common left atrial pressure and cause circulatory compromise. After performing the modified right-sided maze procedure, we isolated the tricuspid valve

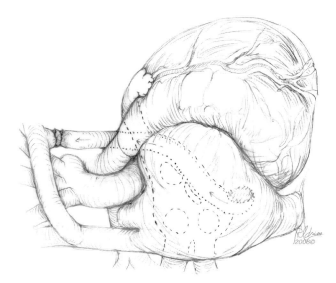

Figure 41.29 Drawing of a patient with double-inlet left ventricle, bulboventricular foramen, and L-transposition of the great arteries with bilateral superior venae cavae. The patient underwent ligation of the left superior vena cava in preparation for an eventual atriopulmonary Fontan without prior knowledge of orifice atresia of the coronary sinus. Lack of ebb flow from the coronary sinus caused sinus dilatation and obstruction of the left pulmonary veins as noted. (Reproduced with permission from Mavroudis *et al.* [85].)

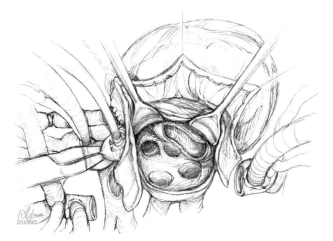

Figure 41.30 Left atrial view of a patient described in Figure 41.12. The large coronary sinus was unroofed, thereby establishing proper coronary sinus drainage and relief of the left pulmonary vein stenosis. (Reproduced with permission from Mavroudis *et al.* [85].)

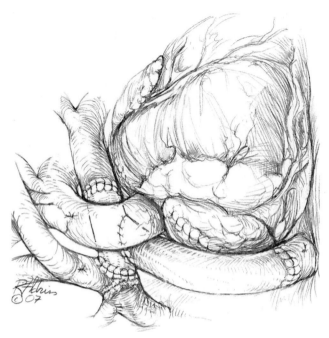

Figure 41.31 Artist's representation of a patient who previously had a classic Glenn shunt to the right pulmonary artery connection who had reconnection of the pulmonary arteries using a Gore-Tex interposition graft and an extracardial inferior vena cava to pulmonary artery connection. Homografts are not used to avoid stimulation of preformed antibodies which could complicate cardiac transplantation should it become necessary. (Reproduced with permission from Mavroudis *et al.* [85].)

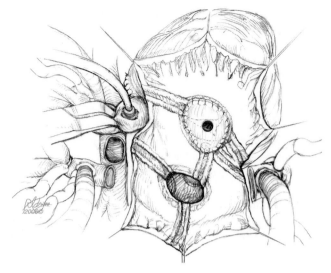

Figure 41.32 Right atrial view of a patient with pulmonary atresia and intact ventricular septum who had a prior atriopulmonary Fontan and presents now with arrhythmias and suprasystemic right ventricular pressure. The cryoablation lines are noted for the modified right-sided maze procedure as well as the fenestrated tricuspid valve isolation patch. The idea of the fenestration is to limit the inflow to the right ventricle in diastole, which will decrease the developed pressure of the right ventricle in systole. (Reproduced with permission from Mavroudis *et al.* [85].)

with a fenestrated (8 mm) Gore-Tex patch, which restricted blood flow into the right ventricle and decreased developed pressure by volume unloading the right ventricle. The fenestration also allowed blood egress into the common atrium during diastole (Figure 41.32) [85]. The developed right ventricular pressure in both patients postoperatively was significantly reduced and had no effect on the pulmonary venous atrial pressure.

Right Atrial Reduction in the Setting of a Systemic Right Ventricle Leading to Pulmonary Vein Stenosis

Right atrial wall reduction can be performed without hesitancy in patients with tricuspid atresia as long as the resultant anterior and posterior sides align without distortion [85]. The pulmonary veins are rarely compromised under these circumstances. However, complications can arise from overzealous right atrial wall reduction when the right ventricle is the dominant ventricle. Under these conditions, the right atrium must be large enough to direct blood flow from the pulmonary veins/left atrium, through the atrial septal defect, and then into the tricuspid valve. We have experience with one patient in whom an aggressive right atrial wall reduction (Figure 41.33) resulted in atrial septal defect compression and turbulence of pulmonary venous

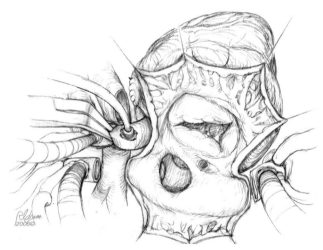

Figure 41.33 Global view of the right atrium and single right ventricle after an overzealous right atrial wall reduction was performed. (Reproduced with permission from Mavroudis *et al.* [85].)

flow into the right ventricle (Figure 41.34) noted by transesophageal echocardiography [85]. The distortion was immediately repaired by a large Gore-Tex patch that relieved the turbulence and obstruction (Figure 41.35) [85]. We experienced a second case where we suspected the same problem would occur not from overzealous resection, but because of limited atrial tissue following the removal of a prosthetic anterior patch of the atriopulmonary con-

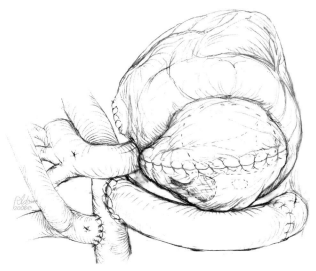

Figure 41.34 Global view of a completed extracardiac Fontan in a patient with a dominant right ventricle and tricuspid valve. The overzealous right atrial wall resection resulted in atrial septal compression and pulmonary venous obstruction to the right ventricle that was noted on transesophageal echocardiography. The compression of the atrial septum is noted within the right atrium. (Reproduced with permission from Mavroudis *et al.* [85].)

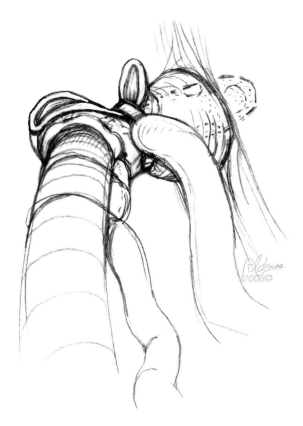

Figure 41.36 Artist's representation of a partially retracted transected cannulated inferior vena cava below the Rummel tourniquet. The end-to-end anastomosis between the extracardiac Gore-Tex tube and the inferior vena cava cannot be performed under these circumstances. (Reproduced with permission from Mavroudis *et al.* [85].)

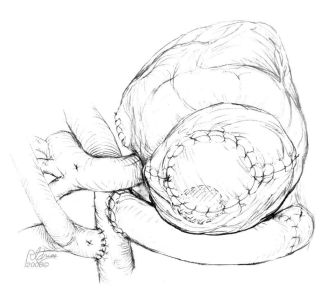

Figure 41.35 Global view of a Gore-Tex augmentation patch that was used to enlarge the right atrium that eliminated the atrial septal defect compression as noted within the right atrium. (Reproduced with permission from Mavroudis *et al.* [85].)

nection. We placed an augmenting Gore-Tex patch prophylactically during atrial closure with no pulmonary venous flow obstruction noted.

Unwanted Inferior Vena Cava Retraction During the Extracardiac Connection

Occasionally, the transected inferior vena cava orifice retracts inferiad to the caval tourniquet making the end-to-end anastomosis impossible to perform unless the tourniquet is released (Figure 41.36) [85]. This problem is easily solved by clamping the inferior vena cava cannula, releasing the tourniquet, establishing sucker bypass, and performing an open end-to-end anastomosis (Figure 41.37) [85]. Once the anastomosis is completed the inferior vena cava catheter can be purged of air, the tourniquet can be replaced, and venous drainage can be resumed (Figure 41.38) [85]. We have found that this complication can be largely avoided by staged vena cava transection and strategic placement of traction sutures during the anastomosis,

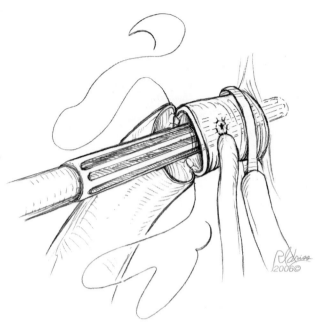

Figure 41.37 Artist's depiction of tourniquet removal, establishing of sucker bypass, and the end-to-end anastomosis in progress. (Reproduced with permission from Mavroudis *et al.* [85].)

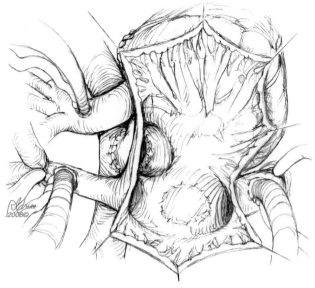

Figure 41.39 Right atrial view of a patient who underwent atriopulmonary Fontan by moving the atrial septum posteriorly which realigned the outflow of the right atrium to conform to the more posterior main pulmonary artery. This "dropped atrial septum" required a suture line in the left atrium which caused scarring and an area of slow conduction leading to atrial re-entry tachycardia. In addition, when this anastomosis was taken down, a significant moiety was created which required attention lest pulmonary venous obstruction be created. (Reproduced with permission from Mavroudis *et al.* [85].)

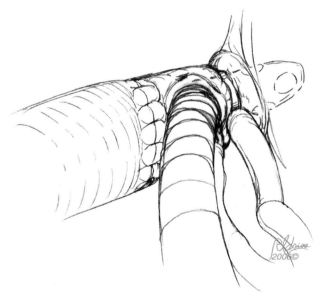

Figure 41.38 Artist's view of the completed inferior vena cava to Gore-Tex graft anastomosis, recannulation, and tourniquet application. (Reproduced with permission from Mavroudis *et al.* [85].)

which will prevent inferior vena cava retraction beyond the caval tourniquet.

Surgical Translocation of Atrial Septal Alignment

Some surgeons hypothesized that because the pulmonary artery was more posterior to the right atrium, aligning the pulmonary artery directly with a revised translocated atrial outflow into the pulmonary artery would optimize blood flow [85]. Resecting a portion of the superior atrial septum and anastomosing the confluence of pulmonary arteries to the dome of the right and left atrium was performed in a subset of patients. The separation of the circulations was accomplished by a synthetic septal patch that in effect dropped the atrial septum into the left atrial dome, thereby aligning the pulmonary artery with the newly formed systemic atrium (Figure 41.39) [85]. We call this the "dropped atrial septum" technique, which has important arrhythmia implications. Some of these patients will have left atrial re-entry tachycardia based on the suture lines in the dome of the left atrium. Arrhythmia surgery in this setting will require left atrial resection with cryoablation lesions delivered in the left atrium. Atrial reconstruction will require a

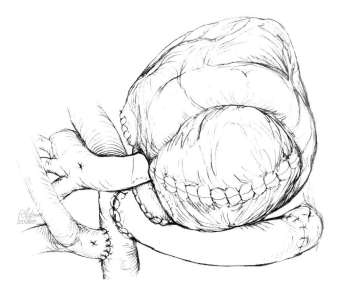

Figure 41.40 Global view of the corrected patient in Figure 41.39. A Gore-Tex patch was inserted in the dome of the left, now common, atrium to prevent pulmonary vein obstruction. (Reproduced with permission from Mavroudis *et al.* [85].)

Gore-Tex patch in the dome of the left atrium to prevent pulmonary vein stenosis (Figure 41.40) [85].

The Modified Right-Sided Maze Procedure for Various Single-Ventricle Pathology

Different types of modified right-sided maze procedures are performed based on the varying types of single-ventricle anatomy. The modified ablation lesions based on anatomy have been previously published [38]. Important variations include the presence of a right-sided atrioventricular valve, a common atrioventricular valve, and the absence of a coronary sinus associated with heterotaxy syndrome [85]. These conditions require modification of the right-sided maze procedure simply because the landmarks that determine the ablation lesions may or may not be present to interrupt the macro-re-entry circuits [59]. Figure 41.8 shows the cryoablation lesions that are used for tricuspid atresia patients with right atrial macro re-entry tachycardia [85]. Because there is no tricuspid valve, the standard lesion cannot be placed to connect the inferior vena cava os with the tricuspid valve. However, there are anatomic variants in which one can identify a "tricuspid valve dimple," which is thought to be a remnant of the tricuspid valve. It would seem intuitive to place the standard lesion from the inferior vena cava os to the tricuspid valve dimple. The difficulty with this action is that the atrioventricular node is in close proximity to this tricuspid valve dimple and therefore will likely cause heart block. We do not recommend placing this lesion for these reasons. Also noted in Figure 41.8 is a new lesion that con-

nects the coronary sinus os with the atrial septal defect [85]. The rationale for this lesion is to interrupt any macro re-entrant circuits that may traverse this area. The other two lesions are standard and have been described before [38]. Figure 41.9 shows the right-sided lesions used in patients who have a dominant right ventricle and tricuspid valve [85]. In the presence of a right-sided atrioventricular valve, all the standard lesions can be performed. Figure 41.10 shows the right-sided lesions used in patients with a common atrioventricular valve and a present coronary sinus [85]. Some of these patients have heterotaxy syndrome and therefore may have absence of the coronary sinus. Under these circumstances, the usual lesion from the coronary sinus os to the inferior vena cava os cannot be performed. There can be other circumstances in which the modified right-sided maze procedure will have to be changed to accommodate the anatomic findings. In general, anatomic areas between large orifices tend to be involved with slowing of the atrial electrical impulse, which is a substrate for a re-entry circuit to take place. These areas will require cryoablation as long as the atrioventricular node is not in danger of injury. Figure 41.12 shows the cryoablation lesions and surgical incisions/excisions necessary for the left-sided maze procedure [85]. When the right- and left-sided lesions are performed in concert, we call this the modified Cox-maze III procedure. The lesion from the confluence of pulmonary veins to the mitral valve must align with the lesion placed on the epicardial surface of the coronary sinus to avoid recurrent atrial tachycardia caused by conduction via fibers within the coronary sinus. Therefore, we have changed the location of the intracardiac lesion from the confluence of the pulmonary veins to the mitral valve posterior leaflet middle scallop (P2 location) to the confluence of the pulmonary veins to the mitral valve posterior leaflet medial scallop (P3 location). Using this approach we have had no patient who has presented with recurrent atrial fibrillation.

Patient Population

From December 1994 until April 2009, 132 patients have undergone conversion from an atriopulmonary to a total cavopulmonary artery extracardiac Fontan with concomitant arrhythmia surgery and pacemaker placement at our institutions. All patients underwent preoperative cardiac catheterization with hemodynamic assessment and angiography for anatomic definition. Most underwent preoperative intracardiac electrophysiologic mapping; patients with atrial fibrillation, atrial thrombus, or poor vascular access were omitted. In the first nine procedures in our series isthmus cryoablation was used for arrhythmia control. The next 123 consecutive cases had variations of the modified right atrial maze for macro re-entrant atrial tachycardia and the Cox-maze III procedure for atrial fibrillation and left macro re-entrant atrial tachycardia.

Results

There were three (3/132, 2.3%) early and 12 (12/132, 9.1%) late deaths. Seven patients (7/132, 5.3%) required cardiac transplantation after Fontan conversion with arrhythmia surgery. Two patients (1.5%) underwent re-exploration for postoperative bleeding, mediastinitis occurred in three patients (2.3%), and nine patients (6.8%) had acute renal failure. The mean duration of chest tube placement was 9.0 ± 4.8 days. The mean postoperative hospital stay was 14.0 ± 12.0 days. The Kaplan-Meier curve (Plate 41.5, see plate section opposite p. 594) shows freedom from death in 126 patients who underwent Fontan conversion with arrhythmia surgery from 1994–2009 [37].

Atrioventricular Nodal Re-Entry Tachycardia

Mechanism

Atrioventricular nodal re-entry tachycardia is a re-entrant circuit in the area between the atrioventricular node, coronary sinus, and inferior vena cava associated with unidirectional block in one direction and an area of slowed conduction in the other (Plate 41.6, see plate section opposite p. 594) [37,41]. Atrioventricular conduction encounters unidirectional block in the normal fast pathway fibers superior to the atrioventricular node. The electrical wave front is redirected toward the atrial isthmus (between the coronary sinus and tricuspid valve) and encounters the slow pathway fibers of the atrioventricular node. After the impulse exits the isthmus, conduction now re-enters the fast pathway, anteriorly and superiorly, and establishes the re-entrant circuit. Cryoablation of the inferior isthmus region interrupts the re-entrant circuit.

Ablation of Atrioventricular Nodal Re-Entry Tachycardia

The concept that the perinodal region could be modified in patients with AVNRT was found inadvertently during an unsuccessful attempt at atrioventricular nodal ablation, which preserved nodal function but abolished the nodal tachycardia [4]. Holman and associates [5,95] subsequently showed that discrete cryolesions near the atrioventricular node could interrupt the tachycardia circuit while preserving atrioventricular conduction. Further support of this idea came from Ross and associates [96], who separated the perinodal connections from the compact node by dissection instead of cryoablation with excellent results. Extensive catheter ablation experience has demonstrated that an anatomic approach to slow pathway modification effectively treats AVNRT. Lesions are delivered inferior and anterior to the os of the coronary sinus, with slow pullback from the tricuspid annulus toward the inferior vena cava.

Currently, either the cryoablation or radiofrequency technique for patients with AVNRT is used [97]. A linear lesion is placed from the posterior inferior rim of the coronary sinus os to the inferior vena cava. In the presence of a right-sided atrioventricular valve, a linear lesion from the valve to the posterior os of the coronary sinus is delivered. The approach in a beating nonworking heart using discrete cryolesions [98,99] around the coronary sinus is no longer used. Results of radiofrequency catheter modification of the atrioventricular node slow pathway in the region of the coronary sinus os indicate that it is not desirable to attain prolongation of the PR interval as previously performed. The surgical cryoablation modification of the atrioventricular node as described previously requires less than 3 minutes. In patients with prior Mustard or Senning procedures undergoing reoperation, we have elected to perform ablation of AVNRT directly intraoperatively and avoid the retrograde catheter approach to the pulmonary venous atrium.

Focal (Automatic) Atrial Tachycardia

Mechanism

Focal atrial tachycardia is a localized area of electrical impulse generation [37] which may be due to either discrete micro re-entry or an automatic focus. Either form of focal tachycardia results in tachycardia occurring, independently of normal sinus function, which is inhibited (Plate 41.7, see plate section opposite p. 594) [37,41]. Electrical impulse conduction is propagated over the body of the atria, which results in stimulation of the atrioventricular node and ventricles. Cryoablative therapy and resection is used to obliterate or isolate this localized discrete area.

Ablation of Focal/Automatic Atrial Tachycardia

Surgical treatment of tachycardia localized to the atria may involve resection or cryoablation of atrial tissue; wider areas of focal tachycardia may require isolation. Some authors had good results with simple cryoablation and excision of automatic foci when found [100–102]. Multiple ectopic foci arrhythmia recurrence led surgeons to apply more extensive techniques [103] such as pulmonary vein isolation, left atrial isolation [104], right atrial isolation (Figure 41.41) [105], and His bundle cryoablation with pacemaker insertion in difficult cases. Automatic atrial foci, often localized to the right atrial appendage, may be directly resected intraoperatively. We have successfully resected automatic atrial tachycardia sites from the right atrial appendage in a neonate undergoing a Norwood procedure for hypoplastic left heart syndrome and in an older child undergoing closure of a primum atrial septal defect. In addition, a teenager presenting with cardiogenic shock secondary to tachycardia was taken to the operating room emergently for placement of a mechanical assist device; a focal right atrial tachycardia originating in the right atrial appendage was identified and resected, resulting in sinus

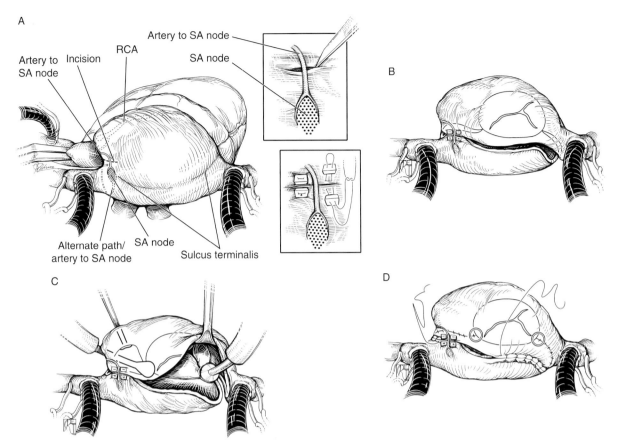

Figure 41.41 Right atrial isolation. **A**, The sinoatrial node (SAN) artery is dissected free from the atrial tissue 5 mm anterior to the crista terminalis. A 2-cm incision parallel to the crista terminalis is placed beneath the artery. **B**, The incision beneath the SAN artery is closed with a continuous nonabsorbable suture, and care is taken not to damage the artery. Small pledgets are used above and below the artery to reinforce the incision. The right atriotomy is then extended to a point anterior to the junction of the superior vena cava and the base of the right atrial appendage. **C**, The atriotomy is extended along the anterior limbus of the fossa ovalis to the anteromedial tricuspid valve annulus, just anterior to the membranous interatrial septum. **D**, Caudad extension of the right atriotomy around the posterior right atrial–inferior vena caval junction to the posterior–lateral tricuspid valve annulus. A cryolesion (−60 °C for 2 minutes) is placed at the end of the incision to ensure complete interruption of connecting atrial muscle fibers between the body of the right atrium and the remainder of the heart. The atriotomy is closed with a continuous 4-0 nonabsorbable suture. (Modified with permission from Harada *et al.* [105].)

rhythm. We avoided placement of an assist device in this patient, who was discharged within a week, and recovered normal ventricular function over a period of weeks. In general, refractory cases are rare and require an individualized treatment plan for accurate diagnosis and ablation.

Atrial Fibrillation

Mechanism

Atrial fibrillation is characterized by uncoordinated atrial activation with consequent deterioration of atrial mechanical function. On ECG, consistent P waves are replaced by rapid oscillations or fibrillatory waves that vary in amplitude, shape, and timing, associated with an irregular, frequently rapid ventricular response with variable atrioventricular conduction.

Ablation of Atrial Fibrillation

Atrial fibrillation typically occurs in markedly dilated left atria, usually with significant mitral regurgitation, either due to ventricular dysfunction or valve abnormalities. In adults with unoperated atrial septal defects, atrial flutter and fibrillation occurs in 14–22% of patients [106–108]. Atrial fibrillation will recur in a high percentage of patients following surgery [106–108] if direct arrhythmia intervention is not performed [109,110]. Performance of right atrial arrhythmia surgery is ineffective in preventing recurrence of atrial fibrillation. Therefore, careful evaluation of older patients undergoing atrial surgery is necessary to determine the presence of atrial fibrillation and to assess the need for left atrial arrhythmia surgery. As described previously, the Cox-maze III procedure is designed to eliminate atrial fibrillation while preserving intact atrioventricular nodal conduction and atrial contractility. This procedure prevents atrial fibrillation recurrence in over 90% of adult patients, often in association with mitral valve repair [111–114], atrial septal defect closure [109,110], or coronary artery bypass surgery [115]. We have incorporated successfully the Cox-maze III procedure into repair of complex congenital heart disease, such as the Fontan conversion, atrial septal defect closure, and mitral valve repair in a 4-year-old girl with cardiomyopathy. We have had no late recurrence of atrial fibrillation in our patient population, using no antiarrhythmic medications. Use of a linear cryoablation probe or radiofrequency catheter intraoperatively instead of making atrial incisions shortens surgical time considerably. Attempts to duplicate these results using the transvenous catheter approach at electrophysiologic study are the subject of intense effort. Pulmonary vein stenosis is an infrequent but serious complication of this technique.

Ventricular Tachycardia

Mechanism

Ventricular tachycardia is an abnormal ventricular rhythm with a rate greater than 120 bpm in adolescents or adults, or a rate greater than 150 bpm in children [37]. This arrhythmia arises from various locations in either the left or right ventricles, and is usually re-entrant in nature. As there is no specific localized origin of ventricular tachycardia, treatment with cryoablative lesions or endocardial/epicardial resection must be individualized to the patient.

Surgery for Ventricular Tachycardia

Patients with ventricular tachycardia refractory to medications and transvenous catheter ablation techniques as well as patients undergoing concomitant repair of structural heart disease are considered for intraoperative ablation of ventricular tachycardia.

Structurally Normal Hearts

Incessant life-threatening ventricular tachycardia in infancy is associated with ventricular hamartomas or histiocytosis [116–118]. Before the availability of intravenous amiodarone, such infants underwent surgical resection of the left ventricular endomyocardium with some success [116–118]. In older patients, usually adolescents, idiopathic ventricular tachycardia in the ostensibly normal heart typically arises from either the right ventricular outflow tract (left bundle branch block, normal to rightward QRS axis morphology) or the septal surface of the left ventricle (right bundle branch block, left axis morphology). Both forms of idiopathic ventricular tachycardia are amenable to catheter ablation techniques, with success rates of 70–80% [26,119–

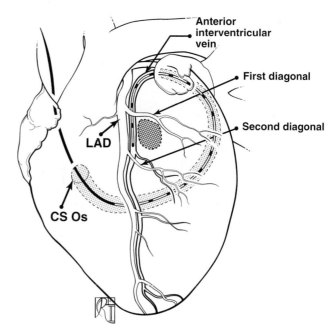

Figure 41.42 Ventricular tachycardia originating from epicardial surface of left ventricular outflow tract. Tachycardia could not be ablated successfully using endocardial catheter approach. Note proximity of tachycardia focus to left anterior descending (LAD) coronary artery. (CS, coronary sinus.) (Reproduced with permission from Deal *et al.* [59].)

121]. Rarely, ventricular tachycardia may originate from the epicardial surface of either the left or right ventricle, making the catheter ablation approach challenging.

Figure 41.42 illustrates the epicardial focus of ventricular tachycardia on the left ventricular outflow tract in a young boy with recurrent exertional syncope [59]. This rapid ventricular tachycardia was refractory to numerous medication combinations, and catheter ablations attempted at three institutions failed. Preoperative mapping using a small-diameter catheter in the anterior interventricular vein identified the epicardial origin on the high anterior left septal surface. Successful surgical cryoablation of the well circumscribed tachycardia focus was performed, using cardiopulmonary bypass to protect the left anterior descending artery. The patient has remained arrhythmia free without medication for over 14 years. Detailed preoperative and intraoperative mapping of the arrhythmia focus is essential to the successful performance of such procedures.

Structural Heart Disease

Patients with postoperative tetralogy of Fallot or double-outlet right ventricle are known to have late postoperative sustained ventricular tachycardia, with an incidence of 5–8% [30,122,123] and with a risk of late sudden death of 2–6% [124–126]. Risk factors for ventricular tachycardia include older age at initial repair, residual right ventricular hypertension, right ventricular outflow tract patch or aneurysm, significant pulmonary regurgitation, prolonged QRS duration over 180 msec on resting electrocardiogram, abnormal signal-averaged electrocardiogram, and longer duration of follow-up [30,122–126]. At least 15% of patients with repaired tetralogy of Fallot undergo reoperation for residual defects or late pulmonary valve regurgitation [127–129]. Because these patients are at increased risk for sustained ventricular tachycardia, they should undergo preoperative assessment for significant atrial and ventricular arrhythmias, with ambulatory electrocardiographic monitoring and exercise testing. Electrophysiologic studies are indicated for patients with symptoms of palpitations, syncope, cardiac arrest, sustained wide-QRS tachycardia, or QRS prolongation greater than 180 msec. Sustained ventricular tachycardia may be ablated preoperatively; should catheter ablation fail, direct endocardial resection and cryoablation may be performed intraoperatively. Physicians at our center and others [129–133] have performed surgical revision of residual hemodynamic abnormalities in the adult patient with tetralogy of Fallot at the same time as resection and cryoablation of the focus of ventricular tachycardia, sometimes eliminating the need for antiarrhythmic drugs or an implanted defibrillator. Careful preoperative and intraoperative mapping of tachycardia is necessary; common sites of arrhythmia origin are related to the ventriculotomy, outflow tract patch, and perimeter of the ventricular septal defect. Postoperative ventricular stimulation is necessary to determine efficacy, with defibrillator implantation performed if sustained ventricular tachycardia remains inducible. Successful surgical treatment of ventricular tachycardia in this setting ranges from 50–70% [37,123].

Rarely, patients with congenital heart disease may have sustained ventricular tachycardia before surgical repair. Two young patients with a membranous ventricular septal defect had recurrent ventricular tachycardia associated with syncope in one and dizziness in the other. During electrophysiologic study, the tachycardia was mapped to the anterior septal surface of the right ventricular outflow tract, opposite the jet of the ventricular shunt. Because surgical closure of the ventricular septal defect was necessary, catheter ablation was not performed. During surgery, large white plaque lesions were found, resected, and cryoablated. Ventricular tachycardia was not inducible during postoperative study in either patient.

Ventricular Tachycardia Associated with Ion Channelopathies

Mechanism

Ventricular tachycardia, either torsades des pointes due to long QT syndrome or catecholaminergic polymorphic ventricular tachycardia (CPVT) are inherited arrhythmogenic diseases due to ion channelopathies, typically due to sodium or potassium channel disorders (long QT syndrome); ryanodine receptors (RYR2) and calsequestrin (CASQ2) are identified causes of CPVT. Genetic testing is now commercially available and may identify the causative genes in up to 70% of patients currently. Tachycardia is characterized by episodic syncope that occurs during exercise or in association with an acute emotional response, startle, or during sleep in patients without structural cardiac abnormalities. Patients can undergo spontaneous recovery when these arrhythmias self-terminate or the arrhythmia may morph into ventricular fibrillation and sudden death. These forms of tachycardia may account for 10% of cases of sudden infant death syndrome and frequently present in the second decade of life. The mean age of onset of CPVT is between 7 and 9 years, although onset into the fourth decade of life has been reported [134–136]. Exercise stress testing or epinephrine infusion may reproduce the arrhythmia, with characteristic ECG features, which include an alternating 180 degree-QRS axis on a beat-to-beat basis, and an irregular polymorphic ventricular tachycardia without a stable QRS vector alternans. The two genes currently known to be associated with CPVT are RYR2 and CASQ2.

Medical and Surgical Therapeutic Options

Beta-blockers are the medical therapy of choice for most arrhythmias due to ion channel disorders. Implantable automatic internal cardio-defibrillators (AICD) have been used for primary or secondary prevention of cardiac arrest, or recurrent syncope. Left cardiac sympathetic denervation (LCSD) has been used to ablate the left thoracic sympathetic chain in order to reduce the surge of catecholamines due to sympathetic nervous system activation. Wilde and associates [137] have shown that LCSD proved to be effective in their three patients whose symptoms were not controlled by beta-blockade [137]. This surgical therapy can be considered for patients with intractable ventricular tachycardia in order to reduce the incidence of tachycardia episodes and limit the number of AICD shocks.

Prophylactic Arrhythmia Surgery

Initial concerns over the development of late arrhythmias following congenital heart disease focused on the risk of sudden death due to ventricular tachycardia in the tetralogy of Fallot population, occurring in 2–7% of patients. Over the last two decades, it has become clear that the risk of atrial tachycardia, while not typically fatal, occurs in a much higher percentage of patients following repair of congenital heart disease as their survival improves. Atrial tachycardia may result in syncope, congestive heart failure, atrial thrombi, thromboembolic events, and sudden death, and is the most common reason for hospitalization among older patients with repaired congenital heart disease. The incidence of late atrial tachycardia ranges from 15% in patients with prior atrial septal defect closures, over 30% in repaired tetralogy of Fallot or atrial switch repairs for transposition of the great arteries, and is highest (over 50%) among patients with atriopulmonary Fontan repairs and Ebstein anomaly of the tricuspid valve. Many of these patients will undergo repeat surgeries over time. It is clear that efforts to reduce the incidence of late atrial tachycardia will result in major improvements in quality of life in patients with congenital heart disease, and efforts to minimize the opportunity for tachycardia development either at the initial or redo surgery should become routine. As described above, surgical arrhythmia techniques in the right atrium can reduce the recurrence of atrial macro re-entrant tachycardia in over 90% of patients. Efforts to limit the development of tachycardia include alteration or limitation of atrial incisions, prophylactic ablation of identified inducible atrial re-entrant circuits, atrial maze procedures or atrioventricular node modification in patients with clinical arrhythmias, and earlier pacing strategies to avoid bradycardia-related tachycardia.

Advances in surgical techniques have improved survival in patients undergoing a Fontan type repair of complex single-ventricle anatomy, with surgical mortality now less than 7–10% [138]. Early postoperative tachycardia is a significant contributor to early postoperative death, and the incidence of late atrial arrhythmia in Fontan patients escalates at 7–10 years of follow-up [139–141]. Staging procedures such as the hemi-Fontan may increase the incidence of sinus node dysfunction [142,143]. Variations in the surgical technique have been made in an attempt to decrease the incidence of late arrhythmia. Although initial results with the total cavopulmonary connection appear favorable compared with the atriopulmonary connection [144–146], the incidence of arrhythmia with longer-term follow-up may be similar [147].

Results of arrhythmia studies in both the animal model [148,149] and Fontan patients [36,69,75] have identified several anatomic and surgical barriers or incisions, which are critical to the atrial macro re-entrant tachycardia circuit. Critical sites included the atriotomy incision, the inferior right atrial isthmus between the coronary sinus os and atrioventricular valve or groove, the rim of the atrial septal defect, the site of the atriopulmonary connection, and the crista terminalis [36,69,75,148–151]. Studies in the dog model with lateral tunnel suture lines showed that extending the atriotomy scar with an incision to the right atrioventricular groove prevented the induction of atrial flutter postoperatively [149]. Performing this incision at the time of initial lateral tunnel repair might reduce the incidence of re-entry around the free wall atriotomy incision, although this lesion may also be arrhythmogenic by creating an additional zone of slowed conduction. In patients large enough to accommodate an extracardiac conduit, this approach is used in an attempt to limit atrial incisions and

extensive suture lines [152]. In addition, because the re-entrant circuit involves the inferior isthmus, and preoperative studies may provoke atrial re-entry tachycardia in as many as 15% of patients [153], "prophylactic" cryoablation lesions can be made between the posterior rim of the coronary sinus and the inferior vena cava, and between the inferior vena cava and atrioventricular valve or groove in patients undergoing initial lateral tunnel cavopulmonary connections. Similarly, adult survivors of other forms of repaired congenital heart disease, such as tetralogy of Fallot and atrial septal defects, have a substantial incidence of late atrial tachycardia [64,106-108]. Should such patients undergo a repeat intracardiac repair, consideration should be given to surgical cryoablation of the inferior right atrial isthmus in an attempt to avoid episodes of typical atrial flutter. Karamlou and colleagues have shown that incorporation of atrial arrhythmia surgery into conduit revision surgery significantly reduces the incidence of late atrial tachycardia [154]. Adult patients undergoing surgical closure of atrial septal defects have a high incidence of atrial fibrillation, particularly if present before surgery [106–108]. Specific consideration should be given to the performance of the Cox-maze III procedure for atrial fibrillation at the time of atrial septal defect closure in older patients or those with a history of atrial tachycardia [108–110].

Finally, there is evidence that late postoperative bradycardia contributes to the milieu for the development of atrial tachycardia, providing a regular atrial rhythm significantly decreases the incidence of problematic atrial tachycardia [155]. In a large series of Fontan patients, pacemakers have been implanted in 7–10% of patients owing to sinus bradycardia or atrioventricular block. At present, there are no data showing that prophylactic maintenance of a regular atrial rhythm following initial surgeries will prevent or reduce the incidence of late atrial tachycardia in high-risk patient populations. Nonetheless, due to the difficulty of implanting pacemakers late after Fontan repairs, it is our policy to implant epicardial atrial (and often ventricular) bipolar pacing leads at the time of initial Fontan repair (or at the time of ventricular septal defect closure in patients with congenitally corrected transposition of the great arteries) and implantation of a pacemaker generator if there is preexisting or operative evidence of sinus node dysfunction or chronotropic incompetence. Should bradycardia develop postoperatively, the atrial pacing lead simplifies pacemaker implantation in patients with limited venous access and prior thoracotomy.

Pacemaker and Device Therapy

Utilization of device therapy in children and patients with congenital heart disease is expected to increase substantially as survival to adolescence and adulthood increases, with attendant sequelae of heart failure. Device options have expanded with lead advancements, antitachycardia therapies, cardiac resynchronization therapy, and the availability of epicardial or subcutaneous defibrillator leads. Technologic improvements have shifted attention from focusing on lead and generator longevity to issues of optimizing conduction characteristics, owing to the recognition of the development of myocardial dysfunction from chronic right ventricular apical pacing. Defibrillator therapy for primary and secondary prevention of sudden death includes populations with repaired congenital heart disease, dilated cardiomyopathies, and, with increasing frequency, electrical myopathies without structural heart disease. The psychologic impact of pacemaker or device implantation on children and particularly adolescents is frequently significant and requires a careful educational approach, and emotional support from all involved personnel. Restrictions from engaging in blunt contact sports after pacemaker implantation often involve a major change in lifestyle among adolescents.

Pacemakers

Antibradycardia Pacing

The most common indication for pacemaker implantation in the United States is sinus node dysfunction following surgical repair of congenital heart disease, followed by postoperative atrioventricular block, congenital atrioventricular block, and isolated sick sinus syndrome in the absence of structural heart disease [156]. Guidelines for implantation of cardiac pacemakers and antiarrhythmia devices have been published by the American College of Cardiology/American Heart Association Task Force on Practice Guidelines [157], and the pediatric indications are summarized in Table 41.5 [53,157,158]. Symptomatic sinus bradycardia or tachycardia–bradycardia syndrome following atrial surgery, such as Senning, Mustard, and Fontan procedures [159], constitutes the most common indication for implantation. Indications for pacing in congenital complete atrioventricular block include a wide QRS escape rhythm, ventricular dysfunction, and a resting ventricular rate less than 50–55 bpm in the infant with a normal heart or less than 70 bpm in the infant with structural heart disease. In older children with congenital block, an average heart rate less than 50 bpm, or abrupt pauses two to three times the basic cycle length indicate a need for pacing. Per a multicenter long-term follow-up study, pacemaker implantation is recommended in older adolescents to avoid ventricular dysfunction, syncope, or sudden death in adulthood [160]. Surgical atrioventricular block (complete or advanced second-degree block) persisting beyond 7–10 days postoperatively is a class I indication for pacing. Without pacing, 53–65% of these patients will die suddenly [161,162]. Surgery involving ventricular septal defect closure, particularly in infants weighing less than 10 kg, or atrioventricular valve replacement accounts for most cases of surgically acquired heart block. In the setting of postoperative atrioventricular block, up to 65% of patients will recover normal conduction, with the majority resolving by the eighth postoperative day [163]; pacemaker implantation is generally delayed until this time in most patients.

There is a bimodal age curve for device implantation, with implantation in infancy for profound congenital or surgical atrioventricular block or sinus bradycardia, often associated with complex anatomy, with a second group receiving device implantation in childhood. The age at device implantation outside of infancy is typically 5-6 years of age [164,165]; this age has substantially decreased from earlier studies, where the median age ranged from 11–17 years [166]. Issues relative to pacing in infants include the optimal route, transvenous versus epicardial, and the mode of pacing. The availability of thin transvenous leads, 4 Fr or smaller, allows transvenous implantation in infancy, with improved pacing thresholds compared to epicardial leads [167,168], although utilization of steroid-eluting epicardial leads narrows the difference in lead longevity and function between the two approaches [93]. Disadvantages of transvenous lead placement in small children include acute complications of lead dislodgement and hemothorax, generator erosion, venous occlusion in patients with life-long need for pacing, tricuspid regurgitation exacerbated by the need to loop the lead within the atrium to accommodate patient growth, and the subsequent need for lead extraction with its attendant risks. Epicardial systems have the potential for generator migration or wound dehiscence, and an increased risk of lead fracture with activity. In most centers, current practice is to implant epicardial systems in infants and small children, and in children undergoing surgery for structural heart disease, maintaining this approach as long as the leads remain viable. The transvenous approach is used primarily at weights over approximately 35 kg, although many centers transition at lower weights. Using a subxiphoid incision, dual-chamber pacing can be accomplished in the majority of infants [169], although there are no data suggesting superiority of dual-chamber pacing versus rate responsive ventricular pacing in the small child without coexisting heart disease. Illustrations of our technique for epicardial pacing in a newborn are shown in Plates 41.8 and 41.9 (see plate section opposite p. 594), with the resultant chest radiograph in Figure 41.43 [169]. In patients with complex heart disease, the benefit of atrial contractility to cardiac output and arrhythmia avoidance provides a distinct rationale for dual-chamber pacing. Nonetheless, patients undergoing pacemaker implantation as neonates have a high mortality, reported as 30% within the first year [169,170]. An alternative approach in the very small newborn with atrioventricular block is pacing with temporary leads until the child has grown and matured enough for an implanted permanent pacemaker [171].

Technical issues related to transvenous lead access are present in patients with congenital heart disease, particularly single-ventricle patients following Fontan type repairs,

Table 41.5 Indications for permanent pacing in children and adolescents. (AV, atrioventricular.) (Adapted from Gregoratos *et al.* [157].)

SINUS NODE DYSFUNCTION

Class	Indication
I	Sinus node dysfunction with correlation of symptoms during age-inappropriate bradycardia Definition of bradycardia varies with patient's age and expected heart rate
IIa	Asymptomatic sinus bradycardia in child with complex congenital heart disease with resting heart rate <35 bpm or pauses in ventricular rate >3 seconds
IIa	Bradycardia-tachycardia syndrome with need for long-term antiarrhythmic treatment other than digitalis
IIb	Asymptomatic sinus bradycardia in adolescent with congenital heart disease with resting heart rate <35 bpm or pauses in ventricular rate >3 seconds
III	Asymptomatic sinus bradycardia in adolescent with longest RR interval <3 seconds and minimum heart rate >40 bpm

ATRIOVENTRICULAR CONDUCTION DISORDERS

Congenital heart block

I	Congenital third-degree AV block in infant with ventricular rate <50–55 bpm or with congenital heart disease and a ventricular rate <70 bpm
I	Congenital third-degree AV block with a wide QRS escape rhythm or ventricular dysfunction
IIa	Congenital third-degree AV block beyond the first year of life with an average heart rate <50 bpm or abrupt pauses in ventricular rate which are 2 or 3 times the basic cycle length
IIb	Congenital third-degree AV block in asymptomatic neonate, child, or adolescent with an acceptable rate, narrow QRS complex, and normal ventricular function

Postoperative AV block

I	Postoperative advanced second-degree or third-degree AV block that is not expected to resolve or persists at least 7 days after cardiac surgery
IIb	Transient postoperative third-degree AV block that reverts to sinus rhythm with residual bifascicular block
III	Transient postoperative AV block with return of normal AV conduction within 7 days
III	Asymptomatic postoperative bifascicular block with or without first-degree AV block

Other conduction disorders

I	Advanced second-degree or third-degree AV block associated with symptomatic bradycardia, congestive heart failure, or low cardiac output
III	Asymptomatic type I second-degree AV block

LONG QT OR VENTRICULAR TACHYCARDIA

I	Sustained pause-dependent ventricular tachycardia, with or without prolonged QT, in which efficacy of pacing is documented thoroughly
IIa	Long QT syndrome with 2:1 AV or third-degree AV block

transposition of the great arteries following atrial repairs, and congenitally corrected transposition of the great arteries [172]. The presence of a right-to-left intracardiac shunt favors an epicardial approach, or chronic anticoagulation. Although transvenous pacing can be accomplished in patients with atriopulmonary Fontan repairs, sluggish flow predisposes to clot formation on the lead even in the presence of anticoagulation; we have removed a 4 × 6 cm dense thrombus from one such patient at the time of Fontan con-

version; this patient had suffered a prior stroke. In patients with prior atrial baffle repairs for transposition, systemic venous baffle constriction may require stent placement to allow passage of a pacing lead. In congenitally corrected transposition, the incidence of developing atrioventricular block approaches 40%; the smooth trabeculations of the subpulmonary left ventricle may require active fixation leads [172]. Prior resection of atrial appendages may require alternate atrial pacing sites. Venous occlusions due to inter-

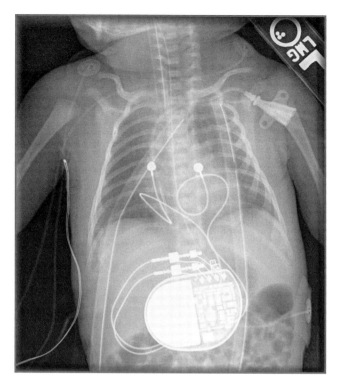

Figure 41.43 Babygram in a 2.2-kg infant shows the typical postoperative appearance after placement of a dual-chamber epicardial pacemaker. The left pleural space has been drained by a left chest tube. The right pleural space and mediastinum are drained by a chest tube passed through the right pleural space. The ventricular lead is on the high right ventricular outflow tract. Coils of the lead are placed within the pericardium to allow for growth. In a similar fashion, a coil is placed within the pacemaker pocket. The size of the dual-chamber pacemaker in comparison to the baby is quite evident, illustrating the need for implantation beneath both rectus muscles. (Reproduced with permission from Kelle *et al.* [169].)

ventional or surgical procedures are not uncommonly present. For most patients, venous angiograms to clarify anatomy and access are advisable, although cardiac magnetic resonance imaging or computerized tomography may be suitable.

Left ventricular dysfunction secondary to chronic right ventricular apex pacing has been reported in approximately 10% of patients with congenital atrioventricular block [164,173]. Ventricular remodeling based on the abnormal sequence of contractility is the presumed cause [174]. Several studies have attempted to identify the optimal location for right ventricular leads, without identification of a single optimal site [175,176]. The anterior right ventricular free-wall appears to result in the most desynchrony, and should be avoided; the left ventricular free-wall may be optimal. Alternate site pacing may produce a narrower QRS, although this finding does not predict improved con-

tractility. For the individual patient, optimization of pacing site may require assessments intraoperatively of indices of cardiac contractility, ejection fraction, and blood pressure.

Antitachycardia Pacing

Newer generators and leads that can detect SVT and deliver antitachycardia pacing to terminate tachycardia are available, and are particularly suitable for patients with repaired congenital heart disease [177]. Limitations include an inability to terminate tachycardia with 1:1 atrioventricular conduction (without specialized software), and limitation of the peak programmable heart rate to 150 bpm (versus 210 bpm in other generators). Electrophysiologic testing to determine the accuracy of tachycardia detection, the efficacy and safety of termination protocols, and an assessment of the peak sinus rate in response to catecholamines is mandatory. A typical protocol recognizes atrial rates greater than 200 bpm, and the device delivers a train of six to eight atrial impulses at 80% of the tachycardia cycle length to terminate. The termination algorithm is programmed to continue pacing automatically at faster rates until termination is achieved or to a predetermined minimum paced cycle length. To avoid initiating inappropriate pacing therapy, tachycardia detection criteria need to account for sinus tachycardia at rates up to 200 bpm in pediatric patients. Beta-blocker therapy is frequently advisable to ensure that sinus rates do not exceed 160–180 bpm.

Lead Extraction

The increased usage of transvenous leads in small children, the incidence of lead failure and recall, and improved longevity of patients with repaired congenital heart disease, has resulted in the increasing need for lead extraction in children and patients with congenital heart disease. Laser lead extraction is presently performed, with success rates of 90%, and complications of 6% [178]. Complications may be life threatening, including vessel laceration and cardiac perforation with potential for exsanguination [179,180].

Cardiac Resynchronization Therapy

The efficacy of cardiac resynchronization therapy in improving symptoms of heart failure and longevity has been established in adult patients with dilated or ischemic cardiomyopathies, ventricular dilatation, and QRS prolongation. In these adult patients, guidelines for resynchronization include a left ventricular ejection fraction ≤35%, QRS duration ≥120 msec, and symptoms of heart failure despite optimal medical treatment with NYHA class III–IV [181,182]. The principle of therapy is to correct ventricular mechanical desynchrony, usually with biventricular pacing, although atrial pacing with optimization of atrioventricular delay and spontaneous ventricular activation is also used

[183,184]. Biventricular or multisite pacing requires electrical and spatial separation between pacing leads, with one lead placed in or on the subpulmonary ventricle and the other lead located over the systemic ventricular free-wall. Efforts to identify the appropriate pediatric or congenital heart disease population likely to benefit from this approach have been ongoing, and include patients with failing systemic right ventricles, right bundle branch block, and desynchrony without significant QRS prolongation [185]. Populations likely to benefit from this approach include patients with ventricular dysfunction, secondary chronic right ventricular pacing for congenital heart block, patients with dilated cardiomyopathy, and patients with systemic right ventricles or complex ventricular anatomy [186,187]. In some cases, improvement in ventricular dysfunction has been dramatic, allowing removal from listing for heart transplantation [187]. Sophisticated measures of ventricular synchrony are needed, including tissue Doppler imaging.

Automatic Implantable Defibrillators

Implantable defibrillators have demonstrated their efficacy in preventing sudden death in patients surviving cardiac arrest, and in adult patients with low ejection fractions [188]. Defibrillator implantations in children and patients with congenital heart disease account for fewer than 1% of all ICD recipients, with limited prospective data available. Improvements in lead technology, smaller implantable generators (weight <75 g), incorporation of antibradycardia and antitachycardia pacing capability, and device diagnostic memory, have led to dramatic expansion of defibrillator use in pediatric patients over the last decade [189–195].

The epicardial approach to pediatric cardioverter defibrillator placement has changed in the past several years. In the initial epicardial placements a large subcutaneous patch was placed along the upper left chest or along the left edge of the pericardium adjacent to the ventricle. The subcutaneous patch however is quite bulky and not easy to place. It is susceptible to crinkling and an increase in defibrillation thresholds. Recently we have been using the transvenous lead "coil" and placing the "coil" in either the transverse pericardial sinus or in the subcutaneous tissue of the left chest wall. The atrial and ventricular epicardial leads are placed in the usual fashion and connected to the defibrillator device. The cardioverter defibrillator is placed beneath the right rectus muscle. This provides an excellent vector across the myocardial mass for defibrillation. This can be performed with a subxiphoid incision without a full sternotomy. Obviously if the patient was having a simultaneous open cardiac procedure the sternotomy exposure is used.

Excellent results with the transverse sinus technique have been reported by Hsia and associates from the Medical University of South Carolina [193]. In that series of seven children all implantations were performed through a small subxiphoid incision without a full sternotomy. The coil lead was actively fixated in the transverse sinus under fluoroscopic guidance. We have used this technique in a 3-month-old, 6 kg child. Bove and associates have reported similar results with the subcutaneous coil placed along the left chest wall [196]. In pediatric and congenital heart disease patients, data from the registry of defibrillator implantation in the United States shows the majority of implants in the following three types of heart disease: 1) repaired congenital heart disease (>45%), most commonly tetralogy of Fallot and transposition of the great arteries following atrial repairs [197,198]; 2) primary electrical disease (long QT syndromes, Brugada syndrome, idiopathic ventricular fibrillation, >30%); and 3) cardiomyopathies (26%) [190]. The threshold for implanting defibrillators in pediatrics has decreased, and data are available on 443 pediatric and congenital heart disease patients with defibrillators implanted in the US between 1992 and 2004, at a median age of 16 years and median weight of 61 kg [190]. Acute implantation complications occur in 12% and chronic complications are reported in 29% of pediatric or congenital heart disease patients, almost all related to lead issues, including insulation breaches, lead fractures, and oversensing. Inappropriate shocks occur in at least 24% of pediatric patients, significantly higher than the 14% reported in adults [190]. Appropriate shocks are reported in 23% of pediatric patients and are more common in patients with defibrillators for secondary prevention (32%) versus primary prevention (18%) [190]. Mortality in the multicenter registry was 4%, mainly owing to progressive heart failure, with only 1% attributable to fatal arrhythmia [190].

Over time, the indications for implantation of defibrillators have become more commonly primary prevention (52%) versus secondary prevention (48%) [190]. Primary prevention refers to implantation in at-risk patients who have not yet experienced an episode of sustained ventricular tachycardia, venticular fibrillation, or resuscitated cardiac arrest. Secondary prevention refers to implantation following resuscitation from cardiac arrest or sustained ventricular arrhythmia. Secondary prevention indications also include patients with congenital heart disease and recurrent syncope of undetermined origin in the presence of ventricular dysfunction or inducible ventricular tachycardia, or associated with advanced ventricular dysfunction without identifiable etiology for syncope after thorough invasive and noninvasive evaluation [199]. Data establishing efficacy of defibrillators for primary prevention in patients with ejection fractions less than 35% is derived from adult populations with ischemic or nonischemic cardiomyopathy; comparable data are not available for the congenital heart disease populations. This is confounded by the difficulty in assessing ventricular function in the systemic right or univentricular heart, and the contribution to risk from multiple scars of prior surgeries, subendocardial ischemia, and coronary abnormalities. Appropriate candidates for primary prevention in congenital heart disease may include patients with a failing systemic ventricle with an ejection fraction less than 30% in addition to other indicators of high risk, such as marked QRS prolongation, nonsustained ventricular tachycardia, and elevated end-diastolic pressure greater than 12 mmHg [200].

Defibrillator implantation may be used as a bridge to cardiac transplantation in patients with severe ventricular dysfunction and ventricular arrhythmias or syncope.

Management of Acute Perioperative Arrhythmias

Early postoperative arrhythmias in pediatric patients following repair of congenital heart disease occur in approximately 30–47% of patients [201,202]. Intraoperative procedural factors are directly associated with the development of arrhythmias, as well as the postoperative milieu characterized by excess catecholamines, elevated atrial pressures, intra-atrial monitor lines, pericardial inflammation, autonomic imbalance, and neurohormonal changes [203]. An excellent review of guidelines for postoperative arrhythmia management in adults has been published by van Mieghem [203], and that approach is summarized in Table 41.6 [53,203]. Appropriate therapy for postoperative SVT begins with establishing the mechanism of tachycardia as summarized in Table 41.7 [53]. The acute administration of adenosine has become the default acute treatment of choice due to ease of administrations and may be diagnostic even when not therapeutic. Caveats regarding the use of adenosine include recognition of the potential for provoking torsades des pointes or atrial fibrillation with rapid conduction requiring immediate defibrillation; patients following heart transplantation may experience profound asystole.

Determination of the mechanism of tachycardia may be facilitated by recording atrial electrograms, particularly when P waves are not readily apparent on the electrocardiogram (Figure 41.44A) [53]. Atrial activity should be clearly visible, allowing the atrial-to-ventricular relationship to be defined [204]. Administration of adenosine while recording electrograms may unmask rapid atrial activity with 2:1 or variable atrioventricular conduction (Figure 41.44B) [53] indicating a primary atrial tachycardia, such as atrial flutter. A 1:1 ventricular-to-atrial (VA) relationship (ventricular electrogram precedes atrial electrogram) indicates either junctional tachycardia with retrograde conduction or an atrioventricular re-entry tachycardia (utilizing an accessory connection). Measurement of the VA interval further defines the mechanism of tachycardia. A VA interval longer than 70 msec suggests orthodromic reciprocating tachycardia, while a VA interval shorter than 70 msec is consistent with either junctional tachycardia or AVNRT. Atrial overdrive pacing may then be performed to terminate tachycardia when appropriate. Atrial overdrive pacing is initiated at 120–150% of the atrial cycle length, or 20–30 bpm faster than the tachycardia rate, and continued for four beats or up to 30 seconds (Figure 41.44C,D) [53]. Pacing output of approximately 5 mA for temporary atrial wires, or 10–20 mA for esophageal leads, is required. Pacing will effectively terminate up to 95% of re-entry tachycardias.

Table 41.6 Guidelines for postoperative arrhythmia management. (Adapted from van Mieghem [203].)

1. Establish mechanism of tachycardia
2. Consider precipitating or aggravating causes
3. Evaluate hemodynamic consequences
4. Estimate natural course
5. Define therapeutic goal:
   a. Terminate arrhythmia
   b. Slow ventricular rate
   c. Correct precipitating mechanism

Table 41.7 Therapy for early postoperative supraventricular tachycardia. (ORT, orthodromic reciprocating tachycardia; AVNRT, atrioventricular nodal re-entry tachycardia; AV, atrioventricular.)

Mechanism	Adenosine	Atrial pacing	Other medications
ORT	•	•	Procainamide, esmolol or oral beta-blocker, digoxin
AVNRT	•	•	Digoxin, diltiazem
Atrial flutter		•	Ibutilide, amiodarone, procainamide, diltiazem for rate control
Atrial fibrillation			Ibutilide, direct current cardioversion, amiodarone, procainamide, esmolol or diltiazem for rate control
Sinus bradycardia		•	Isoproterenol, dobutamine
Junctional ectopic tachycardia		Overdrive for AV synchrony	Procainamide, amiodarone, diltiazem

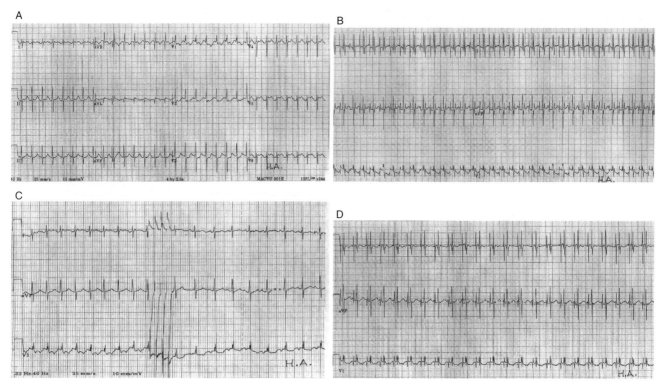

Figure 41.44 A, Postoperative atrial electrogram obtained in a 4-week-old infant after repair of anomalous left coronary artery arising from the pulmonary artery. Heart rate had been persistent at 180 bpm without variation for 12 hours. **B,** Esophageal electrogram in infant in **A** showing atrial tachycardia with 2:1 atrioventricular conduction. Atrial activity is indicated by the smaller spikes in the second lead, ventricular activity by the tall spikes. Atrial cycle length is 210 msec. **C,** Atrial overdrive pacing using esophageal lead. Four extrastimuli at 160 msec are delivered, resulting in conversion to sinus rhythm with 1:1 AV conduction. **D,** Atrial esophageal electrogram postconversion shows sinus rhythm with 1:1 AV conduction.

Junctional Ectopic Tachycardia

In childhood, the most frequent acute postoperative arrhythmia other than premature ventricular contraction is junctional ectopic tachycardia, present in 5–10% of pediatric patients, followed by atrioventricular block (2–4%), ventricular tachycardia (2%), and SVT [201,202,205]. Junctional ectopic tachycardia is defined as tachycardia originating from the His bundle, usually narrow complex, at rates greater than 170 bpm, often with atrioventricular dissociation [206]. The mechanism is presumed to be abnormal automaticity of the atrioventricular node, as the rhythm does not respond to cardioversion and may be due to either direct trauma or stretch of tissues near the atrioventricular junction. The median postoperative time for development of junctional ectopic tachycardia is in the first 24 hours, ranging up to 6 days with median rate of 195 bpm; duration ranges from 1–13 days postoperatively [207]. Anatomic lesions and younger age at repair are risk factors for the development of junctional ectopic tachycardia, which is associated with transient intraoperative or postoperative atrioventricular block [208], increased mortality, and prolonged length of stay [205,209]. Junctional ectopic tachycardia occurs most commonly in patients <24 months of age, particularly following repair of atrioventricular septal defect (47%), tetralogy of Fallot (35%), ventricular septal defects (30%), and arterial switch repair [201,202]. Prolonged bypass time and aortic cross-clamp time are risk factors for arrhythmia [201,202,210], as well as postoperative infusion of dopamine [210]. Magnesium supplementation during cardiopulmonary bypass may reduce the incidence of junctional ectopic tachycardia [211]. Treatment is necessary in 40–60% of patients with junctional ectopic tachycardia due to hemodynamic instability [205,210]; the goal of therapy is to achieve heart rates under 180 bpm. Current treatment strategies include cessation of dopamine infusion, normothermia, volume support, and intravenous amiodarone or procainamide infusion [208,212]. Atrial pacing using either temporary atrial pacing wires or an esophageal catheter at rates faster than the tachycardia may augment cardiac output, particularly when the junctional rate can be slowed by amiodarone infusion.

Atrial Fibrillation

Although atrial fibrillation occurs postoperatively in 20–40% of adult patients undergoing cardiac surgery [203,213], it occurs uncommonly in pediatric patients. However, as the number of older patients with congenital heart disease undergoing repeat surgeries increases, this arrhythmia will be encountered more frequently. Direct current cardioversion using high energy (1–2 J/kg) is used when prompt termination of hemodynamically significant atrial fibrillation is necessary. Conversion of atrial fibrillation to sinus rhythm may be achieved pharmacologically with ibutilide or amiodarone. Intravenous diltiazem or esmolol are effective for rapid rate control of atrioventricular conduction. In patients thought to be at high risk for developing atrial fibrillation, such as patients with enlarged left atria with mitral valve disease, a short prophylactic perioperative course of amiodarone may be useful [214–216].

Ventricular Arrhythmias

Early postoperative ventricular arrhythmias often are associated with ventricular dysfunction, severe hypertrophy, coronary insufficiency, electrolyte abnormalities, and excess catecholamines. Patients known to have episodes of sustained ventricular tachycardia preoperatively should be considered for operative mapping and ablation of the tachycardia focus intraoperatively. Certain patients at high risk for ventricular arrhythmias postoperatively, such as patients with hypertrophic cardiomyopathy or severe left ventricular outflow tract obstruction, may benefit from amiodarone infusion at the conclusion of cardiopulmonary bypass and during the early postoperative course. Postoperatively, correcting or minimizing the predisposing arrhythmogenic factors is essential. Maintaining the serum potassium greater than 3.5 mEq/L and magnesium greater than 2.0 g/dL, as well as decreasing the degree of inotropic support when possible, will decrease the potential for triggering sustained tachycardia. In patients thought to be at risk for developing sustained arrhythmias, a prophylactic lidocaine infusion is effective. Lidocaine is less efficacious than amiodarone or procainamide in terminating a sustained ventricular tachycardia [217,218]. For termination of sustained ventricular tachycardia, direct current cardioversion using 1 J/kg is indicated where acute hemodynamic compromise is present; otherwise amiodarone or procainamide infusions may be effective [217].

References

1. Cobb FR, Blumenschein SD, Sealy WC, *et al.* (1968) Successful surgical interruption of the bundle of Kent in a patient with Wolff-Parkinson-White syndrome. Circulation 38, 1018–1029.
2. Cox JL, Gallagher JJ, Cain ME. (1985) Experience with 118 consecutive patients undergoing operation for the Wolff-Parkinson-White syndrome. J Thorac Cardiovasc Surg 90, 490–501.
3. Guiraudon GM. (1994) Surgical treatment of Wolff-Parkinson-White syndrome: a "retrospectroscopic" view. Ann Thorac Surg 58, 1254–1261.
4. Pritchett EL, Anderson RW, Benditt DG, *et al.* (1979) Reentry within the atrioventricular node: surgical cure with preservation of atrioventricular conduction. Circulation 60, 440–446.
5. Holman WL, Ikeshita M, Lease JG, *et al.* (1982) Elective prolongation of atrioventricular conduction by multiple discrete cryolesions: a new technique for the treatment of paroxysmal supraventricular tachycardia. J Thorac Cardiovasc Surg 84, 554–559.
6. Cox JL, Gallagher JJ, Ungerleider RM. (1982) Encircling endocardial ventriculotomy for refractory ischemic ventricular tachycardia. IV. Clinical indication, surgical technique, mechanism of action, and results. J Thorac Cardiovasc Surg 83, 865–872.
7. Guiraudon G, Fontaine G, Frank R, *et al.* (1978) Encircling endocardial ventriculotomy: a new surgical treatment for life-threatening ventricular tachycardias resistant to medical treatment following myocardial infarction. Ann Thorac Surg 26, 438–444.
8. Cox JL, Boineau JP, Schuessler RB, *et al.* (1995) Modification of the maze procedure for atrial flutter and atrial fibrillation. I. Rationale and surgical results. J Thorac Cardiovasc Surg 110, 473–484.
9. Cox JL, Boineau JP, Schuessler RB, *et al.* (1995) Electrophysiologic basis, surgical development, and clinical results of the maze procedure for atrial flutter and atrial fibrillation. Adv Card Surg 6, 1–67.
10. Cox JL, Jaquiss RD, Schuessler RB, *et al.* (1995) Modification of the maze procedure for atrial flutter and atrial fibrillation. II. Surgical technique of the maze III procedure. J Thorac Cardiovasc Surg 110, 485–495.
11. Cox JL, Ferguson TB Jr. (1989) Surgery for the Wolff-Parkinson-White syndrome: the endocardial approach. Semin Thorac Cardiovasc Surg 1, 34–46.
12. Guiraudon GM, Klein GJ, Sharma AD, *et al.* (1986) Closed-heart technique for Wolff-Parkinson-White syndrome: further experience and potential limitations. Ann Thorac Surg 42, 651–657.
13. Guiraudon GM, Klein GJ, Sharma AD, *et al.* (1989) Surgery for the Wolff-Parkinson-White syndrome: the epicardial approach. Semin Thorac Cardiovasc Surg 1, 21–33.
14. Lowe JE. (1986) Surgical treatment of the Wolff-Parkinson-White syndrome and other supraventricular tachyarrhythmias. J Card Surg 1, 117–134.
15. Mahomed Y, King RD, Zipes DP, *et al.* (1988) Surgical division of Wolff-Parkinson-White pathways utilizing the closed-heart technique: a 2-year experience in 47 patients. Ann Thorac Surg 45, 495–504.
16. Mavroudis C, Deal BJ, Backer CL. (2004) Surgery for arrhythmias in children. Int J Cardiol 97(Suppl 1), 39–51.
17. Guiraudon GM, Klein GJ, Sharma AD, *et al.* (1986) Surgical treatment of supraventricular tachycardia: a five-year experience. Pacing Clin Electrophysiol 9, 1376–1380.

18. Josephson ME. (2003) Electrophysiology of ventricular tachycardia: an historical perspective. J Cardiovasc Electrophysiol 14, 1134–1148.

19. Ashburn DA, Harris L, Downar EH, et al. (2003) Electrophysiologic surgery in patients with congenital heart disease. Semin Thorac Cardiovasc Surg Pediatr Card Surg Annu 6, 51–58.

20. Bottoni N, Tomasi C, Donateo P, et al. (2003) Clinical and electrophysiological characteristics in patients with atrioventricular reentrant and atrioventricular nodal reentrant tachycardia. Europace 5, 225–229.

21. Dobreanu D, Micu S, Toma O, et al. (2007) Intraprocedural predictors of successful ablation of slow pathway for atrioventricular nodal reentrant tachycardia. Rom J Intern Med 45, 35–46.

22. Foldesi C, Pandozi C, Peichl P, et al. (2003) Atrial flutter: arrhythmia circuit and basis for radiofrequency catheter ablation. Ital Heart J 4, 395–403.

23. Goldberger J, Kall J, Ehlert F, et al. (1993) Effectiveness of radiofrequency catheter ablation for treatment of atrial tachycardia. Am J Cardiol 72, 787–793.

24. Jackman WM, Beckman KJ, McClelland JH, et al. (1992) Treatment of supraventricular tachycardia due to atrioventricular nodal reentry, by radiofrequency catheter ablation of slow-pathway conduction. N Engl J Med 327, 313–318.

25. Jackman WM, Wang XZ, Friday KJ, et al. (1991) Catheter ablation of accessory atrioventricular pathways (Wolff-Parkinson-White syndrome) by radiofrequency current. N Engl J Med 324, 1605–1611.

26. Klein LS, Shih HT, Hackett FK, et al. (1992) Radiofrequency catheter ablation of ventricular tachycardia in patients without structural heart disease. Circulation 85, 1666–1674.

27. Lee PC, Chen SA, Hwang B. (2009) Atrioventricular node anatomy and physiology: implications for ablation of atrioventricular nodal reentrant tachycardia. Curr Opin Cardiol 24, 105–112.

28. Lesh MD, Van Hare GF, Epstein LM, et al. (1994) Radiofrequency catheter ablation of atrial arrhythmias. Results and mechanisms. Circulation 89, 1074–1089.

29. Khositseth A, Danielson GK, Dearani JA, et al. (2004) Supraventricular tachyarrhythmias in Ebstein anomaly: management and outcome. J Thorac Cardiovasc Surg 128, 826–833.

30. Gatzoulis MA, Till JA, Somerville J, et al. (1995) Mechano-electrical interaction in tetralogy of Fallot. QRS prolongation relates to right ventricular size and predicts malignant ventricular arrhythmias and sudden death. Circulation 92, 231–237.

31. Deal BJ, Mavroudis C, Backer CL. (2003) Beyond Fontan conversion: Surgical therapy of arrhythmias including patients with associated complex congenital heart disease. Ann Thorac Surg 76, 542–553; discussion 553–554.

32. Mavroudis C, Deal BJ, Backer CL. (2003) Arrhythmia surgery in association with complex congenital heart repairs excluding patients with fontan conversion. Semin Thorac Cardiovasc Surg Pediatr Card Surg Annu 6, 33–50.

33. Deal BJ, Mavroudis C, Backer CL. (2002) Beyond Fontan: surgical therapy of arrhythmias in young patients. Presented at the 38th Annual Meeting, Society of Thoracic Surgeons; Fort Lauderdale, FLA; January 30, 2002.

34. Backer CL, Tsao S, Deal BJ, et al. (2008) Maze procedure in single ventricle patients. Semin Thorac Cardiovasc Surg Pediatr Card Surg Annu 44–48.

35. Deal BJ, Mavroudis C, Backer CL. (2007) Arrhythmia management in the Fontan patient. Pediatr Cardiol 28, 448–456.

36. Deal BJ, Mavroudis C, Backer CL, et al. (1999) Impact of arrhythmia circuit cryoablation during Fontan conversion for refractory atrial tachycardia. Am J Cardiol 83, 563–568.

37. Mavroudis C, Backer CL, Deal BJ. (2008) Late reoperations for Fontan patients: state of the art invited review. Eur J Cardiothorac Surg 34, 1034–1040.

38. Mavroudis C, Backer CL, Deal BJ, et al. (2001) Total cavopulmonary conversion and maze procedure for patients with failure of the Fontan operation. J Thorac Cardiovasc Surg 122, 863–871.

39. Mavroudis C, Backer CL, Deal BJ, et al. (1998) Fontan conversion to cavopulmonary connection and arrhythmia circuit cryoblation. J Thorac Cardiovasc Surg 115, 547–556.

40. Mavroudis C, Deal BJ, Backer CL, et al. (1999) The favorable impact of arrhythmia surgery on total cavopulmonary artery Fontan conversion. Semin Thorac Cardiovasc Surg Pediatr Card Surg Annu 2, 143–156.

41. Mavroudis C, Deal BJ, Backer CL, et al. (2008) Arrhythmia surgery in patients with and without congenital heart disease. Ann Thorac Surg 86, 857–868; discussion 868.

42. Cox JL. (1983) Surgery for cardiac arrhythmias. Curr Probl Cardiol 8, 1–60.

43. Langberg JJ, Man KC, Vorperian VR, et al. (1993) Recognition and catheter ablation of subepicardial accessory pathways. J Am Coll Cardiol 22, 1100–1104.

44. Cappato R, Schluter M, Weiss C, et al. (1996) Radiofrequency current catheter ablation of accessory atrioventricular pathways in Ebstein's anomaly. Circulation 94, 376–383.

45. Reich JD, Auld D, Hulse E, et al. (1998) The Pediatric Radiofrequency Ablation Registry's experience with Ebstein's anomaly. Pediatric Electrophysiology Society. J Cardiovasc Electrophysiol 9, 1370–1377.

46. Dubin AM, Van Hare GF. (2000) Radiofrequency catheter ablation: indications and complications. Pediatr Cardiol 21, 551–556.

47. Van Hare GF. (1997) Indications for radiofrequency ablation in the pediatric population. J Cardiovasc Electrophysiol 8, 952–962.

48. Chiou CW, Chen SA, Chiang CE, et al. (1995) Radiofrequency catheter ablation of paroxysmal supraventricular tachycardia in patients with congenital heart disease. Int J Cardiol 50, 143–151.

49. Levine JC, Walsh EP, Saul JP. (1993) Radiofrequency ablation of accessory pathways associated with congenital heart disease including heterotaxy syndrome. Am J Cardiol 72, 689–693.

50. Van Hare GF, Lesh MD, Ross BA, *et al.* (1996) Mapping and radiofrequency ablation of intraatrial reentrant tachycardia after the Senning or Mustard procedure for transposition of the great arteries. Am J Cardiol 77, 985–991.

51. Van Hare GF, Lesh MD, Stanger P. (1993) Radiofrequency catheter ablation of supraventricular arrhythmias in patients with congenital heart disease: results and technical considerations. J Am Coll Cardiol 22, 883–890.

52. Cox JL. (1990) The surgical management of cardiac arrhythmias. In: Sabiston DC Jr, Spencer FC, eds. *Surgery of the Chest*, 5th ed. Philadelphia, PA: WB Saunders.

53. Deal BJ, Mavroudis C, Backer CL. (2003) Surgical therapy of cardiac arrhythmias. In: Mavroudis C, Backer CL, eds. *Pediatric Cardiac Surgery*, 3rd ed. Philadelphia, PA: Mosby Inc.

54. WHO/ISC Task Force. (1978) Definition of terms related to cardiac rhythm. Am Heart J 95, 796–806.

55. Deal BJ, Jacobs JP, Mavroudis C. (2000) Congenital Heart Surgery Nomenclature and Database Project: arrhythmias. Ann Thorac Surg 69 (Suppl), S319–S331.

56. Deal BJ, Mavroudis C, Jacobs JP, *et al.* (2008) Arrhythmic complications associated with the treatment of patients with congenital cardiac disease: consensus definitions from the Multi-Societal Database Committee for Pediatric and Congenital Heart Disease. Cardiol Young 18(Suppl 2), 202–205.

57. Theodoro DA, Danielson GK, Porter CJ, *et al.* (1998) Right-sided maze procedure for right atrial arrhythmias in congenital heart disease. Ann Thorac Surg 65, 149–153; discussion 153–154.

58. Deal BJ, Mavroudis C, Backer CL. (2008) The role of concomitant arrhythmia surgery in patients undergoing repair of congenital heart disease. Pacing Clin Electrophysiol 31(Suppl 1), S13–S16.

59. Deal BJ, Mavroudis C, Backer CL, *et al.* (2000) New directions in surgical therapy of arrhythmias. Pediatr Cardiol 21, 576–583.

60. Gatzoulis MA, Walters J, McLaughlin PR, *et al.* (2000) Late arrhythmia in adults with the mustard procedure for transposition of great arteries: a surrogate marker for right ventricular dysfunction? Heart 84, 409–415.

61. Puley G, Siu S, Connelly M, *et al.* (1999) Arrhythmia and survival in patients >18 years of age after the mustard procedure for complete transposition of the great arteries. Am J Cardiol 83, 1080–1084.

62. Ghai A, Harris L, Harrison DA, *et al.* (2001) Outcomes of late atrial tachyarrhythmias in adults after the Fontan operation. J Am Coll Cardiol 37, 585–592.

63. Peters NS, Somerville J. (1992) Arrhythmias after the Fontan procedure. Br Heart J 68, 199–204.

64. Roos-Hesselink J, Perlroth MG, McGhie J, *et al.* (1995) Atrial arrhythmias in adults after repair of tetralogy of Fallot. Correlations with clinical, exercise, and echocardiographic findings. Circulation 91, 2214–2219.

65. Kannankeril PJ, Fish FA. (2005) Management of intra-atrial reentrant tachycardia. Curr Opin Cardiol 20, 89–93.

66. Samii SM, Cohen MH. (2004) Ablation of tachyarrhythmias in pediatric patients. Curr Opin Cardiol 19, 64–67.

67. Kanter RJ, Papagiannis J, Carboni MP, *et al.* (2000) Radiofrequency catheter ablation of supraventricular tachycardia substrates after mustard and senning operations for d-transposition of the great arteries. J Am Coll Cardiol 35, 428–441.

68. Baker BM, Lindsay BD, Bromberg BI, *et al.* (1996) Catheter ablation of clinical intraatrial reentrant tachycardias resulting from previous atrial surgery: localizing and transecting the critical isthmus. J Am Coll Cardiol 28, 411–417.

69. Triedman JK, Saul JP, Weindling SN, *et al.* (1995) Radiofrequency ablation of intra-atrial reentrant tachycardia after surgical palliation of congenital heart disease. Circulation 91, 707–714.

70. Triedman JK, Bergau DM, Saul JP, *et al.* (1997) Efficacy of radiofrequency ablation for control of intraatrial reentrant tachycardia in patients with congenital heart disease. J Am Coll Cardiol 30, 1032–1038.

71. Gandhi SK. (2007) Atrial arrhythmia surgery in congenital heart disease. J Interv Card Electrophysiol 20, 119–125.

72. Kanter RJ, Garson A Jr. (1997) Atrial arrhythmias during chronic follow-up of surgery for complex congenital heart disease. Pacing Clin Electrophysiol 20, 502–511.

73. Dorostkar PC, Cheng J, Scheinman MM. (1998) Electroanatomical mapping and ablation of the substrate supporting intraatrial reentrant tachycardia after palliation for complex congenital heart disease. Pacing Clin Electrophysiol 21, 1810–1819.

74. Schumacher B, Wolpert C, Lewalter T, *et al.* (2000) Predictors of success in radiofrequency catheter ablation of atrial flutter. J Interv Card Electrophysiol 4(Suppl 1), 121–125.

75. Triedman JK, Jenkins KJ, Colan SD, *et al.* (1997) Intra-atrial reentrant tachycardia after palliation of congenital heart disease: characterization of multiple macroreentrant circuits using fluoroscopically based three-dimensional endocardial mapping. J Cardiovasc Electrophysiol 8, 259–270.

76. Lesh MD, Kalman JM, Saxon LA, *et al.* (1997) Electrophysiology of "incisional" reentrant atrial tachycardia complicating surgery for congenital heart disease. Pacing Clin Electrophysiol 20, 2107–2111.

77. Balaji S, Johnson TB, Sade RM, *et al.* (1994) Management of atrial flutter after the Fontan procedure. J Am Coll Cardiol 23, 1209–1215.

78. Conte S, Gewillig M, Eyskens B, *et al.* (1999) Management of late complications after classic Fontan procedure by conversion to total cavopulmonary connection. Cardiovasc Surg 7, 651–655.

79. Kao JM, Alejos JC, Grant PW, *et al.* (1994) Conversion of atriopulmonary to cavopulmonary anastomosis in management of late arrhythmias and atrial thrombosis. Ann Thorac Surg 58, 1510–1514.

80. Kreutzer J, Keane JF, Lock JE, *et al.* (1996) Conversion of modified Fontan procedure to lateral atrial tunnel cavopulmonary anastomosis. J Thorac Cardiovasc Surg 111, 1169–1176.

81. McElhinney DB, Reddy VM, Moore P, *et al.* (1996) Revision of previous Fontan connections to extracardiac or intraatrial conduit cavopulmonary anastomosis. Ann Thorac Surg 62, 1276–1282; discussion 1283.

82. van Son JA, Mohr FW, Hambsch J, *et al.* (1999) Conversion of atriopulmonary or lateral atrial tunnel cavopulmonary anastomosis to extracardiac conduit Fontan modification. Eur J Cardiothorac Surg 15, 150–157; discussion 157–158.

83. Vitullo DA, DeLeon SY, Berry TE, *et al.* (1996) Clinical improvement after revision in Fontan patients. Ann Thorac Surg 61, 1797–1804.

84. Mavroudis C, Deal BJ, Backer CL, *et al.* (2007) J. Maxwell Chamberlain Memorial Paper for congenital heart surgery. 111 Fontan conversions with arrhythmia surgery: surgical lessons and outcomes. Ann Thorac Surg 84, 1457–1465; discussion 1465–1466.

85. Mavroudis C, Backer CL, Deal BJ, *et al.* (2007) Evolving anatomic and electrophysiologic considerations associated with Fontan conversion. Semin Thorac Cardiovasc Surg Pediatr Card Surg Annu 136–145.

86. Hillman ND, Mavroudis C, Backer CL. (2003) Adult congenital heart disease. In: Mavroudis C, Backer CL, eds. *Pediatric Cardiac Surgery*, 3rd ed. Philadelphia, PA: Mosby Inc.

87. Bridges ND, Lock JE, Castaneda AR. (1990) Baffle fenestration with subsequent transcatheter closure. Modification of the Fontan operation for patients at increased risk. Circulation 82, 1681–1689.

88. Marcelletti C, Corno A, Giannico S, *et al.* (1990) Inferior vena cava-pulmonary artery extracardiac conduit. A new form of right heart bypass. J Thorac Cardiovasc Surg 100, 228–232.

89. Mavroudis C, Zales VR, Backer CL, *et al.* (1992) Fenestrated Fontan with delayed catheter closure. Effects of volume loading and baffle fenestration on cardiac index and oxygen delivery. Circulation 86(5 Suppl), II85–II92.

90. Puga FJ, Chiavarelli M, Hagler DJ. (1987) Modifications of the Fontan operation applicable to patients with left atrioventricular valve atresia or single atrioventricular valve. Circulation 76, III53–III60.

91. Hoyer MH, Beerman LB, Ettedgui JA, *et al.* (1994) Transatrial lead placement for endocardial pacing in children. Ann Thorac Surg 58, 97–101; discussion 102.

92. Johnsrude CL, Backer CL, Deal BJ, *et al.* (1999) Transmural atrial pacing in patients with postoperative congenital heart disease. J Cardiovasc Electrophysiol 10, 351–357.

93. Dodge-Khatami A, Johnsrude CL, Backer CL, *et al.* (2000) A comparison of steroid-eluting epicardial versus transvenous pacing leads in children. J Card Surg 15, 323–329.

94. Deal BJ, Mavroudis C, Backer CL, *et al.* (2002) Comparison of anatomic isthmus block with the modified right atrial maze procedure for late atrial tachycardia in Fontan patients. Circulation 106, 575–579.

95. Holman WL, Ikeshita M, Lease JG, *et al.* (1986) Cryosurgical modification of retrograde atrioventricular conduction. Implications for the surgical treatment of atrioventricular nodal reentry tachycardia. J Thorac Cardiovasc Surg 91, 826–834.

96. Ross DL, Johnson DC, Denniss AR, *et al.* (1985) Curative surgery for atrioventricular junctional ("AV nodal") reentrant tachycardia. J Am Coll Cardiol 6, 1383–1392.

97. Cox JL, Holman WL, Cain ME. (1987) Cryosurgical treatment of atrioventricular node reentrant tachycardia. Circulation 76, 1329–1336.

98. Cox JL. (1991) Surgery for cardiac arrhythmias. In: Braunwald E, ed. *Heart Disease Update 13 to Heart Disease: A Textbook of Cardiovascular Medicine*, 3rd ed. Philadelphia, PA: WB Saunders.

99. Case CL, Crawford FA, Gillette PC, *et al.* (1988) Successful surgery for atrioventricular reentrant tachycardia in a small child. Am Heart J 116, 187–189.

100. Gillette PC, Smith RT, Garson A Jr, *et al.* (1985) Chronic supraventricular tachycardia. A curable cause of congestive cardiomyopathy. JAMA 253, 391–392.

101. Gillette PC, Wampler DG, Garson A Jr, *et al.* (1985) Treatment of atrial automatic tachycardia by ablation procedures. J Am Coll Cardiol 6, 405–409.

102. Lowe JE, Hendry PJ, Packer DL, *et al.* (1989) Surgical management of chronic ectopic atrial tachycardia. Semin Thorac Cardiovasc Surg 1, 58–66.

103. Prager NA, Cox JL, Lindsay BD, *et al.* (1993) Long-term effectiveness of surgical treatment of ectopic atrial tachycardia. J Am Coll Cardiol 22, 85–92.

104. Williams JM, Ungerleider RM, Lofland GK, *et al.* (1980) Left atrial isolation: new technique for the treatment of supraventricular arrhythmias. J Thorac Cardiovasc Surg 80, 373–380.

105. Harada A, D'Agostino HJ Jr, Schuessler RB, *et al.* (1988) Right atrial isolation: a new surgical treatment for supraventricular tachycardia. I. Surgical technique and electrophysiologic effects. J Thorac Cardiovasc Surg 95, 643–650.

106. Berger F, Vogel M, Kramer A, *et al.* (1999) Incidence of atrial flutter/fibrillation in adults with atrial septal defect before and after surgery. Ann Thorac Surg 68, 75–78.

107. Brandenburg RO Jr, Holmes DR Jr, Brandenburg RO, *et al.* (1983) Clinical follow-up study of paroxysmal supraventricular tachyarrhythmias after operative repair of a secundum type atrial septal defect in adults. Am J Cardiol 51, 273–276.

108. Gatzoulis MA, Freeman MA, Siu SC, *et al.* (1999) Atrial arrhythmia after surgical closure of atrial septal defects in adults. N Engl J Med 340, 839–846.

109. Bonchek LI, Burlingame MW, Worley SJ, *et al.* (1993) Cox/maze procedure for atrial septal defect with atrial fibrillation: management strategies. Ann Thorac Surg 55, 607–610.

110. Kobayashi J, Yamamoto F, Nakano K, *et al.* (1998) Maze procedure for atrial fibrillation associated with atrial septal defect. Circulation 98(19 Suppl), II399–II402.

111. Izumoto H, Kawazoe K, Eishi K, *et al.* (2000) Medium-term results after the modified Cox/Maze procedure combined with other cardiac surgery. Eur J Cardiothorac Surg 17, 25–29.

112. Kawaguchi AT, Kosakai Y, Sasako Y, *et al.* (1996) Risks and benefits of combined maze procedure for atrial fibrillation associated with organic heart disease. J Am Coll Cardiol 28, 985–990.

113. McCarthy PM, Cosgrove DM 3rd, Castle LW, *et al.* (1993) Combined treatment of mitral regurgitation and atrial fibrillation with valvuloplasty and the Maze procedure. Am J Cardiol 71, 483–486.

114. Sandoval N, Velasco VM, Orjuela H, *et al.* (1996) Concomitant mitral valve or atrial septal defect surgery and the modified Cox-maze procedure. Am J Cardiol 77, 591–596.

115. Millar RC, Arcidi JM Jr, Alison PJ. (2000) The maze III procedure for atrial fibrillation: should the indications be expanded? Ann Thorac Surg 70, 1580–1586.

116. Garson A Jr, Gillette PC, Titus JL, et al. (1984) Surgical treatment of ventricular tachycardia in infants. N Engl J Med 310, 1443–1445.

117. Garson A Jr, Smith RT Jr, Moak JP, et al. (1987) Incessant ventricular tachycardia in infants: myocardial hamartomas and surgical cure. J Am Coll Cardiol 10, 619–626.

118. Zeigler VL, Gillette PC, Crawford FA Jr, et al. (1990) New approaches to treatment of incessant ventricular tachycardia in the very young. J Am Coll Cardiol 16, 681–685.

119. Calkins H, Kalbfleisch SJ, el-Atassi R, et al. (1993) Relation between efficacy of radiofrequency catheter ablation and site of origin of idiopathic ventricular tachycardia. Am J Cardiol 71, 827–833.

120. O'Connor BK, Case CL, Sokoloski MC, et al. (1996) Radiofrequency catheter ablation of right ventricular outflow tachycardia in children and adolescents. J Am Coll Cardiol 27, 869–874.

121. Smeets JL, Rodriguez LM, Timmermans C, et al. (1997) Radiofrequency catheter ablation of idiopathic ventricular tachycardias in children. Pacing Clin Electrophysiol 20, 2068–2071.

122. Gatzoulis MA, Balaji S, Webber SA, et al. (2000) Risk factors for arrhythmia and sudden cardiac death late after repair of tetralogy of Fallot: a multicentre study. Lancet 356, 975–981.

123. Harrison DA, Harris L, Siu SC, et al. (1997) Sustained ventricular tachycardia in adult patients late after repair of tetralogy of Fallot. J Am Coll Cardiol 30, 1368–1373.

124. Jonsson H, Ivert T. (1995) Survival and clinical results up to 26 years after repair of tetralogy of Fallot. Scand J Thorac Cardiovasc Surg 29, 43–51.

125. Murphy JG, Gersh BJ, Mair DD, et al. (1993) Long-term outcome in patients undergoing surgical repair of tetralogy of Fallot. N Engl J Med 329, 593–599.

126. Nollert G, Fischlein T, Bouterwek S, et al. (1997) Long-term survival in patients with repair of tetralogy of Fallot: 36-year follow-up of 490 survivors of the first year after surgical repair. J Am Coll Cardiol 30, 1374–1383.

127. Knott-Craig CJ, Elkins RC, Lane MM, et al. (1998) A 26-year experience with surgical management of tetralogy of Fallot: risk analysis for mortality or late reintervention. Ann Thorac Surg 66, 506–511.

128. Oechslin EN, Harrison DA, Harris L, et al. (1999) Reoperation in adults with repair of tetralogy of fallot: indications and outcomes. J Thorac Cardiovasc Surg 118, 245–251.

129. Zhao HX, Miller DC, Reitz BA, et al. (1985) Surgical repair of tetralogy of Fallot. Long-term follow-up with particular emphasis on late death and reoperation. J Thorac Cardiovasc Surg 89, 204–220.

130. Deal BJ, Scagliotti D, Miller SM, et al. (1987) Electrophysiologic drug testing in symptomatic ventricular arrhythmias after repair of tetralogy of Fallot. Am J Cardiol 59, 1380–1385.

131. Downar E, Harris L, Kimber S, et al. (1992) Ventricular tachycardia after surgical repair of tetralogy of Fallot: results of intraoperative mapping studies. J Am Coll Cardiol 20, 648–655.

132. Harken AH, Horowitz LN, Josephson ME. (1980) Surgical correction of recurrent sustained ventricular tachycardia following complete repair of tetralogy of Fallot. J Thorac Cardiovasc Surg 80, 779–781.

133. Misaki T, Tsubota M, Watanabe G, et al. (1994) Surgical treatment of ventricular tachycardia after surgical repair of tetralogy of Fallot. Relation between intraoperative mapping and histological findings. Circulation 90, 264–271.

134. Lehnart SE, Wehrens XH, Laitinen PJ, et al. (2004) Sudden death in familial polymorphic ventricular tachycardia associated with calcium release channel (ryanodine receptor) leak. Circulation 109, 3208–3214.

135. Napolitano C, Priori SG, Bloise R. (2009) Catecholaminergic polymorphic ventricular tachycardia. Gene reviews 2009 cited August 1, 2010.; Available from: http://www.ncbi.nlm.nih.gov/bookshelf/br.fcgi?book=gene&part=cvt&log$=disease_name

136. Priori SG, Napolitano C, Memmi M, et al. (2002) Clinical and molecular characterization of patients with catecholaminergic polymorphic ventricular tachycardia. Circulation 106, 69–74.

137. Wilde AA, Bhuiyan ZA, Crotti L, et al. (2008) Left cardiac sympathetic denervation for catecholaminergic polymorphic ventricular tachycardia. N Engl J Med 358, 2024–2029.

138. Cetta F, Feldt RH, O'Leary PW, et al. (1996) Improved early morbidity and mortality after Fontan operation: the Mayo Clinic experience, 1987 to 1992. J Am Coll Cardiol 28, 480–486.

139. Cromme-Dijkhuis AH, Hess J, Hahlen K, et al. (1993) Specific sequelae after Fontan operation at mid- and long-term follow-up. Arrhythmia, liver dysfunction, and coagulation disorders. J Thorac Cardiovasc Surg 106, 1126–1132.

140. Fishberger SB, Wernovsky G, Gentles TL, et al. (1997) Factors that influence the development of atrial flutter after the Fontan operation. J Thorac Cardiovasc Surg 113, 80–86.

141. Fontan F, Kirklin JW, Fernandez G, et al. (1990) Outcome after a "perfect" Fontan operation. Circulation 81, 1520–1536.

142. Cohen MI, Wernovsky G, Vetter VL, et al. (1998) Sinus node function after a systematically staged Fontan procedure. Circulation 98(Suppl), II352–II358; discussion II358–II359.

143. Manning PB, Mayer JE Jr, Wernovsky G, et al. (1996) Staged operation to Fontan increases the incidence of sinoatrial node dysfunction. J Thorac Cardiovasc Surg 111, 833–839; discussion 839–840.

144. Balaji S, Gewillig M, Bull C, et al. (1991) Arrhythmias after the Fontan procedure. Comparison of total cavopulmonary connection and atriopulmonary connection. Circulation 84(Suppl), III162–III167.

145. Cecchin F, Johnsrude CL, Perry JC, et al. (1995) Effect of age and surgical technique on symptomatic arrhythmias after the Fontan procedure. Am J Cardiol 76, 386–391.

146. Pearl JM, Laks H, Stein DG, et al. (1991) Total cavopulmonary anastomosis versus conventional modified Fontan procedure. Ann Thorac Surg 52, 189–196.

147. Durongpisitkul K, Porter CJ, Cetta F, *et al.* (1998) Predictors of early- and late-onset supraventricular tachyarrhythmias after Fontan operation. Circulation 98, 1099–1107.

148. Gandhi SK, Bromberg BI, Schuessler RB, *et al.* (1996) Characterization and surgical ablation of atrial flutter after the classic Fontan repair. Ann Thorac Surg 61, 1666–1678; discussion 1678–1679.

149. Rodefeld MD, Gandhi SK, Huddleston CB, *et al.* (1996) Anatomically based ablation of atrial flutter in an acute canine model of the modified Fontan operation. J Thorac Cardiovasc Surg 112, 898–907.

150. Chinitz LA, Bernstein NE, O'Connor B, *et al.* (1996) Mapping reentry around atriotomy scars using double potentials. Pacing Clin Electrophysiol 19, 1978–1983.

151. Van Hare GF. (1998) Electrical-anatomic correlations between typical atrial flutter and intra-atrial re-entry following atrial surgery. J Electrocardiol 30(Suppl), 77–84.

152. Amodeo A, Galletti L, Marianeschi S, *et al.* (1997) Extracardiac Fontan operation for complex cardiac anomalies: seven years' experience. J Thorac Cardiovasc Surg 114, 1020–1030; discussion 1030–1031.

153. Blurton DJ, Dubin AM, Chiesa NA, *et al.* (2006) Characterizing dual atrioventricular nodal physiology in pediatric patients with atrioventricular nodal reentrant tachycardia. J Cardiovasc Electrophysiol 17, 638–644.

154. Karamlou T, Silber I, Lao R, *et al.* (2006) Outcomes after late reoperation in patients with repaired tetralogy of Fallot: the impact of arrhythmia and arrhythmia surgery. Ann Thorac Surg 81, 1786–1793; discussion 1793.

155. Silka MJ, Manwill JR, Kron J, *et al.* (1990) Bradycardia-mediated tachyarrhythmias in congenital heart disease and responses to chronic pacing at physiologic rates. Am J Cardiol 65, 488–493.

156. Midwest Pediatric Pacemaker Registry. Gerald Serwer Director cited 2010 August 1.; Available from: http://www.med.umich.edu/pdc

157. Gregoratos G, Abrams J, Epstein AE, *et al.* (2002) ACC/AHA/NASPE 2002 guideline update for implantation of cardiac pacemakers and antiarrhythmia devices: summary article: a report of the American College of Cardiology/American Heart Association Task Force on Practice Guidelines (ACC/AHA/NASPE Committee to Update the 1998 Pacemaker Guidelines). Circulation 106, 2145–2161.

158. Gregoratos G, Cheitlin MD, Conill A, *et al.* (1998) ACC/AHA Guidelines for Implantation of Cardiac Pacemakers and Antiarrhythmia Devices: Executive Summary–a report of the American College of Cardiology/American Heart Association Task Force on Practice Guidelines (Committee on Pacemaker Implantation). Circulation 97, 1325–1335.

159. Rao V, Williams WG, Hamilton RH, *et al.* (1995) Trends in pediatric cardiac pacing. Can J Cardiol 11, 993–999.

160. Michaelsson M, Jonzon A, Riesenfeld T. (1995) Isolated congenital complete atrioventricular block in adult life. A prospective study. Circulation 92, 442–449.

161. Hofschire PJ, Nicoloff DM, Moller JH. (1977) Postoperative complete heart block in 64 children treated with and without cardiac pacing. Am J Cardiol 39, 559–562.

162. Lillehei CW, Sellers RD, Bonnabeau RC, *et al.* (1963) Chronic postsurgical complete heart block with particular reference to prognosis, management, and a new P-wave Pacemaker. J Thorac Cardiovasc Surg 46, 436–456.

163. Weindling SN, Saul JP, Gamble WJ, *et al.* (1998) Duration of complete atrioventricular block after congenital heart disease surgery. Am J Cardiol 82, 525–527.

164. Kim JJ, Friedman RA, Eidem BW, *et al.* (2007) Ventricular function and long-term pacing in children with congenital complete atrioventricular block. J Cardiovasc Electrophysiol 18, 373–377.

165. Sachweh JS, Vazquez-Jimenez JF, Schondube FA, *et al.* (2000) Twenty years experience with pediatric pacing: epicardial and transvenous stimulation. Eur J Cardiothorac Surg 17, 455–461.

166. Webster G, Margossian R, Alexander ME, *et al.* (2008) Impact of transvenous ventricular pacing leads on tricuspid regurgitation in pediatric and congenital heart disease patients. J Interv Card Electrophysiol 21, 65–68.

167. Aellig NC, Balmer C, Dodge-Khatami A, *et al.* (2007) Long-term follow-up after pacemaker implantation in neonates and infants. Ann Thorac Surg 83, 1420–1423.

168. Fortescue EB, Berul CI, Cecchin F, *et al.* (2005) Comparison of modern steroid-eluting epicardial and thin transvenous pacemaker leads in pediatric and congenital heart disease patients. J Interv Card Electrophysiol 14, 27–36.

169. Kelle AM, Backer CL, Tsao S, *et al.* (2007) Dual-chamber epicardial pacing in neonates with congenital heart block. J Thorac Cardiovasc Surg 134, 1188–1192.

170. Kurosaki K, Miyazaki A, Watanabe K, *et al.* (2008) Long-term outcome of isolated congenital complete atrioventricular block pacing since neonatal period: experience at a single Japanese institution. Circ J 72, 81–87.

171. Glatz AC, Gaynor JW, Rhodes LA, *et al.* (2008) Outcome of high-risk neonates with congenital complete heart block paced in the first 24 hours after birth. J Thorac Cardiovasc Surg 136, 767–773.

172. Karpawich PP. (2008) Technical aspects of pacing in adult and pediatric congenital heart disease. Pacing Clin Electrophysiol 31(Suppl 1), S28–S31.

173. Tse HF, Lau CP. (1997) Long-term effect of right ventricular pacing on myocardial perfusion and function. J Am Coll Cardiol 29, 744–749.

174. Karpawich PP, Rabah R, Haas JE. (1999) Altered cardiac histology following apical right ventricular pacing in patients with congenital atrioventricular block. Pacing Clin Electrophysiol 22, 1372–1377.

175. Laske TG, Skadsberg ND, Hill AJ, *et al.* (2006) Excitation of the intrinsic conduction system through his and interventricular septal pacing. Pacing Clin Electrophysiol 29, 397–405.

176. Lieberman R, Grenz D, Mond HG, *et al.* (2004) Selective site pacing: defining and reaching the selected site. Pacing Clin Electrophysiol 27, 883–886.

177. Stephenson EA, Casavant D, Tuzi J, *et al.* (2003) Efficacy of atrial antitachycardia pacing using the Medtronic AT500 pacemaker in patients with congenital heart disease. Am J Cardiol 92, 871–876.

178. Khairy P, Roux JF, Dubuc M, *et al.* (2007) Laser lead extraction in adult congenital heart disease. J Cardiovasc Electrophysiol 18, 507–511.

179. Cooper JM, Stephenson EA, Berul CI, *et al.* (2003) Implantable cardioverter defibrillator lead complications and laser extraction in children and young adults with congenital heart disease: implications for implantation and management. J Cardiovasc Electrophysiol 14, 344–349.

180. Mathur G, Stables RH, Heaven D, *et al.* (2003) Cardiac pacemaker lead extraction using conventional techniques: a single centre experience. Int J Cardiol 91, 215–219.

181. Ng K, Kedia N, Martin D, *et al.* (2007) The benefits of biventricular pacing in heart failure patients with narrow QRS, NYHA class II and right ventricular pacing. Pacing Clin Electrophysiol 30, 193–198.

182. Lubitz SA, Leong-Sit P, Fine N, *et al.* (2010) Effectiveness of cardiac resynchronization therapy in mild congestive heart failure: systematic review and meta-analysis of randomized trials. Eur J Heart Fail 12, 360–366.

183. Janousek J. (2009) Cardiac resynchronisation in congenital heart disease. Heart 95, 940–947.

184. Janousek J, Gebauer RA, Abdul-Khaliq H, *et al.* (2009) Cardiac resynchronisation therapy in paediatric and congenital heart disease: differential effects in various anatomical and functional substrates. Heart 95, 1165–1171.

185. Villain E. (2008) Indications for pacing in patients with congenital heart disease. Pacing Clin Electrophysiol 31 (Suppl 1), S17–S20.

186. Cecchin F, Frangini PA, Brown DW, *et al.* (2009) Cardiac resynchronization therapy (and multisite pacing) in pediatrics and congenital heart disease: five years experience in a single institution. J Cardiovasc Electrophysiol 20, 58–65.

187. Dubin AM, Janousek J, Rhee E, *et al.* (2005) Resynchronization therapy in pediatric and congenital heart disease patients: an international multicenter study. J Am Coll Cardiol 46, 2277–2283.

188. The Antiarrhythmics versus Implantable Defibrillators (AVID) Investigators. (1997) A comparison of antiarrhythmic-drug therapy with implantable defibrillators in patients resuscitated from near-fatal ventricular arrhythmias. N Engl J Med 337, 1576–1583.

189. Bauersfeld U, Tomaske M, Dodge-Khatami A, *et al.* (2007) Initial experience with implantable cardioverter defibrillator systems using epicardial and pleural electrodes in pediatric patients. Ann Thorac Surg 84, 303–305.

190. Berul CI, Van Hare GF, Kertesz NJ, *et al.* (2008) Results of a multicenter retrospective implantable cardioverter-defibrillator registry of pediatric and congenital heart disease patients. J Am Coll Cardiol 51, 1685–1691.

191. Blom NA. (2008) Implantable cardioverter-defibrillators in children. Pacing Clin Electrophysiol 31(Suppl 1), S32–S34.

192. Chun TU, Collins KK, Dubin AM. (2004) Implantable cardioverter defibrillators in children. Expert Rev Cardiovasc Ther 2, 561–571.

193. Hsia TY, Bradley SM, LaPage MJ, *et al.* (2009) Novel minimally invasive, intrapericardial implantable cardioverter defibrillator coil system: a useful approach to arrhythmia therapy in children. Ann Thorac Surg 87, 1234–1238; discussion 1238–1239.

194. Kron J, Oliver RP, Norsted S, *et al.* (1990) The automatic implantable cardioverter-defibrillator in young patients. J Am Coll Cardiol 16, 896–902.

195. Silka MJ, Kron J, Dunnigan A, *et al.* (1993) Sudden cardiac death and the use of implantable cardioverter-defibrillators in pediatric patients. The Pediatric Electrophysiology Society. Circulation 87, 800–807.

196. Bove T, Francois K, De Caluwe W, *et al.* (2010) Effective cardioverter defibrillator implantation in children without thoracotomy: a valid alternative. Ann Thorac Surg 89, 1307–1309.

197. Khairy P, Harris L, Landzberg MJ, *et al.* (2008) Implantable cardioverter-defibrillators in tetralogy of Fallot. Circulation 117, 363–370.

198. Khairy P, Harris L, Landzberg MJ, *et al.* (2008) Sudden death and defibrillators in transposition of the great arteries with intra-atrial baffles: a multicenter study. Circ Arrhythm Electrophysiol 1, 250–257.

199. Epstein AE, DiMarco JP, Ellenbogen KA, *et al.* (2008) ACC/AHA/HRS 2008 Guidelines for Device-Based Therapy of Cardiac Rhythm Abnormalities: a report of the American College of Cardiology/American Heart Association Task Force on Practice Guidelines (Writing Committee to Revise the ACC/AHA/NASPE 2002 Guideline Update for Implantation of Cardiac Pacemakers and Antiarrhythmia Devices): developed in collaboration with the American Association for Thoracic Surgery and Society of Thoracic Surgeons. Circulation 117, e350–e408.

200. Silka MJ, Bar-Cohen Y. (2008) Should patients with congenital heart disease and a systemic ventricular ejection fraction less than 30% undergo prophylactic implantation of an ICD? Patients with congenital heart disease and a systemic ventricular ejection fraction less than 30% should undergo prophylactic implantation of an implantable cardioverter defibrillator. Circ Arrhythm Electrophysiol 1, 298–306.

201. Delaney JW, Moltedo JM, Dziura JD, *et al.* (2006) Early postoperative arrhythmias after pediatric cardiac surgery. J Thorac Cardiovasc Surg 131, 1296–1300.

202. Pfammatter JP, Wagner B, Berdat P, *et al.* (2002) Procedural factors associated with early postoperative arrhythmias after repair of congenital heart defects. J Thorac Cardiovasc Surg 123, 258–262.

203. Van Mieghem W. (1995) The complications of thoracic surgery: prophylaxis and treatment of arrhythmias. Acta Cardiol 50, 381–386.

204. Humes RA, Porter CJ, Puga FJ, *et al.* (1989) Utility of temporary atrial epicardial electrodes in postoperative pediatric cardiac patients. Mayo Clin Proc 64, 516–521.

205. Andreasen JB, Johnsen SP, Ravn HB. (2008) Junctional ectopic tachycardia after surgery for congenital heart disease in children. Intensive Care Med 34, 895–902.

206. Perry JC. (1997) Ventricular tachycardia in neonates. Pacing Clin Electrophysiol 20, 2061–2064.

207. Batra AS, Chun DS, Johnson TR, *et al.* (2006) A prospective analysis of the incidence and risk factors associated with junctional ectopic tachycardia following surgery for congenital heart disease. Pediatr Cardiol 27, 51–55.

208. Walsh EP, Saul JP, Sholler GF, *et al.* (1997) Evaluation of a staged treatment protocol for rapid automatic junctional tachycardia after operation for congenital heart disease. J Am Coll Cardiol 29, 1046–1053.

209. Dodge-Khatami A, Miller OI, Anderson RH, *et al.* (2002) Impact of junctional ectopic tachycardia on postoperative morbidity following repair of congenital heart defects. Eur J Cardiothorac Surg 21, 255–259.

210. Hoffman TM, Bush DM, Wernovsky G, *et al.* (2002) Postoperative junctional ectopic tachycardia in children: incidence, risk factors, and treatment. Ann Thorac Surg 74, 1607–1611.

211. Manrique AM, Arroyo M, Lin Y, *et al.* (2010) Magnesium supplementation during cardiopulmonary bypass to prevent junctional ectopic tachycardia after pediatric cardiac surgery: a randomized controlled study. J Thorac Cardiovasc Surg 139, 162–169.

212. Laird WP, Snyder CS, Kertesz NJ, *et al.* (2003) Use of intravenous amiodarone for postoperative junctional ectopic tachycardia in children. Pediatr Cardiol 24, 133–137.

213. Ommen SR, Odell JA, Stanton MS. (1997) Atrial arrhythmias after cardiothoracic surgery. N Engl J Med 336, 1429–1434.

214. Daoud EG, Strickberger SA, Man KC, *et al.* (1997) Preoperative amiodarone as prophylaxis against atrial fibrillation after heart surgery. N Engl J Med 337, 1785–1791.

215. Guarnieri T, Nolan S, Gottlieb SO, *et al.* (1999) Intravenous amiodarone for the prevention of atrial fibrillation after open heart surgery: the Amiodarone Reduction in Coronary Heart (ARCH) trial. J Am Coll Cardiol 34, 343–347.

216. Katariya K, DeMarchena E, Bolooki H. (1999) Oral amiodarone reduces incidence of postoperative atrial fibrillation. Ann Thorac Surg 68, 1599–1603; discussion 1603–1604.

217. The American Heart Association in collaboration with the International Liaison Committee on Resuscitation. (2000) Guidelines 2000 for Cardiopulmonary Resuscitation and Emergency Cardiovascular Care. Part 6: advanced cardiovascular life support: section 5: pharmacology I: agents for arrhythmias. The American Heart Association in collaboration with the International Liaison Committee on Resuscitation. Circulation 102(8 Suppl), I112–I128.

218. Gorgels AP, van den Dool A, Hofs A, *et al.* (1996) Comparison of procainamide and lidocaine in terminating sustained monomorphic ventricular tachycardia. Am J Cardiol 78, 43–46.

42

Heart Transplantation

Joseph W. Rossano, David L.S. Morales, and Charles D. Fraser Jr

Texas Children's Hospital, Baylor College of Medicine, Houston, TX, USA

History of Heart Transplantation

The genesis of solid organ transplantation dates back to the beginning of the last century with the pioneering work of Alexis Carrel and Charles Guthrie [1]. Carrel and Guthrie improved techniques of suturing vascular structures that enabled them to perform successful experiments of solid organ transplantation in animals [2,3,4,5], earning Carrel the Nobel Prize in Medicine and Physiology in 1912. This work was advanced by others including Frank Mann and colleagues [6] at the Mayo Clinic and Vladimir Demikhov at Moscow State University [7]. Demikhov's work initially went unnoticed in the west, but he performed hundreds of experiments with heart transplantation in animals, initially placing the heart in the neck of the animal but eventually replacing the recipient's heart with that of the donor. The first orthotopic heart transplantation in an animal was performed by Demikhov on Christmas Day in 1951 [7]. Novel work continued around the world by pioneers such as Norman Shumway and Richard Lower *et al.* at Stanford University [8], which culminated in the first human orthotopic heart transplantation being performed on December 3, 1967, by Christiaan Barnard [9]. The first heart transplantation to be performed in a human actually occurred 3 years earlier in 1964 by James Hardy, who transplanted a chimpanzee heart into a 68-year-old man with end-stage heart failure [10]. The patient survived for less than 2 hours, and the operation drew substantial criticism [11].

Just days after Barnard's operation, heart transplantation expanded into the pediatric arena with the first pediatric transplant being performed by Adrian Kantrowitz in a neonate with severe Ebstein anomaly of the tricuspid valve. The infant, however, survived for only several hours. Extending pediatric heart transplantation to the youngest of patients was promoted by Denton Cooley and colleagues, who performed the first successful pediatric heart transplant in 1964 [12], and then by Leonard Bailey and coworkers, who performed the first successful neonatal heart transplant [13]. Today, approximately 450 pediatric heart transplantations are reported to the International Society for Heart and Lung Transplantation (ISHLT) each year [14].

Etiology and Indication for Heart Transplantation in Children

Heart failure is not rare in children; a recent nationwide study from the United States described more than 12 000 admissions for heart failure in children annually [15]. Even though most of these children will never require heart transplantation, a significant number will progress to end-stage heart failure where the only real option is heart transplantation. Other therapies, such as left ventricular assist devices (LVADs) for "destination therapy" (i.e., placing the ventricular assist device where there is no expectation of ventricular recovery or heart transplantation) can be used successfully in selected adults with improved survival and quality of life [16]; however, this has not yet been used in children. Thus, the only therapy that exists to improve survival and quality of life for children with end-stage heart failure is heart transplantation.

Unlike adults, where cardiomyopathy and coronary artery disease account for the majority of patients undergoing heart transplantation, congenital heart disease (CHD) and cardiomyopathy account for the majority of cases in children undergoing transplant [14,17,18]. Infants (<12 months old) make up the largest portion of heart transplantations performed in childhood, accounting for approximately 25% of cases, with the remaining distributed somewhat evenly throughout the remaining childhood years (Plate 42.1, see plate section opposite p. 594) [14].

Some form of CHD is the most common reason for infant heart transplants, accounting for >60% of cases, whereas cardiomyopathy accounts for approximately 30% [14]. In contrast, cardiomyopathy accounts for >60% of transplantations in older children. Retransplantation, an increasing indication for transplantation, now accounts for 5% of the total number of transplants performed.

Complex CHD remains an important indication for transplantation not only in infants but in older children as well. Although in the past heart transplantation was advocated by some centers as a primary management strategy only for some lesions, such as hypoplastic left heart syndrome, this strategy has fallen out of favor as surgical outcomes for complex lesions have improved [19]. In the current era, most children with repaired CHD are suitable for heart transplantation after not having fared well some time after surgical intervention [20].

Dilated cardiomyopathy is the most common cardiomyopathy in children and accounts for the largest percentage of transplants among the types of cardiomyopathies [21,22,23]. While many children with cardiomyopathy will experience improvement and normalization of ventricular size and function with the initiation of medical and occasionally surgical therapy, the overall survival is poor. The transplant-free survival for patients with dilated cardiomyopathy is approximately 50% at 5 years [24,25]. The etiology of dilated cardiomyopathy is important in the patient's overall outcome: for example, fulminant myocarditis has some of the highest reported rates of normalization of ventricular function [26,27], whereas dilated cardiomyopathy from neuromuscular disorders has the worst reported outcomes [24].

Hypertrophic cardiomyopathy is a common cardiomyopathy in children, accounting for 25–42% of cardiomyopathies in childhood [21,22]; however, <5% of these patients will progress to heart transplantation [28,29]. Restrictive cardiomyopathy is the least common type of cardiomyopathy experienced in children [22,30,31]; nevertheless, this condition has an extremely poor prognosis [32]. The transplant-free survival rate is less than 50% at 5 years after diagnosis, and the risk of sudden death and the development of irreversible pulmonary hypertension is high [33,34,35]. Because no known medical therapies effectively alter the natural history of restrictive cardiomyopathy, many centers, including our own, will consider patients for heart transplantation at the time of diagnosis for restrictive cardiomyopathy [36].

Left ventricular noncompaction (LVN) is an increasingly recognized cardiomyopathy in children with and without CHD [37]. While the features and phenotype of LVN are variable, many of these children will have features similar to dilated cardiomyopathy with a dilated and poorly functioning left ventricle [37,38,39,40]. Some of these patients will progress to end-stage heart failure and require trans-

plantation. Arrhythmogenic right ventricular dysplasia/cardiomyopathy is a rare cardiomyopathy diagnosed in childhood. This cardiomyopathy is characterized by a loss of myocytes with fibrofatty infiltration of the right and often the left ventricle [41]. Arrhythmias are common with this condition.

Though overall survival has increased over time for children undergoing heart transplantation, this has been driven almost exclusively by the improvement in surviving the first posttransplant year [23,42]. Unfortunately, there has been little advancement in past two decades for survival after the first posttransplant year, with the current median survival after transplant being 11–18 years depending on the age at transplant [14]. Thus, many patients who have undergone heart transplantation in childhood will either die during childhood or require another heart transplant. The most common reason for late graft failure is transplant coronary artery disease, which will be discussed in a subsequent section. Because of the lack of long-term durability of the cardiac allograft, retransplantation has become an increasing reason for heart transplantation, now accounting for ~5% of the transplants performed annually. Several studies have found similar posttransplant survival in patients undergoing a retransplant compared with a primary heart transplant [43,44,45]. However, data from the United Network for Organ Sharing (UNOS) registry indicated that patients with early primary graft failure had a 1-year survival rate of only 53% [46].

Management of Chronic Heart Failure

Heart failure is generally a chronic, progressive disorder [47]. However, certain types of cardiomyopathies such as LVN can have an undulating phenotype with periods of improvement and/or deterioration in function [37]. Additionally, patients with acute myocarditis, especially the fulminant form, may have complete recovery of function. Guidelines exist for the management of chronic heart failure in adults and children and have been published by the ISHLT, the American College of Cardiology, and the American Heart Association [48,49]. The primary aims of therapy are to reduce symptoms, preserve long-term ventricular performance, and extend survival.

Pharmacologic Agents used for Treatment of Heart Failure

Diuretics
Treating symptoms of "congestion" is critical to the management of heart failure, both in the acute and chronic settings [49], and diuretics are recommended for patients with symptoms of heart failure and evidence of volume overload. However, the long-term use of diuretics may be

detrimental; in adults with heart failure, increasing loop diuretic dose has been identified as an independent predictor of mortality [50]. Thiazide diuretics and loop diuretics, such as furosemide, remain the most commonly used diuretics. In adults, aldosterone antagonists, such as spironolactone, have been shown to improve mortality when added to standard heart failure management [51], though there is an increase in hyperkalemia [52,53].

Angiotensin-Converting Enzyme Inhibitors/Angiotensin Receptor Blockers

Angiotensin-converting enzyme (ACE) inhibitors were the first agents to demonstrate improved survival in adults with symptomatic heart failure. Prospective, randomized, controlled trails of various agents within this class have demonstrated improvement in symptoms with reduced progression of heart failure, decreased hospitalization, and improved survival [54,55,56,57,58,59]. Angiotensin receptor blockers, primarily used in adults who are not tolerant of ACE inhibitors, have also demonstrated an improvement in mortality that is comparable, and possibly superior, to ACE inhibitors [60,61,62]. While there have been no large, randomized, controlled trials of ACE inhibitors in the treatment of pediatric heart failure, several studies have demonstrated hemodynamic and echocardiographic improvements [63,64,65].

Beta Blockers

As with ACE inhibitors, there is an accumulation of evidence from multiple, randomized, controlled trials of beta blockers in adult heart failure patients demonstrating benefits in symptoms, heart function, frequency of hospitalization, and survival [66,67,68,69]. Data on beta blocker use in pediatric heart failure is limited, but most have been supportive. Retrospective studies of metoprolol and carvedilol have demonstrated improved cardiac function [70,71], and a small, randomized, placebo-controlled study found that patients given carvedilol had an improvement in ejection fraction and New York Heart Association (NYHA) class over a 3-month period [72]. However, a multicenter, randomized, placebo-controlled trial of carvedilol failed to demonstrate an improvement in the composite heart failure outcome, ventricular function, or natriuretic peptide levels compared with placebo [73].

Digoxin

Digoxin is one of the oldest medications used for the treatment of heart failure symptoms. While effective in alleviating symptoms of heart failure [74], digoxin has not been shown to improve mortality [75], and higher doses are associated with an increase in mortality [76]. Data on children have been extrapolated from adult studies, and the current recommendations of the ISHLT are to use digoxin for symptomatic patients with the aim of reducing symptoms [48].

Management of Acute Heart Failure

Most patients who present with acute decompensated heart failure (ADHF) have adequate tissue perfusion but require higher filling pressures to achieve it; however, some patients will present in cardiogenic shock. Assessment of cardiac output is an important aspect of the initial and ongoing assessment of patients in heart failure. Indirect measures of cardiac output include mental status, heart rate, temperature of extremities, capillary refill time, and urine output. Laboratory assessment of cardiac output includes measurements of acid-base status and lactic acid. In the absence of intracardiac shunting, superior vena cava (SVC) saturation correlates well to pulmonary artery (PA) saturation [77]. Thus, a central line placed into the SVC can be used to approximate a mixed venous saturation.

Patients with congestion but adequate perfusion are likely the largest group of patients with ADHF and the group that responds best to medical therapy. Diuresis is a critical component of the initial management of these patients and may be the only therapy needed to improve symptoms in patients with adequate perfusion. In studies of adult patients, diuretics were found to increase stroke volume, decrease pulmonary capillary wedge pressure, and decrease systemic vascular resistance [78]. Diuretics combined with vasodilators have also been shown to decrease mitral regurgitation and increase forward ejection fraction [79]. Careful monitoring is warranted with aggressive diuresis, as volume depletion and renal insufficiency may result.

Patients with poor perfusion represent a significant group of patients with ADHF admitted to the intensive care unit. The initial approach to these patients will depend on the degree of circulatory compromise. The cornerstone of therapy for these patients is afterload reduction. Avoiding inotropic agents when possible appears to be beneficial. A review of more than 15000 adults hospitalized for heart failure observed higher in-hospital mortality in patients treated with dobutamine or milrinone compared with patients treated with nitroglycerin or nesiritide [80]. However, inotropic agents may be required to improve perfusion in this group of patients. The decision to use inotropic agents should be based primarily on clinical assessment, not on echocardiography. The goal of acute therapy is to have the patient in a compensated state of heart failure, not to improve echocardiographic measures of systolic function. Many patients can become compensated without the use of inotropic agents.

In adult patients, milrinone use is associated with improved symptoms and decreased filling pressures [81,82]. However, it is not clear that milrinone has an overall beneficial effect in patients with heart failure. In a study of almost 1000 patients evaluating the short-term use of milrinone versus placebo, there was no difference in mortality, hospital length of stay, or hospital readmission [83]. However, there was a significantly increased incidence of hypotension and arrhythmias in the milrinone-treated patients. In a retrospective analysis of this study, short-term milrinone in patients with ischemic cardiomyopathy was associated with increased in-hospital mortality and increased death or rehospitalization at 60 days [84]. Interestingly, patients with nonischemic cardiomyopathy had a decreased rate of death or rehospitalization at 60 days. Other studies have also supported the lack of overall benefit with milrinone. A prospective study of oral milrinone for chronic heart failure found that milrinone-treated patients had increased hospitalization, overall mortality, and cardiovascular mortality [85].

It is our practice to avoid catecholamines, especially at high doses, for the failing myocardium. Epinephrine has dose-dependent actions on alpha (α)- and beta (β)-adrenergic receptors. At low doses, β-adrenergic receptor response predominates, resulting in vasodilation, increased heart rate, and contractility. At higher doses there is α-adrenergic receptor stimulation resulting in vasoconstriction and increased systemic vascular resistance. The increased systemic vascular resistance and contractility may acutely improve perfusion, but will also increase myocardial oxygen consumption and myocardial work. Additionally, high-dose catecholamines for inotropic support will promote tachycardia and proarrhythmic effects, increase myocardial oxygen consumption, and depress the myocardial adrenergic response by downregulating β-adrenergic receptors. Furthermore, prolonged use of high-dose catecholamines may further amplify cardiomyocyte injury, thus aggravating diastolic and systolic ventricular dysfunction [86]. The failing myocardium will likely not tolerate long periods of epinephrine infusions.

In the setting of increased inotropic requirements for the failing myocardium, the situation is dire. Medical therapy is unlikely to return the patient to an asymptomatic state and continuation of therapy will increase the stress on an already stressed myocardium. At this point, mechanical support should be considered. A detailed description of mechanical circulatory support (MCS) is beyond the scope of this chapter, but a variety of options now exist. Total cardiopulmonary support from extracorporeal membrane oxygenation (ECMO), medium-term support with centrifugal pump devices (e.g., RotaFlow), and long-term support with LVADs (e.g., Thoratec, Berlin Heart, DeBakey VAD) are now available and are being used successfully.

The field of mechanical circulatory support for children is maturing; thus, ECMO should no longer be used for heart failure unless the patient is arresting or support is delayed (i.e., late presentation with compromised pulmonary function).

Transplantation Evaluation

All potential recipients of a heart transplant require a thorough pretransplant evaluation to assess the appropriateness of transplantation. The aim of this evaluation is to ensure as much as possible that long-term survival can be achieved. It is not only necessary to ensure the patient is an appropriate candidate from a medical standpoint, but also that there are no significant social or financial barriers that will limit the success of the transplantation.

Medical Evaluation

The medical evaluation is crucial so that transplantation is only offered to patients who are sick enough to benefit from the operation but not so sick with multiorgan system failure that they will not survive transplantation [87]. Table 42.1 includes generally accepted contraindications to heart transplantation [87]. Pediatric patients are quite sick once

Table 42.1 Contraindications. (Adapted with permission from Gajarski *et al.* [87].)

General contraindications

Presence of any noncardiac condition that significantly shortens life expectancy compared with that expected with cardiac transplantation or in conjunction with immunosuppressive requirements importantly reduces the expected survival after transplantation

Specific contraindications

Active infection
Active ulcer disease
Coexisting active neoplasm
Renal insufficiency[a]
Hepatic dysfunction with elevated transaminases[b]
Elevated, nonreactive pulmonary vascular resistance[c]
Recent pulmonary embolic event with infarction
History of or current recreational drug use
History of recurrent medical noncompliance

---

[a]Creatinine >2 times normal for age/body surface area (unless concomitant renal transplantation is planned).
[b]Aspartate aminotransferase/alanine aminotransferase (AST/ALT) out of proportion to that expected with passive congestion and may require liver biopsy for more complete assessment. May also include elevated total bilirubin. The presence of cirrhosis on liver biopsy generally contraindicates transplantation.
[c]Generally, pulmonary vascular resistance >6 Um^2 requires evaluation with vasodilators in the catheterization laboratory to test vascular bed reactivity with a target decrease in pulmonary vascular resistance to ≤4 Um^2.

listed for transplant, and the death rate while waiting for transplantation is high, especially for those with CHD requiring increased support such as mechanical ventilation, ECMO, or dialysis [88,89]. Our approach to recipient evaluation is detailed herein. However, certain portions of the evaluation may be delayed or deferred if the patient's status dictates urgency for listing.

A thorough evaluation of the underlying cardiac disease includes echocardiogram, electrocardiogram, usually cardiac catheterization, and occasionally other modalities such as computed tomography (CT), magnetic resonance imaging (MRI), and exercise testing [90,91]. It is imperative to rule out any residual cardiac disease that, if treated appropriately, could avoid the need for transplantation. This would include conditions such as residual coarctation, anomalous left main coronary artery arising from the PA, ventricular outflow tract obstruction, or unrecognized arrhythmias. Additionally, anatomic details including any systemic and pulmonary venous anomalies must be clarified as they may have implications for surgical technique [92,93]. Cardiac catheterization can reveal anatomic and hemodynamic data. Importantly, pulmonary vascular resistance, which may be elevated in patients with long-standing left atrial hypertension from heart failure, can be determined. Patients with elevated pulmonary vascular resistance are at increased risk for right ventricular failure in the donor graft after transplantation [94,95,96]. While the use of pulmonary vasodilators such as inhaled nitric oxide has improved the course of patients with elevated pulmonary vascular resistance [97,98,99], a pulmonary vascular resistance indexed to body surface area of >6 Woods units with pulmonary vasodilators or a transpulmonary gradient >15 mmHg are generally considered a relative contraindication to heart transplantation [36]. However, these cut-offs are no longer considered absolute, as the chronic use of pulmonary vasodilators, inotropic medications, and/or MCS may decrease the pulmonary vascular resistance and allow heart transplantation in some of these patients [98,100,101,102].

Other components of the medical evaluation include an assessment of other organ systems including neurologic, immunologic, renal, and gastrointestinal. Table 42.2 describes the laboratory data that we obtain as part of our pretransplant evaluation at Texas Children's Hospital. Part of the immunologic evaluation includes an assessment of the presence of antibodies against human leukocyte antigens. Patients with prior blood product or allograft material exposure, which is common in pediatric patients with CHD or MCS, are at increased risk for the development of these antibodies [103]. The presence of these antibodies is typically assessed via panel reactive antibody (PRA) testing; 10% reactivity is generally considered significant [104,105]. Patients with elevated antibodies are at increased risk for acute rejection and early graft loss [105,106,107,

Table 42.2 Transplant evaluation. (EBNA, Epstein-Barr nuclear antigen; Ig, immunoglobulin; PCR, polymerase chain reaction; RSV, respiratory syncytial virus.)

Laboratories	Cardiac evaluation (minimum)
Basic metabolic panel	Echocardiogram
B-type natriuretic peptide	Cardiac catheterization
Uric acid	Electrocardiogram, 24-hour Holter
Amylase	monitor
Lipase	
Total protein	**Consulting services**
Albumin	Infectious diseases
Prealbumin	Immunology
Lipid panel	Nutrition
Aspartate aminotransferase	Dentistry
Alanine aminotransferase	Social work
Gamma-glutamyltransferase	Child life
Alkaline phosphatase	
Lactate dehydrogenase	
Aldolase	
Creatine kinase	
Urinalysis	
Stool sample (culture, ova and parasites, alpha-1 anti-trypsin)	
Complete blood count	
Blood type	
Iron panel	
Reticulocyte count	
Sedimentation rate	
Complement (C3, C4)	
Immunoglobulins (IgG, IgM, IgE)	
Thyroid studies	
Viral hepatitis panel	
Human immunodeficiency virus	
Cytomegalovirus (CMV IgG, IgM, antigenemia, quantitative PCR, urine)	
Epstein-Barr virus (EBV IgG, IgM, EBNA, quantitative PCR)	
Respiratory secretions (viral culture, RSV, influenza)	
Nasal swab for methicillin-resistant *Staphylococcus aureus*	
Purified protein derivative test for tuberculosis	
Varicella (IgG)	
Toxoplasma (IgG)	
Panel of reactive antibodies	

108,109,110,111]. A detailed discussion of the treatment of patients sensitized to human leukocyte antigens is beyond the scope of this chapter. However, there are a number of strategies including avoidance of antigens from the potential donors [112], pretransplant medical therapy to decrease the number of antibodies [103], and posttransplant immunosuppressive strategies [40]. There is no clearly superior strategy or combination of strategies.

Our current strategy in sensitized patients is to avoid potential donor human leukocyte antigens that the recipient makes antibodies against. This is performed by a prospective crossmatch if the potential donor is local or a virtual crossmatch if the donor is not local. If a virtual crossmatch is employed, we have generally performed a volume exchange blood transfusion when cardiopulmonary bypass is initiated for the transplant. If the crossmatch is subsequently positive, we follow a protocol of plasmapheresis, intravenous immunoglobulin (Ig), and anti-CD20 monoclonal antibody (e.g., Rituximab).

An evaluation of active or latent infectious diseases is also important given the lifelong immunosuppression required after transplantation. There is no general agreement about what noncardiac medical issues constitute an absolute contraindication to transplantation. For example, human immunodeficiency virus (HIV) infection has been considered an absolute contraindication; however, there are now reports of successful transplantation in HIV-positive patients [113]. Likewise, significant neurologic injury or neurodevelopmental delay is often considered a contraindication to heart transplantation, but there have been successful transplantations performed in patients with significant neurologic issues. Thus, it is important that each case is considered individually and that the pros and cons of transplantation are evaluated carefully.

Donor Evaluation

There are several factors including donor size and age, distance from the institution, infectious considerations, and cardiac performance, that need to be taken into consideration for proper donor selection. Most importantly, the adequacy of the donor must take into account the state of the recipient. One cannot always wait for an ideal donor if the recipient is a critically ill child or has a limited donor pool (i.e., size <4 kg, PRA >50%). There is some controversy regarding the optimal donor size for pediatric heart transplant patients. Data from the ISHLT registry suggest that there is increased risk with both significantly undersized or oversized donors [114]. The use of oversized donors has been advocated by some centers, especially in cases of pulmonary hypertension, with the thought that the larger graft may decrease postoperative right ventricular failure [115]. The group from Loma Linda University did not find a difference in cardiac performance or days of ventilator support based on donor-to-recipient size. There were, however, more instances of lung collapse when oversized grafts were used [116]. The group has also demonstrated similar long-term outcomes, though their experience is better with over-sized grafts than undersized grafts [117]. A recent study from the UNOS registry did not find a difference on long-term survival based on donor-to-recipient weight ratios in children [118]. Other groups have found increased graft failure with undersized donors [119]. Our general policy has been to match the donor and recipient within 20% of weight; however, this guideline is not rigid and more liberal criteria are used depending on an individual patient's condition.

Donor age and size are generally closely correlated for younger patients, but older donors may be of acceptable size for adolescent patients. The issue of donor age in this group is important, as older patients are more likely to have significant cardiovascular disease, such as coronary artery disease, that may limit graft survival. There have been several studies that donor age is significant factor in long-term survival in pediatric heart transplant patients [14,120,121]. A recent study from UNOS found significantly worse survival when donors over 30 years of age were used for pediatric patients [121].

The distance of the donor from the transplant center is important, predominately for the ability to perform a prospective crossmatch for local donors and for donor heart ischemic times. A crossmatch is performed by testing the donor's tissue, usually lymphocytes, against the recipient's serum and assessing for an antibody-mediated reaction. This ideally is done before transplantation, as patients with a positive crossmatch are at significantly increased risk of acute graft failure. However, this approach limits the donor pool essentially to local donors. A virtual crossmatch may be performed in patients at increased risk for a positive crossmatch by performing tissue typing on the donor and assessing the antibody profile of the patient. A negative virtual crossmatch, however, does not guarantee a negative actual crossmatch. Thus, a crossmatch is still performed posttransplant. If the crossmatch is positive, generally the immunosuppression protocol is augmented. Donors at a long distance from the transplant center will have a longer ischemic time. However, with the advent of pediatric VAD explant and heart transplant, ischemic time is sometimes dictated by the explant procedure. Duration of donor ischemia has been associated with worse outcomes in many [94] but not all pediatric studies [14,122,123]. The group from Loma Linda University has been one of the largest proponents of not limiting potential donors on the basis of prolonged ischemic times. Their group has demonstrated functioning grafts with ischemic times as long as 10 hours [122].

Potential donors are screened for infectious diseases, including hepatitis B virus (HBV), hepatitis C virus (HCV), HIV, Epstein-Barr virus (EBV), and cytomegalovirus (CMV), that could be transmitted to the recipients. Current infection with HBV, HCV, or HIV would be considered a contraindication to transplantation. Cytomegalovirus and EBV may potentiate donor morbidity, such a posttransplant lymphoproliferative disorder and cardiac allograft vasculopathy; however, their presence does not preclude transplant. Most centers will administer prophylaxis against CMV infections posttransplant if either the donor or the recipient has a history of an infection.

Blood type compatibility is of interest in pediatric heart transplantation. Several studies from adult and pediatric patients have demonstrated superior outcomes when the donor and recipient are ABO identical (e.g., an O donor with an O recipient) as compared to ABO compatible (e.g., an O donor with a B recipient) [14,124,125,126]. However, even ABO-incompatible heart transplantation has been performed at times in infants, and reports have shown no decrease in survival [127,128]. While this strategy certainly has the potential to expand the donor pool for infants and thereby decrease waitlist mortality [127], a recent study from UNOS found that infants listed for ABO-incompatible hearts had similar waitlist mortality [129].

Ventricular function is frequently diminished in brain-dead donors and from donors who have undergone prolonged cardiopulmonary resuscitation [130]. Brain deaths are associated with increased catecholamines, altered thyroid hormone, and cortisol levels that can impair cardiac performance [130,131]. The use of inotropic medications is common in donors. It is difficult to quantitate the degree of ventricular dysfunction that precludes transplantation in children. While the use of high-dose inotropic support is considered a contraindication by many centers, a recent study from the Loma Linda University group found that when they accepted donors who had previously been turned down by other centers for donor quality, their long-term outcomes were not diminished [122]. The donor ejection fractions were as low as 37%, and 41% were on high-dose vasopressors [122]. There is a current interest in expanding the potential donor pool from brain-dead donors exclusively to donors after cardiac death. The limited experience with this strategy has demonstrated that transplantation can be successfully performed from donors after cardiac death [132].

Surgical Technique

Even though the right atrial technique developed by Lower and Shumway is still performed in some centers, the majority of programs (67% in the 2007 ISHLT registry) perform a bicaval-left atrial cuff technique. This was described by Sievers and associates in 1994 [133]. Through a standard median sternotomy, aortic and bicaval cannulation is established. High cannulation of the aorta and SVC will allow for adequate recipient cuffs. Also, dissection of the diaphragmatic reflection off the inferior vena cava (IVC) allows for low IVC cannulation and an adequate IVC recipient cuff. Once cardiopulmonary bypass has been established, the patient is cooled to 32 °C. The aorta is cross-clamped and antegrade cardioplegia is given until the heart stops. Caval snares are applied, the SVC is transected, and a large right atrial-IVC cuff is created. The aorta is transected followed by the main PA. Once com-

pleted, the dome of the left atrium is opened just posterior to the great vessels. The left atrial cuff is created being careful to include all four pulmonary veins but not the left atrial appendage. It is important to ensure hemostasis of the left atrial cuff.

Once the recipient field is prepared, the donor heart is removed from the transport cooler and prepared for implantation. The aorta and main PA are separated. The left atrium is prepared by opening the pulmonary veins and then making a uniform circular cuff. The atrial septum is then probed from the left atrial side and the right atrial side via the IVC to identify a patent foramen ovale. If present, it can be closed primarily. If lungs were procured, the left atrial appendage was most likely incised for decompression during the procurement procedure; this must be repaired.

Implantation consists of five anastomoses completed with a running Prolene polypropylene suture in the following order: left atrial cuff, aorta, IVC, SVC, and main PA (Figure 42.1) [134,135]. The three right-sided connections are done with the heart beating on cardiopulmonary bypass. The left atrial anastomosis is preformed first, starting at the base of the left atrial appendage and sewing to the IVC, ensuring that the cuff edges are everted out of the left atrium so that only endocardium is exposed to the blood stream. We believe this to be less thrombogenic. The left atrial anastomosis is not completely finished because a left heart vent is left in place. The aorta is prepared with the idea that it should be the shortest vessel among the SVC and PA so that the donor heart that often is small compared with the pericardial space will "hang" off the aorta. This will ensure that the SVC and PA are not under tension. As the aortic anastomosis is being completed, the left heart vent is turned off and the heart is de-aired. This anastomosis is completed and an anterior aortic vent is placed. The cross-clamp is removed and, once normal sinus rhythm has been established, the IVC anastomosis is completed followed by the SVC anastomosis. It is important, especially with infants, to make the SVC anastomosis tension free, aligned, and free of a purse-string effect. When connecting the main PA, it is important to remember that making it too long is a well described technical error that results in either main PA or branch PA stenosis secondary to buckling of the PA. Therefore, the donor and recipient PAs should be aggressively trimmed, making certain to keep the pulmonary valve and the branch PAs properly aligned. The patient should be completely rewarmed while the PA is anastomosed. We place a transthoracic left atrial line as well as temporary atrial and ventricular pacemaker wires. Before, separating from cardiopulmonary bypass, the heart should be lifted to ensure hemostasis of the left atrial suture line. Separation from bypass is performed under transesophageal echocardiography guidance to ensure excellent

A

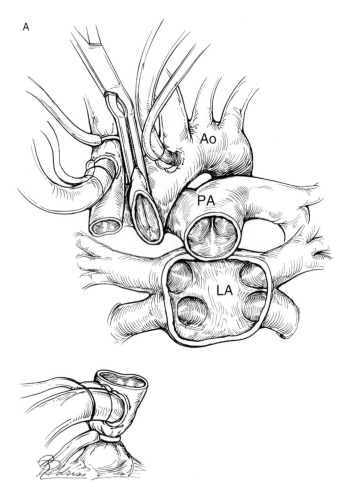

B

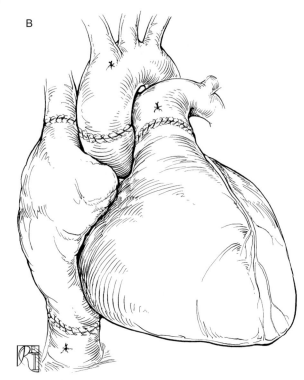

Figure 42.1 "Bicaval" cardiac transplantation. **A,** The recipient cardiectomy has been completed. Note the entire recipient right atrium has been removed. **B,** The completed implant. The sequence of anastomoses is (1) left atrial (LA), (2) aortic (Ao) (cross-clamp removed and heart perfused), (3) inferior vena cava, (4) pulmonary artery (PA), and (5) superior vena cava. (Reproduced with permission Backer *et al.* [135]. Copyright © 2000 Backer and Mavroudis.)

de-airing and to assess post-bypass ventricular and valvar function.

Many anatomic variants require special consideration; however, the vast majority are not a contraindication to heart transplant and can usually be resolved by procuring an adequate amount of tissue from the donor. A left SVC can be anastomosed to a donor innominate vein. Patients who have hypoplastic left heart syndrome can have their arch reconstructed with the donor aorta and the recipient arch vessels taken as a patch and sewn into the donor arch. An anatomic variant that can make transplant difficult occurs when all the pulmonary veins drain far to the right of the vertebral column. When anastomosed to the left atrium, these tend to become draped over the vertebral column causing obstruction. Left VAD explant and heart transplant is becoming a more frequent procedure in children and can prove challenging with regard to adhesions and aortic cannulation. Cannulae often are substernal. Techniques to avoid unwanted cavitary entry should be employed in consideration of future resternotomy. Also, enough ascending aorta may not be available to cannulate and cross-clamp at the time of transplant, especially in the smaller child with a VAD. Therefore, we often cannulate a shunt anastomosed to the innominate artery, which allows for a cross-clamp, an adequate aortic cuff, and the avoidance of circulatory arrest.

Postoperative Recovery

One of the clear distinctions between children recovering after heart transplantation compared with children with other forms of CHD is the need for immunosuppression. The cornerstone of immunosuppression at many centers has been triple drug immunosuppression with corticosteroids, a calcineurin inhibitor (e.g., cyclosporine or tacrolimus), and an antiproliferative agent (e.g., azathioprine or mycophenolate mofetil). This has been modified by many centers with steroid weaning or avoidance, and occasionally calcineurin inhibitor monotherapy. Other agents such as proliferation signal inhibitors (e.g., sirolimus or everolimus) may have a role in the prevention of coronary allograft vasculopathy; however, there is an increased risk of wound healing problems with these agents if used in the first few weeks after transplant [136]. Many centers will use additional agents at the time of transplant that are not part of the chronic immunosuppressive regimen, so-called induction therapy. Medications such as antithymocyte globulin and interleukin-2 receptor antagonists have been used for induction therapy. Some believe that with induction therapy the incidence of acute rejection can be diminished and that the initiation of calcineurin inhibitors, and their associated toxicities, can be delayed. While more than half of pediatric centers report the use of induction therapy, the use of therapy has not clearly been associated with decreased episodes of rejection or survival in the ISHLT registry [14]. As discussed previously, the presence of antibodies against donor antigens places the patient at increased risk for acute or hyperacute rejection and primary graft failure. This can have devastating effects in the early postoperative period. Treatment may include intensive immunosuppression and MCS, which has been used successfully for primary graft failure [137].

Patients with longstanding heart failure or certain CHD often have elevation in pulmonary vascular resistance (PVR). This can lead to donor right ventricular dysfunction and failure in the immediate postoperative period as the donor heart may respond poorly to the increased afterload. Medical therapy with pulmonary vasodilators such as inhaled nitric oxygen, isoproterenol, milrinone, and prostacyclin can be helpful in this clinical scenario [138,139]. These new therapies have clouded the limits of pretransplant PVR that would exclude transplant. Most patients with elevated PVR before heart transplantation will improve over time after transplantation [140].

It is important to note that the transplanted heart does not have the normal sympathetic innervation and thus may not respond in the usual manner to sympathetic stimulation. It has been our practice to use isoproterenol or cardiac pacing to avoid significant bradycardia in the immediate postoperative period. Partial reinnervation may occur over time [141,142]. Patients are also at risk for tachyarrhythmias, including ventricular tachycardia, likely occurring secondary to myocardial ischemia.

Long-Term Outcomes and Follow-Up

After heart transplantation, children require a lifetime of immunosuppression and are at risk for serious complications including graft rejection, cardiac allograft vasculopathy, infections, and malignancy. While there has been significant improvement in overall survival, this has been mostly from improved early survival. Patients who survive the first year posttransplant have good overall survival with >70% alive at 7 years after transplantation (Plate 42.2, see plate section opposite p. 594) [14].

The largest contributor to decreased graft longevity is the development of cardiac allograft vasculopathy; however, acute rejection remains an important cause of death even late after transplantation [14,143]. Cardiac allograft vasculopathy is a form of atherosclerosis distinct from the typical coronary artery disease in adults and consists initially of intimal proliferation and eventual luminal obstruction. Multiple immunologic and nonimmunologic factors likely contribute to the development of cardiac allograft vasculopathy including viral infection (e.g., CMV), rejection episodes, hypertension, hyperlipidemia, and diabetes [144].

Heart transplant patients are at an increased risk of multiple chronic comorbidities including hypertension, renal insufficiency, hyperlipidemia, cognitive difficulties, and psychological problems [14,145,146]. Fortunately, however, most are without major functional limitations. Data from the ISHLT indicates that more than 90% of patients have no limitations in physical activities [14].

Heart transplant for children remains the safest and most efficient therapy for children with end-stage heart failure.

References

1. Meine TJ, Russell SD. (2005) A history of orthotopic heart transplantation. Cardiol Rev 13, 190–196.
2. Carrel A. (1907) Heterotransplantation of blood vessels preserved in cold storage. J Exp Med 9, 226–228.
3. Carrel A. (1907) The surgery of blood vessels, etc. Johns Hopkins Hospital Bulletin 18, 18–28.
4. Carrel A, Guthrie CC. (1905) Functions of a transplanted kidney. Science 22, 473.
5. Carrel A, Guthrie CC. (1906) Successful transplantation of both kidneys from a dog into a bitch with removal of both normal kidneys from the latter. Science 23, 394–395.
6. Mann FC, Priestley JT, Markowitz J, *et al.* (1933) Transplantation of the intact mammalian heart. Arch Surg 26, 219–224.
7. Konstantinov IE. (1998) A mystery of Vladimir P. Demikhov: the 50th anniversary of the first intrathoracic transplantation. Ann Thorac Surg 65, 1171–1177.
8. Lower RR, Stofer RC, Shumway NE. (1961) Homovital transplantation of the heart. J Thorac Cardiovasc Surg 41, 196–204.
9. Barnard CN. (1967) The operation. A human cardiac transplant: an interim report of a successful operation performed at Groote Schuur Hospital, Cape Town. S Afr Med J 41, 1271–1274.
10. Hardy JD, Kurrus FD, Chavez CM, *et al.* (1964) Heart transplantation in man. Developmental studies and report of a case. JAMA 188, 1132–1140.

11. Aru GM, Call KD, Creswell LL, *et al.* (2004) James D. Hardy: a pioneer in surgery (1918 to 2003). J Heart Lung Transplant 23, 1307–1310.

12. Cooley DA, Frazier OH, Van Buren CT, *et al.* (1986) Cardiac transplantation in an 8-month-old female infant with subendocardial fibroelastosis. JAMA 256, 1326–1329.

13. Bailey LL, Nehlsen-Cannarella SL, Doroshow RW, *et al.* (1986) Cardiac allotransplantation in newborns as therapy for hypoplastic left heart syndrome. N Engl J Med 315, 949–951.

14. Kirk R, Edwards LB, Aurora P, *et al.* (2009) Registry of the International Society for Heart and Lung Transplantation: Twelfth Official Pediatric Heart Transplantation Report – 2009. J Heart Lung Transplant 28, 993–1006.

15. Rossano JW, Zafar F, Graves DE, *et al.* (2009) Prevalence of heart failure related hospitalizations and risk factors for mortality in pediatric patients: an analysis of a nationwide sampling of hospital discharges. Circulation 120, S586 (abstr).

16. Rose EA, Gelijns AC, Moskowitz AJ, *et al.* (2001) Long-term mechanical left ventricular assistance for end-stage heart failure. N Engl J Med 345, 1435–1443.

17. Kirk R, Edwards LB, Aurora P, *et al.* (2008) Registry of the International Society for Heart and Lung Transplantation: eleventh official pediatric heart transplantation report– 2008. J Heart Lung Transplant 27, 970–977.

18. Taylor DO, Stehlik J, Edwards LB, *et al.* (2009) Registry of the International Society for Heart and Lung Transplantation: Twenty-Sixth Official Adult Heart Transplant Report –2009. J Heart Lung Transplant 28, 1007–1022.

19. Bailey LL. (2009) The evolution of infant heart transplantation. J Heart Lung Transplant 28, 1241–1245.

20. Hsu DT, Quaegebeur JM, Michler RE, *et al.* (1995) Heart transplantation in children with congenital heart disease. J Am Coll Cardiol 26, 743–749.

21. Lipshultz SE, Sleeper LA, Towbin JA, *et al.* (2003) The incidence of pediatric cardiomyopathy in two regions of the United States. N Engl J Med 348, 1647–1655.

22. Nugent AW, Daubeney PE, Chondros P, *et al.* (2003) The epidemiology of childhood cardiomyopathy in Australia. N Engl J Med 348, 1639–1646.

23. Morales DL, Dreyer WJ, Denfield SW, *et al.* (2007) Over two decades of pediatric heart transplantation: how has survival changed? J Thorac Cardiovasc Surg 133, 632–639.

24. Towbin JA, Lowe AM, Colan SD, *et al.* (2006) Incidence, causes, and outcomes of dilated cardiomyopathy in children. JAMA 296, 1867–1876.

25. Redfield MM, Gersh BJ, Bailey KR, *et al.* (1994) Natural history of incidentally discovered, asymptomatic idiopathic dilated cardiomyopathy. Am J Cardiol 74, 737–739.

26. McCarthy RE 3rd, Boehmer JP, Hruban RH, *et al.* (2000) Long-term outcome of fulminant myocarditis as compared with acute (nonfulminant) myocarditis. N Engl J Med 342, 690 695.

27. Amabile N, Fraisse A, Bouvenot J, *et al.* (2006) Outcome of acute fulminant myocarditis in children. Heart 92, 1269–1273.

28. Nugent AW, Daubeney PE, Chondros P, *et al.* (2005) Clinical features and outcomes of childhood hypertrophic cardio-

myopathy: results from a national population-based study. Circulation 112, 1332–1338.

29. Decker JA, Rossano JW, Smith EO, *et al.* (2009) Risk factors and mode of death in isolated hypertrophic cardiomyopathy in children. J Am Coll Cardiol 54, 250–254.

30. Andrews RE, Fenton MJ, Ridout DA, *et al.* (2008) New-onset heart failure due to heart muscle disease in childhood: a prospective study in the United kingdom and Ireland. Circulation 117, 79–84.

31. Malcic I, Jelusic M, Kniewald H, *et al.* (2002) Epidemiology of cardiomyopathies in children and adolescents: a retrospective study over the last 10 years. Cardiol Young 12, 253–259.

32. Rivenes SM, Kearney DL, Smith EO, *et al.* (2000) Sudden death and cardiovascular collapse in children with restrictive cardiomyopathy. Circulation 102, 876–882.

33. Russo LM, Webber SA. (2005) Idiopathic restrictive cardiomyopathy in children. Heart 91, 1199–1202.

34. Kimberling MT, Balzer DT, Hirsch R, *et al.* (2002) Cardiac transplantation for pediatric restrictive cardiomyopathy: presentation, evaluation, and short-term outcome. J Heart Lung Transplant 21, 455–459.

35. Weller RJ, Weintraub R, Addonizio LJ, *et al.* (2002) Outcome of idiopathic restrictive cardiomyopathy in children. Am J Cardiol 90, 501–506.

36. Canter CE, Shaddy RE, Bernstein D, *et al.* (2007) Indications for heart transplantation in pediatric heart disease: a scientific statement from the American Heart Association Council on Cardiovascular Disease in the Young; the Councils on Clinical Cardiology, Cardiovascular Nursing, and Cardiovascular Surgery and Anesthesia; and the Quality of Care and Outcomes Research Interdisciplinary Working Group. Circulation 115, 658–676.

37. Pignatelli RH, McMahon CJ, Dreyer WJ, *et al.* (2003) Clinical characterization of left ventricular noncompaction in children: a relatively common form of cardiomyopathy. Circulation 108, 2672–2678.

38. Stanton C, Bruce C, Connolly H, *et al.* (2009) Isolated left ventricular noncompaction syndrome. Am J Cardiol 104, 1135–1138.

39. Koh C, Lee PW, Yung TC, *et al.* (2009) Left ventricular noncompaction in children. Congenit Heart Dis 4, 288–294.

40. Fazio G, Pipitone S, Iacona MA, *et al.* (2007) The noncompaction of the left ventricular myocardium: our paediatric experience. J Cardiovasc Med (Hagerstown) 8, 904–908.

41. Maron BJ, Towbin JA, Thiene G, *et al.* (2006) Contemporary definitions and classification of the cardiomyopathies: an American Heart Association Scientific Statement from the Council on Clinical Cardiology, Heart Failure and Transplantation Committee; Quality of Care and Outcomes Research and Functional Genomics and Translational Biology Interdisciplinary Working Groups; and Council on Epidemiology and Prevention. Circulation 113, 1807–1816.

42. Boucek MM, Edwards LB, Keck BM, *et al.* (2005) Registry of the International Society for Heart and Lung Transplantation: eighth official pediatric report–2005. J Heart Lung Transplant 24, 968–982.

43. Michler RE, Edwards NM, Hsu D, *et al.* (1993) Pediatric retransplantation. J Heart Lung Transplant 12, S319–S327.

44. Dearani JA, Razzouk AJ, Gundry SR, *et al.* (2001) Pediatric cardiac retransplantation: intermediate-term results. Ann Thorac Surg 71, 66–70.

45. Kanter KR, Vincent RN, Berg AM, *et al.* (2004) Cardiac retransplantation in children. Ann Thorac Surg 78, 644–649.

46. Mahle WT, Vincent RN, Kanter KR. (2005) Cardiac retransplantation in childhood: analysis of data from the United Network for Organ Sharing. J Thorac Cardiovasc Surg 130, 542–546.

47. Mann DL. (1999) Mechanisms and models in heart failure: A combinatorial approach. Circulation 100, 999–1008.

48. Rosenthal D, Chrisant MR, Edens E, *et al.* (2004) International Society for Heart and Lung Transplantation: Practice guidelines for management of heart failure in children. J Heart Lung Transplant 23, 1313–1333.

49. Hunt SA, Abraham WT, Chin MH, *et al.* (2005) ACC/AHA 2005 Guideline Update for the Diagnosis and Management of Chronic Heart Failure in the Adult: a report of the American College of Cardiology/American Heart Association Task Force on Practice Guidelines (Writing Committee to Update the 2001 Guidelines for the Evaluation and Management of Heart Failure): developed in collaboration with the American College of Chest Physicians and the International Society for Heart and Lung Transplantation: endorsed by the Heart Rhythm Society. Circulation 112, e154–e235.

50. Eshaghian S, Horwich TB, Fonarow GC. (2006) Relation of loop diuretic dose to mortality in advanced heart failure. Am J Cardiol 97, 1759–1764.

51. Pitt B, Zannad F, Remme WJ, *et al.* (1999) The effect of spironolactone on morbidity and mortality in patients with severe heart failure. Randomized Aldactone Evaluation Study Investigators. N Engl J Med 341, 709–717.

52. Pitt B, Williams G, Remme W, *et al.* (2001) The EPHESUS trial: eplerenone in patients with heart failure due to systolic dysfunction complicating acute myocardial infarction. Eplerenone Post-AMI Heart Failure Efficacy and Survival Study. Cardiovasc Drugs Ther 15, 79–87.

53. Svensson M, Gustafsson F, Galatius S, *et al.* (2004) How prevalent is hyperkalemia and renal dysfunction during treatment with spironolactone in patients with congestive heart failure? J Card Fail 10, 297–303.

54. The CONSENSUS Trial Study Group. (1987) Effects of enalapril on mortality in severe congestive heart failure. Results of the Cooperative North Scandinavian Enalapril Survival Study (CONSENSUS). N Engl J Med 316, 1429–1435.

55. Cohn JN, Johnson G, Ziesche S, *et al.* (1991) A comparison of enalapril with hydralazine-isosorbide dinitrate in the treatment of chronic congestive heart failure. N Engl J Med 325, 303–310.

56. The SOLVD Investigators. (1991) Effect of enalapril on survival in patients with reduced left ventricular ejection fractions and congestive heart failure. N Engl J Med 325, 293–302.

57. Pfeffer MA, Braunwald E, Moye LA, *et al.* (1992) Effect of captopril on mortality and morbidity in patients with left ventricular dysfunction after myocardial infarction. Results of the survival and ventricular enlargement trial. The SAVE Investigators. N Engl J Med 327, 669–677.

58. Packer M, Poole-Wilson PA, Armstrong PW, *et al.* (1999) Comparative effects of low and high doses of the angiotensin-converting enzyme inhibitor, lisinopril, on morbidity and mortality in chronic heart failure. ATLAS Study Group. Circulation 100, 2312–2318.

59. The SOLVD Investigators. (1992) Effect of enalapril on mortality and the development of heart failure in asymptomatic patients with reduced left ventricular ejection fractions. N Engl J Med 327, 685–691.

60. Sharma D, Buyse M, Pitt B, *et al.* (2000) Meta-analysis of observed mortality data from all-controlled, double-blind, multiple-dose studies of losartan in heart failure. Losartan Heart Failure Mortality Meta-analysis Study Group. Am J Cardiol 85, 187–192.

61. Hamroff G, Katz SD, Mancini D, *et al.* (1999) Addition of angiotensin II receptor blockade to maximal angiotensin-converting enzyme inhibition improves exercise capacity in patients with severe congestive heart failure. Circulation 99, 990–992.

62. Wong M, Staszewsky L, Latini R, *et al.* (2002) Valsartan benefits left ventricular structure and function in heart failure: Val-HeFT echocardiographic study. J Am Coll Cardiol 40, 970–975.

63. Bengur AR, Beekman RH, Rocchini AP, *et al.* (1991) Acute hemodynamic effects of captopril in children with a congestive or restrictive cardiomyopathy. Circulation 83, 523–527.

64. Stern H, Weil J, Genz T, *et al.* (1990) Captopril in children with dilated cardiomyopathy: acute and long-term effects in a prospective study of hemodynamic and hormonal effects. Pediatr Cardiol 11, 22–28.

65. Mori Y, Nakazawa M, Tomimatsu H, *et al.* (2000) Long-term effect of angiotensin-converting enzyme inhibitor in volume overloaded heart during growth: a controlled pilot study. J Am Coll Cardiol 36, 270–275.

66. (1999) The Cardiac Insufficiency Bisoprolol Study II (CIBIS-II): a randomised trial. Lancet 353, 9–13.

67. Hjalmarson A, Goldstein S, Fagerberg B, *et al.* (2000) Effects of controlled-release metoprolol on total mortality, hospitalizations, and well-being in patients with heart failure: the Metoprolol CR/XL Randomized Intervention Trial in congestive heart failure (MERIT-HF). MERIT-HF Study Group. JAMA 283, 1295–1302.

68. Packer M, Coats AJ, Fowler MB, *et al.* (2001) Effect of carvedilol on survival in severe chronic heart failure. N Engl J Med 344, 1651–1658.

69. Poole-Wilson PA, Swedberg K, Cleland JG, *et al.* (2003) Comparison of carvedilol and metoprolol on clinical outcomes in patients with chronic heart failure in the Carvedilol Or Metoprolol European Trial (COMET): randomised controlled trial. Lancet 362, 7–13.

70. Shaddy RE, Tani LY, Gidding SS, *et al.* (1999) Beta-blocker treatment of dilated cardiomyopathy with congestive heart failure in children: a multi-institutional experience. J Heart Lung Transplant 18, 269–274.

71. Bruns LA, Chrisant MK, Lamour JM, *et al.* (2001) Carvedilol as therapy in pediatric heart failure: an initial multicenter experience. J Pediatr 138, 505–511.

72. Azeka E, Franchini Ramires JA, Valler C, *et al.* (2002) Delisting of infants and children from the heart

transplantation waiting list after carvedilol treatment. J Am Coll Cardiol 40, 2034–2038.

73. Shaddy RE, Boucek MM, Hsu DT, *et al.* (2007) Carvedilol for children and adolescents with heart failure: a randomized controlled trial. JAMA 298, 1171–1179.

74. Lee DC, Johnson RA, Bingham JB, *et al.* (1982) Heart failure in outpatients: a randomized trial of digoxin versus placebo. N Engl J Med 306, 699–705.

75. The Digitalis Investigation Group. (1997) The effect of digoxin on mortality and morbidity in patients with heart failure. N Engl J Med 336, 525–533.

76. Rathore SS, Curtis JP, Wang Y, *et al.* (2003) Association of serum digoxin concentration and outcomes in patients with heart failure. JAMA 289, 871–878.

77. Freed MD, Miettinen OS, Nadas AS. (1979) Oximetric detection of intracardiac left-to-right shunts. Br Heart J 42, 690–694.

78. Wilson JR, Reichek N, Dunkman WB, *et al.* (1981) Effect of diuresis on the performance of the failing left ventricle in man. Am J Med 70, 234–239.

79. Stevenson LW, Brunken RC, Belil D, *et al.* (1990) Afterload reduction with vasodilators and diuretics decreases mitral regurgitation during upright exercise in advanced heart failure. J Am Coll Cardiol 15, 174–180.

80. Abraham WT, Adams KF, Fonarow GC, *et al.* (2005) In-hospital mortality in patients with acute decompensated heart failure requiring intravenous vasoactive medications: an analysis from the Acute Decompensated Heart Failure National Registry (ADHERE). J Am Coll Cardiol 46, 57–64.

81. Anderson JL. (1991) Hemodynamic and clinical benefits with intravenous milrinone in severe chronic heart failure: results of a multicenter study in the United States. Am Heart J 121, 1956–1964.

82. Seino Y, Momomura S, Takano T, *et al.* (1996) Multicenter, double-blind study of intravenous milrinone for patients with acute heart failure in Japan. Japan Intravenous Milrinone Investigators. Crit Care Med 24, 1490–1497.

83. Cuffe MS, Califf RM, Adams KF Jr, *et al.* (2002) Short-term intravenous milrinone for acute exacerbation of chronic heart failure: a randomized controlled trial. JAMA 287, 1541–1547.

84. Felker GM, Benza RL, Chandler AB, *et al.* (2003) Heart failure etiology and response to milrinone in decompensated heart failure: results from the OPTIME-CHF study. J Am Coll Cardiol 41, 997–1003.

85. Packer M, Carver JR, Rodeheffer RJ, *et al.* (1991) Effect of oral milrinone on mortality in severe chronic heart failure. The PROMISE Study Research Group. N Engl J Med 325, 1468–1475.

86. Singh K, Communal C, Sawyer DB, *et al.* (2000) Adrenergic regulation of myocardial apoptosis. Cardiovasc Res 45, 713–719.

87. Gajarski RJ, Pearce BF. (2007) Recipient evaluation: medical and psychosocial morbidities. In: Canter CE, Kirklin JK, eds. *ISHLT Monograph Series: Pediatric Heart Transplantation.* Philadelphia, PA: Elsevier, pp. 19–32.

88. Almond CS, Thiagarajan RR, Piercey GE, *et al.* (2009) Waiting list mortality among children listed for heart transplantation in the United States. Circulation 119, 717–727.

89. Mital S, Addonizio LJ, Lamour JM, *et al.* (2003) Outcome of children with end-stage congenital heart disease waiting for cardiac transplantation. J Heart Lung Transplant 22, 147–153.

90. Mancini DM, Eisen H, Kussmaul W, *et al.* (1991) Value of peak exercise oxygen consumption for optimal timing of cardiac transplantation in ambulatory patients with heart failure. Circulation 83, 778–786.

91. O'Neill JO, Young JB, Pothier CE, *et al.* (2005) Peak oxygen consumption as a predictor of death in patients with heart failure receiving beta-blockers. Circulation 111, 2313–2318.

92. Doty DB, Renlund DG, Caputo GR, *et al.* (1990) Cardiac transplantation in situs inversus. J Thorac Cardiovasc Surg 99, 493–499.

93. Razzouk AJ, Gundry SR, Chinnock RE, *et al.* (1995) Orthotopic transplantation for total anomalous pulmonary venous connection associated with complex congenital heart disease. J Heart Lung Transplant 14, 713–717.

94. Huang J, Trinkaus K, Huddleston CB, *et al.* (2004) Risk factors for primary graft failure after pediatric cardiac transplantation: importance of recipient and donor characteristics. J Heart Lung Transplant 23, 716–722.

95. Bourge RC, Naftel DC, Costanzo-Nordin MR, *et al.* (1993) Pretransplantation risk factors for death after heart transplantation: a multiinstitutional study. The Transplant Cardiologists Research Database Group. J Heart Lung Transplant 12, 549–562.

96. Hoskote A, Carter C, Rees P, *et al.* (2010) Acute right ventricular failure after pediatric cardiac transplant: predictors and long-term outcome in current era of transplantation medicine. J Thorac Cardiovasc Surg 139, 146–153.

97. Gajarski RJ, Towbin JA, Bricker JT, *et al.* (1994) Intermediate follow-up of pediatric heart transplant recipients with elevated pulmonary vascular resistance index. J Am Coll Cardiol 23, 1682–1687.

98. Kao B, Balzer DT, Huddleston CB, *et al.* (2001) Long-term prostacyclin infusion to reduce pulmonary hypertension in a pediatric cardiac transplant candidate prior to transplantation. J Heart Lung Transplant 20, 785–788.

99. Khan TA, Schnickel G, Ross D, *et al.* (2009) A prospective, randomized, crossover pilot study of inhaled nitric oxide versus inhaled prostacyclin in heart transplant and lung transplant recipients. J Thorac Cardiovasc Surg 138, 1417–1424.

100. Perez-Villa F, Cuppoletti A, Rossel V, *et al.* (2006) Initial experience with bosentan therapy in patients considered ineligible for heart transplantation because of severe pulmonary hypertension. Clin Transplant 20, 239–244.

101. Salzberg SP, Lachat ML, von Harbou K, *et al.* (2005) Normalization of high pulmonary vascular resistance with LVAD support in heart transplantation candidates. Eur J Cardiothorac Surg 27, 222–225.

102. Morris CD, Smith RD, Kar B, *et al.* (2009) Successful cardiac transplantation in a patient with elevated pulmonary vascular resistance: a relative contraindication to transplantation. Heart Surg Forum 12, E59–E60.

103. Mehra MR, Uber PA, Uber WE, *et al.* (2003) Allosensitization in heart transplantation: implications and management strategies. Curr Opin Cardiol 18, 153–158.

104. Kerman RH, Susskind B, Kerman D, *et al.* (1998) Comparison of PRA-STAT, sHLA-EIA, and anti-human globulin-panel reactive antibody to identify alloreactivity in pretransplantation sera of heart transplant recipients: correlation to rejection and posttransplantation coronary artery disease. J Heart Lung Transplant 17, 789–794.

105. Kobashigawa JA, Sabad A, Drinkwater D, *et al.* (1996) Pretransplant panel reactive-antibody screens. Are they truly a marker for poor outcome after cardiac transplantation? Circulation 94, II294–II297.

106. Nwakanma LU, Williams JA, Weiss ES, *et al.* (2007) Influence of pretransplant panel-reactive antibody on outcomes in 8,160 heart transplant recipients in recent era. Ann Thorac Surg 84, 1556–1562; discussion 1562–1563.

107. Przybylowski P, Balogna M, Radovancevic B, *et al.* (1999) The role of flow cytometry-detected IgG and IgM anti-donor antibodies in cardiac allograft recipients. Transplantation 67, 258–262.

108. Bishay ES, Cook DJ, El Fettouh H, *et al.* (2000) The impact of HLA sensitization and donor cause of death in heart transplantation. Transplantation 70, 220–222.

109. Holt DB, Lublin DM, Phelan DL, *et al.* (2007) Mortality and morbidity in pre-sensitized pediatric heart transplant recipients with a positive donor crossmatch utilizing perioperative plasmapheresis and cytolytic therapy. J Heart Lung Transplant 26, 876–882.

110. Jacobs JP, Quintessenza JA, Boucek RJ, *et al.* (2004) Pediatric cardiac transplantation in children with high panel reactive antibody. Ann Thorac Surg 78, 1703–1709.

111. Rossano JW, Morales DL, Denfield SW, *et al.* (2009) Impact of panel-reactive antibodies on long-term outcome in pediatric heart transplant patients: an analysis of the United Network of Organ Sharing Databse. J Heart Lung Transplant 28, S232 (abstr).

112. Zangwill S, Ellis T, Stendahl G, *et al.* (2007) Practical application of the virtual crossmatch. Pediatr Transplant 11, 650–654.

113. Uriel N, Jorde UP, Cotarlan V, *et al.* (2009) Heart transplantation in human immunodeficiency virus-positive patients. J Heart Lung Transplant 28, 667–669.

114. Boucek MM, Waltz DA, Edwards LB, *et al.* (2006) Registry of the International Society for Heart and Lung Transplantation: ninth official pediatric heart transplantation report–2006. J Heart Lung Transplant 25, 893–903.

115. Bernstein D, Parisi F. (2007) The pediatric heart donor: evaluation of age, size, cause of death, donor heart function, and vitality. In: Canter CE, Kirklin JK, editors. *ISHLT Monograph Series: Pediatric Heart Transplantation*. Philadelphia: Elsevier. pp. 71–81.

116. Fullerton DA, Gundry SR, Alonso de Begona J, *et al.* (1992) The effects of donor-recipient size disparity in infant and pediatric heart transplantation. J Thorac Cardiovasc Surg 104, 1314–1319.

117. Razzouk AJ, Johnston JK, Larsen RL, *et al.* (2005) Effect of oversizing cardiac allografts on survival in pediatric patients with congenital heart disease. J Heart Lung Transplant 24, 195–199.

118. Davies RR, Russo MJ, Mital S, *et al.* (2008) Predicting survival among high-risk pediatric cardiac transplant recipients: An analysis of the United Network for Organ Sharing database. J Thorac Cardiovasc Surg. 135, 147–155.

119. Tamisier D, Vouhe P, Le Bidois J, *et al.* (1996) Donor-recipient size matching in pediatric heart transplantation: a word of caution about small grafts. J Heart Lung Transplant 15, 190–195.

120. Chin C, Miller J, Robbins R, *et al.* (1999) The use of advanced-age donor hearts adversely affects survival in pediatric heart transplantation. Pediatr Transplant 3, 309–314.

121. Morales DL, Zafar F, Rossano JW, *et al.* (2009) Pediatric cardiac graft survival is reduced when donors are over 30 years old. Circulation 120, S596–S597 (abstr).

122. Bailey LL, Razzouk AJ, Hasaniya NW, *et al.* (2009) Pediatric transplantation using hearts refused on the basis of donor quality. Ann Thorac Surg 87, 1902–1908; discussion 1908–1909.

123. Morgan JA, John R, Park Y, *et al.* (2005) Successful outcome with extended allograft ischemic time in pediatric heart transplantation. J Heart Lung Transplant 24, 58–62.

124. Nakatani T, Aida H, Frazier OH, *et al.* (1989) Effect of ABO blood type on survival of heart transplant patients treated with cyclosporine. J Heart Transplant 8, 27–33.

125. McKenzie FN, Tadros N, Stiller C, *et al.* (1987) Influence of donor-recipient lymphocyte crossmatch and ABO status on rejection risk in cardiac transplantation. Transplant Proc 19, 3439–3441.

126. Kocher AA, Schlechta B, Ehrlich M, *et al.* (2001) Effect of ABO blood type matching in cardiac transplant recipients. Transplant Proc 33, 2752–2754.

127. West LJ, Pollock-Barziv SM, Dipchand AI, *et al.* (2001) ABO-incompatible heart transplantation in infants. N Engl J Med 344, 793–800.

128. Patel ND, Weiss ES, Scheel J, *et al.* (2008) ABO-incompatible heart transplantation in infants: analysis of the united network for organ sharing database. J Heart Lung Transplant 27, 1085–1089.

129. Everitt MD, Donaldson AE, Casper TC, *et al.* (2009) Effect of ABO-incompatible listing on infant heart transplant waitlist outcomes: analysis of the United Network for Organ Sharing (UNOS) database. J Heart Lung Transplant 28, 1254–1260.

130. Power BM, Van Heerden PV. (1995) The physiological changes associated with brain death–current concepts and implications for treatment of the brain dead organ donor. Anaesth Intensive Care 23, 26–36.

131. Cooper DK, Novitzky D, Wicomb WN. (1989) The pathophysiological effects of brain death on potential donor organs, with particular reference to the heart. Ann R Coll Surg Engl 71, 261–266.

132. Boucek MM, Mashburn C, Dunn SM, *et al.* (2008) Pediatric heart transplantation after declaration of cardiocirculatory death. N Engl J Med 359, 709–714.

133. Sievers HH, Leyh R, Jahnke A, *et al.* (1994) Bicaval versus atrial anastomoses in cardiac transplantation. Right atrial dimension and tricuspid valve function at rest and during exercise up to thirty-six months after transplantation. J Thorac Cardiovasc Surg 108, 780–784.

134. Backer CL, Mavroudis C, Pahl E. (2003) Heart transplantation. In: Mavroudis C, Backer CL, eds. *Pediatric Cardiac Surgery*, 3rd ed. Philadelphia, PA: Mosby Inc.

135. Backer CL, Mavroudis C (2000) Pediatric transplantation, Part A: Heart transplantation. In: Stuart FP, Abecassis MM, Kaufman DB, eds. *Organ Transplantation*. Georgetown, TX: Landes Bioscience.

136. Kuppahally S, Al-Khaldi A, Weisshaar D, *et al.* (2006) Wound healing complications with de novo sirolimus versus mycophenolate mofetil-based regimen in cardiac transplant recipients. Am J Transplant 6, 986–992.

137. Tissot C, Buckvold S, Phelps CM, *et al.* (2009) Outcome of extracorporeal membrane oxygenation for early primary graft failure after pediatric heart transplantation. J Am Coll Cardiol 54, 730–737.

138. Kieler-Jensen N, Lundin S, Ricksten SE. (1995) Vasodilator therapy after heart transplantation: effects of inhaled nitric oxide and intravenous prostacyclin, prostaglandin E1, and sodium nitroprusside. J Heart Lung Transplant 14, 436–443.

139. De Broux E, Lagace G, Chartrand C. (1992) Efficacy of isoproterenol on the failing transplanted heart during early acute rejection. Ann Thorac Surg 53, 1062–1067.

140. Tenderich G, Koerner MM, Stuettgen B, *et al.* (2000) Preexisting elevated pulmonary vascular resistance: long-term hemodynamic follow-up and outcome of recipients after orthotopic heart transplantation. J Cardiovasc Surg (Torino) 41, 215–219.

141. Bernardi L, Bianchini B, Spadacini G, *et al.* (1995) Demonstrable cardiac reinnervation after human heart transplantation by carotid baroreflex modulation of RR interval. Circulation 92, 2895–2903.

142. Bengel FM, Ueberfuhr P, Schiepel N, *et al.* (2001) Effect of sympathetic reinnervation on cardiac performance after heart transplantation. N Engl J Med 345, 731–738.

143. Zuppan CW, Wells LM, Kerstetter JC, *et al.* (2009) Cause of death in pediatric and infant heart transplant recipients: review of a 20-year, single-institution cohort. J Heart Lung Transplant 28, 579–584.

144. Valantine H. (2004) Cardiac allograft vasculopathy after heart transplantation: risk factors and management. J Heart Lung Transplant 23, S187–S193.

145. Uzark K, Spicer R, Beebe DW. (2009) Neurodevelopmental outcomes in pediatric heart transplant recipients. J Heart Lung Transplant 28, 1306–1311.

146. Wray J, Pot-Mees C, Zeitlin H, *et al.* (1994) Cognitive function and behavioural status in paediatric heart and heart-lung transplant recipients: the Harefield experience. BMJ 309, 837–841.

CHAPTER 43

Pediatric Lung and Heart-Lung Transplantation

Dewei Ren, George B. Mallory Jr, David L.S. Morales, and Jeffrey S. Heinle

Texas Children's Hospital, Houston, TX, USA

Introduction

Lung and heart-lung transplantation have become accepted therapeutic modalities for end-stage pulmonary and pulmonary vascular diseases. In the past two decades more than 25 000 adult and 1200 pediatric lung transplantations were performed worldwide [1,2]. This life-saving procedure has been applied to a small but significant number of infants, children, and adolescents in a relatively small number of centers around the world. Over the last 10 years the number of lung transplants per year worldwide has ranged from 59 to 93 in recipients less than 18 years of age with the majority of these performed in adolescent patients (12–17 years) (Figure 43.1) [1]. This is in comparison to approximately 1000–2000 transplants performed annually in adults [2]. The number of infant transplants has continued to remain low, with less than 10 procedures performed each year since 1997 [1].

The number of centers performing pediatric lung transplants has been rising, with 32 centers reporting pediatric transplants in 2006, and 36 centers reporting transplants in 2007 [1]. A majority of these 36 centers are adult programs performing occasional lung transplants in adolescents. However, over the past 5 years, less than 10 pediatric centers report performing more then five transplants per year and no single pediatric center is consistently performing more than 20 transplants per year, while 38 adult centers are performing greater than 20 transplants per year [1,2]. Of these pediatric centers, only two centers have averaged more than 10 transplants per year from 2002 to 2009 [1,2].

To date, more than 549 pediatric heart-lung transplants (HLTs) have been performed [1]. The volume of pediatric HLT procedures has decreased since a peak in 1989 to recent years with only eight pediatric HLTs performed in 2007. This finding is probably because single-/double-lung transplantation offers potential advantages over HLT, including shorter waiting time and improved efficiency of organ utilization. High death rates on the waiting list [3] and poor long-term survival posttransplant may also be a limiting factor for HLT candidates.

Historical Background

The first human lung transplantation was performed by Hardy and his team in 1963 [4]. The patient was a 58-year-old male with severe emphysema and left lung carcinoma. Single-lung transplant was successfully performed, but the recipient died from renal failure and malnutrition on the 18th postoperative day. In 1967, Denton Cooley and associates performed HLT in a 2½-year-old girl with an atrioventricular canal defect and pulmonary hypertension [5]. The patient died 14 hours after the procedure. In 1969, Lillehei and colleagues transplanted a heart-lung block to a 43-year-old man, who expired 8 days later [6].

Between 1963 and 1980, multiple attempts at lung transplants were performed around the world with no real success. Most of these transplants were performed on debilitated patients as "rescue" attempts after the development of acute respiratory failure. Challenges presumably related to immunosuppression and healing of the airway anastomoses prevented successful application of lung and HLT until the early 1980s. The advent of cyclosporine and vascular anastomotic techniques led to the first successful HLT [7]. In 1981, Reitz performed the first successful HLT in a 45-year-old woman with idiopathic pulmonary hypertension [8]. She did well for more then 5 years after the transplantation. This was soon followed by the first successful single-lung transplant in 1983 and the first successful double-lung transplant in 1986, both performed by

Pediatric Cardiac Surgery, Fourth Edition. Edited by Constantine Mavroudis and Carl L. Backer.
© 2013 Blackwell Publishing Ltd. Published 2013 by Blackwell Publishing Ltd.

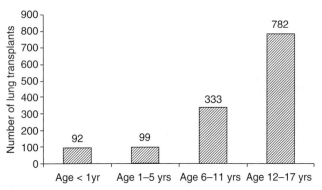

Figure 43.1 Pediatric lung transplantation age distribution and number, from January 1990 to June 2008. (Data from Aurora *et al.* [1].)

Table 43.1 Indication for pediatric lung transplantation by age group, January through June 2008. (Data from Aurora *et al.* [1].)

Diagnosis	<1 year	1–5 years	6–11 years	12–17 years
Cystic fibrosis (%)	2.4	5.1	53.0	69.2
Idiopathic pulmonary arterial hypertension (%)	13.4	22.2	10.7	7.6
Retransplant (%)	3.7	8.1	6.4	5.5
Congenital heart disease (%)	25.6	8.1	1.7	1.3
Pulmonary vascular disease (%)	9.8	5.1	3.0	0.2
Surfactant protein B deficiency (%)	13.4	4.0		
Other (%)	31.6	47.4	25.2	16.2

Cooper and his team at University of Toronto [9]. The first reported pediatric lung transplantation was performed in Toronto in 1987 in a 16-year-old boy with familial pulmonary fibrosis [10]. These practices have since been successfully employed to provide selected children with end-stage lung disease with years of improved quality of life.

In 1966 Shinoi and colleagues at Tokyo Medical College performed the world's first human lobar transplant [11]. However, the transplanted lobe was removed on postoperative day 18 because of graft failure. This attempt by Shinoi and team advanced knowledge and interest in lobar transplantation and foreshadowed the development of living donor lobar transplantation. The disparity between available donors and potential recipients of lung transplants remains a significant limitation to pediatric lung transplantation. Living donor lobar transplant has been tried as a partial solution to the problem of donor graft availability. Starnes and colleagues first introduced living donor lobar transplantation in 1993 [12]. Since most children are best treated with bilateral lung transplantation, living-donor lobar transplantation involves two suitable adult donors each donating a single lower lobe. Despite over 300 procedures having been performed worldwide, application of this technique has generally fallen out of favor, the number dramatically falling from a peak of 14 in both 1998 and 1999 to only three total procedures from 2005 to 2007 in the United States [1]. Recently, Date and colleagues have demonstrated impressive success with this technique with reported survival of 94% at 54 months in 31 patients [13].

Indications for Transplantation

The indication for lung transplantation is end-stage pulmonary parenchymal or vascular disease that is not amenable to any further medical or surgical therapy. Patients being considered for transplantation are generally those who are expected to die of their primary disease within 1–2 years.

Diseases leading to pediatric lung transplantation are distinct from those seen in adults. The primary indications for adult lung transplant are chronic obstructive pulmonary disease/emphysema, idiopathic pulmonary fibrosis, and cystic fibrosis (CF), while the indications in children depend on the age of the recipients. According to the Registry of the International Society for Heart and Lung Transplantation (ISHLT): Twelfth Official Pediatric Lung and Heart/Lung Transplantation Report – 2009 [1], the great majority of lung transplants in children greater than 5 years of age are performed for CF, whereas, in infants and preschool children, the most common indications are idiopathic pulmonary arterial hypertension, congenital heart disease, and surfactant dysfunction syndromes. A breakdown of these diagnoses by age group is listed in Table 43.1 [1]. Lung retransplant for severe graft dysfunction was the indication for 6% of lung transplants in children [1]. The total number of transplants reported to the Registry has remained relatively constant with approximately 50–60 pediatric lung transplants performed per year; this number was slightly higher in recent years with 87 transplants performed in 2006 and 93 transplants performed in 2007. The majority were performed in adolescent patients (Figure 43.1) [1] owing to CF or pulmonary hypertension.

For CF patients, bilateral lung transplantation, or occasionally, HLT, is indicated. Because end-stage pulmonary insufficiency in this disease has a significant infectious component, single-lung transplant has no practical role. Heart-lung transplantation is rarely performed for CF anymore, especially in North America, unless left ventricular function is significantly decreased. Patients with CF are considered for lung transplantation secondary to poor pulmonary function as indicated by a combination of the following: a forced expiratory volume in 1 second (FEV_1) below 30% of predicted normal value, hypercarbia, hypoxemia with requirement for supplemental oxygen, decreased 6-minute walk, or need for noninvasive ventilation. The level of pulmonary insufficiency warranting a lung transplantation consult usually results in a poor quality of life with a life expectancy of 1 year or less. More recently, unremitting infection requiring repeated hospitalizations and/or continuous intravenous antibiotics causing a poor quality of life has also become an indication for transplant in some patients. Patients with CF may benefit more from transplantation than other transplant groups [14].

The child with end-stage pulmonary hypertension is hemodynamically fragile and tends to follow an aggressive course with high pretransplant mortality [15,16]. Idiopathic pulmonary hypertension can be approached with single-lung, double-lung, or heart-lung transplantation depending on left ventricular function. Double-lung transplantation is now performed more often than single-lung or heart-lung transplantation for this indication without an increase in mortality or morbidity [17]. However, idiopathic pulmonary artery hypertension and congenital heart disease resulting in pulmonary vascular disease represent the most frequent indication for pediatric HLT over the past 8 years in North America [1].

Living donor lobar lung transplantation (LDLT) developed in 1993 [12] and became an accepted alternative to deceased donor lung transplantation in a few transplant centers in select patients with end-stage lung disease. One-year survival rate for LDLT recipients has been reported at 81% [18], which compared favorably with ISHLT average of 75% for pediatric transplant. Living donor lobar lung transplantation has also been reported to reduce the incidence of bronchiolitis obliterans in pediatric patients [19]. Complication rates in living donors have been reported to be as high as 20% [20], and prospective donors need to be informed of the potential morbidity and mortality associated with lobectomy. In retransplant patients, Kozower and colleagues have demonstrated that LDLT offers potential advantages over deceased donor donation and may be the preferred method of retransplantation for this high-risk group [21].

In properly selected patients, HLT provides a viable therapeutic option in those children with uncorrectable congenital heart disease and pulmonary vascular disease who are unresponsive to conventional management. Patients with surgically irreparable complex congenital heart disease with a systemic ventricular ejection fraction less than 35% and end-stage pulmonary disease or Eisenmenger's syndrome are candidates for HLT [22]. Gorler and associates reported 16 pediatric HLTs performed at Hannover Medical School, Germany [23]. Among them, nine patients had congenital heart disease with Eisenmenger syndrome, four patients had underlying pulmonary hypertension, and three with other diseases [23]. Another German group has performed 51 HLTs since 1983 with eleven patients younger than 14 years old [24]. Among these pediatric patients, idiopathic pulmonary hypertension was the indication for transplant in 55% of patients, pulmonary

atresia with severe pulmonary artery hypoplasia in 27%, and CF and cardiomyopathy with fixed pulmonary hypertension in 9% [24].

Contraindications to Transplantation

Medical and surgical contraindications to lung transplantation in children are listed in Table 43.2. In the current era, many of the contraindications can be viewed as relative and not necessarily absolute. Over time, the surgical contraindications to transplantation have narrowed at many centers. For example, several centers, including our own institution, have successfully performed thoracic organ transplantation in select children with significant scoliosis. A tracheostomy alone generally would not be considered a contraindication because early posttransplant decannulation could obviate the problem of a long-term portal of entry for microorganisms into the lower airway. In previously operated patients with pulmonary atresia and nonconfluent pulmonary arteries, transplantation is generally

Table 43.2 Medical and surgical contraindications to pediatric lung transplantation. (BID, twice daily; CF, cystic fibrosis.)

Absolute
1. Pan-resistant Gram-negative or mycobacterial lung and/or sinus infection in CF
2. Uncontrolled seizure disorder
3. Severe mental retardation
4. Current/history of substance or alcohol abuse
5. Positive serum pregnancy test at the time of evaluation
6. HIV infection
7. Chronic hepatitis B and C
8. Acute active viral infection
9. Multiorgan failure*
10. *Burkholderia cenocepacia* (genomovar 3) lower respiratory infection in patient with CF
11. Severe scoliosis or thoracic cage deformity
12. Poorly controlled diabetes mellitus
13. Active neoplasm
14. Serious and untreatable psychiatric disorder on the part of patient or primary caretaker
15. Severe tracheomalacia

Relative
1. Symptomatic osteoporosis or osteopenia
2. Pneumonectomy (unless volume-occupying device in place)
3. Panresistant microorganisms within the respiratory tract
4. Other *Burkholderia cenocepacia* complex lower respiratory infection
5. Daily systemic corticosteroids (>60 mg/day BID)
6. Severe malnutrition
7. Talc pleurodesis

*Multi-organ transplantation such as liver-lung, renal-lung or heart-lung transplantation might be an appropriate option.

contraindicated [25]. Pulmonary blood flow depends exclusively on collateral arterial supply, and in the context of previous thoracotomy, there may also be diffuse arterial connections across the pleura. In the early experience at St. Louis Children's Hospital, this particular clinical scenario predisposed to diffuse small arterial bleeding, which led to the early demise of several patients [25].

Issues of active infection are generally straightforward. It appears that outcome after lung transplantation in CF patients infected with the most virulent and transmissible form of *Burkholderia cepacia* infection is poor with an early mortality from infection approaching 50% [26,27]. Recently, *Burkholderia cepacia* complex has been differentiated into distinct species, of which *B. cenocepacia* [genomovar 3] appears to be the most virulent species post transplantation; we consider this organism to be an absolute contraindication to transplant.

Nonmedical contraindications include financial and psychosocial factors. Inability to attend follow-up visits or recalcitrant medical nonadherence are contraindications to transplant. It would seem obvious that serious mental health disorders or disability that would obviate cooperation with the administration of medication and/or follow-up testing are strong contraindications to transplantation. A thorough evaluation of the child and family by a child psychologist, pediatric social worker, and the team of transplant caregivers should be required before accepting or rejecting any individual candidate.

Timing of Referral

The timing of the referral and listing of patients for lung transplantation remains a difficult decision. The careful consideration of the natural history and prognosis of the underlying primary disease needs to be weighed against the projected survival time post transplant. Quality of life with and without a transplant and the waiting time for the patient while on the transplant list also need to be factored into the timing of the listing. The ultimate goals remain obtaining "maximal mileage" from the patient's native lung, conferring a greater chance of survival with a new lung, and avoiding death while waiting on the transplant list [28]. It is generally recommended to consider transplantation when the patient is symptomatic during activities of daily living (New York Heart Association class III or IV) and survival is expected to be limited to 1–2 years. Ultimately, life expectancy and quality of life issues are commonly used by referring physicians as determinants of when to refer [29]. Table 43.3 [29] outlines the general recommendation for timing of referral.

Allocation of Organs

Like their adult counterparts in the United States, pediatric candidates for lung transplantation used to be listed by ABO blood group, height range, and the date of initial listing. Waiting period was and remains highly variable

Table 43.3 Recommendations regarding timing of referral. (FEV, forced expiratory volume in 1 second; NYHA, New York Heart Association.) (Reproduced with permission from Sweet [29].)

	Timing of referral
Surfactant dysfunction disorders	Patients with SP-B deficiency and ABCA3 deficiency with refractory respiratory failure should be referred immediately
	Patients with SP-C deficiency and less severe forms of ABCA3 deficiency may respond to medical therapy and should be referred when unrelenting progression of disease develops
Idiopathic pulmonary hypertension	Patients who present in NYHA class III or IV or have evidence of right heart failure should be referred immediately
	Patients who fail to respond adequately to vasodilator therapy should also be referred
Eisenmenger syndrome	Refer when the trajectory of pulmonary hypertension appears to be worsening with impaired exercise tolerance and worsening quality of life
Other pulmonary vascular disorders (pulmonary vein stenosis, alveolar capillary dysplasia)	These patients should be referred immediately since they typically do not respond to medical management and are at risk for sudden death
Cystic fibrosis	Patients with percent predicted FEV_1 values less than 30%, frequent hospitalizations, refractory hypoxemia or hypercapnia should be referred for transplant
Bronchopulmonary dysplasia	Refer patients with recurrent or severe episodes of respiratory failure or evidence for progressive pulmonary hypertension and absence of significant comorbidities
Diffuse parenchymal lung disease	Patients without evidence for systemic disease that could affect outcome should be referred early

Waiting list deaths to transplants

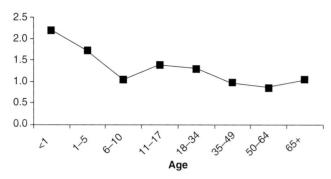

Figure 43.2 Ratio of the number of waiting list deaths to the number of transplants for each age group. (Reproduced with permission from Sweet [30].)

Table 43.4 Standard lung donor selection criteria.

Age <55 years

ABO blood group compatibility

Clear chest radiograph

Normal bronchoscopic examination

No history of pulmonary disease

Adequate gas exchange (PaO$_2$ >300 mmHg on FiO$_2$ 1.0 and PEEP 5 cmH$_2$O or PaO$_2$ 120 mmHg on FiO$_2$ 0.4 and PEEP 5 cmH$_2$O)

Absence of pulmonary contusion

Size matching

Negative serologic screening for hepatitis B, C and HIV

<20-pack-year smoking history

from region to region and center to center owing to a variety of factors. According to the data from Organ Procurement and Transplantation Network (OPTN) and the Scientific Registry of Transplant Recipients (SRTR), the incidence of waiting list deaths to transplants was higher in pediatric candidates than in most adults (Figure 43.2) [30], and post-transplant survival of adolescent lungs in adolescent recipients may be better than the survival of adolescent lungs transplanted into adults [30]. Therefore, allocation policies for potential recipients 12 years of age and older changed in May 2005 [30]. The new lung allocation scoring system (LAS) is based on waiting list urgency and measure of predicted transplant benefit. The score is calculated by multiple clinical measures, some of which are forced vital capacity (FVC), age, body mass index, 6-minute walk distance, diagnosis, and current use of mechanical ventilation. The LAS is currently being used only in patients 12 years of age and older because there were not enough data to generate a reliable LAS in younger candidates. Candidates 11 years of age and younger are still listed by date of listing and a simplified two-level status designation. Finally, OPTN recently prioritized lungs from pediatric donors to be preferentially offered to pediatric recipients in the local area before being offered to adults. With over 3 years since implementation, the LAS system has resulted in smaller waiting lists, shorter waiting times, and a shift in the predominant diagnosis group receiving transplantation [31]. While preliminary results on the effects of the new system on waiting list mortality and long-term survival have recently been published and showed no significant effects, more time is needed to assess its impact on organ allocation [32].

Donor Selection

Organ shortage is particularly significant for lung transplantation because less than 20% of suitable organ donors have lungs that meet the standard donor lung criteria [31].

Donor and recipient ABO compatibility is essential. Donor and recipient human leukocyte antigen (HLA) matching is not routinely required. Size considerations are important for pediatric recipients and donors because of the wide variability in size of the thorax and lungs during the span of childhood. Undersizing of the donor lung is to be avoided. Although some authors have expressed preference for donors less than 35 years old [33], there is no objective data to support this practice and recent data suggest that lungs from donors over 55 years of age have acceptable short- and intermediate-term success [34]. Satisfactory gas exchange of the donor lungs is confirmed by a PaO$_2$ to FiO$_2$ ratio of 300 or greater. A recent chest radiograph should show clear lung fields without evidence of infiltrates or contusion. Bronchoscopic assessment is performed to confirm normal airway anatomy and to identify and characterize any secretions and confirm the ease of clearance with suction. If mucopurulent secretions are present, easily cleared with suction and do not reaccumulate, the lungs may function acceptably after implantation. However, evidence of aspiration or persistent purulent secretions would be a contraindication to transplantation of that lung [35]. Standard donor lung criteria are outlined in Table 43.4.

Anesthetic and Operative Considerations

The pediatric anesthesiologist must be aware of the individual characteristics of each transplant recipient and their important comorbidities. Pediatric patients, especially infants, are more likely to be in the intensive care unit (ICU) at the time that organs become available than adult candidates. The transition from the ICU to the operating room should be managed with careful attention to timing of donor organ recovery and the condition and therapy of the child. Close coordination with the procurement team is critical to minimize donor lung ischemic time. As a rule, the recipient is moved to the operating suite 2 hours before the donor operation, allowing time for induction of anesthesia, line placement, and positioning without increasing ischemic time. Once the donor lungs are visualized and felt to be of acceptable quality, the recipient operation is begun. Furthermore, in our institution, a thoracic epidural catheter is inserted in most patients before surgery for intraoperative and postoperative infusion of local anesthetic.

Although single-lung transplantation is still a relatively common option in adult lung transplantation, most pediatric lung transplants involve bilateral lung transplantation and are performed with the use of cardiopulmonary bypass (CPB). Bilateral lung transplantation is preferred in most centers in children because of growth considerations, for CF patients because of irreversible bacterial infection in both lungs, and because there are usually two lungs available for most pediatric patients. Cardiopulmonary bypass provides adequate perfusion and oxygenation during the recipient pneumonectomy and donor implantation, aids in exposure and dissection of the hilar structures, allows both native lungs to be removed thereby minimizing contamination of the donor organ, provides the ability to cleanse (with instillation of antibiotic irrigation) the proximal tracheobronchial airway, and potentially minimizes ischemic time. The use of CPB also allows for gradual and controlled reperfusion of the implanted donor lungs to limit reperfusion injury and early graft dysfunction. The potential disadvantages of CPB include the associated coagulopathy owing to anticoagulation and hemodilution and the potential inflammatory effects of bypass.

Operative Technique

Organ Procurement

Following arrival at the donor hospital, the procurement team confirms appropriate brain-death notification, donor consents, and ABO compatibility. Serial arterial blood gas and chest radiograph results are reviewed. Flexible bronchoscopy via the endotracheal tube is performed to confirm normal anatomy and clear the airway of secretions. A final assessment is made by gross inspection of the lungs. The donor is ventilated throughout the recovery at an FiO$_2$ of 0.5 and a tidal volume 10 mL/kg. The administration of large fluid boluses is avoided. Airway heaters and heating blankets are discontinued.

Most commonly, the lung procurement is performed in conjunction with heart and abdominal organ procurement. The mediastinal organs are exposed via a median sternotomy which is continuous with a midline laparotomy for the abdominal organ procurement. Both pleural spaces are opened widely with care being taken to avoid injuring the lungs and creating an air leak. The lungs are visually inspected and palpated. Areas of atelectasis are recruited

by manual ventilation by the anesthesiologist under the surgeon's direct view. Throughout the procedure, over-inflation of the lungs must be avoided because distention is strongly associated with reperfusion injury. If the lungs are found to be acceptable, the implant team is notified of suitability and the anticipated donor cross-clamp time.

A pericardial well is created and the heart is inspected by the heart procurement team. The ascending aorta is mobilized to allow for placement of the aortic cross-clamp. The aorta and superior vena cava (SVC) are mobilized from the right pulmonary artery. The innominate vein and artery are mobilized to expose the trachea superior to the aortic arch. The trachea is circumferentially dissected to allow for later stapling with care being taken to avoid injury to the membranous portion during posterior dissection. Once thoracic and abdominal dissection is completed, the donor is systemically heparinized with 300 units/kg of heparin. A cardioplegia cannula is placed in the ascending aorta and a large bore cannula is placed in the distal main pulmonary artery (MPA) at the level of the bifurcation. A prostaglandin E1 bolus (500 µg mixed in 9 mL sterile water) is instilled into the MPA. The SVC is clamped, the left atrial appendage is amputated/incised to vent the left heart, the inferior vena cava (IVC) is transected, and the aortic cross-clamp is applied. The lungs are flushed antegrade with 50–60 mL/kg of cold (4 °C) flush solution given over approximately 5 minutes at low pressure. Our preferred lung preservation solution is an extracellular low potassium dextran (LPD) solution (Perfadex; Vitrolife, Goteborg, Sweden) shown clinically and experimentally to enhance graft preservation [36–38]. It is buffered with THAM and modified to include calcium chloride and sodium nitroprusside. Prostaglandin E1 (500 µg) is added to the first perfusate bag. The lungs are topically cooled with iced saline slush solution placed in the mediastinum and pleural spaces. Gentle ventilation is continued until the time of tracheal stapling. Care is taken to avoid effluent from the abdominal organs draining into the right pleural space and warming the lung. A suction catheter is placed in the incised IVC (or alternatively, the abdominal team may place a drainage catheter through the abdominal IVC) to capture the effluent. Clear Perfadex solution should be seen draining from the left atrial appendage. Complete decompression of the left heart should be confirmed during the administration of the flush solution.

After the cardioplegia and pulmonary flush are completed, the cannulae are removed and the heart is separated from the lungs. The IVC is divided and posterior pericardial attachments are divided to the level of the inferior pulmonary vein. The SVC is divided and separated from the right pulmonary artery. The MPA is divided at the level of the bifurcation. The distal ascending aorta is transected. The left atrium is divided with the heart and lung teams working together to insure adequate cuffs for both teams. The left atrium is incised inferiorly midway between the coronary sinus and pulmonary veins. The right and left

Table 43.5 Pediatric lung preservation protocol. (Adapted with permission from de Perrot *et al.* [39].)

Preservation solution: Perfadex®

Volume of antegrade flush solution: 50–60 mL/kg

Volume of retrograde flush solution: 250 mL per pulmonary vein, or 5 mL/kg for donor <40 kg

Pulmonary artery pressure during flush delivery: 10–15 mm Hg

Temperature of flush solution: 4 °C

Ventilator settings: FiO$_2$ 0.5, V$_T$ 10 cc/kg, PEEP 5 cmH$_2$O, airway pressure 15–20 cm H$_2$O

Storage temperature: 4 °C

pulmonary veins are visualized and the atrium divided leaving a cuff of left atrial tissue around the pulmonary vein orifices. The heart is removed from the field. Retrograde pulmonary flush is then delivered through the individual pulmonary veins (250 mL/vein for donors >40 kg or 5 mL/kg for donors <40 kg) to flush out thrombi or other material that may have embolized to the pulmonary arteries and to provide uniform flush of the capillary beds. The inferior pulmonary ligament is divided and the posterior mediastinal pleura are incised bilaterally. The endotracheal tube is withdrawn slightly and the trachea is stapled well above the bifurcation with the lungs expanded at approximately end-tidal volume. Care is taken to avoid over-inflation of the lungs during the final stages of recovery and transport. The trachea is divided and posterior dissection anterior to the esophagus is performed. The pericardium is excised anterior to the hilum. The pericardium at the diaphragm is incised to the level of the spine and the dissection is carried superiorly to the level of tracheal dissection. The lungs are removed to the back table and prepared for transport. They are immersed in lung preservation solution, triple bagged, and transported in ice. Donor lungs safely sustain an ischemic time up to 8 hours under these conditions. A summary of the authors' current protocol for lung preservation is outlined in Table 43.5 [39].

Deceased Donor Lung Transplantation

As noted, the vast majority of lung transplantations performed in children and adolescents use two donor lungs and CPB support. At the authors' institution, all pediatric transplants, with the exception of HLT, have been performed in this manner. The patients are intubated with a large single-lumen endotracheal tube and arterial and central venous accesses are obtained. A thoracic epidural catheter is placed preoperatively for perioperative pain management. The patient is positioned supine and padded appropriately. Although access to the lungs can be obtained

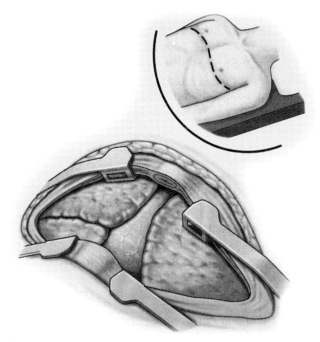

Figure 43.3 Transverse sternotomy with bilateral thoracotomy (clamshell incision). (Reproduced with permission from Nigro *et al.* [40].)

via sternotomy, bilateral anterior thoracotomies, or a bilateral thoracosternotomy incision (the so-called "clamshell" incision), we most commonly use the bilateral thoracosternotomy incision (Figure 43.3) [40] because of the excellent exposure of the mediastinal and hilar structures and both pleural spaces.

Once the donor lungs are confirmed to be of good quality, the recipient operation begins. The bilateral thoracosternotomy is performed in the fourth or fifth intercostal space. Initial chest wall dissection is carried out, dividing pleural adhesions with electrocautery. We perform the majority of the dissection on CPB. A pericardial well is created, the patient is heparinized, and the patient is cannulated for bypass using a single venous cannula via the right atrial appendage. If an intracardiac procedure is planned, direct bicaval venous cannulation is used. Bypass is established and the patient is cooled to 32–34 °C. An active vent is placed into the MPA. Ventilation is discontinued. For patients undergoing transplant for septic lung disease, tracheal secretions are aspirated and tobramycin irrigation is instilled into the airway. The remaining pleural adhesions are divided with electrocautery.

Bilateral recipient pneumonectomies are carried out. The inferior pulmonary ligament is divided. The hilar structures are mobilized with care being taken to identify and avoid injuring the phrenic and vagus nerves. The pulmonary veins are mobilized into the lung. The pulmonary arteries are dissected distal to the upper lobe takeoff and are controlled proximally with atraumatic snares. The pulmonary veins are divided individually between staple lines preserving a length of vein for the eventual atrial cuff. Dividing the veins first aids in exposure to the pulmonary artery. The pulmonary artery is ligated distally and divided. On the right side, the upper lobe artery is ligated and divided and the pulmonary artery is divided distal to the upper lobe branch. Tracheal secretions and the tobramycin irrigation are aspirated and a suction catheter is left in the airway. The bronchus is transected with care being taken to avoid contaminating the pleural space with residual tracheobronchial secretions. Large bronchial collateral arteries, common in recipients with CF, are controlled with hemoclips. The lungs are removed, and the pleural spaces irrigated with an appropriate antibiotic solution based on preoperative respiratory cultures with antibiotic susceptibility testing. Traction is placed on the pulmonary vein stumps and the pericardium is circumferentially incised around the veins exposing the left atrium. Meticulous hemostasis is obtained at this point as visualization of the posterior mediastinum and chest wall is difficult following implantation of the graft.

Bilateral sequential lung transplantation is then carried out. The donor lungs are brought onto the field and prepared. They are kept cold with iced saline sponges during the preparation. Bilateral atrial (pulmonary venous) cuffs are prepared. The pulmonary artery is transected. The left bronchus is stapled proximally and divided. Donor secretions are sent for culture. The right lung is returned to the cold preservative solution, still inflated while the left lung is implanted. The donor bronchus is trimmed to within several millimeters of the upper lobe bronchus. The lung is placed into the pleural space and kept cold with iced saline sponges. The bronchial anastomosis is performed first followed by the pulmonary venous anastomosis and finally the pulmonary artery anastomosis. An end-to-end bronchial anastomosis is performed using a running absorbable monofilament suture (polydioxanone) for the membranous portion and simple interrupted polydioxanone sutures on the cartilaginous portion (Figure 43.4) [40]. This technique allows for any size discrepancy and permits for future growth. The suction catheter is advanced into the left bronchus and left to low continuous suction. The pulmonary veins are retracted and a large vascular clamp is placed across the left atrium at the base of the veins. The staple lines are excised and a common pulmonary venous cuff created. An end-to-end pulmonary venous anastomosis is performed with running polypropylene suture (Figure 43.5). [40]. Before completing the anterior suture line, the pulmonary artery is flushed with iced preservative solution to de-air the pulmonary veins. The suture line is completed, the pulmonary veins controlled with an atraumatic snare, and the venous clamp removed. The donor pulmonary artery is trimmed to prevent kinking

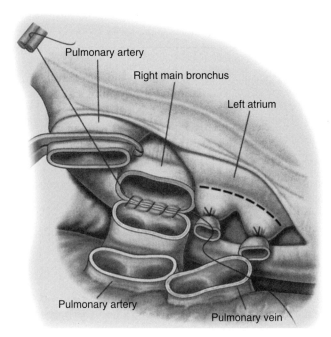

Figure 43.4 End-to-end right bronchial anastomosis. (Reproduced with permission from Nigro *et al.* [40].)

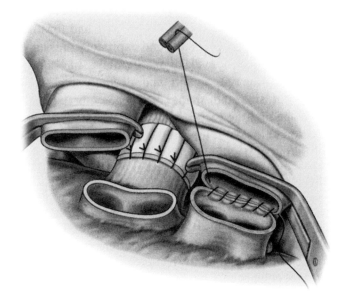

Figure 43.5 End-to-end right pulmonary vein anastomosis. (Reproduced with permission from Nigro *et al.* [40].)

of the artery owing to excessive length and end-to-end anastomosis performed with running fine polypropylene suture (Figure 43.6) [40]. Care is taken to avoid pursestringing of the anastomosis. The lung is packed in iced saline and in a similar fashion the right lung is implanted. Occasionally, the right pulmonary artery anastomosis is

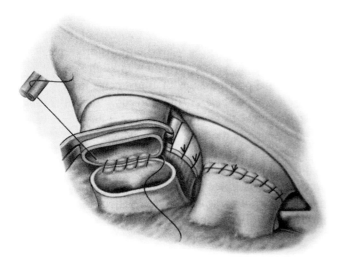

Figure 43.6 End-to-end right pulmonary artery anastomosis. (Reproduced with permission from Nigro *et al.* [40].)

performed distal to the recipient upper lobe branch based on relative diameter of the bronchi.

During the final anastomosis, the patient is rewarmed and bronchoscopy is performed by the anesthesiologist to clear the airway of secretions and blood and to confirm patency of the airway. An active vent is placed in the ascending aorta, the pulmonary artery vent is removed, and the pulmonary vein and artery snares removed. The lungs are ventilated with an FiO$_2$ of 0.5 and recruitment maneuvers performed keeping peak airway pressures less than 30 cm H$_2$O. Donor appropriate tidal volumes are used with a positive end-expiration pressure of 5 cm H$_2$O and peak inspiratory pressures less than 25 cm H$_2$O. Prostaglandin (0.025 μg/kg/min), dopamine and vasopressin infusions are begun as indicated by blood pressure, and the patient is slowly weaned from bypass over a 10–15-minute period to minimize reperfusion injury. Inhaled nitric oxide is frequently used to improve ventilation-perfusion mismatch during this phase of surgery and generally continued in the ICU. When graft function and hemodynamics are satisfactory, the patient is decannulated, heparin is reversed, and hemostasis is achieved. The mediastinum and pleural spaces are irrigated with antibiotic saline irrigation. Bilateral anterior and posterior chest tubes are inserted and placed to suction drainage. The sternum is reapproximated with stainless steel wires and the rib edges are reapproximated with interrupted, absorbable pericostal sutures. The soft tissues are closed in layers and the skin edges reapproximated with a running absorbable suture.

Living Donor Lobar Lung Transplantation

In 1990, Starnes introduced living donor lung transplantation (LDLT) [12]. In the most common form of LDLT, the recipient undergoes bilateral pneumonectomy and then receives implantation of lower lobes from each of two healthy adult donors. Given the size of even the shortest adults, LDLT is not a realistic option for children younger than 6 years of age [41]. Ideally, the donors should be taller than the recipient so that the donor lobe can readily fill the recipient hemithorax. There are important differences in performing a lobectomy for lobar transplantation in comparison with that for cancer or infection. The lobe must be removed with an adequate cuff of bronchus and pulmonary artery and vein to allow for successful implantation into the recipient [42]. Despite concerns of potential donor morbidity and mortality, Barr and Starnes and colleagues reported no perioperative or long-term mortality and a low morbidity rate following lobectomy for living lobar lung transplantation [43]. At the time of LDLT, three simultaneous thoracic operations are carried out – a requirement of resources that may be more than most transplant centers can mobilize. Although the most recent results achieved by Starnes in adults and children were acceptable, technical considerations and survival rates have been a problem in other institutions. We have not performed LDLT in our institution and readers are referred to Barr *et al.* [42] for a more detailed description of the operative technique.

Heart-Lung Transplantation

Sternotomy is frequently used in performing HLT. However, a bilateral thoracosternotomy (clamshell) is a useful alternative especially if significant adhesions are expected or if major bronchopulmonary or aortopulmonary collaterals are expected. However, bicaval cannulation can prove challenging via a clamshell incision as can the IVC anastomosis, both of which are easily achieved via sternotomy. The clamshell incision can be associated with more postoperative pain and prolonged respiratory insufficiency than the sternotomy. However, the use of an epidural catheter in these patients can greatly help with these issues and improve postoperative mobility. The clamshell incision is performed through the fourth or fifth intercostal spaces. When choosing where to transverse the sternum, we feel that it can be helpful to look at the preoperative computed tomography (CT) scan and chest X-ray to determine the level of the hilum, whether it is high or low in the thoracic cage.

The heart is cannulated for CPB using bicaval venous drainage. However, if the patient has significant aortopulmonary collaterals, which if excessive may be a contraindication to HLT, then they must be controlled so that adequate perfusion can be achieved with bypass. Once stable on bypass, the patient is cooled to nasopharyngeal temperature of 30 °C. The phrenic nerves are identified, and incisions in the mediastinal pleural reflection posterior to the phrenic nerves are created bilaterally. It is important that these pericardial windows are large enough to place the new lungs without having to put undue stress on the phrenic nerves. The ascending aorta is cross-clamped, and cardiac arrest is achieved with cardioplegia. The caval tourniquets are secured, and superior and inferior venae cavae are transected. The ascending aorta is transected as proximally as possible. The heart is excised leaving the pulmonary vein cuff behind and transecting the MPA. The hilum of the left lung is dissected out and the left pulmonary artery is transected, leaving a small button of the pulmonary artery at the insertion of the ligamentum arteriosum. This is done to protect the left recurrent laryngeal nerve. Once the phrenic nerve and vagus nerves have been clearly dissected off the hilum, the left atrial cuff is divided, followed by the left bronchus, allowing the left lung to be removed. The hilum of the right lung is dissected out, the right bronchus is transected, and the right lung removed. If there is an infectious component to the recipient's clinical history, one may choose to transect the airways after applying a thoracoabdominal stapler. The trachea is dissected to right above the carina and transected. One should minimize tracheal dissection especially laterally. The best opportunity to establish meticulous hemostasis of the posterior mediastinum is following completion of the recipient explantation as this area will be inaccessible after graft implantation.

The heart-lung donor block is brought onto the field and inspected. Once the block is placed in the chest with both pulmonary hila being posterior to the phrenic nerves, the trachea is cut one ring above the carina. An end-to-end tracheal anastomosis is accomplished using a running polydioxanone suture circumferentially or alternatively, running polydioxanone posteriorly with interrupted simple polydioxanone sutures anteriorly. The latter is a preferred technique when there is a significant size discrepancy between the airways. The donor and recipient aorta are tailored appropriately and an end-to-end aortic anastomosis is accomplished using a running polypropylene suture. After ensuring the absence of a donor patent foramen ovale, rewarming begins, the heart is de-aired, and the aortic cross-clamp is removed. After establishing a normal sinus rhythm, both caval anastomoses are created using a running polypropylene suture. Weaning off CPB is similar to that after bilateral lung transplantation.

Postoperative Management

Important immediate postoperative issues are graft function, bleeding, and stabilization of a critically ill patient after a major operation. Patients are initially managed in an ICU setting. A thorough physical examination, initial chest radiograph, continuous monitoring of blood pressure, central venous pressures, and gas exchange, and assessment of urine output are critical in assessing graft function and organ perfusion on arrival in the intensive

care unit. Fluid administration including the administration of blood products (always treated to eliminate all white blood cells) and inotropic agents are administered according to cardiac status and renal function. Judicious use of fluids is essential to avoid volume overload and pulmonary dysfunction in the early postoperative period. Inotropic agents and vasopressin are begun in the operating room to maintain adequate cardiac output and blood pressure in an effort to limit the use of volume bolus infusions to treat hypotension. A prostaglandin (alprostadil) infusion is begun before weaning from bypass and is continued for 48–72 hours postoperatively to promote pulmonary vasodilation and perfusion of pulmonary capillary beds. Inhaled nitric oxide is frequently employed in the early postoperative period to improve ventilation-perfusion mismatch. Flexible bronchoscopy is performed in the first 6–24 hours to inspect the bronchial anastomosis and the vascular supply of the bronchial mucosa just distal to the anastomosis and to perform bronchoalveolar lavage (BAL) to clear the airways and for the diagnosis of infection. Once hemostasis is assured and hemodynamics are satisfactory, weaning from ventilatory support should proceed as quickly as graft function permits. More than half of our pediatric patients are able to be weaned from ventilatory support within the first 24 hours postoperatively. We have used thoracic epidural anesthesia for postoperative pain control in our older patients to minimize the dosing of opiate therapy and to assist in mucus clearance and early mobilization of these patients.

For HLT, the postoperative management of these patients is almost identical to patients undergoing double-lung transplant at our institution. Their postoperative management is coordinated between the heart and lung transplant teams. However, immunosuppression and antimicrobial prophylaxis and therapy are managed by the lung transplant team. The postoperative course and complications are usually driven by the lungs. The surveillance for graft dysfunction, graft rejection, and infection is coordinated between the heart and lung transplant teams. In our institution, transbronchial biopsies and endomyocardial biopsies are routinely performed during the same anesthetic procedure at 2 weeks, 6 weeks, and 3, 6, 9, and 12 months after surgery.

Immunosuppression

With the introduction of cyclosporine into routine clinic practice nearly 30 years ago, early success in lung and heart-lung transplantation was achieved in pioneering centers, especially Toronto, Stanford, and Harefield in the United Kingdom. By 1990, these procedures became established treatment for adult and pediatric patients with advanced heart and lung disease. Most lung and heart-lung transplant programs rely on a triple-drug immunosuppression regimen consisting of a calcineurin inhibitor, an antimetabolite, and corticosteroids (cyclosporine/ tacrolimus, azathioprine/mycophenolate mofetil, and prednisone/prednisolone). The number of patients currently receiving tacrolimus is approximately double the number of those reported receiving cyclosporine and the majority of patients receive mycophenolate rather than azathioprine [1]. More than 95% of recipients remain on maintenance corticosteroids at 1 year and 5 years after transplantation [1].

In 2007, the International Pediatric Lung Transplant Collaborative (IPTLC), a consortium of pediatric lung transplant centers in the United States, Europe, Australia, and Canada, adopted an immunosuppression regimen consisting of tacrolimus, mycophenolate, and steroids for all pediatric lung transplants performed after January 1, 2007. Our immunosuppression protocol is based on the IPTLC consensus and is outlined in Table 43.6.

Induction Immunosuppression

Although induction therapy has been used to decrease the incidence and severity of acute rejection in solid organ transplantation, there are conflicting results from multiple studies regarding the effectiveness of induction therapy [44–49].

The most recent ISHLT registry [1] reports approximately 45% of pediatric lung transplants are recipients receiving induction immunosuppression. Interleukin-2 receptor (IL-2) antagonists (e.g., basiliximab and daclizumab) were used in approximately 30% of recipients while polyclonal anti-lymphocyte globulin (e.g., thymoglobulin or ATGAM®) was used in 10%. The IPTLC has concluded that no definitive long-term survival benefit or reduced incidence of bronchiolitis obliterans syndrome (BOS) has yet been demonstrated and no consensus regarding the use of induction therapy has been reached. We continue to use basiliximab as an induction agent in our practice (Table 43.6).

Perioperative Antimicrobial Prophylaxis

Antibiotic treatment before and after transplantation is not, in the strictest sense, prophylaxis. Most donor lungs, if cultured, grow one or more potential pathogens [35]. Cystic fibrosis patients have intrathoracic airways, including the proximal trachea and bronchi, which probably remain colonized and *in situ* after transplantation. Therefore, it is universal practice to choose an antibiotic regimen before, during, and immediately after lung transplantation tailored to the most recently cultured respiratory pathogens.

Table 43.6 Pediatric lung transplant immunosuppression protocol.

Preoperative

Tacrolimus: 0.05–0.1 mg/kg orally 2 hours before surgery

Basiliximab: 10 mg if less than 35 kg, 20 mg if greater than 35 kg intravenous (IV) before surgery

Mycophenolate mofetil (MMF): 600 mg/m² or 800 mg/m²

Intraoperative

Methylprednisolone: 10 mg/kg IV at skin incision

Postoperative (within the first two hours)

Tacrolimus: 0.05–0.15 mg/kg by nasogastric tube or gastrostomy tube and continue every 12 hours

MMF: IV infusion 30 mg/kg every 12 hours (maximum dose 1500 mg twice daily)

Methylprednisolone: 5 mg/kg IV every12 hours for 4 doses, then 1 mg/kg every 12 hours

Postoperative (beyond 2 hours)

Methylprednisolone: transition to oral prednisone when able to take medication orally

MMF: convert to oral when oral intake established (check MMF blood trough level weekly for first 6 weeks with target trough level 1.0–5.0 µg/mL)

Tacrolimus: convert to oral when oral intake established; daily morning blood trough assays (target trough level 12–15 ng/mL) are mandatory in the first days after transplantation when oral absorption, renal and hepatic drug metabolism, and clearance are dynamic

Basiliximab: same IV dose as preoperative on day 4

Maintenance

Prednisone: wean slowly to 1 mg/kg once daily by 2 weeks posttransplant, 0.5 mg/kg daily by 3 months, 0.25 mg/kg by 6 months, and 0.1–0.15 mg daily by 1 year posttransplant

Tacrolimus: target trough will be 12–15 ng/mL through the first 6 months, then if doing well without significant rejection, 10 ng/mL until 1 year, then 6–10 ng/mL depending on record of allograft rejection and renal function

MMF: titrated to blood trough levels (range as noted above) and white blood cell on serial determinations

Initial antibiotic choice in non-CF patients is usually limited to vancomycin and ceftazidime. In CF patients, at least two intravenous antipseudomonal antibiotics are chosen based on the most recent respiratory microbiological specimen. Other agents are chosen if *Pseudomonas aeruginosa* is either not present or not the exclusive pathogen. Two agents are chosen to obtain synergism between antibiotics and to lessen the chance of emergence of antibiotic-resistant organisms. Because of the severe morbidity of inapparent early graft fungal infection, antifungal therapy with inhaled amphotericin B and enteral voriconazole has become our practice in all transplant recipients. Depending on the clinical course and the results of respiratory cultures at transplant and the first bronchoalveolar lavage culture, amphotericin B is usually discontinued after 1–2 weeks. Virtually all patients remain on oral voriconazole titrated to therapeutic drug level for weeks to months after transplantation.

Lung transplant recipients who have circulating antibody for cytomegalovirus (CMV) before transplantation or who receive an organ from a donor with positive CMV serology are treated with intravenous ganciclovir for the first days posttransplant. As soon as the oral route has been established, oral valganciclovir is begun and continued for 5 months posttransplantation.

Trimethoprim-sulfamethoxazole is commenced the first week after transplantation as prophylaxis for *Pneumocystis jiroveci* pneumonia (PCP). Some programs continue PCP prophylaxis long-term; others discontinue after 3 months of therapy. Oral nystatin is commonly prescribed to reduce the likelihood of clinically significant oral candidiasis. Oral acyclovir is used in some programs routinely as prophylactic treatment for herpes simplex infection although this has not been a routine part of our perioperative protocol.

Outcome

Survival

One and 5-year survival rates for recipients transplanted in the most recent era (2002–2007) are 83% and 50%, respectively, compared with 67% and 43% for recipients transplanted between 1988 and 1994 [1]. The majority of this survival advantage is owing to improvement in early posttransplant survival likely owing to advances in donor and recipient selection, surgical technique, and postoperative management. Expected operative survival is now greater than 95%; however, conditional long-term survival is relatively unchanged over the different eras [1]. The most recent data from the ISHLT reveals an average survival for pediatric lung transplant similar to that for adult lung transplant: half-life of 4.5 years and 5.2 years, respectively

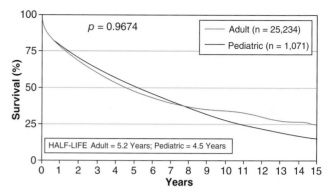

Figure 43.7 Kaplan-Meier survival by age group (pediatric vs. adult) for lung transplant performed from January 1990 through June 2007. (Reproduced with permission from Aurora *et al.* [1].)

(Figure 43.7) [1]. Among pediatric age groups, children under 1 year of age have survival half-life of 6.4 years compared with 5.7 years in children ages 1–11 years, and 4.2 years in adolescents. Children aged 1–11 years have a trend toward better survival than children aged 12–17 years at time of transplant. Outcomes for infants may be limited by a relatively higher incidence of early death. When early deaths are excluded (Figure 43.8) [1], infants have a trend toward better survival than adolescents, although there is no statistically significant difference between the two groups [1].

The causes of recipient death at different time points posttransplant are presented in Figure 43.9 [1]. Graft failure, technical issues, and infection are the most common cause of death in the early posttransplant period. Chronic rejection (bronchiolitis obliterans) is the most common cause of later death. Bronchiolitis obliterans syndrome has been reported in more than 40% of deaths at long-term follow-up posttransplant and is the most significant factor limiting long-term survival.

Pediatric HLT in the modern era, 1999 through June of 2007 [n = 122], has a graft half-life of 3.8 years. It appears that patients receiving HLT for idiopathic pulmonary artery hypertension (half-life 4.0 years) do significantly better than for other diagnoses like congenital heart disease (half-life 1.8 years). Infant HLT have been rare over the past two decades (n = 20) and have had disappointing outcomes (half-life 0.2 years). Early and late graft loss mimic those seen in lung transplantation with graft failure and infection dominating early graft loss and infection but predominately bronchiolitis obliterans being responsible for late graft loss. Overall survival analysis of pediatric heart-lung transplant recipients reveals at 5-year survival of 45% in the most recent era [1].

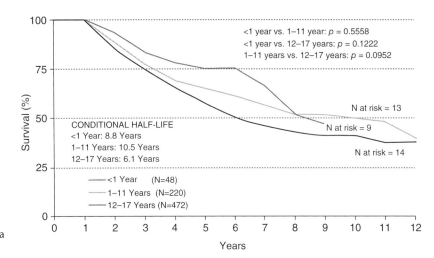

Figure 43.8 Conditional Kaplan-Meier survival by pediatric age group for lung transplants performed from January 1990 through June 2007. (Reproduced with permission from Aurora *et al.* [1].)

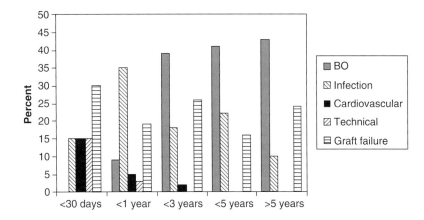

Figure 43.9 Cause of death after pediatric lung transplantation from January 1992 to June 2008. (BO, bronchiolitis obliterans.) (Data from Aurora *et al.* [1].)

Quality of Life After Lung Transplantation

Increasing attention has been given to assessments of the quality of survival following lung transplantation. Health-related quality of life (HRQL) has been defined on the basis of physical, psychological, and social function. Health-related quality of life has been reported by several authors to improve significantly in the physical and psychological components after lung transplantation [50–53]. Patients have reported better overall HRQL, higher level of energy and mobility, and decreased feelings of anxiety and depression compared with before transplantation. Furthermore, the functional status of long-term survivors of pediatric lung transplantation is good with 84% of children surviving 5 years after lung transplantation reporting no limitations in their activity [1]. However, BOS has a strong negative impact on quality of life, particularly on the physical component [53].

Acute and Chronic Rejection

Despite the introduction of improved immunosuppressive agents for use in transplantation, acute rejection affects up to 55% of lung transplant recipients within the first year after transplant [54]. Timely surveillance and accurate diagnosis of allograft rejection is central to the post-transplant care of children. Clinical presentation of acute rejection is usually without symptoms but may include fever, dyspnea, hypoxemia, leukocytosis, perihilar interstitial infiltrate on chest radiograph, and decline in FEV_1. Most frequently acute rejection is diagnosed in the absence of clinical signs in patients undergoing surveillance biopsy. Routine surveillance bronchoscopy with bronchoalveolar lavage and transbronchial biopsy is performed in lung and heart-lung transplant patients at 2 weeks, 6 weeks, and then every 3 months during the first year following transplantation in our program. Bronchoscopic biopsy allows acute rejection to be distinguished from other potential etiologies of allograft dysfunction such as airway stenosis or infection, and routinely is accompanied by bronchoalveolar lavage with viral, fungal, and quantitative bacterial cultures. The diagnosis of acute rejection is based on the histopathologic evaluation of the transbronchial biopsy specimen. The characteristic histologic appearance of rejection is the perivascular and interstitial mononuclear infiltrate with airway inflammation. Recent evidence

Table 43.7 Histologic grading of pulmonary allograft rejection. (Reproduced with permission from Stewart *et al.* [56].)

A: Acute rejection
    Grade A0 (none)
    Grade A1 (minimal)
    Grade A2 (mild)
    Grade A3 (moderate)
    Grade A4 (severe)
B: Small airways inflammation: lymphocytic bronchiolitis
    Grade B0 (none)
    Grade B1R (low grade)
    Grade B2R (high grade)
    BX (ungradeable)
C: Chronic rejection: obliterative bronchiolitis
    Present (C1)
    Absent (C0)
D: Chronic vascular rejection: Accelerated graft vascular sclerosis

Table 43.8 Refractory acute allograft rejection immunosuppression protocol from Texas Children's Hospital. (IV, intravenous; MMF, mycophenolate mofetil.)

Methylprednisolone 10 mg/kg IV for 3 consecutive days plus 10 days of IV Atgam or Thymoglobulin
or
Methotrexate 0.15–0.25 mg/kg orally 6-week course of once weekly
or
Sirolimus 3 mg/m^2 orally as single loading dose followed by 1 mg/m^2 orally once daily, follow serum trough levels aiming for 5-20 ng/mL
or
Push MMF dosing higher by up to 50% and follow blood trough levels
or
Total lymphoid irradiation

demonstrates that peribronchiolar mononuclear inflammation (also known as lymphocytic bronchiolitis) or even a single episode of minimal perivascular inflammation significantly increases the risk for bronchiolitis obliterans syndrome [55]. The internationally accepted classification for pulmonary rejection was revised in 2006 (Table 43.7) [56].

The first episode of grade A2 or greater acute rejection is treated with three consecutive days intravenous methylprednisolone at a dose of 10 mg/kg. Uncertainty remains whether to treat grade A1 and isolated B-grade airway inflammation. In light of recent evidence that grade A1 rejection and lymphocytic bronchiolitis are risk factors for BOS, treatment seems prudent. Most patients respond promptly to corticosteroids. For recurrent and/or persistent acute rejection of grade A2 or greater, the majority of programs will alter the immunosuppressant program in addition to intravenous methylprednisolone. Alternatives commonly considered include a course of cytolytic therapy, an intermediate course of weekly oral methotrexate, or substituting sirolimus for mycophenolate (Table 43.8).

Despite a shift toward more potent immunosuppressive regimens that incorporate tacrolimus and mycophenolate, the development of chronic allograft rejection, as manifested by BOS, continues to have a negative impact on the long-term survival of lung and heart-lung transplant recipients. Bronchiolitis obliterans is the major factor limiting prolonged survival in lung and heart-lung transplant recipients, and affects more than half of pediatric patients who survive transplantation for 5 years [1]. Bronchiolitis obliterans is a fibroproliferative process of the small airways that results in multifocal bronchiolar obliteration. Although the diagnosis of BOS is based on histologic findings, a tissue diagnosis via transbronchial or open lung biopsy may not always be possible. The ISHLT has proposed the use of a spirometric definition for the clinical diagnosis

Table 43.9 Bronchiolitis obliterans syndrome scoring system. (BOS, bronchiolitis obliterans syndrome; FEV, forced expiratory volume in 1 second.) (Reproduced with permission from Cooper *et al.* [57].)

0. No significant abnormality: FEV_1 >80% of the best postoperative value
1. Mild BOS: FEV_1 66–80% of the best postoperative value
2. Moderate BOS: FEV_1 50–65% of the best postoperative value
3. Severe BOS: FEV_1 <50% of the best postoperative value

of chronic allograft dysfunction based on serial lung function testing [57]. The term of BOS was established by the ISHLT [58] for patients with an unexplained and sustained decline in FEV_1 by a greater than 20% decrease from baseline and/or a greater than 25% decline in FEV 25 to 75 (FEV_{25-75}) without acute rejection or infection [58,59]. The severity of BOS is graded based on the recommendations of the ISHLT (Table 43.9) [57]. The prevalence of bronchiolitis obliterans increases steadily with time post-transplant (Figure 43.10) [1]. Clinical symptoms at onset (dyspnea, wheezing, exercise intolerance) are nonspecific or even absent. The diagnosis of BOS is based on serial lung function testing. Bronchoscopy with transbronchial and endobronchial biopsies is performed when a diagnosis of BOS is being considered to rule out airway stenosis or active, treatable infection and to assess via transbronchial biopsy the presence or absence of active lymphocytic inflammation within the airways suggesting active immune response, which might respond to augmentation of immunosuppression.

Once the diagnosis of BOS is established, first-line therapy is short-course corticosteroids and intravenous

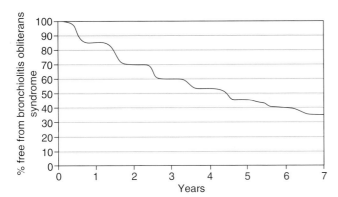

Figure 43.10 Freedom from bronchiolitis obliteran syndrome for pediatric lung recipients followed from April 1994 through June 2008. (Reproduced with permission from Aurora *et al.* [1].)

ATGAM or thymoglobulin or oral sirolimus. On occasion, alemtuzumab may be used. Because of the progressive nature of the disease, the average survival following onset of BOS is only 50% at 3 years [60]. For progressive BOS not responding to the above measures, retransplantation may be considered in select patients.

Only a minority of HLT recipients die as the result of cardiac disease or cardiac rejection [61]. Therefore, posttransplant surveillance and immunosuppression are based on the surveillance for pulmonary rejection.

Infection

Pediatric recipients are immunologically vulnerable to infections. Respiratory infections result in significant morbidity and mortality in lung and heart-lung transplant recipients in children. Infection has been reported for approximately 60–90% of recipients [62,63]. Infection is the leading cause of death among children who died between 1 month and 1 year posttransplant, accounting for almost 28% of deaths [1].

Bacterial infection is a serious infectious complication in lung and heart-lung transplant patients. Among all diagnosed infections, 35–66% are bacterial and 50–85% of patients present with at least one infectious episode [64]. Cystic fibrosis patients after lung or heart-lung transplant are particularly challenging. Their airway and sinuses are colonized with large numbers of virulent organisms, often multiresistant and pan-resistant Gram-negative organisms especially *Pseudomonas* species. As discussed previously, CF patients infected with *Burkholderia cenocepacia* have worse outcomes [65].

Cytomegalovirus has historically been the second most frequent cause of infectious complications following lung or heart-lung transplantation. Despite the use of various preventive strategies, the risk of developing CMV disease

in lung transplant recipients is over 30% during the first year [66]. Donor or recipient CMV seropositivity is associated with increased risk of CMV episodes. One recent study suggests that extended prophylactic regimens may be more efficacious in reducing CMV-related events [67].

Fungal pathogens most often responsible for infections in lung or heart-lung transplant recipients are *Candida* species, *Aspergillus* species, and *Cryptococcus neoformans*, although other fungi may also cause infection in these patients. Overall, *Aspergillus* species are the most common cause of fungal infection in lung or heart-lung transplant population [68], and the associated mortality rate is high [68,69]. It has been estimated that 9.3% of deaths after lung transplantation result from fungal pathogens [70,71]. The threat of serious fungal infection after lung transplantation has led many institutions to utilize some form of prophylactic or preemptive antifungal management. A variety of prophylactic protocols have been used for the prevention of aspergillosis under these circumstances. Most commonly oral itraconazole has been used. Recently, aerosolized amphotericin B, followed by an indefinite maintenance period on oral itraconazole [72] has been used with some success. We prefer oral voriconazole because of its extended antifungal spectrum and better bioavailability compared with itraconazole. We use therapeutic drug monitoring to titrate the dose of voriconazole.

Posttransplant Lymphoproliferative Disorders

The incidence of posttransplant lymphoproliferative disease (PTLD) are higher in children than in adults [73], and there are additional data suggesting that primary Epstein-Barr virus infection after transplantation is a related risk factor [74]. Posttransplant lymphoproliferative disease encompasses a wide spectrum of disease manifestations, ranging from a benign plasmacytic hyperplasia and infectious mononucleosis-like PTLD to an aggressive monoclonal lymphoma that leads to high morbidity and significant mortality. Most cases are Epstein-Barr virus–related B-cell tumors resulting from impaired immunity owing to immunosuppressive therapy. Approximately 15% of children will develop a lymphoproliferative malignancy by 5 years posttransplantation [1]. The most common treatment of PTLD has included decreasing immunosuppression and the use of rituximab often in combination with chemotherapy; radiation and antiviral agents are less commonly used [75–77]. A higher risk of graft rejection is associated with PTLD [75–78].

Morbidity

Other long-term complications related to immunosuppressive agents such as hypertension, renal dysfunction,

Table 43.10 Morbidity at 1, 5, and 7 years of follow-up from April 1994 to June 2008. (Data from Aurora *et al.* [1].)

Outcome	% within 1 year	% within 5 years	% within 7 years
Hypertension	43	69	71
Renal dysfunction	11	22	35
Hyperlipidemia	5	11	5
Diabetes	27	33	34
Bronchiolitis obliterans	14	37	36

hyperlipidemia, and diabetes mellitus are common in survivors (Table 43.10) [1]. Hypertension is highly prevalent in lung transplantation and increases steadily with time posttransplant. With the introduction of calcineurin inhibitors as immunosuppressive drugs, acute allograft rejection episodes have been significantly reduced. However, cardiovascular complications have become an important cause of morbidity and mortality. Treating cardiovascular risk factors such as diabetes, dyslipidemia, and hypertension is important in the routine posttransplant management of lung transplant recipients.

Summary

Experience has shown definitively that lung transplantation can be successfully performed in infants, children, and adolescents. With improvements in selection and management, survival continues to improve. However, this survival is driven by an improvement in short-term (1 year) survival. Long-term survival for pediatric lung transplantation has not changed in over two decades. The basic indication for lung transplantation is end-stage lung disease not amenable to other forms of therapy, but the specific disease entities vary by age group. There is a strong preference for bilateral lung transplantation using CPB in pediatric patients. Donor organ availability and waiting list mortality remain serious issues. At present, the paucity of pediatric lung transplant centers severely limits the options for infants, children, and adolescents with end-stage lung and pulmonary vascular disease. Postoperative management requires attention to early graft function, acute and chronic rejection, and infection. Bronchiolitis obliterans continues to be a significant obstacle limiting long-term survival. Despite the recognized complications of transplantation, quality of life improves significantly posttransplant and the functional status of the great majority of long-term survivors is very good.

References

1. Aurora P, Edwards LB, Christie JD, *et al.* (2009) Registry of the International Society for Heart and Lung Transplantation: Twelfth Official Pediatric Lung and Heart/Lung Transplantation Report – 2009. J Heart Lung Transplant 28, 1023–1030.
2. Christie JD, Edwards LB, Aurora P, *et al.* (2009) The Registry of the International Society for Heart and Lung Transplantation: Twenty-sixth Official Adult Lung and Heart-Lung Transplantation Report – 2009. J Heart Lung Transplant 28, 1031–1049.
3. Horslen S, Barr ML, Christensen LL, *et al.* (2007) Pediatric transplantation in the United States, 1996–2005. Am J Transplant 7, 1339–1358.
4. Hardy JD, Webb WR, Dalton ML Jr, *et al.* (1963) Lung homotransplantation in man. JAMA 186, 1065–1074.
5. Cooley DA, Bloodwell RD, Hallman GL, *et al.* (1967) Organ transplantation for advanced cardiopulmonary disease. Ann Thorac Surg 8, 30–42.
6. Wildevuur CR, Benfield JR. (1970) A review of 23 human lung transplantations by 20 surgeons. Ann Thorac Surg 9, 489–515.
7. Reitz BA, Burton NA, Jamieson SW, *et al.* (1980) Heart and lung transplantation: autotransplantation and allotransplantation in primates with extended survival. J Thorac Cardiovasc Surg 80, 360–372.
8. Reitz BA, Wallwork JL, Hunt SA, *et al.* (1982) Heart-lung transplantation: successful therapy for patients with pulmonary vascular disease. N Engl J Med 306, 557–564.
9. Toronto Lung Transplant Group. (1986) Unilateral lung transplantation for pulmonary fibrosis. N Engl J Med 314, 1140–1145.
10. Mendeloff EN. (2002) The history of pediatric heart and lung transplantation. Pediatr Transplant 6, 270–279.
11. Shinoi K, Hayata Y, Aoki H, *et al.* (1966) Pulmonary lobe homotransplantation in human subjects. Am J Surg 111, 617–628.
12. Starnes VA, Barr ML, Cohen RG. (1994) Lobar transplantation. Indications, technique, and outcome. J Thorac Cardiovasc Surg 108, 403–410; discussion 410–411.
13. Toyooka S, Yamane M, Oto T, *et al.* (2008) Favorable outcomes after living-donor lobar lung transplantation in ventilator-dependent patients. Surg Today 38, 1078–1082.
14. Hosenpud JD, Bennett LE, Keck BM, *et al.* (1998) Effect of diagnosis on survival benefit of lung transplantation for end-stage lung disease. Lancet 351, 24–27.
15. Bridges ND, Clark BJ, Gaynor JW, *et al.* (1996) Outcome of children with pulmonary hypertension referred for lung or heart and lung transplantation. Transplantation 62, 1824–1828.
16. Bridges ND, Mallory GB Jr, Huddleston CB, *et al.* (1995) Lung transplantation in children and young adults with cardiovascular disease. Ann Thorac Surg 59, 813–820; discussion 820–821.
17. Kamler M, Pizanis N, Aleksic I, *et al.* (2005) [Pulmonary hypertension and lung transplantation]. Herz 30, 281–285.
18. Woo MS, MacLaughlin EF, Horn MV, *et al.* (1998) Living donor lobar lung transplantation: the pediatric experience. Pediatr Transplant 2, 185–190.
19. Woo MS, MacLaughlin EF, Horn MV, *et al.* (2001) Bronchiolitis obliterans is not the primary cause of death in pediatric living donor lobar lung transplant recipients. J Heart Lung Transplant 20, 491–496.

20. Bowdish ME, Barr ML, Schenkel FA, *et al.* (2004) A decade of living lobar lung transplantation: perioperative complications after 253 donor lobectomies. Am J Transplant 4, 1283–1288.

21. Kozower BD, Sweet SC, de la Morena M, *et al.* (2006) Living donor lobar grafts improve pediatric lung retransplantation survival. J Thorac Cardiovasc Surg 131, 1142–1147.

22. Bando K, Armitage JM, Paradis IL, *et al.* (1994) Indications for and results of single, bilateral, and heart-lung transplantation for pulmonary hypertension. J Thorac Cardiovasc Surg 108, 1056–1065.

23. Gorler H, Struber M, Ballmann M, *et al.* (2009) Lung and heart-lung transplantation in children and adolescents: a long-term single-center experience. J Heart Lung Transplant 28, 243–248.

24. Reichart B, Gulbins H, Meiser BM, *et al.* (2003) Improved results after heart-lung transplantation: a 17-year experience. Transplantation 75, 127–132.

25. Grady RM, Gandhi S, Sweet SC, *et al.* (2009) Dismal lung transplant outcomes in children with tetralogy of Fallot with pulmonary atresia compared to Eisenmenger syndrome or pulmonary vein stenosis. J Heart Lung Transplant 28, 1221–1225.

26. Aris RM, Routh JC, LiPuma JJ, *et al.* (2001) Lung transplantation for cystic fibrosis patients with Burkholderia cepacia complex. Survival linked to genomovar type. Am J Respir Crit Care Med 164, 2102–2106.

27. Chaparro C, Maurer J, Gutierrez C, *et al.* (2001) Infection with Burkholderia cepacia in cystic fibrosis: outcome following lung transplantation. Am J Respir Crit Care Med 163, 43–48.

28. Nathan SD. (2005) Lung transplantation: disease-specific considerations for referral. Chest 127, 1006–1016.

29. Sweet SC. (2009) Pediatric lung transplantation. Proc Am Thorac Soc 6, 122–127.

30. Sweet SC. (2009) Update on pediatric lung allocation in the United States. Pediatr Transplant 13, 808–813.

31. McCurry KR, Shearon TH, Edwards LB, *et al.* (2009) Lung transplantation in the United States, 1998–2007. Am J Transplant 9, 942–958.

32. Lingaraju R, Blumenthal NP, Kotloff RM, *et al.* (2006) Effects of lung allocation score on waiting list rankings and transplant procedures. J Heart Lung Transplant 25, 1167–1170.

33. Spray TL. (1998) Lung and heart-lung transplantation in children. In: Kaiser LR, Kron IL, Spray TL, eds. *Mastery of Cardiothoracic Surgery*, 1st ed. Philadelphia, PA: Lippincott-Raven.

34. Pizanis N, Heckmann J, Tsagakis K, *et al.* (2010) Lung transplantation using donors 55 years and older: is it safe or just a way out of organ shortage? Eur J Cardiothorac Surg 38, 192–197.

35. Mallory GB Jr, Schecter MG, Elidemir O. (2009) Management of the pediatric organ donor to optimize lung donation. Pediatr Pulmonol 44, 536–546.

36. Fischer S, Matte-Martyn A, de Perrot M, *et al.* (2001) Low-potassium dextran preservation solution improves lung function after human lung transplantation. J Thorac Cardiovasc Surg 121, 594–596.

37. Struber M, Wilhelmi M, Harringer W, *et al.* (2001) Flush perfusion with low potassium dextran solution improves early graft function in clinical lung transplantation. Eur J Cardiothorac Surg 19, 190–194.

38. Thabut G, Vinatier I, Brugiere O, *et al.* (2001) Influence of preservation solution on early graft failure in clinical lung transplantation. Am J Respir Crit Care Med 164, 1204–1208.

39. de Perrot M, Keshavjee S. (2003) Lung preservation. Chest Surg Clin N Am 13, 443–462.

40. Nigro JJ, Bart RD, Starnes VA. (2006) Pediatric lung transplantation. In: Stark JF, de Leval M, Tsang VT, eds. *Surgery for Congenital Heart Defects*, 3rd ed. Chichester, England: John Wiley & Sons, Ltd.

41. Mallory GB Jr, Cohen AH. (1997) Donor considerations in living-related donor lung transplantation. Clin Chest Med 18, 239–244.

42. Barr ML, Baker CJ, Schenkel FA, *et al.* (2001) Living donor lung transplantation: selection, technique, and outcome. Transplant Proc 33, 3527–3532.

43. Barr ML, Schenkel FA, Bowdish ME, *et al.* (2005) Living donor lobar lung transplantation: current status and future directions. Transplant Proc 37, 3983–3986.

44. Ailawadi G, Smith PW, Oka T, *et al.* (2008) Effects of induction immunosuppression regimen on acute rejection, bronchiolitis obliterans, and survival after lung transplantation. J Thorac Cardiovasc Surg 135, 594–602.

45. Brock MV, Borja MC, Ferber L, *et al.* (2001) Induction therapy in lung transplantation: a prospective, controlled clinical trial comparing OKT3, anti-thymocyte globulin, and daclizumab. J Heart Lung Transplant 20, 1282–1290.

46. Burton CM, Andersen CB, Jensen AS, *et al.* (2006) The incidence of acute cellular rejection after lung transplantation: a comparative study of anti-thymocyte globulin and daclizumab. J Heart Lung Transplant 25, 638–647.

47. Garrity ER Jr, Villanueva J, Bhorade SM, *et al.* (2001) Low rate of acute lung allograft rejection after the use of daclizumab, an interleukin 2 receptor antibody. Transplantation 71, 773–777.

48. Hachem RR, Chakinala MM, Yusen RD, *et al.* (2005) A comparison of basiliximab and anti-thymocyte globulin as induction agents after lung transplantation. J Heart Lung Transplant 24, 1320–1326.

49. Waddell TK, Borro J, Roman A, *et al.* (2006) A double-blind randomized trial comparing basiliximab to placebo in lung transplantation. J Heart Lung Transplant 25(suppl 1), S114 (abstract).

50. Kugler C, Fischer S, Gottlieb J, *et al.* (2005) Health-related quality of life in two hundred-eighty lung transplant recipients. J Heart Lung Transplant 24, 2262–2268.

51. Rodrigue JR, Baz MA, Kanasky WF Jr, *et al.* (2005) Does lung transplantation improve health-related quality of life? The University of Florida experience. J Heart Lung Transplant 24, 755–763.

52. Vermeulen KM, van der Bij W, Erasmus ME, *et al.* (2004) Improved quality of life after lung transplantation in individuals with cystic fibrosis. Pediatr Pulmonol 37, 419–426.

53. Vermeulen KM, van der Bij W, Erasmus ME, *et al.* (2007) Long-term health-related quality of life after lung transplan-

tation: different predictors for different dimensions. J Heart Lung Transplant 26, 188–193.

54. Trulock EP, Christie JD, Edwards LB, *et al.* (2007) Registry of the International Society for Heart and Lung Transplantation: twenty-fourth official adult lung and heart-lung transplantation report-2007. J Heart Lung Transplant 26, 782–795.

55. Sharples LD, McNeil K, Stewart S, *et al.* (2002) Risk factors for bronchiolitis obliterans: a systematic review of recent publications. J Heart Lung Transplant 21, 271–281.

56. Stewart S, Fishbein MC, Snell GI, *et al.* (2007) Revision of the 1996 working formulation for the standardization of nomenclature in the diagnosis of lung rejection. J Heart Lung Transplant 26, 1229–1242.

57. Cooper JD, Billingham M, Egan T, *et al.* (1993) A working formulation for the standardization of nomenclature and for clinical staging of chronic dysfunction in lung allografts. International Society for Heart and Lung Transplantation. J Heart Lung Transplant 12, 713–716.

58. Estenne M, Maurer JR, Bochler A, *et al.* (2002) Bronchiolitis obliterans syndrome 2001: an update of the diagnostic criteria. J Heart Lung Transplant 21, 297–310.

59. Nathan SD, Barnett SD, Wohlrab J, *et al.* (2003) Bronchiolitis obliterans syndrome: utility of the new guidelines in single lung transplant recipients. J Heart Lung Transplant 22, 427–432.

60. Reichenspurner H, Girgis RE, Robbins RC, *et al.* (1996) Stanford experience with obliterative bronchiolitis after lung and heart-lung transplantation. Ann Thorac Surg 62, 1467–1472; discussion 1472–1473.

61. Lim TT, Botas J, Ross H, *et al.* (1996) Are heart-lung transplant recipients protected from developing transplant coronary artery disease? A case-matched intracoronary ultrasound study. Circulation 94, 1573–1577.

62. Kramer MR, Marshall SE, Starnes VA, *et al.* (1993) Infectious complications in heart-lung transplantation. Analysis of 200 episodes. Arch Intern Med 153, 2010–2016.

63. Maurer JR, Tullis DE, Grossman RF, *et al.* (1992) Infectious complications following isolated lung transplantation. Chest 101, 1056–1059.

64. Gavalda J, Roman A. (2007) [Infection in lung transplantation]. Enferm Infecc Microbiol Clin 25, 639–649; quiz 650.

65. Egan TM, Detterbeck FC, Mill MR, *et al.* (2002) Long term results of lung transplantation for cystic fibrosis. Eur J Cardiothorac Surg 22, 602–609.

66. Danziger-Isakov LA, Worley S, Michaels MG, *et al.* (2009) The risk, prevention, and outcome of cytomegalovirus after pediatric lung transplantation. Transplantation 87, 1541–1548.

67. Thomas LD, Milstone AP, Miller GG, *et al.* (2009) Long-term outcomes of cytomegalovirus infection and disease after lung or heart-lung transplantation with a delayed ganciclovir regimen. Clin Transplant 23, 476–483.

68. Singh N, Husain S. (2003) Aspergillus infections after lung transplantation: clinical differences in type of transplant and implications for management. J Heart Lung Transplant 22, 258–266.

69. Tollemar JG. (1998) Fungal infections in solid-organ transplant recipients. In: Bowden RA, Ljungman P, Paya CV, eds. *Transplant Infections*, 1st ed. Philadelphia, PA: Lippincott-Raven, pp. 339–350.

70. Paterson DL, Singh N. (1999) Invasive aspergillosis in transplant recipients. Medicine (Baltimore) 78, 123–138.

71. Singh N. (2000) Antifungal prophylaxis for solid organ transplant recipients: seeking clarity amidst controversy. Clin Infect Dis 31, 545–553.

72. Palmer SM, Drew RH, Whitehouse JD, *et al.* (2001) Safety of aerosolized amphotericin B lipid complex in lung transplant recipients. Transplantation 72, 545–548.

73. Cohen AH, Sweet SC, Mendeloff E, *et al.* (2000) High incidence of posttransplant lymphoproliferative disease in pediatric patients with cystic fibrosis. Am J Respir Crit Care Med 161, 1252–1255.

74. Boyle GJ, Michaels MG, Webber SA, *et al.* (1997) Posttransplantation lymphoproliferative disorders in pediatric thoracic organ recipients. J Pediatr 131, 309–313.

75. Aurora P, Whitehead B, Wade A, *et al.* (1999) Lung transplantation and life extension in children with cystic fibrosis. Lancet 354, 1591–1593.

76. Metras D, Viard L, Kreitmann B, *et al.* (1999) Lung infections in pediatric lung transplantation: experience in 49 cases. Eur J Cardiothorac Surg 15, 490–494; discussion 495.

77. Sweet SC, Spray TL, Huddleston CB, *et al.* (1997) Pediatric lung transplantation at St. Louis Children's Hospital, 1990–1995. Am J Respir Crit Care Med 155, 1027–1035.

78. Starnes VA, Woo MS, MacLaughlin EF, *et al.* (1999) Comparison of outcomes between living donor and cadaveric lung transplantation in children. Ann Thorac Surg 68, 2279–2283; discussion 2283–2284.

44

Infective Endocarditis

Muhammad Ali Mumtaz,[1] Lara Danziger-Isakov,[2] Constantine Mavroudis,[3] and Carl L. Backer[4]

[1]Children's Hospital of the King's Daughters, Norfolk, VA, USA
[2]Cleveland Clinic Children's Hospital, Cleveland Clinic Lerner College of Medicine of Case Western Reserve University, Cleveland, OH, USA
[3]Florida Hospital for Children, Orlando, FL, USA
[4]Ann & Robert H. Lurie Children's Hospital of Chicago, formerly Children's Memorial Hospital, Chicago, IL, USA

Definition

Infective endocarditis (IE) is the infection of the endothelial lining of the heart. In addition, the term is very commonly used to include infection of the patent ductus arteriosus and the proximal great arteries and veins, though histologically there is no endocardium present in these structures. The condition commonly involves the cardiac valves leading to valvar dysfunction. The process starts with damage to the endothelium. Fibrin and platelet deposition ensues along with bacterial growth of the deposits to form clumps of exudative and proliferative material termed "vegetations." Further deposition of fibrin and platelets allows vegetation growth, isolating the microorganisms from leukocytes and antibiotics in a zone of "agranulocytosis" [1]. Vegetations are responsible for the remote effects from micro and macro emboli. Diagnosis of IE focuses mainly on the epidemiologic risk, culture results, and imaging. Most cases are successfully treated with prolonged antimicrobial management; however, surgical intervention may be necessary for complex or unresponsive cases.

Epidemiology

Infective endocarditis is less common in children than adults, accounting for ~1 in 1300 to ~1 in 3000 pediatric hospital admissions [2–4]. However, the incidence of IE appears to be increasing [3,5,6]. Previously, complications of rheumatic heart disease accounted for a significant proportion of endocarditis episodes in children, but recent studies estimate the contribution of rheumatic heart disease to IE at <10% in the developed world [2,7]. The surgical advances in the treatment of congenital heart disease (CHD) increase the risk for IE for several reasons. First, surgical repair creates physiology within the heart that may predispose to endocarditis. Second, surgical techniques frequently require implantation of prosthetic materials including conduits, shunts, and patches [8]. The use of nonsurgical repair with intracardiac devices, including coils, also continues to rise and poses a potential risk. Finally, with improved survival, lifetime cumulative risk of IE increases despite the potential decrease in risk related to surgical intervention.

In 2007, the American Heart Association (AHA) revised guidelines for the prevention of IE [9] including the risk stratification based on underlying CHD. The new guidelines focus on providing prophylaxis based on the risk of adverse outcome with IE rather than lifetime risk of IE acquisition. Conditions considered to be high risk for adverse outcomes related to IE include unrepaired or palliated cyanotic CHD, repaired CHD with residual defects adjacent to prosthetic material, and completely repaired CHD with implanted device or prosthetic material for the first 6 months after repair. Heart transplant recipients with cardiac valvulopathy and patients with prosthetic valves are also categorized as high risk. Many common CHDs (e.g., patent ductus arteriosus, ventricular septal defect [VSD]) have increased risk of IE, yet prophylaxis is no longer recommended owing to the lack of efficacy data. Patients who are more than 6 months after their repair with no residual defects are considered to have the same risk as the general population.

The incidence of IE in patients without CHD has also increased. Immunosuppression secondary to malignancy and transplantation with or without the use of long-term indwelling catheters are risk factors for IE. The incidence of IE in neonates is also rising. Advances in the care of premature and other critically ill neonates, who have substantially improved neonatal survival, rely on the prolonged use of arterial and venous indwelling catheters,

Pediatric Cardiac Surgery, Fourth Edition. Edited by Constantine Mavroudis and Carl L. Backer.
© 2013 Blackwell Publishing Ltd. Published 2013 by Blackwell Publishing Ltd.

which has been associated with an increased risk of IE even in the absence of CHD [10–12].

Pathophysiology

The primary event leading to the development of IE is damage to the epithelial lining of the heart followed by bacteremia with organisms capable of adhering to the damaged endothelial tissue. Several dynamics create the potential for endothelial damage. Turbulent blood flow from high- to low-pressure areas creates trauma to the endothelium. Injury may also be mediated by intracardiac catheters and intracardiac surgical or transcatheter repair. The damage to endothelial lining of the heart allows formation of nonbacterial thrombotic endocarditis (NBTE), which results from the deposition of fibrin and platelets on the damaged endothelium. Prosthetic materials including shunts, patches, valve, conduits, and intracardiac catheters provide additional sites for the deposition of fibrin and platelets. Once vegetations form, transiently circulating bacteria adhere to the fibrin-platelet aggregate to propagate the infection. Transient bacteremia occurs frequently with daily activities including brushing teeth or chewing food that cause local trauma to mucosal surfaces. Additional episodes of bacteremia can occur with dental or select surgical procedures [9]. The ability of the bacteria to adhere to the sterile vegetation influences the risk of IE after transient bacteremia. Gram-positive bacteria have specific factors that promote their ability to adhere to NBTE. Staphylococcal species have adhesin proteins and some viridans streptococci have FimA protein, which promotes adherence [13–15]. Once the bacteria attach to the platelet-fibrin aggregate they multiply. Although the adherence factors are immunogenic in animal studies [16], once the bacteria embed in the vegetation they become sequestered from the circulating host immune defenses avoiding clearance of the infection. Additional layers of platelet and fibrin deposit over the bacteria. Therefore, prolonged antibiotic therapy is recommended to penetrate the vegetation and kill the bacteria.

Microbiology

The span of organisms identified as causative agents in IE continues to grow, especially with the availability of molecular diagnostic techniques. However, Gram-positive cocci, with their identified adherence factors, remain the dominant causative organisms of IE in children [2,3,5]. Streptococci have previously been reported as the most common organisms in pediatric IE with viridans streptococci reported most frequently. However, in the most recent reports, *Staphylococcus aureus* has emerged as the most common overall cause of IE in children [2,8]. Although it is less common than *Staphylococcus aureus*, coagulase-

negative *Staphylococcus* is also a significant contributor. Other organisms including Gram-negative bacteria, *Candida* species, and fungi are rare but may pose increased risk to children without underlying structural heart defects, including neonates and immunocompromised hosts.

Endocarditis related to prosthetic valves or other implanted foreign material requires special consideration. For children with CHD, more than 50% with IE have had previous corrective or palliative surgery. Both early and late postsurgical infections have been reported. Early infections, within a few months of surgery, may be related to surgical contamination or invasive postsurgical monitoring [1]. *Staphylococcus aureus* and coagulase-negative *Staphylococcus* are commonly recovered early after interventions [2]. In addition, less commonly reported organisms include *Klebsiella*, *Pseudomonas aeruginosa*, diphtheroids, and *Candida*. Reports of IE from anaerobic bacteria in pediatrics are rare [17]. The organisms recovered more than one year after surgical intervention reflect the organisms recovered before or without surgery. In a significant proportion of cases, an organism is not identified despite aggressive evaluation. Culture-negative endocarditis occurs in 5–20% of cases of IE [5,7,18].

Diagnosis

Combined information from clinical, laboratory, and imaging areas assist in the diagnosis of IE.

Clinical Manifestations

The clinical manifestations of IE are variable but include systemic symptoms relating to persistent bacteremia. The presentation for persistent bacteremia ranges from simple fever with malaise to fulminant sepsis with multiorgan system failure. Fever is the most common symptom in patients outside of the neonatal age. Fever and other symptoms may be subtle, delaying the diagnosis [4,7]. In the absence of fever, IE should be considered in patients with signs and symptoms of a systemic illness especially for neonates who may not mount an appropriate fever response. Additional nonspecific systemic symptoms include malaise, anorexia, weight loss, and arthralgia.

Cardiac manifestations of IE also vary and are dependent on the site of infection within the heart. Valvar lesions may lead to regurgitation or the perforation of the valve leaflet. Subvalvar lesions can cause rupture of the cordae tendineae or papillary muscles with subsequent severe valvar dysfunction. Lesions near the valve annulus may invade the myocardium resulting in cardiac conduction disturbances. Additionally, annular abscess and valve rupture occur with infection at the annulus. Large vegetations may produce mechanical obstruction mimicking valvar stenosis. Clinical manifestations of cardiac dysfunction include congestive heart failure (CHF), tachycardia, and arrhythmia. Functional changes in murmur quality occur in the patient with underlying CHD. Fever without a source in the presence of underlying valvar disease or CHD should prompt investigation for IE.

Embolic phenomena depend greatly on the site of infection as well. Areas of embolization primarily include the lung and brain. However, embolization to kidney, spleen, liver, skin, and coronary arteries has been reported [4,7,19]. Pulmonary embolization principally occurs with right-sided vegetations that enter the pulmonary circulation resulting in infarction and lung abscess. Early in its presentation, IE may masquerade as pneumonia after unrealized pulmonary embolization.

Neurologic manifestations complicate a significant number of cases. Involvement likely results from embolic events and can include isolated papilledema, altered sensorium, paresis, seizures, cranial nerve palsies, stroke, and coma [7,20]. Mycotic aneurysms may develop after septic embolization from a vegetation leading to rupture and death in rare cases. Infections with *Staphylococcus aureus* are associated with increased risk of neurologic complications with IE [21].

Renal manifestations, including glomerulonephritis, are also fairly common with IE. The etiology for renal involvement is multifactorial, including the deposition of immune complexes within the kidney, hypoperfusion secondary to CHF and sepsis, or deposition of septic emboli. Clinical evaluation for gross and microscopic hematuria should be considered.

Skin manifestations can be either from emboli or deposition of immune complexes and are relatively rare in children. Janeway lesions, which present as flat painless lesions on the palms and soles, result from hemorrhage around microabscesses from septic emboli. Alternatively, Osler nodes, which present as painful, red lesions, develop after immune-mediated infiltration around the dermal vessels. Roth spots found on the retina and subungual splinter hemorrhages on the digits may also occur.

Laboratory Investigations

Diagnosis of IE relies primarily on recovery of a pathogen with a positive blood culture. A positive blood culture with a causative pathogen, in the absence of a pathologic diagnosis from positive histology or culture from vegetation, is one of the major conditions in the modified Duke criteria for IE diagnosis. Increased numbers and volumes of blood culture improve the yield of organisms in the diagnosis of IE. Generally, three or more individual cultures are sent in a 24-hour period aiming to meet the Duke criteria for IE. Blood volumes for pediatric patients may not meet volumes recommended for adults (10–20 mL of blood per culture)

owing to restrictions in specimen collection, but volumes of at least 3 mL per sample are generally acceptable in small children, although smaller volumes may be collected in neonates. To avoid confusion with skin flora contamination, sterile preparation at the time of sample collection is essential. Administration of antibiotics before specimen collection decreases the yield of positive blood cultures by up to 40% [22]. Several additional techniques to improve pathogen recovery exist. Antimicrobial absorbent resins improve bacterial recovery in patients exposed to antibiotics before cultures are obtained [23]. Prolonged incubation of blood cultures for up to 2 weeks is also recommended to evaluate for fastidious organisms. These organisms include the HACEK organisms (*Haemophilus, Actinobacillus, Cardiobacterium hominis, Eikenella corrodens, Kingella kingae*) and nutritionally deficient *Streptococcus*. Emerging molecular technologies have the potential to further improve organism identification, potentially limiting the diagnosis of culture-negative endocarditis, both in patients who received antibiotics before cultures were obtained and also in patients with endocarditis attributed to organisms that are extremely difficult to grow in conventional culture. These techniques have improved recovery of organisms in adult and pediatric patients but require further standardization and are not considered a major criterion in the Duke classification [24–26]. Availability of molecular diagnostics and other techniques to improve recovery of pathogens should be discussed with specialists in infectious diseases and microbiologists in complicated cases.

Additional laboratory findings support the diagnosis of IE and may include elevated erythrocyte sedimentation rate and C-reactive protein and positive rheumatoid factor. Decreased serum complement and hematuria from glomerulonephritis are immunologic phenomena that may be present; glomerulonephritis is one of the minor criteria for IE. Leukocytosis may be present; however, severe sepsis from IE may present with leukopenia. Additionally, anemia from chronic illness can be masked by relative polycythemia secondary to cyanotic CHD.

Imaging Studies

Imaging is the mainstay of defining intracardiac disease in IE, and it is key in guiding therapy and prognosis. Findings of vegetations, intracardiac abscess, new partial dehiscence of a prosthetic valve, or new valvar regurgitation are included as major criteria for the diagnosis of IE [27]. Furthermore, progression of disease and valvar dysfunction can also be followed echocardiographically. Transthoracic echocardiography (TTE) has a poor sensitivity but is usually the first test performed [28]. Transesophageal echocardiography (TEE) typically provides more detailed information [29,30], especially when small vegetations and intramyocardial abscesses are suspected. Reynolds *et al.*

[30] found the sensitivity of TTE in detecting vegetations to be only 55% when compared with TEE. Li *et al.* [27] found TEE to be positive in 19% of cases where the TTE was negative. Limitations of echocardiographic imaging include the difficulty in distinguishing old healed vegetations from active infection. Also, it is difficult to differentiate small vegetations from uninfected clots related to suture material and pledgets. Interference from prosthetic materials such as valves and patches makes it difficult to look for vegetations around these structures with echocardiography. Repeat studies are very helpful to evaluate progression of disease.

Other imaging modalities may be used to assess IE. Magnetic resonance imaging (MRI) can occasionally be helpful in assessing ventricular and valvar function. Its value along with contrast-enhanced computed tomography (CT) scanning is more for detection of remote emboli and distinguishing between infarction, hemorrhage, and abscess. Interestingly, a recent study showed that CT scan was more accurate than TEE in detecting perivalvar extent of endocarditis, but all cases of leaflet perforations were missed [31]. Fluoroscopy may play a role in detecting valvar dysfunction in prosthetic valves by demonstrating impaired disc excursion. Angiography is rarely needed except in detection of aneurysms in the affected area, especially intracranial mycotic aneurysms. Coronary angiography is occasionally performed in children with unexplained ventricular dysfunction.

Antimicrobial Therapy

Treatment of IE depends on prolonged antimicrobial therapy with or without surgical intervention. The prolonged duration of antibiotics recommended is a function of the relatively slow metabolism of the organisms in the vegetation as well as the structure of the vegetation with the pathogenic organisms deeply embedded in the fibrin-platelet aggregate. Duration of antimicrobial therapy depends on the organism recovered, and counting should begin from the date of the first negative culture. Antibiotics should ideally be tailored to the organism, but empiric therapy after multiple cultures are obtained can be directed at the most likely causative organisms pending results, especially in the case of a critically ill patient. Generally, treatment recommendations for duration range from 4–6 weeks or longer depending on the clinical scenario, with longer durations for patients with implanted prosthetic materials. Empiric therapy for presumed viridans *Streptococcus* relies on penicillin G or ceftriaxone, while penicillinase-resistant penicillin (nafcillin, oxacillin) should be used for possible staphylococcal endocarditis. For penicillin-allergic patients and in areas with a high prevalence of methicillin-resistance *S. aureus*, vancomycin is recommended. The use of an aminoglycoside for synergy is considered optional in most recent recommendations from the AHA, secondary to reports of renal toxicity without increased benefit with aminoglycoside use, although some experts recommend its use in fulminant cases [32–34]. Aminoglycosides are recommended for 2 weeks along with rifampin for the duration of therapy in addition to the primary antimicrobial in patients with staphylococcal infections who have prosthetic materials. Empiric therapy for culture-negative endocarditis depends on the clinical course and epidemiologic aspects including pretreatment with antimicrobial agents and the presence of and time since placement of prosthetic materials. Current recommendations include ampicillin-sulbactam plus an aminoglycoside for 6 weeks for native valve IE. For patients with prosthetic material, vancomycin is recommended with the addition of a broad-spectrum cephalosporin if IE occurs within 2 months of valve placement [32]. Early surgical intervention should be considered if the patient is unresponsive to empiric therapy.

Fungal endocarditis is primarily caused by *Candida* species, with *Aspergillus* species occurring less frequently [35]. Morbidity and mortality related to fungal endocarditis is high. Early surgical intervention is suggested by many experts, and medical therapy with an amphotericin B-containing product is suggested for at least 6 weeks.

Indications for Surgery

Traditionally, surgery was reserved as a means of last resort. However, early surgery is recommended with increasing frequency [36,37]. The goal of surgery is removing the infected material, improving valvar function, repairing anatomic complications, and decreasing mortality [18,37,38]. Data and recommendations specific for children are not available separately, but AHA guidelines [39] recommend surgical intervention in native valve endocarditis in the presence of:
1. heart failure (especially related to valvar dysfunction);
2. worsening valvar function;
3. recurrent emboli;
4. evidence of intramyocardial infection (such as abscess formation, heart block, and intracardiac fistula formation);
5. infections from resistant organisms.

The decision to proceed to surgery is frequently subject to much discussion. In the absence of specific recommendations for children, it is important to take all factors into consideration, including the clinical status of the patient, chances of recovery from a neurologic event, the microorganism involved, prospects of valve repair or replacement, and the AHA guidelines [39]. Also, it is recommended that these factors be assessed as a continuum rather than only at a single point in the clinical course of a patient (Table 44.1).

Table 44.1 Indications for consideration of surgery in infective endocarditis. (IE, infective endocarditis.)

Congestive heart failure despite medical therapy

Deterioration of valve function (regurgitation from leaflet perforation or dehiscence, stenosis from vegetation)

Mechanical intracardiac complications (ventricular septal defect, fistula, pseudoaneurysm, mycotic aneurysm formation, etc.)

Evidence of myocardial infection (annular or myocardial abscess, heart block)

Recurrent embolization or single episode while on adequate therapy

Large vegetation or growth of vegetations while on adequate medical therapy

Failure of medical therapy (as evidence by persistent bacteremia, fever, growth of vegetations)

Endocarditis owing to resistant or difficult to treat organisms (fungal IE, Gram-negative bacilli)

Early prosthetic valve endocarditis

Late prosthetic valve endocarditis with prosthetic dysfunction

---

Congestive Heart Failure

This is perhaps the most important consideration in surgical therapy as it is the most common predictor of mortality [40]. Congestive heart failure in IE is frequently related to the added burden of sepsis on the underlying valvar lesion. For example, a patient with preexisting aortic stenosis without heart failure may decompensate into CHF because of associated fever, anemia, and sepsis. Under such circumstances, correction of these associated factors may improve CHF. Heart failure from acute valvar dysfunction, destructive intracardiac lesions, and uncorrected shunting lesions is more likely to need surgical intervention. Early surgery for endocarditis is associated with reduced mortality in patients with CHF when compared with medical treatment alone [37].

Valvar Dysfunction

Stable patients with valvar dysfunction and no other complications can frequently be treated with antibiotics alone until the acute infection has cleared. Subsequently, patients can be assessed for intervention if the usual surgical indications exist for valvar dysfunction. However, acute valvar dysfunction from leaflet perforation or valve stenosis owing to vegetations is frequently associated with CHF and is unlikely to improve with antibiotics alone. Renal and other organ dysfunction is commonly present. Surgery in this group of patients can frequently improve cardiac function by treating valvar dysfunction. In mitral valve endocarditis, early surgery makes repair more likely than valve replacement [39].

Mechanical Intracardiac Complications

Intracardiac complications of fistula and abscess formation are frequently associated with CHF and have a high mortality with medical treatment alone. Periannular or myocardial abscess may be a precursor of mechanical complication. New-onset atrioventricular (AV) block is indicative of myocardial infection. These are indications to proceed with surgery even without significant CHF [39]. The size of vegetations alone is difficult to interpret in small children. While, a 5-mm vegetation on the tricuspid valve in a teenager may not be significant, a similar-sized vegetation on the mitral valve of a newborn may be quite significant. Furthermore, a small embolus in a child may result in ischemia of a large territory. In adults with IE, vegetation >10 mm is felt to be a risk factor for remote emboli, especially stroke [41]. Similarly, patients with mobile vegetations or those that increase in size while on adequate therapy, are at risk of remote emboli. Such factors should be taken into consideration during decision making for surgery.

Remote Embolic Complications

Embolic stroke frequently leads to cerebral abscess formation or intracranial mycotic aneurysm formation. Occurrence of two or more episodes of major embolism during adequate medical treatment is commonly considered an indication for surgery. However, the presence of large vegetations with a single episode or new stroke, especially during adequate therapy, are reasonable indications for surgical intervention. Mortality of IE with a cerebral embolus is higher [37,41]. Some studies report *S aureus* and *Candida* endocarditis to be more commonly associated with embolic stroke [41–43]. At least half the strokes in adults are not apparent clinically and are discovered by MRI [42]. Because of the possibility of intracranial hemorrhage, the presence of a recent stroke is frequently of concern when using cardiopulmonary bypass. As a result, many surgeons prefer to wait for a few days, or up to 3 weeks if possible, before proceeding to surgery [44]. However, a low incidence of postoperative stroke has been reported in adults in the absence of hemorrhagic infarction [42,45].

Failure of Adequate Medical Therapy

Persistent fever or bacteremia, failure of the indices of infection to resolve, and progression of echocardiographic evidence of disease are considerations leading to a decision about failed medical therapy. Evidence of organisms that are frequently resistant to antibiotics or failure to clear with antibiotics alone, such as methicillin-resistant *S. aureus*, fungal endocarditis, and Gram-negative endocarditis, especially with a prosthetic valve, fall into this category [39,43].

Culture-Negative Endocarditis

In cases of culture-negative endocarditis, a detailed examination of all parameters of the disease must be considered, as organisms resistant to commonly used therapy may be the causative agents. Progression of anatomic disease on echocardiography, such as large or growing vegetations, evidence of emboli, and persistent indices of inflammation all point to failure of medical therapy. Culture-negative endocarditis has a higher chance of complications and need for surgery [46].

Prosthetic Valve/Device Endocarditis

Intracardiac prosthetic materials are not well endothelialized within the first 2 months. Bacteremia early after surgery may be more likely to cause infection of the prosthesis, necessitating its removal. Furthermore, endocarditis on a recently placed prosthetic valve is more likely to lead to annular abscess. Hence, presence of even mild heart failure and early staphylococcal endocarditis of a prosthetic valve is sufficient to warrant surgery [39]. Indications for surgery in late prosthetic valve endocarditis are similar to the ones discussed previously.

Timing of Surgery

Timing of surgery in IE should not be based on duration of preoperative antibiotics alone, but rather on clinical status of the patient. In stable patients, without progressive valve destruction or other complications, a complete course of antibiotics followed by re-evaluation for possible need for surgical therapy is appropriate. Very unstable patients will frequently require a period of resuscitation in the intensive care unit (ICU) before surgery. However, in the presence of severe sepsis, or severe CHF, prolonged delay before surgery for controlling sepsis is unnecessary. Patients with cerebral infarction are not necessarily at a higher risk of postoperative stroke [36,45]. However, if possible, it is prudent to wait 2–3 weeks after the stroke before proceeding to cardiac surgery [45]. Hemorrhagic stroke presents with a more difficult situation. Cardiopulmonary bypass in face of a hemorrhagic stroke from a ruptured mycotic aneurysm is associated with a significant chance of extending the stroke. A multidisciplinary approach with involvement of the neurosurgery service is recommended. Though postoperative hemorrhage from a previously unruptured mycotic aneurysm has been reported [47], it is generally felt that cardiopulmonary bypass does not increase the immediate risk of rupture [48]. Furthermore, mycotic aneurysms related to IE may have a lower propensity to rupture

as opposed to atherosclerotic aneurysms [49]. Ruptured mycotic aneurysm with subarachnoid hemorrhage presents a prohibitive risk to cardiopulmonary bypass. Many of these patients require craniotomy. Based on their experience, Gillinov *et al.* [44] recommended waiting 2–3 weeks after craniotomy before proceeding with open heart surgery.

Surgical Procedures

The procedure of choice for treatment of IE varies with the underlying pathology. The primary surgical principles include:
1. Complete debridement and removal of infected material. This includes vegetations, myocardial abscess, and infected prosthesis. The infected area is commonly irrigated with povidone-iodine solution, though the efficacy of this technique has not been studied.
2. Restoration of hemodynamic abnormality. Intracardiac defects are repaired and the underlying malformation can also be addressed. An exception may be made in case of infected Blalock-Taussig (BT) shunts. The underlying pathology may not be ready to be repaired. In such a situation, a new shunt, preferably in a new location, removal of the old shunt, and repair of the underlying vessels can be carried out. If a new site is not available or preferred, the old shunt needs to be completely debrided. Vegetations are commonly adherent to the suture lines. As a result the native blood vessels may need debridement and reconstruction and then a new shunt is reconstructed.
3. Repair using autologous tissues such as pericardium.
4. Use of biologic tissues. There is lack of evidence to show that biologic tissues have a lower incidence of reinfection [50]. However, we find that homograft material is easier to handle in the face of extensive debridement and possibly reduces the chance of postoperative hemorrhage [51].

Technique of Cardiopulmonary Bypass

Our preferred technique of cardiopulmonary bypass includes aortic and bicaval cannulation, systemic hypothermia, use of cold blood antegrade/retrograde cardioplegia, and modified ultrafiltration on completion of surgical repair. If cardiac perforation is suspected, carotid or femoral cannulation in small children and axillary or femoral cannulation in teenagers should be considered, as catastrophic fatal hemorrhage may ensue when opening the chest. Remote arterial cannulation can be aided by sewing in a tube graft in end-to-side fashion to the carotid, axillary, or femoral artery. This allows the use of larger cannula in a smaller artery with reduced risk of arterial damage. Furthermore, with this technique the distal vessel does not have to be clamped, thus avoiding distal ischemia. Bicaval cannulation allows inspection of all intracardiac structures, as the extent of pathology is frequently underestimated during preoperative assessment. Smaller catheters for retrograde cardioplegia allow its use even in small babies. Patients with IE frequently have overt renal dysfunction; in these cases modified ultrafiltration is recommended.

Aortic Valve Endocarditis

Aortic valve endocarditis occurs with similar incidence as mitral valve endocarditis, though some series have reported it being more common [30,40]. Vegetations on the leaflets should be debrided and leaflets can frequently be preserved. Perforation of a leaflet can frequently be repaired using fresh or glutaraldehyde-treated autologous pericardium. Infection extending to the common annulus with the mitral valve can similarly be debrided and the aortic and mitral continuity reconstructed without valve replacement. However, infection into the myocardium or a frank annular abscess necessitates complete debridement of the aortic root and subsequent reconstruction. Though such reconstruction is facilitated with the use of an aortic homograft in teenagers and adults [52], this prosthesis has dismal durability in smaller children. We prefer the Ross procedure in younger children [53–55]. However, a mechanical valved conduit can also be used for aortic root replacement. There does not appear to be a difference in recurrence rates between biologic and mechanical prostheses [50]. As the durability of biologic prosthesis in small children is quite disappointing, we prefer to use a mechanical prosthesis if the Ross procedure is not feasible. In females, the use of mechanical prosthesis must be weighed against the issues of potential subsequent pregnancy. Root reconstruction may be facilitated by using fresh autologous pericardium to buttress or reconstruct the debrided areas. More complex techniques using coronary bypass grafts are rarely applicable to children.

Mitral Valve Endocarditis

Mitral valve endocarditis was previously felt to be more frequently associated with systemic emboli, though recent studies show equal incidence of emboli from aortic and mitral valve endocarditis [41]. Earlier surgery may allow a higher likelihood of repair and also, possibly decrease the risk of recurrent systemic emboli. A variety of repair techniques have been used [18,56]. Debridement of the vegetation may be all that is needed [18]. Defects in the mitral leaflets can be repaired using a pericardial patch or by performing a primary repair. Homograft material can be used as an alternative to pericardium. Chordal reattachment or chordal transfer can be performed for ruptured chords. Ring annuloplasty is typically not required and is certainly contraindicated in growing children, but localized annuloplasty can be performed, especially in the posterior annulus, if a portion of posterior mitral leaflet is excised. Presence of annular or ring abscess does not pre-

clude repair if the leaflets and chordae are intact. In this situation, leaflets can be detached and annular abscess can be completely debrided. The annulus is then reconstructed using fresh autologous pericardium or a pulmonary homograft, and the leaflet can be reattached. If the mitral valve is not amenable to repair, then a mechanical valve is our prosthesis of choice in young children. This is because of diminished durability of biologic valves in this position in children [57]. Homograft mitral valves have been used. However, they are difficult to place, with unpredictable function. In a sick patient with endocarditis, an expedient operation with a competent valve is more likely to be successful.

Tricuspid Valve

Isolated tricuspid endocarditis is frequently associated with indwelling catheters. It is also more commonly involved in fungal infection especially in premature babies and newborn who require long-term venous catheters [35,43]. Mortality from surgery for fungal endocarditis is high. However, in the presence of usual indications, surgery should not be delayed. Surgical treatment should include removal of the associated catheter and atrial mass if present. Vegetations on the tricuspid valve should be excised and tricuspid valve should be repaired in the usual fashion. Residual VSD or primary VSD should be repaired using preferably a pericardial patch, especially in cases of active endocarditis. Excision of the tricuspid valve is not well tolerated in young children and infants; however, it may be considered in a teenager. If the tricuspid valve is not amenable to repair, a bioprosthesis is our preference.

Pulmonary Valve

Native pulmonary valve endocarditis is rare in children. In almost all cases in children, insertion of a pulmonary valve can be avoided. The infection is debrided, even if this means removal of all leaflets [58]. In patients with poor cardiac function, tricuspid regurgitation or high pulmonary vascular resistance, where a competent valve may be desired, insertion of pulmonary homograft or bioprosthesis is safe.

Ventricular Septal Defect

Many infections associated with VSD can be treated with antibiotics, and surgery can be performed at a time when infection is cleared. This is also true for infections occurring in residual VSDs late (>2 months) after surgery. Early postoperative infections in the presence of the usual surgical indications are approached with the goal of removing the VSD patch and all associated pledgets. The VSD is subsequently repaired with glutaraldehyde-treated or fresh pericardium. Aortic homograft material is another option to use for VSD closure. It is important to avoid even small residual VSDs in this situation.

Patent Ductus Arteriosus

Infections associated with patent ductus arteriosus (PDA) are rare. The vegetation is typically on the pulmonary artery opposite the opening of the PDA, though involvement of the aortic valve has been reported [58,59]. Urgent surgery is rarely needed. At the time of surgery, debridement of the vegetation should be strongly considered unless it can be demonstrated that it is sterile and not mechanically obstructive. In the absence of active infection, the PDA can simply be closed in the usual fashion without the use of cardiopulmonary bypass.

Systemic-to-Pulmonary Artery Shunts

Infections in the BT shunts are rare. In some cases the infection can be cleared with antibiotics alone. It is difficult to clear documented infections of BT shunts with vegetations or pseudoaneurysm with medical treatment alone. Infection of the shunt can result in increased cyanosis by decreasing pulmonary blood flow. Surgery typically involves complete removal of the shunt and either repair of the underlying cardiac defect or insertion of a new shunt from a different source vessel to a new site on the pulmonary artery. As there is insertion of new prosthetic material there is the potential for reinfection. Thus, it is important to have adequate serum levels of appropriate antimicrobials. If a new source blood vessel is not possible, complete removal of the old shunt with removal of any visible disease followed by insertion of a new shunt may be acceptable.

Infections in Prosthetic Valves

Early (<2 months) infection in a prosthetic valve is commonly treated surgically with removal of the prosthesis and replacement with a new prosthetic valve [51]. Diagnosing prosthetic valve endocarditis may be quite challenging. Presence of alternative sources of bacteremia (e.g., central venous catheters), difficulty of echocardiogram to confirm vegetations owing to presence of pledgets, and shadowing from the mechanical valve, possibility of thrombi at intracardiac suture lines causing remote emboli, are some of the challenges that are frequently encountered. Serial echocardiograms and TEE may help resolve some controversial issues. In the absence of the usual indications for surgery, especially if no vegetations are confirmed and if there is no prosthetic valvar dysfunction, it is acceptable to treat with a course of antibiotics. Rapid clearance of bacteremia, stable heart function, and good prosthetic valve function, indicate successful treatment and possibly error in the initial diagnosis. Otherwise, reoperation with removal and debridement of the prosthetic valve is warranted. It is important to remove the old sewing ring and pledgets used at the original surgery. The valve is replaced with a new prosthesis. Surprisingly the incidence of recurrent infection is low. Indications for surgery in late prosthetic valve infection are similar to those for native valve endocarditis, but the surgical technique remains the same.

Results

Infective Endocarditis in Children

Very few series of surgical treatment of endocarditis are reported in children in the recent era. Surgical mortality has been reported from 8–25%. Mavroudis et al. [18] reported a series of 16 patients with endocarditis undergoing surgery. Surgical mortality was 25%. In half of the patients, excision of vegetations was the only procedure needed. More recently, Niwa et al. from Japan [60] reported 119 patients with CHD who were diagnosed with endocarditis; 43.1% of the patients underwent surgery. Total mortality in the series was 8.8%. Mortality was 11.1% in patients who underwent surgery in the acute phase, but there were no deaths in the group who could undergo surgery after the infection was cleared with antibiotics. The mortality in patients undergoing medical treatment alone was 8%. Another pediatric series from the United Kingdom by Alexiou et al. [61] reported a 6.25% surgical mortality, and only one patient had late recurrence of endocarditis. Interestingly, 68% of patients underwent valve replacement, and the median time to surgery was 21 days.

Early Surgery

A number of studies demonstrate the advantage of early surgical treatment within the first month of starting antibiotics [36,37]. Chu et al. [62] reported a mortality of 14% in patients undergoing surgery versus 20% in patients undergoing medical treatment alone. Tleyjeh et al. [63] performed a systematic review of observational studies, which included propensity score analysis. They found surgical advantage on mortality from two observational studies only. Other studies yielded inconclusive results. Interestingly, despite having advanced disease in patients undergoing surgery, none of the studies showed a survival disadvantage of surgery. Thuny et al. [36] reported on 291 patients undergoing surgery within 1 week of starting antibiotics. Surgical mortality was 15%. Interestingly only one of the 10 patients with a preoperative stroke had worsening of the neurologic status, whereas two patients had a new postoperative stroke, and 12% of the patients had recurrence of endocarditis within 1 year of surgery. Prosthetic valve endocarditis was a risk factor for mortality. A number of studies in adults show a survival benefit [36,37].

Table 44.2 Risk factors for mortality.

Authors	Year	Adults vs. children	Risk factors for mortality
Mavroudis et al. [18]	1992	Children	Age <2 years
Chen et al. [64]	1994	Children	Age <2 Native valve endocarditis
Hill et al. [41]	2008	Adults	Vegetation >10 mm *Staphylococcus aureus* Multiple emboli
Nadji et al. [37]	2008	Adults	Heart failure *Staphylococcus aureus* Major neurologic event Prosthetic valve endocarditis
Thuny et al. [36]	2008	Adults	Periannular extension
Chu et al. [62]	2008	Adults	*Staphylococcus aureus* Embolic event APACHE II score

However, there is lack of randomized data. In a review by Tleyjeh et al. [63], two studies showed benefit of surgical therapy and two revealed conflicting results.

Risk Factors for Death

A number of risk factors have been related to mortality and morbidity (Table 44.2) [18,36,37,41,62,64]. Both Rhodes and Mavroudis found age <2 years to be a risk factor for death after surgery in children [18,65]. Fungal endocarditis [35,66] and culture-negative endocarditis [46] have been implicated in higher mortality in children. A large series from adult patients with endocarditis report *S. aureus* endocarditis, large vegetation size (>10 mm), and multiple emboli to be associated with death [41]. Similarly, prosthetic valve endocarditis, uncontrolled sepsis, CHF, and periannular extension of infection have all been associated with mortality [36,37].

Summary

Infectious endocarditis is rare in children. The risk is increased in those with untreated CHD or those with residual lesions post repair. Cyanotic children are particularly at risk. Routine antibiotic prophylaxis is no longer recommended by new AHA guidelines except in high-risk cases. Gram-positive organisms are the most common cause of infection, but fungal infections occur with increasing incidence, especially in premature babies and immunocompromised children. A prolonged course of antibiotic treatment is needed. We advocate early consideration of surgery in patients with appropriate indications to avoid valve replacement and reduce mortality and morbidity.

References

1. Karl T, Wensley D, Stark J, et al. (1987) Infective endocarditis in children with congenital heart disease: comparison of selected features in patients with surgical correction or palliation and those without. Br Heart J 58, 57–65.
2. Day MD, Gauvreau K, Shulman S, et al. (2009) Characteristics of Children Hospitalized With Infective Endocarditis. Circulation 119, 865–870.
3. Ferrieri P, Gewitz MH, Gerber MA, et al. (2002) Unique features of infective endocarditis in childhood. Pediatrics 109, 931–943.
4. Van Hare GF, Ben-Shachar G, Liebman J, et al. (1984) Infective endocarditis in infants and children during the past 10 years: a decade of change. Am Heart J 107, 1235–1240.
5. Martin JM, Neches WH, Wald ER. (1997) Infective endocarditis: 35 years of experience at a children's hospital. Clin Infect Dis 24, 669–675.
6. Saiman L, Prince A, Gersony WM. (1993) Pediatric infective endocarditis in the modern era. J Pediatr 122, 847–853.
7. Johnson DH, Rosenthal A, Nadas AS. (1975) A forty-year review of bacterial endocarditis in infancy and childhood. Circulation 51, 581–588.
8. Weber R, Berger C, Balmer C, et al. (2008) Interventions using foreign material to treat congenital heart disease in children increase the risk for infective endocarditis. Pediatr Infect Dis J 27, 544–550.
9. Wilson W, Taubert KA, Gewitz M, et al. (2007) Prevention of infective endocarditis: guidelines from the American Heart Association: a guideline from the American Heart Association Rheumatic Fever, Endocarditis, and Kawasaki Disease Committee, Council on Cardiovascular Disease in the Young, and the Council on Clinical Cardiology, Council on Cardiovascular Surgery and Anesthesia, and the Quality of Care and Outcomes Research Interdisciplinary Working Group. Circulation 116, 1736–1754.
10. Daher AH, Berkowitz FE. (1995) Infective endocarditis in neonates. Clin Pediatr (Phila) 34, 198–206.
11. Opie GF, Fraser SH, Drew JH, et al. (1999) Bacterial endocarditis in neonatal intensive care. J Paediatr Child Health 35, 545–548.
12. Pearlman SA, Higgins S, Eppes S, et al. (1998) Infective endocarditis in the premature neonate. Clin Pediatr (Phila) 37, 741–746.
13. Burnette-Curley D, Wells V, Viscount H, et al. (1995) FimA, a major virulence factor associated with Streptococcus parasanguis endocarditis. Infect Immun 63, 4669–4674.
14. Gould K, Ramirez-Ronda CH, Holmes RK, et al. (1975) Adherence of bacteria to heart valves in vitro. J Clin Invest 56, 1364–1370.
15. Piroth L, Que YA, Widmer E, et al. (2008) The fibrinogen- and fibronectin-binding domains of Staphylococcus aureus fibronectin-binding protein A synergistically promote endothelial invasion and experimental endocarditis. Infect Immun 76, 3824–3831.

16. Viscount HB, Munro CL, Burnette-Curley D, *et al.* (1997) Immunization with FimA protects against Streptococcus parasanguis endocarditis in rats. Infect Immun 65, 994–1002.

17. Myers C, Aggoun Y, Gervaix A, *et al.* (2007) Postoperative gram-negative anaerobic bacterial endocarditis. Pediatr Infect Dis J 26, 369.

18. Citak M, Rees A, Mavroudis C. (1992) Surgical management of infective endocarditis in children. Ann Thorac Surg 54, 755–760.

19. Sulayman RF, Giri N, Chiemmongkoltip P. (1975) Myocardial infarction complicating bacterial endocarditis in rheumatic heart disease. Report of a case and review of the literature. J Pediatr 86, 59–62.

20. Venkatesan C, Wainwright MS. (2008) Pediatric endocarditis and stroke: a single-center retrospective review of seven cases. Pediatr Neurol 38, 243–247.

21. Salgado AV, Furlan AJ, Keys TF, *et al.* (1989) Neurologic complications of endocarditis: a 12-year experience. Neurology 39, 173–178.

22. Washington JA. (1987) The microbiological diagnosis of infective endocarditis. J Antimicrob Chemother 20(Suppl A), 29–39.

23. Callihan DR, Migneault PC, Nolte FS. (1984) Clinical and bacteriologic evaluation of BACTEC resin-containing blood culture medium. Am J Clin Pathol 82, 465–469.

24. Goldenberger D, Kunzli A, Vogt P, *et al.* (1997) Molecular diagnosis of bacterial endocarditis by broad-range PCR amplification and direct sequencing. J Clin Microbiol 35, 2733–2739.

25. Pitchford CW, Creech CB 2nd, Peters TR, *et al.* (2006) *Bartonella henselae* endocarditis in a child. Pediatr Cardiol 27, 769–771.

26. Gauduchon V, Chalabreysse L, Etienne J, *et al.* (2003) Molecular diagnosis of infective endocarditis by PCR amplification and direct sequencing of DNA from valve tissue. J Clin Microbiol 41, 763–766.

27. Li JS, Sexton DJ, Mick N, *et al.* (2000) Proposed modifications to the Duke criteria for the diagnosis of infective endocarditis. Clin Infect Dis 30, 633–638.

28. Aly AM, Simpson PM, Humes RA. (1999) The role of transthoracic echocardiography in the diagnosis of infective endocarditis in children. Arch Pediatr Adolesc Med 153, 950–954.

29. Karalis DG, Bansal RC, Hauck AJ, *et al.* (1992) Transesophageal echocardiographic recognition of subaortic complications in aortic valve endocarditis. Clinical and surgical implications. Circulation 86, 353–362.

30. Reynolds HR, Jagen MA, Tunick PA, *et al.* (2003) Sensitivity of transthoracic versus transesophageal echocardiography for the detection of native valve vegetations in the modern era. J Am Soc Echocardiogr 16, 67–70.

31. Feuchtner GM, Stolzmann P, Dichtl W, *et al.* (2009) Multislice computed tomography in infective endocarditis: comparison with transesophageal echocardiography and intraoperative findings. J Am Coll Cardiol 53, 436–444.

32. Baddour LM, Wilson WR, Bayer AS, *et al.* (2005) Infective endocarditis: diagnosis, antimicrobial therapy, and management of complications: a statement for healthcare professionals from the Committee on Rheumatic Fever, Endocarditis, and Kawasaki Disease, Council on Cardiovascular Disease in the Young, and the Councils on Clinical Cardiology, Stroke, and Cardiovascular Surgery and Anesthesia, American Heart Association: endorsed by the Infectious Diseases Society of America. Circulation 111, e394–e434.

33. Buchholtz K, Larsen CT, Hassager C, *et al.* (2009) Severity of gentamicin's nephrotoxic effect on patients with infective endocarditis: a prospective observational cohort study of 373 patients. Clin Infect Dis 48, 65–71.

34. Fowler VG Jr, Boucher HW, Corey GR, *et al.* (2006) Daptomycin versus standard therapy for bacteremia and endocarditis caused by Staphylococcus aureus. N Engl J Med 355, 653–665.

35. Millar BC, Jugo J, Moore JE. (2005) Fungal endocarditis in neonates and children. Pediatr Cardiol 26, 517–536.

36. Thuny F, Beurtheret S, Gariboldi V, *et al.* (2008) Outcome after surgical treatment performed within the first week of antimicrobial therapy during infective endocarditis: a prospective study. Arch Cardiovasc Dis 101, 687–695.

37. Nadji G, Goissen T, Brahim A, *et al.* (2008) Impact of early surgery on 6-month outcome in acute infective endocarditis. Int J Cardiol 129, 227–232.

38. Normand J, Bozio A, Etienne J, *et al.* (1995) Changing patterns and prognosis of infective endocarditis in childhood. Eur Heart J 16(Suppl B), 28–31.

39. Bonow RO, Carabello BA, Chatterjee K, *et al.* (2006) ACC/AHA 2006 guidelines for the management of patients with valvular heart disease: a report of the American College of Cardiology/American Heart Association Task Force on Practice Guidelines (writing Committee to Revise the 1998 guidelines for the management of patients with valvular heart disease) developed in collaboration with the Society of Cardiovascular Anesthesiologists endorsed by the Society for Cardiovascular Angiography and Interventions and the Society of Thoracic Surgeons. J Am Coll Cardiol 48, e1–e148.

40. Jault F, Gandjbakhch I, Rama A, *et al.* (1997) Active native valve endocarditis: determinants of operative death and late mortality. Ann Thorac Surg 63, 1737–1741.

41. Hill EE, Herijgers P, Claus P, *et al.* (2008) Clinical and echocardiographic risk factors for embolism and mortality in infective endocarditis. Eur J Clin Microbiol Infect Dis 27, 1159–1164.

42. Snygg-Martin U, Gustafsson L, Rosengren L, *et al.* (2008) Cerebrovascular complications in patients with left-sided infective endocarditis are common: a prospective study using magnetic resonance imaging and neurochemical brain damage markers. Clin Infect Dis 47, 23–30.

43. Baddley JW, Benjamin DK Jr, Patel M, *et al.* (2008) Candida infective endocarditis. Eur J Clin Microbiol Infect Dis 27, 519–529.

44. Gillinov AM, Shah RV, Curtis WE, *et al.* (1996) Valve replacement in patients with endocarditis and acute neurologic deficit. Ann Thorac Surg 61, 1125–1129; discussion 1130.

45. Ting W, Silverman N, Levitsky S. (1991) Valve replacement in patients with endocarditis and cerebral septic emboli. Ann Thorac Surg 51, 18–21; discussion 22.

46. Zamorano J, Sanz J, Moreno R, *et al.* (2001) Comparison of outcome in patients with culture-negative versus culture-positive active infective endocarditis. Am J Cardiol 87, 1423–1425.

47. Soeda A, Sakai N, Murao K, *et al.* (2003) [Management strategy for infectious cerebral aneurysms: report of four cases]. No Shinkei Geka 31, 319–324.

48. Morawetz RB, Karp RB. (1984) Evolution and resolution of intracranial bacterial (mycotic) aneurysms. Neurosurgery 15, 43–49.

49. Kannoth S, Iyer R, Thomas SV, *et al.* (2007) Intracranial infectious aneurysm: presentation, management and outcome. J Neurol Sci 256, 3–9.

50. Fedoruk LM, Jamieson WR, Ling H, *et al.* (2009) Predictors of recurrence and reoperation for prosthetic valve endocarditis after valve replacement surgery for native valve endocarditis. J Thorac Cardiovasc Surg 137, 326–333.

51. Drinkwater DC Jr, Laks H, Child JS. (1996) Issues in surgical treatment of endocarditis including intraoperative and postoperative management. Cardiol Clin 14, 451–464.

52. Sabik JF, Lytle BW, Blackstone EH, *et al.* (2002) Aortic root replacement with cryopreserved allograft for prosthetic valve endocarditis. Ann Thorac Surg 74, 650–659; discussion 659.

53. Kato Y, Tsutsumi Y, Kawai T, *et al.* (2008) [Ross operation and mitral valve repair for active infective endocarditis]. Kyobu Geka 61, 982–985.

54. Okada K, Tanaka H, Takahashi H, *et al.* (2008) Aortic root replacement for destructive aortic valve endocarditis with left ventricular-aortic discontinuity. Ann Thorac Surg 85, 940–945.

55. Bohm JO, Botha CA, Hemmer W, *et al.* (2001) The Ross operation as a combined procedure and in complicated cases–is there an increased risk? Thorac Cardiovasc Surg 49, 300–305.

56. Frank MW, Mavroudis C, Backer CL, *et al.* (1998) Repair of mitral valve and subaortic mycotic aneurysm in a child with endocarditis. Ann Thorac Surg 65, 1788–1790.

57. Karamlou T, Jang K, Williams WG, *et al.* (2005) Outcomes and associated risk factors for aortic valve replacement in 160 children: a competing-risks analysis. Circulation 112, 3462–3469.

58. Aggarwal SK, Barik R. (2007) Infective endocarditis of a patent arterial duct in an adult, with vegetations extending to the aortic and pulmonary valves. Cardiol Young 17, 565–566.

59. Touze JE, Ekra A, Bertrand E. (1986) Isolated pulmonary valve endocarditis with patent ductus arteriosus. A report of a case. Acta Cardiol 41, 313–318.

60. Niwa K, Nakazawa M, Tateno S, *et al.* (2005) Infective endocarditis in congenital heart disease: Japanese national collaboration study. Heart 91, 795–800.

61. Alexiou C, Langley SM, Monro JL. (1999) Surgery for infective valve endocarditis in children. Eur J Cardiothorac Surg 16, 653–659.

62. Chu VH, Cabell CH, Benjamin DK Jr, *et al.* (2004) Early predictors of in-hospital death in infective endocarditis. Circulation 109, 1745–1749.

63. Tleyjeh IM, Kashour T, Zimmerman V, *et al.* (2008) The role of valve surgery in infective endocarditis management: a systematic review of observational studies that included propensity score analysis. Am Heart J 156, 901–909.

64. Chen SC, Hsieh KS, Wang YJ, *et al.* (1994) Infective endocarditis in infants and children during the past ten years. Zhonghua Yi Xue Za Zhi (Taipei) 53, 109–115.

65. Johnson CM, Rhodes KH. (1982) Pediatric endocarditis. Mayo Clin Proc 57, 86–94.

66. Coward K, Tucker N, Darville T. (2003) Infective endocarditis in Arkansan children from 1990 through 2002. Pediatr Infect Dis J 22, 1048–1052.

CHAPTER 45

Pediatric Mechanical Circulatory Support

Brian W. Duncan[1,2]

[1]BioEnterprise, Cleveland, OH, USA
[2]Arboretum Ventures, Cleveland, OH, USA

Introduction

Mechanical circulatory support has become standard therapy for adults with medically refractory heart failure. Several device options are available for adults for most clinically relevant indications including bridge to transplantation, bridge to myocardial recovery, or destination therapy. Historically, these same options have been unavailable for children. The main cause for limited device availability for pediatric circulatory support is clear—the small number of affected children makes it difficult for manufacturers to justify the expense and other resources required for the limited pediatric market. In addition, anatomic limitations imposed by patient size and physiologic limitations imposed by the nature of pediatric cardiovascular disease make many devices used for adult circulatory support unsuitable for children. During the past several decades, extracorporeal membrane oxygenation (ECMO) has been the therapeutic mainstay for pediatric mechanical circulatory support; at many centers in the United States, it remains the only available option. However, ECMO is suitable only for short-term support, significantly limiting its effectiveness as a bridge to transplantation or recovery for children. These limitations are particularly significant for the youngest patients; infants with unrecoverable cardiac failure who require mechanical circulatory support often die if a donor heart does not become available within a few weeks. Lack of availability of ventricular assist devices (VADs) and other circulatory support technologies designed to meet the specific requirements of children remains a major therapeutic gap in the management of pediatric heart failure [1–24].

Over the last few years, significant advances have been made suggesting that the outlook for the field of pediatric mechanical circulatory support is brighter. These advances, over a variety of subdisciplines, include educational activities (medical conferences with dedicated content), increased pediatric experience with a number of new devices, and research funding for the development of innovative circulatory support systems aimed specifically at the pediatric population (Table 45.1) [25]. This broad range of activities is important in that the therapeutic approach has been substantially broadened to address current clinical needs, and development and educational activities ensure that a pipeline of innovative technologies will continue to have a positive effect in the future.

As the experience with pediatric circulatory support has increased, the greater number of devices available for children has required increased understanding of which device is most suitable in a given clinical setting. Currently available devices for which there is significant clinical experience include ECMO, the Bio-Pump (Medtronic Corp., Minneapolis, Minnesota), a number of adult devices that have been successfully used in children, the DeBakey VAD *Child* (MicroMed Cardiovascular, Inc., Houston, Texas), and the Berlin Heart VAD (Berlin Heart Inc, The Woodlands, Texas) (Figure 45.1) [7,26]. Based on the clinical circumstances, each device possesses certain advantages and limitations; therefore, thorough understanding of the unique characteristics of each device is critical to appropriate device selection for a given clinical case.

Available Devices for Pediatric Mechanical Circulatory Support

Extracorporeal Membrane Oxygenation

Extracorporeal membrane oxygenation remains the most commonly used form of pediatric mechanical circulatory support in the United States; well over 3500 cases of pediatric cardiac ECMO have been recorded in the registry of the Extracorporeal Life Support Organization [1,3,6,23,27–37]. Extracorporeal membrane oxygenation is flexible in its ability to provide support for even the smallest patients and

Pediatric Cardiac Surgery, Fourth Edition. Edited by Constantine Mavroudis and Carl L. Backer.
© 2013 Blackwell Publishing Ltd. Published 2013 by Blackwell Publishing Ltd.

its ability to be instituted via peripheral cannulation. This flexibility and the extensive experience in pediatric hospitals using ECMO in the management of newborn respiratory failure has led to its widespread use in the treatment of children with heart failure. In fact, until recently, ECMO was the only available form of mechanical circulatory support capable of treating newborns and infants at many pediatric hospitals in the United States. Because of the presence of an oxygenator, ECMO remains the only option for support when significant hypoxemia and respiratory failure contribute to the underlying pathophysiology. Ease of cannulation via sternotomy or via peripheral sites makes it particularly useful as an acute resuscitative tool [38–40].

However, ECMO also has a number of limitations; its use is restricted to short-term applications making it a poor

Table 45.1 Important recent advances in pediatric mechanical circulatory support. (VAD, ventricular assist device.)

Advance	Year
Funding for National Heart, Lung, and Blood Institute Pediatric Circulatory Support Program begins	2004
First Annual International Conference on Pediatric Mechanical Circulatory Support Systems and Pediatric Cardiopulmonary Perfusion	2004
Humanitarian device exemption status granted to MicroMed DeBakey VAD *Child*	2005
Clinical trial begins in the United States for pediatric use of Berlin Heart VAD	2007
US Food and Drug Administration approves Berlin Heart VAD as bridge for transplant	2011

choice for long-term bridge to transplantation. Perhaps most important is that its large size as usually configured and its extracorporeal design limit attempts at ambulation and effective physical rehabilitation during support. In addition, the presence of an oxygenator and long tubing lengths that are usually employed damage blood elements and activate the inflammatory cascade. Historically, survival to discharge for pediatric cardiac patients supported with ECMO has been in the range of 40–50% [35]. If successfully supported in the short term, long-term survival of pediatric cardiac patients who require ECMO has been reported to exceed 90% after discharge; however, some degree of neurologic impairment in most patients has also been reported [13].

Extracorporeal membrane oxygenation retains an important role in pediatric mechanical circulatory support and has saved thousands of lives of pediatric cardiac patients who otherwise would have died without the availability of this modality; however, the shortcomings cited above are significant and have been well documented (Table 45.2) [26]. In the current era, ECMO continues to play a particularly important role when respiratory failure is present, in addition to cardiac failure and for the rescue of children who suffer cardiorespiratory arrest. As an extension of its role as a resuscitation tool, it is anticipated that ECMO will increasingly be used as a bridge to bridge, similar to its use in adult patients where it has been very useful in providing a period of support after acute resuscitation during which time decision making and evaluation can occur [41]. If cardiac dysfunction is quickly reversible, these patients can be weaned, and patients without prompt cardiac recovery can be transitioned to a device capable of providing long-term support if other end-organ function appears to be recoverable.

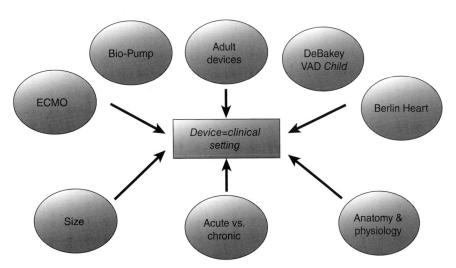

Figure 45.1 Appropriate selection of a device should match the needs of the clinical setting for a given case of pediatric heart failure. (Reproduced with permission from Duncan [26].)

Table 45.2 Extracorporeal membrane oxygenation characteristics. (Reproduced with permission from Duncan [26].)

Advantages	Disadvantages
Versatile	Short-term support only
Track record	Complex circuit
Peripheral/percutaneous cannulation	Complications
	Bleeding
Can be used in patients of any size	Thromboembolic
	Extracorporeal
Biventricular support	No ambulation/rehabilitation potential during support

Table 45.3 Bio-Pump characteristics. (BVAD, biventricular assist device; LVAD, left ventricular assist device; RVAD, right ventricular assist device.) (Reproduced with permission from Duncan [26].)

Advantages	Disadvantages
Track record	Short-term support only
Can be used in patients of any size	Complications
	Bleeding
LVAD, RVAD, BVAD	Thromboembolic
	Extracorporeal
	No ambulation/rehabilitation potential during support

The Bio-Pump

Historically, centrifugal pump-based systems have been the most commonly used form of VAD support for children. The Bio-Pump (Medtronic Bio-Medicus, Minneapolis, Minnesota) employs a constrained vortex design that provides nonpulsatile flow, which is both preload and afterload sensitive. The VAD circuit based on this pump employs short tubing lengths to connect the pump to the venous and aortic cannulas, which results in smaller priming volumes compared with ECMO and makes the system easy to maintain (Table 45.3) [8,14,26,40,42–47]. Similar to ECMO, the Bio-Pump can be used to support patients of all ages and can be used as a right, left, or biventricular assist device (RVAD, LVAD, or BVAD). Despite its simplicity and proven track record, the Bio-Pump is limited to short term support, usually ranging from days to at most a few weeks. As is the case for ECMO, the relatively large size and extracorporeal configuration of the Bio-Pump limits ambulation and rehabilitation potential during support (Table 45.3) [26]. With the availability of newer VADs designed specifically for children, the role of the Bio-Pump for pediatric applications is likely to decline in the future.

Adult Systems Used for Pediatric Support

A number of devices designed for adults have been used successfully to support older children and adolescents with results that are at least as good as those reported for adults [48]. These devices include the Thoratec and Heartmate VADs (Thoratec Corp; Pleasanton, California), the BVS 5000 (ABIOMED, Inc; Danvers, Maine), and the NovaCor LVAS (WorldHeart Inc; Oakland, California). The Thoratec VAD has had the greatest use in children, with a worldwide experience that exceeds 200 pediatric implants [48–50]. As

Table 45.4 Adult device characteristics. (BVAD, biventricular assist device; LVAD, left ventricular assist device; RVAD, right ventricular assist device.) (Reproduced with permission from Duncan [26].)

Advantages	Disadvantages
Chronic support	Use limited to older children
Usually paracorporeal	Decreased washout in smallest patients leads to high incidence of thromboembolic complications
Allows ambulation/rehabilitation during support	
Excellent performance	
LVAD, RVAD, BVAD	

in adults, these devices are capable of providing long-term circulatory support in children, making them suitable for use as a bridge to transplantation. In addition, the Thoratec VAD and similar paracorporeal systems allow children to ambulate and facilitate rehabilitation during support with the same salutary effects as seen in the adult population. The chief limitation for these systems is their large size, which restricts their use to large children and adolescent patients (Table 45.4) [26]. The relatively large stroke volumes of these pulsatile systems require their operation at nonphysiologic, low pump rates for all but the largest children, limiting pump wash-out, which leads to increased thromboembolic risk [42,51].

Recently, Blume and colleagues summarized a 10-year, multicenter experience with VADs as a bridge to heart transplantation in children [48]. Most of the patients in this report were older than 10 years of age, which is reflective of VAD use patterns in North America during that period when the majority of the pediatric bridge to transplant experience was limited to older children who could be supported with devices designed for adults. Seventy-seven percent of these patients were successfully bridged to transplantation, with 86% successfully bridged in the most recent cohort. Hill and Reinhartz reported the worldwide pediatric experience from the Thoratec registry in 2006 that included 209 pediatric patients with a mean age of 14.5 years (range, 5–18 years) and a mean body surface area (BSA) of $1.6\,m^2$ (range, $0.73–2.3\,m^2$) [50]. Fifty-three percent of these patients were supported with BVAD, and 42% were supported with LVAD. The mean support period was 44 days, with the longest duration of support greater than 430 days. More than 68% of the patients survived to heart transplantation or native heart recovery.

The MicroMed DeBakey VAD Child

In the spring of 2004, the DeBakey VAD Child (MicroMed Cardiovascular, Inc; Houston, Texas) was granted Humanitarian Device Exemption (HDE) status by the FDA for use in children [52]. The pediatric version employs the same axial-flow pump used in the adult system, with design modifications aimed at reducing the lateral space requirements to make implantation easier in small children. These modifications include a shortened, more acutely angled inflow cannula, a shortened plastic outflow graft protector, and reduced size of the flow probe on the outflow graft (Plate 45.1, see plate section opposite p. 594). Under the current HDE, the VAD Child is limited to use as a bridge to cardiac transplantation for children from 5–16 years of age with a BSA greater than $0.7\,m^2$ and less than $1.5\,m^2$ and is designed to be fully implantable in this size range, which allows ambulation and rehabilitation during support (Table 45.5) [26]. Fraser and colleagues summarized a six-patient experience with the VAD Child with an average age of 11.3 years (range, 6–15 years) and a BSA of $0.8–1.7\,m^2$ [53]. The average duration of support was 39 days, with 84 days being the longest duration of support. Three of these patients were successfully transplanted, and three died during support, before transplantation.

Table 45.5 DeBakey VAD *Child* characteristics. (LVAD, left ventricular assist device.) (Reproduced with permission from Duncan [26].)

Advantages	Disadvantages
Implantable	Limited age range (5–16 years)
Allows ambulation/rehabilitation during support	Implantation difficult in smallest patients
Long-term support	LVAD only
	Limited indications

The DeBakey VAD Child was the first VAD designed specifically for children available in the United States, and its development represented a true breakthrough in the field of pediatric mechanical circulatory support. However, the restricted patient size range for which the device is suitable has contributed to its relatively limited pediatric experience to date [53].

The Berlin Heart VAD

The Berlin Heart VAD (Berlin Heart Inc, The Woodlands, Texas) is a pulsatile, paracorporeal VAD that is suitable for the entire size range of pediatric patients, including neonates [2,12,17,18,21,49,54–63]. The Berlin Heart VAD employs pneumatically driven, thin membrane pumps to provide pulsatile flow and is available in a variety of pump sizes (10–80 mL), with the smallest pump sizes suitable for infant support (Plate 45.2, see plate section opposite p. 594). The Berlin Heart VAD has been an important tool in the management of heart failure in children for more than a decade in European centers, and a number of reports exist detailing these results [57,64,65]. Of particular benefit, this pulsatile paracorporeal system allows extubation and ambulation, providing an opportunity for rehabilitation during support. Improvement in a patient's physiologic status during support is commonly seen in adults but has only recently been attainable for small children; the Berlin Heart is almost singularly responsible for this revolutionary improvement in pediatric patient management. The Berlin Heart VAD is superior to ECMO in providing moderate- to long-term support, while preserving the options of bridging to transplantation or recovery (Table 45.6) [26,66].

The chief impediment to more widespread use of the Berlin Heart VAD in the United States was its limited availability, which until recently was limited to emergency compassionate use. In 2007, the Berlin Heart was approved for a US multicenter trial in pediatric patients. Early US experience with the Berlin Heart includes a report by Rockett and

Table 45.6 Berlin Heart VAD characteristics. (BVAD, biventricular assist device; LVAD, left ventricular assist device; RVAD, right ventricular assist device.) (Reproduced with permission from Duncan [26].)

Advantages	Disadvantages
Can be used in patients of any size	Availability for use in US centers limited to emergency basis or as part of clinical trial
Paracorporeal	
Allows ambulation/rehabilitation during support	
Excellent performance	
Chronic support LVAD, RVAD, BVAD	

colleagues, with a survival rate during support to transplant or recovery in excess of 80% [62]. Malaisrie and colleagues reported a small experience, with more than 60% successful bridge to transplantation [59]. Both of these studies reported a significant number of neurologic complications because of thromboembolic phenomena during support. A previous report has suggested that the Berlin Heart VAD may have fewer bleeding complications compared with ECMO, with decreased blood product use during support [64]. One recent report notes improving results for infants in the latest cohort of patients, with survival rates now approaching those achieved in adults [65].

Other Devices

There is increasing but still limited pediatric experience with a number of other devices. The MEDOS HIA-VAD (MEDOS Medizintechnik AG; Stollberg, Germany) is a pulsatile, paracorporeal system that is available in a variety of pump sizes capable of providing support for pediatric patients of all sizes from newborns to adolescents [49,67–72]. The Levitronix CentriMag LVAS (Levitronix LLC; Waltham, Maine) employs a magnetically suspended rotor without bearings and has been used in children; and a version intended specifically for pediatrics, the PediVAS, is in development [67,73]. In addition, TandemHeart (CardiacAssist, Inc; Pittsburgh, Pennsylvania) and the VentrAssist LVAD (VentraCor Ltd; Sydney, Australia) have had limited pediatric use [74,75].

Despite their widespread use in the management of heart failure and ischemic heart disease in adults, there has been relatively limited clinical experience with intra-aortic balloon pumps (IABP) in children [76–79]. The general view in pediatrics has been that effective circulatory support with IABP is limited because of greater elasticity of the aorta and the inability of the device to track high heart rates seen in pediatric practice. Complications from insertion in significantly smaller femoral vessels have been a particular limitation to more widespread adoption. Despite these limitations, a number of centers have developed reasonably large experiences with pediatric IABP, and technologic developments aimed at addressing specific needs in children may lead to greater use in the future.

Decision Matrix to Guide Device Selection for Pediatric Circulatory Support

The increased number of available devices for mechanical circulatory support may lead to uncertainty in pediatric practice regarding which device is most suitable for a given case of medically refractory heart failure. As described above, each of the available devices has unique characteristics that affect their use; on the other side of the equation are the unique needs presented by the specific clinical situation.

A decision support tool has been developed that provides a graphical representation of the key clinical components, namely patient size and the intended duration of support on a 2 × 2 matrix to guide selection from among the available devices currently available for pediatric use [26].

Graphical Depiction of the Clinical Setting on the Decision Matrix

Patient size is obviously an important issue in device selection; in pediatrics, the need for devices that are suitable over a wide range of patient sizes from newborns to adolescents is the single greatest difference compared with the practice of mechanical circulatory support in adults. The anticipated duration of support is also a critical determinant of the overall clinical setting. Perioperative cardiac arrest after congenital heart surgery may be rescued with rapid resuscitation devices and may require only brief periods of support for conditions that are quickly reversible (electrolyte imbalance, transient pulmonary hypertension) [38–40]. At the other end of the spectrum, medically refractory heart failure occurring in end-stage dilated cardiomyopathy may require months of support waiting for a suitable donor organ as a bridge to cardiac transplantation.

Figure 45.2 depicts a 2 × 2 graph that defines the clinical setting in which heart failure occurs in terms of patient size and anticipated duration of support [26]. On this graph, patient age is a surrogate for patient size and is plotted on the vertical axis while the anticipated duration of support is plotted on the horizontal axis. The clinical setting may

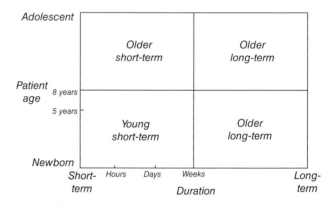

Figure 45.2 Graphical representation of the clinical setting in which pediatric heart failure occurs, determined by patient age (vertical axis) and the anticipated duration of support (horizontal axis). The four clinically relevant clinical settings are depicted as belonging to one of four quadrants: (1) young patients requiring short-term support, (2) young patients requiring long-term support, (3) older children/adolescents requiring short-term support and (4) older children/adolescents requiring long-term support. (Reproduced with permission from Duncan [26].)

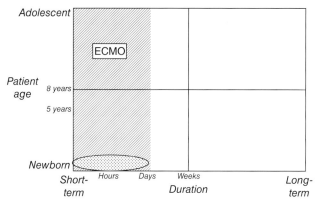

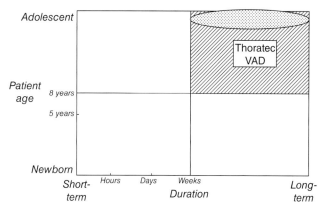

Figure 45.3 Graphical representation of postoperative cardiorespiratory failure in an infant. This patient may recover after relatively short periods of support demonstrated by the stippled oval in the young patient/short term support quadrant. Extracorporeal membrane oxygenation (EMCO) works well in this setting being capable of providing support for newborns and being limited to short term support only (cross-hatched area). In addition, it is the only device capable of providing respiratory support. (Reproduced with permission from Duncan [26].)

Figure 45.4 Graphical representation of advanced heart failure in an adolescent with cardiomyopathy. This patient will most likely require extended support as a bridge to transplantation (stippled oval in the older patient/long-term support quadrant). Devices primarily designed for adults such as the Thoratec ventricular assist device (VAD) have demonstrated good results for this indication (cross-hatched area). (Reproduced with permission from Duncan [26].)

then be considered to belong to one of four quadrants: (1) young patients requiring short-term support, (2) young patients requiring long-term support, (3) older children and adolescents requiring short-term support, and (4) older children and adolescents requiring long term support.

All of the available devices can then be placed on this graph that defines the clinical setting based on suitability for patient size and intended duration of support. Colocation of the patient characteristics and the device on the matrix then identifies the appropriate device for that patient in the relevant clinical setting. Figure 45.3 demonstrates this matching process for a device and patient for a hypothetical case of postoperative cardiorespiratory failure in an infant [26]. Extracorporeal membrane oxygenation is suitable for patients of all sizes and therefore spans the entire vertical axis; however, ECMO is limited to short-term use, which accounts for spanning the horizontal axis from days to weeks. The graphical representation of an infant who suffers cardiorespiratory failure is appropriately placed on the vertical axis close to the origin. Regarding the anticipated duration of support, lung disease in this setting may not respond as promptly as other causes of pediatric cardiorespiratory failure [8]; therefore, the anticipated duration of support may range from days to weeks, as demonstrated by the span of the patient marker on the horizontal axis. The colocation of the device and the patient graphically demonstrates that ECMO is the best choice for support in this case. This example also demonstrates how underlying anatomy and physiology can override all other considerations; for patients suffering from respiratory and cardiac failure, ECMO is the only appropriate choice.

Figure 45.4 [26] provides another example: devices that are designed primarily for adults but which may be used in older children and adolescents, such as the Thoratec VAD, occupy the older child/long-term support quadrant on the graph. These patients would colocate with devices such as the Thoratec, Berlin Heart or Heartmate VADs, which would all be reasonable choices for support.

The National Heart, Lung, and Blood Institute Pediatric Circulatory Support Program

The National Heart, Lung and Blood Institute (NHLBI) Pediatric Circulatory Support Program is another recent landmark development in this field. This program was established to fund stage development of novel pediatric circulatory support devices. Included in the technical requirements of the original solicitation were the following objectives for applicant devices [80]:
1. capable of being instituted in less than 1 hour after the decision to initiate support;
2. minimal priming volumes;
3. cannulation strategies that accommodate potential variations in patient anatomy commonly encountered in pediatric practice;
4. minimized blood product exposure;
5. minimized risks of infection, bleeding, hemolysis, and thrombosis;

Table 45.7 Devices supported by the National Heart, Lung, and Blood Institute Pediatric Circulatory Support program. (pCAS, pediatric cardiopulmonary assist system; PVAD, pediatric ventricular assist device; VAD, ventricular assist device.)

Device	Institution	Characteristics
PediaFlow VAD	University of Pittsburgh	Implantable mixed-flow VAD
PediPump	Cleveland Clinic	Implantable mixed-flow VAD
pCAS	Ension, Inc.	Integrated cardiopulmonary assist system
Pediatric Jarvik 2000	Jarvik Heart, Inc.	Implantable axial-flow VAD
PVAD	Penn State University	Pulsatile VAD

6. capable of providing support for up to 6 months, depending on the intended application.

In the spring of 2004, five contracts were awarded by the NHLBI to support preclinical development of a range of pediatric VADs and similar circulatory support systems (Table 45.7). The pediatric circulatory support devices funded by the NHLBI Pediatric Circulatory Support Program are described below.

The PediaFlow Ventricular Assist Device

The PediaFlow ventricular assist device (VAD; Ension, Inc; Pittsburgh, Pennsylvania) is an implantable, magnetically suspended mixed-flow turbodynamic blood pump [81–83]. The PediaFlow VAD is intended to provide chronic (6 months) of circulatory support for neonates to toddlers (3–15 kg body weight) with congenital or acquired heart disease (Plate 45.3, see plate section opposite p. 594). Anticoagulation therapy while on the device is intended to be limited to antiplatelet medications. The device is designed to provide a flow rate range from 0.3–1.5 L/ minute, with a device weight of 30 g, a maximum volume of 5 mL, and a maximum priming volume 0.5 mL to help achieve the goal of being fully implantable. The design includes the requirement for only a single percutaneous lead crossing the skin for energy transmission.

The PediPump

The PediPump VAD (Cleveland Clinic; Cleveland, Ohio) is a magnetic bearing-supported, rotary dynamic blood pump designed specifically for children [84–88]. Because its capabilities are packaged into a small size, the resulting basic pump design provides support for the entire range of patient sizes encountered in pediatrics. The pump rotating assembly consists of an impeller in the front, front and rear radial mag-

netic bearings, and a motor rotor magnet in its center. Blood enters axially at the inlet and is turned to exit the pump at an intermediate angle through the pump's outside diameter. The use of passive, radial magnetic bearings to support the rotor is anticipated to result in exceptional device durability. In its latest iteration, the PediPump prototype measures approximately $10.5\,mm \times 64.5\,mm$ with a priming volume of 0.6 mL, imparting less than 10% of the physical displacement of currently available axial flow pumps.

Pediatric Cardiopulmonary Assist System

The goal of Ension's Pediatric Cardiopulmonary Assist System (pCAS; Ension, Inc; Pittsburgh, Pennsylvania) development program is to improve on the performance of currently used ECMO leading to decreased clinical complications and increased opportunity for parent-child contact and bonding during support [89,90]. The paracorporeal design of the pCAS system affords modularity, allowing a separate device for each target patient population and the possibility of device exchange during the support period. Such modularity also permits the patient to be "upgraded" from a device appropriate for a neonate to one appropriate for an older child as growth or support needs change (Plate 45.4, see plate section opposite p. 594). In addition to steady flow, the pCAS system will include an option to deliver pulsatile flow at the higher heart rates of the intended patient population [91].

The Pediatric Jarvik 2000

The design of the Pediatric Jarvik 2000 device (Jarvik Heart, Inc; New York) is based on the Jarvik 2000 VAD, which has been implanted in more than 200 patients in the United States, Europe, and Asia. Two pediatric axial flow blood pumps are being developed for the Pediatric Jarvik 2000. These small child and infant Jarvik 2000 models are intended to be versatile and despite the similarity in appearance, are not simply scaled down models of the adult device (Plate 45.5, see plate section opposite p. 594) [92]. The pediatric models have incorporated new blade designs for the lower flow and pressure requirements of children and infants. The encouraging clinical performance of the adult Jarvik 2000 VAD has resulted in high expectations for the Pediatric Jarvik 2000 models; based on the design and clinical results to date for the adult device, the reliability of the pediatric Jarvik 2000 VAD is targeted to exceed 10 years.

Penn State Pediatric VAD

The Penn State Infant VAD (PVAD; Pennsylvania State University, Hershey, Pennsylvania) is a pulsatile, pneumatically actuated blood pump based on the design principles of the adult-sized Pierce-Donachy VAD, which was

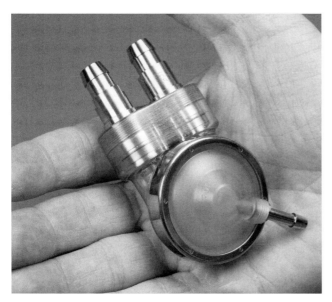

Figure 45.5 The Penn State Infant VAD is a pneumatically actuated pulsatile pump with a dynamic stroke volume of 12–14 mL that utilizes Bjork-Shiley monostrut valves to minimize thrombus formation. (Courtesy of William J Weiss, Pennsylvania State University, Hershey, PA, USA.)

developed at Pennsylvania State University and is now known as the Thoratec VAD [93]. The PVAD, which underwent initial development in 1986 under the direction of William S. Pierce, MD, in collaboration with 3M Corporation, is intended to be used as an LVAD, RVAD, or BVAD for up to 6 months [24,94,95]. The device is intended primarily for paracorporeal placement but will also be implantable for bridge to transplantation applications [96]. The PVAD is being developed in two sizes: a 12 mL dynamic stroke volume size for infants ranging in weight from 5–15 kg and a 25 mL stroke volume size for children weighing 15–35 kg (Figure 45.5). The flow rate ranges of the infant and child-size devices are 0.5–1.3 L/min and 1.3–3.3 L/min, respectively. Each of the pumps consists of a seamless segmented polyether polyurethane urea blood sac positioned within a rigid titanium case, mechanical heart valves, and cannulae connectors. The pump shape encourages the development of a vortex flow pattern, which efficiently maintains high wall shear rates to help prevent thrombus formation. The PVAD is controlled by a new portable biventricular pneumatic driver, which is based on actuator technology developed by Pennsylvania State University for electrically powered implantable blood pumps.

The NHLBI Pediatric Circulatory Support Program's 5-year period of funding ended in March 2009. All five funded projects made important progress throughout the program. All programs were successful in satisfying the primary objectives originally established by the NHLBI, namely to make progress in development of these innova-

tive devices through a rigorous preclinical testing program. All five projects gained considerable understanding of the engineering and other technical aspects of these devices in the pediatric setting. Substantial progress was also made in determining the physiologic impact of these systems, particularly documenting low levels of hemolysis and minimal thromboembolic potential during support. Of particular importance, progress was made during in vivo preclinical testing; all five programs established robust survival animal test programs and documented satisfactory performance of each of these devices during prolonged in vivo support.

Future Directions

In the spring of 2009, the NHLBI made funds available for clinical development projects to support activities necessary to obtain Investigational Device Exemptions (IDEs) from the US Food and Drug Administration (FDA) for investigational circulatory assist devices for infants and small children [97]. These activities include preclinical testing, development of manufacturing processes, and collaboration to develop IDE clinical studies to support Humanitarian Device Exemption (HDE) applications to market the devices as Humanitarian Use Devices (HUDs). Selected developers are asked to conduct all necessary activities with documentation necessary for the IDE in the first 3 years of the contract. During the third year, the developers will generate the clinical studies for their individual projects in partnership with a Data Coordinating Center and complete the requirements for FDA approval of their IDE. Following IDE approval, the contractors will provide regulatory, technical and clinical support for the investigational device during the clinical study, hopefully leading to devices that are clinically available as HUDs [97].

The PumpKIN solicitation represents yet another important milestone in the field of pediatric mechanical circulatory support. As stated in the introduction, educational and scientific progress during the last 5 years in the field of pediatric mechanical circulatory support will hopefully translate into improved clinical results for children with advanced heart failure. Although VADs and similar circulatory support technology had undergone relatively little progress for pediatric applications until recently, these exciting new clinical and research developments suggest that the near future will be a time of significant advances for mechanical circulatory support in children. While immediate prospects for device availability are improving with the introduction of devices such as the DeBakey VAD *Child* and increasing worldwide use of the Berlin Heart VAD for children, support of early stage development of a variety of devices under the NHLBI-funded pediatric circulatory support initiatives will expand treatment options in the future.

Acknowledgment

The PediPump has been funded in whole or in part with federal funds from the National Heart, Lung and Blood Institute, National Institutes of Health, under Contract No.HHSN268200448188C.

References

1. Black MD, Coles JG, Williams WG, *et al.* (1995) Determinants of success in pediatric cardiac patients undergoing extracorporeal membrane oxygenation. Ann Thorac Surg 60, 133–138.

2. Cooper DS, Jacobs JP, Moore L, *et al.* (2007) Cardiac extracorporeal life support: state of the art in 2007. Cardiol Young 17 (Suppl 2), 104–115.

3. del Nido PJ. (1996) Extracorporeal membrane oxygenation for cardiac support in children. Ann Thorac Surg 61, 336–339; discussion 340–341.

4. Duncan BW, ed. (2001) *Mechanical Circulatory Support for Cardiac and Respiratory Failure in Pediatric Cardiac Patients.* New York: Marcel Dekker.

5. Duncan BW. (2002) Mechanical circulatory support for infants and children with cardiac disease. Ann Thorac Surg 73, 1670–1677.

6. Duncan BW. (2005) Pediatric mechanical circulatory support. ASAIO J 51, ix–xiv.

7. Duncan BW. (2006) Pediatric mechanical circulatory support in the United States: past, present, and future. ASAIO J 52, 525–529.

8. Duncan BW, Hraska V, Jonas RA, *et al.* (1999) Mechanical circulatory support in children with cardiac disease. J Thorac Cardiovasc Surg 117, 529–542.

9. Fiser WP, Yetman AT, Gunselman RJ, *et al.* (2003) Pediatric arteriovenous extracorporeal membrane oxygenation (ECMO) as a bridge to cardiac transplantation. J Heart Lung Transplant 22, 770–777.

10. Gajarski RJ, Mosca RS, Ohye RG, *et al.* (2003) Use of extracorporeal life support as a bridge to pediatric cardiac transplantation. J Heart Lung Transplant 22, 28–34.

11. Goldman AP, Cassidy J, de Leval M, *et al.* (2003) The waiting game: bridging to paediatric heart transplantation. Lancet 362, 1967–1970.

12. Hetzer R, Stiller B. (2006) Technology insight: Use of ventricular assist devices in children. Nat Clin Pract Cardiovasc Med 3, 377–386.

13. Ibrahim AE, Duncan BW, Blume ED, *et al.* (2000) Long-term follow-up of pediatric cardiac patients requiring mechanical circulatory support. Ann Thorac Surg 69, 186–192.

14. Khan A, Gazzaniga AB. (1996) Mechanical circulatory assistance in paediatric patients with cardiac failure. Cardiovasc Surg 4, 43–49.

15. Kirshbom PM, Bridges ND, Myung RJ, *et al.* (2002) Use of extracorporeal membrane oxygenation in pediatric thoracic organ transplantation. J Thorac Cardiovasc Surg 123, 130–136.

16. Kolovos NS, Bratton SL, Moler FW, *et al.* (2003) Outcome of pediatric patients treated with extracorporeal life support after cardiac surgery. Ann Thorac Surg 76, 1435–1441; discussion 1441–1442.

17. Pauliks LB, Undar A. (2008) New devices for pediatric mechanical circulatory support. Curr Opin Cardiol 23, 91–96.

18. Potapov EV, Stiller B, Hetzer R. (2007) Ventricular assist devices in children: current achievements and future perspectives. Pediatr Transplant 11, 241–255.

19. Sidiropoulos A, Hotz H, Konertz W. (1998) Pediatric circulatory support. J Heart Lung Transplant 17, 1172–1176.

20. Thiagarajan RR, Nelson DP. (2005) Should we be satisfied with current outcomes for cardiac extracorporeal life support? Pediatr Crit Care Med 6, 89–90.

21. Throckmorton AL, Chopski SG. (2008) Pediatric circulatory support: current strategies and future directions. Biventricular and univentricular mechanical assistance. ASAIO J 54, 491–497.

22. Undar A, McKenzie ED, McGarry MC, *et al.* (2004) Outcomes of congenital heart surgery patients after extracorporeal life support at Texas Children's Hospital. Artif Organs 28, 963–966.

23. Walters HL 3rd, Hakimi M, Rice MD, *et al.* (1995) Pediatric cardiac surgical ECMO: multivariate analysis of risk factors for hospital death. Ann Thorac Surg 60, 329–336; discussion 336–337.

24. Weiss WJ. (2005) Pulsatile pediatric ventricular assist devices. ASAIO J 51, 540–545.

25. Duncan BW. (2005) Pediatric mechanical circulatory support: a new golden era? Artif Organs 29, 925–926.

26. Duncan BW. (2006) Matching the mechanical circulatory support device to the child with heart failure. ASAIO J 52, e15–e21.

27. Aharon AS, Drinkwater DC Jr, Churchwell KB, *et al.* (2001) Extracorporeal membrane oxygenation in children after repair of congenital cardiac lesions. Ann Thorac Surg 72, 2095–2101; discussion 2101–2102.

28. Anderson HL 3rd, Attorri RJ, Custer JR, *et al.* (1990) Extracorporeal membrane oxygenation for pediatric cardiopulmonary failure. J Thorac Cardiovasc Surg 99, 1011–1019; discussion 1019–1021.

29. del Nido PJ, Armitage JM, Fricker FJ, *et al.* (1994) Extracorporeal membrane oxygenation support as a bridge to pediatric heart transplantation. Circulation 90, II66–II69.

30. Duncan BW. (2006) Mechanical cardiac support in the young. Short-term support: ECMO. Semin Thorac Cardiovasc Surg Pediatr Card Surg Annu 75–82.

31. Jaggers JJ, Forbess JM, Shah AS, *et al.* (2000) Extracorporeal membrane oxygenation for infant postcardiotomy support: significance of shunt management. Ann Thorac Surg 69, 1476–1483.

32. Klein MD, Shaheen KW, Whittlesey GC, *et al.* (1990) Extracorporeal membrane oxygenation for the circulatory support of children after repair of congenital heart disease. J Thorac Cardiovasc Surg 100, 498–505.

33. Kulik TJ, Moler FW, Palmisano JM, *et al.* (1996) Outcome-associated factors in pediatric patients treated with extracorporeal membrane oxygenator after cardiac surgery. Circulation 94(9 Suppl), II63–II68.

34. Levi D, Marelli D, Plunkett M, *et al.* (2002) Use of assist devices and ECMO to bridge pediatric patients with cardio-

myopathy to transplantation. J Heart Lung Transplant 21, 760–770.

35. Extracorporeal Life Support Organization. (2007) ECLS Registry Report International Summary. Ann Arbor, MI.

36. Raithel SC, Pennington DG, Boegner E, et al. (1992) Extracorporeal membrane oxygenation in children after cardiac surgery. Circulation 86(5 Suppl), II305–II310.

37. Ziomek S, Harrell JE Jr, Fasules JW, et al. (1992) Extracorporeal membrane oxygenation for cardiac failure after congenital heart operation. Ann Thorac Surg 54, 861–867; discussion 867–868.

38. del Nido PJ, Dalton HJ, Thompson AE, et al. (1992) Extracorporeal membrane oxygenator rescue in children during cardiac arrest after cardiac surgery. Circulation 86(5 Suppl), II300–II304.

39. Duncan BW, Ibrahim AE, Hraska V, et al. (1998) Use of rapid-deployment extracorporeal membrane oxygenation for the resuscitation of pediatric patients with heart disease after cardiac arrest. J Thorac Cardiovasc Surg 116, 305–311.

40. Jacobs JP, Ojito JW, McConaghey TW, et al. (2000) Rapid cardiopulmonary support for children with complex congenital heart disease. Ann Thorac Surg 70, 742–749; discussion 749–750.

41. Smedira NG, Moazami N, Golding CM, et al. (2001) Clinical experience with 202 adults receiving extracorporeal membrane oxygenation for cardiac failure: survival at five years. J Thorac Cardiovasc Surg 122, 92–102.

42. Ashton RC Jr, Oz MC, Michler RE, et al. (1995) Left ventricular assist device options in pediatric patients. ASAIO J 41, M277–M280.

43. Chang AC, Hanley FL, Weindling SN, et al. (1992) Left heart support with a ventricular assist device in an infant with acute myocarditis. Crit Care Med 20, 712–715.

44. Ferrazzi P, Glauber M, Di Domenico A, et al. (1991) Assisted circulation for myocardial recovery after repair of congenital heart disease. Eur J Cardiothorac Surg 5, 419–423; discussion 424.

45. Karl TR, Horton SB. (2001) Centrifugal pump ventricular assist device in pediatric cardiac surgery. In: Duncan BW, ed. *Mechanical Support for Cardiac and Respiratory Failure in Pediatric Patients*. New York: Marcel Dekker, pp. 21–47.

46. Karl TR, Horton SB, Brizard C. (2006) Postoperative support with the centrifugal pump ventricular assist device (VAD). Semin Thorac Cardiovasc Surg Pediatr Card Surg Annu 83–91.

47. Langley SM, Sheppard SV, Tsang VT, et al. (1998) When is extracorporeal life support worthwhile following repair of congenital heart disease in children? Eur J Cardiothorac Surg 13, 520–525.

48. Blume ED, Naftel DC, Bastardi HJ, et al. (2006) Outcomes of children bridged to heart transplantation with ventricular assist devices: a multi-institutional study. Circulation 113, 2313–2319.

49. Arabia FA, Tsau PH, Smith RG, et al. (2006) Pediatric bridge to heart transplantation: application of the Berlin Heart, Medos and Thoratec ventricular assist devices. J Heart Lung Transplant 25, 16–21.

50. Hill JD, Reinhartz O. (2006) Clinical outcomes in pediatric patients implanted with Thoratec ventricular assist device.

Semin Thorac Cardiovasc Surg Pediatr Card Surg Annu 115–122.

51. Ishino K, Loebe M, Uhlemann F, et al. (1997) Circulatory support with paracorporeal pneumatic ventricular assist device (VAD) in infants and children. Eur J Cardiothorac Surg 11, 965–972.

52. Morales DL, Dibardino DJ, McKenzie ED, et al. (2005) Lessons learned from the first application of the DeBakey VAD Child: an intracorporeal ventricular assist device for children. J Heart Lung Transplant 24, 331–337.

53. Fraser CD Jr, Carberry KE, Owens WR, et al. (2006) Preliminary experience with the MicroMed DeBakey pediatric ventricular assist device. Semin Thorac Cardiovasc Surg Pediatr Card Surg Annu 109–114.

54. Alexi-Meskishvili V, Hetzer R, Weng Y, et al. (2001) The use of the Berlin Heart in children. In: Duncan BW, ed. *Mechanical Circulatory Support for Cardiac and Respiratory Failure in Pediatric Patients*. New York: Marcel Dekker, pp. 287–314.

55. Gandhi SK, Huddleston CB, Balzer DT, et al. (2008) Biventricular assist devices as a bridge to heart transplantation in small children. Circulation 118(14 Suppl), S89–S93.

56. Hetzer R, Alexi-Meskishvili V, Weng Y, et al. (2006) Mechanical cardiac support in the young with the Berlin Heart EXCOR pulsatile ventricular assist device: 15 years' experience. Semin Thorac Cardiovasc Surg Pediatr Card Surg Annu 99–108.

57. Hetzer R, Hennig E, Schiessler A, et al. (1992) Mechanical circulatory support and heart transplantation. J Heart Lung Transplant 11, S175–S181.

58. Kirklin JK. (2008) Mechanical circulatory support as a bridge to pediatric cardiac transplantation. Semin Thorac Cardiovasc Surg Pediatr Card Surg Annu 80–85.

59. Malaisrie SC, Pelletier MP, Yun JJ, et al. (2008) Pneumatic paracorporeal ventricular assist device in infants and children: initial Stanford experience. J Heart Lung Transplant 27, 173–177.

60. Merkle F, Boettcher W, Stiller B, et al. (2003) Pulsatile mechanical cardiac assistance in pediatric patients with the Berlin heart ventricular assist device. J Extra Corpor Technol 35, 115–120.

61. Potapov EV, Hetzer R. (2006) Pediatric Berlin Heart Excor. Ann Thorac Cardiovasc Surg 12, 155.

62. Rockett SR, Bryant JC, Morrow WR, et al. (2008) Preliminary single center North American experience with the Berlin Heart pediatric EXCOR device. ASAIO J 54, 479–482.

63. Stiller B, Lemmer J, Schubert S, et al. (2006) Management of pediatric patients after implantation of the Berlin Heart EXCOR ventricular assist device. ASAIO J 52, 497–500.

64. Stiller B, Lemmer J, Merkle F, et al. (2004) Consumption of blood products during mechanical circulatory support in children: comparison between ECMO and a pulsatile ventricular assist device. Intensive Care Med 30, 1814–1820.

65. Stiller B, Weng Y, Hubler M, et al. (2005) Pneumatic pulsatile ventricular assist devices in children under 1 year of age. Eur J Cardiothorac Surg 28, 234–239.

66. Imamura M, Dossey AM, Prodhan P, et al. (2009) Bridge to cardiac transplant in children: Berlin Heart versus extracorporeal membrane oxygenation. Ann Thorac Surg 87, 1894–1901; discussion 1901.

67. Cassidy J, Haynes S, Kirk R, *et al.* (2009) Changing patterns of bridging to heart transplantation in children. J Heart Lung Transplant 28, 249–254.

68. El-Banayosy NR, Arusoglu L, Kleikamp G, *et al.* (2003) Recovery of organ dysfunction during bridging to heart transplantation in children and adolescents. Int J Artif Organs 26, 395–400.

69. Grinda JM, Chevalier P, D'Attellis N, *et al.* (2004) Fulminant myocarditis in adults and children: bi-ventricular assist device for recovery. Eur J Cardiothorac Surg 26, 1169–1173.

70. Guldner NW, Siemens HJ, Schramm U, *et al.* (1996) First clinical application of the Medos-HIA ventricular support system: monitoring of the thrombotic risk by means of the biomarker prothrombin fragment F1 + 2 and scanning electron microscopy evaluation. J Heart Lung Transplant 15, 291–296.

71. Konertz W, Hotz H, Schneider M, *et al.* (1997) Clinical experience with the MEDOS HIA-VAD system in infants and children: a preliminary report. Ann Thorac Surg 63, 1138–1144.

72. Martin J, Sarai K, Schindler M, *et al.* (1997) MEDOS HIA-VAD biventricular assist device for bridge to recovery in fulminant myocarditis. Ann Thorac Surg 63, 1145–1146.

73. Dasse KA, Gellman B, Kameneva MV, *et al.* (2007) Assessment of hydraulic performance and biocompatibility of a MagLev centrifugal pump system designed for pediatric cardiac or cardiopulmonary support. ASAIO J 53, 771–777.

74. Ricci M, Gaughan CB, Rossi M, *et al.* (2008) Initial experience with the TandemHeart circulatory support system in children. ASAIO J 54, 542–545.

75. Ruygrok PN, Esmore DS, Alison PM, *et al.* (2008) Pediatric experience with the VentrAssist LVAD. Ann Thorac Surg 86, 622–626.

76. Akomea-Agyin C, Kejriwal NK, Franks R, *et al.* (1999) Intraaortic balloon pumping in children. Ann Thorac Surg 67, 1415–1420.

77. Hawkins JA, Minich LL. (2001) Intra-aortic balloon counterpulsation for children with cardiac disease. In: Duncan BW, ed. *Mechanical Support for Cardiac and Respiratory Failure in Pediatric Patients*. New York: Marcel Dekker, pp. 49–60.

78. Minich LL, Tani LY, Hawkins JA, *et al.* (2001) Intra-aortic balloon pumping in children with dilated cardiomyopathy as a bridge to transplantation. J Heart Lung Transplant 20, 750–754.

79. Pinkney KA, Minich LL, Tani LY, *et al.* (2002) Current results with intraaortic balloon pumping in infants and children. Ann Thorac Surg 73, 887–891.

80. National Heart, Lung, and Blood Institute. (2002) Pediatric Circulatory Support Program.

81. Borovetz HS, Badylak S, Boston JR, *et al.* (2006) Towards the development of a pediatric ventricular assist device. Cell Transplant 15(Suppl 1), S69–S74.

82. Noh MD, Antaki JF, Ricci M, *et al.* (2008) Magnetic design for the PediaFlow ventricular assist device. Artif Organs 32, 127–135.

83. Wearden PD, Morell VO, Keller BB, *et al.* (2006) The PediaFlow pediatric ventricular assist device. Semin Thorac Cardiovasc Surg Pediatr Card Surg Annu 92–98.

84. Duncan BW, Dudzinski DT, Gu L, *et al.* (2006) The PediPump: development status of a new pediatric ventricular assist device: update II. ASAIO J 52, 581–587.

85. Duncan BW, Dudzinski DT, Noecker AM, *et al.* (2005) The pedipump: development status of a new pediatric ventricular assist device. ASAIO J 51, 536–539.

86. Duncan BW, Lorenz M, Kopcak MW, *et al.* (2005) The PediPump: a new ventricular assist device for children. Artif Organs 29, 527–530.

87. Saeed D, Weber S, Ootaki Y, *et al.* (2007) Initial acute in vivo performance of the Cleveland Clinic PediPump left ventricular assist device. ASAIO J 53, 766–770.

88. Weber S, Dudzinski DT, Gu L, *et al.* (2007) The PediPump: a versatile, implantable pediatric ventricular assist device-update III. ASAIO J 53, 730–733.

89. Fill B, Gartner M, Johnson G, *et al.* (2008) Computational fluid flow and mass transfer of a functionally integrated pediatric pump-oxygenator configuration. ASAIO J 54, 214–219.

90. Pantalos GM, Horrell T, Merkley T, *et al.* (2009) In vitro characterization and performance testing of the ension pediatric cardiopulmonary assist system. ASAIO J 55, 282–286.

91. Pantalos GM, Giridharan G, Colyer J, *et al.* (2007) Effect of continuous and pulsatile flow left ventricular assist on pulsatility in a pediatric animal model of left ventricular dysfunction: pilot observations. ASAIO J 53, 385–391.

92. Kilic A, Nolan TD, Li T, *et al.* (2007) Early in vivo experience with the pediatric Jarvik 2000 heart. ASAIO J 53, 374–378.

93. Pierce WS, Rosenberg G, Donachy JH, *et al.* (1987) Postoperative cardiac support with a pulsatile assist pump: techniques and results. Artif Organs 11, 247–251.

94. Cooper BT, Roszelle BN, Long TC, *et al.* (2008) The 12 cc Penn State pulsatile pediatric ventricular assist device: fluid dynamics associated with valve selection. J Biomech Eng 130, 041019.

95. Roszelle BN, Cooper BT, Long TC, *et al.* (2008) The 12 cc Penn State pulsatile pediatric ventricular assist device: flow field observations at a reduced beat rate with application to weaning. ASAIO J 54, 325–331.

96. Daily BB, Pettitt TW, Sutera SP, *et al.* (1996) Pierce-Donachy pediatric VAD: progress in development. Ann Thorac Surg 61, 437–443.

97. National Heart, Lung and Blood Institute. (2008) Pumps for Kids, Infants and Neonates (PumpKIN). National Heart, Lung and Blood Institute.

46

Adult Congenital Heart Disease

Stamatia Prapa,[1,2] Konstantinos Dimopoulos,[1,2] Darryl F. Shore,[1,2] Mario Petrou,[1] and Michael A. Gatzoulis[1,2]

[1]Royal Brompton Hospital, London, UK
[2]Imperial College London, London, UK

The successful management and correction of congenital heart defects (CHD) during infancy has resulted in an increasing number of adults with CHD. Due to medical and surgical advances, 85% of children born with CHD now survive to adulthood [1]. It is imperative that this group of young adults is not lost to follow-up. Smooth transition of these individuals from pediatric to adult care is an essential but often difficult process for both the clinician and the patient. Important issues such as residual hemodynamic lesions, arrhythmia management, endocarditis prophylaxis, career, and family planning should be addressed in an appropriate and timely fashion [2]. In fact, as this population ages, long-term complications become more frequent posing a significant burden and challenge on healthcare [3].

Adults with CHD may be divided into those with previous repair or palliation and those with unrepaired lesions. While patients with repaired lesions are more likely to have had relief of the hemodynamic burden posed by the original cardiac defect, residual hemodynamic lesions and sequelae from surgery, such as scar-related arrhythmias, are frequent. Follow-up is thus essential in all, even the most stable, adult CHD (ACHD) patients. Patients with unrepaired lesions are those with a delayed or missed diagnosis and those in whom repair was impossible or considered too high-risk at the time. Those with persistent unrepaired lesions may at times undergo palliative procedures as a definitive approach or a bridge to repair, even though the latter is rare in adult life. Certain lesions may be amenable to late repair (e.g., atrial septal defects [ASD]), but long-term complications are frequent even after successful repair. In specialist ACHD centers, approximately one half of operations are first repairs, while the other half are reoperations following reparative or palliative proce-

dures [4]. The number of operations on ACHD patients has increased dramatically in recent years and reflects the increasing number of patients and the increasing complexity of patients reaching adulthood (Plate 46.1, see plate section opposite p. 594).

General Considerations

There are numerous issues to be considered when caring for ACHD patients, many of which are unique to this population. Uncorrected lesions can lead to volume overload, heart failure, arrhythmias, or chronic cyanosis. Previously repaired or palliated patients are likely to require reoperations with an inherently higher risk (e.g., repeat sternotomy, adhesions, thrombotic or air embolism related to retrosternal conduits). Finally, as this population ages, the risk of acquired heart disease (e.g., coronary artery disease, valvar disease) increases and its burden superimposes to the congenital defect, accelerating deterioration.

Heart Failure

Heart failure is defined as symptoms of exercise intolerance and signs of fluid retention in the presence of a cardiac defect [5]. Exercise intolerance is common in ACHD and may result from a variety of mechanisms, both cardiac and extracardiac. A persistent or residual defect or hemodynamic lesion can result in chronic volume or pressure overload and ventricular dysfunction. Coronary anomalies, pericardial disease, arrhythmias, chronotropic incompetence, and myocardial injury during surgery may also affect cardiac function and output. Extracardiac factors include pulmonary parenchymal and vascular disease,

Pediatric Cardiac Surgery, Fourth Edition. Edited by Constantine Mavroudis and Carl L. Backer.
© 2013 Blackwell Publishing Ltd. Published 2013 by Blackwell Publishing Ltd.

cyanosis and pulmonary arterial hypertension (PAH), skeletal abnormalities, and detraining.

Subjective evaluation of exercise intolerance using the New York Heart Association (NYHA) classification appears to underestimate the severity of functional impairment in ACHD [6]. In fact, asymptomatic ACHD patients often have subnormal exercise capacity and a high prevalence of asymptomatic ventricular dysfunction [7]. Objective assessment of exercise capacity with cardiopulmonary exercise testing and regular cardiac imaging by echocardiography and cardiovascular magnetic resonance (CMR) are a fundamental part of the preoperative assessment, perioperative management, and long-term follow-up. In particular, CMR imaging is considered ideal for quantifying right ventricular function, which is commonly affected in ACHD [8].

The primary aim when managing an ACHD patient with signs and symptoms of heart failure is to identify and treat residual hemodynamic lesions, especially those potentially amenable to surgical or percutaneous repair. These could be valve lesions (e.g., pulmonary valve regurgitation after repair of tetralogy of Fallot or tricuspid regurgitation in patients with congenitally corrected [L-] transposition of great arteries) or other obstructive lesions (e.g., baffle stenosis in patients with previous Mustard or Senning repair) [9]. While there is mounting evidence to suggest common pathophysiologic mechanisms between acquired heart failure and ACHD, including neurohormonal activation, established heart failure therapies counteracting neurohormonal activation are still not widely in use in ACHD. This is because of the lack of evidence supporting the efficacy and safety of these therapies in ACHD, which has prevented the establishment of evidence-based guidelines for the pharmacologic treatment of these patients. Few studies have examined the effect of angiotensin-converting enzyme (ACE)-inhibitors and beta-blockers in CHD, all of which were limited by a small sample size [10]. Current practice is still based on extrapolation from trials in acquired heart disease. This approach, however, ignores important differences between the two conditions and the unique characteristics of the individual with CHD, which could affect dosage, tolerability, and effectiveness [11]. Finally, new therapeutic approaches such as cardiac resynchronization have been reported in patients with severe left ventricular dysfunction associated with tetralogy of Fallot and could be considered in selected patients [12]. As the CHD adult population ages and increases in number, randomized controlled trials are urgently needed to rationalize treatment of heart failure in these patients.

Pulmonary Arterial Hypertension

Despite advances in cardiac surgery that have allowed repair of CHD at an early age, it is estimated that approxi-mately 5–10% of patients with CHD develop PAH [13,14]. The current definition of PAH relies on the presence of mean pulmonary arterial pressure exceeding 25 mmHg at rest, a left atrial pressure or left ventricular end-diastolic pressure below 15 mmHg, and resting pulmonary vascular resistance above 3 Wood units [15,16]. According to the Venice classification, congenital systemic-to-pulmonary shunts associated with PAH can be divided into: 1) simple shunts, such as ASD, ventricular septal defect (VSD), patent ductus arteriosus, and unobstructed total or partial anomalous pulmonary venous return; 2) combined shunts; and 3) complex shunts such as truncus arteriosus, single ventricle with unprotected pulmonary circulation, and atrioventricular septal defects (AVSD) [15,17]. Ventricular septal defects are the most frequent simple defects causing PAH, with an estimated 10% of all VSDs and 50% of large VSDs having the potential to cause Eisenmenger syndrome if not repaired by age 2 [18,19].

Eisenmenger syndrome is the extreme manifestation of the spectrum of PAH secondary to CHD. It includes patients with large left-to-right shunts, which result in significant PAH (systemic or near-systemic levels) and subsequent reversal of the shunt, which may become right-to-left or bidirectional, and ultimately leads to cyanosis. Currently, approximately 4% of ACHD patients followed in tertiary centers have Eisenmenger syndrome, as opposed to 8% in previous eras when early diagnosis and repair were not available [20].

The clinical manifestations of PAH secondary to CHD can vary depending on the underlying heart defect, patient age, repair status, and degree and direction of shunting. Common nonspecific symptoms include breathlessness on exertion or at rest, chest pain, and syncope [20]. Exercise intolerance is the cardinal symptom of PAH and patients with significant PAH have greatly reduced exercise tolerance, which affects their functional status and quality of life [21]. Eisenmenger patients, in particular, have been found to have the lowest exercise capacity of all ACHD patients, followed by patients with complex cardiac anatomy and univentricular circulation. This is attributable to a combination of PAH and cyanosis, both of which contribute to a significant increase in physiologic dead space.

Eisenmenger syndrome also has important systemic effects. Long-standing hypoxia results in hematologic phenomena, such as secondary erythrocytosis with thrombocytopenia and coagulation disorders. Moreover, patients with Eisenmenger syndrome have a high prevalence of peripheral organ dysfunction such as renal disease and hepatic dysfunction as a result of long-standing hypoxia, on which we will expand later in this chapter.

Patients with PAH secondary to CHD are at increased perioperative risk for cardiac and noncardiac surgery, both major and minor. Routine and preoperative evaluation of these patients should include a chest radiograph, electrocardiogram, measurement of arterial oxygen saturations at rest and during exercise, formal exercise testing, and echocardiography. Cardiac catheterization is often necessary to establish the diagnosis and severity of PAH as well as to assess pulmonary vasoreactivity. Routine laboratory testing should focus on hemoglobin concentration, platelet count, and the detection of iron deficiency. Finally, CMR imaging and high-resolution chest computed tomography (CT) may provide additional information on right ventricular size and function as well as on the pulmonary vascular bed [20].

The general care of patients with PAH consists of preservation of fluid balance, management of secondary erythrocytosis, appropriate iron supplementation, and abolition of routine venesections. Anticoagulation may be indicated, especially for patients with documented pulmonary thrombosis and embolic phenomena, in the absence of prior severe hemoptysis.

Recently, new pharmacologic options became available for patients with PAH, including those with CHD [15,20]. Based on the results of the BREATHE 5 (the only randomized trial in this cohort) and other nonrandomized trials, advanced pulmonary hypertension therapy is currently indicated for highly symptomatic patients with Eisenmenger syndrome (NYHA functional class III or IV) [15]. Advanced PAH therapies have also been used to reduce the risk of developing postoperative PAH and for treating this in patients undergoing surgical repair of CHD or acquired valve disease [22,23]. Whether such therapies could be used to treat and subsequently repair congenital defects that have already led to the development of pulmonary hypertension remains unclear [24]. In fact, the long-term efficacy and safety of advanced therapies in PAH related to CHD warrants further investigation. Moreover, available data on closure of intra- or extracardiac communications in the presence of severe PAH, with or without the use of advanced therapies, are scarce and limited to case reports [24]. Currently, reparative surgery is indicated only in patients with evidence of pulmonary arterial reactivity and/or at least 1.5:1 left-to-right shunting [25].

Arrhythmias

Arrhythmias are a prominent cause of morbidity and mortality in adolescents and adults with CHD [26]. Arrhythmias in ACHD are the result of sudden hemodynamic changes, or more commonly reflect the chronic interplay between the cardiac defects, hemodynamic lesions, and postoperative scarring (Table 46.1) [5]. The entire spectrum of rhythm abnormalities can be encountered in adults

Table 46.1 Rhythm disturbances in adults with congenital heart disease. (ASD, atrial septal defect; AV, atrioventricular; VSD, ventricular septal defect.) (Reproduced with permission from Warnes et al. [5].)

Rhythm disturbance	Associated lesions
Tachycardias	
Wolff-Parkinson-White syndrome	Ebstein anomaly
	Congenitally corrected transposition
Intra-atrial re-entrant tachycardia (atrial flutter)	Postoperative Mustard
	Postoperative Senning
	Postoperative Fontan
	Tetralogy of Fallot
	Other
Atrial fibrillation	Mitral valve disease
	Aortic stenosis
	Tetralogy of Fallot
	Palliated single ventricle
Ventricular tachycardia	Tetralogy of Fallot
	Aortic stenosis
	Other
Bradycardias	
Sinus node dysfunction	Postoperative Mustard
	Postoperative Senning
	Postoperative Fontan
	Sinus venosus ASD
	Heterotaxy syndrome
Spontaneous AV block	AV septal defects
	Congenitally corrected transposition
Surgically induced AV block	VSD closure
	Subaortic stenosis relief
	AV valve replacement

with CHD. Supraventricular arrhythmias are more frequent in patients with atrial dilatation (e.g., atriopulmonary Fontan) and those with history of surgery involving extensive atrial incisions (e.g., Mustard, Senning, or Fontan procedures).

The type of arrhythmia most commonly encountered in ACHD patients is intra-atrial re-entry tachycardia. This is usually initiated and sustained by viable myocardial fibers embedded within areas of scar tissue [27]. Macro re-entrant circuits are also responsible for ventricular arrhythmias and are encountered in patients with repaired tetralogy of Fallot. In this case, the circuit involves the isthmus between the outflow tract patch and the tricuspid annulus [28]. Atrial fibrillation is common in ACHD, especially in patients with significant atrial dilatation due to unrepaired lesions or residual hemodynamic burden.

Bradyarrhythmias are also commonly encountered in ACHD patients, and their incidence and timing depend on the type of cardiac defect and/or previous palliation/

repair. Sinus node dysfunction can be present at birth due to congenital abnormalities such as sinus venosus ASD and atrioventricular (AV) discordance with left atrial isomerism. Sinus node dysfunction may also occur following cardiac surgery (Mustard, Senning, or Fontan procedures). Very often, loss of sinus rhythm in postoperative cases is gradual, suggesting a chronic hemodynamic process rather than an occurrence of direct surgical injury of the sinus node [29].

An AV block can occur spontaneously, especially in congenital defects with conduction system abnormalities (e.g., AVSD and congenitally corrected transposition) or postoperatively. Surgery commonly associated with acquired AV block includes closure of VSD, relief of subaortic stenosis, replacement or repair of an AV valve, and tetralogy of Fallot repair. Surgical manipulation of the ventricular septum may cause AV block because of either direct injury or secondary damage of the interventricular conduction system associated with an inflammatory response [29].

The clinical manifestations of arrhythmia in patients with CHD range from completely asymptomatic to rapid deterioration or sudden cardiac death. The onset of arrhythmia often heralds a hemodynamic decline and contributes to a vicious cycle of progressive clinical deterioration. Persistent atrial tachycardia may also lead to intracavity thrombus formation and thromboembolic events [30]. Most importantly, sudden cardiac death secondary to documented or presumed arrhythmia is the leading cause of mortality in adult patients with CHD, with a higher risk in patients with unrepaired cyanotic or left-sided obstructive lesions [31,32].

The first and most effective step in the management of recurrent or persistent arrhythmias in ACHD is identification and correction of hemodynamic abnormalities. Correction of hemodynamic lesions is usually accompanied, in our practice, by electrophysiologic mapping and ablation in the catheter laboratory, mostly before surgery. Catheter ablation and surgical interventions are, in fact, increasingly used in ACHD for both supraventricular and ventricular arrhythmias. Today, new three-dimensional mapping techniques and increasing expertise allow mapping and ablation of complex arrhythmogenic circuits. The rationale for preoperative ablation is that it reduces hemodynamic burden perioperatively, especially in the presence of persistent supraventricular tachycardia, by lowering the risk of hemodynamic instability during anesthesia induction. Moreover, preoperative targeted transcatheter ablation prevents the creation of unnecessary surgical scars that, in themselves, may provide the substrate for tachycardias. Therefore, our current practice is that supraventricular tachycardias should be treated by mapping and ablation in the catheter laboratory before surgery. If ablation fails to address the arrhythmia, surgical ablation becomes a viable alternative.

Patients with episodes of documented or strongly suspected ventricular tachycardia (VT) should also undergo preoperative mapping and ablation if possible. Implantable cardioverter defibrillators (ICD) are also increasingly used in patients with CHD, despite a lack of solid evidence to support this approach. Risk stratification is essential for identifying patients at a high risk of sudden death who would benefit from implantation of an automatic ICD or invasive electrophysiologic studies. Several predictors of sudden cardiac death have been proposed for patients with tetralogy of Fallot, including a prolonged QRS duration, presence of symptomatic dysrhythmias, and inducible VT on electrophysiologic study [33,34]. Currently, according to guidelines by the American College of Cardiology, the European Society of Cardiology and the American Heart Association, implantation of ICDs is recommended in patients with CHD who have survived a cardiac arrest, those with spontaneous VT that could not be ablated, and in patients with inducible VT, concomitant unexplained syncope, and impaired right or left ventricular function [5,35,36]. In our practice, patients with tetralogy of Fallot and poor left or right ventricular function, evidence of extensive scarring on CMR imaging and prolonged QRS duration, are referred for ICD implantation. While patients with preserved ventricular function, narrow QRS complex, and minimal scarring are not candidates for ICD implantation, there remains a group of patients of moderate severity who may be at risk of sudden death and for whom the indication for ICD implantation remains unclear.

Antiarrhythmic agents are often used in ACHD, but most have proved to be disappointing, especially long-term. Amiodarone and beta-blockers are the most commonly used drugs, with amiodarone being the most effective [35]. However, significant long-term amiodarone toxicity makes ablative treatment even more important.

Patients with atrial tachycardia will often require long-term anticoagulation to prevent thrombus formation. This is especially true in patients with a Fontan circulation and those with intracardiac communications. However, anticoagulation may prove problematic in Eisenmenger patients who are prone to hemoptysis and in patients with vascular malformations.

Pacing for bradyarrhythmias can prove challenging in ACHD patients. Limited access to the heart owing to congenital venous anomalies or acquired venous occlusion, surgical obstacles such as conduits and baffles, and the presence of intracardiac shunts with a significant thromboembolic risk may preclude endocardial lead placement and require an epicardial approach [37].

Cyanosis

Cyanosis can be defined as bluish coloration of the skin and mucous membranes that is a consequence of an increased quantity of desaturated hemoglobin or derivates of hemoglobin, in the vessels of those districts [38]. Cyanosis is "peripheral" when it is secondary to slow peripheral flow of normally saturated blood, leading to increased oxygen extraction, and "central" when it is secondary to desaturation of arterial blood.

Persistent right-to-left shunting through unrepaired CHD results in central cyanosis. Shunting leading to cyanosis may occur through intracardiac (ASD or VSD) or extracardiac (e.g., patent ductus arteriosus) communications in the presence or absence of pulmonary hypertension (e.g., VSD, pulmonary stenosis). Cyanosis may also occur due to AV malformations within the lung or other organ segments [39].

Long-standing cyanosis is a multisystem disorder, causing multiorgan failure and a range of hematologic, neurologic, and metabolic disorders [40]. Chronic hypoxia results in an increase in erythropoietin production and an isolated rise in red blood cell count (secondary erythrocytosis). This a physiologic adaptation phenomenon to chronic hypoxia aimed at improving oxygen transport. The term "polycythemia" is often inappropriately used to describe this phenomenon. However, polycythemia implies proliferation of all three cell lines (red and white blood cells and the platelets). In chronic cyanosis, there is no increase in white cell count and the platelet count is normal or, most often, decreased [38,41,42]. Moreover, while polycythemic patients may benefit from regular venesections, this is not true for cyanotic ACHD patients with secondary erythrocytosis. Routine prophylactic phlebotomies in cyanotic patients pose the potential hazard of iron deficiency, cerebrovascular events, and decreased exercise tolerance [43–45]. In fact, venesections are hardly ever necessary today [46]. Hyperviscosity symptoms in cyanotic patients are often caused by iron deficiency or dehydration [47]. Hyperviscosity symptoms include headache, light-headedness, dizziness, blurred or double vision, paresthesias, altered cognitive functions, fatigue, tinnitus, and restlessness.

Venesection should not exceed 1 unit of blood and should always be accompanied by volume replacement [42]. In fact, dehydration may exacerbate the hyperviscous state and aggressive volume replacement should be undertaken when hyperviscosity symptoms occur. The beneficial effects of phlebotomy are usually evident within 24 hours and reflect the increase in systemic blood flow induced by isovolumetric reduction in erythrocyte mass [41].

Cyanotic ACHD patients are prone to iron deficiency because of increased iron requirements [42,45], recurrent phlebotomies, and blood loss (e.g., gastrointestinal, hemoptysis, menses) due to abnormal hemostasis (see below). Iron deficiency can increase blood viscosity through the production of microcytic hypochromic red blood cells, which are rigid and resistant to deformation [48]. Moreover,

iron deficiency may limit the physiologic rise in hemoglobin (relative anemia), resulting in impaired oxygen-carrying capacity. Annual screening for iron deficiency is, thus, important and is best performed by measuring serum ferritin and transferrin saturation [45]. Oral or intravenous iron can be used to treat iron deficiency, with close monitoring of hemoglobin levels to avoid excessive erythrocyte production.

Hemostatic Dysfunction

Cyanotic patients are at increased risk of both thrombotic events and bleeding. Hemostatic defects in cyanotic ACHD patients include thrombocytopenia, primary fibrinolysis, coagulation factor deficiencies, and disseminated intravascular coagulation (DIC) [47]. Bleeding in cyanotic patients can occur spontaneously (gingival bleeding, epistaxis, hemoptysis, or menorrhagia) or perioperatively/periprocedurally. Hemoptysis is especially common in Eisenmenger syndrome and is the cause of death in 11–30% of patients, even though in most occasions they are not severe [49].

Low-normal platelet counts and thrombocytopenia are common in cyanotic patients [50]. The reduced platelet count can be caused by increased peripheral platelet consumption and decreased platelet life. It has also been suggested that megakaryocytes delivered into the systemic arterial circulation through right-to-left shunting cannot release platelets by cytoplasmic fragmentation, which would have normally occurred in the pulmonary circulation [50]. Moreover, there are data suggesting that platelet function is abnormal (thrombasthenia) and that this improves with surgical repair of the underlying cardiac defect. Nevertheless, bleeding time in these patients is not increased, possibly due to the high blood viscosity and marked platelet activation [47].

Disseminated intravascular coagulation has also been proposed as a mechanism responsible for the hemostatic abnormalities in cyanotic patients [47]. The increased viscosity caused by the erythrocytosis may lead to a reduction in tissue perfusion and stasis. Widespread intravascular deposition of fibrin and platelets may lead to factor and platelet consumption and an increased risk of hemorrhage. Intravascular coagulation is probably nongeneralized but localized to specific districts such as the pulmonary microcirculation. The reported increase in factor levels after heparin administration supports DIC as an important mechanism for increased bleeding diathesis in cyanotic ACHD patients.

Cyanotic CHD often results in congestive heart failure that may affect liver function and influence the production of coagulation factors. Even in the presence of normal liver function, gastrointestinal absorption of vitamin K could be impaired and affect production of factors II, VII, IX, and X. In the latter case, intramuscular administration of vitamin

K could increase factor levels, whereas, in the presence of abnormal liver function, this will have little effect [46,47].

Primary fibrinolysis has been reported in few cyanotic patients, but its role is uncertain. Recently, evidence of increased sensitivity of cyanotic patients to activated protein C was reported, which could predispose patients to bleeding [51]. Other authors reported suppression of the thrombomodulin-protein C–protein S pathway that could predispose towards thrombosis in the microcirculation and subsequent DIC phenomena [52].

Thrombosis in cyanotic heart disease is often a consequence of blood stasis occurring in dilated chambers, arrhythmias (atrial fibrillation or flutter), and prosthetic material (valves, pacemaker leads, conduits) [46]. Massive thrombosis of the pulmonary arteries was found in 29% of Eisenmenger patients in one study [53], and thrombosis of the proximal pulmonary arteries was found in 21% of patients in another study [54]. Female sex and lower arterial saturations were associated with the risk of thrombosis in the pulmonary arteries. Pulmonary infarction appears to be the most common cause of hemoptysis in these patients [49,55]. The coexistence of hemoptysis and thrombosis make clinical decision on anticoagulation arduous [49].

Treatment of the hemostatic dysfunction is not typically required. Moreover, administration of anticoagulants and antiplatelet agents in this group of patients remains controversial [46]. In our practice, indications for anticoagulation include atrial flutter or fibrillation, recurrent episodes of thromboembolic events in the absence of iron deficiency and dehydration, and the presence of mechanical heart valves or other high-risk anatomy. Monitoring of anticoagulation in these patients should be meticulous.

Cyanotic ACHD patients requiring surgery are at high risk of perioperative bleeding due to the aforementioned hemostatic abnormalities and the presence of fragile mediastinal collateral arteries. Therefore, coagulation parameters should be accurately measured before surgery and fresh frozen plasma and platelets administered accordingly. Special attention should be made when assessing coagulation parameters in cyanotic patients with secondary erythrocytosis. The increased hematocrit results in a decrease in plasma volume per unit of blood. Thus the amount of anticoagulant in the vials used for collection of blood should be adjusted accordingly. Other measurements include administration of aminocaproic acid and tranexamic acid, meticulous hemostasis during sternotomy, application of fibrin glue to suture lines when necessary, and continuous ultrafiltration during cardiopulmonary bypass (CPB) [56].

Stroke

Children less than 4 years of age with iron deficiency are at an increased risk of intracranial venous and sinus throm-bosis [57]. In contrast, cerebral venous thrombosis has not been described in older patients with cyanotic CHD [58].

In adult patients with cyanotic heart disease, the risk of cerebrovascular thrombotic events was estimated at 14% (1/100 patient-years) in one study, whereas in another study no cerebrovascular events occurred (112 patients, 748 patient-years) [43,58]. Daliento and colleagues reported that 8% of Eisenmenger patients had a major cerebrovascular event by age 31 ± 16 years [59]. Systemic arterial hypertension, atrial fibrillation, and microcytosis are independent predictors of cerebrovascular events in cyanotic heart disease [43]. Multiple ischemic changes were identified by magnetic resonance imaging (MRI) in cyanotic patients with heart disease even in the absence of clinical history of major cerebrovascular events, atrial fibrillation, brain abscess, or prosthetic valves [60]. Patients with a hematocrit exceeding 60%, oxygen saturation less than 85%, and decreased protein C activity were at higher risk of subclinical ischemic cerebral changes on MRI. However, Perloff and colleagues [58] found no relation between stroke due to arterial thrombosis and hyperviscosity. In fact, blood viscosity may have less of an effect on flow rates in the adult cerebral microcirculation, and intrinsic autoregulation may preserve blood flow in the face of hyperviscosity [60].

Renal Dysfunction

Chronic cyanotic heart disease is associated with decreased glomerular filtration rate and proteinuria. This is secondary to hypercellular congested glomeruli with segmental sclerosis and basement membrane thickening [61]. In a recent study, 72% of patients with Eisenmenger syndrome were found to have moderate or severe reduction in glomerular filtration rate [62]. Moreover, renal dysfunction is an established marker of adverse outcome in acquired and CHD (Figure 46.1) [62].

Care should be taken when performing cardiac catheterization with angiography in cyanotic patients who are at increased risk for contrast induced nephropathy. Patients requiring cardiac catheterization should be well hydrated prior to the procedure and a minimal amount of contrast agent should be used for imaging. Postcatheterization monitoring of urinary output is required and rehydration should be used judiciously.

Metabolic Complications

Acute gout occurs in 2% of adults with cyanotic heart disease [63]. High uric acid levels require no treatment if gout is absent; acute symptomatic gout may be treated with colchicine. However, colchicine may produce vomiting or diarrhea, which requires discontinuation to prevent dehydration. Nonsteroidal anti-inflammatory agents may be

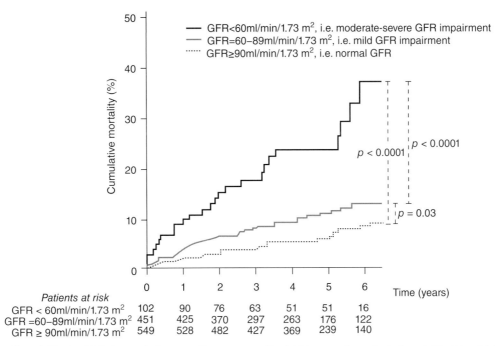

Figure 46.1 Unadjusted (Kaplan-Meier) cumulative mortality curves according to glomerular filtration rate (GFR) group. Patients with moderate or severe GFR reduction (<60 mL/min/1.73 m²) had a five-fold increased unadjusted mortality risk, which was apparent even from the first year of follow-up. (Reproduced with permission from Dimopoulos *et al.* [62].)

used with caution, acknowledging the increased risk of bleeding with their use.

Hemoptysis

Pulmonary infarction due to pulmonary embolus may result in hemoptysis. Hemoptysis may also be caused by rupture of an enlarged friable bronchial artery. Prompt bronchoscopy should be performed to clear the airway and identify the site of the lesion. Measures to protect the contralateral bronchial tree are undertaken. CT or MRI may be beneficial in identifying pulmonary infarction and intraparenchymal hemorrhage. If bleeding persists despite bed rest and correction of coagulopathies, angiography to localize the site of bleeding is indicated. At the time of angiography, embolization of the vessel should be performed. If bleeding cannot be controlled with interventional catheterization techniques, then emergent pulmonary resection is required.

Re-Sternotomy

Re-sternotomy in patients who have undergone prior palliative or corrective procedures carries an increased risk. Lying just beneath or adherent to the posterior sternal table may be a dilated thin-walled right atrium, an enlarged right ventricle, a right ventricle-to-pulmonary artery conduit, the aorta (in patients with transposition of great arteries), or a markedly dilated aorta (common, for example, in tetralogy of Fallot). Meticulous review of the previous operative note, posteroanterior and lateral chest X-ray, CMR, and cardiac catheterization can aid in planning the re-sternotomy.

The groin should be prepped and draped into the operative field should rapid access be required during re-sternotomy. The femoral vessels can be dissected before the re-sternotomy for rapid cannulation and institution of CPB if risk of injury to the right-sided heart chambers appears high. Alternatively, femoral cannulation with institution of CPB may be accomplished before re-sternotomy to allow decompression of the heart, reducing the risk of injury. Peripheral cardiopulmonary artery bypass can be converted to central atrial–aortic bypass once the heart has been dissected free from the surrounding structures. This provides more effective venous drainage and reduces the risk of compartment syndrome due to reduced arterial flow in the limb.

Some authors prefer to develop a dissection plane just behind the posterior sternal table under direct visualization before sternotomy is attempted. Once the sternum has been successfully opened, early identification of the aorta and atrium should be achieved so that rapid institution of CPB may be accomplished in the event of mishap during dissection of the heart. During the course of the operation the dissection plane should remain medial to the pericardium to avoid injury to the phrenic nerve. In many cases, the pericardium has previously been harvested for intracardiac repair; therefore, the phrenic nerves are at increased risk for injury. Entry into the cardiac chambers is to be avoided to reduce the risk of paradoxical air embolus occurring through residual intracardiac shunts. If entry into the cardiac chambers occurs, suture closure of the defect should be performed. Also during dissection, attention should be paid to the patient's hemodynamics. Cardiac output is reliant on adequate volume loading of the heart. Most patients are volume depleted secondary to their nothing by mouth status. In addition, retraction on the heart during dissection may result in severe hemodynamic instability. If exposure for dissection is difficult, then institution of CPB should be considered. With careful preoperative planning and great care during re-sternotomy, poor outcomes can be avoided.

Collateral Vessels

Chronic cyanosis may lead to the development of multiple thin-walled mediastinal collateral vessels. These vessels may become problematic at the time of sternotomy and during the operation. They do not coagulate well and may need to be sutured to avoid unnecessary persistent blood loss during preparation of the heart for CPB.

During the operation, systemic to pulmonary collaterals may produce excessive pulmonary venous return making visualization of intracardiac anatomy difficult and may result in myocardial distention and wash out of cardioplegic solution and myocardial rewarming. In these circumstances a left atrial vent will be required. Occasionally, systemic cooling and periods of low-flow CPB will be required.

Large collateral vessels identified on preoperative cardiac catheterization should be occluded at the time of cardiac catheterization (transcatheter coil occlusion). If cardiac catheterization is not performed or coil occlusion is unsuccessful, suture ligation of the collaterals should be performed during the initial stages of the operation to avoid complications during the course of the procedure.

Pregnancy and Heart Disease

As female patients with CHD reach reproductive age, the issue of pregnancy and labor naturally arises. Preconceptual counseling should start in adolescence, especially for high-risk patients. Patients should be educated about the risks and the precautions to be taken, allowing them to make informed decisions with regards to family planning. An important step in the management of ACHD patients who wish to become pregnant is prepregnancy assessment of cardiac status and counseling on the risks of pregnancy, intervention required before becoming pregnant, and the need for close follow-up during and after pregnancy and labor. The risk of maternal death is less than 1% for the

majority of parturients with CHD. Certain conditions, however, are associated with significantly higher risk. These include all cyanotic defects and those associated with pulmonary hypertension, poor systemic ventricular function, severe left heart obstructive lesions, Marfan syndrome with dilated aortic root, previous repair of coarctation with a Dacron patch, and women with history of peripartum cardiomyopathy [64]. It is imperative that such women use highly effective methods of contraception appropriately tailored to the severity of their condition and possible adverse effects of contraception.

Inevitably, some women, regardless of the risks to their health, will decide to become pregnant. Minimization of risk by optimization of cardiac function before pregnancy is, thus, essential. This may include catheter or surgical intervention before gestation, surgical or medical treatment of arrhythmias, and appropriate management of medication, including anticoagulation and ACE inhibitors, which may harm the fetus. Patients with left-sided obstructive lesions should be recognized and considered for balloon valvotomy or surgery before pregnancy. The choice of bioprosthetic or mechanical valve requires careful discussion with the patients. Some reports suggest accelerated degeneration of bioprostheses during pregnancy [65,66]; however, this was not confirmed by several large series [67,68]. Nevertheless, it has been suggested that the appearance of accelerated degeneration associated with pregnancy might reflect the well established deterioration of bioprostheses in younger patients [69]. Mechanical prostheses are more problematic than tissue valves during gestation due to the increased risk of clotting [70]. Careful pregestation assessment of aortic root size is important in women with Marfan syndrome, bicuspid aortic valve, and aortic coarctation associated with hypertension. Elective aortic root replacement should be considered in patients with large or enlarging aortic roots [71]. Likewise, women with repaired tetralogy of Fallot, pulmonary regurgitation, and right ventricular enlargement may be considered for pulmonary valve replacement before pregnancy. In fact, recent studies have demonstrated an increase in right ventricular size with pregnancy, which persists after labor [72,73].

Arrhythmia is a frequent complication of pregnancy in women with CHD and may cause significant hemodynamic compromise to both the mother and the fetus [74]. DIC cardioversion is safe during pregnancy whereas antiarrhythmic drug therapy may have adverse effects and should be used with great care [75,76]. The management of anticoagulation is often problematic, especially in women with prosthetic heart valves. Warfarin is a more effective anticoagulant in pregnancy but it is also associated with increased fetal loss and embryopathy, especially when used between the 6th and 12th week of pregnancy [77,78]. Our current practice consists of low molecular weight heparin during the first trimester substituted by warfarin during the second and early third trimesters. Warfarin is again replaced by unfractioned heparin at approximately 35 weeks of gestation [79]. The use of aspirin is also recommended until the 35th week of pregnancy in women with increased risk of thromboembolism, such as patients with a Fontan circulation, and in those at risk of paradoxical embolization across an intracardiac defect [80].

The timing of pregnancy is particularly important for women with a systemic right ventricle or a univentricular heart, as they are more likely to tolerate pregnancy earlier rather than later in their lives. In fact, progressive ventricular dysfunction is common and affects the risk and outcome of pregnancy.

Despite all efforts for optimal medical management of pregnancy in CHD, the need for surgical or catheter intervention during pregnancy may still arise. Most interventions involve women with an undiagnosed cardiac lesion, those lost to follow-up, or those with an acute, life-threatening situation. The most common indication for cardiac intervention during pregnancy is valvar heart disease, in particular mitral valve stenosis, which is usually secondary to rheumatic disease [81]. Other indications include severe aortic valve stenosis, pulmonary valve stenosis, acute dissection of the aorta, pacemaker insertion, and insertion of an inferior vena cava filter. CPB is associated with a high risk of fetal loss and should only be considered in women with symptoms refractory to medical treatment, for whom no percutaneous options are available [82].

Surgical Considerations in Patients with Previous Operations

Blalock-Taussig Shunt

The classic Blalock-Taussig shunt involves ligation of the subclavian artery with anastomosis of the subclavian to the pulmonary artery. The radial pulse is absent on the side of the shunt, therefore arterial monitoring must be performed on the contralateral side. The modified Blalock-Taussig shunt is an interposition polytetrafluoroethylene (PTFE) graft between the subclavian or innominate artery and the pulmonary artery. Arterial blood pressure monitoring should be preformed on the opposite side of the shunt. Blood flow through the shunt, and thus the pulmonary blood flow, is dependent on systemic blood pressure. During the induction of anesthesia, care must be taken to prevent systemic hypotension, which can result in both systemic and pulmonary hypoperfusion.

Aspirin is often prescribed in patients with Blalock-Taussig shunts and should be discontinued 5 days before reoperation. The shunt is dissected free from the surrounding tissue before institution of CPB. Injury to the shunt during the dissection may have disastrous consequences if the shunt is the only source of pulmonary blood flow. At the start of CPB, the shunt is ligated and divided to avoid excessive pulmonary blood flow and prevent systemic hypotension during CPB. Pulmonary artery distortion or stenosis may occur at the site of the PTFE–pulmonary artery anastomosis. These anatomic abnormalities are repaired using arterioplasty techniques to restore unobstructed blood flow to the lungs.

Glenn Shunt

The classical Glenn shunt is an end-to-end anastomosis between the divided right pulmonary artery and the superior vena cava. Therefore all superior vena caval blood flow is directed to the right lung. The bidirectional Glenn is an end-to-side anastomosis of the superior vena cava to the superior margin of the right pulmonary artery, thereby maintaining continuity between the right and left main pulmonary arteries. This permits bidirectional flow from the superior vena cava to the right and left lungs.

With both the classical Glenn and the bidirectional Glenn shunt, the inferior vena cava is left intact, resulting in right-to-left shunting and hypoxemia. As previously discussed, chronic hypoxemia leads to erythrocytosis, abnormalities of hemostasis, development of collateral circulation, and systemic-to-pulmonary arterial shunts. If patients with classical Glenn shunts become candidates for the Fontan operation, the classical Glenn shunt is taken down, pulmonary artery continuity is re-established, and a bidirectional Glenn is constructed. During dissection of the Glenn shunt, care must be taken to avoid injury to the phrenic nerve.

Pulmonary Artery Band

Pulmonary artery banding protects the pulmonary circulation from excessive blood flow during infancy, thereby reducing the risk of PAH. A pulmonary artery band results in focal supravalvar stenosis of the main pulmonary artery. At the time of reoperation, repair of the stenosis must be addressed. Repair is typically performed by pericardial or prosthetic patch arterioplasty. If the band has migrated distally on the artery, then bilateral pulmonary artery stenoses or distortion of the pulmonary arteries may occur. The anatomic defect can be repaired with pericardium, homograft, or prosthetic material.

Anesthesia Considerations

Planning for an anesthetic procedure requires in-depth knowledge of the cardiac anatomy and physiology and the patient's medical history. Successful delivery of anesthesia requires modification of techniques to account for specific pathophysiologic states. Adequate premedication is needed to prevent anxiety, tachycardia, and increased myocardial demands. In patients with physiology dependent on preload (Fontan patients) avoidance of myocardial depression, vasodilatation, and hypotension are critical for maintenance of hemodynamic stability. Moreover, large tidal volumes or high levels of positive end-expiratory pressure should be avoided to avoid a reduction in pulmonary blood flow. Hypoxemia and acidosis may also induce pulmonary vascular constriction and, thus, reduce pulmonary blood flow. A balance between pulmonary and systemic blood flow may be obtained by adjusting the fraction of inspired oxygen and ventilation. Patients with increased pulmonary blood flow should be maintained on minimal oxygen, with permissive hypercapnia and mild acidosis to prevent excessive pulmonary blood flow producing dilatation and failure of the systemic ventricle.

Monitoring

The degree of invasive monitoring required during anesthesia depends on the severity of the congenital defect and associated physiology. Continuous electrocardiographic monitoring is essential for identifying arrhythmic or ischemic events, especially during the onset of general anesthesia and before the institution of CPB. Pulse oximetry and end-tidal carbon dioxide (CO_2) monitoring assess the adequacy of oxygenation and ventilation throughout the procedure. Particular attention to the balance between oxygenation and ventilation is important in those patients in whom the pulmonary flow, filling of the systemic ventricle, and cardiac output is dependent on the resistance of the pulmonary vascular bed (i.e., Glenn, Fontan). Systemic arterial catheters provide continuous blood pressure monitoring and arterial access for blood gas analysis throughout the course of the operation. Placement of the catheter may be problematic due to numerous prior cannulations, arterial cut-downs, and the presence of systemic-to-pulmonary shunts (i.e., Blalock-Taussig shunt). Use of the femoral or lower extremity arteries may be limited due to associated coarctation of the aorta.

Central venous pressure monitoring is important for assessing preload and the fluid management in patients who require high central pressures to maintain adequate pulmonary perfusion. Insertion of central venous catheters in ACHD patients may be difficult due to abnormal venous anatomy and thrombosis of previously cannulated central veins. Extreme care should be taken to avoid systemic air embolism during insertion of central lines in patients with right-to-left shunts. Pulmonary artery catheters are not used routinely but may be beneficial in patients with anticipated postoperative hemodynamic instability.

Intracardiac Shunts

Patients with left-to-right shunts may benefit from a mild increase in pulmonary vascular resistance induced through

a low fraction of inspired oxygen (to the lowest acceptable level to maintain sufficient partial pressure of arterial oxygen), and hypercapnia with mild acidosis. This limits excessive pulmonary blood flow and distention of the systemic ventricle during anesthesia.

In patients with right-to-left shunts due to a large intracardiac communication and fixed right ventricular outflow tract (RVOT) obstruction (which protects the pulmonary vascular bed from excessive blood flow) pulmonary blood flow can be improved by increasing systemic vascular resistance.

In patients with PAH resulting from an intracardiac shunt, the maintenance of a balance between systemic and pulmonary vascular resistance during surgery is vital. Factors that may affect that balance include hypercarbia, hypoxia, atelectasis, uncontrolled vasodilation by anesthetics, altered intrathoracic pressures by artificial ventilation, and hypovolemia. A combination of meticulous fluid administration, norepinephrine infusion, and inhaled nitric oxide can preserve a stable circulation.

Tetralogy of Fallot

High catecholamines levels result in increased dynamic right ventricular outflow obstruction resulting in worsening cyanosis in patients with tetralogy of Fallot. Adequate preoperative premedication is required to limit the catecholamine surge associated with anxiety and pain. Use of pre-bypass inotropic agents may also increase the dynamic right ventricular outflow obstruction and result in hemodynamic deterioration. Hypovolemia and vasodilating agents can also worsen right-to-left shunting. Beta-adrenergic antagonists decrease dynamic right ventricular obstruction and can reduce the risk of "tet" spells during the perioperative time period. In severe cases of acute cyanosis, phenylephrine may be used to increase systemic vascular resistance, reducing right-to-left shunting, which may lead to hemodynamic improvement. If supportive and pharmacologic measures fail, rapid institution of CPB is required.

Postoperative Care

On completion of the operation, the patient is transported to the intensive care unit (ICU). It is during this time of decreased monitoring that complications may occur. Portable monitors are used during transport to monitor blood pressure, oxygen saturation, and the electrocardiogram. All intravenous infusions should be maintained during transport. Equipment for reintubation and medication for the treatment of cardiac arrest should be promptly available. On arrival to ICU, mechanical ventilation is reinstituted, temporary monitoring is converted to permanent monitoring, and infusion of medication is established and confirmed. Adequate hand-over is also fundamental for ensuring a smooth transition.

Blood is drawn for routine laboratory tests (e.g., complete blood count, electrolytes, coagulation factors, arterial blood gases). Electrolyte abnormalities and coagulation deficiencies should be corrected promptly. Portable chest X-ray is obtained to confirm proper position of the endotracheal tube and rule out hemothorax or pneumothorax. Adequate warming is begun with warm blankets, forced warm air blankets, or radiant heat lamps, as body is heat is often lost during transport from the operating room to the ICU.

Respiratory Management

The respiratory management of ACHD patients may differ significantly from that of adults undergoing repair of acquired cardiac lesions. In ACHD patients, alterations in respiratory mechanics can have profound effects on hemodynamics. An increase in intrathoracic pressure can affect systemic venous return, right ventricular ejection, left atrial filling, and cardiac output. Postoperative pulmonary arterial vasodilatation is desirable in patients with previous right-to-left shunts and PAH. The goal of ventilator management is to maintain partial pressure of arterial oxygen between 100 to 150 torr, mild respiratory alkalosis with a pH of 7.50 to 7.60, and a CO_2 between 30 to 35 torr. Sedation and analgesia are administered using intermittent or continuous infusions of morphine and midazolam to help prevent transient pulmonary hypertensive crises associated with painful stimulation. In cases of severe pulmonary hypertension, temporary paralysis with pancuronium bromide may be beneficial.

Ventilator strategies differ for patients with shunt-dependent pulmonary blood flow. These patients require a reduction in oxygen saturation (75% to 80%) and an increase in CO_2 (45 to 50 torr). This management protocol improves systemic blood flow by increasing pulmonary vascular resistance, thereby reducing pulmonary blood flow and increasing systemic flow [83, 84]. In patients with a bidirectional Glenn, hypoventilation (PCO_2 48 to 52 torr) has been shown to improve pulmonary blood flow [85]. Hypoventilation results in cerebral vascular vasodilatation thus increasing cerebral blood flow and the volume of blood return to the pulmonary arteries through the superior vena cava. Fontan physiology is dependent on passive pulmonary blood flow. Low tidal volumes, minimal positive end-expiratory pressure, and early extubation minimizes respiratory inhibition of passive pulmonary blood flow [86].

Cardiovascular Monitoring

Close cardiovascular monitoring is required during the initial postoperative period. Hemodynamic changes occur frequently due to rewarming, vasodilatation, variations in acid–base status, and changes in the catecholamine levels in response to the level of sedation and pain control. Continuous monitoring of arterial blood pressure, central venous pressure, cardiac output, oxygen consumption, and body temperature are extremely helpful. Hypotension often occurs during rewarming. Hypovolemia may occur due to fluid shifts from the intravascular space to the extravascular space. Postoperative hypothermia may also cause intravascular volume depletion but can be associated with normal systemic blood pressure due to peripheral vasoconstriction. Crystalloid, colloid, or blood may be used for fluid replacement.

Mild sodium and water retention occurs with CPB resulting in increased bodyweight. Spontaneous mobilization of interstitial fluids and diuresis typically occur once the patient is rewarmed and capillary leak has subsided. Diuretics may be used to enhance the diuretic phase, depending on the patient's clinical status.

Hypokalemia and hypomagnesemia often occur due to hemodilution. Potassium should be replaced through central lines to maintain serum levels above 3.5 mEq/L. Magnesium should be normalized to reduce the incidence of atrial and ventricular arrhythmias [87]. Metabolic acidosis should also be promptly corrected, as it may result in decreased cardiac function, impaired tissue perfusion, and reduced efficacy of inotropic agents. Causes of metabolic acidosis (e.g., hypothermia, hypovolemia, ischemia) should be addressed. Treatment with sodium bicarbonate (1 mEq/kg) may be required while correcting the cause of the acidosis.

Low Cardiac Output

There is no single sign or symptom diagnostic of low cardiac output syndrome. Frequent postoperative assessments and a low threshold of suspicion are imperative. Assessment includes capillary refill time, absent or weak peripheral pulses, cool mottled skin, decreased urinary output, acid–base balance, and core body temperature. Treatment of low cardiac output is based on identification and reversal of the etiology.

Cardiac output is the product of heart rate and stroke volume. Stroke volume is the difference between end-diastolic volume and end-systolic volume. Diastolic volume is dependent on preload and compliance of the ventricle. Systolic ejection is a function of afterload and contractility. Fluctuations in heart rate, preload, afterload, and contractility often occur during the postoperative period. The inter-relationship between the determinants of cardiac output can be manipulated to maintain adequate tissue perfusion. In general low cardiac output may be caused by: 1) alterations in heart rate and rhythm; 2) decreased preload due to hypovolemia, cardiac tamponade, or excessive intrathoracic pressures; 3) increased afterload from PAH and increased systemic vascular resistance; 4) decreased contractility from acidosis, myocardial injury/ischemia due to poor myocardial protection during the operation, ventriculotomy, or acidosis; and 5) pump failure with myocardial injury. Detailed review of each determinant of cardiac output can be found in Chapter 7, *Perioperative Care*.

Mechanical Assist Devices

Mechanical assist devices were initially developed for the treatment of postcardiotomy cardiogenic shock. In recent years, however, they have also been used to provide temporary cardiac support in patients with irreversible cardiomyopathy until a donor heart becomes available for transplantation (i.e., "bridge to transplantation"). Less commonly these devices may be used in patients with reversible heart failure as a "bridge to recovery" by unloading the ventricle while it is in the recovery phase following an acute insult such as viral cardiomyopathy. Destination therapy refers to the use of some of these pumps to permanently support the heart in patients who are not transplant candidates because of major contraindications.

Several types of devices currently exist, and major technological advances in their development have been made in recent years. The basic left ventricular assist device (LVAD) configuration consists of an inflow or drainage cannula placed into the left atrium (via the left atrial appendage or right superior pulmonary vein/left atrial wall junction) or the left ventricle through the apex. The pump, which may lie in the paracorporeal or intracorporeal position, is filled by the inflow cannula and then pumps the blood either in a pulsatile or nonpulsatile manner into the outflow cannula, which is connected directly to the ascending aorta. In cases where the patient has established severe biventricular failure then a biventricular assist device (BIVAD) is used with the inflow cannula of the right-sided (RVAD) device draining the right atrium and the outflow cannula anastomosed to the main pulmonary artery. Similarly, a BIVAD may be required when right ventricular dysfunction or failure becomes unmasked shortly after the start of LVAD support. Once LVAD or BIVAD support has been established and the hemodynamics have been stabilized, catecholamine-based inotropes are weaned off to minimize the oxygen consumption and metabolic stress imposed on the unloaded ventricle, thus facilitating the process of recovery.

Further assessment to determine the likelihood of recovery is made with regular multidisciplinary discussions between the cardiac surgeon, cardiologist, and intensivist. Close monitoring of the central hemodynamics (Swan–Ganz catheter), mixed venous oxygen saturations, end-organ perfusion (renal output), metabolic status, and transesophageal echocardiogram parameters should all be used to determine whether the ventricle is showing convincing signs of recovery. The level of anticoagulation should be intensified during a 6–8-hour period of "low-flows" (<1.2 L) as part of the trial of weaning protocol. Once the decision has been made to remove the device, inotropes are re-established to support the patient in the early postexplant period.

Short-Term Devices

Patients who develop postcardiotomy cardiogenic shock or acute decompensation of background chronic heart failure are often very ill and sometimes in extremis. Such patients can be successfully rescued by the expeditious use of short-term mechanical assist devices. Ideally a simple device is chosen that can be inserted relatively easily and often without the need for CPB support. This helps to minimize the inflammatory response and reduce postoperative bleeding. Furthermore, the management of the pump should be user-friendly for the medical and nursing staff on the ICU.

The ABIOMED, Inc (Danvers, MA) device has in the past been used successfully in patients requiring temporary support (a few days to a few weeks). It provides either univentricular or biventricular pulsatile mechanical support. The pump, which lies extracorporeally, consists of a 100 cc inflow and outflow polyurethane bladder separated by a trileaflet valve. The upper (atrial) chamber fills passively by gravity and as the inflow bladder fills the console detects the displacement of air around the bladder and sends a bolus of compressed air to the lower (outflow) chamber, pumping blood back to the patient. As the upper atrial bladder fills passively by gravity, preload is controlled simply by raising and lowering the level of the ABIOMED pump. Anticoagulation with systemic heparin is mandatory. The recognized complications include bleeding, respiratory failure, renal failure, neurologic deficit, and infection [88]. Several centers have reported good results with this device in the setting of postcardiotomy heart failure, with discharge rates of 50–59% and for bridge to transplantation of 50% [89,90].

More recently the Levitronix (CentriMag®) VAD has been used by many centers to provide temporary support for patients with acute decompensated heart failure. This device consists of a magnetically levitated rotating impeller without any mechanical bearings. This unique design minimizes trauma to the blood elements even at high flows. Cannulation is relatively simple and can often be done without CPB. The cannulae are exteriorized and connected to the pump, which sits at the bedside on a retort stand next to the relatively small console. Potential flow rates of up to 9.9 L/min can be achieved at 5500 rpm. There are no flexing valves, diaphragms, or sacs, and the unique design helps to minimize the risk of blood stagnation, turbulence, and component failure. The degree of hemolysis associated with the CentriMag VAD, as measured by plasma-free hemoglobin levels, has been shown to be significantly lower compared to other similar devices. The CentiMag VAD has been used successfully in the setting of bridge to transplantation [91] and as a bridge to recovery for post-cardiotomy cardiogenic shock [92,93].

Long-Term Devices

The Thoratec Paracorporeal Ventricular Assist Device (PVAD; Thoratec Laboratories, Pleasanton, CA) is a pneumatic driven pulsatile assist device that can be used as an RVAD, LVAD, or BIVAD to provide medium- to long-term support. The pump is paracorporeal lying outside the anterior abdominal wall. The inflow and outflow ports contain a Bjork–Shiley tilting disc valves to maintain unidirectional flow. The device permits the patient to be ambulatory when connected to a mobile pneumatic console and has been used successfully as a bridge to transplantation as shown in many published series [94–96].

The HeartMate XVE® LVAD (Thoratec Laboratories) is a totally implantable pneumatically or electrically driven dual-chamber pump in titanium housing. The pump itself is positioned within the left upper quadrant of the abdomen or preperitoneally without entering the abdomen. The metallic side of the blood chamber is made of sintered titanium microspheres and this surface promotes the development of a neointima, which minimizes clot formation. These patients are therefore given only antiplatelet agents and do not require vitamin K antagonists. This device can generate up to 8 L/min of flow and allows the patient to mobilize and indeed be sent home while waiting for a heart transplant.

The HeartMate II® LVAD (Thoratec Laboratories) is a miniaturized rotary pump with axial flow design and represents a second generation of implantable assist devices. It is designed to be small, portable, and offers reliable long-term outpatient left ventricular support. The system consists of an internal blood pump with a percutaneous lead connected to an external system, driver, and power source. The pump itself is implanted preperitoneally below the left costal margin and under the rectus abdominis muscle. The inflow cannula is placed into the left ventricular apex and tunneled through the diaphragm at the costophrenic angle into the preperitoneal pocket. The outflow cannula traverses across the midline under the sternum and is anastomosed to the ascending aorta. Miller and colleagues [97] reported the results of a prospective multicenter study in 133 patients with end-stage heart failure who were on the waiting list for heart transplantation and were bridged using the HeartMate II device. The survival rate during support was 75% at 6 months and 68% at 12 months. At 3 months there was a significant improvement in functional status and in quality of life. Major adverse events included

postoperative bleeding, stroke, right heart failure, and percutaneous lead infection.

Specific Congenital Heart Defects

Atrial Septal Defects

Atrial septal defects are the third most common ACHD [98]. There are several types of ASD, according to the region of the atrial septum involved. Secundum ASDs are the most common and can be amenable to percutaneous closure, provided that their anatomy is suitable. Primum, sinus venosus, and coronary sinus ASDs all require surgical closure.

Common presenting symptoms in the adult are arrhythmia and exercise intolerance with dyspnea on exertion, while many are identified during routine medical screening. Repair of an ASD is usually indicated when significant left-to-right shunt results in dilatation of the right ventricle. Other indications for closure include documented paradoxical embolism and platypnea–orthodeoxia syndrome [5]. In patients with unrepaired ASD the incidence of atrial arrhythmias increases with age. The incidence of atrial arrhythmias is as high as 83% in patients greater than 50 years of age [99]. Atrial arrhythmias may precipitate atrial thrombosis and the potential for paradoxical emboli. Moreover, as patients become older, the incidence of congestive heart failure due to right heart failure increases. Tricuspid regurgitation has been identified by echocardiogram in 28% of patients greater than 50 years of age and in 50% of patients greater than 60 years of age [99].

Secundum Atrial Septal Defects

Patients with a secundum ASD and adequate rims around the defect are amenable to transcatheter closure of the ASD. The Amplatzer® Septal Occluder (AGA Medical Corporation, Plymouth, MN) has been shown to be safe and effective for this purpose. Chan and colleagues [100] used the Amplatzer Septal Occluder in 100 patients (86 ASD, 7 Fontan fenestrations, and 7 patent foramen ovales [PFOs]), failing to close the defect only in seven. There was one device embolization requiring surgical removal. The immediate total occlusion rate was 20.4%, increasing to 98.9% complete occlusion at 3 months' follow-up. Numerous subsequent reports have confirmed these data [101–103].

Patients who do not meet the criteria for transcatheter closure of the ASD require CPB for closure. Anatomic indications for surgical closure usually include a stretched secundum ASD with a diameter of more than 36 mm, inadequate atrial septal rims, and proximity of the defect to the AV valves, the coronary sinus, or the vena cavae [104]. All patients older than 40 years of age undergoing surgical or transcatheter ASD closure should also be assessed for possible coexistent acquired heart disease, including coronary artery disease [105]. Primary suture closure, autologous pericardial patch closure, or prosthetic patch closure can be used. Minimally invasive direct-access surgery has also been used for ASD closure. Byrne and colleagues [106] reported 34 cases of minimally invasive ASD closure. Access to the mediastinum was obtained through a right parasternal, submammary, or upper hemisternotomy incision. There were no operative deaths, but 12% developed major complications (one adult respiratory distress syndrome, one ASD recurrence, one upper extremity deep venous thrombosis, and one reoperation for bleeding). As experience in minimally invasive cardiac procedures increases, safety and efficacy have improved. Bichell and colleagues [107] reported ASD closure through a 3.5–5.0-cm midline incision with division of the xiphoid process alone or with opening the lower portion of the sternum. No early deaths or major complications were reported, with a very brief hospital stay (mean, 2.7 days).

Standard open median sternotomy remains a safe and effective approach to the mediastinum for ASD closure. Following bicaval cannulation, the patient is cooled to $32\,°C$ and the heart arrested with cold blood antegrade cardioplegia. A right atrial atriotomy is then performed, taking care not to injure the crista terminalis, which may lead to an increased risk of postoperative atrial arrhythmias. For small defects or defects with redundant septum primum, the ASD is closed primarily by a two-layer running suture technique. If the defect is too large, or adequate septum primum is not present for a tension-free primary repair, pericardial or prosthetic patch closure is performed. Once de-airing maneuvers have been accomplished, the patient is weaned from CPB. In patients with associated mitral valve disease, valve repair or replacement is performed through the ASD before closure.

Surgical outcomes of ASD repair in adults are excellent. Perioperative mortality is less than 2% and morbidity (primarily atrial arrhythmias) is 8–13% [99,108,109]. Long-term mortality is 1–2% and morbidity 12–13% for a mean follow-up of 9.6 and 7.5 years, respectively [99,109]. Improvement in NYHA functional class is reported in most patients [99]. Patient age greater than 40 years at the time of closure is considered an independent risk factor for the development of postoperative atrial flutter or fibrillation [110]. Postoperative embolic events have been reported in 4% of patents undergoing either primary or patch closure of ASD [99].

Long-term follow up of adult patients following closure of ASD (mean, 42.2 years of age; range, 18.5–74.9 years), revealed that 22% of late deaths were due to stroke, occurring in patients with atrial flutter or fibrillation [111]. Stroke was also the main cause of death in patients who had undergone closure of ASD after the age of 60 years [112]. Because of the risk of postoperative emboli, anticoagulation should be maintained for 3 months following closure

of ASD. Anticoagulation is continued in patients with persistent atrial arrhythmias. For patients with preoperative atrial flutter or fibrillation, the right-sided maze or Cox-maze III operation has been advocated in addition to ASD closure [113].

The management of adult patients with an ASD is determined by a number of factors, including symptoms, age, size of the defect, associated lesions, and pulmonary vascular resistance. Patients with a significant ASD with signs of right heart dilatation and a pulmonary artery systolic or mean pressure of less than 50% of the corresponding aortic pressures should be offered elective closure, irrespective of age [104]. Young adults and older asymptomatic patients with indications for closure should undergo closure of the ASD on diagnosis to prevent long-term sequelae [110]. If left untreated, the risk of death is 25% by 27 years of age, 50% by 36 years, 75% by 50 years, and 90% by the age of 60 [114]. Death occurs due to the sequelae of prolonged increased pulmonary blood flow, PAH, atrial arrhythmias, embolic events, and congestive heart failure.

The management of unrepaired ASDs in patients of over the age of 60, especially when significant comorbidities exist, remains controversial. A few studies have reported percutaneous closure of ASD in elderly patients, with conflicting results [111,115]. In fact, ASD closure can result in abrupt elevation of left ventricular overload, leading to left ventricular dysfunction and acute pulmonary edema, especially in patients with impaired systolic or diastolic left ventricular function [116,117]. Preexisting left ventricular dysfunction may also be concealed by the presence of left-to-right ventricular shunting at atrial level, which unloads the left ventricle [118]. Yalonetsky and colleagues have reported successful transcatheter ASD closure in elderly patients who presented with normal left ventricular function [115]. Patients who were thought to be at high risk of developing hemodynamic compromise on ASD closure (moderate to severe elevated pulmonary pressure, impaired ventricular diastolic function, and modest left ventricular size) underwent transient balloon occlusion of the ASD with repeated measurements of pulmonary wedged pressure, left ventricular end-diastolic pressure, systemic arterial pressure, and cardiac output. No cases of postoperative acute pulmonary edema were reported.

Patients with an ASD and suspected PAH should undergo right heart cardiac catheterization to measure pulmonary artery pressures. Pulmonary hypertension is a complication of the prolonged increased in pulmonary blood flow due to the ASD. Pulmonary artery hypertension and pulmonary artery resistance increase significantly between the age groups of 18–40 years and 40–60 years, with no further increase in patients over 60 years of age [119]. The incidence of PAH (mean pulmonary artery pressure >25 mmHg) is variable, ranging from 9 to 33% [108,119]. Gatzoulis and colleagues [108] showed that the outcome of surgical repair was independent of pulmonary artery pressure in the presence of a left-to-right atrial shunt. However, the patient with the highest pulmonary artery pressure in their study had a mean pressure of 45 mmHg. In contrast, the experience of Vogel and colleagues [119] with patients who had repair of ASD and PAH was not as encouraging. In their series there was one death (mean pulmonary artery pressure, 68 mmHg, Qp/Qs 1.8:1) and two patients were listed for heart transplantation (mean pulmonary artery pressures, 55 mmHg and 76 mmHg, respectively). Balint and colleagues performed a similar study with patients undergoing percutaneous ASD closure and moderate to severe PAH, defined as moderate (50–59 mmHg) or severe (≥60 mmHg) according to the right ventricular systolic pressure (RVSP) [120]. Early follow-up showed no deaths and an overall decrease of the RVSP from 57 (11) mmHg to 51 (17) mmHg ($p = 0.003$) whereas late follow-up showed a decrease in the overall mean RVSP but only 44% of patients had complete normalization of pressures (defined as RVSP <40 mmHg). In addition, two deaths occurred during late follow-up, one due to bowel obstruction and another due to recurrent pulmonary embolism.

ASD closure in patients with PAH remains a controversial issue. In the past operability in this group of patients was often decided based on lung biopsy. Currently, it relies on cardiac catheterization and the degree of vasoreactivity of the pulmonary circulation by means of inhaled 100% oxygen or nitric oxide, intravenous epoprostenol, or adenosine. In patients with evidence of vasoreactivity during acute testing but high pulmonary vascular resistance and bidirectional shunting, balloon test occlusion may provide additional information on the suitability for closure and the possible post-procedural outcome [24]. Detailed history, physical examination, resting oxygen saturations, chest X-ray, ECG, and echocardiography are also important in the clinical decision [121]. In our practice, left-to-right shunting, that is to say in the absence of reversal of shunting and, thus, absence of resting or exercise-induced cyanosis, is a favorable marker for operation.

Sinus Venosus Atrial Septal Defect

Sinus venosus ASD is a much rarer entity than secundum ASD. Commonly, the defect occurs at the junction between the superior vena cava and the right atrium. Typically there is associated partial anomalous drainage of the right superior pulmonary vein into the lateral aspect of the superior vena cava at the level of the defect. When compared to patients with secundum type ASD, patients with sinus venosus ASD have a three-fold greater incidence of pulmonary hypertension (26% vs. 9%) and a four-fold greater incidence of increased pulmonary artery resistance (16% vs. 4%) [119]. Pulmonary artery hypertension and increased

pulmonary artery resistance occur at an earlier age in patients with sinus venosus type defects than in those with secundum defects [119]. Therefore, adults with sinus venosus ASD should undergo right heart catheterization to rule out severe PAH, which would preclude closure of the defect. Because PAH and increased pulmonary artery resistance occur at an earlier stage, early closure of the sinus venosus ASD is indicated to avoid the consequences of chronic pulmonary hypertension.

Sinus venosus ASD can only be repaired surgically. Intraoperative transesophageal echocardiography can be used to define the anatomy and physiology both before and after the repair. Following median sternotomy, CPB is instituted using aortobicaval cannulation. Once the heart is arrested with antegrade blood cardioplegia, a vertical atriotomy is made from the atrial appendage to the pulmonary vein. This incision improves visualization of the defect, which can be repaired using autologous pericardium. Following de-airing maneuvers, the patient is weaned from CPB. Echocardiography is performed to confirm unobstructed flow from the superior pulmonary vein to the left atrium and to rule out obstruction of superior vena cava flow from the pericardial patch.

Patients should be placed on thromboprophylaxis for 3 months following repair to reduce the risk of postoperative embolic events.

Ostium Primum Atrial Septal Defect

Ostium primum ASD are part of the spectrum of AVSD. With ostium primum ASD, the ventricular septum may be intact or there can be an associated restrictive (partial AVSD) or nonrestrictive inlet VSD (complete AVSD) [122]. In partial AVSD, the defect is adjacent to a common AV junction guarded by a common AV valve. In partial AVSD, the common five-leaflet valve is divided into a trileaflet left and quadrileaflet right AV valve, which differ anatomically to the normal mitral and tricuspid valves. The trileaflet left AV valve has been described as "cleft" mitral valve, as the commissure between the two bridging leaflets may resemble this. However, cleft mitral valve is a different anatomic entity to AVSD and the two should not be confused.

The age of clinical presentation is variable depending on various hemodynamic factors. In fact, the hemodynamic consequences of partial AVSD are similar to those of secundum ASD, with varying degrees of left-to-right shunt depending on the physiology of the left and right ventricles, the presence and severity of left AV valve insufficiency, and the presence and size of a VSD. Many individuals present in the third and fourth decades of life due to atrial arrhythmias or symptoms of congestive heart failure [123]. Atrial arrhythmias occur in 25% of patients by age 30 and in 80% by age 45 [124]. Transthoracic echocardiography is usually sufficient for the diagnosis, based on identification of the anatomic defect and typical left AV valve anatomy. Owing to the high incidence of atrial arrhythmias and hemodynamic sequelae, repair should be undertaken once the diagnosis is made. Cardiac catheterization should be performed in individuals greater then 40 years of age to determine the presence of associated acquired cardiac disease that needs to be repaired at the time of the operation.

Intraoperative transesophageal echocardiogram is used for preoperative assessment of anatomy and function, and postoperatively to determine adequacy of left AV valve repair. The surgical approach includes bicaval cannulation, antegrade blood cardioplegia, and topical cooling. Following cardiac arrest, the right atrium is entered through a longitudinal incision taking care not to injure the crista terminalis. The left AV valve is approached through the ASD. Repair of the "cleft" is accomplished by interrupted suture technique aligning the edges of the anterior leaflet and reapproximating the body of the leaflet. Rarely, inadequate leaflet tissue is present necessitating extensive mitral valve repair or mitral valve replacement. The ASD is closed with an appropriately sized pericardial patch. Prosthetic patches are avoided because of the possibility of residual mitral regurgitation that could cause hemolytic anemia from the jet striking the prosthetic patch. The displaced AV node is avoided during suturing of the ASD patch by staying on the left atrial side and suturing only on valve tissue and the fibrous rim of the defect or by placing the sutures in the right AV valve tissue and circling around the AV node area. If necessary, the patch can be sutured around the coronary sinus leaving the coronary sinus blood flow to the left atrium. Following rewarming and separation from CPB, if normal sinus rhythm is not present, atrial and ventricular pacing wires should be placed due to the risk of developing complete heart block.

Surgical results are excellent, with no patient mortality reported in some recent series [123,125]. The majority of patients undergoing repair show significant improvement in NYHA functional class following operation. Preoperative pulmonary hypertension has not precluded repair. Burke and colleagues [123] reported successful operative outcomes in nine patients with pulmonary artery pressures greater than 25 mmHg and in four patients with a pulmonary vascular resistance of greater than 4 Wood units. They did not find any relationship between elevated pulmonary artery pressures and postoperative mortality. Gatzoulis and colleagues [125] reported on 13 patients with elevated pulmonary artery pressures (pulmonary artery systolic pressure greater than 45 mmHg) who underwent successful repair. However, preoperative pulmonary artery pressures were greater than 50 mmHg in four of the six patients who died. Overall, preoperative systolic pulmonary artery pressure was significantly higher in those who died (56.8 ± 9.1 mmHg) than in survivors (42.7 ± 13.4 mmHg).

Others have also noted an association between late mortality and elevated preoperative pulmonary artery pressures [126].

Atrial arrhythmias occur in up to 30% of patients before operation and typically persist after repair. Increased pulmonary artery pressure is associated with an increased incidence of preoperative atrial arrhythmias that persist postoperatively [126]. Patients with atrial arrhythmias that are refractory to medical therapy should be considered for either the right-sided maze or the Cox-maze III at the time of operation [127]. Following repair, complete AV node block requiring permanent pacemaker implantation has been reported in 2–6% of patients [123,125].

Patients should receive anticoagulation for 3 months after repair due to the risk of thromboembolic events from patch closure of the ASD. Anticoagulation should be continued in those patients who have persistent atrial arrhythmias.

Late complications include left AV valve regurgitation, left ventricular outflow tract (LVOT) obstruction, and residual intracardiac shunts. Reoperation for residual ostium primum defect or left AV valve regurgitation is approximately 6–10% [123,125,126]. Left AV valve replacement is often required under these circumstances. Therefore, these patients require continuous lifelong follow-up.

Fossa Ovalis Membrane Aneurysm

Fossa ovalis membrane aneurysm (FOMA) has been identified in 4–8% of adult patients undergoing echocardiography [128]. FOMA is defined as a greater than 10-mm deviation of the membrane from the atrial septal plane during the cardiac cycle [129]. FOMA has been reported in 5–39% of patients with cerebral ischemic events studied with transesophageal echocardiography [130]. Patients with FOMA and cerebral embolism have an associated interatrial communication more frequently than patients without such embolic events [129]. The degree of foramen ovale membrane redundancy is directly related to the incidence of a PFO; 45% of patients with >15 mm membrane redundancy have a PFO compared with an 8% incidence in patients with <15 mm of redundancy [131].

In patients with a large redundant fossa ovalis membrane, a PFO should be ruled out by transesophageal echocardiography. Injection of microbubbles (agitated saline) into the right atrium improves the identification of the PFO. The association of FOMA and PFO with cerebral embolic events could suggest closure of PFO at the time of identification. However, this finding remains controversial as several other studies have failed to show a higher risk [132,133]. According to the American Heart Association guidelines, due to lack of data, PFO closure may only be considered for patients with recurrent episodes of cryptogenic stroke despite medical therapy [134].

Ventricular Septal Defects

Ventricular septal defect is the most commonly recognized CHD, constituting over 20% of all forms of CHD [135]. Most VSDs are restrictive (< 5 mm in diameter) and undergo spontaneous closure during the first year of life [136]. Mechanisms responsible for spontaneous closure include apposition of tricuspid valve tissue to the defect (with or without formation of a tricuspid pouch), hemodynamic changes resulting in fibrosis of the defect, or hypertrophy of interventricular muscle bundles (muscular VSDs). Prolapse of the right coronary cusp or the noncoronary cusp of the aortic valve may also result in VSD closure. Patients who reach adulthood with restrictive VSDs may experience spontaneous closure of the VSD during any decade of life, but this is less likely. Neumayer and associates [137] observed spontaneous closure of VSDs in 10% of their adult population (a 0.8%/year spontaneous closure rate). However, 25% of the total population experienced complications related to the VSD, including infective endocarditis (11%), aortic regurgitation secondary to leaflet involvement (20%), and symptomatic arrhythmias (8.5%).

Large unrestrictive VSDs may lead to Eisenmenger syndrome. Niwa and colleagues [138] reported an 83% prevalence of Eisenmenger syndrome in adults with nonrestrictive VSD. They also reported a 67% 5-year actuarial survival rate after initial diagnosis of the VSD. Large unrestrictive VSD are usually identified in infancy and require full evaluation with right heart catheterization before closure. If Qp/Qs ratio is greater than 1.5:1.0 and the pulmonary vascular resistance is less than 6 Wood units, closure of the VSD is recommended. The approach to VSD repair depends on the type and size of the VSD, as well as the presence of associated lesions. Following aortobicaval cannulation, systemic cooling, and antegrade cardioplegic arrest of the heart, the right atrium is opened with a linear medial atriotomy. The VSD is usually closed through the tricuspid valve with a Dacron patch and interrupted pledgeted suture technique.

If PAH precludes closure of the VSD, right heart function is evaluated at the time of cardiac catheterization and with the use of CMR imaging and echocardiography. If right heart function is adequate, lung transplantation with concomitant closure of the VSD may be undertaken. If the right heart function is poor, or if significant associated cardiac lesions are present, heart–lung transplantation is recommended. The experience with this approach is limited due to donor availability.

Closure of small restrictive VSD is somewhat controversial because of the 10% spontaneous closure rate. Moreover, most patients with restrictive VSD remain asymptomatic and free of complications. However, with a 25% complication rate, we recommend Dacron patch closure of the VSD. Doubly committed subarterial VSD with prolapse of the aortic valve can be approached through the aortic valve via an aortotomy. Indications to close a restrictive VSD are significant left-to-right shunt causing left ventricular dilation, aortic cusp prolapse with significant aortic regurgitation, recurrent endocarditis, and when patients undergo surgery for other reasons such as double-chambered RV or RVOT obstruction. In the case of aortic cusp prolapse, the aortic valve leaflets are resuspended to alleviate aortic insufficiency after VSD closure. Long-term follow-up is required to evaluate pulmonary artery pressure because pulmonary vascular resistance may continue to rise following closure of a large VSD during adulthood [139,140].

Successful transcatheter closure of multiple muscular VSD has been reported to be safe and effective [141,142]. Percutaneous occluders have also been used for perimembranous VSD. Chessa and colleagues have reported successful transcatheter VSD closure in 40 patients, (28 perimembranous and 12 muscular VSD) with two different Amplatzer devices (the mVSD and pVSD Occluder) [143]. In six patients complications occurred, most commonly conduction and rhythm abnormalities during or immediately after VSD closure (one left transient anterior hemiblock, one transient complete AV block, and two ventricular fibrillations). One month after the procedure, one patient had a residual shunt, one aortic regurgitation, and another tricuspid regurgitation. However, larger controlled studies are needed to assess the effectiveness and safety of the percutaneous closure of perimembranous VSD owing to their proximity to the aortic and tricuspid valves.

Tetralogy of Fallot

Today, complete repair of tetralogy of Fallot is typically performed during infancy. Early repair improves overall survival and long-term ventricular function and reduces the development of late-onset atrial and ventricular arrhythmias [144]. Patients with unrepaired tetralogy of Fallot rarely survive to adulthood: 34% of patients die within the first year of life and only 24% survive until the age of 10 [145]. Mortality is a constant 6.4%/year thereafter [145,146]. The clinical picture of an adult with unrepaired tetralogy of Fallot depends on the severity of the RVOT obstruction. Patients with "pink" tetralogy are those with mild RVOT obstruction, which may not be sufficient to protect the pulmonary circulation from the effects the large VSD. Eisenmenger syndrome may develop as a result. Typically, however, RVOT obstruction is sufficient to protect the pulmonary circulation but results in right-to left shunting and cyanosis. Patients, thus, often present with the sequelae of chronic cyanosis and/or Eisenmenger syndrome: erythrocytosis, coagulation, massive hemoptysis, cerebral vascular accidents secondary to abscesses and emboli, epistaxis, and infective endocarditis [144,147].

Once the echocardiographic diagnosis of tetralogy of Fallot is made, surgical correction should not be delayed. The principles and surgical techniques for complete repair are similar to those adhered to during complete neonatal repair with emphasis on the transatrial transannular approach to avoid a right ventriculotomy and with preservation of pulmonary valve function. Repairs are performed with hypothermic CPB, bicaval cannulation, and cold blood cardioplegic arrest. Systemic to pulmonary artery shunts are ligated. Local stenosis or arterial distortion is dealt with by a variety of arterioplasty techniques. Through a right atriotomy and through the tricuspid valve, parietal and septal muscle bundles are excised to relieve subvalvar stenosis. The size of the RVOT can be evaluated with dilators following resection. The pulmonary artery is incised and a pulmonary valvotomy performed. The pulmonary artery is repaired using a pericardial patch that, when necessary, can be fashioned into a pantaloon shape extending into the sinuses. If annular enlargement is required, a limited incision is performed where possible through an anterior commissure onto the RVOT. If to relieve RVOT obstruction significant pulmonary regurgitation is created, it is our practice in adults to replace the pulmonary valve with a homograft, as in our experience acute pulmonary incompetence is tolerated poorly in the adult with tetralogy undergoing repair.

Contemporary series [147–149] report early mortality in adult patients undergoing complete repair of tetralogy of Fallot to be 2.5–16%. Older age at the time of the initial operation has been shown to be a risk factor for surgical mortality and decreased long-term survival. High early mortality may be due to the negative influences of chronic cyanosis and the development of right ventricular dysfunction [149]. Despite the high mortality, surgical results are superior to the natural history of uncorrected tetralogy of Fallot.

The incidence of perioperative supraventricular and ventricular arrhythmias has been reported to be greater then 35% and may be associated with right ventricular dysfunction at the time of operation [148,150]. Avoidance of right ventricular incisions and earlier repair may reduce the incidence of ventricular arrhythmias.

Patients who survive the first postoperative year have an actuarial 10-, 20-, 30-, and 35-year survival of 94%, 93%, 83%, and 72%, respectively [151]. Long-term survival did not differ significantly from the normal population. The majority of patients report clinical improvement following complete repair; 80–90% of patients are reported to be in NYHA class I or II [147,148,151]. Ventricular arrhythmias following complete repair of tetralogy of Fallot have been reported in 33–35% of patients [144,152] and may occur from 2 months to 21 years postoperatively (mean, 7.3 years) [153]. Ventricular arrhythmias were significantly related to longer follow-up duration, an older age at follow-up, older age at time of operation, and higher postoperative right ventricular systolic and end-diastolic pressures. Right ventriculotomy has been associated with late right ventricular dilatation and subsequent dysfunction leading to increased risk of ventricular ectopy. Misaki and associates identified abnormal histopathology at the site of the prior right ventriculotomy scar [154]. These scar sites were found to be within the region of delayed activation and were part of the re-entry circuit. A site of VT predominantly in the infundibular septum adjacent to the VSD patch has also been described. There is also an association between chronic right ventricular volume overload and ventricular arrhythmias [155,156]. Deal and colleagues studied nine patients with symptomatic ventricular arrhythmias after complete repair of tetralogy of Fallot (mean follow-up after repair, 16 years). They concluded that patients with inducible sustained VT showed improvement with antiarrhythmia drug therapy, whereas patients with right ventricular hypertension and VT were likely to be refractory to drug therapy. Oechslin and colleagues [151] showed a 26% reduction in ventricular arrhythmias after reoperation on patients with prior complete repair of tetralogy of Fallot. Reoperation included intraoperative electrophysiology, mapping, cryoablation of re-entry circuits, and relief of right ventricular volume overloading (repair of RVOT obstruction, reduction of pulmonary insufficiency [PI], or closure of residual VSD).

Ventricular arrhythmias have been associated with sudden death in up to 6% of individuals following complete repair of tetralogy of Fallot [157]. The high incidence of sudden cardiac death has led to an increased utilization of ICDs in repaired tetralogy of Fallot, which should be considered for selected patients [158]. Several factors predicting sudden cardiac death have been proposed, including poor exercise capacity, cardiac enlargement, severe systemic ventricular systolic dysfunction, symptomatic dysrhythmias, prolonged QRS duration, and inducible VT [33,34,159]. In a multicenter study by Khairy and colleagues, indications for ICD therapy in repaired tetralogy of Fallot were primary prevention of sudden cardiac death in high-risk patients with no near-fatal events and secondary prevention in patients with resuscitated cardiac arrest or clinical sustained ventricular arrhythmias [160]. When used in tetralogy of Fallot appropriate ICD shots have been noted for both primary (23.5%) and secondary (30.2%) intervention. However, Witte and colleagues noted an inappropriate shock rate of 20% in a total of 20 patients with repaired tetralogy of Fallot [161] which was considered to be due to the high incidence of atrial arrhythmias.

Right ventricular dysfunction and PI are common following intracardiac repair of tetralogy of Fallot. The need for transannular patch placement or previous large ventriculotomy for relief of RVOT obstruction results in variable degrees of PI. The preservation of pulmonary valve function and avoidance of right ventriculotomy in contemporary surgical management of tetralogy is aimed at reducing the incidence of these important long-term problems.

Shimazaki and colleagues [162] show that despite PI, most patients remained asymptomatic until 30 years of age. Beyond the age of 30–40 years, progressively more patients become symptomatic with onset of right heart failure. In addition to time, the effects of PI are aggravated by additional residual lesions, including pulmonary stenosis, aneurysm of the RVOT or residual VSD. Several reports [163,164] show a correlation between pulmonary valve incompetence with right ventricular volume overload, and significant reduction in cardiovascular response to exercise in the absence of symptoms. Symptoms of increasing fatigue and dyspnea typically result from advanced irreversible myocardial damage. Pulmonary valve insufficiency may also be associated with development of arrhythmias and possible sudden death [156,157,165,166].

Timing of intervention in patients with complete repair of tetralogy of Fallot and PI is controversial. The presence of symptoms, heart size, arrhythmias, evidence of right ventricular dysfunction, QRS prolongation, tricuspid regurgitation, and impaired exercise capacity may all influence the decision. Interval change in one or more of these parameters is an important consideration [56]. Ilbawi and associates [164] showed that once a patient becomes symptomatic, irreversible right ventricular myocardial damage has occurred. Valve insertion did not reverse the RV dysfunction but prevented further progression, supporting the view that valve insertion should occur before the development of symptoms. However, early pulmonary valve replacement in all asymptomatic patients with severe PI would lead to overtreatment of a large proportion of patients and possible future reoperations for a failing prosthetic valve. Meijboom and colleagues, in a long-term follow-up study, showed that 89% of patients with severe PI who were asymptomatic and had not undergone pulmonary valve replacement, had a satisfactory outcome 12 years later [167] but 11% were considered to have had an unsatisfactory result on the basis of prolongation of the QRS complex beyond 180 msec, the development of new arrhythmias or persistent symptoms after pulmonary valve replacement.

Based on the above studies, patients with significant PI and associated residual defects and patients who are symptomatic with significant PI should undergo insertion of a pulmonary valve. Asymptomatic patients should be followed with serial echocardiography and MRI studies, together with exercise stress testing (Plate 46.2, see plate section opposite p. 594) [168]. Cardiac catheterization should be reserved for patients older than 40 years of age referred for surgery or when catheter intervention is contemplated.

Idriss and colleagues [169] reported the first series of patients undergoing pulmonary valve insertion following complete repair of tetralogy of Fallot. Since the initial report, several authors [163,164,170,171] have reported on pulmonary valve insertion after complete repair. These studies confirm the low morbidity and mortality, improvement in NYHA functional class, decrease in right ventricular volume, improved RV function, and tentative reduction of arrhythmias following pulmonary valve insertion.

The type of valve to be inserted into the RVOT is debated; mechanical valve versus bioprosthetic valve versus pulmonary homograft, although few authors advocate the use of mechanical valves. Mechanical valves require long-term anticoagulation with its attendant risks. Kawachi and colleagues [172] compared St. Jude Medical mechanical valves and bioprosthetic valves placed in the RVOT. Thrombotic events occurred in 5.5 ± 2.5%/valve-year versus 0%/valve-year in patients with mechanical versus bioprosthetic valves. Freedom from reoperation rate was 83 ± 9% in mechanical valves versus 94 ± 4% in bioprosthetic valves. There were also more frequent overall valve-related events with mechanical versus bioprosthetic valves (6.6 ± 2.7% versus 1.1 ± 0.6%/valve year).

Long-term durability of the bioprosthetic valve in the pulmonary position has been demonstrated. Ten-year actuarial freedom from reoperation has been reported to be 86% [171]. Ilbawi and associates [164] reported a 10-year complication-free actuarial life of 82% and a functional actuarial life of 84%. Fukada and coworkers [173] reviewed the long-term outcome of 10 patients who underwent pulmonary valve replacement with bioprostheses. They reported no valve dysfunction with a maximal follow-up of 12.2 years. The improved results of the bioprosthetic valve in the RVOT when compared to a similar valve in the LVOT may be due to a reduced hemodynamic load.

Pulmonary homografts have been used successfully for the reconstruction of the RVOT. d'Udekem and colleagues [174] reported on 15 patients who had prior transannular patch repair of tetralogy of Fallot and presented with dyspnea on exertion and fatigue. All patients had insertion of a pulmonary homograft at reoperation. At a mean follow-up of 25 months (range, 3–54 months) there were no deaths, no reoperations, and all patients had decreased RV dilatation and functional recovery of the right ventricle. Long-term durability of pulmonary homografts has been demonstrated after the Ross operation [175]. Freedom from reoperation for homograft obstruction was 94 ± 3% at 8 years' follow-up.

Despite the very good outcomes of surgical pulmonary valve replacement, patients with repaired tetralogy of Fallot who received their first pulmonary valve replacement at a relatively young age may need numerous reoperations in the future. The recent introduction of percutaneous pulmonary valve replacement as an alternative option for carefully selected patients is currently limited by the size of the RVOT [176]. The feasibility of percutaneous pulmonary valve replacement in each patient can be assessed by means of MRI, which provides useful images of the RVOT and its dimensions. Additional CT imaging is required before intervention to assess the anatomy of the proximal coronary arteries and their anatomic relation to the RVOT.

In our center when surgically replacing the pulmonary valve in patients with tetralogy of Fallot, in selected cases we disconnect the right ventricle from the pulmonary artery and use a homograft as a short conduit between these two structures. This policy is based on the theory that as the homograft calcifies and becomes rigid by the time the pulmonary valve fails; this will provide a suitable bed for potential implantation of a stented valve. This policy has been supported by a recent publication describing percutaneous implantation of the pulmonary valve in the RVOT following the Ross procedure [177].

Coarctation of the Aorta

Coarctation of the aorta has a biphasic presentation. Initial presentation is shortly after birth when the ductus begins to close resulting in the sequelae of decreased blood flow distal to the coarctation. The second phase of presentation occurs beyond early childhood when patients present with proximal hypertension and weak and delayed femoral pulses. If left untreated, less than 10% of patients with coarctation of the aorta survive beyond the age of 50 due to cardiovascular or cerebrovascular complications [178], including premature coronary artery disease, congestive cardiac failure, myocardial infarction, intracranial hemorrhage, aortic dissection, and aortic rupture.

The most commonly congenital malformation associated to aortic coarctation is bicuspid aortic valve, seen in 20–40% of patients with coarctation of the aorta [179]. Congenital aneurysm of the circle of Willis is seen less commonly and predisposes to rupture [180].

Following identification of proximal hypertension on physical examination, imaging studies are obtained to define the anatomy of the aortic arch and descending aorta, collateral vessels, and gradients across the coarctation. Advances in imaging techniques provide a variety of methods to evaluate aortic coarctation preoperatively. Angiography remains the standard, providing information regarding anatomy and hemodynamics. Noninvasive imaging with transesophageal echocardiography, high-resolution spiral CT, and magnetic resonance angiography provide similar information and, in some cases, have replaced angiography in the diagnostic stage. Routine coronary angiography should be performed in patients over 40 years of age because of the increased incidence of coro-

nary artery disease. The internal mammary artery is often dilated, with enlarged collateral branches and associated severe atherosclerosis. Significant aortic valve disease (aortic insufficiency and aortic stenosis) occurs in up to 58% of adult patients [181]. Thus, thorough evaluation of aortic valve function is required. Excellent results have been obtained in patients undergoing repair of coarctation and simultaneous myocardial revascularization or aortic valve repair [182].

Treatment for coarctation may be achieved by operation or catheter interventions, including angioplasty and stent implantation. Repair is indicated when the peak to peak coarctation gradient is greater or equal to 20 mmHg or when the peak to peak coarctation gradient is less than 20 mmHg in the presence of significant anatomic obstruction in the presence of left ventricular hypertrophy [5]. Resting gradients may be normal despite significant anatomic stenosis, therefore measurements should be repeated during exercise. In the presence of native discrete coarctation, the choice of catheter versus surgical treatment remains controversial and should be determined jointly between cardiologists and surgeons specialized in ACHD. There is a broad consensus, however, that angioplasty with stenting is the preferred approach to recoarctation or residual stenosis after previous surgery. In patients with previously repaired coarctation, surgical repair should be performed in the presence of concomitant hypoplasia of the aortic arch or long coarctation segment [5].

Surgical repair of coarctation of the aorta is typically approached by a left posterolateral thoracotomy through the fourth or fifth interspace. The patient is positioned so that adequate exposure of the left femoral vessels can be obtained if necessary. Enlarged friable chest wall collateral vessels must be identified and ligated to conserve blood loss during thoracotomy. The aorta is extensively mobilized including the arch, great vessels, and descending aorta. The ligamentum is ligated and divided. Care must be taken during dissection to avoid injury to the recurrent laryngeal and phrenic nerves. Enlarged lymphatics are ligated to prevent subsequent chylothorax. Test occlusion of the aorta is performed to determine the need for distal bypass. Distal pressures are maintained above 40 mmHg during the procedure. If the pressure falls below 40 mmHg, pharmacologic attempts at correction are initially performed. If pharmacologic measures fail, distal bypass is instituted with either atriofemoral bypass or femoral–femoral bypass. Other techniques of spinal cord protection include short cross-clamp times, local and systemic hypothermia, intraoperative monitoring of somatosensory-evoked potentials, cerebral spinal fluid drainage, and pharmacologic intervention. Despite these various techniques, no single method has been shown to impact significantly on the incidence of spinal cord injury. Spinal cord ischemia and motor impairment incidence remains low

(1–2%) but is increased in those patients with poorly developed collaterals [183].

Correction of the coarctation is by resection with end-to-end anastomosis, prosthetic patch aortoplasty, or tube graft. In adults, the usefulness of primary repair (end-to-end anastomosis) is limited due to the immobility of the aorta and the necessity to resect multiple, often enlarged intercostal arteries. Aortotomy with prosthetic patch aortoplasty can be performed with partial occluding vascular clamps therefore avoiding complete occlusion of the aorta during repair. The patch should extend from the proximal origin of the left subclavian artery to 1 cm below the coarctation. Intercostal arteries are temporarily occluded with snares to provide adequate visualization. The coarctation ridge is not resected. Resection of the ridge is associated with a 20% incidence of aneurysm formation at the site of resection [184]. Long-segment stenosis can be repaired with resection and interposition tube graft. This requires cross-clamping of the aorta and the inherent risk of paraplegia. The risk of paraplegia can be reduced with the above-described protective measures and limiting the cross-clamp time. Extra-anatomic bypass grafting with a tube graft from the left subclavian artery to the distal descending aorta can be performed without occlusion of the aorta. The procedure is performed through a left thoracotomy and is especially useful in patients who have undergone previous repair of a coarctation [185,186].

Postoperative hypertension is aggressively treated with sodium nitroprusside. The paradoxical hypertension is due to an initial response to increased circulating catecholamines. Once the catecholamine response subsides, hypertension is sustained owing to elevated levels of norepinephrine and angiotensin. Once oral intake is begun sodium nitroprusside is discontinued and oral antihypertensive agents begun. Severe acute arteritis may occur below the coarctation [187,188]. Mesenteric arteritis may develop leading to ischemic bowel or infarction requiring resection. Therefore, enteral nutrition is withheld for 24 hours following the operation.

The long-term effects of coarctation repair on adult systemic hypertension are debated. It is generally accepted that the risk of postoperative hypertension increases with increasing age at repair and the degree of preoperative hypertension. Late hypertension is more prevalent in patients who have had repair after 1 year of age (27%) when compared to those who have had surgery during infancy (4%) [189]. Despite successful surgical repair of aortic coarctation, Kaemmerer and colleagues [190] showed that in a total of 44 patients who underwent repair as adults, 72% had hypertension at rest, 20% during exercise, and 53% during ambulatory blood pressure monitoring. However, others [185] have shown significant reduction in blood pressure with many patients normotensive without the use of antihypertensives. This difference may be explained by the fact that patients may be normotensive at rest but develop significant hypertension during exercise. Vigano reported that nearly 50% of their patients who were normotensive at rest became hypertensive during exercise [191]. Therefore measurements of blood pressure should be taken during exercise at follow-up visits. Because of the risk of recurrent hypertension, coronary artery disease, and recoarctation, patients with repaired coarctation should be followed closely. Either beta-blockers or ACE inhibitors should be instituted if hypertension occurs. The incidence of recurrent coarctation, after initial repair, is between 5% and 30% [192–194]. The occurrence of recoarctation in the adult population is usually a complex problem associated with cardiovascular disease, including aortic arch hypoplasia, aneurysmal dilatation of the ascending aorta, and valvar disease in the form of bicuspid aortic valve, mitral valve disease, or subvalvar aortic stenosis [195]. Several factors have been sited as possible predictors for aneurysm formation at the site of coarctation repair. Oliver *et al.* looked at predictors for major aortic wall complications, including aortic aneurysm, dissection and acute rupture, and their results indicated advanced age and bicuspid aortic valve as independent risk factors [196]. Aneurysm formation has also been reported to be related to the type of primary surgical repair, with a higher incidence late after previous patch aortoplasty, and to transcatheter relief of the coarctation [197,198]. Both true and false aneurysms occur and if not detected on routine follow-up and left untreated, they may present at the time of rupture with a mortality as high as 36% [199]. Cardiovascular magnetic resonance imaging is the diagnostic modality of choice and, therefore, recommended for all patients with previous coarctation repair. Small aneurysms can be followed by repeated MRI but large aneurysms, those with rapid progression in size, and those producing symptoms, are associated with rupture and should be repaired [200]. The traditional surgical approach for coarctation and recoarctation repair has been through a left thoracotomy. However, postoperative complications of reoperation for recoarctation in the adult through a left thoracotomy are common and include postoperative bleeding, false aneurysm formation, residual coarctation, and recurrent laryngeal nerve palsy [201]. For this reason in cases of complex recoarctation (with hypoplasia of the aortic arch, aortic/mitral valve involvement, or ischemic heart disease), we would consider repair through a median sternotomy placing a conduit between the ascending and descending aorta approached through the posterior pericardium. The advantage of this approach is that it deals effectively with associated arch hypoplasia [202]. It avoids the often difficult dissection of the lung and collateral circulation associated with rethoracotomy and eliminates the risk of damage to the recurrent laryngeal nerve, which is often intimately bound to vascular structures by fibrous tissue at the site of re-coarctation [56].

Approach through a rethoracotomy may still be required for the excision of expanding or ruptured aneurysms associated with recoarctation or occurring at the site of previous coarctation repair. In cases of recoarctation, where the collateral circulation is often inadequate, our preference is to use CPB, either atriofemoral or femoral–femoral, to maintain descending thoracic perfusion during the period of aortic cross-clamping. In the most complex cases of ruptured aortic aneurysm, CPB with hypothermia and circulatory arrest may be required.

In the past years there has been a dramatic increase in the use of endovascular stenting and angioplasty in adults with coarctation, utilized for primary repair, repair of recoarctation, and associated aneurysms [203–205]. However, no prospective, randomized, controlled trial of surgical versus endovascular therapy is available in the adult population, and only two studies have been reported in children [206,207]. Hernandez-Gonzalez and colleagues [207] showed that angioplasty had higher rates of recurrence (50% vs. 21%) and a higher incidence of persistent hypertension (49% vs. 19%) compared to surgery. Cowley and colleagues [206] showed, as well, a higher rate of recurrence with repeat intervention after angioplasty repair but also a higher incidence of aneurysm formation (35% vs. 0%) in patients treated with angioplasty. An extensive review of the different methods for treatment of coarctation in adults has showed that surgical repair has a very low morbidity and mortality that is comparable to transcatheter treatment [203]. However, the shorter hospitalization and lower costs of endovascular repair have increased the use of this method in many centers. Today, the current view is that percutaneous intervention in patients with recoarctation after surgical repair is the preferred approach. However, this requires the absence of complex concomitant features such as aneurysm formation and coarctation affecting the adjoining arch arterial branches [5]. In cases of uncomplicated native coarctation, balloon angioplasty with or without stent placement may be considered as an alternative to surgery, although it is still thought to be a less suitable method for long-segment or tortuous forms of coarctation. In conclusion, each case of adult patient with native or recurrent coarctation should be discussed jointly between surgeons and cardiologists to determine the most appropriate management strategy. A hybrid approach may be considered for patients with coarctation of the aorta and significant concomitant aortic valve disease. Aortic valve replacement in this case may follow suit after endovascular relief of coarctation with primary stenting.

Fontan-Type Repair

The Fontan operation establishes a separation between the pulmonary and systemic circulation by directing right atrial blood flow or total caval blood flow to the pulmonary arteries. The Fontan operation is used for congenital lesions in which biventricular repair is not possible. These lesions include tricuspid atresia (or absent right AV valve connection), double-inlet left ventricle, and other complex anatomic defects. Eligibility criteria for the Fontan operation include normal distal pulmonary artery anatomy, low pulmonary vascular resistance, adequate systolic and diastolic function, and no AV valve insufficiency.

Atriopulmonary Fontan Connection

Atriopulmonary Fontan connections are associated with significant long-term complications. Over time, the right atrium becomes severely dilated and is a source of arrhythmias and thromboembolic events (Figure 46.2) [208]. Moreover, it results in excessive energy dissipation from sluggish blood flow within the cardiac chamber, compromising Fontan hemodynamics. Anatomic obstruction of the right-sided pulmonary veins can also occur due to external mechanical compression by the right atrium [209]. However, arrhythmias are the most common complication,

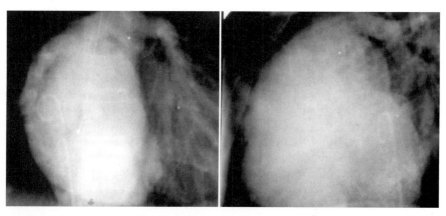

Figure 46.2 Cardiac catheterization of a patient with an atriopulmonary Fontan to the left pulmonary artery and a classic Glenn shunt to the right pulmonary artery. Note the huge dilated right atrium.

the incidence and severity of which increases with time and causes further deterioration in a vicious circle of arrhythmia, right atrial enlargement, and heart failure [210].

Efforts to circumvent these complications have resulted in the present-day modifications of the Fontan procedure. These modifications include total cavopulmonary artery connections using intracardiac (lateral tunnel) or extracardiac techniques with or without fenestration. Encouraging results with total cavopulmonary artery connections have nowadays made the atriopulmonary Fontan connection obsolete. However, there remain a significant number of adult patients with atriopulmonary connection, who require close follow-up and treatment of sequelae and may need further surgical intervention. Therefore it is important for the adult congenital heart surgeon to be familiar with this technique.

Intracardiac Fontan Connection

The intracardiac lateral tunnel connects the inferior vena caval blood flow to the pulmonary artery using an intra-atrial baffle. The baffle, which is constructed of PTFE patch material, is sutured to the lateral wall of the right atrium and directs blood from the inferior vena cava through the cardiac end of the transected superior vena cava, which is anastomosed to the pulmonary artery. The superior vena caval blood flow is directed to the right pulmonary artery through a bidirectional Glenn shunt.

When compared with the atriopulmonary Fontan connection, the intracardiac lateral tunnel minimizes the risk of pulmonary venous obstruction due to dilatation of the right atrium. In addition, the lateral tunnel reduces atrial enlargement by decreasing the right atrial surface area exposed to elevated venous pressures. The lateral tunnel has also been shown to improve the Fontan circuit hemodynamics by allowing laminar flow through the baffle, thus reducing energy loss from turbulent flow within the dilated right atrium [211]. Further improvement in flow dynamics can be obtained by offsetting the superior vena cava–pulmonary artery anastomosis from the inferior vena caval flow and directing the superior vena cava blood flow to the left pulmonary artery by flaring the superior vena cava pulmonary artery anastomosis [212].

The benefit on flow hemodynamics may, however, be lost with the development of atrial arrhythmias due to unidirectional block at the suture line [213]. In addition, extensive dissection and suturing in the region of the sinoatrial node and nodal artery increase the risk of developing postoperative atrial arrhythmias [214–216]. The incidence of late arrhythmias may be reduced by limiting the dissection around the sinoatrial node and nodal artery, avoiding suturing the lateral patch near or to the crista terminalis, and by using multiple shallow bites when suturing the baffle to the atrium rather than broad deep advances [217].

Extracardiac Fontan Connection

The extracardiac total cavopulmonary connection uses a PTFE tube graft to connect the inferior vena cava to the right pulmonary artery. This has several potential advantages when compared to the lateral tunnel intracardiac Fontan connection. Prolonged cardioplegic arrest and extended CPB times with intracardiac Fontan are associated with an increased risk of early postoperative death or failure necessitating takedown of the Fontan circulation [218–220]. Extracardiac total cavopulmonary connection does not require cardioplegic arrest and CPB time is reduced or eliminated completely [221,222] optimizing early postoperative outcomes. Fluid dynamic studies have also shown that the extracardiac connection with offset between the conduit and superior vena cava provides superior hemodynamics compared to the intracardiac lateral tunnel technique [223].

In addition to improved hemodynamics, the extracardiac Fontan may reduce the incidence of supraventricular arrhythmias [224]. Exposure of the right atrium to elevated systemic venous pressures is eliminated. Atrial incision and suture lines are avoided. Dissection in the region of the sinoatrial node and nodal artery is reduced. Ventricular dysfunction due to cardioplegic arrest and prolonged CPB times is minimized. Petrossian and colleagues [224] reported a 10% incidence of new-onset transient supraventricular tachyarrhythmias and an 8% incidence of transient sinus node dysfunction during the early postoperative period in patients undergoing extracardiac Fontan procedures. The extracardiac conduit technique also permits extensive reduction arterioplasty of the right atrium thereby eliminating the dysfunctional and arrhythmogenic right atrial tissue [225]. Although early results are promising, longer follow-up will be necessary to establish the benefits of the extracardiac total cavopulmonary connection.

Arrhythmias Following Fontan Operations

Atrial arrhythmias following the Fontan operation continue to be a source of significant morbidity and mortality. The incidence of arrhythmias following the Fontan operation has been reported to be 14–32% [219,226,227]. The type of Fontan circulation has been identified as an independent risk factor for atrial arrhythmias, with a higher risk after atriopulmonary connection [227–229]. Gelatt and colleagues [230] followed up 228 patients who underwent the Fontan operation for a mean interval of 4.4 years and found that late atrial tachyarrhythmias were noted in 29% of patients who received an atriopulmonary connection and 14% of those who received a total cavopulmonary connection. It has been postulated that, following atriopulmonary connection, the extensive atrial incisions and the exposure of the right atrium to the increased systemic pressure are significant factors predisposing to atrial rhythm disturbances. These factors have lead to a meta-morphosis of the Fontan operation in an attempt to reduce the incidence of late-onset arrhythmias. The intracardiac lateral tunnel reduced the incidence of arrhythmias by decreasing exposure of the right atrium to elevated systemic venous pressures [213–216]. The extracardiac total cavopulmonary connection further reduces the number of atrial incisions and suture lines, which further reduces the substrate for arrhythmias.

The results of medical therapy for recurrent symptomatic arrhythmias in the Fontan population have been disappointing. Amiodarone appears to be the most effective drug, but is associated with significant long-term complications. Moreover, many patients experience recurrent arrhythmic episodes despite treatment with antiarrhythmics. Medical therapy for recurrent symptomatic arrhythmias in the Fontan population is associated with significant morbidity and mortality as high as 22% [231]. Radiofrequency catheter ablation is increasingly being used in Fontan patients but is associated with a relatively low success rate (at most 50%) and a high recurrence rate during short-term follow-up (at least 50%) [232–234]. Abnormal hemodynamics, massive dilation of the right atrium, and a thickened fibrotic atrial wall resulting in suboptimal ablation lesions all contribute to these disappointing results [127]. The use of new mapping techniques may result in a greater short- and long-term success rate of ablation, but this will always be suboptimal as long as the dilating right atrium remains part of the Fontan circuit.

The rationale for reoperation in patients with medically refractory symptomatic arrhythmias is based on the concept that improving flow hemodynamics by reduction atrioplasty and elimination of the high-pressure atrium by lateral tunnel or extracardiac techniques will reduce the arrhythmia burden. However, reoperation for refractory atrial arrhythmias without specific antiarrhythmia intervention is associated with a high incidence of recurrent tachycardia (76% recurrence rate) (Table 46.2) [208,209, 228,231,235–239]. In fact, preexisting Fontan intra-atrial suture lines are the substrate for re-entry atrial tachycardias and should be dealt with by arrhythmia intervention (arrhythmia circuit cryoablation) [214,215].

Takahashi and colleagues [240] demonstrated a reduction in prevalence (95% vs. 28%, $p < 0.0001$) and severity (severity score 7.3 vs. 3.3, $p = 0.001$) of atrial tachyarrhythmias in patients who underwent Fontan conversion with concomitant arrhythmia surgery, in contrast to patients without arrhythmia intervention (47% vs. 53%; 3.3 vs. 3.9, $p = $ NS). Survival at 3 years postoperatively was noted to be 84% in the total patient population, without a significantly different probability of survival between the two groups. Mavroudis et al. [241] have reported a combined technique of Fontan conversion with concomitant arrhythmia surgery in a total of 111 patients from 1994 to 2006. The

Table 46.2 Results of Fontan conversion without arrhythmia surgery.

Author	# Patients	Mortality	Transplant	Arrhythmia recurrence
Balaji et al. [228]	3	33% (1)	–	0/2
Kao et al. [235]	3	0	–	2/3
Vitullo et al. [209]	9	11% (1)	–	3/3
McElhinney et al. [237]	7	14% (1)	14% (1)	3/3
Kreutzer et al. [236]	8	12.5% (1)	12.5% (1)	4/6
Scholl et al. [238]	12	8.3% (1)	–	7/7
van Son et al. [239]	18	11% (2)	11% (2)	9/13
Total	60	12%	7%	76%

first group (nine cases from 1994–1996) underwent isthmus cryoablation for arrhythmia control, the second group (51 patients from 1996–2003) underwent early modified right atrial maze and Cox-maze III and the third group (51 patients from 2003–2006) had recent modifications of the modified right atrial maze and left atrial Cox-maze III procedure for both atrial fibrillation and left macro re-entrant atrial tachycardia (see Figure 41.11) [241]. One (0.9%) early and six (5.4%) late deaths were reported and six patients (5.4%) required cardiac transplantation 1 week and 6, 8, 10, 11, and 33 months after Fontan conversion with arrhythmia surgery. Late recurrence of atrial tachycardia (30 days after surgery) occurred in 13.5% of total patient population. The recurrence rate was 33% in the first group, 15.7% in the second group, and 7.8% in the third group of patients ($p = 0.3$, group 2 versus group 3) (Figure 46.3) [241]. Importantly, cardiac transplantation is not precluded as a significant mode of therapy for the failed Fontan. However, the current metamorphosis of arrhythmia surgery to a modified right-sided maze procedure for right atrial re-entry tachycardia, and to left atrial Cox-maze procedure for atrial fibrillation and left atrial re-entry tachycardia, has made Fontan conversion with arrhythmia surgery an efficacious alternative for Fontan patients with concomitant atrial arrhythmias.

Protein-Losing Enteropathy Following Fontan Operations

Protein-losing enteropathy (PLE) has been reported in up to 20% of patients following the Fontan operation [242,243].

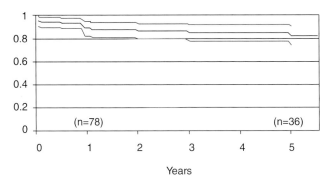

Figure 46.3 Kaplan-Meier curve with 95% confidence interval showing actuarial freedom from arrhythmia recurrence in 111 patients who underwent Fontan conversion with arrhythmia surgery. (Reproduced with permission from Mavroudis *et al.* [241].)

The etiology of PLE is poorly understood, and, as such, PLE treatment remains inadequate. It is thought that chronic venous congestion and persistent elevated pressure in the superior vena cava result in altered lymphatic drainage through the thoracic duct [244]. In addition, increased inferior vena caval and portal pressures lead to intestinal congestion and increased lymphatic production which allows proteins and lymphocytes to leak from the lymphatics [243]. Chronic congestion and enteric loss of proteins can also cause an inflammatory response, which may play a role in the pathogenesis of PLE.

Because the exact pathophysiologic mechanism of PLE remains undefined, several treatment strategies have emerged that can be loosely divided into medical only, surgical, and interventional. In reality, most patients receive a combination of all three approaches as no single approach is effective.

Medical Treatment of PLE
Medical therapy is directed towards the improvement of symptoms (diuretics, intermittent infusion of albumin), hemodynamics (digitalis, ventricular afterload reduction), and the inflammatory response associated with PLE (steroids) as well as prevention of further complications with antiarrhythmics and anticoagulants [243].

Steroids. Suppression of the inflammatory response to chronic enteric protein loss may account for the improvement seen with steroids. Rychik and colleagues [245] reported improvement in two patients following use of steroids. Mertens and colleagues [243], reported near-complete resolution of PLE symptoms in five of 16 patients treated with steroids, while seven had some subjective improvement, and four patients showed no improvement. As no consistent improvement following the addition of steroids has been reported, steroids are used on an individual case-by-case basis.

Heparin. Sulfated glycolsaminoglycans may play an important role in the regulation of vascular and renal albumin loss [246,247]. Murch and colleagues [247] reported three infants with congenital PLE who had complete absence of enterocyte heparan sulfate on histochemistry. These infants had profound enteric protein loss with secretory diarrhea and absorption failure despite having histologically normal intestines. Two of the three infants did not survive. Donnelly and colleagues [246] reported on the use of heparin infusion in three patients with PLE. The decision to use heparin was made after a parent noted that her son's symptoms of PLE improved whenever his anticoagulation therapy was changed from warfarin to intravenous heparin. All three patients showed dramatic improvement in symptoms, marked elevations in serum albumin levels, and quantitative reversal of enteric protein loss within a few weeks of beginning therapy. Each time heparin therapy was discontinued their symptoms recurred and thus daily subcutaneous heparin therapy was continued indefinitely. While heparin may have a role in the treatment of PLE, once again results are inconsistent.

Surgical Treatment of PLE
Several surgical approaches to PLE have been suggested. Initial interventions are directed towards correction and relief of anatomic obstructions within the Fontan circuit. This may be achieved either surgically or through a percutaneous approach. Obstruction may be due to stenosis within the Fontan circuit or the pulmonary arteries. Resolution of PLE symptoms following successful intervention and complete relief of the obstruction has not been consistent [243].

Conversion to total cavopulmonary connection. Conversion of the Fontan circuit (e.g., atriopulmonary to total cavopulmonary connection) has also had varying results on PLE. Identification of patients who will definitely benefit from total cavopulmonary connection conversion remains problematic. Abella *et al.* [248], Conte and colleagues [249], van Son and colleagues [239] have all reported on patients in whom PLE symptoms improved following total cavopulmonary connection conversion, however mortality remains high in this subgroup of patients.

The high perioperative mortality may be due to reluctance to refer these debilitated patients to surgery. Oftentimes, surgery is undertaken after all other efforts to treat the patient have failed. The variable results following total cavopulmonary connection conversion may be explained by differences in flow dynamics between different Fontan circuits and their effect on individual patients [211,212,223]. Total cavopulmonary connection conversion should be undertaken early in this subset of patients before significant ventricular dysfunction and clinical deterioration occur.

Fenestration. Baffle fenestration either surgically or by percutaneous catheter techniques has been reported to improve symptoms of PLE [250–252]. In the Rychik series [252] three of five patients showed significant sustained (greater than 2 years) improvement in PLE symptoms. Improvement was noted when arterial saturations were ≤86%, consistent with diversion of approximately one-third of the systemic venous return through the fenestration [252,253]. Improvement was felt to be due to increased cardiac output resulting in greater blood flow and increased oxygen delivery to the tissues. Mertens and colleagues [243] reported similar encouraging results with percutaneous creation of an intra-atrial fenestration in five patients. Three patients had complete resolution of symptoms while two patients had mild improvement. However, two patients suffered thromboembolic events with neurologic complications. Therefore, anticoagulation before and after fenestration is recommended.

Cardiac transplantation. Cardiac transplantation has also been used for patients with a failing Fontan circulation and PLE. Gamba and colleagues have published a study regarding 14 failed Fontan patients who underwent cardiac transplantation [254]. Seven of them had PLE. They reported a total of 10 late survivors with a mean follow-up of 64 ± 42 months (range, 9.2 to 123 months). In the six surviving patients with PLE, the serum protein levels reached a normal value within 18 months after discharge. Another study by Mertens and colleagues reported 10 Fontan patients with PLE who underwent heart transplantation [255]. Out of seven long-term survivors, one patient had continuous problems with PLE despite excellent graft function and another patient had temporary improvement of PLE with recurrence after 1 year, despite normal graft function. Based on the results of these studies, one concludes that cardiac transplantation is yet another treatment strategy for symptomatic PLE; however postoperative morbidity and mortality remain high.

Medical Versus Surgical Therapy for PLE

In an international multicenter registry [243] of patients with Fontan circulation (35 centers, 3029 patients) the incidence of symptomatic PLE was 4%. Comparison was made between medical and surgical management (Figure 46.4) [208, 243]: patients with PLE following the Fontan operation had a poor prognosis (5-year survival, 59%). Medical therapy alone was associated with a 46% mortality rate and only 25% of patients treated showed improvement. Patients treated surgically did not fare better. There was a 62% mortality rate and only 19% of patients reported symptomatic improvement following surgery, perhaps reflecting late referral to surgery. It is clear that PLE following the Fontan operation is associated with significant morbidity

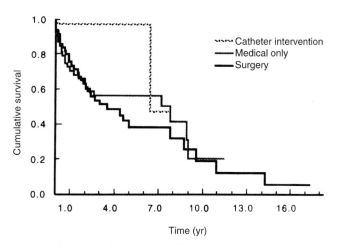

Figure 46.4 Survival analysis of different treatment groups. A Kaplan-Meier analysis of the different treatment subgroups is represented. Time zero represents the date of diagnosis of protein-losing enteropathy. Log rank analysis did not show a significant effect of treatment on survival. (Reproduced with permission from Mertens *et al.* [243].)

and mortality. New approaches to the single ventricle and new treatment strategies are needed.

Features of the Fontan Operation in Adult Patients

In appropriately selected adult patients, the Fontan operation results in a reduction of left ventricle size, normalization of mass-to-volume ratio and an increase in myocardial contractile function [256]. Improvement in NYHA functional class is seen in most patients after the operation. Long-term function is best when a morphologic left rather than right ventricle is present [257].

Extracardiac Fontan reduces the number of atrial incisions and atrial suture lines with the expectation of developing fewer atrial arrhythmias. Despite diversion of blood from the right atrium to the pulmonary artery, atrial arrhythmias can still develop within the dilated high pressure right atrium. Reduction atrioplasty and elimination of the high pressure right atrium have been proposed to control atrial arrhythmias [210,230,242]. Mavroudis [258] and others [236,237] have noted that conversion of an atriopulmonary Fontan to a total cavopulmonary artery connection without arrhythmia surgery continues to be associated with a high incidence of recurrent atrial arrhythmias. Preoperative electrophysiology studies have identified three consistent sites of re-entry circuits that may predispose to the development of atrial arrhythmias. These sites of reentry circuits include 1) the area between the coronary sinus os and the inferior vena cava os; 2) the area between the AV valve annulus and the inferior vena cava; and 3) the lateral atriotomy and its relationship to the length of the crista terminalis, and the region at the superior limbus corresponding to the rim of the prior ASD patch. Mavroudis and coworkers [258] reported a series of 20 patients (mean age, 17.3 ± 6.8 years) who underwent conversion to a total cavopulmonary artery connection. All patients had cryoablation of the re-entry sites at the time of the conversion operation. There were no deaths, and all patients experienced improvement in NYHA class. Pacemakers were placed in all patients as a "back up" in the event future arrhythmias were to occur. Only two patients developed late postoperative arrhythmias that were controlled with long-term antiarrhythmia medication.

Postoperative care following extracardiac Fontan and arrhythmia surgery includes maintenance of adequate preload by the infusion of intravenous fluids at 25% above the calculated maintenance rate. This additional fluid is discontinued on the first postoperative day. Early arrhythmias have been noted despite performance of the right-sided maze operation or the Cox-maze III operation. Aldactone has had some effect on reducing the development of early postoperative atrial arrhythmias. Therefore, aldactone is started in the early postoperative period. The risk of recurrent arrhythmias persists for up to 3 months postoperatively until scarring of the cryoablation lesions develops. To reduce the recurrence of arrhythmias, amiodarone is added in the immediate postoperative time period and weaned during subsequent months. Anticoagulation with coumadin is begun once the chest tubes are removed and titrated to an INR of 2.5 times normal. Anticoagulation should be continued for lifetime to help prevent thrombus formation and subsequent embolic events.

Late Fontan-Type Repair

Originally, Fontan recommended operation in children greater than 4 years of age but less then 15 years old [259]. Currently, definitive repair between the ages of 18 months and 6 years of age is being recommended [260]. Occasionally adult patients with uncorrected cardiac lesions, with or without previous palliative procedures (systemic-to-pulmonary artery shunts, pulmonary artery band) are candidates for a Fontan-type operation. In 1986, Castaneda and colleagues [261] reported on their experience with the Fontan procedure in patients greater than 15 years of age. Their favorable results suggested that age alone should not be a contraindication to the Fontan operation. They identified that pulmonary vascular resistance index >2.0 Um^2 and distorted pulmonary artery anatomy not amenable to repair were the only significant risk factors of poor outcomes following the Fontan operation in adults.

Previous palliative procedures (systemic-to-pulmonary artery shunt, Glenn procedure, or pulmonary artery band) are not a contraindication to the Fontan operation in the presence of favorable hemodynamics. However, anatomic distortion of the pulmonary arteries due to palliative procedures must be repaired at the time of the Fontan operation to reduce postoperative risk.

The outcomes of the Fontan operation performed in adults have been promising (Figure 46.5) [208,262]. Results obtained at the University of California-Los Angeles between 1982 and 1994 are similar to those reported by others [262]. In 21 patients aged 18–40 years who underwent Fontan operation at the University of California between 1982 and 1994, there was a 5% early mortality and 81% survival rate at 12 years. However, almost one-third of patients experienced major perioperative complications, mainly prolonged pleural effusions. Long-term complications include

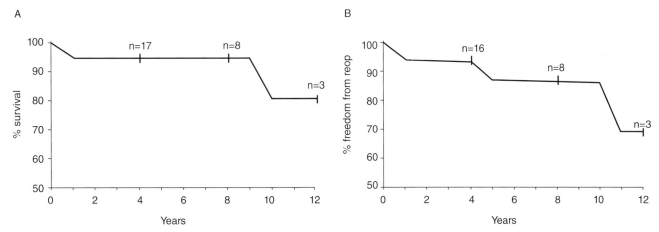

Figure 46.5 A, Actuarial survival after Fontan procedure in 21 adult patients. **B,** Actuarial freedom from reoperation in 19 adult patients after Fontan procedure. (Reproduced with permission from Gates *et al.* [262].)

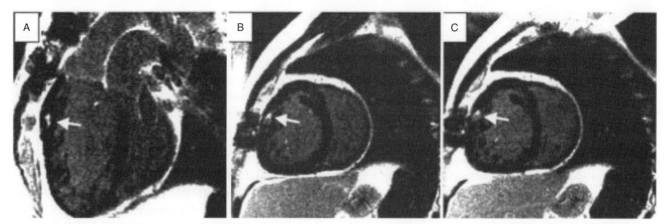

Figure 46.6 A, Inversion recovery cardiovascular magnetic resonance image demonstrating focal late gadolinium enhancement in the trabeculated free-wall of the right ventricle (arrow). **B,** The same region is seen in the short-axis view (arrow) and (**C**) is still present when the phase encoding has been swapped (arrow). There is also subtle enhancement at the junction between the right and left ventricle. (Reproduced with permission from Babu-Narayan *et al.* [8].)

atrial arrhythmias in 24–37% of patients, and PLE in up to 28% of patients [262,263].

Recently Fujii *et al.* [264] reported on the mid- to long-term outcome of total cavopulmonary connection in high-risk adult candidates. Twenty-five consecutive adult patients aged 18 years or more who underwent total cavopulmonary connection had at least two of the following risk factors: age more than 30 years, systemic ventricular ejection fraction of <50%, AV valve regurgitation moderate, pulmonary arterial index <200, mean pulmonary arterial pressure ≥15 mmHg, pulmonary arterial resistance of 2 units or greater, arrhythmia, PLE, NYHA functional class III or greater, previous Fontan procedure, systemic ventricular outflow tract obstruction, and end-diastolic pressure in the systemic ventricle ≥11 mmHg. There were one early death and two late deaths occurring in a mean follow-up period of 57 ± 45 months.

Although the majority of the adult total cavopulmonary connection candidates tolerated the total cavopulmonary connection procedure in the early postoperative period, the accumulation of risk factors influenced late mortality.

Transposition of the Great Arteries

The current treatment of choice for complete (D) transposition of great arteries is the arterial switch operation performed during the neonatal period. However, until the early 1980s, repair of transposition of the great arteries consisted of atrial switch (Mustard or Senning) procedures. With atrial switch operations, venous return is redirected at atrial level by means of an intra-atrial baffle. The Mustard procedure uses either pericardium or Dacron to construct the baffle, whereas the Senning operation uses the native atrial wall. Atrial switch provides physiologic but not anatomic correction of the defect. In fact, while early and intermediate-term results are excellent, the presence of a morphologically right systemic ventricle and extensive atrial scarring account for the significant late morbidity and mortality due to progressive right ventricular dysfunction and high arrhythmic burden (mechanoelectric interaction: interaction between the failing ventricle and arrhythmias) [265–267]. Both intra-atrial re-entrant tachycardia and sinus node dysfunction are common in these patients, the latter being more common late after Mustard (rather than Senning) repair due to direct injury of the sinus node during surgery or progressive fibrosis related to surgical scars (Figure 46.6) [8,268].

Patients with sinus node dysfunction often require pacemaker implantation, with more than 20% of Mustard and Senning patients being paced [269]. Before lead insertion stenosis of the superior vena cava baffle limb and baffle leaks should be identified. Atrial arrhythmias can be treated through catheter ablation or medically. Ablation is increasingly used nowadays with a reported success rate in the region of 80% [270]. In refractory cases, medical therapy with amiodarone is an option, although side effects are a significant issue [271].

Patients with previous Mustard or Senning repair are at high risk of sudden cardiac death, presumably due to rapidly conducted atrial arrhythmias or primary ventricular arrhythmias [272]. Predictors of sudden cardiac death include a history of concomitant VSD, impaired systemic ventricular function, atrial flutter, and increased QT dispersion [266,273,274]. Limited data are available on prophylactic implantation of ICDs in high-risk patients, which currently relies on clinical judgment.

Other late complications of the Mustard or Senning repair include baffle leaks and baffle stenosis. In the case of baffle leaks, percutaneous closure may be achieved using septal occlude devices and/or stents [275]. Baffle obstruction develops most commonly in the systemic venous pathway with a frequency of 5–15% [261], usually affecting the superior vena cava limb. Surgical baffle revision for this complication is, however, uncommon as flow is redirected to the inferior vena cava through collaterals. Transcatheter repair may be achieved with balloon dilatation and stent implantation of the baffle stenosis [276,277]. If acquired atresia has taken place, a Brockenbrough needle or a radiofrequency wire can be used in order to perforate the atretic site, followed by stent implantation to ensure patency of the superior vena cava baffle [276]. In case of pulmonary venous pathway obstruction, transcatheter balloon dilatation can also relief the obstruction successfully [277].

When right ventricular dysfunction occurs, a cycle of right ventricular dilatation and tricuspid insufficiency develops leading to worsening right ventricular function and poor clinical outcomes. Treatment options include conversion to the arterial switch or cardiac transplantation. Arterial switch conversion can be performed in two stages. During the first stage, the left ventricle is prepared to become the systemic ventricle by banding the pulmonary artery. The second stage involves takedown of the baffle, closure of the ASD, removal of the pulmonary artery band and arterial switch. Arterial switch conversion is only possible if the left ventricle can tolerate systemic pressures. In patients with poor left ventricular function unable to tolerate or support systemic pressures following pulmonary artery banding, cardiac transplantation should be considered.

As patients with atrial repair operations become older, identification of suitable candidates for arterial switch conversion and the appropriate timing of the procedure have become problematic [265]. The goal is to identify symptomatic patients who have enough reserve to tolerate the multiple operations required for conversion. Older age has been reported as a significant risk factor for conversion and patients aged 16 years or more appear to be less likely to have a successful conversion [265,278].

Significant improvement after arterial switch conversion has been noted [279,280]. Pulmonary artery banding can significantly reduce tricuspid regurgitation owing to shift of the ventricular septum towards the systemic right ventricle resulting in improved coaptation of the tricuspid valve leaflets [281]. Tricuspid regurgitation is further reduced following the arterial switch. Even when arterial switch is not possible due to inability of the left ventricle to sustain systemic pressures, pulmonary artery banding alone may result in symptomatic improvement [267]. If,

however, functional deterioration occurs, cardiac transplantation should be considered.

Subpulmonary stenosis (LVOT obstruction) is common following atrial switch repair [282] due to deviation of the ventricular septum towards the low-pressure left ventricle. As mentioned above, pulmonary/subpulmonary stenosis may be beneficial in patients with a systemic right ventricle as it allows the subpulmonary left ventricle to maintain a high systolic pressure, thus avoiding excessive deviation of the ventricular septum, which may result in tricuspid incoaptation and insufficiency.

Once selected for the two-stage arterial switch conversion, patients undergo pulmonary artery banding, either through a left thoracotomy or a median sternotomy. Systemic and pulmonary arterial pressure (a reflection of left ventricular pressures) are monitored. The pulmonary artery band is fully tightened occluding the pulmonary artery for 2–3 seconds and maximal left ventricular pressure is recorded. The band is released allowing the heart to fully recover. The band is then tightened until there is a fall in systemic arterial pressure or a rise in systemic venous pressure (typically a proximal peak pressure about 70% of maximal left ventricle pressure) [265]. Intraoperative transesophageal echocardiography is also used to monitor the effect of pulmonary artery banding on right and left ventricular function, ventricular septal deviation, and improvement of tricuspid regurgitation [265]. Intraoperatively, a dopamine infusion (5–10 μg/kg/min) is begun and sodium bicarbonate is administered to correct acidosis that occurs during the perioperative period [283]. Postoperatively the dopamine infusion is continued and the patient is fully ventilated for 24–72 hours. A postoperative transthoracic echocardiogram is obtained to document progression of left ventricular adaptation and guide in the weaning from inotropic support.

The timing of the arterial switch operation following the first-stage pulmonary artery band is variable, determined by the rate at which the left ventricle is retrained to support the systemic circulation. Interval assessment of left ventricular function is made by echocardiography and cardiac catheterization. Most patients require about 1 year for complete training of the left ventricle [265,267]. In general, patients are referred for arterial switch operation when left ventricular systolic pressure is greater than 80% of the right ventricular (systemic) pressure and the left ventricular freewall thickness has returned to normal (indexed for patient age and weight) [265].

Following the arterial switch conversion a high incidence of neoaortic valve insufficiency due to annular dilatation has been reported. Chang and associates [284] reported one of five patients requiring aortic valve replacement 4 months after arterial switch operation. Cochrane and colleagues [265] reported that two of 16 patients undergoing arterial switch operation conversion developed severe

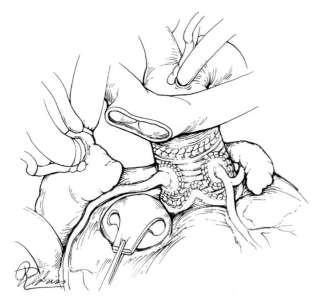

Figure 46.7 Hemashield (Boston Scientific/Medi-tech, Natick, MA) neoaortic valve-sparing reconstruction used to prevent proximal neoaortic dilatation and resultant neoaortic insufficiency. The pulmonary artery wall is removed and the contoured Hemashield graft is sewn into the resected sinuses of Valsalva. Appropriately sized holes are made in the corresponding facing sinuses for coronary reimplantation. The distal Hemashield graft is sutured end-to-end into the ascending aorta, thereby reconstructing the neoaorta. (Reproduced with permission from Mavroudis et al. [267].)

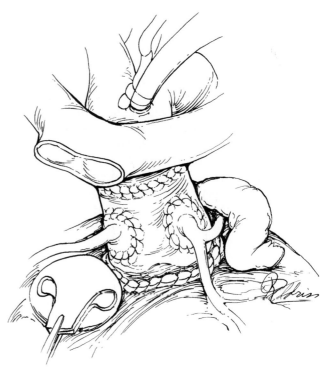

Figure 46.8 Aortic homograft implantation in a patient who had a Senning operation for transposition of the great arteries and moderate pulmonary stenosis. The patient underwent a preparatory pulmonary artery band placement en route to arterial switch operation conversion by neoaortic reconstruction using an aortic homograft because of the poor quality of the existing pulmonary valve (neoaortic valve). (Reproduced with permission from Mavroudis et al. [267].)

neoaortic valve insufficiency and required aortic valve replacement (12%), and an additional five patients (31%) developed mild aortic insufficiency. To address the issue of annular dilatation and subsequent neoaortic valve insufficiency, Mavroudis and Backer [267] have performed neoaortic reconstruction in four of six patients at the time of the initial conversion procedure. In three patients, a Hemashield (Boston Scientific/Medi-tech®, Natick, MA) neoaortic valve-sparing reconstruction was used to prevent proximal neoaortic dilatation (Figure 46.7) [208,267]. The fourth patient had reconstruction of the neoaorta using an aortic homograft because of the poor quality of the existing valve (Figure 46.8) [208,267]. To date, no neoaortic valve insufficiency has been identified in the patients who had neoaorta reconstruction. In addition to neoaortic valve insufficiency, atrial arrhythmias have occurred in patients following arterial switch operations. Atrial arrhythmias occur due to persistent elevation in atrial pressures following conversion. Mavroudis and colleagues [285] have successfully performed the right-sided maze cryoablation procedure in twopatients with atrial re-entry tachycardia and nodal re-entry tachycardia. Initial results of arterial

switch conversion operation are promising. Long-term results remain to be seen.

Left Ventricular Outflow Obstruction

Obstruction of the left ventricular outflow tract covers a wide range of anatomic lesions. Obstruction may be caused by discrete or diffuse subvalvar stenosis, valvar stenosis, or may involve the supravalvar portion of the aorta. In addition, obstruction may occur due to abnormal insertion of the mitral valve, abnormal insertion of the papillary muscles, accessory mitral valve leaflet, and hypertrophied muscle bands within the LVOT or following repair of partial AV canal. Finally, subaortic stenosis may be part of a complex syndrome of multiple levels of left ventricular obstruction (e.g., Shone's complex of mitral stenosis, hypoplastic aortic annulus, and coarctation). Subaortic stenosis is considered a progressive lesion with a variable rate of progression. Patients with subaortic stenosis are at an increased risk of bacterial endocarditis and aortic insufficiency when fibrous strands extend onto the base of the aortic leaflets [286]. Chronic obstruction of the LVOT may lead to left ventricular hypertrophy resulting in congestive heart failure, angina, arrhythmias, and sudden death.

Surgical repair is the mainstay of LVOT obstruction repair. The timing and technique to be used remain, however, controversial. Discrete subaortic membranes may be treated by simple excision with or without myotomy or myectomy. Early excision of discrete subaortic membranes reduces the development of aortic insufficiency but recurrent membrane formation remains a long-term complication [287]. Diffuse subaortic stenosis has been treated with medical therapy, ventricular pacing, and resection with extensive reconstruction of the LVOT. Aortic valve stenosis has been treated with procedures directed towards enlargement of the aortic annulus (Manougian, Konno) and insertion of a larger valve. Detailed discussion of aortic annular stenosis and annular enlargement is beyond the scope of this chapter, but is fully addressed in Chapter 29, *Ebstein Anomaly*. Supravalvar stenosis is the least common form of aortic stenosis. Treatment is directed toward relief of the obstruction.

Discrete Subaortic Stenosis

Discrete subaortic stenosis causes LVOT obstruction and may lead to significant aortic insufficiency if left untreated. In an attempt to identify the etiology of the subaortic membrane, Cape and colleagues [288,289] noted the potential role of mechanical stress and septal shear stress in the development of subaortic stenosis. A small change in the aortoseptal angle produces changes in the septal shear stress. A steepened aortoseptal angle leads to an increase in septal shear stress and results in cellular proliferation and the development of discrete subaortic stenosis. Conventional resection relieves the obstruction but recurrence rate is high. Serraf and associates [287] reported on their 17-year experience of 120 patients with discrete subaortic stenosis. Thirty-nine patients underwent isolated resection of the membrane, 67 had excision of the membrane plus myotomy, and the remaining 14 patients underwent resection of the membrane plus myectomy. Overall there was a 27.1% recurrence rate and 12% required reoperation (5 of 39 with membranectomy, 7 of 67 with membranectomy plus myotomy, 2 of 14 with membranectomy plus myectomy). Two patients developed complete heart block and two patients died following the operation (one each in the membranectomy plus myotomy or myectomy subsets). In this study, coarctation of the aortic isthmus and the quality of the primary surgical relief were independent risk factors for recurrence. They also found a positive correlation between higher early postoperative gradients, and increased rates of recurrence. Therefore they recommend that patients with residual gradients >30 mmHg at the end

of CPB should undergo reoperation with more aggressive resection at the time of the initial procedure. Results from Parry and colleagues [290] support these findings. Thirty-seven patients age 0.5–35 years (median, 7.5 years) underwent aggressive resection of a discrete subaortic membrane. No patients required reoperation for recurrent obstruction at mid-term follow-up (27 months, range 2–59 months). However, long-term results are required to confirm if the benefits of aggressive resection are maintained.

Extensive myectomy increases the risk of heart block and iatrogenic VSD. Use of intraoperative transesophageal echocardiography has been shown to reduce the complications of complete heart block and iatrogenic VSD during the performance of aggressive subaortic resection [291]. Considering the work of Cape and colleagues [288] regarding the importance of the aortoseptal angle and septal sheer stress, it is not surprising that recurrence occurs following resection alone. In addition to aggressive resection of the membrane, development of procedures to relieve the morphologic abnormalities and restore the normal aortoseptal relationship may reduce the recurrence of subaortic stenosis.

Diffuse/Tunnel Subaortic Stenosis

Tunnel subaortic stenosis represents a more severe and more complex form of LVOT obstruction. Tunnel subaortic stenosis is associated with higher mortality rates and higher reoperation rates when compared to less complex forms of LVOT obstruction [287]. Treatment of tunnel subaortic stenosis has been both medical and surgical.

Nonsurgical Therapy

Beta-adrenergic blocking agents and verapamil have been used in the treatment of diffuse subaortic stenosis. Patients who do not initially respond to one class of agent may in fact respond to the other class of agent. Therefore drug selection has not been standardized and is for the most part based on the bias of the clinician [292]. The mechanism by which negative inotropic agents provide therapeutic benefit is poorly understood. Sherrid and colleagues [293] studied the effects of medical therapy in 11 patients with obstructive hypertrophic cardiomyopathy. They concluded that negative inotropic agents decrease the acceleration of left ventricular ejection leading to reduced hemodynamic forces on the mitral valve leaflet. By decreasing the acceleration forces on the mitral valve, anterior motion of the anterior leaflet of the mitral valve towards the interventricular septum is reduced, thereby diminishing the degree of LVOT obstruction. Several studies [293–295] have confirmed the beneficial effects of negative inotropes. Ostman-Smith and colleagues [296] showed that high-dose beta-blockade therapy (propranolol 5–23 mg/kg/day) produced a 5–10-fold reduction in the risk of disease-related deaths. Despite reports supporting medical therapy for the treatment of obstructive cardiomyopathy, LVOT obstruction is not significantly improved in many patients. Seiler and colleagues [297] reported on 139 patients with obstructive hypertrophic cardiomyopathy followed for 8.9 years (range, 1–28 years). Patients were divided into four treatment groups: 1) propranolol, 2) verapamil, 3) verapamil plus surgical myectomy, and 4) surgical myectomy only. They concluded that survival was significantly better in the verapamil plus surgical myectomy group when compared to all other groups. Based on the above studies, patients with obstructive hypertrophic cardiomyopathy who are symptomatic or have failed to respond to medical therapy should undergo surgical treatment.

Dual-Chamber Pacing

The role of dual-chamber pacing for relief of diffuse LVOT obstruction is unclear, with conflicting reports in the literature. Some studies have reported significant clinical improvement and substantial reduction in the LVOT gradient with chronic dual-chamber pacing. Sakai and colleagues [298] reported on their results of chronic dual chamber pacing in 11 patients with obstructive hypertrophic cardiomyopathy. All patients had resolution of their symptoms within 1 month. The LVOT pressure gradient diminished from 99 ± 56 mmHg to 21 ± 13 mmHg at 1 week and 17 ± 12 mmHg at 1 year. There was significant reduction of the septal hypertrophy and disappearance of the systolic anterior motion of the mitral valve. Results from the Mayo Clinic [299] were not as encouraging. Thirty-eight patients with hypertrophic cardiomyopathy received dual chamber pacemakers. At a mean follow-up of 24 ± 14 months, subjective improvement was reported in 47% of the patients and there was no statistically significant improvement noted in maximal oxygen consumption. Ommen and colleagues [300] compared septal myectomy to dual-chamber pacing. Ninety percent of septal myectomy patients experienced symptomatic improvement as compared to 47% of patients in the pacing group. In the myectomy group, exercise duration was significantly greater than for the dual-chamber pacing group. Maximal oxygen consumption increased significantly following myectomy whereas the pacing group did not experience any significant change. Despite early enthusiasm for dual-chamber pacing for the treatment of obstructive hypertrophic cardiomyopathy, recent more carefully controlled investigations have proven pacing to be less favorable then septal myectomy.

Transcoronary Ablation of Septal Hypertrophy

Recently, injection of alcohol into the first major septal coronary artery has been proposed to reduce interventricular septal thickness and diminish LVOT obstruction. Transcoronary ablation of septal hypertrophy (TASH) is based on conventional percutaneous transcoronary angi-

oplasty techniques with the aim of inducing a controlled septal infarction by injection of 97% ethanol into the first septal branch of the left anterior descending artery. This leads to scarring and contraction of the subaortic septum and results in decreased septal bulge and opening of the LVOT. Gietzen and colleagues [301] reported 50 patients who underwent TASH for hypertrophic obstructive cardiomyopathy. TASH led to a reduction in septal wall thickness and eliminated the LVOT pressure gradient (51 ± 41 mmHg vs. 6 ± 41 mmHg) which was sustained at 7 ± 1 months' follow-up. However, 17% of the patients suffered from permanent high-grade AV node block. In addition there was a 4% early mortality rate. Experience with this technique is limited and further prospective randomized trials are required.

Surgical Treatment of Diffuse/Tunnel LVOT Obstruction

Early surgical treatment protocols for diffuse LVOT obstruction included implantation of apical-aortic prosthetic valved conduits. Conduit obstruction due to bioprosthetic valve calcification and a high incidence of reoperation because of conduit valve failure has decreased enthusiasm for this treatment option. Apical-aortic conduit placement has given way to more contemporary procedures that have reduced the need for reoperation.

Konno Procedure

The Konno operation can be used to treat all levels of LVOT obstruction. Tunnel-like subaortic stenosis, diffuse obstructive hypertrophic cardiomyopathy, congenital aortic valve stenosis, and proximal ascending aortic stenosis can all be treated with the Konno operation. The Konno operation was described in 1975 for the treatment of congenital aortic stenosis associated with hypoplasia of the aortic annulus [302]. A longitudinal incision is made on the anterior aspect of the ascending aorta just distal to the aortic valve. The incision is continued to the left of the right coronary artery and into the right ventricle and carried down the interventricular septum below any subvalvar stenosis. A PTFE patch is cut into an appropriately sized ellipse and sutured to the left ventricular side of the VSD. The patch is continued across the aortic annulus and onto the aorta thereby enlarging the aortic annulus. The prosthetic valve is sutured to the native aortic annulus and the synthetic patch neoannulus. The RVOT is then reconstructed with an appropriately shaped prosthetic patch. The Konno operation relieves subaortic stenosis and augments the aortic annulus, which permits the insertion of a larger prosthetic valve than the native annulus would allow [170]. Cobanoglu and colleagues [303] reported on 20 patients at a mean age of 9.2 years (range, 1.7–25.7 years) who underwent a Konno operation for LVOT obstruction. Mean follow-up time was

61.1 ± 31.7 months. Ten-year actuarial survival was 90 ± 7% and the reoperation-free survival was 89 ± 7%. All patients had resolution of their left ventricular hypertrophy with insignificant gradients across the LVOT. Despite current era enthusiasm for homograft and autograft reconstruction of the LVOT, the Konno operation remains among treatment options.

The modified Konno operation permits the enlargement of the LVOT obstruction without the need for insertion of a prosthetic valve. This procedure is used when LVOT obstruction is present in the face of a normal-sized aortic annulus. Vouhe and colleagues [304] used the modified Konno procedure in 11 patients with subaortic stenosis and a normal aortic orifice (six patients with tunnel subaortic stenosis and five patients with diffuse hypertrophic obstructive cardiomyopathy). There were one early death, one reoperation for iatrogenic aortic regurgitation, and one reoperation for residual VSD. At follow-up (mean, 3.8 ± 4.2 years; range 2 months to 10 years) all patients had LVOT gradients of less than 25 mmHg. Jahangiri [305] reported excellent relief of subaortic stenosis in 15 patients and no evidence of iatrogenic injury to the conduction system. The modified Konno operation is advantageous for patients with LVOT obstruction and normal aortic annular size because the native aortic valve is preserved and prosthetic or homograft valves are avoided.

The Ross-Konno operation provides an excellent treatment option for diffuse subaortic stenosis with aortic valve stenosis or insufficiency. In 1987 McKowen and colleagues [306] described the use of a pulmonary allograft for extended aortic root replacement to treat recurrent tunnel stenosis with a hypoplastic aortic annulus. Subsequent reports of excellent results support the Ross-Konno operation as the procedure of choice for the treatment of subaortic stenosis and aortic annular hypoplasia. Daenen [307] reported on the management of 16 patients with complex LVOT obstruction. These patients underwent aortoventriculoplasty and extended aortic root replacement with a pulmonary autograft. There were one early death and one late death due to congestive heart failure. One patient developed complete heart block and another required reoperation 4 years post-procedure for aortic valve insufficiency. At 23 ± 12 months' follow-up, all other patients showed laminar flow in the LVOT and excellent function of the allograft and pulmonary homograft valve. Left ventricular stroke volume was increased after the Ross-Konno operation, van Son and colleagues [308] showed, with improvement in ventricular diastolic function and reduced systolic anterior motion of the mitral valve. The Ross-Konno avoids the use of bioprosthetic tissue valves in the LVOT, which degenerate over time, there is no risk of thromboembolic events due to mechanical valves, and anti-coagulation is avoided. Because of these advantages, the Ross-Konno operation is the procedure of choice for the

treatment of complex LVOT obstruction and annular hypoplasia.

References

1. Gatzoulis MA, Hechter S, Siu SC, et al. (1999) Outpatient clinics for adults with congenital heart disease: increasing workload and evolving patterns of referral. Heart 81, 57–61.
2. Knauth A, Verstappen A, Reiss J, et al. (2006) Transition and transfer from pediatric to adult care of the young adult with complex congenital heart disease. Cardiol Clin 24, 619–629, vi.
3. Webb CL, Jenkins KJ, Karpawich PP, et al. (2002) Collaborative care for adults with congenital heart disease. Circulation 105, 2318–2323.
4. Dore A, Glancy DL, Stone S, et al. (1997) Cardiac surgery for grown-up congenital heart patients: survey of 307 consecutive operations from 1991 to 1994. Am J Cardiol 80, 906–913.
5. Warnes CA, Williams RG, Bashore TM, et al. (2008) ACC/AHA 2008 Guidelines for the Management of Adults with Congenital Heart Disease: Executive Summary: a report of the American College of Cardiology/American Heart Association Task Force on Practice Guidelines (writing committee to develop guidelines for the management of adults with congenital heart disease). Circulation 118, 2395–2451.
6. Dimopoulos K, Diller GP, Piepoli MF, et al. (2006) Exercise intolerance in adults with congenital heart disease. Cardiol Clin 24, 641–660, vii.
7. Piran S, Veldtman G, Siu S, et al. (2002) Heart failure and ventricular dysfunction in patients with single or systemic right ventricles. Circulation 105, 1189–1194.
8. Babu-Narayan SV, Goktekin O, Moon JC, et al. (2005) Late gadolinium enhancement cardiovascular magnetic resonance of the systemic right ventricle in adults with previous atrial redirection surgery for transposition of the great arteries. Circulation 111, 2091–2098.
9. Warnes CA. (2005) The adult with congenital heart disease: born to be bad? J Am Coll Cardiol 46, 1–8.
10. Bolger AP, Coats AJ, Gatzoulis MA. (2003) Congenital heart disease: the original heart failure syndrome. Eur Heart J 24, 970–976.
11. Dimopoulos K. (2008) Trials and tribulations in adult congenital heart disease. Int J Cardiol 129, 160–162.
12. Book WM. (2005) Heart failure in the adult patient with congenital heart disease. J Card Fail 11, 306–312.
13. Engelfriet PM, Duffels MG, Moller T, et al. (2007) Pulmonary arterial hypertension in adults born with a heart septal defect: the Euro Heart Survey on adult congenital heart disease. Heart 93, 682–687.
14. Sachweh JS, Daebritz SH, Hermanns B, et al. (2006) Hypertensive pulmonary vascular disease in adults with secundum or sinus venosus atrial septal defect. Ann Thorac Surg 81, 207–213.
15. McLaughlin VV, Archer SL, Badesch DB, et al. (2009) ACCF/AHA 2009 expert consensus document on pulmonary hypertension a report of the American College of

Cardiology Foundation Task Force on Expert Consensus Documents and the American Heart Association developed in collaboration with the American College of Chest Physicians; American Thoracic Society, Inc.; and the Pulmonary Hypertension Association. J Am Coll Cardiol 53, 1573–1619.

16. Rubin LJ, Badesch DB. (2005) Evaluation and management of the patient with pulmonary arterial hypertension. Ann Intern Med 143, 282–292.

17. Simonneau G, Galie N, Rubin LJ, et al. (2004) Clinical classification of pulmonary hypertension. J Am Coll Cardiol 43(Suppl S), 5S–12S.

18. Beghetti M. (2006) *Pulmonary Arterial Hypertension Related to Congenital Heart Disease*. Munich: Elsevier.

19. Hoffman JI, Rudolph AM. (1965) The natural history of ventricular septal defects in infancy. Am J Cardiol 16, 634–653.

20. Diller GP, Gatzoulis MA. (2007) Pulmonary vascular disease in adults with congenital heart disease. Circulation 115, 1039–1050.

21. Dimopoulos K, Okonko DO, Diller GP, et al. (2006) Abnormal ventilatory response to exercise in adults with congenital heart disease relates to cyanosis and predicts survival. Circulation 113, 2796–2802.

22. Bando K, Turrentine MW, Sharp TG, et al. (1996) Pulmonary hypertension after operations for congenital heart disease: analysis of risk factors and management. J Thorac Cardiovasc Surg 112, 1600–1607; discussion 1607–1609.

23. Miller OI, Tang SF, Keech A, et al. (2000) Inhaled nitric oxide and prevention of pulmonary hypertension after congenital heart surgery: a randomised double-blind study. Lancet 356, 1464–1469.

24. Dimopoulos K, Peset A, Gatzoulis MA. (2008) Evaluating operability in adults with congenital heart disease and the role of pretreatment with targeted pulmonary arterial hypertension therapy. Int J Cardiol 129, 163–171.

25. Therrien J, Warnes C, Daliento L, et al. (2001) Canadian Cardiovascular Society Consensus Conference 2001 update: recommendations for the management of adults with congenital heart disease part III. Can J Cardiol 17, 1135–1158.

26. Somerville J. (1997) Management of adults with congenital heart disease: an increasing problem. Annu Rev Med 48, 283–293.

27. Garson A Jr, Bink-Boelkens M, Hesslein PS, et al. (1985) Atrial flutter in the young: a collaborative study of 380 cases. J Am Coll Cardiol 6, 871–878.

28. Horton RP, Canby RC, Kessler DJ, et al. (1997) Ablation of ventricular tachycardia associated with tetralogy of Fallot: demonstration of bidirectional block. J Cardiovasc Electrophysiol 8, 432–435.

29. Triedman JK. (2002) Arrhythmias in adults with congenital heart disease. Heart 87, 383–389.

30. Deal BJ, Mavroudis C, Jacobs JP, et al. (2008) Arrhythmic complications associated with the treatment of patients with congenital cardiac disease: consensus definitions from the Multi-Societal Database Committee for Pediatric and Congenital Heart Disease. Cardiol Young 18(Suppl 2), 202–205.

31. Oechslin EN, Harrison DA, Connelly MS, et al. (2000) Mode of death in adults with congenital heart disease. Am J Cardiol 86, 1111–1116.

32. Silka MJ, Hardy BG, Menashe VD, et al. (1998) A population-based prospective evaluation of risk of sudden cardiac death after operation for common congenital heart defects. J Am Coll Cardiol 32, 245–251.

33. Alexander ME, Walsh EP, Saul JP, et al. (1999) Value of programmed ventricular stimulation in patients with congenital heart disease. J Cardiovasc Electrophysiol 10, 1033–1044.

34. Gatzoulis MA, Balaji S, Webber SA, et al. (2000) Risk factors for arrhythmia and sudden cardiac death late after repair of tetralogy of Fallot: a multicentre study. Lancet 356, 975–981.

35. Deanfield J, Thaulow E, Warnes C, et al. (2003) Management of grown up congenital heart disease. Eur Heart J 24, 1035–1084.

36. Zipes DP, Camm AJ, Borggrefe M, et al. (2006) ACC/AHA/ESC 2006 guidelines for management of patients with ventricular arrhythmias and the prevention of sudden cardiac death–executive summary: A report of the American College of Cardiology/American Heart Association Task Force and the European Society of Cardiology Committee for Practice Guidelines (Writing Committee to Develop Guidelines for Management of Patients with Ventricular Arrhythmias and the Prevention of Sudden Cardiac Death) Developed in collaboration with the European Heart Rhythm Association and the Heart Rhythm Society. Eur Heart J 27, 2099–2140.

37. Walsh EP, Cecchin F. (2007) Arrhythmias in adult patients with congenital heart disease. Circulation 115, 534–545.

38. Braunwald E. (2008) Hypoxia and cyanosis. In: Fauci AS, Braunwald E, Wilson JD, et al., eds. *Harrison's Principles of Internal Medicine*, 17th ed. New York: McGraw-Hill Medical, pp. 229–231.

39. Colman JM, Oechslin E, Taylor D. (2003) Glossary. In: Gatzoulis MA, Webb GD, Daubeney PEF, eds. *Diagnosis and Management of Adult Congenital Heart Disease*. London: Churchill Livingstone, pp. 497–508.

40. Perloff JK. (1993) Systemic complications of cyanosis in adults with congenital heart disease. Hematologic derangements, renal function, and urate metabolism. Cardiol Clin 11, 689–699.

41. Oechslin E. (2004) Hematological management of the cyanotic adult with congenital heart disease. Int J Cardiol 97(Suppl 1), 109–115.

42. Spence MS, Balaratnam MS, Gatzoulis MA. (2007) Clinical update: cyanotic adult congenital heart disease. Lancet 370, 1530–1532.

43. Ammash N, Warnes CA. (1996) Cerebrovascular events in adult patients with cyanotic congenital heart disease. J Am Coll Cardiol 28, 768–772.

44. Broberg CS, Bax BE, Okonko DO, et al. (2006) Blood viscosity and its relationship to iron deficiency, symptoms, and exercise capacity in adults with cyanotic congenital heart disease. J Am Coll Cardiol 48, 356–365.

45. Diller GP, Dimopoulos K, Broberg CS, et al. (2006) Presentation, survival prospects, and predictors of death

in Eisenmenger syndrome: a combined retrospective and case-control study. Eur Heart J 27, 1737–1742.

46. Oechslin E. (2003) Eisenmenger's syndrome. In: Gatzoulis MA, Webb GD, Daubeney PEF, eds. *Diagnosis and Management of Adult Congenital Heart Disease.* London: Churchill Livingstone, pp. 363–377.

47. Tempe DK, Virmani S. (2002) Coagulation abnormalities in patients with cyanotic congenital heart disease. J Cardiothorac Vasc Anesth 16, 752–765.

48. Linderkamp O, Klose HJ, Betke K, *et al.* (1979) Increased blood viscosity in patients with cyanotic congenital heart disease and iron deficiency. J Pediatr 95, 567–569.

49. Broberg C, Ujita M, Babu-Narayan S, *et al.* (2004) Massive pulmonary artery thrombosis with haemoptysis in adults with Eisenmenger's syndrome: a clinical dilemma. Heart 90, e63.

50. Fyfe A, Perloff JK, Niwa K, *et al.* (2005) Cyanotic congenital heart disease and coronary artery atherogenesis. Am J Cardiol 96, 283–290.

51. Sambasivan A, Tibble A, Donahue BS. (2006) Low arterial saturation is associated with increased sensitivity to activated protein C in children with congenital heart disease. J Cardiothorac Vasc Anesth 20, 38–42.

52. Horigome H, Murakami T, Isobe T, *et al.* (2003) Soluble P-selectin and thrombomodulin-protein C-Protein S pathway in cyanotic congenital heart disease with secondary erythrocytosis. Thromb Res 112, 223–227.

53. Perloff JK, Hart EM, Greaves SM, *et al.* (2003) Proximal pulmonary arterial and intrapulmonary radiologic features of Eisenmenger syndrome and primary pulmonary hypertension. Am J Cardiol 92, 182–187.

54. Silversides CK, Granton JT, Konen E, *et al.* (2003) Pulmonary thrombosis in adults with Eisenmenger syndrome. J Am Coll Cardiol 42, 1982–1987.

55. Canada WJ, Goodale F Jr, Currens JH. (1953) Defect of the interatrial septum, with thrombosis of the pulmonary artery; report of three cases. N Engl J Med 248, 309–316.

56. Shore DF. (2003) Late repair and reoperations in adults with congenital heart disease. In: Gatzoulis MA, Webb GD, Daubeney PEF, eds. *Diagnosis and Management of Adult Congenital Heart Disease.* London: Livingstone Churchill, pp. 73–78.

57. Phornphutkul C, Rosenthal A, Nadas AS, *et al.* (1973) Cerebrovascular accidents in infants and children with cyanotic congenital heart disease. Am J Cardiol 32, 329–334.

58. Perloff JK, Marelli AJ, Miner PD. (1993) Risk of stroke in adults with cyanotic congenital heart disease. Circulation 87, 1954–1959.

59. Daliento L, Somerville J, Presbitero P, *et al.* (1998) Eisenmenger syndrome. Factors relating to deterioration and death. Eur Heart J 19, 1845–1855.

60. Horigome H, Iwasaki N, Anno I, *et al.* (2006) Magnetic resonance imaging of the brain and haematological profile in adult cyanotic congenital heart disease without stroke. Heart 92, 263–265.

61. Spear GS. (1977) The glomerular lesion of cyanotic congenital heart disease. Johns Hopkins Med J 140, 185–188.

62. Dimopoulos K, Diller GP, Koltsida E, *et al.* (2008) Prevalence, predictors, and prognostic value of renal dysfunction in adults with congenital heart disease. Circulation 117, 2320–2328.

63. Warnes C. (2000) Management of erythrocytosis and other long-term complications of cyanosis. Presented at Eleventh Annual Congenital Heart Disease in the Adult – A Combined International Symposium. May 21–24, 2000.

64. Vause S, Thorne SA, Clarke B. (2006) Preconceptual counselling for women with cardiac disease. In: Steer PJ, Gatzoulis MA, Baker P, eds. *Heart Disease and Pregnancy.* London: RCOG Press, pp. 3–8.

65. Badduke BR, Jamieson WR, Miyagishima RT, *et al.* (1991) Pregnancy and childbearing in a population with biologic valvular prostheses. J Thorac Cardiovasc Surg 102, 179-86.

66. Sbarouni E, Oakley CM. (1994) Outcome of pregnancy in women with valve prostheses. Br Heart J 71, 196–201.

67. Avila WS, Rossi EG, Grinberg M, *et al.* (2002) Influence of pregnancy after bioprosthetic valve replacement in young women: a prospective five-year study. J Heart Valve Dis 11, 864–869.

68. Jamieson WR, Miller DC, Akins CW, *et al.* (1995) Pregnancy and bioprostheses: influence on structural valve deterioration. Ann Thorac Surg 60(Suppl), S282–286; discussion S287.

69. Elkayam U, Bitar F. (2005) Valvular heart disease and pregnancy: part II: prosthetic valves. J Am Coll Cardiol 46, 403–410.

70. Elkayam UR. (1996) Anticoagulation in pregnant women with prosthetic heart valves: a double jeopardy. J Am Coll Cardiol 27, 1704–1706.

71. Immer FF, Bansi AG, Immer-Bansi AS, *et al.* (2003) Aortic dissection in pregnancy: analysis of risk factors and outcome. Ann Thorac Surg 76, 309–314.

72. Khairy P, Ouyang DW, Fernandes SM, *et al.* (2006) Pregnancy outcomes in women with congenital heart disease. Circulation 113, 517–524.

73. Uebing A, Arvanitis P, Li W, *et al.* (2010) Effect of pregnancy on clinical status and ventricular function in women with heart disease. Int J Cardiol 139, 50–59.

74. Tateno S, Niwa K, Nakazawa M, *et al.* (2003) Arrhythmia and conduction disturbances in patients with congenital heart disease during pregnancy: multicenter study. Circ J 67, 992–997.

75. Joglar JA, Page RL. (2001) Antiarrhythmic drugs in pregnancy. Curr Opin Cardiol 16, 40–45.

76. Schroeder JS, Harrison DC. (1971) Repeated cardioversion during pregnancy. Treatment of refractory paroxysmal atrial tachycardia during 3 successive pregnancies. Am J Cardiol 27, 445–446.

77. Chan WS, Anand S, Ginsberg JS. (2000) Anticoagulation of pregnant women with mechanical heart valves: a systematic review of the literature. Arch Intern Med 160, 191–196.

78. Hung L, Rahimtoola SH. (2003) Prosthetic heart valves and pregnancy. Circulation 107, 1240–1246.

79. Warnes CA. (2006) Prosthetic heart valves. In: Steer PJ, Gatzoulis MA, Baker P, eds. *Heart Disease and Pregnancy.* London: RCOG Press, pp. 157–168.

80. Klein LL, Galan HL. (2004) Cardiac disease in pregnancy. Obstet Gynecol Clin North Am 31, 429–459, viii.

81. Elkayam U, Bitar F. (2005) Valvular heart disease and pregnancy part I: native valves. J Am Coll Cardiol 46, 223–230.

82. Kafka H, Uemura H, Gatzoulis MA. (2006) Surgical and catheter intervention during pregnancy in women with heart disease. In: Steer PJ, Gatzoulis MA, Baker P, eds. *Heart Disease and Pregnancy.* London: RCOG Press, pp. 95–125.

83. Barnea O, Austin EH, Richman B, *et al.* (1994) Balancing the circulation: theoretic optimization of pulmonary/systemic flow ratio in hypoplastic left heart syndrome. J Am Coll Cardiol 24, 1376–1381.

84. Mosca RS, Bove EL, Crowley DC, *et al.* (1995) Hemodynamic characteristics of neonates following first stage palliation for hypoplastic left heart syndrome. Circulation 92(Suppl), II267–II271.

85. Bradley SM, Simsic JM, Mulvihill DM. (1998) Hyperventilation impairs oxygenation after bidirectional superior cavopulmonary connection. Circulation 98(Suppl), II372–II376; discussion II376–II377.

86. Williams DB, Kiernan PD, Metke MP, *et al.* (1984) Hemodynamic response to positive end-expiratory pressure following right atrium-pulmonary artery bypass (Fontan procedure). J Thorac Cardiovasc Surg 87, 856–861.

87. England MR, Gordon G, Salem M, *et al.* (1992) Magnesium administration and dysrhythmias after cardiac surgery. A placebo-controlled, double-blind, randomized trial. JAMA 268, 2395–2402.

88. Guyton RA, Schonberger JP, Everts PA, *et al.* (1993) Postcardiotomy shock: clinical evaluation of the BVS 5000 Biventricular Support System. Ann Thorac Surg 56, 346–356.

89. Couper GS, Dekkers RJ, Adams DH. (1999) The logistics and cost-effectiveness of circulatory support: advantages of the ABIOMED BVS 5000. Ann Thorac Surg 68, 646–649.

90. Korfer R, El-Banayosy A, Arusoglu L, *et al.* (1999) Temporary pulsatile ventricular assist devices and biventricular assist devices. Ann Thorac Surg 68, 678–683.

91. Haj-Yahia S, Birks EJ, Amrani M, *et al.* (2009) Bridging patients after salvage from bridge to decision directly to transplant by means of prolonged support with the CentriMag short-term centrifugal pump. J Thorac Cardiovasc Surg 138, 227–230.

92. Clough RE, Vallely MP, Henein MY, *et al.* (2009) Levitronix ventricular assist device as a bridge-to-recovery for post-cardiotomy cardiogenic shock. Int J Cardiol 134, 408–409.

93. De Robertis F, Birks EJ, Rogers P, *et al.* (2006) Clinical performance with the Levitronix Centrimag short-term ventricular assist device. J Heart Lung Transplant 25, 181–186.

94. Korfer R, El-Banayosy A, Arusoglu L, *et al.* (2000) Single-center experience with the thoratec ventricular assist device. J Thorac Cardiovasc Surg 119, 596–600.

95. Mavroidis D, Sun BC, Pae WE Jr. (1999) Bridge to transplantation: the Penn State experience. Ann Thorac Surg 68, 684–687.

96. Minami K, El-Banayosy A, Sezai A, *et al.* (2000) Morbidity and outcome after mechanical ventricular support using Thoratec, Novacor, and HeartMate for bridging to heart transplantation. Artif Organs 24, 421–426.

97. Miller LW, Pagani FD, Russell SD, *et al.* (2007) Use of a continuous-flow device in patients awaiting heart transplantation. N Engl J Med 357, 885–896.

98. Dickinson DF, Arnold R, Wilkinson JL. (1981) Congenital heart disease among 160 480 liveborn children in Liverpool 1960 to 1969. Implications for surgical treatment. Br Heart J 46, 55–62.

99. Shibata Y, Abe T, Kuribayashi R, *et al.*. (1996) Surgical treatment of isolated secundum atrial septal defect in patients more than 50 years old. Ann Thorac Surg 62, 1096–1099.

100. Chan KC, Godman MJ, Walsh K, *et al.* (1999) Transcatheter closure of atrial septal defect and interatrial communications with a new self expanding nitinol double disc device (Amplatzer septal occluder): multicentre UK experience. Heart 82, 300–306.

101. Majunke N, Bialkowski J, Wilson N, *et al.* (2009) Closure of atrial septal defect with the Amplatzer septal occluder in adults. Am J Cardiol 103, 550–554.

102. Noble S, Ibrahim R. (2009) Percutaneous interventions in adults with congenital heart disease: expanding indications and opportunities. Curr Cardiol Rep 11, 306–313.

103. Rastogi N, Smeeton NC, Qureshi SA. (2009) Factors related to successful transcatheter closure of atrial septal defects using the Amplatzer septal occluder. Pediatr Cardiol 30, 888–892.

104. Webb G, Gatzoulis MA. (2006) Atrial septal defects in the adult: recent progress and overview. Circulation 114, 1645–1653.

105. Giannakoulas G, Dimopoulos K, Engel R, *et al.* (2009) Burden of coronary artery disease in adults with congenital heart disease and its relation to congenital and traditional heart risk factors. Am J Cardiol 103, 1445–1450.

106. Byrne JG, Adams DH, Mitchell ME, *et al.* (1999) Minimally invasive direct access for repair of atrial septal defect in adults. Am J Cardiol 84, 919–922.

107. Bichell DP, Geva T, Bacha EA, *et al.* (2000) Minimal access approach for the repair of atrial septal defect: the initial 135 patients. Ann Thorac Surg 70, 115–118.

108. Gatzoulis MA, Redington AN, Somerville J, *et al.* (1996) Should atrial septal defects in adults be closed? Ann Thorac Surg 61, 657–659.

109. Horvath KA, Burke RP, Collins JJ Jr, *et al.* (1992) Surgical treatment of adult atrial septal defect: early and long-term results. J Am Coll Cardiol 20, 1156–1159.

110. Gatzoulis MA, Freeman MA, Siu SC, *et al.* (1999) Atrial arrhythmia after surgical closure of atrial septal defects in adults. N Engl J Med 340, 839–846.

111. Murphy JG, Gersh BJ, McGoon MD, *et al.* (1990) Long-term outcome after surgical repair of isolated atrial septal defect. Follow-up at 27 to 32 years. N Engl J Med 323, 1645–1650.

112. John Sutton MG, Tajik AJ, McGoon DC. (1981) Atrial septal defect in patients ages 60 years or older: operative results and long-term postoperative follow-up. Circulation 64, 402–409.

113. Kobayashi J, Yamamoto F, Nakano K, *et al.* (1998) Maze procedure for atrial fibrillation associated with atrial septal defect. Circulation 98(Suppl), II399–II402.

114. Campbell M. (1970) Natural history of atrial septal defect. Br Heart J 32, 820–826.

115. Yalonetsky S, Lorber A. (2007) Percutaneous closure of a secundum atrial septal defect in elderly patients. J Invasive Cardiol 19, 510–512.

116. Holzer R, Cao QL, Hijazi ZM. (2005) Closure of a moderately large atrial septal defect with a self-fabricated fenestrated Amplatzer septal occluder in an 85-year-old patient with reduced diastolic elasticity of the left ventricle. Catheter Cardiovasc Interv 64, 513–518; discussion 519–521.

117. Tomai F, Gaspardone A, Papa M, *et al.* (2002) Acute left ventricular failure after transcatheter closure of a secundum atrial septal defect in a patient with coronary artery disease: a critical reappraisal. Catheter Cardiovasc Interv 55, 97–99.

118. Ewert P, Berger F, Nagdyman N, *et al.* (2001) Masked left ventricular restriction in elderly patients with atrial septal defects: a contraindication for closure? Catheter Cardiovasc Interv 52, 177–180.

119. Vogel M, Berger F, Kramer A, *et al.* (1999) Incidence of secondary pulmonary hypertension in adults with atrial septal or sinus venosus defects. Heart 82, 30–33.

120. Balint OH, Samman A, Haberer K, *et al.* (2008) Outcomes in patients with pulmonary hypertension undergoing percutaneous atrial septal defect closure. Heart 94, 1189–1193.

121. Viswanathan S, Kumar RK. (2008) Assessment of operability of congenital cardiac shunts with increased pulmonary vascular resistance. Catheter Cardiovasc Interv 71, 665–670.

122. Piccoli GP, Gerlis LM, Wilkinson JL, *et al.* (1979) Morphology and classification of atrioventricular defects. Br Heart J 42, 621–632.

123. Burke RP, Horvath K, Landzberg M, *et al.* (1996) Long-term follow-up after surgical repair of ostium primum atrial septal defects in adults. J Am Coll Cardiol 27, 696–699.

124. Somerville J. (1965) Ostium primum defect: factors causing deterioration in the natural history. Br Heart J 27, 413–419.

125. Gatzoulis MA, Hechter S, Webb GD, *et al.* (1999) Surgery for partial atrioventricular septal defect in the adult. Ann Thorac Surg 67, 504–510.

126. Bergin ML, Warnes CA, Tajik AJ, *et al.* (1995) Partial atrioventricular canal defect: long-term follow-up after initial repair in patients > or = 40 years old. J Am Coll Cardiol 25, 1189–1194.

127. Deal BJ, Mavroudis C, Backer CL, *et al.* (1999) Impact of arrhythmia circuit cryoablation during Fontan conversion for refractory atrial tachycardia. Am J Cardiol 83, 563–568.

128. Cabanes L, Mas JL, Cohen A, *et al.* (1993) Atrial septal aneurysm and patent foramen ovale as risk factors for cryptogenic stroke in patients less than 55 years of age. A study using transesophageal echocardiography. Stroke 24, 1865–1873.

129. Mugge A, Daniel WG, Angermann C, *et al.* (1995) Atrial septal aneurysm in adult patients. A multicenter study using transthoracic and transesophageal echocardiography. Circulation 91, 2785–2792.

130. Cujec B, Polasek P, Voll C, *et al.* (1991) Transesophageal echocardiography in the detection of potential cardiac source of embolism in stroke patients. Stroke 22, 727–733.

131. Ilercil A, Meisner JS, Vijayaraman P, *et al.* (1997) Clinical significance of fossa ovalis membrane aneurysm in adults with cardioembolic cerebral ischemia. Am J Cardiol 80, 96–98.

132. Bogousslavsky J, Garazi S, Jeanrenaud X, *et al.* (1996) Stroke recurrence in patients with patent foramen ovale: the Lausanne Study. Lausanne Stroke with Paradoxal Embolism Study Group. Neurology 46, 1301–1305.

133. Homma S, Sacco RL, Di Tullio MR, *et al.* (2002) Effect of medical treatment in stroke patients with patent foramen ovale: patent foramen ovale in Cryptogenic Stroke Study. Circulation 105, 2625–2631.

134. Sacco RL, Adams R, Albers G, *et al.* (2006) Guidelines for prevention of stroke in patients with ischemic stroke or transient ischemic attack: a statement for healthcare professionals from the American Heart Association/American Stroke Association Council on Stroke: co-sponsored by the Council on Cardiovascular Radiology and Intervention: the American Academy of Neurology affirms the value of this guideline. Circulation 113, e409–e449.

135. Wells WJ, Lindesmith GG. (1985) Ventricular septal defect. In: Arciniegas E, ed. *Pediatric Cardiac Surgery*. Chicago, IL: Year Book Medical, pp 141–153.

136. Alpert BS, Mellits ED, Rowe RD. (1973) Spontaneous closure of small ventricular septal defects. probability rates in the first five years of life. Am J Dis Child 125, 194–196.

137. Neumayer U, Stone S, Somerville J. (1998) Small ventricular septal defects in adults. Eur Heart J 19, 1573–1582.

138. Niwa K, Perloff JK, Kaplan S, *et al.* (1999) Eisenmenger syndrome in adults: ventricular septal defect, truncus arteriosus, univentricular heart. J Am Coll Cardiol 34, 223–232.

139. Ikawa S, Shimazaki Y, Nakano S, *et al.* (1995) Pulmonary vascular resistance during exercise late after repair of large ventricular septal defects. Relation to age at the time of repair. J Thorac Cardiovasc Surg 109, 1218–1224.

140. Moller JH, Patton C, Varco RL, *et al.* (1991) Late results (30 to 35 years) after operative closure of isolated ventricular septal defect from 1954 to 1960. Am J Cardiol 68, 1491–1497.

141. Hijazi ZM, Hakim F, Al-Fadley F, *et al.* (2000) Transcatheter closure of single muscular ventricular septal defects using the amplatzer muscular VSD occluder: initial results and technical considerations. Catheter Cardiovasc Interv 49, 167–172.

142. Thanopoulos BD, Tsaousis GS, Konstadopoulou GN, *et al.* (1999) Transcatheter closure of muscular ventricular septal defects with the amplatzer ventricular septal defect occluder: initial clinical applications in children. J Am Coll Cardiol 33, 1395–1399.

143. Chessa M, Butera G, Negura D, *et al.* (2009) Transcatheter closure of congenital ventricular septal defects in adult:

mid-term results and complications. Int J Cardiol 133, 70–73.

144. Presbitero P, Demarie D, Aruta E, *et al.* (1988) Results of total correction of tetralogy of Fallot performed in adults. Ann Thorac Surg 46, 297–301.

145. Bertranou EG, Blackstone EH, Hazelrig JB, *et al.* (1978) Life expectancy without surgery in tetralogy of Fallot. Am J Cardiol 42, 458–466.

146. Rygg IH, Olesen K, Boesen I. (1971) The life history of tetralogy of Fallot. Dan Med Bull 18(Suppl 2), 25–30.

147. Rammohan M, Airan B, Bhan A, *et al.* (1998) Total correction of tetralogy of Fallot in adults–surgical experience. Int J Cardiol 63, 121–128.

148. Perloff JK, Natterson PD. (1995) Atrial arrhythmias in adults after repair of tetralogy of Fallot. Circulation 91, 2118–2119.

149. Presbitero P, Prever SB, Contrafatto I, *et al.* (1996) As originally published in 1988: Results of total correction of tetralogy of Fallot performed in adults. Updated in 1996. Ann Thorac Surg 61, 1870–1873.

150. Nollert G, Fischlein T, Bouterwek S, *et al.* (1997) Long-term results of total repair of tetralogy of Fallot in adulthood: 35 years follow-up in 104 patients corrected at the age of 18 or older. Thorac Cardiovasc Surg 45, 178–181.

151. Oechslin EN, Harrison DA, Harris L, *et al.* (1999) Reoperation in adults with repair of tetralogy of fallot: indications and outcomes. J Thorac Cardiovasc Surg 118, 245–251.

152. Garson A Jr, Randall DC, Gillette PC, *et al.* (1985) Prevention of sudden death after repair of tetralogy of Fallot: treatment of ventricular arrhythmias. J Am Coll Cardiol 6, 221–227.

153. Horowitz LN, Vetter VL, Harken AH, *et al.* (1980) Electrophysiologic characteristics of sustained ventricular tachycardia occurring after repair of tetralogy of fallot. Am J Cardiol 46, 446–452.

154. Misaki T, Tsubota M, Watanabe G, *et al.* (1994) Surgical treatment of ventricular tachycardia after surgical repair of tetralogy of Fallot. Relation between intraoperative mapping and histological findings. Circulation 90, 264–271.

155. Deal BJ, Scagliotti D, Miller SM, *et al.* (1987) Electrophysiologic drug testing in symptomatic ventricular arrhythmias after repair of tetralogy of Fallot. Am J Cardiol 59, 1380–1385.

156. Gatzoulis MA, Till JA, Somerville J, *et al.* (1995) Mechanoelectrical interaction in tetralogy of Fallot. QRS prolongation relates to right ventricular size and predicts malignant ventricular arrhythmias and sudden death. Circulation 92, 231–237.

157. Quattlebaum TG, Varghese J, Neill CA, *et al.* (1976) Sudden death among postoperative patients with tetralogy of Fallot: a follow-up study of 243 patients for an average of twelve years. Circulation 54, 289–293.

158. National Institute for Health and Clinical Excellence (NICE). (2006) Implantable cardioverter defibrillators for arrythmias. London: National Institute for Health and Clinical Excellence (NICE).

159. Garson A Jr, McNamara DG. (1985) Sudden death in a pediatric cardiology population, 1958 to 1983: relation to prior arrhythmias. J Am Coll Cardiol 5(6 Suppl):134B–137B.

160. Khairy P, Harris L, Landzberg MJ, *et al.* (2008) Implantable cardioverter-defibrillators in tetralogy of Fallot. Circulation 117, 363–370.

161. Witte KK, Pepper CB, Cowan JC, *et al.* (2008) Implantable cardioverter-defibrillator therapy in adult patients with tetralogy of Fallot. Europace 10, 926–930.

162. Shimazaki Y, Blackstone EH, Kirklin JW. (1984) The natural history of isolated congenital pulmonary valve incompetence: surgical implications. Thorac Cardiovasc Surg 32, 257–259.

163. Bove EL, Byrum CJ, Thomas FD, *et al.* (1983) The influence of pulmonary insufficiency on ventricular function following repair of tetralogy of Fallot. Evaluation using radionuclide ventriculography. J Thorac Cardiovasc Surg 85, 691–696.

164. Ilbawi MN, Idriss FS, DeLeon SY, *et al.* (1987) Factors that exaggerate the deleterious effects of pulmonary insufficiency on the right ventricle after tetralogy repair. Surgical implications. J Thorac Cardiovasc Surg 93, 36–44.

165. Burns RJ, Liu PP, Druck MN, *et al.* (1984) Analysis of adults with and without complex ventricular arrhythmias after repair of tetralogy of Fallot. J Am Coll Cardiol 4, 226–233.

166. Dietl CA, Cazzaniga ME, Dubner SJ, *et al.* (1994) Life-threatening arrhythmias and RV dysfunction after surgical repair of tetralogy of Fallot. Comparison between trans-ventricular and transatrial approaches. Circulation 90, II7–II12.

167. Meijboom FJ, Roos-Hesselink JW, McGhie JS, *et al.* (2008) Consequences of a selective approach toward pulmonary valve replacement in adult patients with tetralogy of Fallot and pulmonary regurgitation. J Thorac Cardiovasc Surg 135, 50–55.

168. Shinebourne EA, Babu-Narayan SV, Carvalho JS. (2006) Tetralogy of Fallot: from fetus to adult. Heart 92, 1353–1359.

169. Idriss FS, Markowitz A, Nikaidoh H. (1976) Insertion of Hancock valve for pulmonary valve insufficiency in previously repaired tetralogy of Fallot. Circulation 53, II–100 (abstr).

170. Misbach GA, Turley K, Ebert PA. (1983) Pulmonary valve replacement for regurgitation after repair of tetralogy of Fallot. Ann Thorac Surg 36, 684–691.

171. Yemets IM, Williams WG, Webb GD, *et al.* (1997) Pulmonary valve replacement late after repair of tetralogy of Fallot. Ann Thorac Surg 64, 526–530.

172. Kawachi Y, Masuda M, Tominaga R, *et al.* (1991) Comparative study between St. Jude Medical and bioprosthetic valves in the right side of the heart. Jpn Circ J 55, 553–562.

173. Fukada J, Morishita K, Komatsu K, *et al.* (1997) Influence of pulmonic position on durability of bioprosthetic heart valves. Ann Thorac Surg. 64, 1678–1680; discussion 1680–1681.

174. d'Udekem Y, Rubay J, Shango-Lody P, *et al.* (1998) Late homograft valve insertion after transannular patch repair of tetralogy of Fallot. J Heart Valve Dis 7, 450–454.

175. Elkins RC, Knott-Craig CJ, Ward KE, *et al.* (1998) The Ross operation in children: 10-year experience. Ann Thorac Surg 65, 496–502.

176. Mulder BJ, de Winter RJ, Wilde AA. (2007) Percutaneous pulmonary valve replacement: a new development in the lifetime strategy for patients with congenital heart disease. Neth Heart J 15, 3–4.

177. Nordmeyer J, Lurz P, Tsang VT, et al. (2009) Effective transcatheter valve implantation after pulmonary homograft failure: a new perspective on the Ross operation. J Thorac Cardiovasc Surg 138, 84–88.

178. Campbell M. (1970) Natural history of coarctation of the aorta. Br Heart J 32, 633–640.

179. Findlow D, Doyle E. (1997) Congenital heart disease in adults. Br J Anaesth 78, 416–430.

180. Simon AB, Zloto AE. (1974) Coarctation of the aorta. Longitudinal assessment of operated patients. Circulation 50, 456–464.

181. Bergdahl L, Bjork VO, Jonasson R. (1983) Surgical correction of coarctation of the aorta. Influence of age on late results. J Thorac Cardiovasc Surg 85, 532–536.

182. Thomka I, Szedo F, Arvay A. (1997) Repair of coarctation of the aorta in adults with simultaneous aortic valve replacement and coronary artery bypass grafting. Thorac Cardiovasc Surg 45, 93–96.

183. Perloff JK, Child JS. (1998) *Congenital Heart Disease in Adults*, 2nd ed. Philadelphia, PA: WB Saunders.

184. Aebert H, Laas J, Bednarski P, et al. (1993) High incidence of aneurysm formation following patch plasty repair of coarctation. Eur J Cardiothorac Surg 7, 200–204; discussion 205.

185. Aris A, Subirana MT, Ferres P, et al. (1999) Repair of aortic coarctation in patients more than 50 years of age. Ann Thorac Surg 67, 1376–1379.

186. Elkerdany A, Hassouna A, Elsayegh T, et al. (1999) Left subclavian-aortic bypass grafting in primary isolated adult coarctation. Cardiovasc Surg 7, 351–354.

187. Benson WR, Sealy WC. (1956) Arterial necrosis following resection of coarctation of the aorta. Lab Invest 5, 359–376.

188. Lober PH, Lillehei W. (1954) Necrotizing panarteritis following repair of coarctation of aorta; report of two cases. Surgery 35, 950–956.

189. McCrindle BW. (1999) Coarctation of the aorta. Curr Opin Cardiol 14, 448–452.

190. Kaemmerer H, Oelert F, Bahlmann J, et al. (1998) Arterial hypertension in adults after surgical treatment of aortic coarctation. Thorac Cardiovasc Surg 46, 121–125.

191. Vigano M, Ressia L, Gaeta R. (1997) Long-term follow-up after repair of coarctation of the aorta in adults. Ann Thorac Surg 63, 1827–1828.

192. Beekman RH, Rocchini AP, Behrendt DM, et al. (1986) Long-term outcome after repair of coarctation in infancy: subclavian angioplasty does not reduce the need for reoperation. J Am Coll Cardiol 8, 1406–1411.

193. Foster ED. (1984) Reoperation for aortic coarctation. Ann Thorac Surg 38, 81–89.

194. Sweeney MS, Walker WE, Duncan JM, et al. (1985) Reoperation for aortic coarctation: techniques, results, and indications for various approaches. Ann Thorac Surg 40, 46–49.

195. Attenhofer Jost CH, Schaff HV, et al. (2002) Spectrum of reoperations after repair of aortic coarctation: importance of an individualized approach because of coexistent cardiovascular disease. Mayo Clin Proc 77, 646–653.

196. Oliver JM, Gallego P, Gonzalez A, et al. (2004) Risk factors for aortic complications in adults with coarctation of the aorta. J Am Coll Cardiol 44, 1641–1647.

197. Harrison DA, McLaughlin PR, Lazzam C, et al. (2001) Endovascular stents in the management of coarctation of the aorta in the adolescent and adult: one year follow up. Heart 85, 561–566.

198. Mendelsohn AM, Crowley DC, Lindauer A, et al. (1992) Rapid progression of aortic aneurysms after patch aortoplasty repair of coarctation of the aorta. J Am Coll Cardiol 20, 381–385.

199. von Kodolitsch Y, Aydin MA, Koschyk DH, et al. (2002) Predictors of aneurysmal formation after surgical correction of aortic coarctation. J Am Coll Cardiol 39, 617–624.

200. Massey R, Shore DF. (2004) Surgery for complex coarctation of the aorta. Int J Cardiol 97(Suppl 1), 67–73.

201. Barron DJ, Somerville J, de Leval MR, et al. (1999) Surgical management of recurrent coarctation of the aorta in adults. Presented at Society for Cardiothoracic Surgery Annual Meeting. 14–17 March, 1999.

202. Connolly HM, Schaff HV, Izhar U, et al. (2001) Posterior pericardial ascending-to-descending aortic bypass: an alternative surgical approach for complex coarctation of the aorta. Circulation 104(Suppl 1), I133–I137.

203. Anagnostopoulos-Tzifa A. (2007) Management of aortic coarctation in adults: endovascular versus surgical therapy. Hellenic J Cardiol 48, 290–295.

204. Pedra CA, Fontes VF, Esteves CA, et al. (2005) Stenting vs. balloon angioplasty for discrete unoperated coarctation of the aorta in adolescents and adults. Catheter Cardiovasc Interv 64, 495–506.

205. Suarez de Lezo J, Pan M, Romero M, et al. (2005) Percutaneous interventions on severe coarctation of the aorta: a 21-year experience. Pediatr Cardiol 26, 176–189.

206. Cowley CG, Orsmond GS, Feola P, et al. (2005) Long-term, randomized comparison of balloon angioplasty and surgery for native coarctation of the aorta in childhood. Circulation 111, 3453–3456.

207. Hernandez-Gonzalez M, Solorio S, Conde-Carmona I, et al. (2003) Intraluminal aortoplasty vs. surgical aortic resection in congenital aortic coarctation. A clinical random study in pediatric patients. Arch Med Res 34, 305–310.

208. Hillman ND, Mavroudis C, Backer CL. (2003) Adult congenital heart disease. In: Mavroudis C, Backer CL, eds. *Pediatric Cardiac Surgery*, 3rd ed. Philadelphia, PA: Mosby, Inc.

209. Vitullo DA, DeLeon SY, Berry TE, et al. (1996) Clinical improvement after revision in Fontan patients. Ann Thorac Surg 61, 1797–1804.

210. Peters NS, Somerville J. (1992) Arrhythmias after the Fontan procedure. Br Heart J 68, 199–204.

211. de Leval MR, Kilner P, Gewillig M, et al. (1988) Total cavopulmonary connection: a logical alternative to atriopulmonary connection for complex Fontan operations. Experimental studies and early clinical experience. J Thorac Cardiovasc Surg 96, 682–695.

212. Sharma S, Ensley AE, Hopkins K, *et al.* (2001) In vivo flow dynamics of the total cavopulmonary connection from three-dimensional multislice magnetic resonance imaging. Ann Thorac Surg 71, 889–898.

213. Rodefeld MD, Bromberg BI, Schuessler RB, *et al.* (1996) Atrial flutter after lateral tunnel construction in the modified Fontan operation: a canine model. J Thorac Cardiovasc Surg 111, 514–526.

214. Gandhi SK, Bromberg BI, Rodefeld MD, *et al.* (1996) Lateral tunnel suture line variation reduces atrial flutter after the modified Fontan operation. Ann Thorac Surg 61, 1299–1309.

215. Gandhi SK, Bromberg BI, Schuessler RB, *et al.* (1996) Characterization and surgical ablation of atrial flutter after the classic Fontan repair. Ann Thorac Surg 61, 1666–1678; discussion 1678–1679.

216. Manning PB, Mayer JE Jr, Wernovsky G, *et al.* (1996) Staged operation to Fontan increases the incidence of sinoatrial node dysfunction. J Thorac Cardiovasc Surg 111, 833–839; discussion 839–840.

217. Bando K, Turrentine MW, Park HJ, *et al.* (2000) Evolution of the Fontan procedure in a single center. Ann Thorac Surg 69, 1873–1879.

218. Gentles TL, Mayer JE Jr, Gauvreau K, *et al.* (1997) Fontan operation in five hundred consecutive patients: factors influencing early and late outcome. J Thorac Cardiovasc Surg 114, 376–391.

219. Kaulitz R, Ziemer G, Luhmer I, *et al.* (1996) Modified Fontan operation in functionally univentricular hearts: preoperative risk factors and intermediate results. J Thorac Cardiovasc Surg 112, 658–664.

220. Knott-Craig CJ, Danielson GK, Schaff HV, *et al.* (1995) The modified Fontan operation. An analysis of risk factors for early postoperative death or takedown in 702 consecutive patients from one institution. J Thorac Cardiovasc Surg 109, 1237–1243.

221. Burke RP, Jacobs JP, Ashraf MH, *et al.* (1997) Extracardiac Fontan operation without cardiopulmonary bypass. Ann Thorac Surg 63, 1175–1177.

222. McElhinney DB, Petrossian E, Reddy VM, *et al.* (1998) Extracardiac conduit Fontan procedure without cardiopulmonary bypass. Ann Thorac Surg 66, 1826–1828.

223. Lardo AC, Webber SA, Friehs I, *et al.* (1999) Fluid dynamic comparison of intra-atrial and extracardiac total cavopulmonary connections. J Thorac Cardiovasc Surg 117, 697–704.

224. Petrossian E, Reddy VM, McElhinney DB, *et al.* (1999) Early results of the extracardiac conduit Fontan operation. J Thorac Cardiovasc Surg 117, 688–696.

225. Marcelletti CF, Hanley FL, Mavroudis C, *et al.* (2000) Revision of previous Fontan connections to total extracardiac cavopulmonary anastomosis: A multicenter experience. J Thorac Cardiovasc Surg 119, 340–346.

226. Cetta F, Feldt RH, O'Leary PW, *et al.* (1996) Improved early morbidity and mortality after Fontan operation: the Mayo Clinic experience, 1987 to 1992. J Am Coll Cardiol 28, 480–486.

227. Fishberger SB, Wernovsky G, Gentles TL, *et al.* (1997) Factors that influence the development of atrial flutter after the Fontan operation. J Thorac Cardiovasc Surg 113, 80–86.

228. Balaji S, Gewillig M, Bull C, *et al.* (1991) Arrhythmias after the Fontan procedure. Comparison of total cavopulmonary connection and atriopulmonary connection. Circulation 84(Suppl), III162–III167.

229. Gardiner HM, Dhillon R, Bull C, *et al.* (1996) Prospective study of the incidence and determinants of arrhythmia after total cavopulmonary connection. Circulation 94(Suppl), II17–II21.

230. Gelatt M, Hamilton RM, McCrindle BW, *et al.* (1994) Risk factors for atrial tachyarrhythmias after the Fontan operation. J Am Coll Cardiol 24, 1735–1741.

231. Balaji S, Johnson TB, Sade RM, *et al.* (1994) Management of atrial flutter after the Fontan procedure. J Am Coll Cardiol 23, 1209–1215.

232. Kalman JM, VanHare GF, Olgin JE, *et al.* (1996) Ablation of "incisional" reentrant atrial tachycardia complicating surgery for congenital heart disease. Use of entrainment to define a critical isthmus of conduction. Circulation 93, 502–512.

233. Triedman JK, Bergau DM, Saul JP, *et al.* (1997) Efficacy of radiofrequency ablation for control of intraatrial reentrant tachycardia in patients with congenital heart disease. J Am Coll Cardiol 30, 1032–1038.

234. Triedman JK, Saul JP, Weindling SN, *et al.* (1995) Radiofrequency ablation of intra-atrial reentrant tachycardia after surgical palliation of congenital heart disease. Circulation 91, 707–714.

235. Kao JM, Alejos JC, Grant PW, *et al.* (1994) Conversion of atriopulmonary to cavopulmonary anastomosis in management of late arrhythmias and atrial thrombosis. Ann Thorac Surg 58, 1510–1514.

236. Kreutzer J, Keane JF, Lock JE, *et al.* (1996) Conversion of modified Fontan procedure to lateral atrial tunnel cavopulmonary anastomosis. J Thorac Cardiovasc Surg 111, 1169–1176.

237. McElhinney DB, Reddy VM, Moore P, *et al.* (1996) Revision of previous Fontan connections to extracardiac or intraatrial conduit cavopulmonary anastomosis. Ann Thorac Surg 62, 1276–1282; discussion 1283.

238. Scholl FG, Alejos JC, Laks H. (1997) Revision of the traditional atriopulmonary Fontan connection. Adv Card Surg 9, 217–227.

239. van Son JA, Mohr FW, Hambsch J, *et al.* (1999) Conversion of atriopulmonary or lateral atrial tunnel cavopulmonary anastomosis to extracardiac conduit Fontan modification. Eur J Cardiothorac Surg 15, 150–157; discussion 157–158.

240. Takahashi K, Fynn-Thompson F, Cecchin F, *et al.* (2009) Clinical outcomes of Fontan conversion surgery with and without associated arrhythmia intervention. Int J Cardiol 137, 260–266.

241. Mavroudis C, Deal BJ, Backer CL, *et al.* (2007) J. Maxwell Chamberlain Memorial Paper for congenital heart surgery. 111 Fontan conversions with arrhythmia surgery: surgical lessons and outcomes. Ann Thorac Surg 84, 1457–1465; discussion 1465–1466.

242. Driscoll DJ, Offord KP, Feldt RH, *et al.* (1992) Five- to fifteen-year follow-up after Fontan operation. Circulation 85, 469–496.

243. Mertens L, Hagler DJ, Sauer U, *et al.* (1998) Protein-losing enteropathy after the Fontan operation: an international multicenter study. PLE study group. J Thorac Cardiovasc Surg 115, 1063–1073.

244. Hess J, Kruizinga K, Bijleveld CM, *et al.* (1984) Protein-losing enteropathy after Fontan operation. J Thorac Cardiovasc Surg 88, 606–609.

245. Rychik J, Piccoli DA, Barber G. (1991) Usefulness of corticosteroid therapy for protein-losing enteropathy after the Fontan procedure. Am J Cardiol 68, 819–821.

246. Donnelly JP, Rosenthal A, Castle VP, *et al.* (1997) Reversal of protein-losing enteropathy with heparin therapy in three patients with univentricular hearts and Fontan palliation. J Pediatr 130, 474–478.

247. Murch SH, Winyard PJ, Koletzko S, *et al.* (1996) Congenital enterocyte heparan sulphate deficiency with massive albumin loss, secretory diarrhoea, and malnutrition. Lancet 347, 1299–1301.

248. Abella RF, Marianeschi SM, De la Torre T, *et al.* (1998) [The conversion of a modified Fontan procedure to a total extracardiac cavo-pulmonary conduit. The Medico-Surgical Cardiology Group]. G Ital Cardiol 28, 645–652.

249. Conte S, Gewillig M, Eyskens B, *et al.* (1999) Management of late complications after classic Fontan procedure by conversion to total cavopulmonary connection. Cardiovasc Surg 7, 651–655.

250. Jacobs ML, Rychik J, Byrum CJ, *et al.* (1996) Protein-losing enteropathy after Fontan operation: resolution after baffle fenestration. Ann Thorac Surg 61, 206–208.

251. Lemes V, Murphy AM, Osterman FA, *et al.* (1998) Fenestration of extracardiac fontan and reversal of protein-losing enteropathy: case report. Pediatr Cardiol 19, 355–357.

252. Rychik J, Rome JJ, Jacobs ML. (1997) Late surgical fenestration for complications after the Fontan operation. Circulation 96, 33–36.

253. Laks H. (1990) The partial Fontan procedure. A new concept and its clinical application. Circulation 82, 1866–1867.

254. Gamba A, Merlo M, Fiocchi R, *et al.* (2004) Heart transplantation in patients with previous Fontan operations. J Thorac Cardiovasc Surg 127, 555–562.

255. Mertens L, Canter C, Parisi F. (1999) The outcome for heart transplantation for protein-losing enteropathy after the Fontan operation. Circulation 100(suppl 1), 1602 (abstr).

256. Gewillig MH, Lundstrom UR, Deanfield JE, *et al.* (1990) Impact of Fontan operation on left ventricular size and contractility in tricuspid atresia. Circulation 81, 118–127.

257. Matsuda H, Kawashima Y, Kishimoto H, *et al.* (1987) Problems in the modified Fontan operation for univentricular heart of the right ventricular type. Circulation 76, III45–III52.

258. Mavroudis C, Deal BJ, Backer CL, *et al.* (1999) The favorable impact of arrhythmia surgery on total cavopulmonary artery Fontan conversion. Semin Thorac Cardiovasc Surg Pediatr Card Surg Annu 2, 143–156.

259. Choussat A, Fontan F, Besse P, *et al.* (1978) Selection criteria for Fontan's procedure. In: Anderson RH, Shinebourne EA, eds. *Paediatric Cardiology.* Edinburgh: Churchill Livingstone, pp. 559–566.

260. Pearl JM, Laks H, Drinkwater DC, *et al.* (1992) Modified Fontan procedure in patients less than 4 years of age. Circulation 86(5 Suppl), II100–II105.

261. Castaneda AR, Trusler GA, Paul MH, *et al.* (1988) The early results of treatment of simple transposition in the current era. J Thorac Cardiovasc Surg 95, 14–28.

262. Gates RN, Laks H, Drinkwater DC Jr, *et al.* (1997) The Fontan procedure in adults. Ann Thorac Surg 63, 1085–1090.

263. Humes RA, Mair DD, Porter CB, *et al.* (1988) Results of the modified Fontan operation in adults. Am J Cardiol 61, 602–604.

264. Fujii Y, Sano S, Kotani Y, *et al.* (2009) Midterm to long-term outcome of total cavopulmonary connection in high-risk adult candidates. Ann Thorac Surg 87, 562–570; discussion 570.

265. Cochrane AD, Karl TR, Mee RB. (1993) Staged conversion to arterial switch for late failure of the systemic right ventricle. Ann Thorac Surg 56, 854–861; discussion 861–862.

266. Gatzoulis MA, Walters J, McLaughlin PR, *et al.* (2000) Late arrhythmia in adults with the mustard procedure for transposition of great arteries: a surrogate marker for right ventricular dysfunction? Heart 84, 409–415.

267. Mavroudis C, Backer CL. (2000) Arterial switch after failed atrial baffle procedures for transposition of the great arteries. Ann Thorac Surg 69, 851–857.

268. Deanfield J, Camm J, Macartney F, *et al.* (1988) Arrhythmia and late mortality after Mustard and Senning operation for transposition of the great arteries. An eight-year prospective study. J Thorac Cardiovasc Surg 96, 569–576.

269. Puley G, Siu S, Connelly M, *et al.* (1999) Arrhythmia and survival in patients >18 years of age after the mustard procedure for complete transposition of the great arteries. Am J Cardiol 83, 1080–1084.

270. Collins KK, Love BA, Walsh EP, *et al.* (2000) Location of acutely successful radiofrequency catheter ablation of intraatrial reentrant tachycardia in patients with congenital heart disease. Am J Cardiol 86, 969–974.

271. Thorne SA, Barnes I, Cullinan P, *et al.* (1999) Amiodarone-associated thyroid dysfunction: risk factors in adults with congenital heart disease. Circulation 100, 149–154.

272. Kammeraad JA, van Deurzen CH, Sreeram N, *et al.* (2004) Predictors of sudden cardiac death after Mustard or Senning repair for transposition of the great arteries. J Am Coll Cardiol 44, 1095–1102.

273. Janousek J, Paul T, Luhmer I, *et al.* (1994) Atrial baffle procedures for complete transposition of the great arteries: natural course of sinus node dysfunction and risk factors for dysrhythmias and sudden death. Z Kardiol 83, 933–938.

274. Sun ZH, Happonen JM, Bennhagen R, *et al.* (2004) Increased QT dispersion and loss of sinus rhythm as risk factors for late sudden death after Mustard or Senning procedures

for transposition of the great arteries. Am J Cardiol 94, 138–141.

275. Schneider DJ, Moore JW. (2001) Transcatheter treatment of IVC channel obstruction and baffle leak after Mustard procedure for d-transposition of the great arteries using Amplatzer ASD device and multiple stents. J Invasive Cardiol 13, 306–309.

276. Abdulhamed JM, al Yousef S, Khan MA, et al. (1994) Balloon dilatation of complete obstruction of the superior vena cava after Mustard operation for transposition of great arteries. Br Heart J 72, 482–485.

277. MacLellan-Tobert SG, Cetta F, Hagler DJ. (1996) Use of intravascular stents for superior vena caval obstruction after the Mustard operation. Mayo Clin Proc 71, 1071–1076.

278. Prieto LR, Latson LA, Flamm SD, et al. (1998) Conversion from atrial to arterial switch in patients with D-transposition of the great arteries: risk factors for mortality. Circulation 97(suppl), I–61 (abstr).

279. Hagler DJ, Ritter DG, Mair DD, et al. (1978) Clinical, angiographic, and hemodynamic assessment of late results after Mustard operation. Circulation 57, 1214–1220.

280. Tynan M, Aberdeen E, Stark J. (1972) Tricuspid incompetence after the Mustard operation for transposition of the great arteries. Circulation 45(Suppl), I111–I115.

281. van Son JA, Reddy VM, Silverman NH, et al. (1996) Regression of tricuspid regurgitation after two-stage arterial switch operation for failing systemic ventricle after atrial inversion operation. J Thorac Cardiovasc Surg 111, 342–347.

282. Cooper SG, Sullivan ID, Bull C, et al. (1989) Balloon dilation of pulmonary venous pathway obstruction after Mustard repair for transposition of the great arteries. J Am Coll Cardiol 14, 194–198.

283. Wernovsky G, Giglia TM, Jonas RA, et al. (1992) Course in the intensive care unit after "preparatory" pulmonary artery banding and aortopulmonary shunt placement for transposition of the great arteries with low left ventricular pressure. Circulation 86(Suppl), II133–II139.

284. Chang AC, Wernovsky G, Wessel DL, et al. (1992) Surgical management of late right ventricular failure after Mustard or Senning repair. Circulation 86(Suppl), II140–II149.

285. Mavroudis C, Backer CL, Deal BJ, et al. (1998) Fontan conversion to cavopulmonary connection and arrhythmia circuit cryoblation. J Thorac Cardiovasc Surg 115, 547–556.

286. Feigl A, Feigl D, Lucas RV Jr, et al. (1984) Involvement of the aortic valve cusps in discrete subaortic stenosis. Pediatr Cardiol 5, 185–189.

287. Serraf A, Zoghby J, Lacour-Gayet F, et al. (1999) Surgical treatment of subaortic stenosis: a seventeen-year experience. J Thorac Cardiovasc Surg 117, 669–678.

288. Cape EG, Vanauker MD, Sigfusson G, et al. (1997) Potential role of mechanical stress in the etiology of pediatric heart disease: septal shear stress in subaortic stenosis. J Am Coll Cardiol 30, 247–254.

289. Sigfusson G, Tacy TA, Vanauker MD, et al. (1997) Abnormalities of the left ventricular outflow tract associated with discrete subaortic stenosis in children: an echocardiographic study. J Am Coll Cardiol 30, 255–259.

290. Parry AJ, Kovalchin JP, Suda K, et al. (1999) Resection of subaortic stenosis; can a more aggressive approach be justified? Eur J Cardiothorac Surg 15, 631–638.

291. Kuralay E, Ozal E, Bingol H, et al. (1999) Discrete subaortic stenosis: assessing adequacy of myectomy by transesophageal echocardiography. J Card Surg 14, 348–353.

292. Spirito P, Seidman CE, McKenna WJ, et al. (1997) The management of hypertrophic cardiomyopathy. N Engl J Med 336, 775–785.

293. Sherrid MV, Pearle G, Gunsburg DZ. (1998) Mechanism of benefit of negative inotropes in obstructive hypertrophic cardiomyopathy. Circulation 97, 41–47.

294. Pacileo G, De Cristofaro M, Russo MG, et al. (2000) Hypertrophic cardiomyopathy in pediatric patients: effect of verapamil on regional and global left ventricular diastolic function. Can J Cardiol 16, 146–152.

295. Petkow Dimitrow P, Krzanowski M, Nizankowski R, et al. (2000) Effect of verapamil on systolic and diastolic coronary blood flow velocity in asymptomatic and mildly symptomatic patients with hypertrophic cardiomyopathy. Heart 83, 262–266.

296. Ostman-Smith I, Wettrell G, Riesenfeld T. (1999) A cohort study of childhood hypertrophic cardiomyopathy: improved survival following high-dose beta-adrenoceptor antagonist treatment. J Am Coll Cardiol 34, 1813–1822.

297. Seiler C, Hess OM, Schoenbeck M, et al. (1991) Long-term follow-up of medical versus surgical therapy for hypertrophic cardiomyopathy: a retrospective study. J Am Coll Cardiol 17, 634–642.

298. Sakai Y, Kawakami Y, Hirota Y, et al. (1999) Dual-chamber pacing in hypertrophic obstructive cardiomyopathy: a comparison of acute and chronic effects. Jpn Circ J 63, 971–975.

299. Erwin JP 3rd, Nishimura RA, Lloyd MA, et al. (2000) Dual chamber pacing for patients with hypertrophic obstructive cardiomyopathy: a clinical perspective in 2000. Mayo Clin Proc 75, 173–180.

300. Ommen SR, Nishimura RA, Squires RW, et al. (1999) Comparison of dual-chamber pacing versus septal myectomy for the treatment of patients with hypertrophic obstructive cardiomyopathy: a comparison of objective hemodynamic and exercise end points. J Am Coll Cardiol 34, 191–196.

301. Gietzen FH, Leuner CJ, Raute-Kreinsen U, et al. (1999) Acute and long-term results after transcoronary ablation of septal hypertrophy (TASH). Catheter interventional treatment for hypertrophic obstructive cardiomyopathy. Eur Heart J 20, 1342–1354.

302. Konno S, Imai Y, Iida Y, et al. (1975) A new method for prosthetic valve replacement in congenital aortic stenosis associated with hypoplasia of the aortic valve ring. J Thorac Cardiovasc Surg 70, 909–917.

303. Cobanoglu A, Thyagarajan GK, Dobbs J. (1997) Konno-aortoventriculoplasty with mechanical prosthesis in dealing with small aortic root: a good surgical option. Eur J Cardiothorac Surg 12, 766–770.

304. Vouhe PR, Ouaknine R, Poulain H, et al. (1993) Diffuse subaortic stenosis: modified Konno procedures with aortic valve preservation. Eur J Cardiothorac Surg 7, 132–136.

305. Jahangiri M, Nicholson IA, del Nido PJ, *et al.* (2000) Surgical management of complex and tunnel-like subaortic stenosis. Eur J Cardiothorac Surg 17, 637–642.

306. McKowen RL, Campbell DN, Woelfel GF, *et al.* (1987) Extended aortic root replacement with aortic allografts. J Thorac Cardiovasc Surg 93, 366–374.

307. Daenen WJ. (1996) Management of complex left ventricular outflow tract obstruction with pulmonary autografts. Semin Thorac Cardiovasc Surg 8, 358–361.

308. van Son JA, Hambsch J, Bossert T, *et al.* (1999) Operative treatment of hypertrophic obstructive cardiomyopathy and aortic valve disease in infants. J Card Surg 14, 273–278.

Index

Note: Page numbers in *italics* refer to figures. Those in **bold** refer to tables. In cross-references, commas may indicate that the phrase following is a subheading. Thus, "see also abscess, crypt" means "see also the subheading 'crypt' under the main heading 'abscess'". Entries are in word-by-word alphabetical order, ignoring hyphens, so that "fasting" comes after "fast tracking" and "D-shaped" comes after "dropped".

Pediatric Cardiac Surgery, Fourth Edition. Edited by Constantine Mavroudis and Carl L. Backer.
© 2013 Blackwell Publishing Ltd. Published 2013 by Blackwell Publishing Ltd.